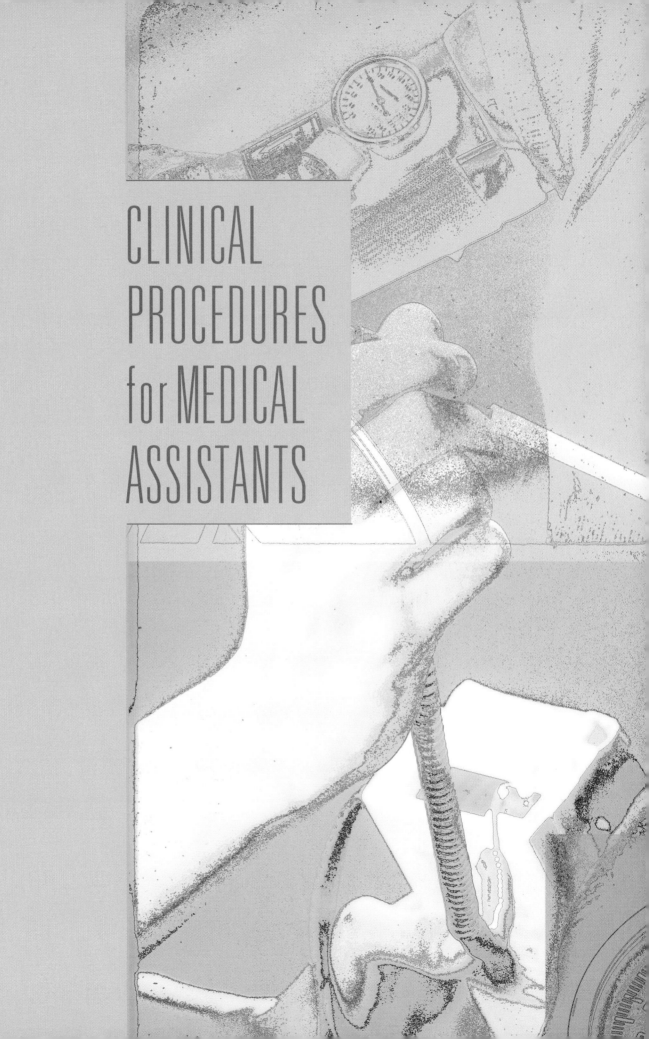

CLINICAL PROCEDURES for MEDICAL ASSISTANTS

CLINICAL PROCEDURES for MEDICAL ASSISTANTS

FIFTH EDITION

Kathy Bonewit-West, B.S., M.Ed., C.M.A.C.

Coordinator and Instructor

Medical Assistant Technology

Curriculum Development

Hocking College

Nelsonville, Ohio

Former Member, Curriculum Review Board of the American Association of Medical Assistants

W.B. SAUNDERS COMPANY

An Imprint of Elsevier Science

Philadelphia London New York St. Louis Sydney Toronto

W.B. SAUNDERS COMPANY
An Imprint of Elsevier Science

The Curtis Center
Independence Square West
Philadelphia, Pennsylvania 19106

Library of Congress Cataloging-in-Publication Data

Bonewit-West, Kathy.

    Clinical procedures for medical assistants / Kathy Bonewit-West,—5th ed.

    p. cm.

    Includes bibliographical references and index.

    ISBN 0-7216-8406-8

    1. Physicians' assistants. 2. Clinical medicine. I. Title.

    [DNLM: 1. Physician Assistants. 2. Clinical Medicine—methods. W 21.5 B712c 2000]

    R697.P45 B66 2000   610.73'7—dc21

DNLM/DLC   99-048210

Editor-in-Chief: Andrew Allen
Acquisitions Editor: Adrianne Williams
Developmental Editor: Scott Weaver/Rachael Zipperlen
Manuscript Editor: Carol DiBerardino
Production Manager: Linda R. Garber
Illustration Specialist: Peg Shaw
Book Designer: Gene Harris
Illustrator: Matt Andrews
Indexer: Dennis Dolan
Manager, Electronic Productions: David Saracco

CLINICAL PROCEDURES FOR MEDICAL ASSISTANTS   ISBN 0-7216-8406-8

Last digit is the print number: 9   8   7   6   5   4   3

To my sister Linda,

for her enduring spirit

and gentle heart

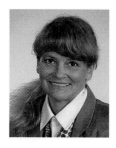

Medical assistants, for many years an integral part of most physicians' staffs, now fulfill an ever-expanding and varied role in the medical office, both clinically and administratively. With increased responsibilities has come a greater need for professional knowledge and skills. This text has been designed to meet that need.

The underlying principle of the text is to provide a format for the achievement of professional competency in clinical skills performed in the medical office and the understanding of their application to real-life or on-the-job situations. When professional competency is achieved in the classroom, less of a gap should exist between the academic and real worlds, and thus the transition from student to practicing medical assistant is made more easily.

Although I have emphasized the book's usefulness to students in medical assisting training programs, the practicing medical assistant will also find this text helpful as a learning and reference source. The organization of the text lends itself well to individualized instruction and convenient reference use.

In this fifth edition, the text has been expanded to encompass additional clinical procedures and the theory relating to each. This additional material will help students and instructors meet the demand for the increasing number and variety of clinical skills required of the practicing medical assistant by providing the most current and up-to-date procedures performed in the medical office. The reader will find that nearly every chapter incorporates new information and illustrations to assist in the educational process. Important additions include current information on the OSHA Bloodborne Pathogens Standards and CLIA regulations, the Hazard Communication Standard and material data safety sheets (MSDS), pulmonary function testing, the procedure for the collection of a 24-hour urine specimen, and the procedure for the butterfly method of venipuncture.

A new chapter, which is entitled The Medical Record focuses on the components of the medical record, medical record documents, medical record formats, legal aspects of medical records, preparing a medical record for a new patient, taking a health history, and charting progress notes. This chapter helps the medical assistant understand the importance of the medical record and how it relates to clinical procedures performed in the medical office.

A very important addition to the fifth edition is the inclusion of three valuable reference sources for each chapter: Medical Practice and the Law, Certification Review, and Resources on the Web. Each of these elements serves an important role in learning and instruction. Medical Practice and the Law provides the student with current legal information pertaining to the chapter. The Certification Review provides the student with a complete overview of the chapter and can be used as an aid in preparing for the certification examination. Resources on the Web allows the student to access web sites containing additional information relating to the chapter.

The organizational format of this edition facilitates the learning process by providing students and educators with detailed objectives and an in-depth study of the most current and up-to-date clinical procedures performed in the medical office. Presented at the beginning of each chapter are a chapter outline, outcomes, educational objectives, and key terminology. The chapter outline provides a quick reference of the cognitive knowledge included in that chapter. Outcomes follow to delineate the task or skill to be mastered by the student. (In the student manual, each outcome is expanded into a detailed performance objective including conditions and standards of acceptable performance.) The educational objectives address the cognitive knowledge required to perform the outcomes. The key terminology list designates the terms and definitions that should be mastered for each chapter.

The knowledge or theory that the student must acquire to perform each skill is presented in a clear and concise manner. Numerous illustrations accompany the theory section to aid the student in acquiring the knowledge relating to each skill. The procedure for each skill follows the theory section and is designed to help the student perform the skill with the level of competency required on the job. Each procedure is presented in an organized step-by-step format, with underlying principles and illustrations accompanying the techniques. A charting example follows each procedure to provide the student with a guide for charting his or her own procedure. Students should find it much easier to acquire competency in charting with these examples.

The student manual that accompanies the textbook greatly enhances the learning value of the textbook. In addition, its outcome-based approach meets the criteria required for outcome-based program accreditation as stipulated by the Curriculum Review Board of the American Association of Medical Assistants.

Continuing education is of utmost importance in such a rapidly changing profession. New techniques and developments in the field of medicine have a direct influence on the medical assisting profession. Continuing education helps the medical assistant maintain and improve existing skills and to learn new skills. The American Association of Medical Assistants (AAMA) is a professional organization for medical assistants that is dedicated to continuing education. Information on the AAMA can be obtained by writing to:

American Association of Medical Assistants
20 N. Wacker Dr., #1575
Chicago, IL 60606–2903
312-899-1500
www.aama-ntl.org

It is the author's hope that individuals who use this approach to medical assisting will view this text not as a stopping place but as a means of opening doors to new paths to be explored in the medical assisting profession.

Kathy Bonewit-West

☐ The completion of the fifth edition of this text permits the opportunity to relay appreciation to the medical assisting educators who so eagerly and enthusiastically use and enjoy this text. To them I am also indebted for their helpful assistance and suggestions for the fifth edition.

The following professionals served as invaluable consultants and reviewers and deserve special recognition and appreciation:

Sharlene K. Aasen, C.M.A.-C., Globe College, Oakdale, Minnesota.

Diana Bennett, R.N., B.S.N., M.A.T., Indiana Vocational Technical College, Indianapolis, Indiana.

Julie A. Benson, A.S., R.M.A., R.Phbt, E.K.G., Medical Program Director, Platt College, Tulsa, Oklahoma.

Lisa Breitbard, A.A., L.V.N., Maric College of Medical Careers, San Diego, California.

Carol S. Champagne, R.M.A., C.M.A.-C., I.C.E.A. C.C.E., Clearwater Family Practice Clinic, Clearwater, Kansas; Chairperson, R.M.A., Continuing Education Committee; Certified Childbirth Education, Private Practice.

Gary A. Clarke, Ph.D., Assistant Professor of Biology, Roanoke College, Salem, Virginia.

Henry G. Croci, M.D., Opthalmology, Riverside Professional Building, Athens, Ohio.

Marlene Donovan, B.S.N., M.S.N., M.Ed., Instructor of Medical Assisting and Nursing, Hocking College, Nelsonville, Ohio.

Beverly G. Dugas, T.N., Douglas College, New Westminster, British Columbia, Canada.

Julie D. Franklin, M.T.(A.S.C.P.), M.H.E., Former Program Director, Medical Office Assisting, Chattanooga State Technical Community College, Chattanooga, Tennessee.

Cathy Goodwin, C.M.A.-A.C., Medical Assistant, San Diego, California

Jeanne Howard, C.M.A., A.A.S., Medical Assisting Technology, El Paso Community College, El Paso, Texas.

Tanya L. Howe, Administrative Assistant, School of Health and Nursing, Hocking College, Nelsonville, Ohio.

Susan K. Ipacs, R.N., M.S., Associate Dean, School of Nursing, Hocking College, Nelsonville, Ohio.

Gail I. Jones, M.S., M.T.(A.S.C.P.), Dettman-Connell School of Medical Technology, Fort Worth, Texas.

Richard W. Kocon, Ph.D., Laboratory Director, Damon Medical Laboratory, Inc., Needham Heights, Massachusetts.

Louis Komarmy, M.D., Clinical Pathologist, Children's Hospital, San Francisco, California.

Miriam Lineberger, R.N., B.S.N., M.Ed., Instructor of Pharmacology, Hocking College, Nelsonville, Ohio.

Albert B. Lowenfels, M.D., Associate Director of Surgery, Westchester County Medical Center, Valhalla, New York.

Susan J. Matthews, R.N., B.S.N., M.Ed., Watterson College, Louisville, Kentucky.

Sharon McCaughrin, C.M.A., Corporate Director of Education, Ross Medical Education Centers, Warren, Michigan.

Deborah Montone, B.S., R.N., R.M.A., L.L.S.-P., R.C.S., Dean of Academics, Hohokus School of Medical Sciences, Ramsey, New Jersey.

Jean Moquin, Ohio University Osteopathic Medical Center, Athens, Ohio.

Sally A. Murdock, B.S.N., M.S., R.N., California Public Health Nursing Certification, Medical Assisting, San Diego Mesa College, San Diego, California.

Kathryn L. Murphy, R.N., C.M.A., Medical Program Director, Department Chair, and Instructor, Springfield College, Springfield, Missouri.

Paulette Nitkiewicz, B.S.N., R.N., C.M.A., Program Director, Medical Assistant Program, and Allied Medical Supervisor, Laurel Business Institute, Uniontown, PA.

Donna F. Otis, L.P.N., Medical Instructor, MAA Program, Metro Business College, Rolla, Missouri.

Raymond E. Phillips, M.D., F.A.C.P., Senior Attending Physician, Phelps Memorial Hospital, North Tarrytown, New York.

Vicki Prater, C.M.A., Concorde Career Institute, San Bernardino, California.

Linda Reed, Indiana Vocational Technical College, Indianapolis, Indiana.

Marjorie J. Reif, P.A.-C., C.M.A., Rochester Community College, Rochester, Minnesota.

Alan M. Rosich, Instructor of Radiologic Technology, Lorain County Community College, Elvira, Ohio.

Kimberly Rubesne, M.A., Median School of Allied Health Careers, Pittsburgh, Pennsylvania.

Lynn G. Slack, C.M.A., ICM School of Business and Medical Careers, Pittsburgh, Pennsylvania.

Robin Snider-Flohr, M.B.A., R.N., C.M.A., Jefferson Community College, Steubenville, Ohio.

Edward R. Stapleton, E.M.T.-P., Assistant Clinical Professor and Director of Prehospital Care and Education, Department of Emergency Medicine, School of Medicine, University Hospital and Medical Center, State University of New York, Stony Brook, New York.

Sandra E. Sterling, M.T.(A.S.C.P.), Boulder Valley Vocational-Technical School, Boulder, Colorado.

Marie Thomas, C.L.T.(N.C.A.), Berdan Institute, Totowa, New Jersey.

Joan K. Werner, P.T., Ph.D., Director, Physical Therapy Program, University of Wisconsin, Madison, Wisconsin.

The photographs in the fifth edition have been redone in color through the efforts of Brian E. Blauser, professional photographer. I am especially indebted to Brian for his careful precision and patience in taking and editing them, thus greatly enhancing the learning value of this text.

Special thanks are also due to Paula Dunham for writing the "Medical Practice and the Law" boxes in each chapter and Debbie Robinson for developing the pronunciations for the key terminology lists.

I would like to gratefully acknowledge the following practicing medical assistants for contributing many hours to be photographed for demonstration of the clinical procedures in the text: Megan Baer, Dawn Bennett, Trudy Browning, Janet Canterbury, Theresa Cline, Marlyne Cooper, Hope Fauber, Dori Glover, Jennifer Hawk, Cammie Lindner, Judy Markins, Korey McGrew, Natalie Morehead, Michelle Parsons, Traci Powell, Linda Proffitt, Latisha Sharpe, Michelle Shockey, Janice Smith, Kara Van Dyke, and Michelle Villers.

I would also like to acknowledge the following individuals who portrayed patients in the text: Brian Adevc, Hollie Bonewit, Phillip Carr, Chloe Cline, Angie Coffin, Chad Cron, Dawn Decaminada, Aja Fox, Connie Hazlett, Gary Hazlett, Isabella Ipacs, Joey Ipacs, Susan Ipacs, Charles Larimer, Pam Larimer, Christopher Mace, Deborah Murray, Delaney Murray, Michael Nkrumah, Nick Palmer, Jan Six, Megan Skidmore, Clinton Swart, Crystal Vamos, Kim van Selm, and Tristen West.

I would like to extend my appreciation to the authors, publishers, and equipment companies who have granted me permission to use their illustrations.

The publication of the fifth edition was accomplished through the capable guidance of many talented individuals at W.B. Saunders. Many thanks to Carol DiBerardino for her careful and excellent editing of the manuscript and to Linda R. Garber for her oustanding production work. This edition could not have attained the same level of excellence without the exceptional capabilities of Rachael Zipperlen, Associate Developmental Editor, and Scott Weaver, Senior Developmental Editor, whom I have come to know as valued friends as much as publishing colleagues. The fifth edition has been completely redesigned through the capable efforts of Gene Harris. I want to relay a very special thank-you to Adrianne Williams, Senior Acquisitions Editor, for her dedication to quality medical assisting education and her encouragement in helping me achieve my very best in this edition.

With warm regard, I would like to recognize those very important individuals—the medical assisting students, graduates, and practicing medical assistants— who continually strive for excellence in meeting the demands and ever-increasing requirements of such a challenging profession. A quote by an unknown author really says it better: "Celebrate your talents, for they are what make you unique."

Kathy Bonewit-West

The **OSHA Standards** must be followed when performing many of the clinical procedures presented in this text. To assist the student in following the **OSHA Standards**, icons have been incorporated into the procedures. An illustration of each icon along with its description is outlined below.

HANDWASHING is an important medical aseptic practice and is crucial in preventing the transmission of pathogens in the medical office. The medical assistant should wash the hands frequently, using the proper handwashing technique. When performing clinical procedures, the hands should always be washed before and after patient contact, before applying gloves and after removing gloves, and after contact with blood or other potentially infectious materials.

CLEAN DISPOSABLE GLOVES should be worn when it is reasonably anticipated that you will have hand contact with the following: blood and other potentially infectious materials, mucous membranes, nonintact skin, and contaminated articles or surfaces.

APPROPRIATE PROTECTIVE CLOTHING such as gowns, aprons, and laboratory coats should be worn when gross contamination can reasonably be anticipated during performance of a task or procedure.

Place infectious waste in **BIOHAZARD CONTAINERS** that are closable, leakproof, and suitably constructed to contain the contents during handling, storage, transport, or shipping. The containers must be labeled or color coded and closed before removal to prevent the contents from spilling.

FACE SHIELDS OR MASKS IN COMBINATION WITH EYE-PROTECTION DEVICES must be worn whenever splashes, spray, spatter, or droplets of blood or other potentially infectious materials may be generated, posing a hazard through contact with your eyes, nose, or mouth.

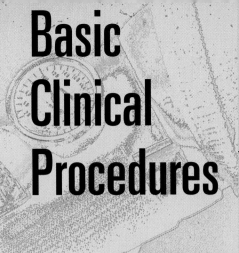

Basic Clinical Procedures

AAMA/CAAHEP COMPETENCIES INCLUDED IN THIS SECTION:

Clinical Competencies

Fundamental Principles

- Perform handwashing
- Dispose of biohazardous materials
- Practice Standard Precautions

Patient Care

- Perform telephone and in-person screening
- Obtain vital signs
- Obtain and record patient history
- Prepare and maintain examination and treatment areas
- Prepare patient for and assist with routine and specialty examinations
- Maintain medication and immunization records

Transdisciplinary Competencies

Communicate

- Respond to and initiate written communications
- Recognize and respond to verbal communications
- Recognize and respond to nonverbal communications
- Demonstrate telephone techniques

Legal Concepts

- Identify and respond to issues of confidentiality
- Perform within legal and ethical boundaries
- Establish and maintain the medical record
- Document appropriately
- Perform risk management procedures

Patient Instruction

- Explain general office policies
- Instruct individuals according to their needs
- Instruct and demonstrate the use and care of patient equipment
- Provide instruction for health maintenance and disease prevention
- Identify community resources

Operational Functions

- Perform an inventory of supplies and equipment
- Perform routine maintenance of administrative and clinical equipment
- Utilize computer software to maintain office systems

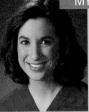

Jennifer Hawk *and I am a Certified Medical Assistant (CMA). I graduated from an accredited medical assisting program and have an associate's degree in Applied Science. I work for a large group of physicians in a multispecialty clinic.*

I have worked as a CMA for a year and a half, obtaining a full-time job right after graduating. Medical assisting graduates are in demand, and I definitely had no problem finding a job. I work in all areas of the office including front office, clinical, and billing. My training in a medical assisting program prepared me to be able to confidently work in all of these office settings. I love that I am able to experience all of these areas of the office, and I definitely never get bored. I love the one-on-one patient contact, as well as the business side of a medical office.

Medical Asepsis and Infection Control

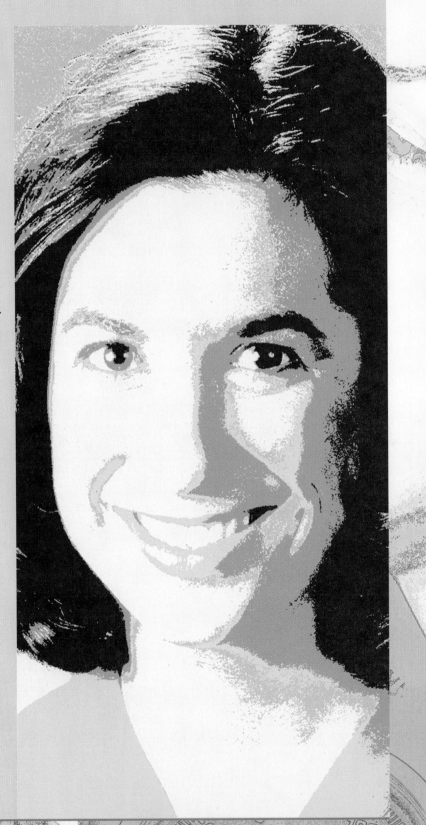

OUTCOMES

After completing this chapter, you should be able to demonstrate the proper procedures to perform the following:

1. Wash hands.
2. Apply and remove clean disposable gloves.
3. Adhere to the OSHA Bloodborne Pathogens Standards.

EDUCATIONAL OBJECTIVES

After completing this chapter, you should be able to do the following:

1. Define the terms listed in Key Terminology.
2. Define a microorganism and give examples of types of microorganisms.
3. Explain the difference between a nonpathogen and a pathogen.
4. List the six basic requirements needed for growth and multiplication of microorganisms.
5. Outline the Infection Process Cycle, including the following:
   a. Give examples of the means of entry of microorganisms into the body.
   b. Give examples of the means of transmission of microorganisms from one person to another.
   c. Give examples of the means of exit of microorganisms from the body.
   d. List and explain five protective mechanisms the body uses to prevent the entrance of microorganisms.
6. Define medical asepsis.
7. Explain the difference between resident flora and transient flora.
8. List and describe the three types of handwashing agents.
9. Identify six medical aseptic practices that should be followed in the medical office.
10. Explain how proper handwashing helps prevent the transmission of microorganisms.
11. Explain the principles underlying each step in the handwashing procedure.
12. Explain the purpose of OSHA.
13. List and describe the elements that must be included in the OSHA Exposure Control Plan.
14. Define and give examples of each of the following: engineering controls, work practice controls, personal protective equipment, and housekeeping procedures.
15. Identify six guidelines that must be followed when using personal protective equipment.
16. Identify the means of transmission of hepatitis B in the health-care setting.
17. Explain the difference between acute and chronic hepatitis B.
18. Describe the treatment for individuals exposed to hepatitis B.
19. List and describe each of the four stages of the AIDS virus infection cycle.
20. List and describe five AIDS-defining conditions.
21. Explain how HIV is transmitted.

1

INTRODUCTION

☐ Medical asepsis and infection control are of critical importance in preventing the spread of disease. The medical assistant should always be sure to practice good medical aseptic techniques to provide a safe and healthy environment in the medical office. The OSHA Bloodborne Pathogens Standards are important in infection control. These standards are required by the federal government to reduce the exposure of employees to infectious diseases. This chapter presents a thorough discussion of medical asepsis, infection control, and the OSHA Bloodborne Pathogens Standards.

MICROORGANISMS

☐ Microorganisms are tiny living plants or animals that cannot be seen with the naked eye but must be viewed with the aid of a microscope. Examples of common types of microorganisms include bacteria, viruses, protozoa, fungi, and animal parasites. Most microorganisms are harmless and do not cause disease. They are termed **nonpathogens.** Other microorganisms, known as **pathogens,** are harmful to the body and can cause disease.

GROWTH REQUIREMENTS FOR MICROORGANISMS

In order for microorganisms to survive, certain growth requirements must be present in the environment. These include the following:

Proper nutrition — Microorganisms that use inorganic or nonliving substances as a source of food are known as **autotrophs.** Microorganisms that use organic or living substances for food are known as **heterotrophs.**

Oxygen — Most microorganisms need oxygen to grow and multiply and are termed **aerobes.** Other microorganisms, known as **anaerobes,** grow best in the absence of oxygen.

Temperature — Each microorganism has a temperature at which it grows best, known as the **optimum growth temperature.** Most microorganisms grow best at 98.6°F (37°C), or body temperature.

Darkness — Microorganisms grow best in darkness.

Moisture — Microorganisms need moisture for cell metabolism and to carry away wastes.

pH — Most microorganisms prefer a neutral pH. If the environment of the microorganisms becomes too acidic or basic, they die.

If growth requirements are taken away from the environment of microorganisms, they are unable to survive. This is one way to reduce the growth and transmission of pathogens in the medical office.

THE INFECTION PROCESS CYCLE

For a pathogen to survive and produce disease, a continuous cycle must be followed; this is known as the Infection Process Cycle (Fig. 1–1). If the cycle is broken at any point, the pathogen dies. The medical assistant has a responsibility to help break this cycle in the medical office by practicing good techniques of medical asepsis. These techniques are discussed in the next section.

PROTECTIVE MECHANISMS OF THE BODY

The body has protective mechanisms to help prevent the entrance of pathogens. These help break the Infection Process Cycle. Protective mechanisms of the body are as follows:

1. The skin is one of the most important defense mechanisms of the body and serves as a protective barrier against the entrance of microorganisms.
2. The mucous membranes of the body, which line the nose, throat, and respiratory, gastrointestinal, and genital tracts, help protect the body from invasion by microorganisms.
3. Mucus and cilia in the nose and respiratory tract. Mucus traps the smaller microorganisms that enter the body, and the hairlike cilia constantly beat toward the outside to remove them from the body.
4. Coughing and sneezing help force pathogens from the body.
5. Tears and sweat are secretions that aid in the removal of pathogens from the body.
6. Urine and vaginal secretions are acidic. Pathogens cannot grow in an acidic environment.
7. The stomach secretes hydrochloric acid, which helps in the process of digestion. This acidic environment discourages the growth of pathogens entering the stomach.

APPLICATION OF MEDICAL ASEPSIS IN THE MEDICAL OFFICE

Medical Asepsis

In the medical office, practices must be employed to reduce the number and hinder the transmission of pathogens. These practices are known as medical asepsis. **Medical asepsis** means that an object or area is clean and free from infection. Nonpathogens will still be present on a clean or medically aseptic substance or surface, but all the pathogens have been eliminated.

Handwashing

Handwashing is an important medical aseptic practice and is crucial in preventing the transmission of pathogens in the medical office. Microorganisms found on the hands are classified into the following categories: resident flora and transient flora. **Resident flora** (also known as normal flora) normally reside and grow in the epidermis and deeper layers of the skin known as the dermis. Resident flora are generally harmless and nonpathogenic. Because resident flora are attached to the deeper skin layers, they are more difficult to remove from the skin and are usually killed only by washing the hands with an antimicrobial agent.

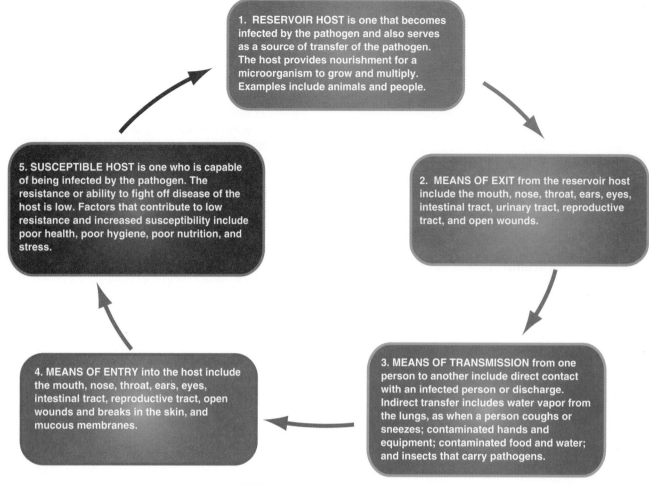

FIGURE 1–1. The infection process cycle.

Transient flora, on the other hand, live and grow on the superficial skin layers, or epidermis. They are picked up on the hands in the course of daily activities. In the medical office, this may include contact with an infected patient, contaminated equipment, or contaminated surfaces. Transient flora are often pathogenic, but because they are attached loosely to the skin, they can be removed easily by washing the hands with soap and water.

Three categories of agents are available for washing the hands: plain soaps, detergents, and antimicrobials. **Soaps** are used to cleanse the skin mechanically. Because of this factor, it is important to use adequate friction when washing the hands with soap and water to ensure the removal of all transient flora. **Detergents** are more effective than soaps because they are able to break down or emulsify dirt and oil present on the skin without relying solely on scrubbing action. **Antimicrobials** are chemical agents that inhibit the

growth of or kill microorganisms. Most antimicrobials also deposit an antibacterial film on the skin that discourages bacterial growth. Examples of antimicrobials include alcohols, chlorhexidine gluconate, and iodophors. For most clinical situations, soap and water is sufficient for effective handwashing; however, if your skin comes in contact with blood or other potentially infectious materials, an antimicrobial may be preferred.

The medical assistant should wash the hands frequently, using the proper handwashing technique. Hands should always be washed in the following situations:

1. On arrival at the medical office.
2. Before and after patient contact.
3. Before applying gloves and after removing gloves.
4. After contact with blood or other potentially infectious materials.
5. After handling contaminated equipment.

6. Before and after eating.
7. After using the rest room.
8. After blowing or wiping the nose.
9. When the hands are obviously soiled.
10. Before leaving the medical office for the day.

Infection Control

In addition to handwashing, other good aseptic practices in the medical office for the control of infection include the following:

1. Following the OSHA Bloodborne Pathogens Standards (presented in this chapter).
2. Keeping the medical office free from dirt and dust, which can collect and carry microorganisms.
3. Making sure that the reception area and examining rooms are well ventilated. Stuffy rooms encourage microorganisms to settle on objects.
4. Keeping the reception area and examining rooms bright and airy. Light discourages the growth of microorganisms.
5. Eliminating insects by the use of insecticides or window screens. Insects are a means of transmission of microorganisms.
6. Carefully disposing of wastes such as urine, feces, and respiratory secretions; all wastes should be handled as if they contained pathogens.

7. Not letting soiled items touch clothing.
8. Avoiding coughs and sneezes of patients. The water vapor expelled from the lungs with coughing and sneezing may contain pathogens.
9. Using discretion in the amount of jewelry worn. Microorganisms can become lodged in the grooves and crevices of jewelry and serve as a means of transmission of pathogens.
10. Teaching patients aseptic practices to control the spread of infection at home.

GLOVES

Clean disposable gloves should be worn when you are likely to come in contact with any body substance such as blood, urine, feces, mucous membranes, and nonintact skin. For example, clean disposable gloves should be worn when administering an injection, performing a venipuncture, and performing a urinalysis. **Sterile gloves** are used to perform sterile procedures such as a dressing change or to assist the physician during minor office surgery, which is described in more detail in Chapter 6 (Minor Office Surgery).

The procedure for the application and removal of clean gloves is presented in this chapter.

1

PROCEDURE

1-1

Handwashing

| EQUIPMENT/SUPPLIES: | Liquid or bar soap | Paper towels |

1. **Procedural Step.** Remove watch or push it up on the forearm so the wrist is clear. Avoid wearing rings. If rings are worn, remove all except a plain wedding band.
   Principle. Microorganisms can lodge in the crevices and grooves of rings.
2. **Procedural Step.** Stand at the sink, making sure clothing does not touch the sink.
   Principle. The sink is considered contaminated, and if the uniform touches the sink, it may pick up microorganisms and transfer them.

3. **Procedural Step.** Turn on the faucets, using a paper towel.
   Principle. The faucets are considered contaminated because they harbor microorganisms.
4. **Procedural Step.** Adjust the water temperature. The water should be warm to make the best suds.
   Principle. Water that is too hot or too cold tends to dry the skin, causing chapping and cracking and making it easy for pathogens to enter the body.

Continued

PROCEDURE 1-1

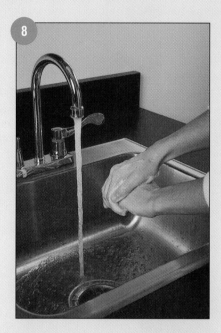

5. **Procedural Step.** Discard the paper towel in the trash receptacle.
   Principle. The paper towel is considered contaminated after touching the faucets.
6. **Procedural Step.** Wet hands and forearms thoroughly with water. The hands should be held lower than the elbows at all times. Be careful not to touch the inside of the sink, as it is also contaminated.
   Principle. By holding the hands lower than the elbows, bacteria and debris will be carried away from the arms and body and into the sink.
7. **Procedural Step.** Apply soap to the hands. If liquid soap is used, apply approximately 1 teaspoon. If bar soap is used, it must be retained in the hands during sudsing up (Note: If the bar soap is accidentally dropped on the floor or in the sink during the handwashing procedure, the medical assistant must repeat the procedure from the beginning.)

Rinse the bar soap before returning to the soap dish. The soap dish should have drainage holes so that the soap can dry out—moisture encourages the growth of microorganisms.
Principle. Microorganisms and debris accumulate on the soap during the handwashing procedure. Rinsing the soap helps carry these away.

8. **Procedural Step.** Wash the palms and backs of the hands with 10 circular motions. Use friction along with the circular motions to wash the palm and back of each hand.
   Principle. Friction helps dislodge and remove microorganisms from the hands.

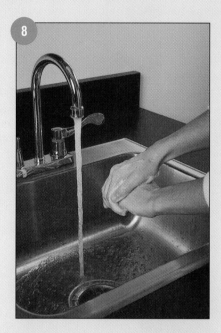

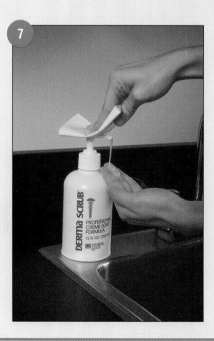

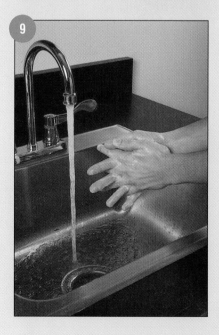

PROCEDURE 1-1

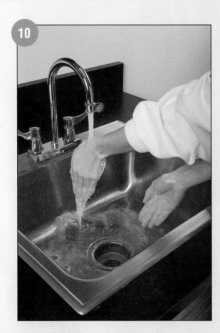

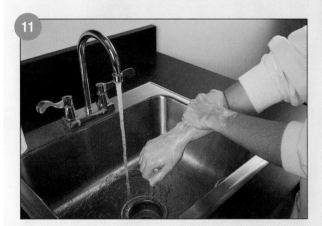

11. **Procedural Step.** Wash wrists and forearms, using friction along with circular motions. (Note: The hands are washed first, as they are the most contaminated; thus organisms and dirt are washed away and not spread to the wrists and forearms.)

12. **Procedural Step.** Rinse arms and hands.
    Principle. The running water rinses away the dirt and microorganisms.

13. **Procedural Step.** Clean the fingernails with a manicure stick. The fingernails should be cleaned at least once daily.

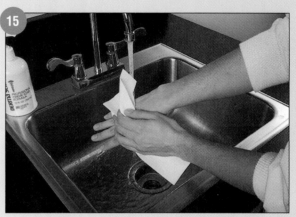

Principle. Dirt and microorganisms collect underneath the fingernails.

14. **Procedural Step.** Repeat the handwashing procedure. For initial handwashing or when the hands come into contact with blood or other potentially infectious materials, the handwashing procedure should be repeated. This is to ensure removal of all pathogens.

15. **Procedural Step.** Dry the hands gently and thoroughly and discard the paper towel.
    Principle. Drying the hands gently prevents them from becoming chapped. Microorganisms can lodge in the crevices of chapped hands. Make sure the hands are dried completely, because wet skin may also cause chapping.

16. **Procedural Step.** Turn off the water, using a paper towel, and discard the paper towel in the trash receptacle.
    Principle. The faucet is considered contaminated, whereas the hands are medically aseptic or clean.

17. **Procedural Step.** Do not touch the sink with the bare hands.
    Principle. The hands are now medically aseptic, and the sink is considered contaminated.

9. **Procedural Step.** Wash the fingers with 10 circular motions. Interlace the fingers and thumbs, and use friction and circular motions while rubbing the fingers back and forth.
   Principle. This kind of movement helps remove microorganisms and debris that have accumulated between the fingers.

10. **Procedural Step.** Rinse well, making sure to hold the hands lower than the elbows.
    Principle. Running water helps rinse away dirt and microorganisms.

1

PROCEDURE

1–2

Application and Removal of Clean Disposable Gloves

EQUIPMENT/SUPPLIES: **Clean disposable gloves**

Applying Clean Disposable Gloves

No special technique is required when clean disposable gloves are applied. This is because the hands are clean and the gloves are clean; therefore, the medical assistant can touch any part of the gloves during application without contaminating them.

1. **Procedural Step:** Remove all rings, and wash the hands.
   Principle: Rings may cause the gloves to tear. The warm, moist environment inside gloves provides ideal growing conditions for the multiplication of transient microorganisms present on the hands. Washing the hands removes these microorganisms and prevents the transmission of pathogens.
2. **Procedural Step:** Choose the appropriate size gloves. Apply the gloves and adjust them so that they fit comfortably.
3. **Procedural Step:** Inspect the gloves for tears. If a tear is present, a new pair of gloves must be applied.

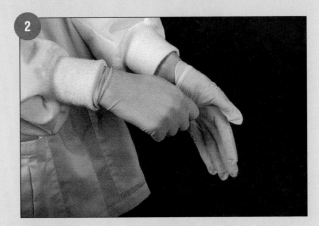

1

Removing Clean Disposable Gloves

Gloves must be removed in a manner that protects the medical assistant from contaminating his or her clean hands with possible pathogens that may be present on the outside of the gloves. This is accomplished by not allowing the bare hands to come in contact with the outside of the gloves.

1. **Procedural Step.** Grasp the outside of the left glove 1 to 2 inches from the top with your gloved right hand. (Note: It does not matter which glove is removed first. You may start with the right glove if you prefer.)
2. **Procedural Step.** Slowly pull the left glove off the hand. It will turn inside out as it is removed from your hand.
3. **Procedural Step.** Pull the left glove free, and scrunch it into a ball with your gloved right hand.
4. **Procedural Step.** Place the index and middle fingers of the left hand on the *inside* of the right glove. Do not allow your clean hand to touch the outside of the glove.

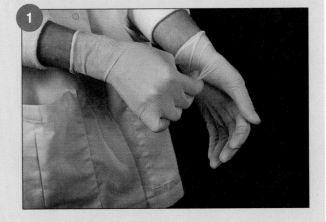

PROCEDURE 1-2

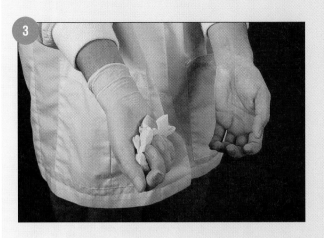

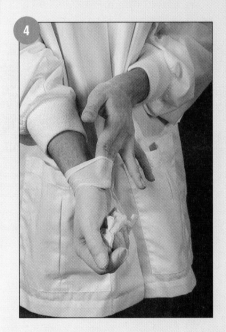

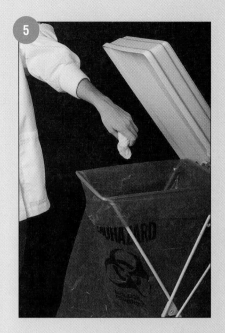

5. **Procedural Step.** Pull the glove off the right hand. It will turn inside out as it is removed from your hand, enclosing the balled-up left glove. Discard both gloves in an appropriate container.
6. **Procedural Step.** Wash hands thoroughly to remove any microorganisms that may have come in contact with your hands.

1

OSHA BLOODBORNE PATHOGENS STANDARDS

The Occupational Safety and Health Administration (OSHA) was established by the federal government to assist employers in providing a safe and healthy working environment for their employees. In 1991, OSHA released a comprehensive set of regulations designed to reduce the risk to employees of exposure to infectious diseases. These regulations are known as the *OSHA Occupational Exposure to Bloodborne Pathogens Standards*, which went into effect in 1992. Failure by employers to comply with the OSHA Standard could result in a citation carrying a maximum penalty of $7,000 for each

violation, and a maximum penalty of $70,000 for repeat violations.

The OSHA Standard must be followed by any employee with occupational exposure, regardless of the place of employment. The following definitions will help clarify terms relating to the OSHA Standard.

■ **Occupational exposure** is defined as reasonably anticipated skin, eye, mucous membrane, or parenteral contact with bloodborne pathogens or other potentially infectious materials that may result from the performance of an employee's duties.

■ **Parenteral** refers to the piercing of the skin barrier or mucous membranes such as through needlesticks, human bites, cuts, and abrasions.

■ **Bloodborne pathogens** means pathogenic microorganisms that are present in human blood and are capable of causing disease, such as the hepatitis B virus (HBV) and the human immunodeficiency virus (HIV); the latter causes AIDS.

■ **Other potentially infectious materials** (OPIM) include
  a. Semen and vaginal secretions
  b. The following body fluids: cerebrospinal, synovial, pleural, pericardial, peritoneal, and amniotic
  c. Any body fluid that is visibly contaminated with blood
  d. Any body fluid the identity of which is unknown
  e. Saliva in dental procedures
  f. Any unfixed human tissue
  g. Any tissue culture, cells, or fluid known to be HIV infected

■ **Contaminated** is defined as the presence or reasonably anticipated presence of blood or other potentially infected materials on an item or surface.

■ **Decontamination** is the use of physical or chemical means to remove, inactivate, or destroy bloodborne pathogens on a surface or item to the point where they are no longer capable of transmitting infectious particles and the surface or item is rendered safe for handling, use, or disposal.

■ **Nonintact skin** is skin that has a break in the surface. It includes, but is not limited to, abrasions, cuts, hangnails, paper cuts, and burns.

■ **Exposure incident** is defined as a specific eye, mouth, other mucous membrane, nonintact skin, or parenteral contact with blood or other potentially infectious materials that results from an employee's duties.

In addition to medical assistants, examples of employees with occupational exposure include physicians, nurses, dentists, dental hygienists, medical laboratory personnel, and emergency medical technicians. Other examples of employees who may have less obvious occupational exposure are correctional and law enforcement officers, fire fighters, hospital laundry workers, morticians, and custodians. The OSHA Standard thoroughly covers all aspects of occupational exposure and is presented here as it pertains to the medical office.

Exposure Control Plan

The OSHA Standard requires that the medical office develop a written Exposure Control Plan designed to eliminate or minimize employee exposure to bloodborne pathogens and other potentially infectious material. The Plan must be made available for review by all medical office staff and updated on an annual basis. The Exposure Control Plan must include the following elements:

1. **An Exposure Determination:** The Exposure Determination must include (a) a list of all job classifications in which *all* employees are likely to have occupational exposure, such as physicians, medical assistants, and laboratory technicians, and (b) a list of job classifications in which only *some* employees have occupational exposure, such as custodians. For the second classification of jobs, the determination must include a list of those tasks in which occupational exposure may occur, such as emptying the trash.

2. **The Method of Compliance:** The Method of Compliance must include specific health and safety measures that are taken in the medical office to minimize the risk of exposure. Because these measures must be closely followed by the medical assistant, they are discussed in more detail later (see Method of Compliance Guidelines).

3. **Post-Exposure Evaluation and Follow-Up Procedures:** The Post-Exposure Evaluation and Follow-Up must specify the procedures to follow in the event of an exposure incident in the medical office, including the method of reporting and investigating the incident and the medical treatment and follow-up that will be made available to the employee. Refer to the OSHA Post-Exposure Evaluation and Follow-Up Standards box for a description of these guidelines.

Communication of Hazards to Employees

According to the OSHA Standard, employers must ensure that all medical office employees with risk of occupational exposure participate in a training program. The program must present the Exposure Control Plan for the medical office, focusing on the measures that are to be taken by employees for their safety. Training must be provided at the time an employee is initially assigned to tasks in which occupational exposure may occur and at least annually thereafter.

Recordkeeping

The OSHA Standard requires that the employer maintain an accurate OSHA record of each medical office employee at risk for occupational exposure. These rec-

OSHA Post-Exposure Evaluation and Follow-up Standards

In the event of an exposure incident to bloodborne pathogens or other potentially infectious materials, OSHA requires the following procedures.

. . . **(3)** *Post-Exposure Evaluation and Follow-Up.* Following a report of an exposure incident, the employer shall make immediately available to the exposed employee a confidential medical evaluation and follow-up, including at least the following elements:

    (i) Documentation of the route(s) of exposure, and the circumstances under which the exposure incident occurred;

    (ii) Identification and documentation of the source individual, unless the employer can establish that identification is infeasible or prohibited by state or local law:

      (A) The source individual's blood shall be tested as soon as feasible and after consent is obtained in order to determine HBV and HIV infectivity. If consent is not obtained, the employer shall establish that legally required consent cannot be obtained. When the source individual's consent is not required by law, the source individual's blood, if available, shall be tested and the results documented.

      (B) When the source individual is already known to be infected with HBV or HIV, testing for the source individual's known HBV or HIV status need not be repeated.

      (C) Results of the source individual's testing shall be made available to the exposed employee, and the employee shall be informed of applicable laws and regulations concerning disclosure of the identity and infectious status of the source individual.

    (iii) Collection and testing of blood for HBV and HIV serologic status:

      (A) The exposed employee's blood shall be collected as soon as feasible and tested after consent is obtained.

      (B) If the employee consents to baseline blood collection, but does not give consent at that time for HIV serologic testing, the sample shall be preserved for at least 90 days. If, within 90 days of the exposure incident, the employee elects to have the baseline sample tested, such testing shall be done as soon as feasible.

    (iv) Post-exposure prophylaxis, when medically indicated, as recommended by the U.S. Public Health Service;

    (v) Counseling; and

    (vi) Evaluation of reported illnesses.

(4) *Information Provided to the Health Care Professional.*

    (i) The employer shall ensure that the health care professional responsible for the employee's Hepatitis B vaccination is provided a copy of this regulation.

Continued

---

ords must be kept confidential except for review by OSHA officials and as required by law.

The record must include the following: employee's name, social security number, hepatitis B vaccination status, including dates of vaccination; results of any post-exposure examinations, medical testing, and follow-up procedures; a copy of the health professional's written evaluation following an exposure incident; and a copy of the exposure incident report.

The employer is required to maintain records for the duration of employment plus 30 years. The employer must also maintain records of the training sessions, which must include presentation dates, content of the sessions, names and qualifications of the trainers, and names and job titles of employees who attended. These records must be maintained for 3 years from the date of the training session.

METHOD OF COMPLIANCE GUIDELINES

The medical assistant must adhere to all guidelines outlined in the OSHA Standard designed to eliminate

OSHA Post-Exposure Evaluation and Follow-up Standards *Continued*

(ii) The employer shall ensure that the health care professional evaluating an employee after an exposure incident is provided the following information:

(A) A copy of this regulation;

(B) A description of the exposed employee's duties as they relate to the exposure incident;

(C) Documentation of the route(s) of exposure and circumstances under which the exposure occurred;

(D) Results of the source individual's blood testing, if available, and

(E) All medical records relevant to the appropriate treatment of the employee including vaccination status, which are the employer's responsibility to maintain.

(5) *Health Care Professional's Written Opinion.* The employer shall obtain and provide the employee with a copy of the evaluating health care professional's written opinion within 15 days of the completion of the evaluation.

(i) The health care professional's written opinion for Hepatitis B vaccination shall be limited to whether Hepatitis B vaccination is indicated for an employee, and if the employee has received such vaccination.

(ii) The health care professional's written opinion for post-exposure evaluation and follow-up shall be limited to the following information:

(A) That the employee has been informed of the results of the evaluation; and

(B) That the employee has been told about any medical conditions resulting from exposure to blood or other potentially infectious materials which require further evaluation or treatment.

(iii) All other findings or diagnoses shall remain confidential and shall not be included in the written report.

From the United States Department of Labor, Occupational Safety and Health Administration: Occupational Exposure to Bloodborne Pathogens: Final Rule. *Federal Register, 29, CFR Part 1910.1030, December 6, 1991.*

1

or minimize the risk of occupational exposure. These guidelines are divided into six categories: engineering controls, work practice controls, personal protective equipment, housekeeping, hepatitis B vaccination, and universal precautions. Each of these categories is discussed next.

Engineering Controls

The medical office must use engineering controls to eliminate or minimize the risk of occupational exposure. **Engineering controls** are physical or mechanical devices that isolate or remove health hazards from the workplace. Examples of these devices include readily accessible handwashing facilities, self-capping needles, biohazard containers and bags, biosafety cabinets, and autoclaves. Engineering controls must be properly maintained or replaced as required to ensure their effectiveness.

Work Practice Controls

Work practice controls reduce the likelihood of exposure by altering the manner in which the technique is performed. It is important that the medical assistant consistently adhere to these safety rules, which include the following:

1. Perform all procedures involving blood or other potentially infectious material in a manner to minimize splashing, spraying, spattering, and generation of droplets of these substances.
2. Observe warning labels on biohazard containers and appliances. Bags or containers that bear a biohazard label (Fig. 1–2) or are color-coded red indicate that they hold blood or other potentially infectious materials. Refrigerators, freezers, or other appliances that contain hazardous materials also bear a biohazard label.
3. Bandage cuts and other lesions on the hands before gloving.

MEMORIES *from* EXTERNSHIP

JENNIFER HAWK: *As a student, I was extremely nervous to go out on externship. I was so scared to think that I was actually going to be in a medical office setting and would have to put everything I had learned into practice. Would I remember everything? Would I do something wrong and hurt the patient? It was such an overwhelming feeling! But to my relief, I had a very good experience. The office staff was so friendly and helpful to me and I surprised myself at how easily everything I had learned stayed with me. It was so exciting to see that I was actually functioning as a team member in the health-care field. I could not have had better training.*

terial, wash the area as soon as possible with soap and water.

6. If your mucous membranes (e.g., mouth, nose) come in contact with blood or other potentially infectious material, flush them with water as soon as possible.

7. Do not bend, break, or shear contaminated needles.

8. A contaminated needle may be removed from its syringe only if required by a specific medical procedure, such as blood gas analysis. Removing the needle must be performed through the use of a mechanical device (Fig. 1–3).

9. A contaminated needle may not be recapped except in unusual circumstances when no other alternative is possible. Such recapping must be performed through the use of a one-handed technique; using a two-handed technique is strictly prohibited. The one-handed recapping technique involves holding the syringe in the dominant hand and using the needle to pick up the cap, using a scooping motion. The cap is then secured onto the needle by pushing it against a hard surface. (Note: Sterile needles may be recapped, such as after the withdrawal of medication from a vial or ampule.)

4. Wash hands as soon as possible after removing gloves.

5. If your hands or other skin surfaces come in contact with blood or other potentially infectious ma-

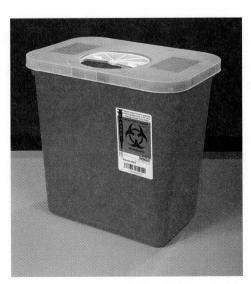

■ **FIGURE 1–2.** Biohazard labels must be fluorescent orange or orange-red, with the biohazard symbol and letters in a contrasting color.

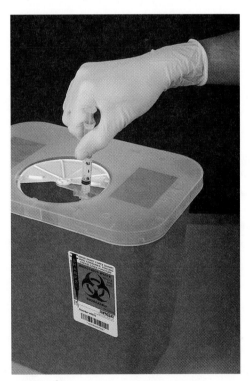

■ **FIGURE 1–3.** Jennifer uses mechanical device to remove a needle from a syringe. This sharps container has a special serrated adapter that mechanically unscrews needles from the syringe.

10. Immediately after use, place contaminated sharps in a puncture-resistant, leakproof container that is appropriately labeled or color-coded. **Contaminated sharps** include any contaminated object that can penetrate the skin, including (but not limited to) needles, lancets, scalpels, broken glass, broken capillary tubes, and exposed ends of dental wires.

11. Do not eat, drink, smoke, apply cosmetics or lip balm, or handle contact lenses in areas where you may be exposed to blood or other potentially infectious materials.

12. Do not store food or drink in refrigerators, freezers, or cabinets or on shelves or countertops where blood or other potentially infectious materials are present.

13. Place blood specimens or other potentially infectious materials in containers that prevent leakage during collection, handling, processing, storage, transport, or shipping. Make sure the containers are closed prior to being stored, transported, or shipped and are labeled or color-coded for easy identification.

14. Before any equipment that might be contaminated is serviced or shipped for repairing or cleaning, such as a centrifuge, it must be inspected for blood or other potentially infectious material. If such material is present, the equipment must be decontaminated. If it cannot be decontaminated, it must be appropriately labeled to clearly indicate the contamination site, to enable those coming into contact with the equipment to take appropriate precautions.

15. If you are exposed to blood or other potentially infectious materials, report the incident immediately to your physician-employer so that post-exposure procedures can be instituted. (Refer to the box entitled OSHA Post-Exposure Evaluation and Follow-Up Standards.) The most obvious exposure incident is a needlestick, but any eye, mouth, or other mucous membrane, nonintact skin, or parenteral contact with blood or other potentially infectious materials constitutes an exposure incident and should be reported.

Personal Protective Equipment

The OSHA Standard specifies that personal protective equipment must be used in the medical office whenever occupational exposure remains after instituting engineering and work practice controls. **Personal protective equipment** is clothing or equipment that protects an individual from contact with blood or other potentially infectious materials; examples include gloves, face shields, masks, protective eyewear, laboratory coats, and gowns. The type of protective equipment appropriate for a given task depends on the degree of exposure that is anticipated, as outlined here:

1. Wear gloves when it is reasonably anticipated that you will have hand contact with the following: blood and other potentially infectious materials, mucous membranes, nonintact skin, and contaminated articles or surfaces (e.g., venipuncture, finger punctures, injections, wound care, assisting with minor office surgery, cleaning contaminated work surfaces and equipment). Gloves will not prevent a puncture, but they could prevent the virus from entering the body through a break in the skin such as a cut, abrasion, burn, or rash.

2. Face shields or masks in combination with eye-protection devices must be worn whenever splashes, spray, spatter, or droplets of blood or other potentially infectious materials may be generated, posing a hazard through contact with your eyes, nose, or mouth (e.g., removing a stopper from a tube of blood, transferring serum from whole blood) (Fig. 1–4).

3. Wear appropriate protective clothing such as gowns, aprons, and laboratory coats when gross contamination can reasonably be anticipated during performance of a task or procedure (e.g., laboratory testing procedure). The type of protective clothing used will depend on the task and degree of exposure anticipated.

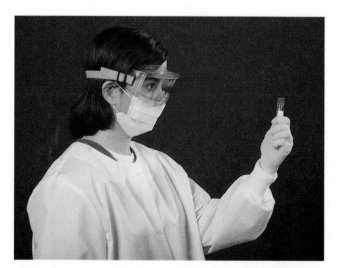

■ **FIGURE 1–4.** Jennifer wears a combination mask and eye-protection device and a laboratory coat to protect against splashes, spray, spatter, or droplets of blood.

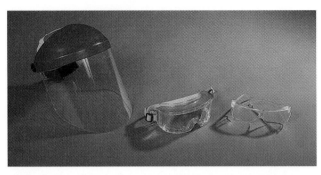

■ **FIGURE 1–5.** Examples of eye protection devices. Face shield (*left*). Goggles (*center*). Glasses with solid side shields (*right*).

Personal Protective Equipment Guidelines

Certain guidelines must be followed when using protective equipment:

1. Protective equipment must not allow potentially infectious material to pass through or reach your work clothes, street clothes, undergarments, skin, eyes, mouth, or other mucous membranes under normal conditions of use and for the duration of time the protective equipment will be used.
2. The employer must provide appropriate personal protective equipment and assure use of the equipment at no cost to you. It must be readily accessible and available in appropriate sizes. In addition, the employer must ensure that the equipment is cleaned, laundered, repaired, replaced, or disposed of as necessary to ensure its effectiveness.
3. If your gloves become contaminated, torn, or punctured, replace them as soon as possible.
4. All eye-protection devices must have solid side shields; therefore face shields, goggles, or glasses with side shields are acceptable, whereas standard prescription eyeglasses are unacceptable (Fig. 1–5).
5. If a garment is penetrated by blood or other potentially infectious materials, it must be removed as soon as possible and placed in an appropriately designated container for washing.
6. All personal protective equipment must be removed prior to leaving the medical office.
7. When protective equipment is removed, it must be placed in an appropriately designated area or container for storage, washing, decontamination, or disposal.
8. Utility gloves may be decontaminated and reused unless they are cracked, peeling, torn, punctured, or no longer provide barrier protection.
9. If you believe using protective equipment would prevent proper delivery of health care or would

pose an increased hazard to your safety or that of a coworker, in extenuating circumstances you may temporarily and briefly decline its use. After such an incident, the circumstances must be investigated to determine whether the situation could be prevented in the future.

HOUSEKEEPING

The OSHA Standard requires that specific housekeeping procedures be followed to ensure that the work site is maintained in a clean and sanitary condition. The medical office must develop and implement a written schedule for cleaning and decontaminating each area where exposure occurs. The method of decontaminating work surfaces must be specified and should be based on the type of surface to be cleaned, the soil present, and the tasks or procedures that occur in that area. Housekeeping procedures include the following:

1. Clean and decontaminate all equipment and work surfaces with an appropriate disinfectant as soon as possible after exposure to blood or other potentially infectious material (Fig. 1–6).
2. Inspect and decontaminate all reusable receptacles, such as bins, pails, and cans, on a regular basis. If contamination is visible, the item must be cleaned and decontaminated as soon as possible.

1

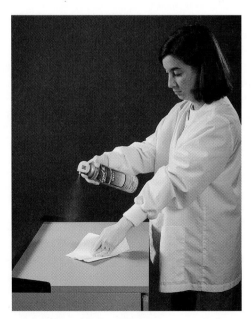

■ **FIGURE 1–6.** Work surfaces should be cleaned with an appropriate disinfectant as soon as possible after exposure to blood or other potentially infectious material.

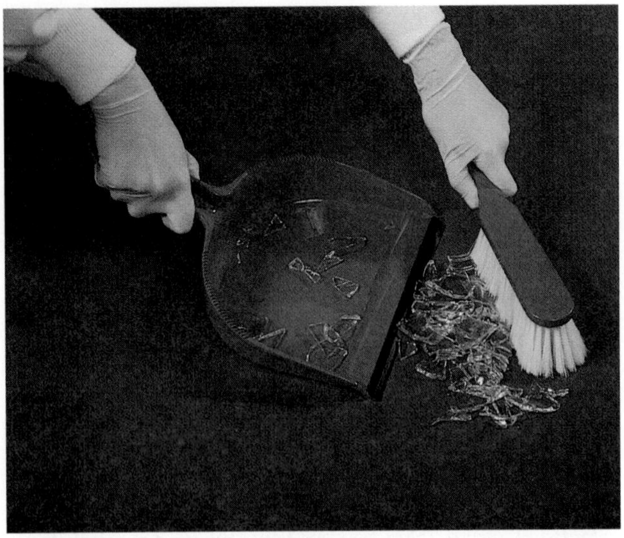

■ **FIGURE 1-7.** Mechanical means must be used to pick up broken glass.

3. Do not pick up broken glassware with your hands, even if you are wearing gloves. Mechanical means should be used, such as a brush and dustpan, tongs, or forceps (Fig. 1–7).
4. Protective coverings such as plastic wrap or aluminum foil may be used to cover work surfaces or equipment, but they must be removed or replaced if contamination occurs.
5. Handle contaminated laundry as little as possible. Place all contaminated laundry in leakproof bags that are properly labeled or color coded. Contaminated laundry must not be sorted or rinsed at the medical office.
6. Handle all regulated waste (also known as infectious waste) with extreme care to prevent exposure incidents. **Regulated waste** is waste containing infectious materials that would pose a substantial threat to health and safety if exposed to the public. Regulated waste includes any waste that contains blood or other potentially infectious materials such as contaminated pathologic laboratory and surgical waste, contaminated sharps, biologic cultures, and live vaccines.
7. Place regulated waste in biohazard containers that are closable, leakproof, and suitably constructed to contain the contents during handling, storage, transport, or shipping. The containers must be labeled or color coded and closed before removal to prevent the contents from spilling. Regulated waste must be disposed of in accordance with all applicable federal, state, and local laws. In general, regulated waste should be either incinerated or autoclaved before

disposal in a sanitary landfill. These methods are discussed more fully at the end of this section.
8. If the outside of any biohazard container becomes contaminated, it must be placed within a second suitable container.
9. Biohazard sharps containers are one of the best ways to prevent cuts and needlesticks from contaminated sharps. To be acceptable, the sharps container must meet these criteria: it must be closable, puncture-resistant, leakproof, and labeled or color coded red to ensure identification of the contents as hazardous. To ensure effectiveness, the following procedures must be observed.
    a. Locate the sharps container as close as possible to the area of use to avoid the hazard of transporting a contaminated needle through the workplace.
    b. Maintain sharps containers in an upright position to keep liquid and sharps inside.
    c. Do not reach into the sharps container with your hand.
    d. Replace sharps containers on a regular basis and do not allow them to overfill.

Highlight on OSHA Standard

The Exposure Control Plan must be made available to OSHA upon request.

OSHA inspectors are responsible for determining whether the medical office meets the OSHA Standard. This is accomplished through a careful review of the Exposure Control Plan, interviews with the medical office employer and employees, and observation of work activities.

The OSHA Standard does not cover stool, urine, sputum, nasal secretions, sweat, tears, or vomitus unless they are visibly contaminated with blood.

Employees are not permitted to launder contaminated clothing at home; rather, it is the responsibility of the employer to have clothing laundered.

General work clothes, such as uniforms, pants, shirts, or blouses, are not intended to function as protection against a hazard and are not considered to be personal protective equipment.

OSHA expects hands to be washed each time gloves are removed, even if that means 50 times a day.

If an employee is allergic to the standard latex gloves, the employer must provide a suitable alternative, such as hypoallergenic gloves, powderless gloves, or glove liners.

e. Close the lid of the sharps container prior to removal or replacement to prevent spillage or protrusion of the contents during handling, storage, transport, or shipping.

f. If there is a chance of leakage from the sharps container, the medical assistant should place it in a second container that is closable, leak-proof, and labeled or color coded.

Hepatitis B Vaccination

The OSHA Standard requires physicians to offer the hepatitis B vaccination series free of charge to all medical office personnel who have occupational exposure. The vaccination must be offered within 10 days of initial assignment to a position with occupational exposure unless the following factors exist: (a) the individual has previously received the hepatitis B vaccination series, (b) antibody testing has revealed that the individual is immune, or (c) the vaccine is contraindicated for medical reasons.

Medical office personnel who decline vaccination must sign a hepatitis B waiver form documenting refusal, which is to be filed in the employee's OSHA record (Fig. 1–8). Employees who decline vaccination may later request the vaccination, which then must be provided by the employer according to the aforementioned criteria.

Universal Precautions

Previous to the release of the OSHA Standard, the U.S. Public Health Service Centers for Disease Control and Prevention (CDC) issued a recommended set of precautions for healthcare workers known as the Universal Precautions. According to the concept of Universal Precautions, all human blood and certain human body fluids are treated as if known to be infectious for HIV, HBV, and other bloodborne pathogens. The OSHA Standard states that the Universal Precautions must be observed, and in fact, these precautions form the heart of the OSHA Standard itself.

Infectious Waste

Infectious waste (also termed **regulated waste** by the CDC) is anything that harbors an infectious agent. This includes any waste that contains blood or other potentially infectious materials and contaminated pathologic laboratory and surgical waste, contaminated sharps, biologic cultures, and live vaccines. Federal and state regulations must be followed in disposing of infectious waste (see Highlight on Infectious Waste Regulations).

Most medical offices use a commercial infectious waste service to dispose of infectious waste. The service is responsible for picking up and transporting the medical waste to an infectious waste treatment facility

HEPATITIS B VACCINE REFUSAL

I understand that due to my occupational exposure to blood or other potentially infectious materials, I may be at risk of acquiring hepatitis B virus (HBV) infection. I have been given the opportunity to be vaccinated with hepatitis B vaccine at no charge to myself. However, I decline hepatitis B vaccination at this time. I understand that by declining this vaccine I continue to be at risk of acquiring hepatitis B, a serious disease. If in the future I continue to have occupational exposure to blood or to other potentially infectious materials and I want to be vaccinated with hepatitis B vaccine, I can receive the vaccination series at no charge to me.

_____
Employee Name (printed)

_____   _____
Employee Signature   Date

_____   _____
Witness Signature   Date

■ **FIGURE 1–8.** Hepatitis B vaccine waiver form. This form must be signed by an employee with occupational exposure who declines hepatitis B vaccination.

for incineration or treatment to render it harmless. To meet federal and state regulations, a series of steps must be followed for handling, packaging, and storing infectious waste for pickup by the service. These steps are directed at minimizing exposure to bloodborne pathogens and other potentially infectious materials and include the following:

1. Separate infectious waste from the general refuse at its point of origin. This means that disposable items containing infectious waste should be placed directly into biohazard containers and not mixed with the regular trash.
2. Make sure that the biohazard containers are closable, leakproof, and suitably constructed to contain the contents during handling, storage, and transport. These containers include biohazard bags and sharps containers.
3. Close the lid of the sharps container before removal or replacement to prevent spillage or protrusion of the contents.
4. Remove full biohazard containers to an area away from patients, using personal protective equipment (e.g., gloves).
5. Securely close biohazard bags and tie them. To provide additional protection, some medical offices double-bag by placing the primary bag inside a second biohazard bag.
6. Put biohazard bags and sharps containers into a receptacle provided by the infectious waste service. The receptacle is usually a cardboard box (Fig. 1–9). The box should be securely sealed with packing tape, and a biohazard label must appear on two opposite sides of the box.
7. Store the biohazard boxes in a locked room inside the facility or outside in a lockable collection container for pickup by the infectious waste service. This step is aimed at preventing unauthorized access to such items as needles and syringes. The infectious waste storage area should be labeled with one of the following:
    a. An "Authorized Personnel Only" sign.
    b. A sign stating "Warning: Infectious Waste."
    c. The international biohazard symbol.
8. The infectious waste cannot be stored for more than 35 days.

BLOODBORNE DISEASES—HEPATITIS B AND AIDS

The biggest threats to health-care workers from occupational exposure are hepatitis B and AIDS. These diseases are discussed in detail on the following pages.

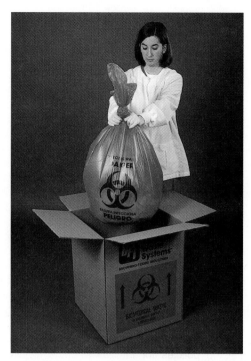

■ **FIGURE 1–9.** Jennifer places a biohazard bag inside a cardboard box in preparation for pickup by the infectious waste service.

Hepatitis B

Hepatitis B is an infection of the liver caused by the hepatitis B virus (HBV). It is the leading occupational bloodborne hazard to health-care workers. Each year, approximately 8700 health-care employees contract hepatitis B in the workplace, and 200 of them die as a result.

The most common means of transmission of the hepatitis B virus in the health-care setting are blood and blood products, such as serum and plasma. The health-care employee is most likely to contract HBV through needlesticks and cuts with contaminated sharps, as well as blood splashes to the eyes, mouth, and nonintact skin, as in lacerations, abrasions, burns, and rashes. The virus also can be spread, but less effectively, through body fluids such as saliva, semen, and vaginal secretions. Therefore, it is important for the medical assistant to carefully follow the OSHA Standard to safeguard against exposure to the hepatitis virus and other bloodborne pathogens.

Acute Viral Hepatitis

The acute phase of hepatitis B occurs after an individual becomes infected. It can last from a few weeks to

Highlight on Infectious Waste Regulations

In the summer of 1988, medical waste—containing syringes and needles—appeared on the beaches along the East Coast. Prompted by this incident as well as mounting pressure from other sources, the federal government enacted legislation aimed at regulating the handling and disposal of infectious medical waste. Anyone who generates infectious waste must comply with these regulations.

Two federal agencies are involved in the process of infectious waste disposal. They include the Environmental Protection Agency (EPA), which is responsible for protecting public health and the environment outside the workplace, and the Occupational Health and Safety Administration (OSHA), which is responsible for ensuring employee health and safety inside the workplace.

Regulations for the management of infectious waste are set down at the federal level by the EPA and OSHA. These federal agencies then delegate to the states the responsibility for developing specific policies and guidelines to meet these regulations. Because of this, the policies for infectious waste disposal vary somewhat from state to state. To avoid noncompliance, it is important to know and understand the infectious waste policies and guidelines set forth in your state.

Any facility that produces infectious waste is referred to by the EPA as a **generator.** The EPA considers anyone who puts out more than 50 pounds of waste per month a large generator, which includes most medical offices. Large generators must register with the EPA and obtain a certificate of registration from the EPA's Division of Solid and Hazardous Waste Management. Small generators produce less than 50 pounds of infectious medical waste in a month; smaller medical offices often fall into this category. The regulations for small generators are not as strict as those for large generators.

Using an infectious waste service meets the regulations required for infectious waste disposal for both large and small generators. Because of this, most medical offices hire such a service for transport and disposal of their infectious waste. Infectious waste treatment facilities must be licensed and hold permits issued by the EPA, allowing them to dispose of infectious waste.

On pickup of the infectious waste at the medical office, a tracking record form must be completed that includes such information as the type and quantity of waste (as weighed in pounds), and where it is being sent. The form must be signed by a representative of both the infectious waste service and the medical office. After the waste has been destroyed, a record documenting disposal is mailed back to the medical office. Tracking records must be retained by the medical office for 3 years and be available for review by the Environmental Protection Agency.

Noncompliance with the regulations governing the disposal of infectious waste could lead to stiff penalties and fines of $10,000 to $25,000; for deliberate violations, a prison sentence of 2 to 4 years is possible. In some states, a generator could be charged with anything from public endangerment to a felony.

1

---

several months. The symptoms of acute viral hepatitis vary greatly in intensity from mild to severe. Approximately one third of all patients who become infected are asymptomatic and not even aware that they have the disease. Another third have relatively mild flulike symptoms that often are mistaken for influenza or similar conditions. The remaining one third of infected patients have such severe symptoms that hospitalization may be required.

The initial symptoms, if present, last from 2 to 14 days and include fatigue, mild fever, nausea, vomiting, malaise, and muscle and joint pain. In patients with severe acute viral hepatitis, these symptoms then progress to dark urine and clay-colored stools, followed several days later by the appearance of jaundice. After the onset of jaundice, the liver enlarges and becomes tender. A very small percentage of patients (0.5 to 2 percent of those infected) develop fulminant hepatitis, which is almost always fatal. Fulminant hepatitis is characterized by a sudden onset of nausea and vomit-ing, chills, high fever, severe and early jaundice, convulsions, coma, and death due to hepatic failure, usually within 10 days after its onset.

There is no specific treatment or drug that kills the hepatitis virus. Rather, supportive care is prescribed to help the patient's own natural defenses overcome the disease; this includes restricted activity, rest, avoidance of alcohol, a well-balanced diet, adequate fluid intake, and precautionary measures to prevent the disease's spread.

Most patients (90 percent) recover fully after the acute phase and acquire life-long immunity to hepatitis B. In some patients, complete recovery may take up to 6 months.

Chronic Viral Hepatitis

The remaining 6 to 10 percent of patients who do not recover from the acute phase go on to develop chronic

1

Highlight on Hepatitis B

Approximately 200,000 to 300,000 new hepatitis B infections occur each year.

It is estimated that over 1 million people in the United States are carriers for hepatitis B and capable of transmitting the disease to others. Many of these individuals do not know that they are carriers.

Hepatitis B is capable of surviving for at least a week in a dried state on environmental surfaces such as contaminated work tables, equipment, and instruments.

Hepatitis B is much easier to transmit than is HIV. After a needlestick injury, health-care workers have a 6 to 30 percent chance of developing hepatitis B and a 1 percent chance of developing AIDS from the same injury.

Hepatitis B is a reportable disease and therefore requires filling out forms for the local public health department.

hepatitis. These individuals are unable to remove the virus from their system and remain infected the rest of their lives. Individuals with chronic hepatitis may or may not experience symptoms; nonetheless, they become carriers of HBV and are capable of transmitting the disease to others. In addition, patients with chronic hepatitis face an increased risk of liver damage, which leaves them vulnerable to developing such diseases as cirrhosis of the liver and liver cancer. A significant number of these patients subsequently die from liver failure.

Post-Exposure Treatment

The treatment of individuals exposed to hepatitis B involves the administration of both a passive and an active immunizing agent. The passive immunizing agent provides temporary immunity to hepatitis B, thereby giving the active agent a chance to take effect. The passive agent is hepatitis B immune globulin (HBIG), which contains antibodies that provide immunity to hepatitis B for a period of 1 to 3 months. It is important to administer HBIG as soon as possible after an exposure incident— preferably within 24 hours, but no later than 7 days after exposure.

The active immunizing agent is the hepatitis B vaccine (Fig. 1–10), which provides immunity for a period of at least 7 years. The hepatitis B vaccine in predominant use is produced from genetically altered yeast

cells; brand names are Recombivax HB and Engerix-B. The hepatitis B vaccine is administered intramuscularly into the deltoid muscle in a series of three doses. The second dose is given 1 month after the first, and the third 6 months after the first (i.e., at 0, 1 month, and 6 months). Mild side effects such as soreness at the injection site may occur, but serious reactions to the vaccine are extremely rare.

As previously discussed, the OSHA Standard recommends that all health-care workers receive the vaccine as a preventive measure against hepatitis B. Therefore, after an exposure incident, a medical assistant who has previously been vaccinated probably will not require further treatment unless laboratory tests reveal that his or her antibody level is low. In this case, a booster dose of the vaccine is recommended.

Other Forms of Viral Hepatitis

In addition to hepatitis B, four other strains that cause viral hepatitis have been identified. They include hepatitis A, C, D, and E. Of these, hepatitis B poses the greatest threat to health-care workers and has already been discussed in detail. Hepatitis A and hepatitis C occasionally have been transmitted to health-care workers but are not considered major occupational

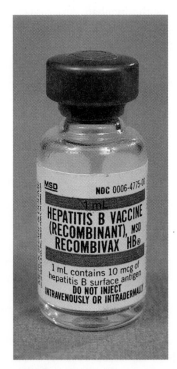

■ **FIGURE 1–10.** Hepatitis B vaccine.

Highlight on Hepatitis B Vaccine

The hepatitis B vaccine is 90-percent effective in providing immunity.

The hepatitis B vaccine is generally well tolerated by most patients, and side effects have not been serious to date. The most common side effect is soreness at the injection site including induration, erythema, and swelling. Occasionally, a low-grade fever, headache, and dizziness may occur.

The hepatitis B vaccine provides immunity for at least 7 years. At the present time, the CDC do not recommend a routine booster dose.

The hepatitis B vaccine is recommended for the following individuals: high-risk health-care workers, clients and staff of institutions for the mentally retarded, hemodialysis patients, homosexually active men, intravenous drug users, hemophiliacs, and household and sexual contacts of hepatitis B carriers.

Treatment of a patient with HBIG and the hepatitis B vaccine is more than 90-percent effective in preventing hepatitis B in exposed persons.

hazards. In all cases of viral hepatitis, the virus invades the liver and causes inflammation, resulting in similar symptoms. The medical assistant should have a general knowledge of each of the forms of viral hepatitis. Table 1–1 outlines the incubation period, means of transmission, characteristics, onset and symptoms, and prognosis for all strains of viral hepatitis.

Acquired Immunodeficiency Syndrome (AIDS)

AIDS is a disorder of the immune system that eventually destroys the body's ability to fight off infection. AIDS is characterized by the presence of severe and life-threatening opportunistic infections and unusual cancers that rarely afflict individuals with healthy immune systems. An **opportunistic infection** is an infection that results from a defective immune system that cannot defend itself from pathogens normally found in the environment. Opportunistic infections are extremely difficult to treat, because the infection tends to recur very quickly once a course of therapy is completed.

AIDS is caused by a retrovirus known as the human immunodeficiency virus (HIV). This virus is transmitted through contaminated body fluids, particularly blood and semen. When HIV gains entrance into the body, it begins to attack and destroy certain white blood cells known as CD4+ T lymphocytes. Over time, more and more CD4+ T lymphocytes are destroyed and the body becomes less able to fight off infection, as well as being more susceptible to opportunistic infections.

The AIDS virus infection cycle has four stages; however, they may not all be experienced by every infected individual. These four stages are described below.

STAGE I: ACUTE HIV INFECTION. An individual infected with HIV may first experience a transient mononucleosis-like illness known as acute HIV infection, which occurs within a month or two after exposure. On the other hand, many people do not develop any symptoms when they first become infected with HIV. Symptoms of acute HIV infection include fever, sweats, fatigue, loss of appetite, diarrhea, pharyngitis, myalgia, arthralgia, and adenopathy. These symptoms usually disappear within a week to a month and are often mistaken for those of another viral infection.

PUTTING IT ALL *into* PRACTICE

▶ JENNIFER HAWK: *The most interesting experience I have had as a CMA is seeing the impact that you make in the patients' lives. Patients rely on you and look to you first for help in their health-care situation. You are most often the first person they come into contact with in the office, and they look to you for understanding and empathy. Especially patients that must come to your office on a regular basis see you as a kind of family member. They appreciate a familiar face and smile. Most often, you are the individual giving the patient instructions concerning testing they will be having done or medication they will be taking. Patients truly do count on your knowledge and assistance throughout their course of care. I was genuinely surprised at what an impact I could have on others.*

1

Forms of Viral Hepatitis

TABLE 1-1

	Hepatitis A	Hepatitis B	Hepatitis C	Hepatitis D	Hepatitis E
Incubation Period	2 to 6 weeks	2 weeks to 6 months	2 weeks to 6 months	2 weeks to 5 months	3 to 6 weeks
Means of Transmission	Transmitted almost exclusively by the fecal-oral route through practices of poor hygiene Also transmitted by the consumption of food and water contaminated with feces	Parenteral exposure to contaminated blood and blood products, such as through accidental needlesticks, IV drug use, and blood transfusions Exposure to contaminated semen and vaginal secretions by personal contact, especially sexual contact Perinatally from an infected mother to her neonate	Parenteral exposure to contaminated blood or blood products, primarily from blood transfusions and occasionally from accidental needlesticks and intravenous drug use	Same as hepatitis B	Fecal-oral route through practices of poor hygiene Consumption of food and water contaminated with feces
Characteristics	Usually occurs in children and young adults, especially in environments of poor sanitation and overcrowding Often a very mild disease with symptoms similar to the flu and lasting 1 to 2 weeks	Symptoms usually last 1 to 4 weeks, but it may be as long as 6 months before the patient fully recovers At greatest risk are health-care workers, fire fighters, law enforcement personnel, intravenous drug users, and people with multiple sexual partners	Affects approximately 170,000 Americans each year, primarily through blood transfusions	Affects only those already infected with hepatitis B A person who has received the hepatitis B vaccine is also protected from hepatitis D	Rare in the United States Generally seen in developing countries Usually occurs in epidemics rather than in sporadic cases
Onset and Symptoms	Acute onset Symptoms include fever, malaise, fatigue, anorexia, nausea, vomiting, and abdominal discomfort, followed in some patients by dark urine, clay-colored stools, and mild jaundice	Insidious (slow and gradual) onset Symptoms include fatigue, mild fever, nausea, vomiting, malaise, and muscle and joint pain, followed in some patients by dark urine, clay-colored stools, and jaundice	Insidious onset Symptoms are similar to those of hepatitis B	Acute onset Occurs as a coinfection or superinfection with hepatitis B and intensifies the symptoms of hepatitis B	Acute onset Symptoms are similar to those of hepatitis B
Prognosis	Most people recover fully within 6 to 10 weeks and become immune to the virus Rarely fatal Chronic hepatitis does not develop Carrier states do not develop	Most people recover fully and become immune to this disease Some patients go on to develop chronic hepatitis and may develop cirrhosis and liver cancer. These patients are also carriers of hepatitis B Approximately 0.5 to 2 percent of those infected develop fulminating hepatitis, which is almost always fatal	Approximately half of all patients infected with hepatitis C develop chronic hepatitis, which may lead to liver damage such as cirrhosis and liver cancer	Frequently leads to chronic hepatitis High fatality rate (as high as 30 percent of chronic hepatitis patients)	Does not progress to chronic hepatitis Hepatitis E is particularly dangerous if contracted by pregnant women (10 to 20 percent fatality rate in these individuals)

PATIENT/TEACHING

ACQUIRED IMMUNODEFICIENCY SYNDROME

Teach patients the ways in which AIDS is transmitted.

Having sex (vaginal, anal, or oral) with someone who is infected with HIV. The virus is most commonly found in semen, blood, and vaginal secretions.

Sharing intravenous drug needles with someone who is infected with HIV.

A woman with HIV can pass it on to her unborn child. Babies born with HIV usually develop AIDS by 2 years of age.

Receiving a blood transfusion or blood products (before 1985) from someone infected with HIV. (In 1985, blood banks began screening blood for AIDS, so this is largely a problem of blood received before then.)

Teach patients how to prevent AIDS:

Know your sexual partner(s) and their past sexual history and drug use.

Use a latex condom during sexual intercourse to minimize the risk of infection. HIV cannot pass through the latex if the condom does not break and is used properly. If a lubricant is used with the condom, it should be water based, such as K-Y Jelly, because an oil-based lubricant, such as petroleum jelly, could break down the latex.

Avoid sexual practices in which the exchange of body fluids, such as semen or vaginal secretions, takes place.

If you think that you could have HIV, never let your blood, semen, or vaginal fluid enter another person's body.

Teach patients to recognize the symptoms of AIDS:

Unexplained fatigue.

Weight loss of 10 to 15 pounds in less than 2 months, but without dieting.

Unexplained fever, chills, and sweating at night for more than 2 weeks.

Unexplained swollen glands for more than a month.

Unexplained diarrhea or bloody stools for more than 2 weeks.

Unexplained persistent dry cough, shortness of breath, or difficulty in breathing.

White patches on the tongue or mouth that cannot be scraped off.

Explain to patients that these symptoms could also be signs of other diseases. However, if they have any of these symptoms they should consider having an HIV test. The earlier the infection is detected, the earlier treatment can begin that may delay the onset of other symptoms.

STAGE 2: ASYMPTOMATIC PERIOD. After these early symptoms have subsided (if they occur at all), the infected individual normally experiences a long incubation period lasting for years, during which he or she is asymptomatic. At that time, the carrier may not realize the HIV infection is present, because the only evidence of HIV infection during this stage is the production by the body of antibodies to HIV that are detectable by blood tests. These HIV antibodies are unable to destroy the virus; however, they are used as a basis for the test procedure to indicate that the HIV infection is present. Because of the length of time required by the body to develop HIV antibodies, however, these tests may fail to detect HIV for as long as 3 to 6 months after an individual has been infected. Since HIV may be transmitted with or without symptoms, it is during this asymptomatic period that the danger of accidental transmission is greatest.

STAGE 3: SYMPTOMATIC PERIOD. Before the development of full-blown AIDS, many HIV-infected individuals experience a series of lesser symptoms. One of the first such symptoms experienced by many people in-

fected with HIV is lymph nodes that remain enlarged for more than 3 months. Other symptoms often experienced months to years before the onset of AIDS include a lack of energy, weight loss, frequent fevers and sweats, persistent or frequent yeast infections (oral or vaginal), persistent skin rashes or flaky skin, pelvic inflammatory disease that does not respond to treatment, or short-term memory loss. Some people develop frequent and severe herpes infections that cause mouth, genital or anal sores, or a painful nerve disease known as shingles.

STAGE 4: AIDS. AIDS is the last stage of the infection cycle that began with HIV infection. As previously described, full-blown AIDS is characterized by the presence of opportunistic infections and unusual cancers known as **AIDS-defining conditions.** These conditions do not usually occur, or produce only mild illness, in individuals with healthy immune systems. For example, a severe and rare type of pneumonia caused by the organism *Pneumocystis carinii* is frequently associated with AIDS patients, as is *Kaposi's sarcoma,* a rare type of cancer. Refer to Table 1–2 for a description of

TABLE 1-2

AIDS-Defining Conditions

Neoplasms

Kaposi's Sarcoma (KS)
Malignant Neoplasm

Kaposi's sarcoma is the most common neoplasm occurring in AIDS patients. It is an aggressive tumor involving multiple body organs but generally occurs initially on the skin. It is characterized by multiple dark red or purplish blotches on the skin. The areas of the body most commonly affected include the trunk, arms, head, and neck. Diagnosis of Kaposi's sarcoma is made by tissue biopsy. Other body sites commonly affected by this neoplasm include the lymph nodes, the lungs, and the gastrointestinal tract. Kaposi's sarcoma is rarely the primary cause of death but does further weaken the AIDS patient, who may succumb eventually to opportunistic infections.

Opportunistic Infections

Pneumocystis carinii Pneumonia (PCP)
Protozoa

Pneumocystis carinii pneumonia is the most common opportunistic infection causing death in individuals with AIDS. This protozoan lung infection was at one time considered rare and in most instances not fatal. PCP occurs at least once in more than 65 percent of all AIDS patients, and 25 percent of those initially infected experience a recurrence. PCP is characterized by moderate-to-severe difficulty in breathing, fever, and a nonproductive cough in the early stages and a productive cough in the later stages of the disease. Death occurs in 30 percent of PCP-infected patients and is generally caused by acute respiratory failure.

Cytomegalovirus Infection (CMV)
Virus

CMV is a virus that belongs to the herpes virus group, which rarely causes disease in healthy adults. The majority of AIDS patients have active cytomegalovirus infection. The most common symptoms of its presence in AIDS patients are spots on the retina that may lead to blindness. This virus also causes pneumonia, esophagitis, and colitis. Specific symptoms may include fever, profound fatigue, muscle and joint aches, night sweats, impaired vision, cough, dyspnea, abdominal pain, and diarrhea.

Herpes Simplex 1 and 2
Virus

Herpes simplex 1 is spread by contact with oral secretions, and herpes simplex 2 is spread by contact with genital secretions. Herpes simplex causes painful vesicular lesions, usually of the nasopharynx, oral cavity, skin, and genital tract. This virus tends to have periods of latency followed by reactivation of symptoms. In AIDS patients, herpes simplex is apt to cause cervical lymphadenopathy and proctitis.

Mycobacterial Infections
Bacteria

Mycobacterial infections are one of the most frequent opportunistic infections in AIDS patients. One strain (*Mycobacterium avium* complex) causes fever, fatigue, weight loss, diarrhea, and malabsorption. Another strain (*Mycobacterium tuberculosis*) causes pulmonary tuberculosis, which is not considered an opportunistic infection. In AIDS patients, tuberculosis is characterized by a productive, purulent cough, fever, dyspnea, fatigue, weight loss, and wasting. The AIDS epidemic appears to be causing a resurgence of tuberculosis in the United States. Because tuberculosis is more contagious than most AIDS-defining conditions, it appears to be spreading beyond AIDS patients and into the general population.

Candidiasis
Yeastlike Fungus

Candida albicans is a fungus that inhabits the oropharynx, large intestine, and skin, causing no harm in individuals with healthy immune systems. Infection with *Candida albicans* is often one of the first signs of a weakened immune system in HIV-infected individuals. It is characterized by a white, patchy growth on the mouth, throat, or esophagus (thrush). AIDS patients develop an extremely severe case of candidiasis that makes eating and swallowing both difficult and painful. In female AIDS patients, this organism causes severe vaginitis.

Cryptosporidiosis
Protozoa

In AIDS patients, this condition usually causes profuse, watery diarrhea along with anorexia, vomiting, fatigue, malaise, and fever. This condition may become chronic, resulting in dehydration and electrolyte imbalance, which in turn leads to weight loss and eventual death.

Toxoplasmosis
Protozoa

Toxoplasmosis is one of the most common causes of encephalitis in AIDS patients, resulting in the following symptoms: headache, altered mental state, visual disturbances, cranial nerve palsy, and motor disorders. Toxoplasmosis may also result in infection of the heart, lungs, skin, stomach, abdomen, and testes.

Cryptococcosis
Fungus

Cryptococcosis is a common cause of meningitis in AIDS patients and includes chronic symptoms of low-grade fever, malaise, and headaches. Other symptoms manifested after these initial symptoms include photophobia, stiff neck, nausea, vomiting, and seizures.

Highlight on AIDS

Scientific evidence shows that HIV is not spread through casual everyday contact. There is no evidence that HIV is spread by sharing facilities or equipment such as telephones, computers, pencils, cups, doorknobs, or bathrooms. Because HIV is not passed through the air, it is not spread through coughing and sneezing.

The majority of individuals who are infected with HIV show no symptoms and may not develop full-blown AIDS for many years. Once infected with HIV, the individual is infected for life.

AIDS was first reported in the United States in 1981. More than 500,000 cases of AIDS have been reported in the United States since 1981, and as many as 900,000 Americans may be infected with HIV. The epidemic is growing most rapidly among minority populations and is a leading killer of black men. According to the CDC, the prevalence of AIDS is six times higher in blacks and three times higher among Hispanics than among whites.

Women can transmit HIV to their fetuses during pregnancy or birth. Approximately one quarter to one third of all untreated pregnant women infected with HIV will pass the infection to their babies. HIV also can be spread to babies through the breast milk of mothers infected with the virus. If the antiretroviral drug zidovudine (AZT) is taken during pregnancy, the chance of transmitting HIV to the baby is reduced significantly.

The enzyme-linked immunosorbent assay (ELISA) test is widely used as a screening test for the presence of HIV. Because of the possibility of a false-positive results, a second ELISA test is always performed if a blood specimen tests positive. If the second ELISA test is also positive, then a more specific test, such as the Western blot test, is performed to confirm the test results. An individual who tests positive for HIV is said to be **seropositive.**

A negative HIV test is not conclusive for the absence of HIV infection. If an individual has recently been infected with HIV, the antibodies may not have had time to develop. It generally takes 3 to 6 months for the antibodies to show up in the blood.

At present, there is no cure for AIDS, nor vaccine to prevent it, but there are methods of treatment for the AIDS-defining opportunistic infections and cancers that occur.

---

these and other AIDS-defining conditions. AIDS is also known to damage the nervous system, which eventually results in varying degrees of dementia and other symptoms. As the HIV infection progresses, the individual becomes overwhelmed by infection and cancer. Because the body is unable to fight back due to a weakened immune system, the patient eventually succumbs to AIDS-defining conditions.

Transmission of AIDS

HIV has been isolated in blood, semen, saliva, tears, breast milk, cerebrospinal fluid, amniotic fluid, urine, and secretions of the female genital tract. However, the only documented transmission of the virus has occurred by exposure to contaminated blood and the exchange of sexual and perinatal fluids. In addition, research has shown that HIV is not transmitted through casual contact or even extensive contact such as occurs among family members of AIDS patients.

Because HIV is not easily transmitted, the risk to health-care workers is low. Still, parenteral exposure to HIV should be considered a definite occupational risk, no matter how small. Studies by the CDC have indicated that even when parenteral exposure to HIV-contaminated blood is known to have occurred, fewer than 1 percent of health-care workers so exposed tested positive for HIV infection. These studies indicate that HIV is inefficiently transmitted, even during accidental needlestick incidents or the exposure of mucous membrane or nonintact skin to contaminated fluids.

Despite the low risk of infection, the serious nature of HIV infection and the likely subsequent development of AIDS warrant the use of the OSHA Standard by all health-care workers. Because most HIV carriers are asymptomatic and may not be aware of their infection, precautions minimizing the risk of exposure to blood and body fluids should be taken with all patients at all times. The precautions are also recommended as a means of protection against other bloodborne pathogens, such as hepatitis B and syphilis.

1

MEDICAL PRACTICE AND THE LAW

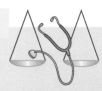

Throughout this book, look for these boxes to give you tips on ethical and legal issues dealing with each chapter topic. These tips are designed to make you think about actions and interactions with patients, and to minimize your risk of being sued.

In general, three behaviors are most important in protecting yourself from a lawsuit.

1. Establish a rapport. If patients believe that you truly care about them and have their best interests at heart, they rarely sue, even if you make a mistake.
2. Follow all procedures according to your procedure manual. If you do everything right and the patient has an adverse outcome, you will not likely be found liable.
3. Document everything you do objectively. Lawsuits often come to court years after the incident, and nobody's memory is as good as written documentation. Document only facts, not your opinion. Be sure to document the patient's reaction to treatments.

Ethics and Law

Ethics is the highest standard of behavior and is loosely based on the golden rule. No law can force you to behave ethically, but most major professions have a written code of ethics, including the American Association of Medical Assistants (AAMA). Ethics uses words such as "should" and "may." If you are angry at someone, ethically, you should not yell at him or her. This is not against the law, but it is unethical.

Law is the lowest standard of behavior, and is enforced by laws and statutes. Laws use words such as "must" and "shall." If you are angry at someone, legally, you must not hit him or her. This is illegal, and you could be charged with assault and battery.

Regarding medical asepsis and infection control, you have a duty and responsibility to protect yourself, your coworkers, and most importantly, your patients. Follow specific guidelines established by OSHA and the CDC to prevent the transmission of pathogens.

CERTIFICATION REVIEW

☐ Microorganisms are tiny living plants or animals that cannot be seen with the naked eye; examples include bacteria viruses, protozoa, fungi, and animal parasites. Microorganisms that do not cause disease are known as nonpathogens. Microorganisms that are harmful to the body and can cause disease are known as pathogens.

☐ Microorganisms that use inorganic substances as a source of food are known as autotrophs, whereas those that use organic substances for food are known as heterotrophs. Aerobes are microorganisms that need oxygen to grow and multiply, and anaerobes are microorganisms that grow best in the absence of oxygen.

☐ The body has protective mechanisms to help prevent the entrance of pathogens and include the following: the skin and mucous membranes, mucus and cilia in the nose and respiratory tract, coughing and sneezing, tears and sweat, urine and vaginal secretions, and hydrochloric acid secreted by the stomach.

☐ Medical asepsis means that an object or area is clean and free from infection. Handwashing is an important medical aseptic practice to prevent the transmission of pathogens in the medical office.

☐ Resident flora, also known as normal flora, normally reside and grow in the epidermis and dermis. Resident flora are generally harmless and nonpathogenic. Transient flora live and grow on the superficial skin layers and are picked up in the course of daily activities. Transient flora are often pathogenic but can be removed easily by washing the hands with soap and water.

☐ Soaps are used to cleanse the skin. Detergents are able to emulsify dirt and oil present on the skin, and antimicrobials are chemical agents that inhibit the growth of or kill microorganisms.

☐ OSHA was established by the federal government to assist employers in providing a safe and healthy working environment for their employees. The OSHA Standard must be followed by any employee with occupational exposure, regardless of the place of employment.

☐ Occupational exposure is defined as reasonably anticipated skin, eye, mucous membrane, or parenteral contact with bloodborne pathogens or other potentially infectious materials that may result from the performance of an employee's duties. Bloodborne pathogens are pathogenic microorganisms that are present in human blood and

Continued

CERTIFICATION REVIEW *Continued*

are capable of causing disease. An exposure incident is a specific eye, mouth, other mucous membrane, nonintact skin, or parenteral contact with blood or other potentially infectious materials that results from an employee's duties.

☐ The OSHA Standard requires that the medical office develop a written Exposure Control Plan designed to eliminate or minimize employee exposure to bloodborne pathogens and other potentially infectious materials.

☐ Engineering controls are physical or mechanical devices (such as readily accessible handwashing facilities, self-capping needles, biohazards containers and bags, and autoclaves) that isolate or remove health hazards from the workplace.

☐ Work practice controls reduce the likelihood of exposure by altering the manner in which the technique is performed and include such practices as bandaging cuts before gloving, washing hands as soon as possible after removing gloves, immediately placing contaminated sharps in a biohazard sharps container, and not eating, drinking, or smoking in areas where you may be exposed to blood or other potentially infectious materials.

☐ Personal protective equipment is clothing or equipment that protects an individual from contact with blood or other potentially infectious materials; examples include gloves, face shields, masks, protective eyewear, laboratory coats, and gowns.

The type of protective equipment appropriate for a given task depends on the degree of exposure that is anticipated.

☐ Regulated waste (also known as infectious waste) is waste containing infectious materials that would pose a substantial threat to health and safety if exposed to the public. Regulated waste includes any waste that contains blood or other potentially infectious materials such as contaminated pathologic laboratory and surgical waste, contaminated sharps, biologic cultures, and live vaccines. Regulated waste must be disposed of in accordance with all applicable federal, state, and local laws.

☐ The biggest threats to health-care workers from occupational exposure are hepatitis B and AIDS. Hepatitis B is an infection of the liver caused by HBV. The most common means of transmission of HBV in the health-care setting are blood and blood products through needlesticks and cuts with contaminated sharps, as well as blood splashes to the eyes, mouth, and nonintact skin.

☐ AIDS is a disorder of the immune system that eventually destroys the body's ability to fight infection. AIDS is characterized by the presence of severe and life-threatening opportunistic infections and unusual cancers. AIDS is caused by HIV. HIV is transmitted through contaminated body fluids, particularly blood and semen.

1

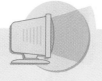

RESOURCES

ON THE WEB

For information on AIDS:

HIV Info Web
www.infoweb.org

AIDS Education Global Info
Service
www.aegis.com

AIDS Research Information
Center
www.critpath.org/aric

The Body—AIDS and HIV
Information Resource
www.thebody.com

Project Inform—HIV Treatment Information
www.projectinform.org

HIV Positive.Com
www.HIVpositive.com

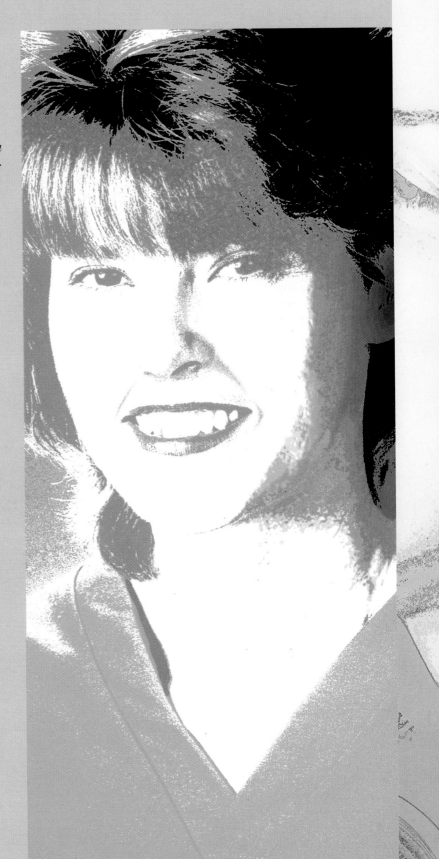

Dawn Bennett *and I graduated from an accredited medical assisting program. I have an associate's degree in Applied Science and I am a Certified Medical Assistant (CMA). I work in a multiphysician family practice medical office. I work in the front area of the office as an administrative supervisor in billing and collections. I have worked as a medical assistant for 3 years and the most fulfilling thing I find about being a medical assistant is helping people.*

OUTCOMES

After completing this chapter, you should be able to demonstrate the proper procedures to perform the following:

1. Obtain patient consent for treatment.
2. Release medical information according to a completed release of information form.
3. Prepare a medical record for a new patient.
4. Complete or assist the patient in completing a health history form.
5. Chart the following: patient symptoms, procedures, administration of medication, specimen collection, laboratory tests, progress notes, and instructions given to the patient.

EDUCATIONAL OBJECTIVES

After completing this chapter, you should be able to do the following:

1. Define the terms listed in the Key Terminology.
2. List and describe the functions served by the medical record.
3. Identify the information contained in each of the following medical office administrative documents: patient registration record and correspondence.
4. Identify the information contained in each of the following medical office clinical documents: health history, physical examination, progress notes, medication record, consultation report, and home health care report.
5. List and describe the information included in the following diagnostic documents: electrocardiogram report, Holter monitor report, sigmoidoscopy report, spirometry report, radiology report, and imaging report.
6. State the purpose of each of the following therapeutic services: physical therapy, occupational therapy, and speech therapy.
7. Identify the information contained in the following hospital documents: history and physical, operative report, discharge summary report, pathology report, and emergency room report.
8. Identify the information contained in the following consent documents: consent to treatment form and consent to release information form.
9. Describe the organization of a source-oriented medical record and a problem-oriented medical record.
10. List and define the four subcategories included in the progress notes of a problem-oriented record (POR).
11. Explain the difference between a paper-based patient record (PPR) and a computer-based patient record (CPR).
12. List and describe the seven parts of the health history.
13. List the guidelines that should be followed in recording the chief complaint.
14. List and describe the guidelines to follow to ensure accurate and concise charting.
15. List and describe the types of progress notes that are charted by the medical assistant.
16. List examples of subjective symptoms and objective symptoms.
17. List and describe common symptoms.

2

KEY TERMINOLOGY

charting: The process of making written entries about a patient in the medical record.

computer-based patient record (CPR): A medical record that is stored on a computer.

consultation report: A narrative report of an opinion about a patient's condition by a practitioner other than the attending physician.

diagnosis (dî-AG-nô-sis): The scientific method of determining and identifying a patient's condition.

diagnostic procedure: A type of procedure performed to assist in the diagnosis, management, and treatment of a patient's condition.

discharge summary report: A brief summary of the significant events of a patient's hospitalization.

familial (FA-mil-yel): Occurring or affecting members of a family more frequently than would be expected by chance.

health history report: A collection of subjective data about a patient.

home health care: The provision of medical and non-medical care in a patient's home or place of residence.

informed consent: Consent given by a patient for a medical procedure after being informed of the nature of his or her condition, the purpose of the procedure, alternative treatments or procedures available, the likely outcome of the procedure, and the risks involved with declining or delaying the procedure.

medical impressions: Conclusions drawn by the physician from an interpretation of data. Other terms for impressions include provisional diagnosis and tentative diagnosis.

medical record: A written record of the important information regarding a patient, including the care of that individual and the progress of the patient's condition.

medical record format: The way a medical record is organized. The two main types of medical record format include the source-oriented record and the problem-oriented record.

objective symptom: A symptom that can be observed by an examiner.

paper-based patient record (PPR): A medical record in paper form.

physical examination report: A report of the objective findings from the physician's assessment of each body system.

problem: Any patient condition that requires further observation, diagnosis, management, or patient education.

prognosis (prog-NÔ-sis): The probable course and outcome of a disease and the prospects of patient recovery.

reverse chronological order: Arranging documents with the most recent document on top, which means that oldest document is on the bottom.

SOAP format: A method of organization for recording progress notes. The SOAP format includes the following categories: subjective data, objective data, assessment, and plan.

subjective symptom: A symptom that is felt by the patient but is not observable by an examiner.

symptom: Any change in the body or its functioning that indicates that a disease is present.

INTRODUCTION

☐ A **medical record** is a written record of the important information regarding a patient, including the care of that individual and the progress of the patient's condition. Medical records are a critical part of a medical practice.

The patient's medical record serves a number of important functions. The physician uses the information in the medical record as a basis for making decisions regarding the patient's care and treatment. The medical record also serves to document the results of treatment and the patient's progress. The medical record provides an efficient and effective method by which information can be shared among members of the medical office.

The medical record also serves as a legal document. The law requires that a record be maintained to document the care and treatment being received by the patient. If something goes wrong, good documentation works to legally protect the physician and the medical staff. On the other hand, incomplete records could be used as evidence in court to show that the patient did not receive the quality of care that meets generally accepted standards.

The medical assistant must always keep in mind that the information contained within the patient's medical record is strictly confidential and must not be read by or discussed with anyone except the physician or medical staff involved with the care of the patient.

COMPONENTS OF THE MEDICAL RECORD

☐ A medical record consists of numerous documents. Each document in the medical record has a specific function or purpose. Most of these documents are on preprinted forms. A large variety of forms are available; the type of form utilized is based upon the specific requirements of each medical office.

Categories of Medical Record Documents

MEDICAL OFFICE ADMINISTRATIVE DOCUMENTS

Patient registration record
Correspondence

MEDICAL OFFICE CLINICAL DOCUMENTS

Health history
Physical examination
Progress notes
Medication record
Consultation report
Home health care report

LABORATORY DOCUMENTS

Hematology report
Clinical chemistry report
Serology report
Urinalysis report
Microbiology report
Parasitology report
Cytology report
Histology report

DIAGNOSTIC PROCEDURE DOCUMENTS

Electrocardiogram report
Holter monitor report
Sigmoidoscopy report
Spirometry report
Radiology report
Imaging report

THERAPEUTIC SERVICE DOCUMENTS

Physical therapy report
Occupational therapy report
Speech therapy report

HOSPITAL DOCUMENTS

History and physical
Operative report
Discharge summary report
Pathology report
Emergency room report

CONSENT DOCUMENTS

Consent to treatment form
Consent to release medical information form

Medical record documents can be classified into categories. Each of these categories is outlined in the box presented on this page, along with the specific documents included in each.

MEDICAL RECORD DOCUMENTS

☐ It is important that the medical assistant have a knowledge of each type of document contained in the medical record. A description of the function or purpose of each medical record document follows (by category), along with the specific information contained in each document.

MEDICAL OFFICE ADMINISTRATIVE DOCUMENTS

☐ Administrative documents contain information needed for the efficient (record-keeping) management of the medical office. Medical office administrative documents include the patient registration record and patient-related correspondence.

PATIENT REGISTRATION RECORD

The patient registration record (Fig. 2–1) consists of patient demographic and billing information. The patient registration form must be completed by all new patients. The procedure for completing a patient registration form is included in Procedure 2–3: Preparing a Medical Record.

In most offices, the data on the patient registration record is entered into a computer. This allows the information to be used for a number of functions such as scheduling appointments, posting patient transactions, and processing patient statements and insurance claims.

Demographic information required on a patient registration form includes the following:

- Full name
- Address
- Phone (home and work)
- Social security number
- Date of birth
- Gender
- Occupation

PATIENT INFORMATION **CONFIDENTIAL**

File no. 10140
Date 11-21-2002

(PLEASE PRINT)

Name Carol (First) H (Middle) Jones (Last) Birthdate 1-20-68 Home phone 740-555-1248

Address 743 Evergreen Terrace City Springfield State OH ZIP 12345

Check appropriate box: ☐ Minor ☐ Single ☒ Married ☐ Divorced ☐ Widowed ☐ Separated

Patient's or parent's Employer Rockford, Inc. Work phone 740-555-1234

Business Address 1 Rockford Place City Shelbyville State OH ZIP 21346

Spouse or parent's name John Employer Self Work phone 740-555-8654

If patient is a student, name of school/college N/A City ____ State ____

Whom may we thank for referring you? Henry Peterson, MD

Person to contact in case of emergency John Jones Phone 740-555-1248

RESPONSIBLE PARTY

Name of person responsible for this account Carol Jones Relationship to patient Self

Address 743 Evergreen Terrace Home phone 740-555-1248

Driver's license number QW123-EIEIO-THX1138 Birthdate 1-20-68 Financial institutions Century National

Employer Rockford, Inc Work phone 740-555-1234

Is this person currently a patient in our office? ☒ Yes ☐ No

INSURANCE INFORMATION

Name of insured Carol Jones Relationship to patient Self

Birthdate 1-20-68 Social Security number 123-45-6789 Date Employed 5-1-79

Name of Employer Rockford, Inc Work phone 740-555-1234

Address of Employer 1 Rockford Place City Shelbyville State OH ZIP 21346

Insurance company Anthem BC/BS Group number 51045 Union or local number —

Insurance company address 521 Anthem Drive City New Haberville State OH ZIP 21436

How much is your deductible? $150 How much have you used? $150 Maximum annual benefit ____

DO YOU HAVE ANY ADDITIONAL INSURANCE? ☒ **YES** ☐ **NO** **IF YES, COMPLETE THE FOLLOWING:**

Name of insured ____ Relationship to patient ____

Birthdate ____ Social Security number ____ Date Employed ____

Name of Employer ____ Work phone ____

Address of Employer ____ City ____ State ____ ZIP ____

Insurance company ____ Group number ____ Union or local number —

Insurance company address ____ City ____ State ____ ZIP ____

How much is your deductible? ____ How much have you used? ____ Maximum annual benefit ____

X Carol Jones

SIGNATURE OF PATIENT OR PARENT IF MINOR

2

■ **FIGURE 2–1.** Patient registration record. (Courtesy of Colwell Systems, Champaign IL.)

- Marital status
- Employer

Billing information is required to bill charges to the patient or an insurance company. Billing information required on a patient information form includes the following:

- Name of responsible party
- Address of responsible party
- Insurance company
- Subscriber's name
- Subscriber's address
- Subscriber's policy and group number

CORRESPONDENCE DOCUMENTS

Correspondence is an important part of the medical record. Correspondence regarding a patient may be received from a number of individuals or facilities. Examples include the patient's insurance company, the patient's attorney, or even the patient himself or herself. Insurance correspondence includes such documents as a precertification authorization for a hospital admission or a request for additional information from the insurance company.

MEDICAL OFFICE CLINICAL DOCUMENTS

☐ Medical office clinical documents include a variety of records and reports that assist the physician in the care and treatment of the patient. Commonly used medical office clinical documents are listed and described next.

HEALTH HISTORY

A health history is a collection of subjective data about the patient. This information may be requested on a preprinted form filled out by the patient or it may be obtained by the physician or medical assistant during an interview.

Along with the physical examination and laboratory and diagnostic tests, the health history is used for the following reasons: to determine the patient's general state of health; to arrive at a diagnosis and prescribe treatment; and to observe any change in a patient's illness after treatment has been instituted.

A thorough history is obtained on a new patient, and subsequent office visits provide additional information regarding changes in the patient's condition or treatment. A complete discussion of the health history is presented later in this chapter.

PHYSICAL EXAMINATION

The physical examination is a report of the findings from the physician's assessment of each body system and is described in detail in Chapter 4: The Physical Examination. The purpose of the physical examination is to provide objective data about the patient, which assists the physician in arriving at a diagnosis. The physical examination includes a patient assessment of the following areas:

- General appearance
- Skin
- Arms and hands
- Head and neck
- Eyes
- Ears
- Nose
- Mouth and pharynx
- Chest and lungs
- Heart
- Breasts
- Abdomen
- Genitalia and rectum

PROGRESS NOTES

Progress notes involve updating the medical record with new information each time the patient visits or telephones the medical office. Progress notes serve to document the patient's health status from one visit to the next. It is important that the date and time be included with each progress note entry along with the signature and credentials of the individual making the entry. A thorough discussion of charting progress notes is presented later in this chapter.

MEDICATION RECORD

A medication record consists of detailed information relating to a patient's medications. The record may include one or more of the following categories: prescription medications; over-the-counter (OTC) medications; medications administered at the medical office.

Most medical offices use one form to record prescription and OTC medications and another form to record medications actually administered to the patient at the medical office (Fig. 2–2).

A medication form for **prescription and OTC medications** includes the following:

- Name of medication
- Dosage
- Frequency of administration of the medication
- Number of refills (prescription medications only)
- Date the patient began taking the medication
- Date the medication was discontinued

A form for recording **medications administered at the medical office** includes the following:

- Date and time of administration
- Name of the medication
- Dosage administered
- Route of administration
- Injection site used
- Manufacturer and lot number
- Any significant observations or patient reactions
- Signature and credentials of the individual administering the medication

IMMUNIZATION RECORD

PATIENT NAME _____ BIRTHDATE _____ PATIENT NUMBER _____

ALLERGIES/SENSITIVITIES _____ PATIENT NUMBER _____

IMMUNIZATION		DATE	SITE	MANUFACTURER	LOT#	INITIALS	COMMENTS/REACTIONS
DTaP	#1						
	#2						
	#3						
	#4						
	#5						
	#6						
OPV IPV	#1						
	#2						
	#3						
	#4						
MMR	#1						
	#2						
MEASLES	#1						
HIB	#1						
	#2						
	#3						
	#4						
VAR							
TETANUS TOXOID	#1						
	#2						
HEPATITIS B	#1						
	#2						
	#3						
PNEUMOCOCCAL	#1						
	#2						
INFLUENZA	#1						
	#2						
	#3						
	#4						
	#5						
OTHER							

TUBERCULIN	Date										
	Type PPD/Tine										
	Result										

FIGURE 2–2. Medication record. (Courtesy of Colwell Systems, Champaign IL.)

2

HAROLD B. COOPER M.D.
6000 MAIN STREET
VENTURA, CA 93003

June 15, 2002

John F. Millstone, M.D.
5302 Main street
Ventura, CA 93003

Dear Dr. Millstone:

RE: Elaine J. Silverman

This 19-year-old woman was seen at your request. The patient was admitted to the hospital yesterday because of chills, fever, and abdominal and back pain.

REVIEW OF HEALTH HISTORY: The history has been reviewed. A prominent feature of the history is the presence of intermittent, severe, shaking chills for four days with associated left lower back pain, left lower quadrant abdominal pain and fever to as high as 103 or 104 degrees. The patient has had hypertension for a number of years and has been managed quite well with Aldomet 250 mg twice a day.

PHYSICAL EXAMINATION: On examination her temperature at this time is 100.6 degrees. The pulse is 110 and regular. Blood pressure is 190/100. The patient has partial bilateral iridectomies, the result of previous cataract surgery. Otherwise, the head and neck are not remarkable. Lung fields are clear throughout. The heart reveals a regular tachycardia, heart sounds are of good quality. No murmurs heard and there is no gallop rhythm present. The abdomen is soft. There is no spasm or guarding. A well-healed surgical scar is present in the right flank area. There is considerable tenderness in the left lower quadrant of the left mid abdomen, but as noted, there is no spasm or guarding present. Bowel sounds are present. Peristaltic rushes are noted and the bowel sounds are slightly high pitched in character. The extremities are unremarkable.

IMPRESSIONS: I believe the patient has acute diverticulitis. She may have some irritation of the left ureter in view of the findings on the urinalysis. She appears to be responding to therapy at this time in that her temperature is coming down and also there has been a slight reduction in the leukocytosis from yesterday.

RECOMMENDATIONS: I agree with the present program of therapy and the only suggestion would be to possibly increase the dose of gentamicin to 60 mg every eight hours, rather than the 40 mg q8h which she is now receiving.

Thank you for asking me to see this patient in consultation.

Sincerely,

Harold B. Cooper

Harold B. Cooper, M.D.

mtf

■ **FIGURE 2–3.** Consultation report. (From Diehl, M. O., Fordney, M. T.: *Medical Keyboarding, Typing, and Transcribing,* 4th ed. Philadelphia, W. B. Saunders, 1997.)

CONSULTATION REPORT

A consultation report is a narrative report of an opinion about a patient's condition by a practitioner other than the attending physician (Fig. 2–3). The consultant is usually a specialist in a certain field of medicine (e.g., cardiology, endocrinology, urology). The consultant's opinion is based on a review of the patient record and an examination of the patient.

The consultation report must include the following:

- Documentation that the consultant reviewed the patient's health history
- Documentation that the consultant examined the patient
- A report of the consultant's impressions
- Any care or treatment provided by the consultant.
- A report of the consultant's recommendations

HOME HEALTH CARE REPORT

Home health care is the provision of medical and nonmedical care in a patient's home or place of residence. The purpose of home health care is to minimize the effect of disease or disability by promoting, maintaining, and restoring the patient's health. There is a growing preference for home health care over equivalent health care options. Research shows that familiar surroundings contribute positively to a patient's emotional and physical well-being.

Home health care must be ordered by the patient's physician and is provided by skilled professionals. Home health care professionals include nurses, home health aides, dietitians, physical therapists, occupational therapists, speech therapists, and social workers. Examples of specialized services available through home health care include cardiac home care, infusion therapy, respiratory care, pain management, diabetes management, rehabilitation, and maternal-child care. Home health care providers must periodically provide a summary report (Fig. 2–4) to the patient's physician that includes the following:

- Observations and evaluations
- Type of care or service provided
- Instructions given to the patient on medications
- Safety measures recommended for the home
- Diet
- Activities permitted

2

Home Health Agency-Visit Report			Date of visit: 11/21/2002	Start: 7	Mileage	Finish: 7
			Patient's name: Clarence Castor			
BP: (L): 160/82	(R): 160/82	T: 97.7	Financial: GH:	VA:	Med. A: Pvt:	Med. B: Other: Hospice
P: (A): 78	(R): 76	W: 151 R: 18	Area:		Diagnosis: Lung cancer	
Pt. Instruction: Continue O$_2$ as needed			Procedures:		Age: 74	

Comments/Observations: (Physical, mental, emotional, activity level, Environ., S/S, Treatments and Effects, Procedures, Med. Effects, Other

Pt. complaining of some difficulty breathing and swelling of his feet. Pt was given Proventil Atrovent neb tx and started on oxygen at 2 liters per nasal cannula following that. Tx was discussed with Dr. Shay.

Plan: Monitor vitals every 2 hrs.

Supplies Used: O$_2$ @ 2 liters

Signature: D. Talley, RN	Next visit: 11/22/2002	RN ✓	PT	HHA	MSN	Other
	Freq of visits: daily ✓					
Supervisory visit:	Travel time:		Service time:			

■ **FIGURE 2–4.** Home health care report. (Courtesy of Briggs, Des Moines, IA.)

LABORATORY DOCUMENTS

☐ A laboratory report is a report of the analysis or examination of body specimens. Its purpose is to relay the results of laboratory tests to the physician to assist in diagnosing and treating disease. A thorough discussion of laboratory documents is presented in Chapter 15: Introduction to the Clinical Laboratory.

The specific categories of laboratory tests follow.

HEMATOLOGY. Laboratory analysis in hematology deals with the examination of blood for the detection of pathologic conditions and includes areas such as blood cell counts, cellular morphology, clotting ability of the blood, and identification of cell types.

CLINICAL CHEMISTRY. Laboratory analysis in clinical chemistry involves detecting the presence of chemical substances or determining the amount of substances present in body fluids, excreta, and tissues (e.g., blood, urine, cerebrospinal fluid). The largest area in clinical chemistry is blood chemistry.

SEROLOGY. Laboratory analysis in serology deals with studying antigen-antibody reactions to assess the presence of a substance or to determine the presence of disease.

URINALYSIS. Laboratory analysis in urinalysis involves the physical, chemical, and microscopic analysis of urine.

MICROBIOLOGY. Laboratory analysis in microbiology deals with the identification of pathogens present in specimens taken from the body (e.g., urine, blood, throat, sputum, wound, urethra, vagina, and cerebrospinal fluid).

PARASITOLOGY. Laboratory analysis in parasitology deals with the detection of the presence of disease-producing human parasites or eggs present in specimens taken from the body (e.g., stool, vagina, blood).

CYTOLOGY. Laboratory analysis in cytology deals with the detection of the presence of abnormal cells.

COLLEGE HOSPITAL

4567 BROAD AVENUE

WOODLAND HILLS, MD 21532

RADIOLOGY REPORT

Examination Date:	June 14, 2002	Patient:	Elaine J. Silverman
Date Reported:	June 14, 2002	X-ray No.:	43200
Physician:	Harold B. Cooper	Patient:	19
Examination:	PA Chest, Abdomen	Hospital No.:	80-32-11

FINDINGS

PA CHEST: Upright PA view of chest shows the lung fields are clear, without evidence of an active process. heart size is normal. There is no evidence of pneumoperitoneum.

IMPRESSION: NEGATIVE CHEST

ABDOMEN: Flat and upright views of the abdomen show a normal gas pattern without evidence of obstruction or ileus. There are no calcifications or abnormal masses noted.

IMPRESSION: NEGATIVE STUDY

RADIOLOGIST:_____

Marian B. Skinner, MD

■ FIGURE 2–5. Radiology report. (From Diehl, M. O., Fordney M. T.: *Medical Keyboarding, Typing, and Transcribing,* 4th ed. Philadelphia, W. B. Saunders, 1997.)

HISTOLOGY. Laboratory analysis in histology deals with the detection of diseased tissues.

DIAGNOSTIC PROCEDURE DOCUMENTS

☐ A diagnostic procedure report consists of a narrative description and interpretation of a diagnostic procedure. A **diagnostic procedure** is a type of procedure performed to assist in the diagnosis, management, and treatment of a patient's condition. The procedure may be performed by a physician, the medical assistant, or a technician specially trained in the procedure. The interpretation of the diagnostic procedure is made by a physician.

ELECTROCARDIOGRAM REPORT

An electrocardiogram (ECG) report is a narrative description of a cardiologist's interpretation of an ECG, including the implications for the patient. The actual graphic tracing is usually included with the report.

HOLTER MONITOR REPORT

A Holter monitor report is a narrative description of the interpretation of an ambulatory electrocardiogram, including the evaluator's impressions. Portions of the actual graphic tracing are usually included with the report.

2

DIAGNOSTIC IMAGING REPORT

Mt. Carmel Hospital, Columbus, OH 43201

DATE REQUESTED	DATE TO BE DONE	TODAY'S DATE	DATE OF BIRTH
6/6/2002	6/10/2002	6/10/2002	8/19/1943

☐ WHEELCHAIR   ☐ PORTABLE   ☐ AMBULATORY   ☐ CART

PATIENT:	INSURANCE:
Vera Ruth	Industrial

SEX	ROOM NO.	RESPONSIBLE PERSON OR EMPLOYER	RADIOLOGIST
F	OP	J.B. Warren, Inc.	Richard W. Adams

CLINICAL INFORMATION AND PROVISIONAL DIAGNOSIS

ATTENDING PHYSICIAN: Dr. Robb

NURSE

Back injury

EXAMINATION REQUESTED (PINPOINT AREA OF CONCERN IF POSSIBLE)
CT LUMBAR SPINE

TECHNIQUE:

CT of the lumbar spine without contrast was performed from L-3 through S-1.

FINDINGS:

The L3-4 level appears satisfactory without evidence of osseous proliferation or disc protrusion.

At the L4-5 level there is some increased density at the disc level which may be more prominent on the left. This is partially obscured due to facet artifact crossing obliquely.

There does appear to be some retention, however, of epidural fat plane. This however, may represent left sided disc bulge or protrusion with the appropriate corresponding clinical appearance Osseous variation at this level is not identified.

At the L5-S1 level, significant variation is not apparent.

IMPRESSION:

Variation at the L4-5 level on the left which may represent annular disc bulge or perhaps protrusion on the left. However, confirmation with myelography and/or Ampaque enhanced computed tomography of the lumbar spine should be suggested prior to any surgical intervention.

Richard W. Adams, MD

■ **FIGURE 2–6.** Diagnostic imaging report (CT scan).

PHYSICAL THERAPY EVALUATION AND TX PLAN

INSTRUCTIONS: This form must be completed by a licensed professional Physical Therapist.

PERTINENT BACKGROUND INFORMATION

Facility __North Side Physical Therapy__

Resident _____ Room no. _____ Admission date __/ /__ D.O.B. __9 /23/ 28__

Medicare No. _____ ☐Part A ☐Part B Other insurance _____

Treatment diagnosis __SIP Ⓛ TKR__ ICD-9 code _____ Onset __/ /__

MD referral and date __Michael Howe__ __9 /15/ 2002__ Date plan established __9 /23/ 2002__

Prior level of function __Ⓘ__

Proir living situation/support system __Lives c̄ spouse__

Describe pertinent medical/social history and/or previous therapy provided: __Hx Ⓛ knee pain x5 yrs; little relief c̄ PT__

MUSCLE STRENGTH/FUNCTIONAL ROM EVALUATION

AREA	STRENGTH RIGHT	STRENGTH LEFT	ACTION	ROM RIGHT	ROM LEFT
Shoulder	5	5	Flex/Extend	5	5
	5	5	Abd./Add.	5	5
	5	5	Int.rot./Ext.rot.	5	5
Elbow	5	5	Flex/Extend	5	5
Forearm	5	5	Sup./Pron.	5	5
Wrist	5	5	Flex/Extend	5	5
Fingers (Grip)	5	5	Flex/Extend	5	5
Hip	5	2 (knee pain)	Flex/Extend	5	3 ~40% to 70%
	5	3	Abd./Add.	5	3
	5	3	Int.rot./Ext.rot.	5	4
Hip	5	2+→3⁻	Flex/Extend	5	3
Ankle	5	3	Plant./Dors.	5	4
Foot	5	3	Inver./Ever.	5	4

FUNCTIONAL INDEPENDENCE/BALANCE EVALUATION

	AREA	ASSIST GRADE	ASSISTIVE DEVICES/ COMMENTS
BED MOBILITY	Roll/turn	Not assessed	2° surgery
	Sit/supine	2	Assist to Ⓛ LE
	Scoot/bridge	2	Uses overhead trapeze
TRANSFERS	Sit/stand	2	
	Bed/wheelchair	2	
	Toilet	2	
	Floor	Not assessed	
	Auto	Not assessed	
BALANCE	Sit Static	5	
	Sit Dynamic	5	
	Stand Static	3	
	Stand Dynamic	3	
W/C SKILLS	Propulsion	N/A	
	Weight shift	N/A	
	Foot rests	N/A	
	Brakes	N/A	

ADDITIONAL SKIN/MUSCLE FUNCTIONAL EVALUATION CRITERIA

TRUNK/NECK POSTURE __FHP__

MUSCLE TONE __Good__

SPECIFIC DEFICITS _____

PALPATION __Knee bandaged__

SKIN CONDITION _____

EDEMA __Mild distal Ⓛ UE/foot__

REHAB POTENTIAL __Good__

PAIN: ☒ Intermittent ☐ Variable ☐ Constant

intensity scale: 1 __Ranges from 2 to 8__ 10

ADDITIONAL FUNCTIONAL EVALUATION CRITERIA

ENDURANCE __Fair__

COGNITION:: ☒ Alert ☐ Oriented x __3__ ☐ Confused

☐ Comatose ☐ Comatose ☐ Lethargic

☒ Good judgement in regards to safety

☐ ST Memory ☐ LT Memory

☒ Follows __full__ step commands

VISION __glasses__ HEARING _____ SPEECH _____

PROPRIOCEPTION __WNL__ COORDINATION __WNL__

GAIT ANALYSIS

ASSIST __Min A +1__ DEVICE __Walker__

ANALYSIS __Pt. able to ambulate normal heel-to-toe pattern, PWB Ⓛ LE__

WEIGHT BEARING STATUS __PWB Ⓛ LE__ LEG LENGTH __N/A__

NAME-Last	First	Middle	Attending Physician	Chart No.
Johnson	Thomas	J.	Michael Howe	

2

■ **FIGURE 2–7.** Physical therapy report. (Courtesy of Briggs, Des Moines, IA.)

SIGMOIDOSCOPY REPORT

A sigmoidoscopy report is a narrative description of the interpretation of a sigmoidoscopic examination, including the practitioner's impressions.

SPIROMETRY REPORT

A spirometry report is a narrative and graphic description of the interpretation of pulmonary function testing.

RADIOLOGY REPORT

A radiology report is a narrative description of a diagnostic or therapeutic radiologic procedure (Fig. 2–5). A radiologist examines the x-ray and provides a written report, which includes a detailed interpretation of the x-ray and his or her impressions. The actual radiograph is kept on file at the radiology department at the hospital but is available for review by the patient's physician.

IMAGING REPORT

An imaging report is a narrative description of a diagnostic imaging procedure (Fig. 2–6). The report includes a detailed interpretation of the diagnostic image along with the practitioner's impressions. Examples of common diagnostc imaging procedures include ultrasonography, computed tomography (CT scan), and magnetic resonance imaging (MRI). The actual diagnostic computer image is kept on file at the hospital but is available for review by the patient's physician.

THERAPEUTIC SERVICE DOCUMENTS

☐ A therapeutic service report documents the assessments and treatments designed to restore patient function. Some examples of therapeutic services that may be ordered by the physician follow.

PHYSICAL THERAPY. This involves the use of exercise, heat, cold, water, electricity, ultrasound, massage, and other physical means to restore the patient to useful activity. Refer to Fig. 2–7 for an example of a physical therapy report.

OCCUPATIONAL THERAPY. This helps the patient learn new skills and adapt to a physical disability to enhance the quality of life and to achieve as much independence as possible.

SPEECH THERAPY. This involves the treatment of defects and disorders of the voice and of spoken and written communication.

MEMORIES *from* **EXTERNSHIP**

DAWN BENNETT: *During my externship as a medical assisting student, I was placed in a family practice clinic. I was very nervous my first day, wondering how in the world I would be able to remember everything I learned in school. My very first patients were an elderly couple. The wife was there for some test results for cancer. I looked at the results and they were positive. After the physician relayed the results, the husband broke down. He had just lost his granddaughter to a heart attack and his son-in-law to a stroke. You could tell that he just could not bear losing his wife too.*

One week later, the elderly man's wife was placed in a nursing home. He came into our office for an appointment. As I was working him up, he was telling me stories about himself and his wife when they were first married. He looked so sad. I sat with him for a few minutes after completing his work-up and gave his stories my full attention. As I was leaving the room, a smile came across his face and he thanked me for listening to him. I realized that working in a physician's office is more than just knowing what we learned in school. Compassion and showing the patients you really do care about them is just as important. I felt good about myself that day.

HOSPITAL DOCUMENTS

☐ Hospital documents are prepared by the physician responsible for the care of a patient while at the hospital. The physician may be the patient's regular physician or a different physician. An example of the latter is a physician attending a patient at an urgent care center or the emergency department of a hospital.

Hospital documents are dictated by the hospital physician and transcribed by the hospital. The original document is filed in the patient's hospital medical record and a copy is sent to the patient's physician. Hospital documents assist the patient's physician in reviewing the patient's hospital visit and in providing follow-up care.

HISTORY AND PHYSICAL
ST. MERCY HOSPITAL

Patient Name: Carol Jacobs   Room #: 215

Physician: Charles Thomas, MD   Hospital #: 5422

Admission Date: 12/14/2002

CHIEF COMPLAINT: Chest pain

HISTORY OF PRESENT ILLNESS: Patient is an 85 year old female complaining of chest pain. Patient was found to have abnormal cardiac enzymes in the Emergency Room consistent with acute myocardial infarction. Patient denied any pain radiating however she did complain of left sided chest pain and lower back pain. Patient did not admit to any shortness of breath, nausea or diaphoresis.

MEDICATIONS: Lasix, Darvocet-N 100, Lisinopril, Lopressor, Glynase, Relafen, Cytotec and Micro K.

ALLERGIES: No drug allergies known.

PAST MEDICAL HISTORY: Significant for Congestive Heart Failure, Chronic Obstructive Pulmonary Disease, Diabetes Mellitus, Type II, Coronary Atherosclerosis and Hypertension and Osteoporosis.

SOCIAL HISTORY: Not a drinker and not a smoker. Patient resides in a Nursing Home.

PAST SURGICAL HISTORY: Unknown.

PHYSICAL EXAMINATION:
General: Patient is in acute distress. She is obese.
HEENT: She has 2 centimeters jugular venous distention. Pupils are equal and reactive to light and accommodation. No evidence of scleral or conjunctival icterus.
Chest: +2 bibasilar rales.
Heart: Regular rate and rhythm. +2/6 systolic ejection murmur in the left sternal border.
Abdomen: Soft, nontender, no splenomegaly and no hepatomegaly and positive bowel sounds.
Extremities: No evidence of edema or deep venous thrombosis.
Neurological: Cranial Nerves II through XII grossly intact.

IMPRESSIONS: Congestive Heart Failure, rule out Myocardial Infarction
Urinary Tract Infection
Uncontrolled Diabetes Mellitus

Charles Thomas

Charles Thomas, MD

■ **FIGURE 2–8.** Hospital history and physical.

HISTORY AND PHYSICAL OF A HOSPITALIZED PATIENT

A health history and physical examination must be performed on a hospitalized patient by the physician responsible for the care of that patient. There is one exception to this; if the history and physical are obtained in the medical office within a week prior to admission, a copy of this document may be used. In the event that a reliable history cannot be obtained from the patient, the history must be obtained from the person best able to relate the facts.

The history and physical consists of a physician's narrative report of the patient history and physical examination along with the physician's medical impressions (Fig. 2–8). **Medical impressions,** or simply impressions, are conclusions drawn from an interpretation of data. In this case, the physician interprets the data in the health history and physical examination and draws conclusions as to the patient's state of health. Other terms for impressions include provisional diagnosis and tentative diagnosis.

OPERATIVE REPORT

An operative report (Fig. 2–9) must be completed for all patients who have had a surgical procedure. This report must be completed and signed by the surgeon performing the operation.

The operative report must include the following:

- Patient identification information
- Name of the surgical procedure
- Date of the surgery

OPERATIVE REPORT
ST. MARY'S HOSPITAL

Name: Natalie Boyer

Hospital #: 291734   Room #: OP

Surgeon: Paul Cain, M.D.   Date of Surgery: 1/6/2002

Anesthesiologist: John Adams, M.D.   Anesthesia: General

PRE-OP DIAGNOSIS: Abnormal Pap smear with history of cervical carcinoma.

POST-OP DIAGNOSIS: Same and awaiting path report.

OPERATION: D & C, laser cone of the cervix.

PROCEDURE: The patient to the operating room, dorsolithotomy position, perineum and vagina were prepped and moist sterile drape was used. Laser precautions all in place. Bimanual examination revealed a uterus which was enlarged with a second degree uterine prolapse. The cervix was dilated. Uterus sounded to around 9 cm. The endocervical canal was dilated and D&C was performed with tissue recovered and submitted to Pathology. The cervix was stained with Iodine and the non-staining area was identified. The laser was brought in, 50 watts of current were utilized to removed laser cone and we submitted that to Pathology. We then vaporized beyond the margins of the cone, 3-4 mm to a depth of 4-5 mm. Hemostasis was adequate. We placed O Vicryl figure-of eight sutures at the 3 and the 9 o'clock position in the cervix and then we put some Monsel solution on the cervix. Hemostasis adequate. Sponge and needle counts correct times two. The patient tolerated the procedure well and she returned to the recovery room in stable condition. She will be discharged home when awake and stable on Cipro 250 mg. twice a day for a week, Darvocet-N 100, #20 as needed for pain. If she continues to have abnormal Pap smears in the future, we will probably want to do a vaginal hysterectomy.

SURGEON: *Paul Cain*
Paul Cain, MD

■ **FIGURE 2–9.** Operative report.

- Full description of the findings at surgery (both normal and abnormal)
- Description of the technique and procedures used during surgery
- Ligatures and sutures used
- Number of packs, drains, and sponges used
- Condition of the patient at the completion of the surgery
- Postoperative diagnosis
- Name of the surgeon

DISCHARGE SUMMARY

Silverman, Elaine J.
97-32-11
July 16, 2002

ADMISSION DATE: June 14, 2002   **DISCHARGE DATE:**   July 15, 2002

HISTORY OF PRESENT ILLNESS:
This 19-year-old black female, nulligravida, was admitted to the hospital on June 14, 2002 with fever of 102°, left lower quadrant pain, vaginal discharge, constipation, and a tender left adnexal mass. Her past history and family history were unremarkable. Present pain had started two to three weeks prior to admission. her periods were irregular, with latest period starting on May 30, 2002 and lasting for six days. She had taken contraceptive pills in the past but had stopped because she was not sexually active.

PHYSICAL EXAMINATION:
She appeared well developed and well nourished, and in mild distress. The only positive physical findings were limited to the abdomen and pelvis. Her abdomen was mildly distended, and it was tender, especially in the left lower quadrant. At pelvic examination, her cervix was tender on motion, and the uterus was of normal size, retroverted, and somewhat fixed. There was a tender cystic mass about 4-5 cm in the left adnexa. Rectal examination was negative.

PROVISIONAL DIAGNOSIS:
1. Probable pelvic inflammatory disease (PID).
2. Rule out ectopic pregnancy.

LABORATORY DATA ON ADMISSION:
Hgb 8.8, Hct 26.5, WBC 8,100 with 80 segs and 18 lymphs. Sedimentation rate 100 mm in one hour. sickle cell prep+ (turned out to be a trait). Urinalysis normal. Electrolytes normal. SMA-12 normal. Chest x-ray negative, 2-hour UCG negative.

HOSPITAL COURSE AND TREATMENT:
initially, she was given cephalothin 2 gm IV q6h, and kanamycin 0.5 gm IM b.i.d. Over the next two days the patient's condition improved. Her pain decreased and her temperature came down to normal in the morning and spiked to 101° in the evening. Repeat CBC showed Hgb 7.8, Hct 23.5. The pregnancy test was negative. On the second night following admission she spiked to 104°. The patient was started on anti-tuberculosis treatment, consisting of isoniazid 300 mg/day, ethambutol 600 mg b.i.d. and rifampin 600 mg. daily. She became afebrile on the sixth postoperative day and was discharged on July 15, 2002 in good condition. She will be seen in the office in one week.

SURGICAL PROCEDURES:
Biopsy of omentum for frozen section; culture specimens.

DISCHARGE DIAGNOSIS:
Genital tuberculosis.

Harold B. Cooper
Harold B. Cooper, MD

■ **FIGURE 2–10.** Discharge summary report. (From Diehl, M. O., Fordney, M. T.: *Medical Keyboarding, Typing, and Transcribing,* 4th ed. Philadelphia, W. B. Saunders, 1997.)

COLLEGE HOSPITAL
4567 BROAD AVENUE
WOODLAND HILLS, MD 21532

PATHOLOGY REPORT

Date:	June 20, 2002	**Pathology No.:**	430211
Patient:	Elaine J. Silverman	**Room No.:**	1308
Physician:	Harold B. Cooper, M.D.		
Specimen Submitted:	Tumor, right axilla		

FINDINGS

GROSS DESCRIPTION:
Specimen A consists of an oval mass of yellow fibroadipose tissue measuring 4 x 3 x 2 cm. On cut section, there are some small, soft, pliable areas of gray apparent lymph node alternating with adipose tissue. A frozen section consultation at time of surgery was delivered as NO EVIDENCE OF MALIGNANCY on frozen section, to await permanent section for final diagnosis. Majority of the specimen will be submitted for microscopic examination.

Specimen B consists of an oval mass of yellow soft tissue measuring 2.5 x 2.5 x 1.5 cm. On cut section, there is a thin rim of pink to tan-brown lymphatic tissue and the mid portion appears to be adipose tissue. A pathological consultation at time of surgery was delivered as no suspicious areas noted and to await permanent sections for final diagnosis. The entire specimen will be submitted for microscopic examination.

MICROSCOPIC DESCRIPTION:
Specimen A sections show fibroadipose tissue and nine fragments of lymph nodes. The lymph nodes show areas with prominent germinal centers and moderate sinus histiocytosis. There appears to be some increased vascularity and reactive endothelial cells seen. There is no evidence of malignancy.

Specimen B sections show adipose tissue and 5 lymph node fragments. These 5 portions of lymph nodes show reactive changes including sinus histiocytosis. There is no evidence of malignancy.

DIAGNOSIS:
A & B: TUMOR, RIGHT AXILLA: SHOWING 14 LYMPH NODE FRAGMENTS WITH REACTIVE CHANGES AND NO EVIDENCE OF MALIGNANCY.

Stanley T. Nason

Stanley T. Nason, MD

■ **FIGURE 2–11.** Pathology report. (From Diehl, M. O., Fordney, M. T.: *Medical Keyboarding, Typing, and Transcribing,* 4th ed. Philadelphia, W. B. Saunders, 1997.)

DISCHARGE SUMMARY REPORT

The discharge summary report is a brief (usually one-page) summary of the significant events of the patient's hospitalization (Fig 2–10). The report is completed and signed by the physician responsible for the care of the hospitalized patient.

The discharge summary report must include the following:

- Patient identification information
- Dates of hospitalization
- Reason for the hospitalization (provisional diagnosis)
- Brief health history
- Significant findings from examinations and tests
- Course of treatment
- Condition of the patient at discharge
- Discharge diagnosis (final diagnosis)
- Prognosis (rehabilitation potential)
- Discharge instructions
- Recommendations and arrangements for follow-up care

PATHOLOGY REPORT

A pathology report consists of a macroscopic (gross) and microscopic description of tissue removed from a patient during surgery or a diagnostic procedure. The report also includes a diagnosis of the patient's condition (Fig. 2–11). A pathologist is required to examine the tissue, complete the report, and sign it.

EMERGENCY ROOM REPORT

The emergency room report is a record of the significant information involved in an emergency room visit (Fig. 2–12). The report is prepared and signed by the

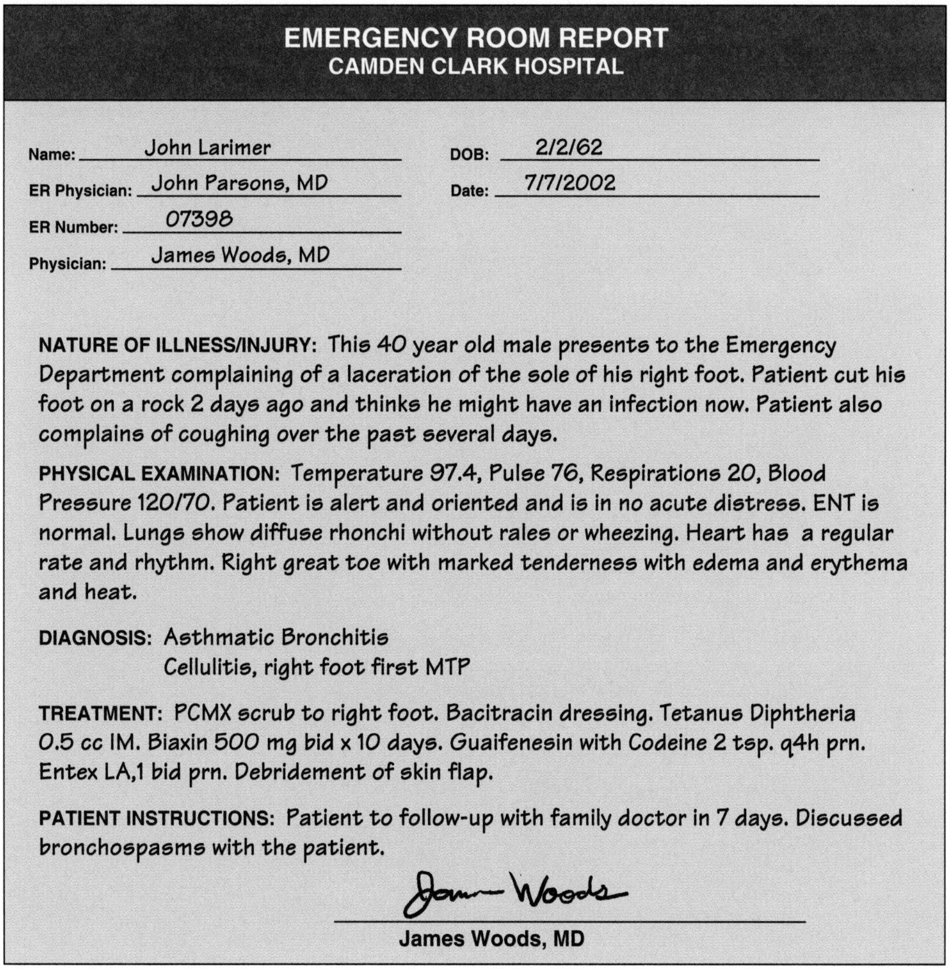

EMERGENCY ROOM REPORT
CAMDEN CLARK HOSPITAL

Name: _John Larimer_　　DOB: _2/2/62_

ER Physician: _John Parsons, MD_　　Date: _7/7/2002_

ER Number: _07398_

Physician: _James Woods, MD_

NATURE OF ILLNESS/INJURY: This 40 year old male presents to the Emergency Department complaining of a laceration of the sole of his right foot. Patient cut his foot on a rock 2 days ago and thinks he might have an infection now. Patient also complains of coughing over the past several days.

PHYSICAL EXAMINATION: Temperature 97.4, Pulse 76, Respirations 20, Blood Pressure 120/70. Patient is alert and oriented and is in no acute distress. ENT is normal. Lungs show diffuse rhonchi without rales or wheezing. Heart has a regular rate and rhythm. Right great toe with marked tenderness with edema and erythema and heat.

DIAGNOSIS: Asthmatic Bronchitis
　　　　　　　 Cellulitis, right foot first MTP

TREATMENT: PCMX scrub to right foot. Bacitracin dressing. Tetanus Diphtheria 0.5 cc IM. Biaxin 500 mg bid x 10 days. Guaifenesin with Codeine 2 tsp. q4h prn. Entex LA,1 bid prn. Debridement of skin flap.

PATIENT INSTRUCTIONS: Patient to follow-up with family doctor in 7 days. Discussed bronchospasms with the patient.

James Woods

James Woods, MD

■ **FIGURE 2–12.** Emergency room report.

2

emergency room physician and a copy is sent to the patient's physician for the purpose of providing follow-up care.

The emergency room report includes the following:

- Date of service
- Patient identification information
- Nature of the illness or injury
- Any laboratory or diagnostic test results
- Procedures performed
- Treatment rendered
- Diagnosis
- Condition of the patient at discharge
- Instructions regarding follow-up care

CONSENT DOCUMENTS

☐ Consent forms are legal documents required in order to perform certain special procedures or to release information contained in the patient's medical record.

CONSENT TO TREATMENT FORM

The completion of a consent to treatment form is required for all surgical operations and nonroutine diagnostic or therapeutic procedures performed in the medical office (e.g., minor office surgery, sigmoidoscopy). The form must be signed by the patient or his or her legally authorized representative and provides written evidence that the patient agrees to the procedure(s) listed on the form (Fig. 2–13).

In order for the patient's consent to be valid, it must be informed consent. **Informed consent** means that the patient is provided with the following information before giving consent:

- the nature of the patient's condition,
- the nature and purpose of the recommended procedure,
- an explanation of any risks involved with the procedure,
- any alternative treatments or procedures available,

2

(attach label or complete blanks)

First name: _____   Last name: _____

Date of Birth: _____ Month _____ Day _____ Year

Account Number: _____

Procedure Consent Form

I, _____ ,hereby consent to have

Dr. _____ , perform _____ .

I have been fully informed of the following by my physician:

1. The nature of my condition.
2. The nature and purpose of the procedure.
3. An explanation of risks involved with the procedure.
4. Alternative treatments or procedures available.
5. The likely results of the procedure.
6. The risks involved with declining or delaying the procedure.

My physician has offered to answer all questions concerning the proposed procedure.

I am aware that the practice of medicine and surgery is not an exact science, and I acknowledge that no guarantees have been made to me about the results of the procedure.

Patient _____   Date _____
     (or guardian and relationship)

Witnessed _____   Date _____

■ **FIGURE 2–13.** Consent to treatment form.

PROCEDURE

2-1

Completion of a Patient Consent to Treatment Form

EQUIPMENT/SUPPLIES: Consent to treatment form

1. **Procedural Step.** Type all required information on the consent to treatment form in the spaces provided (e.g., patient's full name, name of the procedure to be performed and so on.)
2. **Procedural Step.** Ensure that the physician has had an informed consent discussion with the patient. **Principle.** In order for the patient's consent to be valid, it must be informed consent.
3. **Procedural Step.** Greet and identify the patient. Introduce yourself, and explain the purpose of the consent form.
4. **Procedural Step.** Give the consent form to the patient and ask him or her to read it. Ask the patient if he or she has any questions.

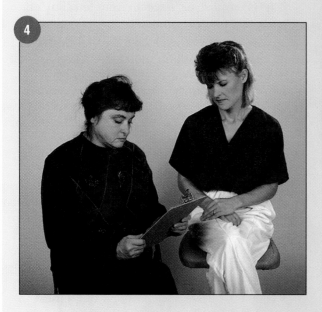

5. **Procedural Step.** Ask the patient to sign the consent form. Witness the patient's signature by signing your name in the appropriate space on the form. Include today's date.

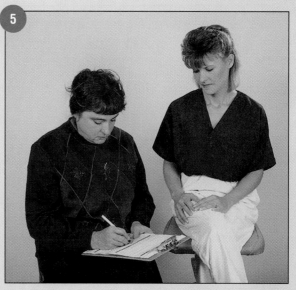

Principle. Witnessing a signature means only that the medical assistant watched the patient sign the form; it *does not* mean that the medical assistant is attesting to the accuracy of the information provided.

6. **Procedural Step.** Provide the patient with a copy of the completed consent form for his or her files.
7. **Procedural Step.** File the original consent to treatment form in the patient's medical record. **Principle.** Maintaining the form provides legal documentation that the patient gave permission for treatment.

2

- the likely outcome (prognosis) of the procedure, and
- the risks involved with declining or delaying the procedure.

The explanation must be in terms the patient can understand, and the patient should be given an opportunity to ask questions regarding the information.

The consent to treatment form should not be signed until the patient has been provided with all necessary information relating to the procedure (as described previously). The patient's signature must be witnessed; this is usually the responsibility of the medical assistant. **Witnessing a signature** means that the medical assistant saw the patient sign the form. If the patient is not someone the medical assistant knows, the patient should be asked to provide a picture identification stating his or her name. Witnessing a signature means only that the medical assistant watched the patient sign the form; it *does not* mean that the medical assistant is attesting to the accuracy of the information provided.

The consent to treatment form outlines the details of the consent discussion with the patient and includes the following information:

- Patient's full name
- Name of the procedure to be performed
- Name of the surgeon
- A statement indicating the patient agrees to receive the procedure
- Acknowledgment that a disclosure of information has been made
- Acknowledgment that all questions asked were answered in a satisfactory manner
- A statement that no guarantee as to the outcome has been made
- Signature of the patient or his or her legal representative
- Signature of the witness

CONSENT TO RELEASE INFORMATION FORM

Except when permitted by law, information from a patient's medical record can only be released upon written request and authorization of the patient. A release of information form (Fig. 2–14) must be completed and signed by the patient requesting the disclosure of medical information. Medical information is most frequently requested by patients for release to the following: the patient's insurance company, another physician providing care for the patient, the patient's attorney, or a professional providing home health care for the patient.

The consent to release information form should stipulate following:

- Name of the medical practice releasing the information
- Name of the individual or facility to receive the information
- Patient's full name
- Specific information to be released
- The purpose of or the need for the information
- Signature of the patient or his or her legal representative
- Date that the consent is signed
- The expiration date of the consent form

Mailed or Faxed Requests for Release of Medical Information

Most medical offices require that the patient come to the office to sign the consent to release information form; however, this may not always be possible. An example is a patient who has moved away and is requesting the transfer of his or her medical records to a new physician. Another example is an elderly patient confined at home who needs medical information released to a home health care agency. In these special instances, the consent to release medical information may be mailed or faxed to your medical office. The procedure for processing this type of request follows.

1. Check the expiration date on the consent to release information form. If the authorization is outdated, a more current release form needs to be signed.
2. Verify the authenticity of the signature on the form. This can be accomplished by comparing the patient's signature on the form with the patient's signature in his or her medical record. If you have any doubt as to the authenticity of the signature, do not release the records.
3. Copy the information requested on the form. Be sure to release **only** the information requested. Include a copy of the completed release form with the medical information.
4. Document what information is being released and the date of the release of the information. Sign the document with your name and credentials.
5. File the release document and the consent to release information form in the patient's medical record.
6. Send the medical information according to your medical office policy.

MEDICAL RECORD FORMATS

☐ Most medical offices rely on the use of paper medical records, known as **paper-based patient records (PPR).** Currently some patient data are maintained on the computer; these include patient registration infor-

CONSENT TO RELEASE MEDICAL INFORMATION

MEDICAL RECORD REQUEST

I hereby request to inspect and/or photocopy information contained in the medical record of

_____Steve Carin_____ compiled during
Print resident name

(his)/her stay at _____St. John's Nursing Home_____
Facility name

from _11/5/2002_ through _12/5/2002_ . The specific information requested shall include the

following items: _____Blood work, x-rays, medication sheet, office notes_____

The reason(s) for this request is: _____Monitor and treatment of Chronic Obstructive_____
_____Pulmonary Disease, HTN, and IDDM_____

Jan Post, MD   _Jan Post MD_   _11/5/2002_
Print name of person requesting information   Signature of person requesting information   Date

St. John's Nursing Home   _(740) 555-3180_
Organization represented   Phone number

PO Box 58725   _Marietta_   _OH_   _45610_
Address   City   State   Zip

RESIDENT REQUEST

I hereby grant authorization to _____Marietta Family Practice_____
Facility

to release the information listed to _____St. John's Nursing Home_____
Name/Organization indicated above

above. In addition, I waive any and all privileges relating to the disclosure hereby authorized.

This consent will expire on _____ or six months after the date shown below. I reserve the right to revoke this consent at any time and further understand that the facility named above is not liable for any records sent prior to such revocation.

X _Steve Carin_   _11/5/2002_
Resident or appropriate resident's representative   Date

If resident's representative signed, complete the following:

_____   _____
Print name   Relationship to resident

Dawn Bennett, CMA   _11/5/2002_
(1) Witness   Date

_____   _____
(2) Witness (Second witness signature required if acknowledged by resident "mark".)   Date

MEDICAL RECORDS OFFICE

Information as requested released: Date _11/5/2002_ Time: _11:50_ AM/PM

Explanation of information released: _Monitor and tx of COPD_

Signature of person accepting information X _Ron Carr, RRA_   _11/6/2002_
Signature of person releasing information X _Ron Carr, RRA_   Date

NAME-Last	First	Middle	Attending Physician	Chart No.
Carin	Steve	W	Dr. Van	4516

■ **FIGURE 2–14.** Release of medical information form. (Courtesy of Briggs, Des Moines, IA.)

2

PROCEDURE

2-2

Release of Medical Information

EQUIPMENT/SUPPLIES: Consent to release medical information form

1. **Procedural Step.** Greet and identify the patient. Introduce yourself, and explain the purpose of the consent to release medical information form.
2. **Procedural Step.** Provide the patient with a consent to release medical information form. Ask the patient to complete the information section on the form. Offer to answer any questions.
   Principle. Information from a patient's medical record can only be released upon written request and authorization of the patient (except when permitted by law).
3. **Procedural Step.** Check to make sure all the requested information on the form has been completed by the patient.
4. **Procedural Step.** Ask the patient to sign the form. Witness the patient's signature by signing your name in the appropriate space on the form. Include today's date. If required by your medical office policy, ask the physician to initial the completed consent to release medical information form.

Principle. In order to release information, the form must be signed by the patient requesting the disclosure of medical information.

5. **Procedural Step.** Provide the patient with a copy of the consent to release medical information form for his or her files.
6. **Procedural Step.** Copy the information requested on the form. Be sure to release **only** the information requested. Include a copy of the completed release form with the medical information.
7. **Procedural Step.** Document what information is being released and the date of the release of the information. Sign the document with your name and credentials.
8. **Procedural Step.** File the release document and the consent to release medical information form in the patient's medical record.
   Principle. Maintaining the form provides legal documentation that the patient gave permission for the release of his or her medical information.
9. **Procedural Step.** Send the medical information to the appropriate site according to your medical office policy.

2

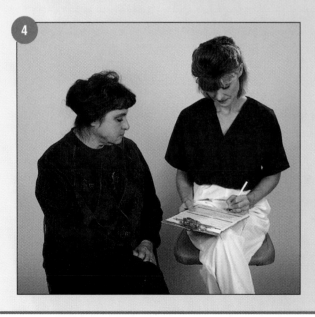

mation and patient charges and payments. As technology advances, a true **computer-based patient record (CPR)** may eventually evolve, meaning that the entire record is stored on the computer, including the history and physical examination, progress notes, laboratory and diagnostic reports, hospital reports, and so on. Since that is not yet the case, this chapter focuses on the paper-based patient record.

The way a PPR medical record is organized is known as its **format.** The two main types of medical record formats include the **source-oriented record** and the **problem-oriented record.** Each of these formats is described next.

SOURCE-ORIENTED RECORD

The source-oriented format is used most often in the medical office for organizing a medical record. The documents in a source-oriented record are organized into sections based on the department, facility, or other source that generated the information (e.g., laboratory, hospital, consultant). Because documents from each source are filed together, it is easier to compare information from laboratory and diagnostic tests results, assessments and treatments, and so on.

Each section in a source-oriented record is separated from the other sections by a chart divider. Attached to each divider is a color-coded tab labeled with the title of its respective section (Fig. 2–15). Within each of these sections, the documents are arranged according to date. Most offices use the reverse chronological order to arrange the documents. **Reverse chronological order** means that the most recent document is placed on top, which means the oldest document is on the bottom of that section.

The titles used to identify each section vary depending on medical office preference; however, typical examples include the following:

- History and physical
- Progress notes
- Medications
- Laboratory reports
- ECG
- X-ray reports
- Consultations
- Rehabilitation therapy
- Home health care
- Hospital reports
- Insurance
- Consents
- Correspondence
- Miscellaneous

PROBLEM-ORIENTED RECORD

The documents in a problem-oriented record (abbreviated **POR** or **POMR** for problem-oriented medical record) are organized by the patient's specific health problems. The advantage of using the POR is that each of the patient's problems can be defined and followed individually. The problem-oriented record is developed in four stages which include the following:

- Establishing a **database**
- Compiling a **problem list**
- Devising a **plan** of action for each problem
- Following each problem with **progress notes**

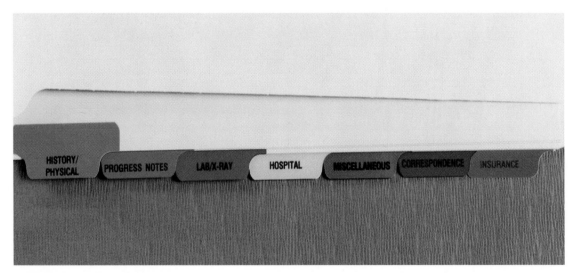

FIGURE 2–15. Chart dividers.

Database

The first step in developing a POR is to establish a database. The **database** consists of a collection of subjective and objective data. These data include the health history, physical examination, and baseline laboratory and diagnostic tests. The information in the database is then used to identify and compile a problem list.

Problem List

The problem list is a crucial part of the POR and is always located in the front of the medical record. The problem list is developed shortly after the database is completed and consists of a list of all patient problems (Fig 2–16). A **problem** is defined as any patient condition that requires further observation, diagnosis, management, or patient education. This includes not only

		PATIENT RECORD							
Name Morani, Betty				ALLERGIES/SENSITIVITY Codeine, Sulfa					
Number		Blood Type: A							
Prob. No.	Date	PROBLEM DESCRIPTION	Date Resolved	Index	Prob. No.	Date	PROBLEM DESCRIPTION	Date Resolved	Index
1	10/95	Hypertension - essential		✓					
2	10/95	Diabetes mellitus (mild)		✓					
3	1/98	L. Retinopathy	see below						
4	4/2002	Atherosclerosis with cerebral vascular insuffic.							
5	4/2002	Hearing loss							
6	1/2002	HBP Non-compliance	2/98						
3	1/2002	Bilat. Grade II Retinopathy							
Prob. No.	CONTINUING MEDICATIONS		Start	Stop	Prob. No.	CONTINUING MEDICATIONS		Start	Stop
1	Sinoserp 1 mg. b.i.d.		10/95	10/99					
2	Orinase 0.5 gm. daily		10/95	10/99					
1	Hydrodiuril 50 mg. A.M.		10/99						
2	1500 cal. diet low Na hi K		2/2002						
Periodic Health Examination	Dates	1/98	4/2000						

■ **FIGURE 2–16.** POR: Problem list. (Courtesy of Miller Communications, Inc., Norwalk, CT.)

PROBLEM ORIENTED-PROGRESS NOTES			
Name Dawn Michaels		**DOB** 9/20/98	**Doctor** Frank Edwards, MD
DATE	**TIME**	**PROBLEM NUMBER**	**FORMAT:** Problem Number and TITLE: S = Subjective O= Objective A = Assessment P= Plan
11/5/2002	9:30 AM	#1	S: Mother states that her child has had a runny nose
			and the back of her throat has been sore for 2 days.
			O: Vital signs: T 98.8 P 108 R 24
			Weight 27 lbs.
			General: alert and active. HEENT: sclera clear.
			TMs negative. Positive clear rhinorrhea. Pharynx benign.
			Heart: regular without murmur. Lungs: clear to
			auscultation and percussion. Abdomen: negative
			tenderness. Positive bowel sounds x4. GU: negative
			Neuro: good tone.
			A: Upper respiratory tract infection.
			P: 1. A prescription for Rondec DM, 1/2 tsp q6h prn
			cough and congestion.
			2. Instructed mother to contact office if child does
			not improve.

2

■ **FIGURE 2–17.** POR: SOAP progress notes. (Courtesy of Briggs, Des Moines, IA.)

medical problems but psychological and social problems as well.

Each problem is numbered and titled and should be thought of as a table of contents for the record. The problem title is stated as a diagnosis, a physiologic finding, a symptom or an abnormal test result. All subsequent data (plans and progress notes) added to the medical record are cross-referenced to these numbered problems.

The problem list is modified as needed. If an additional problem is identified, it is added to the list and dated accordingly. When a problem is resolved, it is marked as such and the date is recorded.

Plan

After examining the problem list, the physician develops the third section of the POR. This involves devising a plan of action for further evaluation or treatment of each problem. Each plan begins with a heading that identifies the number and name of the corresponding problem followed by the plan of action for the problem. This may include plans for laboratory and diagnostic tests, medical or surgical treatment, therapy, and patient education.

Progress Notes

The last stage in the development of the POR is the follow-up for each problem or the progress notes (Fig. 2–17). The progress notes begin with the number and name of the corresponding problem and include the following four categories:

Subjective data: subjective data obtained from the patient

Objective data: objective data obtained by observation, physical examination, diagnostic tests, and so on

Assessment: the physician's interpretation of the current condition based on an analysis of the subjective and objective data

Plan: proposed treatment plan for the patient

The acronym for this process is **SOAP,** and the writing of progress notes in this format is called **soaping.** Some physicians using the source-oriented format have found it advantageous to record progress notes in SOAP format. This structured type of note increases the physician's ability to deal with each problem clearly and to analyze data in an orderly systematic manner.

PUTTING IT ALL *into* PRACTICE

▶ **DAWN BENNETT:** *Working in billing and collections is very challenging and sometimes stressful. It can even be embarrassing. We are a new practice and when we opened, there was no collections system. When it came time to review our accounts, we realized that, like every other business, we needed a collections system. We immediately jumped in and took charge.*

The primary physician at our office is from New York and we were unfamiliar with his family members. One day, he walked into our office with a very puzzled look. I asked him what was wrong. He replied, "You guys are doing a great job with our collection rate. I asked you to be stern, but thoughtful, when sending our patients collection letters—but did you have to send one to my mother-in-law?!" Needless to say, we fixed the error immediately. This incident prompted us to restructure our collections system, and we added a comment screen to our computer system on all of our patient accounts. Going into a medical office that already has a system in place may be easier, but you can learn a lot more by setting up an office system yourself.

PREPARING A MEDICAL RECORD FOR A NEW PATIENT

☐ When a patient comes to the medical office for his or her first visit, a medical record must be prepared for that patient. The method used to prepare the record depends upon the following criteria: the format used to organize the record, and the filing system and type of storage equipment used. Most medical offices use the source-oriented format to organize their medical records, the alphabetic filing system to arrange the records, and shelf filing units to store the medical records. The method used to prepare a medical record is described in the following sections and is based on these criteria.

MEDICAL RECORD SUPPLIES

Certain supplies are required to prepare a medical record. These supplies are categorized and described next.

FILE FOLDERS. A file folder is a protective cover used to hold medical record documents in an organized format. Flexible metal fasteners are typically used to hold documents in the folder. Folders are available with fasteners located on the top or left side of the folder.

Folders are available with tabs. A **tab** is a projection of a folder that extends above the top of the folder and is used to identify its contents. The tab can also be positioned on the side of the folder. If the folder has a tab extending across its complete top or side, it is said to be a **full cut tab.**

In the medical office, file folders with a full cut side tab are typically used to prepare a new patient chart. There are indentations at intervals along the full cut tab to indicate the placement of adhesive labels. This ensures that the labels on all the medical records are affixed at the same place on the file folders.

FOLDER LABELS. Labels are used to identify the medical record and are commercially available in rolls or continuous folded strips for typewriter use. Labels are also available on 8 1/2 × 11-inch sheets for use with a computer system. The most common types of labels used in the medical office include name labels, alphabetic color-coded labels, color-coded year labels, and miscellaneous chart labels.

CHART DIVIDERS. Chart dividers are used to identify each section of the medical record by subject (see Fig. 2–15). Chart dividers consist of a heavy material such as manila card stock. Attached to each divider is a color-coded tab labeled with a subject title; the most frequently used subject titles are illustrated in the following box, along with the documents typically filed under each title.

Chart Divider Subject Titles and Documents Typically Filed Under Each Title

HISTORY AND PHYSICAL

Health history
Physical examination

PROGRESS NOTES

Progress notes
Medication sheet

LAB/X-RAY

Hematology report
Clinical chemistry report
Serology report
Urinalysis report
Microbiology report
Parasitology report
Cytology report
Histology report
Electrocardiogram report
Holter monitor report
Sigmoidoscopy report
Spirometry report
Radiology report
Diagnostic imaging report

HOSPITAL

History and physical
Operative report
Pathology report
Discharge summary report
Emergency room report

CORRESPONDENCE

Consultation reports
Letters from patient
Letters from patient's attorney

INSURANCE

Precertification authorization for hospital admission
Request for additional information from insurance company
Copy of patient's insurance card

MISCELLANEOUS

Consent forms
Home health care report
Physical therapy report
Occupational therapy report
Speech therapy report

TAKING A HEALTH HISTORY

☐ The health history is a collection of data obtained by interviewing the patient. A thorough history is taken for each new patient, and subsequent office visits (in the form of progress notes) provide additional information regarding changes in the patient's illness or treatment. A quiet, comfortable room that allows for

PROCEDURE

2–3

Preparing a Medical Record

The following procedure outlines the method for preparing a medical record for a new patient using the following organization: a source-oriented format stored in shelf files using a color-coded alphabetic filing system.

EQUIPMENT/SUPPLIES:

File folder with a full cut side tab
Metal fasteners
Name labels
Color-coded alphabetic bar labels

Miscellaneous chart labels
Set of chart dividers
Blank preprinted forms
Two-hole punch

2

1. **Procedural Step.** Greet and identify the patient when he or she arrives at the medical office. Introduce yourself, and verify that the patient is a new patient.
2. **Procedural Step.** Ask the patient to complete a patient registration form. Provide the patient with a blank registration form, a pen, and a hard surface (such as a clipboard) on which to write. Offer to answer any questions.
3. **Procedural Step.** When the patient returns the completed registration form, check it for accuracy and make sure that you can read the patient's handwriting. If you have any questions regarding the information on the form, ask the patient for clarification. If required by the medical office policy, ask the patient for his or her insurance card and make a copy of it.
   Principle. A copy of the patient's insurance card is used for third-party billing.
4. **Procedural Step.** Enter the data on the completed registration record into the computer.
5. **Procedural Step.** Assemble supplies needed to prepare the medical record. Type the patient's full name on a name label following these guidelines:
   a. Type the patient's name in transposed order as follows: last name, first name, middle name (or initial).
   b. Type the patient's name at the same distance from the left edge of the label (usually two or three typewritten spaces) and the same distance from the top of the label (usually one space down from the top of the label).
   c. Make sure the patient's name is spelled correctly.
   Principle. Following these guidelines facilitates the accurate and efficient filing of the patient's medical record.
6. **Procedural Step.** Determine the first two letters of the patient's last name and select the appropriate alphabetic color-coded labels. Attach the color-

coded labels to the (full cut) side tab. The labels should be affixed to the folder using the label placement indentations on the tab.

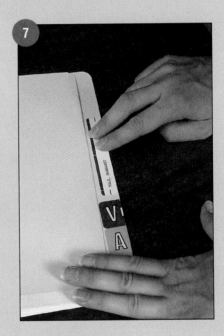

Principle. Using the label placement indentations assures that all labels on medical records are affixed at the same place.

7. **Procedural Step.** Affix the name label immediately above the first color-coded alphabetic label.
8. **Procedural Step.** Attach any additional chart labels, such as a year label and miscellaneous chart labels (e.g., allergy, insurance), to the folder according to the office policy.

PROCEDURE 2–3

9. Procedural Step. Insert the chart dividers onto the metal fasteners of the file folder.

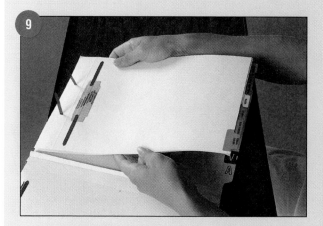

10. Procedural Step. Place the original patient registration form in the front of the medical record. Place the copy of the patient's insurance card in the appropriate section of the record.

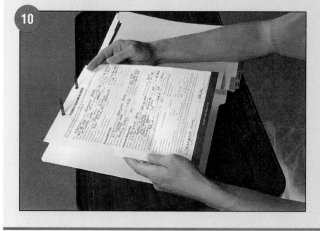

11. Procedural Step. Label preprinted forms to be placed in the record with required information such as the patient's name and date. These forms typically include the medical history form, physical examination form, progress note sheets, and a medication sheet. If the forms are not prepunched, the medical assistant must use a two-hole punch to insert two holes into the top or side of the form.

12. Procedural Step. Insert each form under its proper chart divider. Refer to the earlier box on page 57 for a list of chart divider subject titles and documents typically filed under each title.

13. Procedural Step. Recheck the medical record to ensure that it has been prepared properly.

privacy encourages the patient to communicate honestly and openly. Showing genuine interest in and concern for the patient helps reduce apprehension and facilitates the collection of data.

COMPONENTS OF THE HEALTH HISTORY

The health history is taken before the physical examination, providing the physician the opportunity to compare findings. The health history consists of seven parts or sections, which are listed and described next.

Introductory Data

The introductory or identification data section is included at the beginning of the health history form to obtain basic data on the patient (Fig. 2–18*A*). The introductory data section is completed by the patient.

Chief Complaint

The chief complaint (CC) identifies the patient's reason for seeking care—that is, the symptom causing the patient the most trouble. The chief complaint is used

Text continued on page 65

PATIENT HEALTH HISTORY

IDENTIFICATION DATA   Please print the following information.

Name _____

Address _____

_____   Zip Code

Telephone _____
Home number   Work number

Social Security or Medicare No. _____

Today's date _____   File no. _____

____ Male ____ Female _____ Race Date of Birth_____

____ Married ____ Separated ____ Divorced ____ Widowed ____ Single

Insurance provider _____

Policy number _____

Occupation _____

A

FAMILY HISTORY

For each member of your family, follow the purple or blue line
across the page and check boxes for:
1. Their present state of health
2. Any illnesses they have had

	Good health	Poor health	Deceased	If deceased, write in age and cause of death. Include fatal accidents and suicides.	Allergies or asthma	Anemia	Bleed easily	Diabetes	Cancer or tumor	Epilepsy	Glaucoma	Genetic disease	Alcoholism	Kidney or bladder trouble	Stomach/duodenal ulcer	Nervous breakdown	Rheumatism or arthritis	High blood pressure	Heart trouble	Gout
Father:																				
Mother:																				
Brothers/Sisters:																				
Spouse:																				
Child:																				
Child:																				
Child:																				
Child:																				
Paternal relatives (in each box, write how many affected with) ⟶																				
Maternal relatives (in each box, write how many affected with) ⟶																				

B

PAST HISTORY (begin here with illnesses) ⟶

ADDITIONAL ILLNESSES OR PROBLEMS: mark an X in the box next to any of the following that you have now or have ever had:

☐ Eye infections	☐ Pneumonia	☐ Neuralgia or neuritis	☐ Scarlet fever	☐ Mononucleosis
☐ Thyroid disease	☐ Pancreatitis	☐ Tension/anxiety	☐ Measles	☐ Venereal disease
☐ Eczema	☐ Liver disease	☐ Depression	☐ Mumps	☐ Yellow jaundice
☐ Hives or rashes	☐ Diverticulosis	☐ Childhood hyperactivity	☐ Polio	☐ Tuberculosis
☐ Bronchitis	☐ Hernia	☐ Chicken Pox	☐ Rheumatic fever	☐ _____
☐ Emphysema	☐ Hemorrhoids	☐ German measles	☐ Malaria	☐ _____

Have you ever been turned down for life insurance, military service or employment because of health problems?   ☐ Yes   ☐ No

MAJOR HOSPITALIZATIONS: If you have ever been hospitalized for any major medical illness or operation, write in your most recent hospitalizations below.

Check this box ☐ if you have had more than four such hospitalizations. (Do not include normal pregnancies)

	Year	Operation or illness	Name of hospital	City and state
1st Hospitalization				
2nd Hospitalization				
3rd Hospitalization				
4th Hospitalization				

TESTS AND IMMUNIZATIONS: Mark an X next to those that you have had. Enter the year when you last were given the tests or "shots".

Year		Year	
☐ 19___ chest x-ray		☐ 19___ smallpox "shots"	
☐ 19___ kidney x-ray		☐ 19___ tetanus "shots"	
☐ 19___ G.I. series		☐ 19___ polio series	
☐ 19___ colon x-ray		☐ 19___ typhoid "shots"	
☐ 19___ gallbladder x-ray		☐ 19___ flu injections	
☐ 19___ electrocardiogram		☐ 19___ mumps "shots"	
☐ 19___ TB test		☐ 19___ measles "shots"	
☐ 19___ sigmoidoscopy		☐ 19___ _____	

MEDICINES: Mark an X in the box next to any medicines that you are now taking, or that you are sensitive or allergic to:

Taking	Allergic to:	Taking	Allergic to:
☐	antibiotics	☐	aspirin
☐	penicillin	☐	diet pills
☐	sulfa	☐	antacids
☐	opiates/codeine	☐	laxatives
☐	diuretics/water pills	☐	cold tablets
☐	sedatives	☐	_____
☐	stimulants/caffeine	☐	_____
☐	Demerol	☐	_____
☐	Blood pressure medicine		

C

■ **FIGURE 2–18.** Example of a health history form.

2

SOCIAL HISTORY

EDUCATION

_____ Years elementary   _____ Years high school   _____ Years college, technical, business, etc.

Occupation _____   Years _____

Previous occupation _____   Years _____

Military services _____

Overseas? _____

Have you ever been exposed to any of the following in your work environment?

☐ Excess dust (coal, lime, rock)   ☐ Cleaning fluids/solvents   ☐ Radiation   ☐ Other toxic materials

☐ Sand   ☐ Hair spray   ☐ Insecticides

☐ Chemicals   ☐ Smoke or auto exhaust fumes   ☐ Paints

Please answer the following questions by placing an X in the box in front of the word Yes or No, except where your are asked for specific information. If a question doesn't apply, skip it and go on to the next one. This information is obviously highly confidential and will be released to other health professionals or insurance carriers ONLY with your signed consent.

DIET HISTORY/EXERCISE

1. Do you eat a good breakfast? ☐ Yes ☐ No
2. Do you snack between meals (soft drinks, chips, candy bars)? ☐ Yes ☐ No
3. Do you eat fresh fruits and vegetables each day? ☐ Yes ☐ No
4. Do you eat whole grain breads and cereals? ☐ Yes ☐ No
5. Is your diet high in fat content? ☐ Yes ☐ No
6. Is your diet high in cholesterol content? ☐ Yes ☐ No
7. Is your diet high in salt content? ☐ Yes ☐ No
8. Do you habitually use laxatives? ☐ Yes ☐ No

9. Do you exercise on a regular basis? ☐ Yes ☐ No
10. Does your job require strenuous, sustained, physical work? ☐ Yes ☐ No
11. Are you allergic to any foods? ☐ Yes ☐ No
12. How many glasses of milk do you drink each day? ☐ Yes ☐ No
13. How many glasses of water do you drink each day? ☐ Yes ☐ No
14. How would you describe your overall eating habits? ☐ Excellent ☐ Good ☐ Fair ☐ Poor

SOCIAL HISTORY/EXERCISE

15. Are you very nervous around strangers? ☐ Yes ☐ No
16. Do you find it hard to make decisions? ☐ Yes ☐ No
17. Do you find it hard to concentrate or remember? ☐ Yes ☐ No
18. Do you usually feel lonely or depressed? ☐ Yes ☐ No
19. Do you often cry? ☐ Yes ☐ No
20. Would you say you have a hopeless outlook? ☐ Yes ☐ No
21. Do you have difficulty relaxing? ☐ Yes ☐ No
21. Do you have a tendency to worry a lot? ☐ Yes ☐ No
23. Are you troubled by frightening dreams or thoughts? ☐ Yes ☐ No
24. Do you have a tendency to be shy or sensitive? ☐ Yes ☐ No
25. Do you have a strong dislike for criticism? ☐ Yes ☐ No
26. Do you lose your temper often? ☐ Yes ☐ No
27. Do little things often annoy you? ☐ Yes ☐ No
28. Are you disturbed by any work or family problems? ☐ Yes ☐ No
29. Are you having sexual difficulties? ☐ Yes ☐ No
30. Have you ever considered committing suicide? ☐ Yes ☐ No
31. Have you ever desired or sought psychiatric help? ☐ Yes ☐ No
32 Have you gained or lost much weight recently? ☐ Yes ☐ No
33. Do you have a tendency to be too hot or too cold? ☐ Yes ☐ No
34. Have you lost your interest in eating lately? ☐ Yes ☐ No
35. Do you always seem to be hungry? ☐ Yes ☐ No

36. Are you more thirsty than usual lately? ☐ Yes ☐ No
37. Are there any swellings in your armpits or groin? ☐ Yes ☐ No
38. Do you seem to feel exhausted or fatigued most of the time? ☐ Yes ☐ No
39. Do you have difficulty either falling asleep or staying asleep? ☐ Yes ☐ No
40. Do you participate in physical activity or exercise less than three times a week? ☐ Yes ☐ No
41. How much do you smoke per day? ☐ Cigarettes ☐ Cigars/pipes ☐ Don't smoke
42. Do you take two or more alcoholic drinks per day? ☐ Yes ☐ No
43. Do you drink six or more cups of coffee or tea per day? ☐ Yes ☐ No
44. Are you a regular user of sleeping pills, marijuana, tranquilizers, pain killers, etc.? ☐ Yes ☐ No
45. Have you ever used heroin, cocaine, LSD, PCP, etc? ☐ Yes ☐ No
46. Do you drive a motor vehicle more than 25,000 miles a year? ☐ Yes ☐ No
47. How often do you use seat belts when riding in cars? ☐ Never ☐ Sometimes ☐ Always
48. List any country outside the USA you have visited in the past six months? _____
49. Do you live in: (A) an apartment (B) a house (C) a trailer (D) other _____
50. When did you have your last physical examination? _____

D

■ **FIGURE 2–18** *Continued*

2

Name _____   Date _____

Doctor's notes _____

_____

_____

REVIEW OF SYSTEMS

HEAD AND NECK
92. ____ frequent headaches
93. ____ neck and pains
94. ____ neck lumps or sweating

EYES
95. ____ wears glasses
96. ____ blurry vision
97. ____ eyesight worsening
98. ____ sees double
99. ____ sees halo
100. ____ eye pains or itching
101. ____ watering eyes
102. ____ eye trouble

EARS
103. ____ hearing difficulties
104. ____ earaches
105. ____ running ears
106. ____ buzzing in ears
107. ____ motion sickness

MOUTH
108. ____ dental problems
109. ____ swellings on gums or jaws
110. ____ sore tongue
111. ____ taste changes

NOSE AND THROAT
112. ____ congested nose
113. ____ running nose
114. ____ sneezing spells
115. ____ headcolds
116. ____ nose bleeds
117. ____ sore throat
118. ____ enlarged tonsils
119. ____ hoarse voice

RESPIRATORY
120. ____ wheezes or gasps
121. ____ coughing spells
122. ____ coughs up phlegm
123. ____ coughed up blood
124. ____ chest colds
125. ____ excessive sweating, night sweats

CARDIOVASCULAR
126. ____ high blood pressure
127. ____ racing heart
128. ____ chest pains
129. ____ dizzy spells
130. ____ shortness of breath
131. ____ shortness of breath at night
132. ____ more pillows to breathe
133. ____ swollen feet or ankles
134. ____ leg cramps
135. ____ heart murmur

DIGESTIVE
heartburn ____ 49.
bloated stomach ____ 50.
belching ____ 51.
stomach pains ____ 52.
nausea ____ 53.
vomited blood ____ 54.
difficulty swallowing ____ 55.
constipation ____ 56.
loose bowels ____ 57.
black stools ____ 58.
grey stools ____ 59.
pain in rectum ____ 60.
rectal bleeding ____ 61.

URINARY
night frequency ____ 62.
day frequency ____ 63.
wets pants or bed ____ 64.
burning on urination ____ 65.
brown, black or bloody urine ____ 66.
difficulty starting urine ____ 67.
urgency ____ 68.

MALE GENITAL
weak urine stream ____ 69.
prostate trouble ____ 70.
burning or discharge ____ 71.
lumps on testicles ____ 72.
painful testicles ____ 73.

FEMALE GENITAL
last menstrual period __/__/__ 74.
post-menopausal or hysterectomy ____ 75.
noticed vaginal bleeding ____ 76.

abnormal LMP ____ 77.
heavy bleeding during periods ____ 78.
bleeding between periods ____ 79.
bleeding after intercourse ____ 80.
recent vaginal itching/discharge ____ 81.
no monthly breast exam ____ 82.
lump or pain in breasts ____ 83.
complications with birth control ____ 84.
last Pap test __/__/__ 85.

OBSTETRIC HISTORY
gravida ____ 86.
para ____ 87.
pre-term ____ 88.
miscarriages ____ 89.
still births ____ 90.
has had an abortion ____ 91.

MUSCULOSKELETAL
1. ____ aching muscles
2. ____ swollen joints
3. ____ back or shoulder pains
4. ____ painful feet
5. ____ handicapped

SKIN
6. ____ skin problems
7. ____ itching or burning skin
8. ____ bleeds easily
9. ____ bruises easily

NEUROLOGICAL
10. ____ faintness
11. ____ numbness
12. ____ convulsions
13. ____ change in handwriting
14. ____ trembles

MOOD
15. ____ nervous with strangers
16. ____ difficulty in making decisions
17. ____ lack of concentration or memory
18. ____ lonely or depressed
19. ____ cries often
20. ____ hopeless outlook
21. ____ difficulty relaxing
22. ____ worries a lot
23. ____ frightening dreams or thoughts
24. ____ shy or sensitive
25. ____ dislikes criticism
26. ____ loses temper
27. ____ annoyed by little things
28. ____ work or family problems
29. ____ sexual difficulties
30. ____ considered suicide
31. ____ desired psychiatric help

GENERAL
32. ____ weight changes
33. ____ tends to be hot or cold
34. ____ loss of interest in eating
35. ____ always hungry
36. ____ more thirsty lately
37. ____ armpits or groin swelling
38. ____ fatigue
39. ____ sleeping difficulties
40. ____ exercises less than 3 times per week
41. ____ cigarettes ____ cigars/pipes ____ don't smoke
42. ____ two or more alcoholic drinks per day
43. ____ over 6 cups of coffee/tea per day
44. ____ uses sleeping pills, marijuana, tranquilizers
45. ____ has used hard drugs
46. ____ drives vehicle over 25,000 miles per year
47. ____ never ____ sometimes ____ always uses seat belts
48. ____ visited in the last 6 months

Special problems or symptoms _____

_____

_____

_____

PATIENT'S SIGNATURE _____

E

■ **FIGURE 2–18** *Continued*

Name _____ Age _____

Occupation _____ Social Security Number _____

	BLOOD PRESSURE	VISION	DIAGNOSTIC TESTS	RESULTS

Height _____

Weight _____

Build _____

(Sm. Med. Lg. Obese)

Pulse _____

Resp. _____

Temp. _____

BLOOD PRESSURE

Sitting

R   /   :L   /

Standing

R   /   :L   /

Lying

R   /   :L   /

VISION

Without glasses

Far   R^{20}/   :L^{20} /

Near   R /   :L   /

With glasses

Far   R^{20}/   :L^{20} /

Near   R /   :L   /

Tonometry R___ L___

Colorvision _____
(Ishihara plates missed)

Peripheral fields R___ L___

	250	500	1000	2000	4000	8000
AUDIOMETRIC TESTING	R___	R___	R___	R___	R___	R___
	L___	L___	L___	L___	L___	L___

Gross hearing _____

F

PULMONARY FUNCTIONS

CHIEF COMPLAINT AND PRESENT ILLNESS _____

_____

_____

_____

_____

_____

_____

_____

_____

_____

_____

_____

_____

_____

_____

_____

_____

_____

_____

_____

_____

_____

Employment status _____ Physician's signature _____

Date _____

G

■ **FIGURE 2–18** *Continued*

Highlight on Cultural Diversity

Culture is the shared values, beliefs, and practices of a particular group of people. Culture is deeply rooted and is passed on from one generation to the next through communication. It includes areas such as religion, dietary practices, family lines of authority, family life patterns, beliefs, and health practices.

As the demographics of the United States continue to change, the medical assistant is faced with the challenge of providing care to an increasing number of cultural groups. Therefore, it is important for the medical assistant to learn as much as possible about the cultural values of the patients coming to the medical office.

This is known as **cultural awareness** and can be accomplished by carefully observing and listening to patients to acquire knowledge of their cultural values.

Cultural sensitivity is the respect and appreciation for cultural diversity, whereas **cultural competence** is understanding and using the cultural background of a patient to assist with the resolution of a problem. Because health practices are part of a patient's culture, changing them may have a negative impact on the patient. Whenever possible, the medical assistant should incorporate factors from a patient's cultural background into his or her health care.

Guidelines for Achieving Cultural Competence

The following guidelines will help the medical assistant in developing cultural awareness and sensitivity and in achieving cultural competence:

1. Respect the patient's values, beliefs, and practices. Even if you do not agree with them, it is important to respect the patient's right to hold these values and not dismiss them as being strange or odd. Cultural values play an important role in a patient's lifestyle. For example, patients from some cultures believe that losing blood depletes the body's strength and provides a route for the soul to leave the body. If a blood specimen is needed, these patients may become highly distressed or refuse to have their blood drawn. Members of some cultural groups believe that illness results when the body's natural balance or harmony is disturbed. To restore the balance, alternative forms of medicine are used such as herbal remedies and aromatherapy.

2. Refrain from cultural stereotypes. Realize that not all people of a cultural group have the same beliefs, practices, and values. Assuming that all members of a cultural group are alike is known as **stereotyping** and should be avoided. Just as one would never assume that all Americans like hamburgers and baseball, each individual must be approached according to his or her specific beliefs and practices.

3. Always address patients by their last names (and Mr., Mrs., Miss, Ms.) unless they give you permission to use other names. In most cultures, using a first name to address anyone other than family or friends is considered disrespectful. For example, most older Americans dislike being called by their first name and feel it shows a lack of respect.

4. Communicating with a patient may be difficult if the patient has a limited knowledge of English. With these patients, you should speak slowly and clearly in a normal tone and volume of voice. Speaking loudly does not help the patient understand any better and may even be offensive to the patient.

5. Show respect for cultural lines of authority. In many cultures, respect is given based on age (older) and gender (male). For example, in certain cultures, elders are considered the holders of the culture's wisdom and are highly respected. In other cultures, youth is valued over age. In certain cultures, the male dominates and women have very little status. Because of this, a male patient from this type of culture may not accept instructions from a female medical assistant.

6. Use appropriate eye contact. In most cultures, direct eye contact is regarded as important and generally shows that the other is attentive and listening. It conveys self-confidence, openness, interest, and honesty while the lack of eye contact may be interpreted as secretiveness, shyness, guilt, or lack of interest. Other cultures may view eye contact as impolite or an invasion of privacy, hence these patients show respect by avoiding direct eye contact.

7. The conditions under which an individual assumes the role of a (sick) patient and the way he or she performs in that role vary with culture. For example, individuals of some cultures resist the sick role and blame sickness on external forces as a means of punishment. These individuals may deny their illness and fail to provide much information when the medical assistant takes their symptoms. In other cultures, individuals take an optimistic view of the outcome of health care and, because of this, are more likely to follow the physician's instructions.

8. Learn to appreciate the richness of diversity as an asset rather than as a hindrance to communication and effective patient interaction.

as a foundation for the more detailed information that will be obtained in the Present Illness and Review of Systems sections of the health history. The medical assistant is usually responsible for obtaining the chief complaint from the patient and recording it in the patient's chart. In most offices, this information is recorded on a preprinted, lined form (see Fig. 2–18G). Certain guidelines must be followed in obtaining and recording the chief complaint:

- An open-ended question should be used to elicit the chief complaint from the patient. Examples:
    What seems to be the problem?
    How can we help you today?
    What can we do for you today?
- The chief complaint should be limited to one or two symptoms and should refer to a specific, rather than vague, symptom.
- The chief complaint should be recorded concisely and briefly, using the patient's own words as much as possible.
- The duration of the symptom (onset) should be included in the chief complaint.
- The medical assistant should avoid using names of diseases or diagnostic terms to record the chief complaint.

RECORDING CHIEF COMPLAINTS. The following are correct and incorrect examples of recording chief complaints.

Correct Examples
- Burning during urination that has lasted for 2 days.
- Pain in the shoulder that started 2 weeks ago.
- Shortness of breath for the past month.

Incorrect Examples
- Has not felt well for the past 2 weeks. (This statement refers to a vague, rather than a specific, complaint.)
- Ear pain and fever. (The duration of the symptoms is not listed.)
- Pain upon urination indicative of a urinary tract infection. (Names of diseases should not be used to record the chief complaint; the duration of the symptom is not listed.)

Present Illness

The present illness (PI) is an expansion of the chief complaint and includes a full description of the current status of the patient's illness, from the time of its onset. To complete this section of the health history, the patient is asked questions to obtain a detailed description of the symptom causing the greatest problem. This information is recorded on the same form used to record the chief complaint (see Fig. 2–18G). The medical assistant is often responsible for completing this section of the health history. Much skill and practice in asking the proper questions are required to obtain more detailed information. A general guide for obtaining further information on symptoms is presented in Procedure 2–4 (Obtaining and Recording Patient Symptoms), whereas a more thorough study for analyzing a symptom is included in the *Student Mastery Manual* (Chapter 2: Taking Patient Symptoms).

Past History

The past medical history is a review of the patient's past medical status (see Fig. 2–18C). Obtaining information on past medical care assists the physician in providing optimal patient care for the current problem. Most medical offices ask the patient to complete this section of the health history through a checklist type of form. The medical assistant should assist the patient with this section, as necessary, by offering to answer any questions regarding the information required. The past history includes the following areas:

- Major illnesses
- Childhood diseases
- Unusual infections
- Injuries and accidents
- Hospitalizations and operations
- Previous medical tests
- Immunizations
- Allergies
- Medications, past and present

Family History

The family history is a review of the health status of the patient's blood relatives (see Fig. 2–18B). This section of the health history focuses on diseases that tend to be familial. A **familial** disease is one that occurs in or affects blood relatives more frequently than would be expected by chance. Examples of familial diseases include hypertension, heart disease, allergies, and diabetes mellitus. The patient usually completes this section of the health history and is asked to provide the following information on each blood relative:

- Age
- State of health
- Presence of any significant disease
- If deceased, cause of death

Social/Occupational History

This section of the health history includes information on the patient's lifestyle, including daily routine, health habits, family situation, and living environment (see Fig. 2–18D). The social/occupational history is impor-

2

tant because the patient's lifestyle may have an impact on the condition of that individual as well as influence the course of treatment or therapy chosen by the physician. The social/occupational history also provides the physician with information regarding the effect that the illness may have on the patient's daily living pattern. If it is necessary for the individual to make a major lifestyle adjustment (e.g., stop smoking, reduce working hours), the physician may recommend available support services to assist in this transition. This section of the history is usually completed by the patient and includes the following areas:

- Education
- Occupation (past and present)
- Diet history
- Exercise
- Health habits

Review of Systems

A review of systems (ROS) is a systematic review of each body system in order to detect any symptoms that have not yet been revealed. The importance of the review of systems is that it assists in identifying symptoms that might otherwise remain undetected. The physician usually completes the review of systems by asking a series of detailed and direct questions relating to each body system; the results of this section of the health history assist the physician in a preliminary assessment of the type and extent of physical examination required. Refer to Figure 2–18E for an example of a review of systems form.

CHARTING IN THE MEDICAL RECORD

☐ **Charting** is the process of making written entries about a patient in the medical record and is performed by individuals in the medical office involved directly with the health care of the patient. The medical record is considered a legal document; therefore, the information must be charted as completely and accurately as possible. Developing good charting skills requires a thorough knowledge of charting guidelines combined with much repeated practice. To provide guidance in attaining this important skill, charting guidelines are presented in this section, and examples of proper charting entries are provided here and at the end of each procedure in the text.

CHARTING GUIDELINES

To ensure accurate and concise charting, specific guidelines must be followed. These are listed and described as follows:

1. *Check the name on the chart before making an entry to be sure you have the correct chart.* If the medical assistant records in the wrong patient's chart by mistake, information such as a procedure that was performed on a patient may be excluded from that individual's record. As previously stated, from a legal standpoint, a procedure not documented was not performed.

2. *Use dark ink (black or dark blue) to make entries in the patient's chart.* Dark ink must be used to provide a permanent record. In addition, entries made in dark ink are easier to reproduce, should the record be duplicated for insurance company purposes, patient referral, microfilming, and so on.

3. *Write in legible handwriting.* For the medical record to be meaningful to others, the medical assistant must be sure to chart information legibly. If the medical assistant's cursive script is not legible, the information should be printed.

4. *Chart information accurately, using phrases or sentences.*
   a. The medical assistant should be brief but complete and should avoid vagueness and duplication of information.
   b. It is not necessary to include the patient's name in the entry, because the entire medical record centers on one patient; it is therefore assumed the information refers to that patient.
   c. Each phrase or sentence should begin with a capital letter and end with a period.
   d. Each new entry should begin on a separate line and be dated with the month, day, year, and time (either a.m./p.m. or military time).
   e. Standard abbreviations, medical terms, and symbols should be used to help save time and space. It is important, however, that the medical assistant first check the office policy to determine those abbreviations, medical terms, and symbols that are commonly used in that office to avoid confusing others reading the chart. A list of abbreviations and symbols commonly used in the medical office are presented in the following boxes. Abbreviations used for charting medications are presented in Chapter 7: Administration of Medication.
   f. Correct spelling is essential for accuracy in charting. If you are in doubt about the spelling of a word, check a dictionary.

5. *Chart immediately after performing procedures.* Once a procedure has been performed, it should be charted without delay. If a time lapse occurs between performing the procedure and charting it, the medical assistant may not remember certain aspects of the procedure, such as the results of the treatment or the patient's reaction. Procedures should never be charted in advance. The individual performing the

Abbreviations and Symbols Commonly Used in the Medical Office

ABBREVIATIONS USED TO CHART SYMPTOMS

AM	before noon	NB	newborn
amt	amount	N/C	no complaints
approx	approximately	neg	negative
aq	water	NKA	no known drug allergies
ASAP	as soon as possible	NMP	normal menstrual period
BC	birth control	noct	nocturnal
BM	bowel movement	N & V	nausea and vomiting
c̄	with	OB	obstetrics
CC	chief complaint	occ	occasionally
ck	check	OPV	oral polio vaccine
CMA	Certified Medical Assistant	OT	occupational therapy
c/o	complains of	OTC	over the counter
dc	discontinue	OV	office visit
dec	decrease	peds	pediatrics
def	deficiency	per	by or through
DOB	date of birth	PM	afternoon
DOI	date of injury	po	by mouth
dsg	dressing	postop	postoperative
D & V	diarrhea and vomiting	prep	preparation
DSD	dry sterile dressing	PT	physical therapy
ea	each	pt	patient
EDD	expected date of delivery	qns	quantity not sufficient
GYN	gynecology	RMA	Registered Medical Assistant
H₂O	water	Rx	prescription
lac	laceration	s̄	without
liq	liquid	sigmoid	sigmoidoscopy
LMP	last menstrual period	sl	slight
meds	medications	SOB	shortness of breath
MMR	measles, mumps, and rubella	spec	specimen
mod	moderate	stat	immediately
n	normal		

2

Abbreviations Used to Chart Body Parts and Locations

abd	abdomen
AD	right ear
AS	left ear
AU	in each ear
EENT	eye, ears, nose, and throat
GI	gastrointestinal
GU	genitourinary
LA	left arm
LL	left leg
LLQ	lower left quadrant
LRQ	lower right quadrant
lt or Ⓛ	left
LUQ	left upper quadrant
OD	right eye
OS	left eye
OU	both eyes
RA	right arm
RL	right leg
RLE	right lower extremity
RLQ	right lower quadrant
rt or Ⓡ	right
RUQ	right upper quadrant

Abbreviations Used to Chart Measurement

C	Celsius or centigrade
cc	cubic centimeter
cm	centimeter
F	Fahrenheit
g	gram
kg	kilogram
L	liter
l	length
lb	pound
m	meter
mg	milligram
ml	milliliter
mm	millimeter
qt	quart

Abbreviations Used to Chart Procedures

AP	apical pulse
BP	blood pressure
DVA	distance visual acuity
HC	head circumference
ht	height
ID	intradermal
IM	intramuscular
IV	intravenous
NVA	near visual acuity
P	pulse
R	respiration
SC	subcutaneous
T	temperature
TPR	temperature, pulse, and respiration
VS	vital signs
wt	weight

Symbols

>	greater than
<	less than
↑	increase
↓	decrease
♀	female
♂	male
°	degree
×	times
@	at
Ⓡ	rectal temperature
Ⓐ	axillary temperature
"	inches
'	feet

Miscellaneous Abbreviations

PATIENT EXAMINATION

Dx	diagnosis
H & P	history and physical
H/O	history of
Hx	history
MHx	medical history
PE	physical examination
prog	prognosis
Tx	treatment

CONDITIONS

CAD	coronary artery disease
CHF	congestive heart failure
COPD	chronic obstructive pulmonary disease
CVA	cerebrovascular accident
HT	hypertension
MI	myocardial infarction
OM	otitis media
STD	sexually transmitted disease
TB	tuberculosis
URI	upper respiratory infection
UTI	urinary tract infection

DIAGNOSTIC PROCEDURES

ECG (EKG)	electrocardiogram
Echo	echocardiogram
EEG	electroencephalogram
IVP	intravenous pyelogram
US	ultrasound

LABORATORY TESTS

BG	Blood glucose
Bx	biopsy
C & S	culture and sensitivity
CBC	complete blood count
Diff	differential
FBS	fasting blood sugar
GTT	glucose tolerance test
Hct	hematocrit
Hgb	hemoglobin
PT	prothrombin time
RBC	red blood count
RBS	random blood sugar
UA	urinalysis
U/C	urine culture
WBC	white blood count

procedure should be the one to chart it; in other words, never chart for someone else.

6. *Each charting entry should be signed by the person making it.* The signature should include the medical assistant's first initial, full last name, and title (e.g., D. Bennett, CMA). The following title abbreviations are often used for medical assistants:

CMA Certified Medical Assistant
RMA Registered Medical Assistant
MA Medical Assistant
SMA Student Medical Assistant

7. *Never erase or obliterate an entry.* If an error is made in charting, the medical assistant must never erase or obliterate it. Should the physician or medical staff be involved in litigation, erased or obliterated entries tend to reduce credibility. If incorrect information is charted, the medical assistant should draw a single line through the incorrect information, thus permitting it to remain legible. The word "error" is then written above the incorrect data, including the date and the medical assistant's initials. Some medical offices may request that the reason for the change also be recorded. The correct information is then inserted immediately following the error (Fig. 2–19).

The medical assistant should always take the time to chart properly in the patient's medical record. Good charting helps coordinate efforts in the medical office and leads to high-quality patient care.

		error 10/15/2002 —— D. Bennett, CMA	
10/15/2002	9:30 am	OPV, 0.5 ml, ~~IM~~ —— D. Bennett, CMA	
		p.o.	

■ **FIGURE 2–19.** Proper method for correcting an error in the patient's medical record.

CHARTING PROGRESS NOTES

☐ After completion of the initial health history, a system is needed to update the medical record with new information each time the patient visits the medical office. Most offices use progress notes to fulfill this function. Progress notes document the patient's health status, as well as the care and treament being received by the patient, in chronological order. Progress notes provide effective communication among members of the medical office and also serve as a legal document.

Common Symptoms

INTEGUMENTARY SYSTEM

Diaphoresis	Excessive perspiration
Flushing	A red appearance to the skin, which generally affects the face and neck. A flushed appearance is commonly present with a fever
Jaundice	A yellow appearance to the skin, first evident in the whites of the eyes
Rash	An eruption on the skin

CIRCULATORY SYSTEM

Bradycardia	An abnormally slow pulse rate
Dehydration	A decrease in the amount of water in the body. The patient will have a flushed appearance, dry skin, and a decreased output of urine
Edema	The retention of fluid in the tissues, resulting in swelling. The skin over the area is tight. Edema is most easily observed in the extremities
Tachycardia	An abnormally fast pulse rate

GASTROINTESTINAL SYSTEM

Anorexia	The patient has a loss of appetite and a lack of interest in food
Constipation	A condition in which the stool becomes hard and dry, resulting in difficult passage from the rectum. The consistency of the stool, rather than the frequency of defecation, is used as a guide in determining the presence of constipation. (Frequency of bowel movements varies with the individual. Some people have a bowel movement only every 2 to 3 days but are not constipated.) Other symptoms of constipation include headache, nausea, and general malaise
Diarrhea	The passage of an increased number of loose, watery stools. The fecal material moves rapidly through the intestinal tract, resulting in decreased absorption by the body of water, electrolytes, and nutrients. Other symptoms usually associated with diarrhea are intestinal cramping and general weakness
Flatulence	The presence of excessive gas in the stomach or intestines
Nausea and vomiting	Nausea is a sensation of discomfort in the stomach with a feeling that vomiting may occur. Vomiting is the ejection of the stomach contents through the mouth, also known as *emesis*. The ejected content is known as *vomitus*

RESPIRATORY SYSTEM

Cough	An involuntary and forceful exhalation of air followed by a deep inhalation. A cough may be productive (meaning a discharge is produced) or nonproductive (no discharge is present)
Cyanosis	A bluish discoloration of the skin due to a lack of oxygen
Dyspnea	Labored or difficult breathing
Epistaxis	Hemorrhaging from the nose or a nosebleed

NERVOUS SYSTEM

Chill	A feeling of coldness accompanied by shivering. Chills are generally present with a fever
Convulsion	Involuntary contractions of the muscles
Fever or pyrexia	A body temperature that is higher than normal
Headache	A feeling of pain or aching in the head. It is a common symptom that accompanies many illnesses. Tension, fatigue, and eye strain can result in a headache
Pain	Irritation of pain receptors, resulting in a feeling of distress or suffering. Pain is an important indication that a part of the body is not working properly
Pruritus	Severe itching
Vertigo	A feeling of dizziness or lightheadedness

2

The medical assistant is frequently responsible for charting progress notes in the medical record. Progress notes are usually charted on special preprinted lined sheets known as progress note sheets. These sheets have a column for the date and a column for charting information.

Types of progress notes that are often charted by the medical assistant are presented next along with a charting example of each.

PATIENT SYMPTOMS

The medical assistant takes patient symptoms during office visits and telephone conversations. Information conveyed during a telephone conversation helps determine whether the patient needs to be seen and the immediacy of the situation.

A **symptom** is any change in the body or its functioning that indicates the presence of disease. Symptoms can be classified as subjective or objective. A **sub-jective symptom** is one that is felt by the patient and cannot be observed by another person. Pain, pruritus, vertigo, and nausea are examples of subjective symptoms. An **objective symptom** is one that can be observed by another person as well as by the patient. Rash, coughing, and cyanosis are objective symptoms. The medical assistant should have a thorough knowledge of common symptoms and be able to recognize them. The following box lists and describes some common symptoms.

Taking patient symptoms during an office visit consists of: (1) obtaining a chief complaint (refer to page 65), and (2) obtaining additional information about the chief complaint. For example, if the patient complains of pain in the abdomen that has lasted for 2 days (chief complaint), additional information is needed to describe the pain, including the type, specific location, onset, intensity, precipitating factors, and duration of the pain. The procedure for taking patient symptoms during an office visit is outlined in Procedure 2–4. Additional skill and practice on taking patient symptoms is included in Chapter 2 of the *Student Manual*.

PROCEDURE 2

2–4

Obtaining and Recording Patient Symptoms

EQUIPMENT/SUPPLIES: Medical record of the patient to be interviewed   Dark blue or black pen

1. **Procedural Step.** Assemble the equipment. Make sure you have the correct patient record and a dark blue or black pen for charting patient symptoms.
   Principle. Dark ink must be used to provide a permanent record.
2. **Procedural Step.** Go to the waiting room and ask the patient to come back.
3. **Procedural Step.** Escort the patient to a quiet, comfortable room that allows for privacy, such as an examination room.
   Principle. Patient symptoms should be taken in a room that encourages communication.
4. **Procedural Step.** Greet and identify the patient. Introduce yourself to the patient using a calm and friendly manner.

   Principle. A warm introduction sets a positive tone for the remainder of the interview.
5. **Procedural Step.** Ask the patient to be seated. You should seat yourself so that you face the patient at a distance of 3 to 4 feet.
   Principle. This type of seating arrangement facilitates open communication.
6. **Procedural Step.** Use good communication skills to interact with the patient. These include the following:
   a. Use the patient's name of choice.
   b. Demonstrate genuine interest and concern for the patient.
   c. Maintain appropriate eye contact.
   d. Use terminology the patient can understand.
   e. Listen carefully and attentively to the patient.

f. Pay attention to the patient's nonverbal messages.

g. Avoid judgmental comments.

h. Avoid rushing the patient.

7. **Procedural Step.** Locate the progress note sheet in the patient's medical record. Chart the date and time and the abbreviation for chief complaint (CC).

8. **Procedural Step.** Use an open-ended question to elicit the chief complaint, such as: "What seems to be the problem?"

   Principle. An open-ended question allows the patient to verbalize freely.

9. **Procedural Step.** Chart the chief complaint following the Charting Guidelines outlined on page 65. In addition, these guidelines should be followed:

   a. Limit the chief complaint to one or two symptoms and refer to a specific, rather than a vague symptom.

   b. Chart the chief complaint concisely and briefly, using the patient's own words as much as possible.

   c. Include the duration of the symptom (onset) in the chief complaint.

   d. Avoid using names of diseases or diagnostic terms to record the chief complaint.

10. **Procedural Step.** Obtain additional information regarding the chief complaint using "what," "when," and "where" questions. Chart this information after the chief complaint following proper charting guidelines.

    What Questions:
    What exactly is experienced by the patient?
    Does the symptom occur suddenly or gradually?
    Does anything make it worse?

    Where Question:
    Where is the symptom located?

When Questions:
When did the symptom first occur?
How long does it last after occurring?
Does anything precipitate it?

Principle. This information provides a complete description of the chief complaint.

11. **Procedural Step.** Thank the patient and proceed to the next step in the patient work-up. (This usually includes measuring vital signs and height and weight and preparing the patient as needed for the physical examination as will be presented in the next two chapters.)

12. **Procedural Step.** Inform the patient the physician will be with him or her soon.

13. **Procedural Step.** Place the patient's medical record in the appropriate location as designated by the medical office policy.

    Principle. The physician will want to review the patient's medical record before examining the patient.

CHARTING EXAMPLE

Date	
6/30/2002	3:15 p.m. CC: Intense pain in the (L) ear for the past 2 days. Pt states pain is sharp and continuous. Pt noted sl yellow discharge from (L) ear. Fever of 101° F began last night about 9 p.m. Took Tylenol, 2 tabs, @ 8 a.m. this morning. ———— D. Bennett, CMA

OTHER ACTIVITIES THAT NEED TO BE CHARTED

PROCEDURES. The medical assistant frequently charts procedures performed on the patient; examples include vital signs, weight and height, visual acuity, and ear irrigations. Procedures should be charted immediately after being performed; from a legal standpoint, a procedure that is not documented was not performed. In general, the following information should be included: the date and time, the type of procedure, the outcome, and the patient reaction. The specific information to be recorded is included with each procedure presented in this text.

CHARTING EXAMPLE

Date	
6/30/2002	9:15 a. m. Irrigated (R) ear c̄ 200 ml of normal saline @ 98.6° F. Mod amt of cerumen in returned solution. Pt states can hear better. ———— D. Bennett, CMA

ADMINISTRATION OF MEDICATION. Charting medications administered to the patient is an important responsibility in the medical office. Included in the recording should be the date and time, the name of the medication, the dosage given, the route of administration, the injection site used (for parenteral medication), and any significant observations or patient reactions.

CHARTING EXAMPLE

Date	========
6/30/2002	10:15 a.m. Bicillin, 900,00 units, IM, (L) dorsogluteal. ——————— D. Bennett, CMA

SPECIMEN COLLECTION.   Each time a specimen is collected from a patient, the medical assistant should chart the date and time of the collection, the type of specimen, and the area of the body from which the specimen was obtained. If the specimen is to be sent to an outside laboratory for testing, this information also should be charted, including the test(s) requested and the date the specimen was sent. In this way, the physician will know that the specimen was collected and sent to the laboratory when test results are not back yet.

2

CHARTING EXAMPLE

Date	========
6/30/2002	1:30 p.m. Venous blood spec collected from R arm. Sent to Ross Lab for CBC and diff on 6/30/2002 ——————— D. Bennett, CMA
Date	========
6/30/2002	2:00 p.m. Throat spec collected. Sent to Ross Lab for C & S on 6/30/2002 ——————— D. Bennett, CMA

DIAGNOSTIC PROCEDURES AND LABORATORY TESTS.   Diagnostic procedures and laboratory tests ordered for a patient should always be charted in the medical record. If the patient does not undergo the test, documented proof exists that the test was ordered. Charting diagnostic procedures and laboratory tests protects the physician legally and refreshes the physician's memory of the procedures and tests being run on the patient when results are not yet back from the testing facility. Information to include in the charting entry are the date and time, the type of procedure or test(s) ordered, and the scheduling date.

CHARTING EXAMPLE

Date	========
6/30/2002	10:15 a.m. Mammography scheduled for 7/5/2002 at Grant Hospital. ——————— D. Bennett, CMA
Date	========
6/30/2002	11:30 a.m. Pt given lab request for GTT at Ross Lab. ——————— D. Bennett, CMA

RESULTS OF LABORATORY TESTS.   It is usually not necessary to chart results from laboratory reports returned from outside laboratories, because the report itself is filed in the patient's record. In cases of a stat request or critical findings, however, the test results are telephoned to the medical office, thus requiring the medical assistant to record the results on a report form. Careful recording is essential to avoid errors, which in turn could affect the patient's diagnosis. Results of those laboratory tests performed by the medical assistant in the office should be charted in the medical record and must include the date and time, name of the test, and test results.

CHARTING EXAMPLE

Date	========
6/30/2002	8:00 a.m. FBS: 110 mg/dl. ——————— D. Bennett, CMA
Date	========
6/30/2002	4:15 p.m. Monospot: neg ——————— D. Bennett, CMA

INSTRUCTIONS GIVEN TO THE PATIENT REGARDING MEDICAL CARE.   Many times it is necessary to relay instructions to a patient regarding medical care (e.g., wound care, cast care, care of sutures). The medical assistant should chart this information, making sure to include the date and the type of instructions relayed to the patient. Many medical offices have printed instruction sheets that are given to the patient. The patient is asked to sign a form, which is then filed in the patient's record, indicating that he or she has read and understands the instructions (Fig. 2–20). The form should also be signed by the medical assistant, who functions as a witness. This protects the physician legally in the event that the patient fails to follow the instructions and causes further harm or damage to a body part.

Other areas in which the medical assistant is responsible for charting in the medical record include missed or canceled appointments, telephone calls from patients, medication refills, and changes in medication or dosage by the physician.

CHARTING EXAMPLE

Date	========
6/30/2002	11:15 a.m. Pt telephoned office. States that swelling in the Ⓡ ankle is almost gone. ——————— D. Bennett, CMA
Date	========
6/30/2002	1:15 p.m. Missed appointment scheduled for 6/30/2002 @ 1:00 p.m. —— D. Bennett, CMA

CHARTING EXAMPLE

Date	========
6/30/2002	9:30 a.m. Provided instructions for reading and reporting Tine test results ——————— ——————— D. Bennett, CMA
Date	========
6/30/2002	10:25 a.m. Provided instructions for applying a heating pad to the lower back ——————— ——————— D. Bennett, CMA

PATIENT INSTRUCTIONS FOR WOUND CARE

Name of patient: _____

Follow the instructions indicated below for care of your wound:

1. Use ice bag and elevate to reduce swelling and pain. Elevate higher than your heart.
2. You may take aspirin/Tylenol for pain.
3. Keep the dressing clean and dry.
4. Replace the dressing within _____ days.
5. Discard the dressing within _____ days.
6. Cleanse the wound daily as instructed.
7. Stitches should be removed in _____ days.
8. Despite the greatest of care any wound can become infected. If your wound becomes red or swollen, shows pus or red streaks, or feels more sore instead of less sore, contact the physician **immediately.**

I have received and understand the above instructions:

Patient (or representative): _____

Relationship to patient: _____

Witness: _____   Time and date: _____

■ **FIGURE 2–20.** Patient instruction sheet.

MEDICAL PRACTICE AND THE LAW

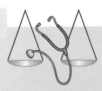

Documentation can be a deciding factor in a legal case. Everything you do for a patient should be documented in a factual manner in the medical record or "chart." When a legal issue arises, often it is several years before it comes to trial. If you are involved, you will be asked detailed questions as to your actions on a particular day, for a particular patient. Few people have accurate memories for that long. Juries will give more credibility to documentation performed at the time of the action than to a memory of years ago. Ethically, you owe the patient thorough documentation in order to provide optimal continuity of care. Remember that all patient information is confidential.

Proper charting is a critical skill for a medical assistant to master. Although proper documentation will not prevent a lawsuit, it may determine the outcome. Pay particular attention to the rules for consents and charting guidelines outlined in this chapter, and follow them to the letter.

CERTIFICATION REVIEW

☐ The patient registration record must be completed by all new patients and consists of patient demographic and billing information.

☐ The health history (along with the physical examination and laboratory and diagnostic tests) is used to determine the patient's general state of health; to arrive at a diagnosis and prescribe treatment; and to observe any change in a patient's illness after treatment has been instituted.

☐ The physical examination is a report of the findings from the physician's assessment of each body system.

☐ The medication record consists of detailed information relating to a patient's medications and includes one or more of the following categories: prescription medications; over-the-counter (OTC) medications; medications administered at the medical office.

☐ A consultation report is a narrative report of an opinion about a patient's condition by a specialist and is based on a review of the patient record and an examination of the patient.

☐ Home health care provides medical and nonmedical care in a patient's home or place of residence to minimize the effect of disease or disability.

☐ A laboratory report is a report of the analysis or examination of body specimens. Its purpose is to relay the results of laboratory tests to the physician to assist him or her in diagnosing and treating disease.

☐ A diagnostic procedure report consists of a narrative description and interpretation of a diagnostic procedure and includes the following reports: electrocardiogram, Holter monitor, sigmoidoscopy, spirometry, radiology, and imaging.

☐ A therapeutic service report documents the assessments and treatment designed to restore patient function such as physical therapy, occupational therapy, and speech therapy.

☐ Hospital documents are prepared by the physician responsible for the care of a patient while at the hospital and include the history and physical of a hospitalized patient, operative report, discharge summary report, pathology report, and emergency room report.

☐ A consent to treatment form is required for all surgical operations and nonroutine diagnostic or therapeutic procedures performed in the medical office. The form must be signed by the patient and provides written evidence that the patient agreed to the procedure(s) listed on the form.

☐ A source-oriented medical record is organized into sections based on the department, facility, or other source that generated the information. Each section in a source-oriented record is separated from the other by a chart divider labeled with the title of its respective section.

☐ The documents in a problem-oriented medical record (POMR or POR) are organized by the patient's specific health problems and include a database, problem list, plan of action for each problem, and progress notes. Progress notes for a POR include four categories: subjective data, objective data, assessment, and plan (SOAP).

☐ A health history consists of the following components: introductory data, chief complaint, present illness, past history, family history, social/occupational history, and review of systems. A health history is taken for each new patient, and subsequent office visits (in the form of progress notes)

CERTIFICATION REVIEW *Continued*

provide additional information regarding changes in the patient's illness or treatment.

☐ Charting is the process of making written entries about a patient in the medical record. The medical record is a legal document and the information must be charted as completely and accurately as possible, following established charting guidelines.

☐ Progress notes update the medical record with new information each time the patient visits or telephones the medical office. Types of progress notes often charted by the medical assistant include patient symptoms, procedures, administration of medication, specimen collection, diagnostic procedures and laboratory tests ordered on a patient, results of laboratory tests, instructions given to the patient regarding medical care, missed or canceled appointments, telephone calls from patients, medication refills, and changes in medication or dosage by the physician.

2

Vital Signs

Janice Smith, *and I'm a Certified Medical Assistant. I graduated from an accredited medical assisting program and have an associate's degree in Applied Science.*

I work in a large clinic that is associated with a medical school. At present, I work in family medicine, but I have also worked in dermatology, obstetrics and gynecology, and internal medicine.

I have worked as a medical assistant for 16 years and have always found it to be very rewarding. Family medicine has been my favorite area because of the wide variety of tasks that are performed. There is rarely a dull moment.

I focus primarily on clinical medical assisting. Taking vital signs is a big part of my job responsibilities. It is the routine at my clinic to take height, weight, blood pressure, pulse, and respiration on every patient seen at the clinic, no matter what the reason for their visit. I also assist the doctor with various procedures, exams, and minor office surgery, as well as administering injections, running electrocardiograms, and performing various laboratory tests.

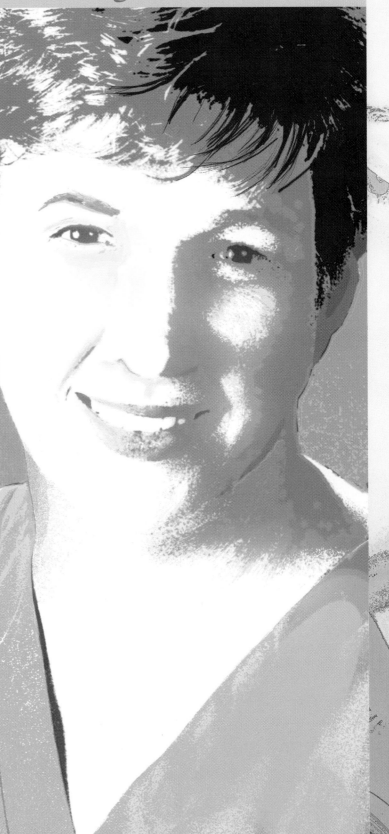

CHAPTER 3

CHAPTER OUTLINE

Body Temperature
Regulation of Body Temperature
Assessment of Body Temperature
Pulse
Mechanism of the Pulse
Assessment of Pulse
Respiration
Mechanism of Respiration
Assessment of Respiration
Blood Pressure
Mechanism of Blood Pressure
Assessment of Blood Pressure

OUTCOMES

After completing this chapter, you should be able to demonstrate the proper procedures to perform the following:

1. Measure oral body temperature.
2. Measure rectal body temperature.
3. Measure axillary body temperature.
4. Measure aural body temperature.
5. Clean glass thermometers.
6. Measure radial pulse.
7. Measure apical pulse.
8. Measure respiration.
9. Measure blood pressure.
10. Determine systolic pressure by palpation.

EDUCATIONAL OBJECTIVES

After completing this chapter, you should be able to do the following:

1. Define a vital sign.
2. Explain the purpose for taking vital signs.
3. Define the terms listed in the Key Terminology.
4. Explain how body temperature is maintained.
5. Give examples of four ways in which heat is produced in the body and four ways in which heat is lost from the body.
6. State the normal body temperature range and the average body temperature.
7. List and explain four factors that can cause a variation in the body temperature.
8. List and describe the three stages of a fever.
9. List the four sites for taking body temperature and explain why these sites are used.
10. List and describe the four types of thermometers.
11. List and describe the guidelines that should be followed when using a tympanic membrane thermometer.
12. Explain the principles underlying each step in the body temperature procedures.
13. Explain the mechanism of pulse.
14. List and explain four factors that affect the pulse rate.
15. Identify one use of each of the eight pulse sites.
16. State the normal range for pulse rate for each of the various age groups.
17. Explain the difference between pulse rhythm and pulse volume.
18. Explain the principles underlying each step in the radial and apical pulse procedures.
19. Explain the purpose of respiration.
20. State what occurs during inhalation and exhalation.
21. State the normal respiratory rate for each of the various age groups.
22. List and explain three factors that affect the respiratory rate.
23. Explain the difference between the rhythm and depth of respiration.
24. Describe the character of the following abnormal breath sounds; stertor, stridor, crackles, gurgles, wheezes, and pleural friction rub.
25. Explain the principles underlying each step in the procedure for measuring respiration.
26. Define blood pressure.
27. State the normal range for blood pressure for an adult.
28. List and describe four factors that affect the blood pressure.
29. Identify the different parts of a stethoscope and a sphygmomanometer.
30. Identify the Korotkoff sounds.
31. Explain how to prevent errors in blood pressure measurement.
32. Explain the principles underlying each step in the blood pressure procedure.

3

KEY TERMINOLOGY

afebrile (â-FÊB-ril): Without fever; the body temperature is normal.

alveolus (pl. alveoli) (al-VÊ-ô-lus): A thin-walled air sac of the lungs in which the exchange of oxygen and carbon dioxide takes place.

antecubital space (ANT-ta-CÛ-bit-al spâs): The space located at the front of the elbow.

antipyretic (ANTÎ-pî-RET-ik): An agent that reduces fever.

aorta (â-OR-ta): The major trunk of the arterial system of the body. The aorta arises from the upper surface of the left ventricle.

apnea (AP-nê-a): The temporary cessation of breathing.

arrhythmia (â-RYTH-mê-a): An irregular rhythm. (Also termed dysrhythmia.)

axilla (AX-il-la): The armpit.

bounding pulse: A pulse with an increased volume that feels very strong and full.

bradycardia (BRÂ-da-car-DÊ-a): An abnormally slow heart rate (below 60 beats per minute).

bradypnea (brad-IP-NÊ-a): An abnormal decrease in the respiratory rate of less than 10 respirations per minute.

Centigrade or Celsius thermometer: A thermometer on which the freezing point of water is 0° and the boiling point of water is 100°.

conduction: The transfer of energy, such as heat, from one object to another.

convection: The transfer of energy, such as heat, through air currents.

crisis: A sudden falling of an elevated body temperature to normal.

cyanosis (SÎ-in-ÔS-is): A bluish discoloration of the skin and mucous membranes.

diastole (DÎ-as-stol-ê): The phase in the cardiac cycle in which the heart relaxes between contractions.

diastolic pressure (DÎ-as-STOL-ic PRESH-ur): The point of lesser pressure on the arterial wall, which is recorded during diastole.

disinfectant (DIS-in-FEK-tant): A substance that kills disease-producing organisms.

dyspnea (disp-NÊ-a): Labored or difficult breathing.

eupnea (ÛP-nê-a): Normal respiration.

exhalation (X-hal-ÂSH-on): The act of breathing out.

Fahrenheit thermometer: A thermometer on which the freezing point of water is 32° and the boiling point of water is 212°.

febrile (FÊ-bril): Pertaining to fever.

fever: A body temperature that is above normal. Synonym for pyrexia.

frenulum linguae (FREN-u-lum LING-gwa): The midline fold that connects the undersurface of the tongue with the floor of the mouth.

hyperpnea (hî-PERP-nê-a): An abnormal increase in the rate and depth of respiration.

hyperpyrexia (hî-PER-pî-REX-êa): An extremely high fever.

hypertension (hî-PER-ten-shun): High blood pressure.

hyperventilation (hî-PER-vent-a-LÂ-shun): An abnormally fast and deep type of breathing usually associated with acute anxiety or emotional tension.

hypopnea (hî-POP-nê-a): An abnormal decrease in the rate and depth of respiration.

hypotension (hî-PÔ-ten-shun): Low blood pressure.

hypothermia (hî-PÔ-THER-mê-a): A body temperature that is below normal.

hypoxia (hî-POX-ê-a): A reduction in the oxygen supply to the tissues of the body.

inhalation (IN-hal-Â-shun): The act of breathing in.

intercostal (IN-ter-CAUS-tal): Between the ribs.

Korotkoff sounds (KÔ-rot-kauf sounds): Sounds heard during the measurement of blood pressure which are used to determine the systolic and diastolic blood pressure readings.

lysis (LÎ-sis): The gradual return of the body temperature to normal.

manometer (MUN-OM-it-er): An instrument for measuring pressure.

meniscus (MU-NIS-kus): The curved surface on a column of liquid in a tube.

orthopnea (orth-OP-nê-a): The condition in which breathing is easier when an individual is in a standing or sitting position.

pulse pressure: The difference between the systolic and diastolic pressures.

pulse rhythm: The time interval between heart beats.

pulse volume: The strength of the heart beat.

pyrexia (pîrex-Ê-a): A body temperature that is above normal. Synonym for fever.

radiation: The transfer of energy, such as heat, in the form of waves.

sphygmomanometer (SFIG-mô-mun-om-it-er): An instrument for measuring arterial blood pressure.

stethoscope (STETH-a-skôp): An instrument for amplifying and hearing sounds produced by the body.

systole (SIS-tô-lê): The phase in the cardiac cycle in which the ventricles contract, sending blood out of the heart and into the aorta and pulmonary aorta.

systolic pressure (sis-TAUL-ik PRESH-ur): The

point of maximum pressure on the arterial walls, which is recorded during systole.

tachycardia (TAK-a-CAR-dê-a): An abnormally fast heart rate (over 100 beats per minute).

tachypnea (TAK-ip-nê-a): An abnormal increase in the respiratory rate of more than 20 respirations per minute.

thready pulse: A pulse with a decreased volume that feels weak and thin.

INTRODUCTION

☐ Vital signs indicate a patient's condition; they are objective guideposts, indicating that life is present. The four vital signs are temperature, pulse, and respiration (TPR) and blood pressure (BP).

The normal ranges of the vital signs are finely adjusted, and any deviation from normal may indicate disease. During the course of an illness, variations in the vital signs may take place. The medical assistant should be alert to any significant changes and report them to the physician because they may indicate a change in the patient's condition. When patients visit the medical office, vital signs are routinely checked to establish each patient's usual state of health or baseline measurements against which future measurements can be compared. The medical assistant should have a thorough knowledge of the vital signs and attain proficiency in taking them to ensure accurate findings.

General guidelines that should be followed by the medical assistant when measuring the vital signs are as follows.

1. Be familiar with the normal ranges for all vital signs. The medical assistant should keep in mind that normal ranges vary based on the individual age group (infant, child, adult elder).
2. Make sure that all equipment for measuring vital signs is in proper working condition to ensure accurate findings.
3. Attempt to eliminate or minimize factors that may affect the vital signs, such as exercise, food and beverage consumption, and emotional states.
4. Use an organized approach when measuring the vital signs. The vital signs are usually measured starting with temperature. If a glass thermometer is being used, the pulse and respiration should be measured during the temperature-registering time period, followed by the measurement of blood pressure.

BODY TEMPERATURE
REGULATION OF BODY TEMPERATURE

Body temperature is maintained within a fairly constant range by the hypothalamus, which is located in the brain. The hypothalamus functions as the thermostat of the body. It normally allows the body temperature to vary only about 1 to 2° Fahrenheit (F) throughout the day.

Body temperature is maintained through a balance of the heat produced in the body and the heat lost from the body (Fig. 3–1). A constant temperature

3

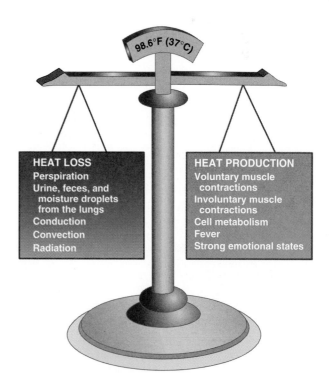

98.6°F (37°C)

HEAT LOSS
Perspiration
Urine, feces, and
    moisture droplets
    from the lungs
Conduction
Convection
Radiation

HEAT PRODUCTION
Voluntary muscle
    contractions
Involuntary muscle
    contractions
Cell metabolism
Fever
Strong emotional states

■ **FIGURE 3–1.** Body temperature represents a balance between the heat produced in the body and the heat lost from the body.

range must be maintained for the body to function properly. When minor changes in the temperature of the body occur, the hypothalamus senses this and makes adjustments as necessary to ensure that the body temperature stays within a normal and safe range. For example, if an individual is playing tennis on a hot day, the body's heat-cooling mechanism is activated to remove excess heat from the body through perspiration.

Heat Production

Most of the heat produced in the body is through voluntary and involuntary muscle contractions. Voluntary muscle contractions involve the muscles over which the person has control, for example, the moving of legs or arms. Involuntary muscle contractions involve the muscles over which the person has no control; physiologic processes such as digestion, the beating of the heart, and shivering are examples of this.

Body heat is also produced by cell metabolism. Heat is produced when nutrients are broken down in the cells. Fever and strong emotional states increase heat production in the body.

Heat Loss

Heat is lost from the body through the urine and feces and in water vapor from the lungs. Perspiration also contributes to heat loss. Perspiration is the excretion of moisture through the pores of the skin. When the moisture evaporates, heat is released and the body is cooled.

Radiation, conduction, and convection all cause loss of heat from the body. **Radiation** is the transfer of heat in the form of waves; body heat is continually radiating into cooler surroundings. **Conduction** is the transfer of heat from one object to another; heat can be transferred by conduction from the body to a cooler object it touches. **Convection** is the transfer of heat through air currents; cool air currents can cause the body to lose heat. These processes are illustrated in Figure 3–2.

Body Temperature Range

The purpose of measuring body temperature is to establish the patient's baseline recording and to monitor an abnormally high or low body temperature. The normal body temperature range is 97 to 99°F (36.1 to 37.2°C), the average temperature being 98.6°F, which is equal to 37° centigrade or Celsius (C). Body temperature is usually recorded using the Fahrenheit system of measurement. Table 3–1 illustrates comparable Fahrenheit and centigrade temperatures, and explains how temperatures are converted from one scale to the other.

Alterations in Body Temperature

A body temperature above 100.4°F (38°C) indicates a **fever,** or **pyrexia.** If the temperature exceeds 100.4°F (38°C), the heat being produced in the body is greater than the heat being lost. A temperature reading above 105.8°F (41°C) is known as **hyperpyrexia.** Hyperpy-

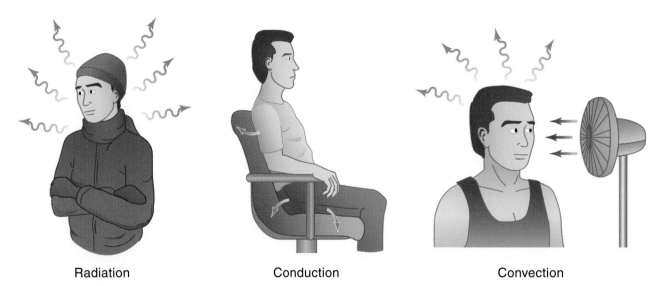

■ **FIGURE 3–2.** Heat loss from the body. **Radiation**—the body gives off heat in the form of waves to the cooler outside air. **Conduction**—the chair becomes warm from heat being transferred from the individual to the chair. **Convection**—the patient will feel cooler as air currents move heat away from the body.

TABLE 3–1

Equivalent Fahrenheit and Centigrade Temperatures

Fahrenheit	Centigrade	Fahrenheit	Centigrade
93.2	34	101.3	38.5
95	35	102.2	39
96.8	36	104	40
97.7	36.5	105.8	41
98.6	37	107.6	42
99.5	37.5	109.4	43
100.4	38	111.2	44

Temperature Conversion

1. Centigrade to Fahrenheit: To convert centigrade to Fahrenheit, multiply by 9/5 and add 32.

$$°F = (°C \times 9/5) + 32.$$

2. Fahrenheit to Centigrade: To convert Fahrenheit to centigrade, subtract 32 and multiply by 5/9.

$$°C = (°F - 32) \times 5/9.$$

rexia is a serious condition, and a temperature above 109.4°F (43°C) is generally fatal.

A body temperature below 97°F (36°C) is classified as subnormal, or **hypothermia.** This means that the heat being lost from the body is greater than the heat being produced. An individual usually cannot survive with a subnormal temperature of less than 93.2°F (34°C). Terms used to describe alterations in body temperature are illustrated in Fig. 3–3.

Variations in Body Temperature

Normal variations may occur in the day-to-day activities of an individual, causing fluctuations in the body temperature. Rarely does the body temperature stay the same throughout the course of a day. The medical assistant should take the following points into consideration when evaluating a patient's temperature:

Age — Infants and young children normally have a higher body temperature than adults because their thermoregulatory system is not yet fully established. Elderly people usually have a lower body temperature owing to factors such as loss of subcutaneous fat, lack of exercise, and loss of thermoregulatory control (Table 3–2).

Diurnal variations — During sleep, body metabolism slows down, as do muscle contractions. The temperature of the body is lowest in the morning before metabolism and muscle contractions begin speeding up.

Exercise — Vigorous physical exercise causes an increase in voluntary muscle contractions, which raises the body temperature.

Emotional states — Strong emotions, such as crying or extreme anger, can increase the body temperature. This is important to consider when working with young children, who frequently cry during examination procedures or when they are ill.

Environment — Cold weather tends to decrease the body temperature, whereas hot weather increases it.

Patient's normal body temperature — Some patients normally run a low or high temperature. The medical assistant should review the patient's past vital sign recordings.

Pregnancy — Cell metabolism increases during pregnancy, which in turn raises body temperature.

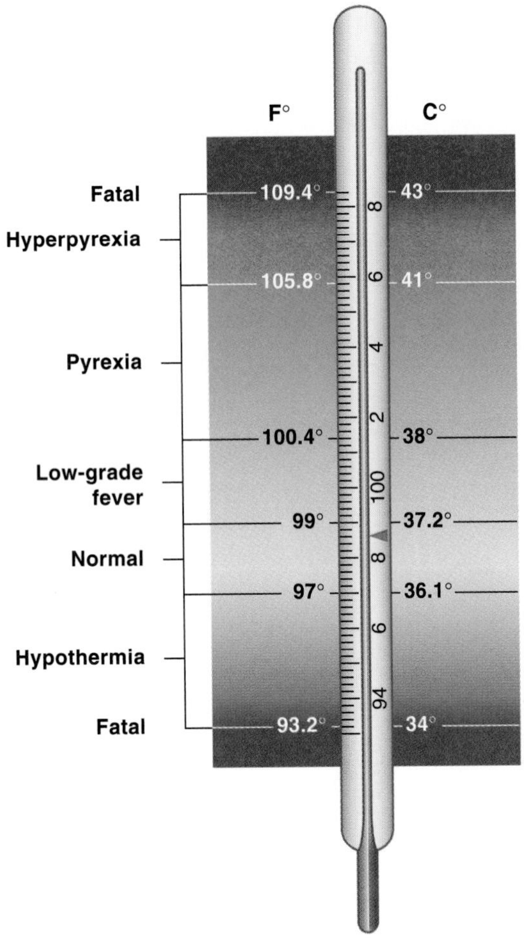

FIGURE 3–3. Terms used to describe alterations in body temperature (adult oral temperature).

3

Fever

Fever, or pyrexia, denotes that a patient's temperature has risen above 100.4°F (38°C). A temperature reading between 99°F (37.2°C) and 100.4°F (38°C) is known as a **low-grade fever.** An individual who has a fever is said to be **febrile;** one who does not is **afebrile.**

Fever is a common symptom of illness, particularly inflammation and infection. When there is an infection in the body, the invading pathogen functions as a **pyrogen,** which is any substance that produces fever. Pyrogens reset the hypothalamus at a higher temperature, causing the body temperature to rise above normal. Fever is not an illness in itself but, rather, a sign that the body may have an infection. An individual with a fever feels hot to the touch and has a flushed appearance. Other symptoms that often occur with a fever include loss of appetite, headache, chills, increased perspiration, thirst, and general malaise. Most fevers are self-limiting, meaning that the body temperature returns to normal after the disease process is completed.

Stages of a Fever

A fever can be divided into the following three stages:

1. The **onset** is when the temperature first begins to rise. The rise may be slow or sudden.
2. During the **course of a fever,** the temperature rises and falls in one of the following three patterns: continuous, intermittent, or remittent. These patterns are described and illustrated in Table 3–3.
3. The **subsiding stage** is when the temperature returns to normal. It can return to normal gradually (known as *lysis*) or suddenly (known as a *crisis*).

ASSESSMENT OF BODY TEMPERATURE

Assessment Sites

There are four sites for measuring body temperature: **oral** (by mouth), **rectal** (by rectum), **axillary** (by axilla),

TABLE 3–2	Variations in Body Temperature by Age		
Age	**Site**	**Average Temperature**	
Newborn	Axillary	97–100°F	36.1–37.7°C
1 year	Oral	99.7°F	37.7°C
5 years	Oral	98.6°F	37°C
Adult	Oral	98.6°F	37°C
	Rectal	99.6°F	37.6°C
	Axillary	97.6°F	36.4°C
	Aural	98.6°F	37°C
Elderly (over 70 yrs)	Oral	96.8°F	36°C

TABLE 3–3

The Course of a Fever

Pattern	Description	Illustration
Continuous fever	The body temperature fluctuates minimally but always remains elevated. Occurs with: Scarlet fever Pneumococcal pneumonia	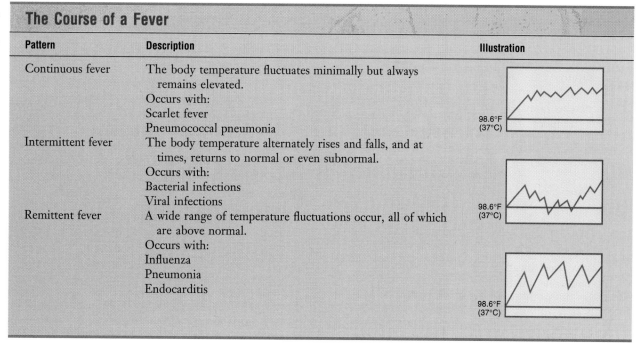 98.6°F (37°C)
Intermittent fever	The body temperature alternately rises and falls, and at times, returns to normal or even subnormal. Occurs with: Bacterial infections Viral infections	98.6°F (37°C)
Remittent fever	A wide range of temperature fluctuations occur, all of which are above normal. Occurs with: Influenza Pneumonia Endocarditis	98.6°F (37°C)

Highlight on Fever

Although most fevers indicate an infection, not all do. Noninfectious causes of fever include heat stroke, drug hypersensitivity, neoplasms, and central nervous system damage.

A fever is usually not harmful if it remains below 102°F (38.9°C). In fact, research suggests that fever may serve as a defense mechanism to destroy pathogens that are unable to survive above the normal body temperature range.

The level of the fever isn't necessarily related to the seriousness of the infection. A patient with a temperature of 104°F (40°C) may not be any sicker than a patient with a temperature of 102°F (38.9°C).

In children, fever often appears as one of the first signs of illness and has a tendency to become highly elevated. In elderly patients, on the other hand, fever may be elevated only 1 to 2° above normal, even with a severe infection.

During a fever, the body's basal metabolism increases 7 percent for each degree of temperature elevation. Heart and respiratory rates also increase to meet this metabolic demand.

Chills during a fever result when the hypothalamus has been reset at a higher temperature. In an attempt to reach this temperature, involuntary muscle contractions occur (chills), which produce heat, causing the temperature of the body to go up. After the higher temperature has been reached, the chills subside and the individual then feels warm.

Increased perspiration during a fever occurs when the hypothalamus has been reset at a lower temperature—for example, after taking an antipyretic or after the cause of the fever has been removed. In order to cool the body and reach this lower temperature, the body perspires, often profusely; profuse perspiration is known as **diaphoresis.**

3

and **aural** (by ear). The sites used for taking temperature must be located in a space as closed as possible to prevent air currents from interfering with the temperature reading. The sites should also have an abundant blood supply, so that the temperature of the entire body is obtained, and not just the temperature of only a part of the body. The site chosen for measuring a patient's temperature depends on the patient's age, condition, and state of consciousness; the type of thermometer being used; and the medical office policy.

Oral Temperature

The oral method is the most convenient and the most commonly used means for measuring body temperature. When the medical assistant records a temperature, the physician assumes it has been taken through the oral route, unless it is otherwise noted. There is a rich blood supply under the tongue in the area located on either side of the frenulum linguae. The thermometer should be placed in this area to receive the most accurate reading. The patient must keep his or her mouth closed during the procedure to provide a closed space for the thermometer.

Rectal Temperature

The rectal temperature is the most accurate measurement of body temperature because few factors can alter the results. The rectum is highly vascular and, of the four sites, provides the most closed cavity. The temperature obtained through the rectal route measures approximately 1°F higher than the same temperature taken through the oral route (see Table 3–2). The medical assistant should make a notation on the patient's chart if the temperature has been taken rectally.

The rectal method is generally used for infants and young children, unconscious patients, and mouth-breathing patients and when greater accuracy in body temperature is desired. The rectal site should not be used with newborns owing to the danger of rectal trauma.

Axillary Temperature

Axillary temperature has long been considered less accurate than the rectal or oral method. Research shows that there is no significant difference in accuracy between axillary temperature measurement and rectal temperature measurement. Because of this, the axilla is recommended as a site for measuring temperature in toddlers and preschoolers who are not yet old enough to understand how to hold a thermometer in their mouths. The axillary site also should be used for mouth-breathing patients and for patients with oral inflammation or who have had oral surgery.

The temperature obtained through the axillary method measures approximately 1°F lower than the same temperature taken through the oral route (see Table 3–2). As with the rectal method, the medical assistant should make a notation to tell the physician that the temperature was taken through the axillary route.

Aural Temperature

The aural (ear) site is used with the tympanic membrane thermometer. This site is discussed with tympanic membrane thermometers.

Types of Thermometers

The four types of thermometers available for measuring body temperature include electronic thermometers, tympanic membrane thermometers, mercury glass thermometers, and chemical thermometers. They are discussed in detail on the following pages.

Electronic Thermometer

An electronic thermometer is often used in the medical office to measure oral, rectal, and axillary body temperature. An electronic thermometer takes less time to measure temperature than does a mercury glass thermometer; the time varies between 10 and 60 seconds, depending on the manufacturer. In addition, it is easier to read the results because the temperature measurement is digitally displayed on a screen.

An electronic thermometer consists of interchangeable oral and rectal probes attached to a battery-operated portable unit that sits in a rechargeable base. A disposable soft plastic cover is placed over the probe to prevent the transmission of microorganisms between patients. Depending on the method of taking temperature, the probe is inserted in the mouth, rectum, or axilla and is left in place until a beep is emitted from the thermometer. When the beep sounds, the patient's temperature in degrees Fahrenheit is displayed on the screen. The plastic cover is then removed from the probe and properly disposed of in a biohazard waste container.

Text continued on page 86

3–1

Measuring Body Temperature—Electronic Thermometer

EQUIPMENT/SUPPLIES: Electronic thermometer
Appropriate probe (oral, axillary, or rectal)
Plastic probe cover
Biohazard waste container

1. **Procedural Step.** Wash the hands, and assemble the equipment.

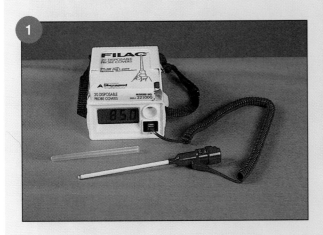

2. **Procedural Step.** Attach the proper probe to the thermometer unit. Next, insert the probe into the face of the thermometer. The probe collars are color coded as follows.

   Blue-collared probe: To take oral and axillary temperature.
   Red-collared probe: To take rectal temperature.
   Principle. The probe collars are color coded for ease in identifying them.

3. **Procedural Step.** Greet and identify the patient. Introduce yourself and explain the procedure. If the patient has recently ingested hot or cold food or beverages, or has been smoking, the medical assistant must wait 15 to 30 minutes before taking the temperature.
   Principle. Ingestion of hot or cold food or beverages and smoking could result in an inaccurate reading.

4. **Procedural Step.** Remove the thermometer unit from its rechargeable base. Grasp the probe by the collar, and remove it from the face of the

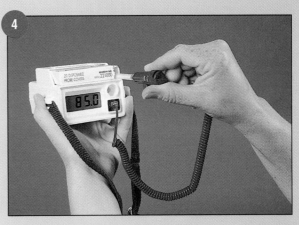

thermometer. Firmly attach a disposable plastic probe cover to the probe.
Principle. Removing the probe from the thermometer automatically turns on the thermometer. The probe cover prevents the transfer of microorganisms from one patient to another.

5. **Procedural Step.** Take the patient's temperature by inserting the probe as follows:

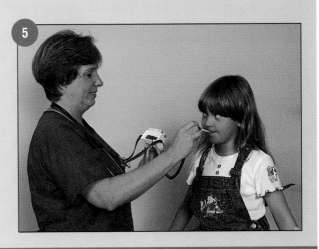

Continued

PROCEDURE 3–1

3

Oral—Place the probe under the tongue in the pocket located on either side of the frenulum linguae.

Axillary—Place the probe in the center of the axilla, and instruct the patient to hold the arm tightly against the chest.

Rectal—Lubricate the end of the probe up to a level of 1 inch. Apply gloves. Spread the buttocks and place the probe approximately 1½ inches into the rectum for adults, 1 inch for children, and ½ inch for infants. (Note: Some rectal probes do not require lubrication. Check with the instruction manual for the manufacturer's recommendation.)

6. **Procedural Step.** Hold the probe in place until the audible tone is heard. At that time, the patient's temperature appears as a digital display on the screen. (The temperature indicated on this thermometer is 98.6°F, or 37°C.)

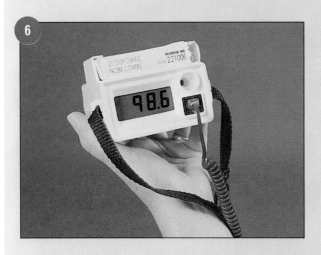

7. **Procedural Step.** Remove the probe from the mouth, axilla, or rectum, and discard the probe cover in in a biohazard waste container by pushing the ejection button. Do not allow your fingers to come in contact with the probe cover.

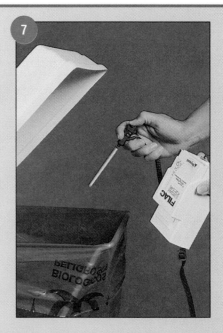

Principle. The probe cover should not be touched, to prevent the transfer of microorganisms from the patient to the medical assistant.

8. **Procedural Step.** Return the probe to its stored position in the thermometer unit.

Principle. Returning the probe to the unit automatically turns off and resets the thermometer.

9. **Procedural Step.** Wash the hands, and chart the results. Include the date and time, the temperature reading, and the site used if other than oral.

Principle. Patient data should be properly recorded to aid the physician in the diagnosis and to provide future reference.

10. **Procedural Step.** Store the thermometer unit in the base, which recharges the unit.

CHARTING EXAMPLE	
Date	
10/15/2002	2:15 p.m. T: 98.6° F. ——— J. Smith, CMA

Tympanic Membrane Thermometer

The tympanic membrane thermometer is used with the aural site. This site provides a closed cavity that is easily accessible. Tympanic membrane thermometers provide instantaneous results, are easy to use, and offer patient comfort, making it easier to measure temperature in children younger than 6 years of age, uncooperative patients, and patients who are unable to have their temperature taken orally.

The tympanic membrane thermometer functions by detecting thermal energy that is naturally radiated from the body. As with the rest of the body, the tympanic membrane and surrounding ear canal give off heat waves known as infrared waves. The tympanic thermometer functions like a camera by taking a "picture" of these infrared waves, which are considered a documented indicator of body temperature (Fig. 3–4). The thermometer then calculates the body temperature from the energy generated by the waves and converts it to an oral or rectal equivalent.

The tympanic membrane thermometer consists of a small hand-held device with a sensor probe; brand names include Thermoscan PRO-1 Instant Thermometer (Thermoscan), Diatek (Welch Allyn), and Core-Check (IVAC). Most are battery operated and rechargeable. To operate the thermometer, the probe is covered with a disposable probe cover and placed in the outer third of the external ear canal. An activation button is depressed momentarily, and the results are displayed in 1 to 2 seconds on a digital screen. The probe cover is then removed and properly disposed of in a biohazard waste container.

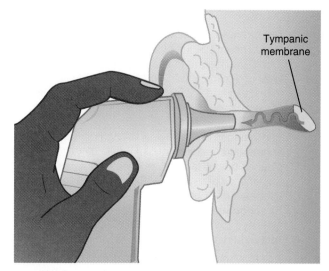

Tympanic membrane

■ **FIGURE 3–4.** Tympanic membrane thermometer. This thermometer functions by detecting thermal energy that is naturally radiated from the body.

Guidelines for Using a Tympanic Membrane Thermometer

The following guidelines help ensure accurate aural temperature measurement with a tympanic membrane thermometer.

1. **Determine if a tympanic thermometer can be used to measure the patient's temperature.** The tympanic thermometer should not be used on a patient with inflammation of the external ear canal (e.g., otitis externa) or when the ear contains a discharge such as blood or pus. The presence of otitis media does not significantly affect the temperature reading, nor does a normal amount of cerumen. However, impacted cerumen can result in a falsely low temperature reading.

2. **Select the proper temperature mode.** Tympanic membrane thermometers can be set to oral or rectal equivalent modes. This means that the thermometer translates the tympanic membrane temperature into a more familiar frame of reference for interpretation. The mode selected depends on the age of the patient. To take the temperature of an adult or child over 3 years of age, the mode should be set to the oral equivalent (ORAL). To take the temperature of a child younger than 3 years of age, the mode should be set to the rectal equivalent (RECTAL). The manufacturer's instructions should be followed carefully to change the temperature mode.

3. **Select the temperature measurement system desired.** The temperature of a tympanic membrane thermometer can be displayed in degrees Fahrenheit or degrees Celsius. Follow the manufacturer's instructions to change from one measurement to the other.

4. **Place the probe properly in the patient's ear.** The most important factor in obtaining an accurate temperature is the proper placement of the probe in the patient's ear as outlined below.

   Straighten the ear canal: The ear canal has an S-shape that obstructs the view of the tympanic membrane. To obtain an accurate temperature measurement, the ear canal must be straightened before inserting the probe. This allows the probe sensor to obtain a clear picture of the tympanic membrane.

   Seal the opening of the ear: The probe must be inserted tightly enough to seal the opening of the ear without causing patient discomfort. If the probe does not seal the ear canal, cooler external air can cause the thermometer to register a lower temperature.

   Correctly position the probe. Position the tip of the probe toward the opposite temple (approximately midway between the opposite ear and eyebrow). This allows the sensor to obtain the best possible picture of the tympanic membrane. If the tip is positioned incorrectly, it may be aimed at the ear canal, which results in a falsely low reading.

5. **Verify the accuracy of the temperature reading, if needed.** If you need to take the patient's temperature again, you can use the other ear. There are slight but insignificant differences between the temperature readings in the right ear and the left ear. Before using the same ear, however, you must wait 2 minutes to allow the aural temperature to stabilize.

Continued

3

6. **Check the probe lens before taking the temperature.** The end of the probe is covered with a lens that is transparent to heat waves. To assure a high level of accuracy, it is very important to keep this lens clean and intact. Before taking temperature, always check to make sure the lens is shiny and clear. Fingerprints, cerumen, and dust reduce the transparency of the lens, resulting in falsely low temperature readings. If the lens is dirty, it must be cleaned before taking the patient's temperature. If the lens is damaged, the thermometer cannot be used and must be repaired.

7. **Respond appropriately to digital messages.** A message to alert the user is displayed in the digital screen under the following circumstances:

An attempt is made to take a temperature without changing the cover after the last temperature.

An attempt is made to take a temperature with no probe cover in place.

The battery is low.

The thermometer is in need of repair.

8. **Care for the tympanic thermometer properly.**

Probe Lens: Dust and other minute particles of environmental debris can build up on the probe lens during normal use. The lens should be cleaned as part of routine maintenance or when it becomes dirty. To clean the lens, gently wipe its surface with an alcohol wipe and immediately wipe it dry with a cotton swab. After cleaning, allow at least 5 minutes for the lens to dry before taking a temperature.

Thermometer Casing: Clean the casing of the thermometer periodically by wiping it dry with a soft cloth slightly dampened with warm water and a mild detergent or germicidal cleaner.

Make sure the cloth is damp but not wet to prevent the cleaning solution from running inside the thermometer, which could damage it.

9. **Store the thermometer properly.** Keep the thermometer away from temperature extremes, which could damage the thermometer. The thermometer should not be exposed to excessive heat (more than 95°F or 35°C) or excessive cold (less than 60°F or 15.6°C).

---

3 PROCEDURE

3–2

Measuring Aural Body Temperature—Tympanic Membrane Thermometer

EQUIPMENT/SUPPLIES: Thermoscan PRO-1 Instant Thermometer
Probe cover
Biohazard waste container

1. **Procedural Step.** Wash the hands, and assemble the equipment.
   Principle. The hands should be clean and free from contamination.
2. **Procedural Step.** Greet and identify the patient. Introduce yourself and explain the procedure.
   Principle. It is important to explain what you will be doing, because body temperature may be higher in a fearful or apprehensive patient.
3. **Procedural Step.** Remove the thermometer from its base. Check to make sure the probe lens is clean and intact. Check the display screen to make sure the thermometer is set on the proper mode for the patient's age. To take the temperature of an adult or a child older than 3 years of age, the thermometer should be set on ORAL mode. To take the temperature of children younger than 3 years of age, the thermometer should be set to RECTAL mode. If the mode desired is not displayed, change the setting according to the manufacturer's instructions.
   Principle. A dirty or damaged probe lens could result in a falsely low temperature reading. Tympanic membrane thermometers are set on different modes depending on the age of the patient.
4. **Procedural Step.** Place a cover on the probe by pressing the probe tip straight down into the cover box. You will be able to see and feel the cover snap securely into place on the probe. This procedure automatically turns the thermometer on.

PROCEDURE 3-2

Principle. The probe cover protects the lens and provides infection control. The cover must be seated securely on the probe to activate the thermometer.

5. **Procedural Step.** Pull the probe straight up from the cover box. When the thermometer is ready, it will display the word "READY" on the digital screen. Do not take a temperature until the word READY is displayed.

6. **Procedural Step.** Hold the thermometer in your dominant hand If you are right handed, you should take the temperature in the patient's right ear. If you are left handed, take the temperature in the patient's left ear.

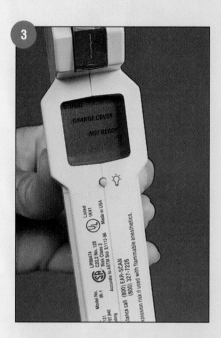

Principle. Taking the temperature with the dominant hand assists in the proper placement of the probe in the patient's ear.

7. **Procedural Step.** Straighten the patient's external ear canal with your nondominant hand as follows:
Adults and children older than 3 years of age: Gently pull the ear pinna upward and backward.
Children younger than 3 years of age: Gently pull the ear pinna downward and backward.
Principle. Straightening the ear canal allows the probe sensor to obtain a clear picture of the tympanic membrane resulting in an accurate temperature measurement.

8. **Procedural Step.** Insert the probe into the patient's ear canal tightly enough to seal the opening but without causing patient discomfort. Point the tip of the probe toward the opposite temple (approximately midway between the opposite ear and eyebrow).
Principle. Sealing the ear canal prevents cooler external air from entering the ear, which could re-

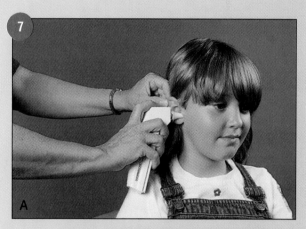

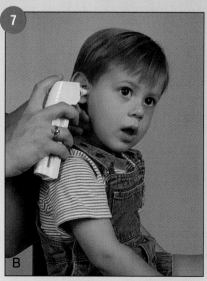

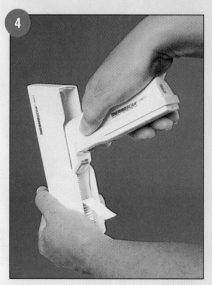

Continued

sult in a falsely low reading. Correct positioning of the probe optimizes the sensor's view of the tympanic membrane, leading to an accurate temperature reading.

9. **Procedural Step.** Ask the patient to remain still. Hold the thermometer steady and depress the activation button. Hold the button down for 1 full second and then release it.
   Principle. The thermometer cannot take a temperature unless the activation button is depressed for one full second. When the button is depressed, the infrared sensor in the probe scans the thermal energy radiated by the tympanic membrane.

10. **Procedural Step.** Turn the digital display of the thermometer toward you, and read the temperature. If the temperature appears to be too low, repeat the procedure to ensure that you have used the proper technique.
    Principle. The temperature remains on the display screen until another cover is inserted on the probe. Improper technique can result in a falsely low temperature reading.

11. **Procedural Step.** Dispose of the probe cover by ejecting it into a biohazard waste container.

12. **Procedural Step.** Replace the thermometer in its base.
    Principle. The thermometer should be stored in its base to protect the probe lens from damage and dirt.

13. **Procedural Step.** Wash the hands.

14. **Procedural Step.** Chart the results. Include the date and time, the aural temperature reading, and which ear was used to take the temperature (AD: right ear; AS: left ear).

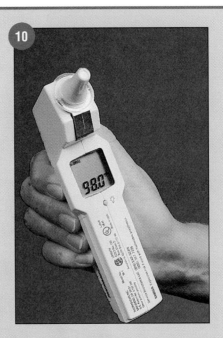

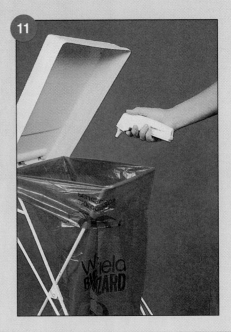

CHARTING EXAMPLE

Date	
10/15/2002	3:00 p.m. T: 98° F. (AD) — J. Smith, CMA

Mercury Glass Thermometer

The mercury glass thermometer is used in the medical office and by patients at home for taking body temperature (Fig. 3–5). It consists of two parts—the **bulb** and the **stem.** Mercury is contained in the bulb of the thermometer. Mercury is a metal that expands when exposed to heat, and it rises in a sealed column located in the center of the thermometer.

The bulb has a constriction that does not allow the mercury to fall back once it has risen in the sealed column. It is necessary to shake the thermometer with a snapping wrist motion to make the mercury return to the bulb. The mercury should be at a level of 96°F

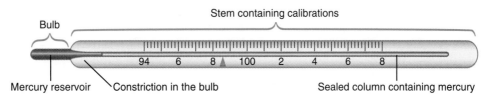

FIGURE 3–5. The parts of a mercury glass thermometer.

(36°C) or below, before a patient's temperature is taken; otherwise, the reading may be inaccurate.

The stem of the thermometer contains calibrations, which are divided into two tenths of a degree (0.2°) on the Fahrenheit thermometer and into one tenth of a degree (0.1°) on the Celsius thermometer. The temperature range on the Fahrenheit thermometer is 94 to 108°, and on the Celsius thermometer it is 34 to 42° (Fig. 3–6). A body temperature above or below these ranges is rare.

The bulb of an oral thermometer is long and slender to provide a greater surface area for contact with the vascular tissues of the mouth or axilla. The bulb of the rectal thermometer is short and blunt for easier insertion into the rectum (Fig. 3–6). An oral thermometer should not be used to take a rectal temperature, because the long, slender bulb may puncture the rectal mucosa. The medical assistant should store oral and rectal thermometers in separate containers. Thermometers are usually color coded at the stem end to facilitate identifying them; the oral thermometer has a blue tip, and the rectal thermometer has a red tip.

If the thermometer breaks, the medical assistant should take care to make sure that the pieces are carefully disposed of, to avoid injury. Mercury is best picked up by brushing the beads onto a piece of paper, without allowing the mercury to touch the skin, and then properly disposing of it in a biohazard container.

TEMPERATURE SHEATHS. A temperature sheath is a clear, plastic disposable cover that fits over the bulb and stem of a thermometer (Fig. 3–7). Temperature sheaths can be used for the measurement of oral, rectal, and axillary temperature. The rectal sheaths are prelubricated for easier insertion. The thermometer must be shaken down before the sheath is applied so that the calibrations can be clearly read. The sheath is applied according to the manufacturer's instructions, which are usually listed on the label (Fig. 3–7A). The medical assistant should make sure that the sheath completely encases the thermometer and is not torn (Fig. 3–7B); if tearing occurs, a new sheath should be applied. The patient's temperature is measured according to the oral, rectal, or axillary body temperature procedures presented on the following pages. Once the temperature has been measured, the sheath is removed. As it is pulled off the stem, the sheath inverts, thereby enclosing secretions and bacteria and reducing the transmission of microorganisms (Fig. 3–7C). To ensure an accurate temperature reading, the thermometer must be read after removing the plastic sheath, which should then be properly discarded in a biohazard waste container.

CLEANING GLASS THERMOMETERS   Hot water cannot be used to clean a glass thermometer, because it causes the mercury to expand too far in the sealed column, and the thermometer could break.

The following procedure is used to clean glass thermometers:

1. Wash the thermometer in cool sudsy water to remove surface dirt. Either soap or detergent can be used.
2. Rinse the thermometer under cold running water.

FIGURE 3–6. Mercury glass thermometers illustrating the difference in the shape of the bulb between rectal and oral thermometers.

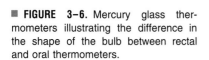

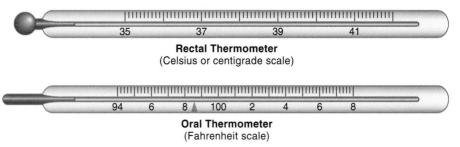

Rectal Thermometer
(Celsius or centigrade scale)

Oral Thermometer
(Fahrenheit scale)

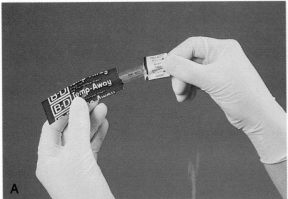
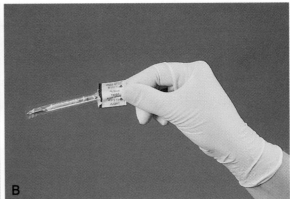

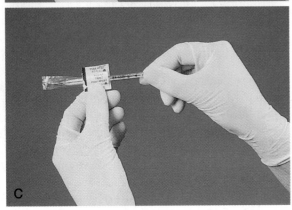

■ **FIGURE 3-7.** Application and removal of a temperature sheath. *A,* The sheath is applied according to the manufacturer's instructions. *B,* The sheath should completely encase the thermometer. *C,* As the sheath is pulled off the stem, it inverts, which encloses secretions and bacteria.

3. Dry the thermometer thoroughly. If the thermometer is wet when immersed in the chemical solution, the water decreases the strength of the chemical by diluting it.
4. Immerse the thermometer in a chemical disinfectant such as benzalkonium chloride (Zephiran

Chloride) or alcohol. A period of at least 20 minutes is usually recommended for this step.
5. Rinse the thermometer again under cold running water to remove all traces of disinfectant.
6. Place the thermometer in its proper storage container.

Text continued on page 97

PROCEDURE

3-3

Measuring Body Temperature—Oral/Mercury Glass Thermometer

EQUIPMENT/SUPPLIES: **Oral thermometer**
Oral temperature sheath
Disposable gloves
Biohazard waste container

1. **Procedural Step.** Wash the hands and assemble the equipment.
   Principle. The hands should be clean and free

from contamination so that pathogens will not be transferred to the patient.
2. **Procedural Step.** Greet and identify the patient. In-

troduce yourself and explain the procedure. If the patient has recently ingested hot or cold food or beverages or has been smoking, the medical assistant must wait 15 to 30 minutes before taking the temperature.

Principle. Ingestion of hot or cold food or beverages and smoking could result in an inaccurate reading.

3. **Procedural Step.** Check the level of the mercury in the thermometer. Hold the thermometer horizontally at eye level and rotate it slowly, to obtain the best reading.

4. **Procedural Step.** If the level of mercury is above 96°F (36°C), it needs to be shaken down, in order to obtain an accurate temperature reading. Hold the thermometer firmly between the thumb and forefinger. Shake the thermometer downward with a snapping wrist movement. Repeat this motion until the mercury is below 96°F. Do not allow the thermometer to hit a hard object during this process to prevent breaking the thermometer.

Principle. The constriction in the bulb prevents the mercury from falling on its own.

5. **Procedural Step.** Apply gloves. Apply the temperature sheath to the thermometer according to the manufacturer's instructions.

Principle. The temperature sheath promotes infection control by reducing the transmission of microorganisms.

6. **Procedural Step.** Place the bulb of the thermometer in the patient's mouth in the pocket located on either side of the frenulum linguae.

Principle. The long slender bulb provides for good contact with the rich blood supply located in the tissue under the tongue.

7. **Procedural Step.** Instruct the patient to keep the mouth closed and to hold the thermometer in place with the lips.

Principle. If the mouth is not closed tightly cooler air from the outside affects the temperature reading. The thermometer must be held in place with the lips—not the teeth—to prevent the patient from biting down on it and breaking it.

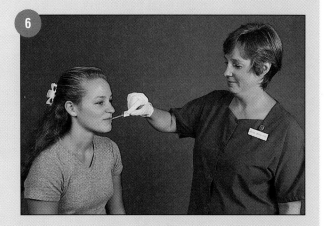

8. **Procedural Step.** Leave the thermometer in place for 2 to 3 minutes. The medical assistant should remain in the room to reassure the patient and to remove the thermometer as soon as the body temperature has registered. The pulse and respiration may be taken during this time.

Principle. The thermometer must remain in the mouth long enough for an accurate temperature reading to register.

9. **Procedural Step.** Remove the thermometer from the patient's mouth. Remove the temperature sheath, and dispose of it in a biohazard waste container.

10. **Procedural Step.** Read the thermometer. To obtain the best reading, hold the thermometer horizontally and rotate it slowly at eye level until the column of silver mercury is clearly visible. The temperature is read at the point at which the mercury level ends. Each long line represents 1° and each short line represents 0.2° on a Fahrenheit thermometer. Read to the nearest 0.2° (The temperature indicated on this thermometer is 101.4°F.)

11. **Procedural Step.** Place the used thermometer in the designated container for cleansing and disinfecting. Oral and rectal thermometers should be stored in separate containers.

12. **Procedural Step.** Remove gloves, and wash the hands.

3

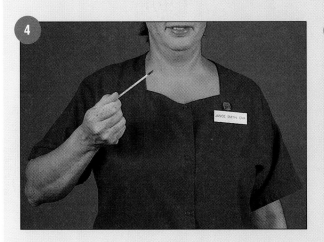

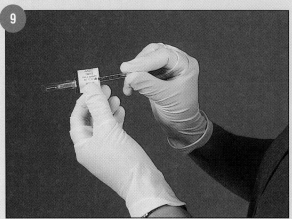

Continued

PROCEDURE 3-3

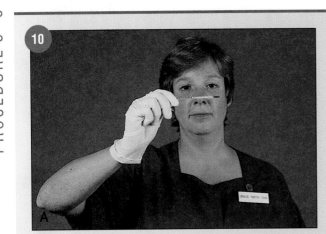

10

A

Principle. Microorganisms from the patient may have been transferred to the medical assistant's hands.

13. **Procedural Step.** Chart the results. Include the date and time, and the oral temperature reading.
Principle. Patient data should be properly recorded to aid the physician in the diagnosis and to provide future reference.

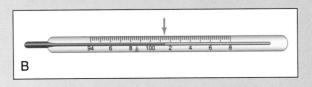

CHARTING EXAMPLE

Date	
10/15/2002	10:30 a.m. T: 101.4° F. ——— J. Smith, CMA

B

3

PROCEDURE

3-4

Measuring Body Temperature—Rectal/Mercury Glass Thermometer

EQUIPMENT/SUPPLIES: Rectal thermometer   Soft tissues
Rectal temperature sheath   Biohazard waste container
Disposable gloves

1. **Procedural Step.** Wash the hands, and assemble the equipment.
Principle. The hands should be clean and free from contamination.

2. **Procedural Step.** Greet and identify the patient. Introduce yourself and explain the procedure.
Principle. It is important to explain what you will be doing, because body temperature may be higher in a fearful or apprehensive patient.

3. **Procedural Step.** Position the patient. *Adults and children:* Position the patient in the Sims position, and drape the patient to expose only the anal

area. *Infants:* Position the infant on his or her abdomen.
Principle. Correct positioning allows for clear viewing of the anal opening and provides for proper insertion of the thermometer. Draping reduces patient embarrassment and provides warmth.

4. **Procedural Step.** Check the level of the mercury in the thermometer. Hold the thermometer horizontally at eye level and rotate it slowly, to obtain the best reading.

5. **Procedural Step.** If the level of mercury is above 96°F (36°C), it will need to be shaken down, in

PROCEDURE 3–4

order to obtain an accurate temperature reading. Hold the thermometer firmly between the thumb and forefinger. Shake the thermometer downward with a snapping wrist movement.

Principle. The constriction in the bulb prevents the mercury from falling on its own.

6. **Procedural Step.** Apply gloves. Apply the prelubricated rectal temperature sheath to the thermometer according to the manufacturer's instructions.

Principle. Gloves protect the medical assistant from microorganisms in the anal area and feces. A lubricated thermometer can be inserted more easily and does not irritate the delicate rectal mucosa. The temperature sheath promotes infection control by reducing the transmission of microorganisms.

7. **Procedural Step.** Spread the buttocks to expose the anal opening and carefully insert the lubricated bulb of the thermometer approximately 1½ inches into the rectum for adults, 1 inch for children, and ½ inch for infants. Do not force insertion of the thermometer. Allow the buttocks to fall back in place. Instruct the patient to lie still. The thermometer should be held in place until the temperature registers.

Principle. The thermometer must be inserted correctly to prevent injury to the tissue of the anal opening. The thermometer should be held in place to prevent damage to the rectal mucosa.

8. **Procedural Step.** Leave the thermometer in place for 2 to 3 minutes. Having the patient breathe through the mouth will help relax the individual.

Principle. The thermometer must remain in the rectum long enough for an accurate temperature reading to register.

9. **Procedural Step.** Carefully remove the thermometer

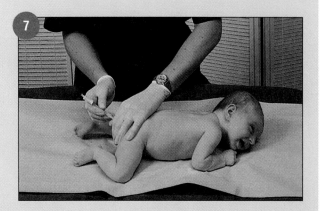

in the same manner as that in which it was inserted. Remove the temperature sheath, and dispose of it in a biohazard waste container.

Principle. The lubricant and any fecal matter must be wiped away to provide for easier reading of the thermometer.

10. **Procedural Step.** Read the thermometer at eye level.

11. **Procedural Step.** Place the used thermometer in the designated container for cleaning and disinfecting. Oral and rectal thermometers should be stored in separate containers.

12. **Procedural Step.** Wipe the anal area with tissues to remove excess lubricant. Dispose of the tissues in a biohazard waste container.

Principle. Wiping the anal area provides patient comfort. Contaminated items must be disposed of properly to prevent the transmission of infection.

13. **Procedural Step.** Remove gloves, and wash the hands.

Principle. Gloves and handwashing reduce the transmission of infection.

14. **Procedural Step.** Chart the results. Include the date and time, and the rectal temperature. The symbol Ⓡ must be charted next to the temperature reading to tell the physician that a rectal reading was taken.

Principle. Patient data should be recorded properly to aid the physician in the diagnosis and to provide for future reference.

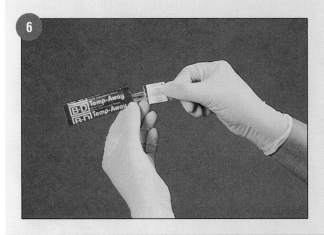

3

CHARTING EXAMPLE	
Date	
10/15/2002	11:15 a.m. T: 99.8° F Ⓡ ——J. Smith, CMA

PROCEDURE

3–5

Measuring Body Temperature—Axillary/Mercury Glass Thermometer

Note: Many of the principles for taking temperature have already been stated and are not included in this procedure.

EQUIPMENT/SUPPLIES: **Axillary thermometer**
Oral temperature sheath
Waste container

1. **Procedural Step.** Wash the hands and assemble the equipment.
2. **Procedural Step.** Greet and identify the patient. Introduce yourself and explain the procedure.
3. **Procedural Step.** Remove clothing from the patient's shoulder and arm. Make sure the axilla is dry. If it is wet, pat it dry with a clean cloth.
   Principle. Clothing removal provides optimal exposure of the axilla for proper placement of the thermometer. Rubbing the axilla causes an increase in the temperature in that area due to friction, resulting in an inaccurate temperature reading.
4. **Procedural Step.** Check the level of the mercury in the thermometer.
5. **Procedural Step.** Shake the mercury to a level of 96°F (36°C) or below, if necessary.
6. **Procedural Step.** Apply the temperature sheath to the thermometer according to the manufacturer's instructions. Place the bulb of the thermometer in

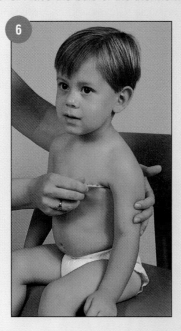

the center of the axilla, and instruct the patient to hold the arm close to the body, with the forearm across the chest. The thermometer and arm should be held in place for small children and any other patients who cannot maintain the position themselves.
   Principle. Interference from outside air currents is reduced when the arm is held in the proper position; in addition, the thermometer is prevented from falling and breaking.
7. **Procedural Step.** Leave the thermometer in place for 5 to 10 minutes.
   Principle. The thermometer must remain in the axilla long enough for an accurate temperature reading to register. The axilla is not as closed a space as the mouth or rectum and therefore is more subject to the influence of air currents.
8. **Procedural Step.** Remove the thermometer from the patient's axilla. Remove the temperature sheath, and dispose of it in a waste container.
9. **Procedural Step.** Read the thermometer at eye level.
10. **Procedural Step.** Place the used thermometer in the designated container for cleansing and disinfecting.
11. **Procedural Step.** Wash the hands.
12. **Procedural Step.** Chart the results. Include the date and time, and the axillary temperature reading. The symbol Ⓐ must be charted next to the temperature reading to tell the physician that an axillary reading was taken.

CHARTING EXAMPLE

Date	
10/15/2002	9:30 a.m.　T: 101.6° F Ⓐ —J. Smith, CMA

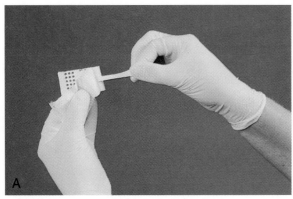

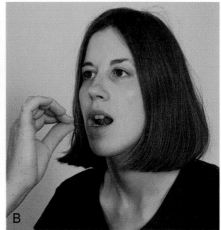

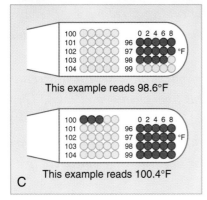

This example reads 98.6°F

This example reads 100.4°F

■ FIGURE 3–8. Disposable chemical single-use thermometers. *A,* The thermometer is removed from the wrapper by pulling on the handle. *B,* The thermometer is inserted under the tongue and left in place for 60 seconds. *C,* The thermometer is read by noting the highest reading among the dots that have changed color.

Chemical Thermometers

Chemical thermometers are used most often by patients at home to measure body temperature and include disposable chemical single-use thermometers and temperature-sensitive strips. They are less accurate than other types of thermometers, but they assist in providing a general assessment of body temperature. Because of their chemical make-up, they should be stored in a cool area, preferably less than 86°F (30°C) and should not be exposed to direct sunlight, because heat may cause the thermometer to register temperature. Each type of chemical thermometer is described here.

DISPOSABLE CHEMICAL SINGLE-USE THERMOMETERS. This type of thermometer has small chemical dots at one end that respond to body heat by changing color (Fig. 3–8*A* and *B*). Each thermometer comes in its own individual wrapper. The protective wrapper must be peeled back to expose the handle of the thermometer. The thermometer is removed from the wrapper by pulling on the handle, being careful not to touch the dotted area. The thermometer is then inserted under the tongue and left in place for the duration of time recommended by the manufacturer (generally 60 seconds). After removal of the thermometer, the dots are

observed for a change in color. The thermometer is read by noting the highest reading among the dots that have changed color. The thermometer is then discarded after use.

3

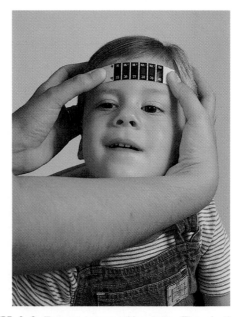

■ FIGURE 3–9. Temperature-sensitive tape. The plastic strip is pressed onto the forehead and held in place until the color stops changing (generally 15 seconds). The results are read by observing the color change and noting the corresponding temperature indicated on the strip.

TEMPERATURE-SENSITIVE STRIPS. A temperature-sensitive strip consists of a reusable plastic strip containing heat-sensitive liquid crystals designed to measure body temperature. Brand names include Fever Scan and Clini-temp. The plastic strip is pressed onto the forehead and held in place until the colors stop changing, generally 15 seconds. The results are read by observing the color change and noting the corresponding temperature indicated on the strip. (Fig. 3–9).

PULSE

MECHANISM OF THE PULSE

When the left ventricle of the heart contracts, blood is forced from the heart into the aorta. The aorta is already filled with blood and must expand to accept the blood being pushed out of the left ventricle. The elastic tissue in the wall of the aorta allows it to expand to accommodate the new supply of blood. When the heart relaxes, the aorta recoils to its original size. The expansion and recoiling of the aorta send a wave of vibration from the aorta through the walls of the arterial system. This vibration, known as the *pulse*, can be felt as a light tap by an examiner. The pulse rate is measured by counting the number of beats per minute. The contraction and relaxation of the heart, or heart
3 rate, can thus be determined by taking the pulse rate.

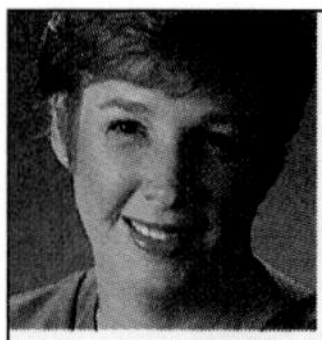

MEMORIES *from* EXTERNSHIP

JANICE SMITH: *Times have changed since I did my externship. I graduated from medical assistant school in 1976. For one of my externships, I was assigned to a small town doctor's office. The entire staff was made up of one doctor and two registered nurses. The nurses shared both the clinical and administrative duties in the office.*

The equipment used at that time was very different from what is used today. There were very few disposable products, and almost everything was reused. Even needles and syringes used for injections were autoclaved and used over again.

At that time no one had ever heard of ear and chemical thermometers. Glass thermometers were all that were available. After being washed, they were stored in alcohol to be used again and again.

Factors Affecting Pulse Rate

Pulse rate can vary, depending on a number of factors. The medical assistant should take each of the following into consideration when measuring pulse:

Age	The pulse varies inversely with age. As the age increases, the pulse rate gradually decreases. Refer to Table 3–4 for the pulse rates of the various age groups.
Gender	Women tend to have a slightly faster pulse rate than men.
Exercise	Physical activity, such as jogging or swimming, increases the pulse rate.
Emotional states	Strong emotional states, such as anxiety, fear, excitement, or anger, increase the pulse rate.

TABLE 3–4 **Pulse Rates of Various Age Groups**

Age Group	Pulse Range (beats/minute)	Average Pulse (beats/minute)
Newborn to 1 month	80–180	130
1 month to 12 months	80–140	120
12 months to 2 years	80–130	110
2 years to 6 years	75–120	100
6 years to 12 years	75–110	95
Adolescence to adult	60–100	80

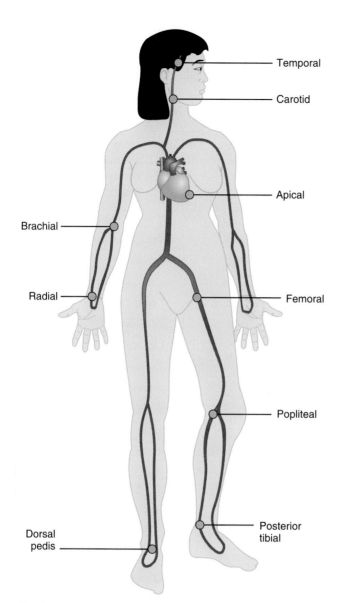

■ **FIGURE 3–10.** Pulse sites.

Radial	The most common site for measuring the pulse is the radial artery, which is located on the inner aspect of the wrist just below the thumb. The radial pulse is easily accessible, and the pulse rate can be measured with no discomfort to the patient.
Apical	The apical pulse has a stronger beat and is more easily heard than the other pulse sites. If the medical assistant is having difficulty feeling the pulse or if the pulse is irregular or abnormally slow or rapid, the apical pulse should be taken. This pulse site is often used to measure pulse in infants and in children up to 3 years of age because the other sites are difficult to palpate accurately in these age groups. The apical pulse is measured using a stethoscope. The chestpiece of the stethoscope is placed lightly over the apex of the heart, which is located in the fifth intercostal space at the junction of the left midclavicular line (Fig. 3–11).
Brachial	The brachial pulse is located in the antecubital space and is used when taking blood pressure. This site is also used to measure pulse in infants during cardiac arrest.
Temporal	The temporal pulse is located in front of the ear and just above eye level. This site is used to measure pulse

3

| Metabolism | Increased body metabolism, such as occurs during a fever or pregnancy, increases the pulse rate. |
| Medications | Medications may alter the pulse rate. For example, digitalis decreases the pulse rate and epinephrine increases it. |

Pulse Sites

The pulse is felt most strongly when a superficial artery is held against a firm tissue, such as bone. The locations of the sites used for measuring the pulse are shown in Figure 3–10 and described later.

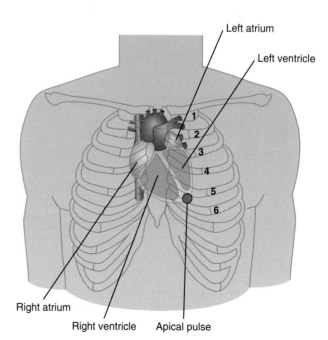

■ **FIGURE 3–11.** Location of the apical pulse. The apical pulse is found over the apex of the heart, which is located in the fifth intercostal space at the junction of the left midclavicular line.

Carotid   when the radial pulse is not accessible. The carotid pulse is located on the anterior side of the neck, slightly to one side of the midline, and is the best site to use to find a pulse quickly. This site is used to measure pulse in infants and in adults during cardiac arrest and to assess circulation to the brain. The carotid site is also commonly used by individuals to monitor pulse during exercise.

Femoral   The femoral pulse is located in the middle of the groin. This site is used to measure pulse in infants and children and in adults during cardiac arrest, as well as to assess circulation to a lower extremity.

Popliteal   The popliteal pulse is located at the back of the knee and is most easily detected when the knee is slightly flexed. This site is used to measure blood pressure when the brachial pulse is not accessible and to assess circulation to a lower extremity.

Dorsalis pedis   The dorsalis pedis pulse is located on the upper surface of the foot, between the first and second metatarsal bones. This site is used to assess circulation to the foot.

ASSESSMENT OF PULSE

The purpose of measuring pulse is to establish the patient's baseline recording and to assess the pulse rate following special procedures, medications, or disease processes that affect heart functioning. Pulse is measured using palpation at all of the pulse sites except the apical site. A pulse is palpated by applying moderate pressure with the sensitive pads located on the tips of the three middle fingers. Excessive pressure should not be applied when measuring pulse because it could obliterate, or close off, the pulse. On the other hand, it may not be possible to detect the pulse if too little pressure is applied. An accurate assessment of pulse includes a determination of the pulse rate, the pulse rhythm, and the pulse volume.

Pulse Rate

The pulse rate is the number of heart pulsations that occur in a minute; therefore, pulse rate is measured in beats per minute. Normal pulse rates vary widely in the various age groups, as shown in Table 3–4. For the healthy adult, the normal resting pulse rate ranges from 60 to 100 beats per minute, with the average falling between 70 and 80 beats per minute.

An abnormally fast heart rate of more than 100 beats per minute is known as **tachycardia.** Tachycardia may indicate disease states such as hemorrhaging or

3

PROCEDURE

3-6

Measuring Radial Pulse

EQUIPMENT/SUPPLIES: **Watch (with a second hand)**

1. **Procedural Step.** Wash the hands. Greet and identify the patient. Introduce yourself and explain the procedure.

   Observe the patient for any signs that may result in an increase or decrease in the pulse rate.
   Principle. Pulse rate can vary, according to the factors listed on page 98.

2. **Procedural Step.** Position the patient in a sitting position. The patient's arm should be placed alongside the body in a comfortable position with the palm of the hand facing downward. The forearm should be slightly flexed, in order to relax the muscles and tendons over the pulse site.
   Principle. Relaxed muscles and tendons over the pulse site make it easier to palpate the pulse.

3. **Procedural Step.** Place the three middle fingertips over the radial pulse site. The medical assistant should not take the pulse with the thumb.
   Principle. The thumb has a pulse of its own, and using the thumb results in a measurement of the medical assistant's pulse and not the patient's pulse.

4. **Procedural Step.** Apply moderate, gentle pressure directly over the site until the pulse can be felt.
   Principle. A normal pulse can be felt with moderate pressure. Too much pressure applied to the radial artery closes it off, and no pulse is felt.

5. **Procedural Step.** Count the pulse for 30 seconds, and multiply by 2. The rhythm and volume of the pulse should also be noted. If any abnormalities occur in the rhythm or volume, count the pulse for 1 full minute.
   Principle. A longer time period ensures an accurate assessment of abnormalities.

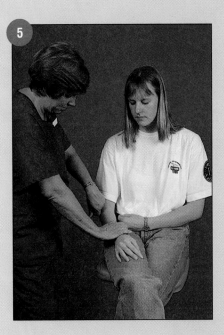

6. **Procedural Step.** Chart the results. Include the date and time, and the pulse rate, rhythm, and volume.

CHARTING EXAMPLE

Date	
10/15/2002	2:30 p.m. P: 78. Reg and strong. ——————————————— J. Smith, CMA

3

PROCEDURE

3–7

Measuring Apical Pulse

EQUIPMENT/SUPPLIES: Watch (with a second hand)
Stethoscope
Antiseptic wipe

3

1. **Procedural Step.** Wash the hands. Greet and identify the patient. Introduce yourself and explain the procedure.
2. **Procedural Step.** Assemble the equipment. Clean the earpieces of the stethoscope with an antiseptic wipe.
   Principle. Cleaning the earpieces helps prevent the transmission of the microorganisms.
3. **Procedural Step.** Position the patient in a lying (supine) or sitting position.
   Principle. A supine or sitting position allows for access to the apex of the heart.
4. **Procedural Step.** Warm the chestpiece of the stethoscope with your hand. Insert the earpieces of the stethoscope into your ears, with the earpieces directed slightly forward, and place the chestpiece over the apex of the heart. The apex of the heart is located in the fifth intercostal space at the junction of the left midclavicular line.
   Principle. Warming the chestpiece helps reduce the discomfort of having a cold object placed on the chest. In addition, a cold chestpiece could startle the patient, resulting in an increase in the pulse rate. The earpieces should be directed forward, permitting them to follow the direction of the ear canal, which facilitates hearing.
5. **Procedural Step.** Listen for the heart beat and count the number of beats for 30 seconds (and multiply by 2) if the rhythm and volume are normal or if the apical pulse is being taken on an infant or child. If any abnormalities occur in the rhythm or volume, count the pulse for 1 full minute. The medical assistant will hear a "lubb-dupp" sound through the stethoscope. This sound occurs as a result of the closing of the valves of the heart. Each "lubb-dupp" is counted as one beat.

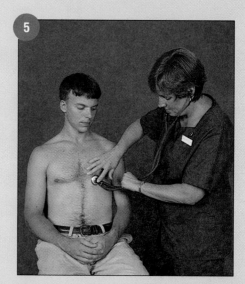

6. **Procedural Step.** Chart the results. Include the date and time, and the apical pulse rate, rhythm, and volume.
   Principle. Good recording techniques provide for a more complete patient record.
7. **Procedural Step.** Clean the earpieces of the stethoscope with an alcohol wipe.

CHARTING EXAMPLE

Date	
10/15/2002	10:15 a.m. AP: 78. Reg and strong. ———— ———————————————— J. Smith, CMA

PATIENT/TEACHING

AEROBIC EXERCISE PROGRAM
■ Answer questions patients have about aerobic exercise.

What Is Aerobic Exercise?
Aerobic exercise raises, sustains, and lowers your pulse through a steady, nonstop activity such as walking, jogging, cycling, or swimming.

What Are the Benefits of an Aerobic Exercise Program?
The benefits of an aerobic exercise program include strengthening of the heart, a slower resting pulse rate, reduction of stress, and lowering of body fat. The key to a safe and effective aerobic exercise program is your target heart rate. (THR).

What Is Target Heart Rate?
Your THR is a safe and effective exercise pulse that indicates you are exercising at the right level for your age and current level of fitness, and for what you are trying to accomplish with exercise. Exercising at a level below your THR does little to promote fitness, whereas exercising at a level above your THR may not be safe.

How Do I Determine My Target Heart Rate?
The following formula is used to determine your THR:

1. Take 220 and subtract your age to determine your maximum heart rate—the fastest your heart can beat safely for your age.

Example: 220 − 30 years old = 190
(maximum heart rate)

2. Choose your current level of fitness and specific goals for exercising from *one* of the following:
   a. Beginning exerciser and to reduce the risk of chronic illness: 50 to 60 percent
   b. Intermediate exerciser and to burn calories and lose weight: 60 to 70 percent
   c. Competitive athlete and to improve aerobic conditioning: 75 to 85 percent
3. To determine your THR, multiply your maximum heart rate by the percentage chosen above.

Example: 190 × 0.70 = 130 (target heart rate)

How Often Should Aerobic Exercise Be Performed?
Aerobic exercise provides the most benefits if it is performed 3 to 5 times per week for a duration of 20 to 30 minutes at your target heart rate. Workouts should be spaced throughout the week to allow your muscles time to rest and recover. Each workout should include a warm-up and cool-down period of at least 5 minutes each. This is to prevent muscle or joint injuries.

3

---

heart disease. However, an individual's pulse rate may normally exceed 100 beats per minute during vigorous exercise or in strong emotional states.

Bradycardia is an abnormally slow heart rate, below 60 beats per minute. Normally, a pulse rate below 60 may occur during sleep; trained athletes often have low pulse rates. If a patient is exhibiting tachycardia or bradycardia, the apical pulse should also be measured.

Rhythm and Volume

In addition to measuring the pulse rate, the medical assistant should also determine the rhythm and volume of the pulse.

The **pulse rhythm** denotes the time interval between heart beats, a normal rhythm having the same time interval between each two beats. Any irregularity in the heart's rhythm is known as an **arrhythmia** (also termed **dysrhythmia**) and is characterized by unequal or irregular intervals between the heart beats. If an arrhythmia is detected, diagnostic tests are often ordered by the physician, such as an electrocardiogram or Holter monitoring.

The **pulse volume** refers to the strength of the heart beat. The amount of blood pumped into the aorta by each contraction of the left ventricle should remain constant, making the pulse feel strong and full. If the blood volume decreases, the pulse feels weak and may be difficult to detect. This type of pulse is usually accompanied by a fast heart rate and is described as a **thready pulse.** An increase in the blood volume results in a pulse that feels extremely strong and full, this is known as a **bounding pulse.**

Any abnormalities occurring in the rhythm or volume of the pulse should be recorded accurately in the patient's chart by the medical assistant. A pulse that has a normal rhythm and volume is recorded as being regular and strong.

PUTTING IT ALL *into* PRACTICE

▶ **JANICE SMITH:** *Taking vital signs and length and weight on small children can be very challenging at times. Some children start to cry as soon as they are put on the scale. Taking a temperature on a squirming, crying infant can be very difficult. This is when the newer and faster acting thermometers come in handy.*

I like to try to calm the patient as much as possible, and for good behavior I give a lot of praise. Candy and stickers are also great rewards for cooperative behavior. Usually, when small children learn that they can trust you, they are not as frightened by the whole experience. It is rewarding when a child learns not to be afraid of being evaluated for routine vital signs.

3 RESPIRATION

MECHANISM OF RESPIRATION

The purpose of respiration is to provide for the exchange of oxygen and carbon dioxide between the atmosphere and the blood. Oxygen is taken into the body to be used for vital body processes, and carbon dioxide is given off as a waste product.

Each respiration is divided into two phases: **inhalation** and **exhalation** (Fig. 3–12). During inhalation or inspiration, the diaphragm descends and the lungs expand, causing air containing oxygen to move from the atmosphere into the lungs. Exhalation, or expiration, involves the removal of carbon dioxide from the body. The diaphragm ascends and the lungs return to their original state, so that air containing carbon dioxide is expelled. One complete respiration is composed of one inhalation and one exhalation.

Respiration may be classified as either **external** or **internal.** External respiration involves the exchange of oxygen and carbon dioxide between the alveoli of the lungs and the blood (Fig. 3–13). The blood, located in small capillaries, comes in contact with the alveoli, picks up oxygen, and carries it to the cells of the body. At this point, the oxygen is given off to the cells and

carbon dioxide is picked up by the blood to be transported as a waste product to the lungs. The exchange of oxygen and carbon dioxide between the body cells and the blood is known as internal respiration.

Control of Respiration

The medulla oblongata, located in the brain, is the control center for involuntary respiration. A build-up of carbon dioxide in the blood sends a message to the medulla, which then triggers respiration to occur automatically.

To a certain extent, respiration is also under voluntary control. An individual can control respiration during activities such as singing, laughing, talking, eating, and crying. Voluntary respiration is ultimately under the control of the medulla oblongata. The breath can be held for only a certain length of time, after which carbon dioxide begins to build up in the body, resulting in a stimulus to the medulla that causes respiration to occur involuntarily. Small children may voluntarily hold their breath during a temper tantrum. A parent who does not understand the principles of respiration may be concerned that the child will cease breathing. The medical assistant should be able to explain that involuntary respiration will eventually occur, and the child will resume breathing.

ASSESSMENT OF RESPIRATION

Because an individual can control his or her respiration, the medical assistant should measure respirations without the patient's knowledge. Patients may change their respiratory rate unintentionally if they are aware that they are being tested. An ideal time to measure respiration is before or after the pulse is taken.

Respiratory Rate

The respiratory rate of a normal healthy adult ranges from 16 to 20 respirations per minute, although wider variations may occur in healthy adults. With most adults, there is a ratio of one respiration for every four pulse beats. For example, if the respiratory rate is 18, the pulse rate would be approximately 72 beats per minute. An abnormal increase in the respiratory rate of more than 20 respirations per minute is referred to as **tachypnea.** An abnormal decrease in the respiratory rate of less than 10 respirations per minute is known as **bradypnea.**

There are certain factors that the medical assistant should take into consideration when measuring the respiratory rate. These include age, physical activity, strong emotions, illness, and drugs. As age increases,

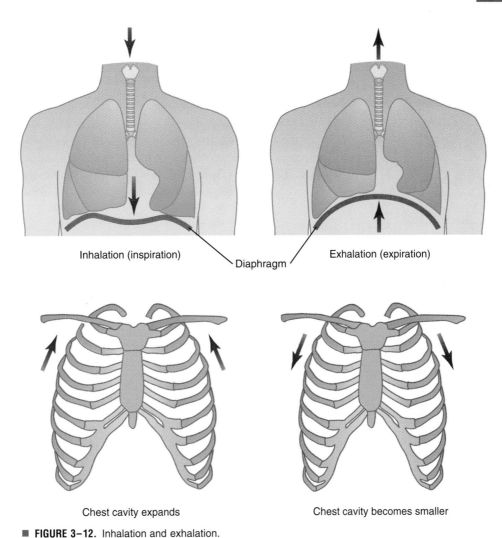

Inhalation (inspiration) Diaphragm Exhalation (expiration)

Chest cavity expands Chest cavity becomes smaller

■ **FIGURE 3–12.** Inhalation and exhalation.

the respiratory rate decreases. Therefore, we would expect the respiratory rate of a child to be faster than that of an adult. Refer to Table 3–5 for a chart of the respiratory rates for the various age groups. Physical activity and strong emotional states increase the respiratory rate. Also, a patient with a fever has an increased respiratory rate: one of the ways heat is lost from the body is through the lungs; therefore, a fever causes an increased respiratory rate as the body tries to rid itself of the excess heat.

Certain medications may increase the respiratory rate, whereas others may decrease it. The medical assistant who is unsure of what effect a particular drug may have should consult a drug reference such as the *Physician's Desk Reference* (PDR).

Rhythm and Depth of Respiration

Both the **rhythm** and **depth** should be noted when measuring respiration. Normally, the rhythm should be even and regular, and the pauses between inhalation and exhalation should be equal.

The depth of respiration indicates the amount of air that is inhaled or exhaled during the process of breathing. Respiratory depth is generally described as normal, deep, or shallow and is determined by observing the amount of movement of the chest. For normal respirations, the depth of each respiration in a resting state is approximately the same. Deep respirations are those in which a large volume of air is inhaled and exhaled, whereas shallow respirations involve the exchange of a small volume of air.

Some illnesses result in an abnormal increase both in the rate and depth of the respirations. This condition is known as **hyperpnea** and occurs normally with exercise. A patient with hyperpnea exhibits a very rapid and panting type of respiration. *Hyperventilation* is an abnormally fast and deep type of breathing that is usually associated with acute anxiety or emotional tension. In contrast, a patient's respiration may show an abnor-

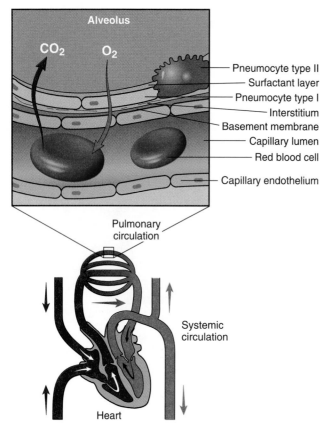

Alveolus

CO_2 O_2

— Pneumocyte type II
— Surfactant layer
— Pneumocyte type I
— Interstitium
— Basement membrane
— Capillary lumen
— Red blood cell

Capillary endothelium

Pulmonary
circulation

Systemic
circulation

Heart

■ **FIGURE 3–13.** Exchange of oxygen and carbon dioxide between the alveoli of the lungs and the blood.

3

mal decrease in the rate and depth; this condition is termed **hypopnea.** The depth is approximately one half that of normal respiration. Normal respiration is referred to as **eupnea.** The rate is approximately 16 to 20 respirations per minute, the rhythm is even and regular, and the depth is normal.

Color of the Patient

The patient's color should also be observed while the respiration is being measured. A lack of oxygen (hypoxia) results in a condition known as **cyanosis,** which causes a bluish discoloration of the skin and mucous membranes. Cyanosis is first observed in the nailbeds and lips, because these are areas in which the blood vessels lie close to the surface of the skin.

Apnea refers to a temporary absence of respiration. Apnea is a serious condition if breathing ceases for more than 4 to 6 minutes, because this problem could result in brain damage and death.

Respiratory Abnormalities

A patient who is having labored or difficult breathing has a condition known as **dyspnea.** Asthma, emphysema, and vigorous physical exertion can result in dyspnea. The patient with dyspnea may find it easier to breathe while in a sitting or standing position. This state is called **orthopnea,** and it is also a common symptom of congestive heart failure.

Breath Sounds

Breath sounds are caused by air moving through the respiratory tract. Normal breath sounds are quiet and barely audible. Abnormal breath sounds are referred to as **adventitious sounds** and generally signify the presence of a respiratory disorder. The cause and character of abnormal breath sounds are presented in Table 3–6.

TABLE 3–5	Respiratory Rates of Various Age Groups		
	Age Group	**Average Respiratory Range (respirations/minute)**	**Respiratory Average**
	Newborn	30–80	35
	1 year	20–40	30
	2 to 10 years	20–30	25
	10 to 16 years	17–22	20
	16 to 18 years	16–20	18
	Adult	16–20	18

3–8

Measuring Respiration

1. **Procedural Step.** Make sure that the patient is unaware that respirations are being monitored. This can be accomplished in the following manner: After taking the pulse, the medical assistant should continue to hold three fingers on the patient's wrist with the same amount of pressure and measure the respirations.
   Principle. If the patient is aware that respiration is being taken, the breathing may change.
2. **Procedural Step.** Observe the rise and fall of the patient's chest as the patient inhales and exhales.
   Principle. One complete respiration includes one inhalation and one exhalation.
3. **Procedural Step.** Count the number of respirations for 30 seconds and multiply by 2; note the rhythm and depth of the respiration. Also observe the patient's color. The respiratory rate should be counted for a full minute if any abnormalities occur in the rhythm or depth.
4. **Procedural Step.** Chart the results. Include the date and time, and the respiratory rate, rhythm, and depth.

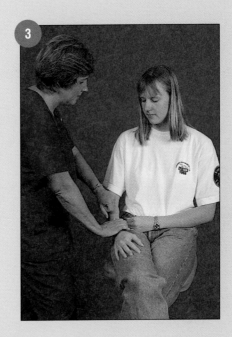

CHARTING EXAMPLE

Date	
10/15/2002	1:30 p.m. R: 18. Reg and strong. ———————— J. Smith, CMA

3

TABLE 3 – 6

Abnormal Breath Sounds

Type	Cause	Character
Stertor	Partial obstruction of the upper airway due to secretions	Noisy, snoring respirations
Stridor	Narrowing of the upper airway, such as occurs with laryngitis, croup, or the lodging of a foreign body in the lung	Shrill, harsh, high-pitched crowing sound heard during inspiration
Crackles* (formerly called rales)	Air moving through airways that contain fluid	Dry or wet intermittent sounds that vary in pitch (this sound can be duplicated by rubbing the hair together next to the ear)
Gurgles* (formerly called rhonchi)	Thick secretions that partially obstruct air flow through the large upper airways	Continuous, low-pitched, wheezing or whistling sounds more audible during expiration
Wheezes	Severely narrowed airways due to partial obstruction in the smaller bronchi and bronchioles; a common symptom of asthma	Continuous, high-pitched, whistling musical sounds
Pleural friction rub*	Inflamed pleura rubbing together	Grating sound similar to rubbing leather pieces together, heard on both inspiration and expiration

*Audible only through a stethoscope.

PATIENT/TEACHING

CHRONIC OBSTRUCTIVE PULMONARY DISEASE (COPD)

■ Answer questions that patients have about COPD:

What Is COPD?

COPD is a chronic airway obstruction that results from emphysema, chronic bronchitis, or asthma, or any combination of these conditions.

How Many People Are Affected with COPD?

COPD affects an estimated 17 million Americans, and its incidence is rising. It is ranked second only to heart disease as the leading cause of disability in men over 40 years of age.

What Causes COPD?

Heavy cigarette smoking is the leading cause of COPD. Other causes include air pollution and occupational exposure to irritating inhalants, such as noxious dusts, fumes, or vapors.

What Types of Tests Might the Physician Order?

Respiratory tests used to diagnose COPD include chest x-ray films, arterial blood gas studies, and pulmonary function tests.

What Treatment Might the Physician Prescribe?

Treatment is focused on improving breathing difficulties and may include bronchodilator aerosol therapy (inhalers), breathing exercises, chest physiotherapy (postural drainage, chest percussion and vibration), and intermittent positive-pressure breathing (IPPB) treatments.

■ Encourage patients with COPD to comply with the therapy prescribed by the physician.

■ Provide the patient with educational materials on smoking, asthma, emphysema, and chronic bronchitis available from the American Lung Association, American Heart Association, and American Cancer Society.

BLOOD PRESSURE

MECHANISM OF BLOOD PRESSURE

Blood pressure measures the pressure or force exerted by the blood on the walls of the arteries in which it is contained. Each time the ventricles contract, blood is pushed out of the heart and into the aorta and pulmonary aorta, exerting pressure on the walls of the arteries. This phase in the cardiac cycle is known as **systole,** and it represents the highest point of blood pressure in the body, or the **systolic pressure.** The phase of the cardiac cycle in which the heart relaxes between contractions is referred to as **diastole.** The **diastolic pressure** (recorded during diastole) is lower, owing to the relaxation of the heart. Thus, contraction and relaxation of the heart result in two different pressures, systolic and diastolic.

Interpretation of Blood Pressure

Blood pressure is abbreviated BP, and its measurement is expressed as a fraction. The numerator represents the systolic pressure and the denominator is the diastolic pressure. Blood pressure is measured in millimeters of mercury, abbreviated mm Hg. A blood pressure reading of 120/80 means that there was enough force

to raise a column of mercury 120 mm during systole and 80 mm during diastole.

The average blood pressure of a healthy adult is 120/80 mm Hg, and the generally accepted range for blood pressure is 110/60 mm Hg to 140/90 mm Hg (Table 3–7). Blood pressure should be taken during each office visit to allow the physician to compare the patient's readings over a period of time. This is a good preventive measure in guarding against serious illness. A single blood pressure reading taken on one occasion does not characterize an individual's blood pressure accurately. Several readings, taken on different occasions, are needed to provide a good index of an individual's baseline blood pressure.

TABLE 3–7	Average Blood Pressure of Various Age Groups	
	Age	**Average Blood Pressure (mm Hg)**
	1 year	95/65
	2 to 7 years	100/65
	8 to 13 years	110/72
	14 to 17 years	120/76
	Adult	120/80

Blood pressure readings always should be interpreted using a patient's baseline blood pressure. A rise or fall of 20 to 30 mm Hg in a patient's baseline blood pressure is significant, even if it is still within the normal accepted blood pressure range.

The most common condition causing an abnormal blood pressure reading is high blood pressure, or **hypertension.** Hypertension results from excessive pressure on the walls of the arteries. Hypertension is determined by a sustained systolic blood pressure reading of 140 or higher or a sustained diastolic reading of 90 or higher. Refer to Table 3–8 for the specific classifications of elevated blood pressure measurements. **Hypotension** results from reduced pressure on the arterial walls. Hypotension is determined by a blood pressure reading below 95/60 mm Hg.

Pulse Pressure

The difference between systolic and diastolic pressure is the **pulse pressure.** It is determined by subtracting the smaller number from the larger. For example, if the blood pressure is 120/80, the pulse pressure would be 40 mm Hg. A pulse pressure between 30 and 50 is considered to be within normal range.

Factors Affecting Blood Pressure

Blood pressure does not remain at a constant value. Numerous factors may affect it throughout the course of the day. An understanding of these factors will help ensure an accurate interpretation of blood pressure readings.

Age — Age is an important consideration when determining whether or not a patient's blood pressure is normal. As age increases, the blood pressure gradually increases: a 6-year-old child may have a normal reading of 90/60, whereas a young, healthy adult generally will have a blood pressure reading of approximately 120/80, and it would not be unusual for a 60-year-old man to have a reading of 140/90. Refer to Table 3–7 for the average blood pressure of various age groups.

Gender — Following puberty, women usually have a lower blood pressure than men of the same age.

Diurnal variations — Fluctuations in an individual's blood pressure are normal during the course of a day. When one awakens, the blood pressure is lower as a result of the decreased metabolism and physical activity that occur during sleep. As metabolism and activity increase during the day, the blood pressure rises.

Emotional states — Strong emotional states, such as anger, fear, or excitement increase the blood pressure. If the medical assistant observes such a reaction, an attempt should be made to calm the patient before taking blood pressure. Other factors that may increase the blood pressure include pain, a recent meal, smoking, and bladder distention.

Exercise — Physical activity temporarily increases the blood pressure. A patient who has been involved in physical activity should be given an opportunity to rest for 20 to 30 minutes before blood pressure is measured to ensure an accurate reading.

3

TABLE 3–8

Classifications of Blood Pressure Measurements (For adults, ages 18 years or older)			
Classification	**Systolic (mm Hg)**	**Diastolic (mm Hg)**	**Follow-Up Recommended**
Normal	Less than 130	Less than 85	Recheck in 2 years
High normal	130–139	85–89	Recheck in 1 year and discuss lifestyle modifications
Hypertension			
Stage 1 (Mild)	140–159	90–99	Confirm within 2 months
Stage 2 (Moderate)	160–179	100–109	Evaluate or refer within 1 month
Stage 3 (Severe)	180–209	110–119	Evaluate or refer within 1 week
Stage 4 (Very Severe)	210 or higher	120 or higher	Evaluate or refer immediately

From the 1992 Report of The Joint National Committee on Detection, Evaluation, and Treatment of High Blood Pressure. National Heart, Lung, and Blood Institute. U.S. Department of Health and Human Services. NIH Publication, 1992.

Body position   In some cases, the blood pressure of a patient who is in a lying or standing position may be different from that measured when the patient is in a sitting position. A notation should be made on the patient's chart if the reading was obtained in any position other than sitting, using the following abbreviations: *L* (lying) and *St* (standing).

Medications   Many medications may either increase or decrease the blood pressure. Because of this factor, it is important to record all medications that the patient is taking in his or her chart.

ASSESSMENT OF BLOOD PRESSURE

The equipment needed to measure blood pressure includes a stethoscope and a sphygmomanometer. The **stethoscope** amplifies sounds produced by the body and allows the medical assistant to hear them.

The most common type of stethoscope used in the medical office is the acoustical stethoscope. It consists of four parts: earpieces, sidepieces known as binaurals, plastic or rubber tubing, and a chestpiece (Fig. 3–14A). Examples of chestpieces include a **diaphragm,** which is a large flat disc, and a **bell,** which has hollowed, curved appearance (Fig. 3–14B). The chestpiece of a stethoscope may be a diaphragm, a bell, or both.

The diaphragm chestpiece is more useful for hearing high-pitched sounds like lung and bowel sounds, whereas the bell chestpiece is more useful for hearing low-pitched sounds such as those produced by the heart and vascular system. Because of this factor, the bell chestpiece works best for measuring blood pressure, although the diaphragm is adequate and frequently used. Before using a stethoscope, the medical assistant should make sure that it is in proper working condition.

The **sphygmomanometer** is an instrument that measures the pressure of blood within an artery. It consists of a manometer containing a scale for registering the pressure of the air within the bladder, an inflatable rubber bladder surrounded by a covering known as the cuff, and a pressure bulb with a control valve to inflate and deflate the rubber bladder (Fig. 2–15).

The two types of sphygmomanometer are the mercury and the aneroid. The **mercury sphygmomanometer** is more accurate, whereas the aneroid sphygmomanometer is portable. It has a vertical tube calibrated in millimeters that is filled with mercury (Fig. 3–15).

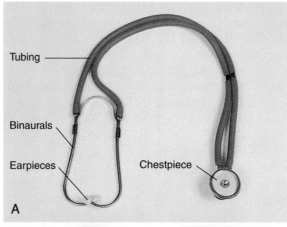
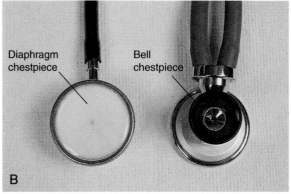

FIGURE 3–14. The parts of a stethoscope.

Before the blood pressure reading is obtained, the mercury must be even with the zero level at the base of the calibrated tube. Pressure created by inflation of the rubber bladder causes the mercury to rise in the tube. The top portion of the mercury column curves slightly upward and is known as the **meniscus.** The blood pressure should be read at the top of the meniscus, with the eye at the same level as the meniscus of the mercury column.

The **aneroid sphygmomanometer** has a round dial calibrated in millimeters, with a needle that points to the calibrations (Fig. 3–16). To ensure an accurate reading, the needle must be positioned initially at zero. An aneroid sphygmomanometer requires regular recalibration, at least once a year, against a mercury manometer.

The manometer must be placed in the correct position for proper viewing. The medical assistant should be no farther than 3 feet from the scale of the manometer. The portable mercury manometer should be placed on a flat surface so that the mercury column is in a vertical position. The wall model mercury manometer is mounted securely against a wall, thereby placing the mercury column in a vertical position. The aneroid manometer should be placed so that it may be viewed directly.

Blood pressure cuffs are available in three different sizes: pediatric, adult, and thigh (Fig. 3–17). To ensure an accurate reading, the proper cuff size should always be used. The diameter of the limb determines the size of cuff to use; the width of the cuff should be 20 percent greater than the diameter of the limb. Pediatric cuffs are used for children and for adults with small arms. The adult cuff is used for the average-sized adult arm, and the thigh cuff is used for taking blood pressure from the thigh or for adults with large arms. If the cuff is too small, the reading may be falsely high, as, for example, when an adult cuff is used on a patient with a large arm. On the other hand, if the cuff is too large, the reading may be falsely low, as when an adult cuff is used with a child or a patient with a thin arm. The cuff should fit snugly and should be applied so that the center of the inflatable bag is directly over the artery to be compressed. The cuff has an interlocking, self-sticking substance (Velcro) that allows for easy closure.

Korotkoff Sounds

Korotkoff sounds are used to determine the systolic and diastolic blood pressure readings. When the cuff is inflated, the brachial artery is compressed, so that no audible sounds are heard through the stethoscope. As the cuff is deflated, at a rate of 2 to 3 mm of mercury (mm Hg) per heart beat, the sounds become audible until the blood flows freely and they can no longer be heard (Table 3–9).

The medical assistant should practice listening to these sounds and be able to identify the various phases.

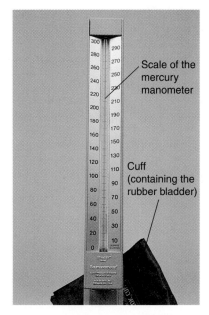

■ **FIGURE 3–15.** The parts of a mercury sphygmomanometer.

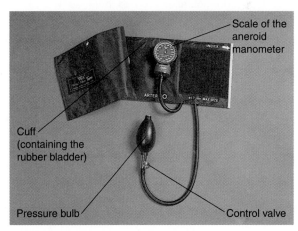

■ **FIGURE 3–16.** The parts of an aneroid sphygmomanometer.

3

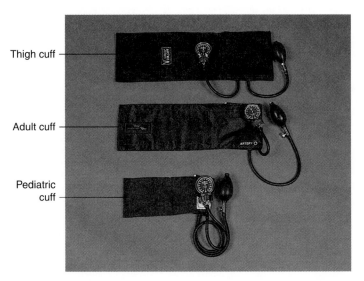

■ **FIGURE 3–17.** Blood pressure cuffs are available in three different sizes: pediatric, adult, and thigh.

Highlight on Stethoscopes

The stethoscope was first introduced in the 1800s by a French physician named Rene Laennec. This early stethoscope consisted of a simple wooden tube with a bell-shaped opening at one end.

The selection of a stethoscope is an individual decision. You will hear sounds differently when using different stethoscopes. The primary consideration in choosing a stethoscope should be that it is well made and fits well in your ears. Stethoscopes are available from uniform shops and medical supply companies.

The usual length of tubing on a stethoscope is 12 to 14 inches, but you may prefer the longer 22-inch tubing. An argument against long tubing is that it transmits sound less efficiently. Research has shown however, that 6 to 8 more inches of tubing does not significantly alter the transmission of most sounds.

The stethoscope should have metal binaurals. The binaurals should allow you to angle the earpieces firmly to follow the direction of your ear canal. Binaurals that are too tight are uncomfortable and binaurals that are too loose do not allow you to hear as well as you should.

The earpieces should fit comfortably and snugly in the ear canal. If you can understand what someone is saying in the same room, they are too loose, which will interfere with effective auscultation. Some stethoscopes come with removable ear tips in different sizes. This offers the advantage of selecting an ear tip that best fits your ear canal. Flexible ear tips of soft rubber are usually more comfortable than nonflexible tips of hard rubber or plastic.

The chestpiece should be a key factor in the selection of a stethoscope. A stethoscope with both a diaphragm and a bell offers the most versatility for listening to different types of sounds. Many stethoscopes have a rubber or plastic nonchill rim around the diaphragm and bell to avoid chilling the patient with a cold chestpiece and to decrease air leaks between the chestpiece and the patient.

The most common problem occurring with stethoscopes is air leak. Air leaks interfere with effective sound transmission and also allow environmental noise to enter the stethoscope. Air leaks may result from a cracked earpiece, a cracked or chipped chestpiece, or a break in the tubing.

3

Korotkoff Sounds

Phase	Description	Illustration
	Inflation of the cuff compresses and closes off the brachial artery so that no blood flows through the artery. The pressure in the cuff is released at a moderate steady rate of 2 to 3 mm Hg per second.	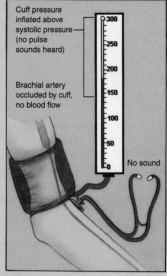
Phase I	Phase I is when the first faint but clear tapping sound is heard that gradually increases in intensity. The first tapping sound is the **systolic pressure.**	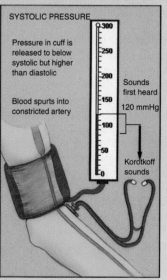
Phase II	As the cuff continues to deflate, Phase II occurs, in which the sounds have a murmuring or swishing quality.	
Phase III	Further deflation results in Phase III, when the sounds become crisper and increase in intensity.	
Phase IV	During Phase IV, the sounds become muffled and have a soft, blowing quality. According to the American Heart Association, the onset of the muffled sounds is regarded as the best index of the diastolic pressure in children.	
Phase V	Phase V is the point at which the sounds disappear. This is typically recorded as the **diastolic pressure** for an adult. Some authorities believe that the adult diastolic pressure falls midway between Phases IV and V; therefore, some physicians may want the medical assistant to record both Phases IV and V as the diastolic pressure (e.g., 128/76/72).	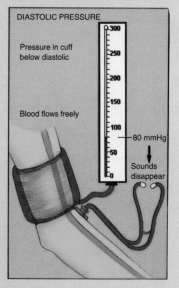

3

3

Prevention of Errors in Blood Pressure Measurement

The following guidelines should be followed to prevent errors in blood pressure measurement.

1. **Always use the proper cuff size.** If the cuff is too small, the reading may be falsely high, and if the cuff is too large, the reading may be falsely low. The width of the cuff should be 20 percent greater than the diameter of the limb.

2. **Never take blood pressure over clothing.** Roll up the patient's sleeve approximately 5 inches above the elbow. If the sleeve is too tight after being rolled up, remove the sleeve from the arm. A tight sleeve causes partial compression of the brachial artery, resulting in an inaccurate reading.

3. **Properly position the patient's arm.** Position the arm at heart level, and make sure it is well supported with the palm facing upward. If the arm is above heart level, the blood pressure reading may be falsely low.

4. **Avoid extraneous sounds from the cuff.** Position the cuff approximately 1 inch above the bend in the elbow. The cuff should be up far enough to prevent the stethoscope from touching it; otherwise extraneous sounds, which could interfere with an accurate measurement, may be picked up.

5. **Compress the brachial artery completely.** Center the rubber bladder of the cuff directly over the artery to be compressed. Most cuffs are labeled with an arrow indicating the center of the bladder. Centering the rubber bladder allows for complete compression of the brachial artery.

6. **Apply equal pressure over the brachial artery.** The cuff should be applied so that it fits smoothly and snugly around the patient's arm. This prevents bulging or slipping and permits application of an equal pressure over the brachial artery.

7. **Position the earpieces so the sounds can be heard clearly.** Place the earpieces of the stethoscope in your ears with the earpieces directed slightly forward. This allows the earpieces to follow the direction of the ear canal, which facilitates hearing.

8. **Avoid extraneous sounds from the stethoscope.** Make sure the tubing of the stethoscope hangs freely and is not permitted to rub against any object. If the stethoscope tubing rubs against an object, extraneous sounds may be picked up with could interfere with an accurate measurement.

9. **Properly position the chestpiece.** Palpate the brachial pulse to provide good positioning of the chestpiece over the brachial artery. Place the chestpiece firmly, but gently, over the brachial artery to assist in transmitting clear and audible sounds. Do not allow the chestpiece to touch the cuff to prevent extraneous sounds from being picked up which could interfere with an accurate measurement.

10. **Release the pressure at a moderate steady rate.** Release the pressure in the cuff at a rate of 2 to 3 mm Hg per second to ensure an accurate blood pressure measurement. Releasing the pressure too quickly or too slowly could cause a falsely low systolic reading and a falsely high diastolic reading.

11. **Avoid venous congestion.** If you need to take the blood pressure again, wait 1 to 2 minutes to allow blood trapped in the veins (venous congestion) to be released. Venous congestion can result in a falsely high systolic reading and a falsely low diastolic reading.

 PATIENT/TEACHING

HYPERTENSION
■ Answer questions patients have about hypertension.

What Is High Blood Pressure?
Blood pressure is the force of blood against the walls of the arteries. High blood pressure, also called **hypertension,** means the pressure in the arteries is consistently above the normal range, resulting in excessive pressure on the walls of the arteries.

What Are the Symptoms of High Blood Pressure?
Approximately half of all individuals with high blood pressure are not aware of it because there are few or no symptoms. Hypertension is the most common of all life-threatening diseases among Americans. It is estimated that 1 in 4 Americans has high blood pressure. The only way to know for sure whether you have high blood pressure is to have your blood pressure checked on a regular basis.

What Causes High Blood Pressure?
In about 90 percent of cases, the precise cause of high blood pressure is unknown. Certain factors, however, seem to increase the risk of developing hypertension. These include

Heredity: A family history of high blood pressure increases an individual's risk of developing high blood pressure.

What Causes High Blood Pressure?

Weight: Individuals who are overweight are two to six times more likely to develop high blood pressure.

Race: Research has shown that more black than white Americans develop high blood pressure.

Age: Blood pressure normally increases as you grow older.

Sodium intake: Sodium found in salt and processed, canned, and most snack foods can aggravate high blood pressure. The average American consumes 10 to 20 grams of sodium a day. This is equivalent to 2 to 4 teaspoons of salt. The body actually requires only 200 milligrams of sodium each day, which is about one tenth of a teaspoon of salt.

Stress: Research indicates that people who are under continuous stress tend to develop more heart and circulatory problems than those who are not under stress.

Smoking: Smoking constricts blood vessels, causing an increase in blood pressure.

Alcohol consumption: Heavy alcohol consumption may increase the blood pressure.

What Can Happen if High Blood Pressure Is Not Treated?

If high blood pressure is not brought under control, it can cause severe damage to vital organs such as the heart, brain, kidneys, or eyes, resulting in a heart attack or heart failure, stroke, kidney failure, or blindness. Early detection and treatment of high blood pressure can prevent these complications.

Can High Blood Pressure Be Cured?

High blood pressure cannot be cured, but a number of treatments are used to bring it under control. These include modifications in diet and lifestyle, such as weight reduction, limiting salt intake, regular aerobic exercise, cessation of smoking, and limiting alcohol consumption. If diet and lifestyle changes alone are not enough, medications are available for lowering blood pressure, allowing the patient to lead a normal, healthy, active life.

How Long Will I Undergo Treatment?

Treatment is usually a life-long process. Even if you feel fine, you'll probably have to continue treatment for the rest of your life to keep your blood pressure down. If you discontinue your diet and lifestyle changes or stop taking your medication, your blood pressure will go up again.

■ Encourage patients with hypertension to adhere to the treatment prescribed by the physician. Help patients remember to take their medication by telling them to associate their medication schedule with a daily routine, such as brushing their teeth or mealtimes.

■ Provide the patient with educational materials on high blood pressure available from sources such as the American Heart Association.

3

PROCEDURE

3–9

Measuring Blood Pressure

EQUIPMENT/SUPPLIES: Stethoscope
Sphygmomanometer
Antiseptic wipe

1. **Procedural Step.** Wash the hands, and assemble the equipment. Be sure to select the proper cuff size. Clean the earpieces of the stethoscope with the antiseptic wipe.

2. **Procedural Step.** Greet and identify the patient. Introduce yourself and explain the procedure. While explaining the procedure, observe the patient for any signs that would influence the reading, such as anger, fear, pain, recent physical activity, and others. If it is not possible to reduce or eliminate these influences, list them in the patient's chart.

3. **Procedural Step.** Position the patient comfortably in a sitting position. Roll up the patient's sleeve approximately 5 inces above the the elbow. If the sleeve does not roll up or is too tight after being

Continued

3

rolled up, remove the sleeve from the arm. The arm should be positioned at heart level and well supported, with the palm facing upward. Make a notation in the patient's chart if the lying or standing position was used to take blood pressure. Abbreviations that can be used are L (lying) and St (standing).

Principle. A tight sleeve causes partial compression of the brachial artery, resulting in an inaccurate reading. The position of the arm allows easy access to the brachial artery. Placing the arm above heart level may cause the reading to be falsely low.

4. **Procedural Step.** Place the cuff on the patient's arm so that the lower edge of the cuff is approximately 1 inch above the bend in the elbow. The rubber bladder should be centered over the brachial artery. (Most cuffs are labeled with an arrow indicating the center of the bladder.)

Principle. The cuff should be placed high enough to prevent the stethoscope from touching it; otherwise, extraneous sounds, which could interfere with an accurate measurement, may be picked up. Centering the rubber bladder allows for complete compression of the brachial artery.

5. **Procedural Step.** Wrap the cuff smoothly and snugly around the patient's arm, and secure the end of it.

Principle. Applying the cuff properly prevents it from bulging or slipping. This technique permits application of an equal pressure over the brachial artery.

6. **Procedural Step.** Position the manometer for direct viewing and at a distance of no more than 3 feet.

Principle. The medical assistant may have trouble seeing the scale on the manometer if it is placed more than 3 feet away.

7. **Procedural Step.** Place the earpieces of the stethoscope in your ears, with the earpieces directed slightly forward. During the blood pressure measurement, the tubing of the stethoscope should hang freely and should not be permitted to rub against any object.

Principle. The earpieces should be directed forward permitting them to follow the direction of the ear canal, which facilitates hearing. If the stethoscope tubing rubs against an object, extraneous sounds may be picked up, which will interfere with an accurate measurement.

8. **Procedural Step.** Making sure the arm is well extended, palpate the brachial pulse with the fingertips and place the chestpiece of the stethoscope (bell or diaphragm) firmly but gently over the artery where the pulse is felt. Do not allow the chestpiece to touch the cuff.

Principle. Locating the brachial pulse allows for good positioning of the chestpiece over the brachial artery. A well-extended arm allows for easier palpation of the brachial pulse. Good con-

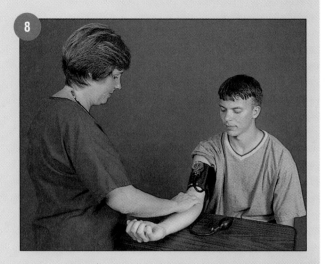

tact of the chestpiece with the skin helps transmit clear and audible Korotkoff sounds through the earpieces of the stethoscope. If the chestpiece touches the cuff, extraneous sounds may be picked up, which will interfere with an accurate measurement.

9. **Procedural Step.** Close the valve on the bulb by turning the thumbscrew in a clockwise direction until it feels tight. Pump air into the cuff as rapidly as possible, up to a level of approximately 20 to 30 mm Hg above the palpated or previously measured systolic pressure. Explain to the patient that this will cause a numbing and tingling sensation in the arm.

Principle. Inflation of the cuff compresses and closes off the brachial artery so that no blood flows through the artery. A preliminary determination of the systolic pressure, by palpation, allows the medical assistant to estimate how high to inflate the cuff. The procedure for palpating the systolic pressure is explained in Procedure 3–10. If the patient has had the blood pressure measured previously at the medical office, the recorded systolic pressure can be used to determine how high to inflate the cuff.

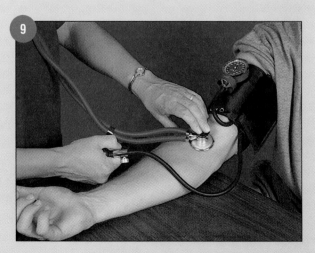

10. **Procedural Step.** Release the pressure at a moderately steady rate of 2 to 3 mm Hg per second by slowly turning the thumbscrew in a counterclockwise direction. This opens the valve and allows the air in the cuff to escape slowly. Listen for the first clear tapping sound (Phase I of the Korotkoff sounds). This represents the systolic pressure. Note this point on the scale of the manometer.

Principle. The systolic pressure is the point at which the blood first begins to spurt through the artery as the cuff pressure begins to decrease; it represents the pressure that occurs on the walls of the arteries during systole.

11. **Procedural Step.** Continue to deflate the cuff while listening to the Korotkoff sounds. Listen for the

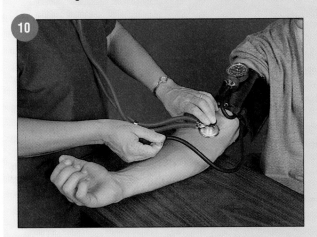

onset of the muffled sound that occurs during Phase IV and note this point on the scale of the manometer. If Phase V is to be recorded, continue to deflate the cuff and note the point on the scale at which the sound ceases.

Principle. Phase IV marks the diastolic pressure (which represents the pressure that occurs on the walls of the arteries during diastole); the cuff pressure is reduced, and blood is flowing freely through the brachial artery.

12. **Procedural Step.** Quickly and completely deflate the cuff to zero. If you could not obtain an accurate blood pressure reading, wait 1 to 2 minutes and repeat the blood pressure measurement procedure outlined previously. Remove the earpieces of the stethoscope from your ears, and carefully remove the cuff from the patient's arm.

Principle. Venous congestion results when blood pressure is taken, which will alter a second reading if it is taken too soon.

13. **Procedural Step.** Chart the results. Include the date and time, and the blood pressure reading.

14. **Procedural Step.** Clean the earpieces with an antiseptic wipe and replace the equipment properly.

CHARTING EXAMPLE

Date	
10/20/2002	2:30 p.m. BP: 124/86. ———J. Smith, CMA

3

3-10

Determining Systolic Pressure by Palpation

1. **Procedural Step.** Locate the radial pulse with the fingertips.
2. **Procedural Step.** Close the valve on the bulb and pump air into the bulb until the pulsation ceases.
3. **Procedural Step.** Release the valve at a moderate rate of 2 to 3 mm Hg per heart beat while palpating the artery with the fingertips.
4. **Procedural Step.** Record the point at which the pulsation reappears as the palpated systolic pressure.
5. **Procedural Step.** Deflate the cuff completely, and wait 15 to 30 seconds before checking the blood pressure.

MEDICAL PRACTICE
AND THE LAW

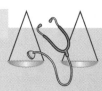

Measurement of vital signs is standard procedure for almost every patient in the physician's office. Because vital sign measurements are performed so frequently, the medical assistant may tend to minimize their importance. Changes in vital signs may be the first indicator of disease or illness, so meticulous attention must be paid to the performance and documentation of vital signs, as well as comparing the current measurements with past measurements for each patient.

Most patients want to know their vital signs, especially their blood pressure or temperature if febrile. Although the patient owns the information that you collect, be aware that you may not give this information to family members without the patient's consent. Some offices have a policy of what information to give the patient when they ask; some physicians prefer to discuss this information themselves.

Often, vital sign measurements are the first contact the patients have with the medical assistant. The most important factor determining whether or not a patient will sue is not the skill of the practitioner, but establishment of a rapport with the patient. In everything you do, convey the feeling of caring and concern to each patient.

CERTIFICATION REVIEW

BODY TEMPERATURE

☐ Body temperature is maintained within a fairly constant range by the hypothalamus, which is located in the brain.

☐ Body temperature is maintained through a balance of the heat produced in the body and the heat lost from the body. Heat is produced in the body by voluntary and involuntary muscle contractions, cell metabolism, and strong emotional states. Heat is lost from the body through perspiration; in the urine, feces, and moisture droplets from the lungs; and through conduction, convection, and radiation.

☐ The normal body temperature range is 97° to 99°F (36.1° to 37.2°C), with the average body temperature being 98.6°F (37°C). Pyrexia is used to describe a temperature above normal, and hypothermia is used to describe a temperature below normal.

☐ Factors affecting body temperature include age, diurnal variations, exercise, emotional states, environmental factors, the patient's normal body temperature, and pregnancy.

☐ An individual with a fever is said to be febrile, while one without a fever is afebrile. The course of a fever rises and falls in one of the following patterns: continuous, intermittent, or remittent.

☐ The four sites for taking body temperature are oral, rectal, axillary, and aural. The site chosen for measuring a patient's temperature depends on the patient's age, condition, and state of consciousness; the type of thermometer being used; and the medical office policy.

☐ The temperature obtained through the rectal route measures approximately 1°F higher than the same temperature taken through the oral route. The axillary temperature measures approximately 1°F lower than the same temperature taken through the oral route.

☐ An electronic thermometer consists of interchangeable oral (red) and rectal (blue) probes attached to a battery-operated portable unit that sits in a rechargeable base. A disposable cover is placed over the probe to prevent the transmission of microorganisms between patients.

☐ The tympanic membrane thermometer is used with the aural site and provides results within 1 to 2 seconds. The thermometer detects thermal energy given off by the tympanic membrane in the form of infrared waves.

☐ The mercury glass thermometer consists of a bulb and stem. Mercury is contained in the bulb; the bulb of an oral thermometer is long and slender, and the bulb of a rectal thermometer is short and blunt. The stem contains calibrations that are divided into two tenths of a degree (0.2°) on the Fahrenheit thermometer and into one tenth of a degree (0.1°) on the Celsius thermometer.

☐ Chemical thermometers are less accurate than other types of thermometers and are often used by patients at home to provide a general assessment of body temperature.

PULSE

☐ The contraction and relaxation of the heart sends a wave of vibration from the aorta through the walls of the arterial system known as the pulse.

☐ Pulse rate can vary due to age, gender, exercise,

3

emotional states, metabolism, and medications.

☐ The most common site for measuring pulse is the radial artery, located on the inner aspect of the wrist just below the thumb. The apical pulse is more easily heard than other sites and is located in the fifth intercostal space at the junction of the left midclavicular line. Other pulse sites include the brachial, temporal, carotid, femoral, popliteal, and dorsalis pedis.

☐ The normal resting pulse rate for an adult ranges from 60 to 100 beats per minute. A pulse rate of more than 100 beats per minute is known as tachycardia and a pulse rate below 60 beats per minute is known as bradycardia.

☐ The pulse rhythm is the time interval between heart beats. An irregularity in the heart's rhythm is known as an arrhythmia (or dysrhythmia). The pulse volume refers to the strength of the heart beat. A pulse that feels weak and thin is termed a thready pulse, and a pulse that feels very strong and full is termed a bounding pulse.

RESPIRATION

☐ One respiration consists of one inhalation and one exhalation. During inhalation, the diaphragm descends and the lungs expand; during exhalation, the diaphragm ascends and the lungs return to their original state.

☐ The respiratory rate of an adult ranges from 16 to 20 respirations per minute. An abnormal increase in the respiratory rate is known as tachypnea, and an abnormal decrease is known as bradypnea.

☐ Normally, the rhythm should be even and regular, and the pauses between inhalation and exhalation should be equal. The depth of each respiration should be the same. Hyperpnea denotes a very rapid and panting type of respiration. Hyperventilation is an abnormally fast and deep type of breathing usually associated with acute anxiety or emotional tension. Hypopnea is an abnormal decrease in the rate and depth of respiration.

☐ Dyspnea, or difficult breathing, can be caused by asthma, emphysema, and vigorous physical exertion. Orthopnea means the patient can breathe easier in a sitting or standing position.

BLOOD PRESSURE

☐ Blood pressure measures the pressure exerted by the blood on the walls of the arteries. The systolic pressure is the highest pressure and the diastolic pressure is the point of lesser pressure on the arterial walls.

☐ The average blood pressure of an adult is 120/80 and ranges from a systolic pressure of 110 to 140 and a diastolic pressure of 60 to 90. A single blood pressure reading taken on one occasion does not characterize an individual's blood pressure; several readings must be taken on different occasions.

☐ Hypertension is excessive pressure on the walls of the arteries and refers to a sustained systolic pressure of 140 or higher or a sustained diastolic reading of 90 or higher

☐ Factors affecting blood pressure include age, gender, diurnal variations, emotional states, exercise, body position, and medication.

3

ON THE WEB

The Physical Examination

Hope Fauber, *and I am a Certified Medical Assistant. I graduated from an accredited medical assisting program and have an associate's degree in Applied Science. I work in a teaching facility with a family medicine department of 10 established physicians and 10 residents and interns. I have worked in the field of medical assisting for 12 years. My duties cover a broad spectrum, from pediatrics to geriatrics, with prenatal care, allergy injections, minor office surgery, electrocardiograms, colposcopies, immunizations, and wound care. Some days I am assigned to the desk to answer patient questions, advise patients of laboratory results, schedule referrals and call prescriptions into pharmacies. The variety helps keep the job interesting. Because this is a teaching facility, there is an emphasis on learning, and physicians are eager to discuss patient diagnosis and care with the medical assistants.*

Before I became a medical assistant, I was a stay-at-home mom. I wanted to have some sort of training that would be flexible for my family situation. I chose not to pursue a career as a nurse because of the shift hours I would have to work. I find that medical assisting is fulfilling and flexible.

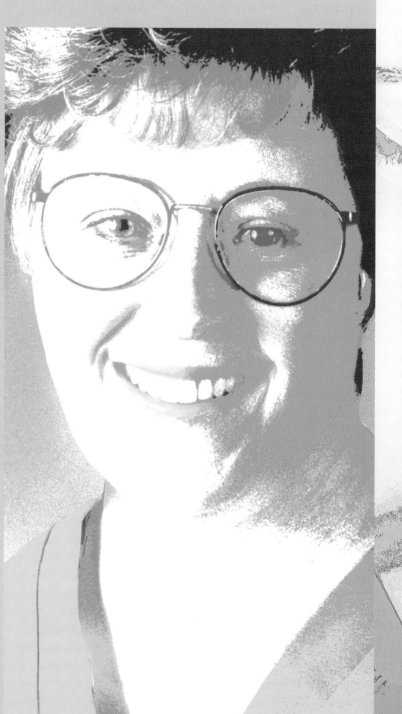

━━━ OUTCOMES

After completing this chapter, you should be able to demonstrate the proper procedure to perform the following:

1. Prepare the examining room.
2. Operate and care for equipment and instruments used during the physical examination, according to the manufacturer's instructions.
3. Prepare a patient for a physical examination.
4. Measure weight and height.
5. Position and drape a patient in the following positions: sitting, supine, prone, dorsal recumbent, lithotomy, Sims, knee-chest, and Fowler's.
6. Assist the physician during the physical examination.

━━━ EDUCATIONAL OBJECTIVES

After completing this chapter, you should be able to do the following:

1. Define the terms listed in the Key Terminology.
2. Identify the three components of a complete patient examination.
3. List the guidelines that should be followed in preparing the examining room.
4. Identify equipment and instruments used during the physical examination.
5. Explain the purpose of measuring weight.
6. List the guidelines that should be followed when measuring weight and height.
7. Explain the purpose of positioning and draping.
8. List and define the four techniques of examining the patient. State an example of the use of each during the physical examination.

KEY TERMINOLOGY

audiometer (a-DÊ-OM-it-er): An instrument used to measure hearing.

auscultation (Aus-kul-TÂ-shun): The process of listening to the sounds produced within the body to detect any signs of disease.

charting: The process of making written entries about a patient in the medical record.

clinical diagnosis: A tentative diagnosis of a patient's condition obtained through the evaluation of the health history and the physical examination, without the benefit of laboratory or diagnostic tests.

conjunctiva (kun-JUNK-tiv-a): The mucous membrane that lines the eyelids and covers the eyeball, except for the cornea.

diagnosis (dî-AG-nô-sis): The scientific method of determining and identifying a patient's condition.

differential diagnosis: A determination of which of two or more diseases with similar symptoms is producing the patient's symptoms

inspection: The process of observing a patient to detect any signs of disease.

medical record: A written record of the important aspects regarding a patient, his or her care, and the progress of his or her illness (also known as "the chart").

mensuration (MEN-sa-RÂ-shun): The process of measuring the patient.

ophthalmoscope (off-THAL-ma-skôp): An instrument for examining the interior of the eye.

otoscope (ô-ta-skôp): An instrument for examining the external ear canal and tympanic membrane.

palpation (PAL-pâ-shun): The process of feeling with the hands to detect signs of disease.

percussion (per-KUSH-n): The process of tapping the body to detect signs of disease.

percussion hammer (per-KUSH-n HAM-er): An instrument with a rubber head, used for testing reflexes.

prognosis (prog-NÔ-sis): The probable course and outcome of a patient's condition and the prospects of patient recovery.

retina (RET-in-a): The interior structure of the eye, which picks up and transmits light impulses to the optic nerve.

speculum (SPEK-û-lem): An instrument for opening a body orifice or cavity for viewing.

symptom: Any change in the body or its functioning that indicates that a disease is present.

tympanic membrane (tim-PAN-ik mem-BRÂN): A thin, semitransparent membrane located between the external ear canal and middle ear that receives and transmits sound waves. Also known as the eardrum.

4

INTRODUCTION

☐ A complete patient examination consists of three parts: the **health history,** the **physical examination** of each body system, and **laboratory and diagnostic tests.** The results are used by the physician to determine the patient's general state of health, to arrive at a diagnosis and prescribe treatment, and to observe any change in a patient's illness after treatment has been instituted.

An important and frequent responsibility of the medical assistant is to assist with a physical examination. Because health-promotion and disease-prevention activities have become an important focus of health care, individuals are becoming more aware of the need for a yearly physical examination to detect early signs of illness and to prevent serious health problems. Also, a physical examination is often a prerequisite for employment and for entering the military service and schools.

The physical examination is explained in detail in this chapter. The health history and collecting specimens and performing laboratory and diagnostic tests are discussed in other chapters.

DEFINITION OF TERMS

The medical assistant should have a knowledge of the following terms relating to the patient examination.

Diagnosis	The term diagnosis, often called the final diagnosis, refers to the scientific method of determining and identifying a patient's condition through the evaluation of the health history, the physical examination, and laboratory tests and diagnostic procedures. The importance of establishing a final diagnosis is to provide a

	logical basis for treatment and prognosis.
Clinical Diagnosis	The clinical diagnosis is an intermediate step in establishing a final diagnosis. The clinical diagnosis of a patient's condition is obtained through the evaluation of the health history and the physical examination without the benefit of laboratory or diagnostic tests. Outside laboratories provide a space for specifying the clinical diagnosis on the laboratory request form to assist the laboratory in correlating the clinical laboratory data with the needs of the physician. Once the test results have been analyzed by the physician, a final diagnosis can usually be established from the clinical diagnosis.
Differential Diagnosis	Two or more diseases may have similar symptoms. The differential diagnosis involves determining which of these diseases is producing the patient's symptoms so that a final diagnosis can be established. For example, both streptococcal sore throat and pharyngitis have similar symptoms. A differential diagnosis is made by obtaining a throat specimen and performing a strep test.
Prognosis	The prognosis is the probable course and outcome of a patient's condition and the prospects of patient recovery.
Risk Factor	A risk factor is one that increases the probability that an individual will develop a particular condition, such as genetic factors, habits, environmental conditions, and physiologic conditions. The presence of a risk factor does not mean that a condition will develop; it means only that the chances are increased of the patient developing a particular condition. For example, cigarette smoking is a risk factor for developing lung cancer and heart disease.
Acute Illness	An acute illness is characterized by symptoms that have a rapid onset, are usually severe and intense, and subside after a relatively short period of time. In some cases, the acute episode progresses into a chronic illness. Examples of acute illness include influenza, strep throat, and chickenpox.
Chronic Illness	A chronic illness is characterized by symptoms that persist for more than 3 months and show little change over a long period of time. Examples of chronic illness include diabetes mellitus, hypertension, and emphysema.
Therapeutic Procedure	A therapeutic procedure is curative in nature and is performed to treat a patient's condition. Examples of therapeutic procedures include the administration of medication, ear and eye irrigations, and therapeutic ultrasound. Procedures should be recorded immediately after being performed; from a legal standpoint, a procedure that is not documented was not performed.
Diagnostic Procedure	A type of procedure performed to assist in the diagnosis of a patient's condition; examples include electrocardiography, x-ray examination, and sigmoidoscopy.
Laboratory Testing	The analysis and study of materials, fluid, or tissues obtained from patients to assist in diagnosing and treating disease.

PREPARATION OF THE EXAMINING ROOM

☐ Proper preparation of the examining room provides a comfortable and healthy environment for the patient and facilitates the physical examination. The following guidelines should be followed in preparing the examining room:

- The examining room should be free of clutter and well lit.
- The medical assistant should check the examining rooms daily to make sure there are ample supplies. Supplies that are getting low should be restocked as needed.
- Waste receptacles should be emptied frequently.
- The room should be well ventilated, and air freshener should be kept on hand to eliminate odors.

Highlight on Health Screening

The chance of developing certain diseases is greater at different ages. Periodic health screening is recommended for the detection and early treatment of disease.

Test or Procedure	Gender	Frequency
Beginning at age 20 years, the following are recommended:		
Blood pressure	M & F	Every year
Cholesterol level	M & F	Every 5 years
Blood glucose level	M & F	Every 3 to 5 years
Breast self-exam	F	Every month
Breast physical examination (by a physician)	F	Every 3 years and then every year beginning at age 40 years
Pap test and pelvic examination	F	An annual Pap test and pelvic examination starting at the onset of sexual activity or at age 18 years, whichever is earlier. After a woman has tested negative for three or more consecutive examinations, the Pap test may be performed less frequently at the discretion of her physician
Testicular self-exam	M	Every month beginning at age 14 years

Test or Procedure	Gender	Frequency
In addition, the following are recommended at the age specified:		
Digital rectal examination	M & F	Every year beginning at age 40 years
Occult blood test	M & F	Every year starting at age 50 years
Sigmoidoscopy	M & F	Beginning at age 50 years, every 3 to 5 years after two negative examinations 1 year apart
Prostate examination	M	Every year beginning at age 50 years
Mammography	F	Baseline between ages 35 and 40 years and then every 1 to 2 years between the ages of 40 to 49 years; every year after age 50 years
Electrocardiogram	M & F	One baseline recording starting at age 40 years

4

- A proper temperature should be maintained, keeping in mind that a temperature that is comfortable for a fully clothed patient may be too cold for one who has disrobed.
- Countertops and faucets should be cleaned frequently and dust removed from furniture and towel dispensers.
- The examining table paper should be changed after each patient by unrolling a fresh length. The medical assistant should check to make sure there is an ample supply of gowns and drapes ready for use.
- Patient privacy should be ensured. The medical assistant is responsible for making sure that the door is closed during the examination.
- Equipment, instruments, and supplies used for patient examinations should be appropriately cleaned and prepared, ready for use by the physician. Table 4–1 lists the equipment and supplies, along with their uses, that may be employed during a physical examination.
- Equipment and instruments must be checked on a regular basis for proper working condition. This protects the patient from harm caused by faulty equipment.
- The medical assistant should have the equipment and supplies ready for the examination. They should be arranged for easy access by the physician. The equipment and supplies needed for the physical examination vary according to the type of examination and physician's preference (Fig. 4–1).
- The medical assistant should know how to operate and care for each piece of equipment and each instrument. The manufacturer includes an instruction manual, which should be read carefully and thoroughly.

PREPARATION OF THE PATIENT

☐ It is the responsibility of the medical assistant to prepare the patient for the physical examination. At this time, the medical assistant takes vital signs and measures weight and height. The results of these procedures are charted in the patient's medical record.

Equipment and Supplies for the Physical Examination

Item	Description and Purpose
Patient examination gown	A gown made of disposable paper or cloth and used to provide patient modesty, comfort, and warmth
Drapes	Drapes are made of disposable paper or cloth and are used to reduce patient exposure
Sphygmomanometer	An instrument used to measure blood pressure
Stethoscope	An instrument used to auscultate body sounds, such as blood pressure and lung and bowel sounds
Thermometer	An instrument used to measure body temperature
Upright balance scale	A device used to measure weight and height
Otoscope	A lighted instrument with a lens, used to examine the external ear canal and tympanic membrane
Tuning fork	A small metal instrument consisting of a stem and two prongs, used to test hearing acuity
Ophthalmoscope	A lighted instrument with a lens, used for examining the interior of the eye
Tongue depressor	A flat wooden blade used to depress the patient's tongue during examination of the mouth and pharynx
Antiseptic wipe	A disposable pad saturated with an antiseptic such as alcohol which is used to cleanse the skin
Tape measure	A flexible device calibrated in inches on one side and centimeters on the other side. It is used to measure the patient (e.g., diameter of a limb, head circumference)
Percussion hammer	An instrument with a rubber head, used for testing neurologic reflexes
Speculum	An instrument for opening a body orifice or cavity for viewing (e.g., an ear speculum, nasal speculum, or vaginal speculum)
Disposable gloves	Gloves are used to provide protection from bloodborne pathogens and other potentially infectious materials
Lubricant	An agent that is applied to the physician's gloved hand or to a speculum that reduces friction between parts and provides for easier insertion
Specimen container	A container in which a body specimen is placed for transport to the laboratory
Tissues	Tissues are used for wiping body secretions
Cotton-tipped applicator	A small piece of cotton wrapped around the end of a slender wooden stick, for the collection of a specimen from the body
Gooseneck lamp	A light mounted on a flexible movable stand to focus light on an area for good visibility
Basin	A container in which used instruments are deposited
Biohazard container	A specially made container used for receiving items that contain infectious waste
Waste receptacle	A container used for depositing disposable articles that do not contain infectious waste

4

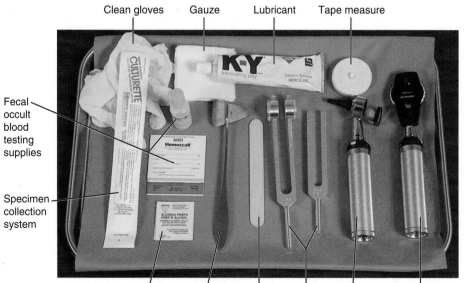

■ **FIGURE 4–1.** Examples of common instruments and supplies used for the physical examination.

PATIENT/TEACHING

HEALTH PROMOTION AND DISEASE PREVENTION

Teach patients the essentials of health promotion and disease prevention. Help patients become aware of the following patterns of behavior that promote and support health.

Keeping up to date with immunizations.
Eating nutritiously from the food pyramid.
Exercising on a regular basis.
Maintaining normal weight.
Managing stress.
Maintaining high self-esteem.

Avoiding tobacco and drugs.
Using alcohol wisely.
Understanding how the environment affects health and taking appropriate action to improve it.
Knowing the facts about cardiovascular disease, cancer, infections, sexually transmitted diseases, and accidents and using this knowledge to protect against them.
Understanding the changes that take place through the natural process of aging.
Developing a sense of responsibility for health by taking an active role toward healthy lifestyles.

Highlight on Patient Teaching

The purpose of patient teaching is to help the patient develop habits, attitudes, and skills that enable the individual to maintain and improve his or her own health.

FACT: Patients who are active, informed participants in their health care are more apt to follow the physician's instructions, as opposed to those who are passive recipients of medical services.

ACTION: Provide patients with information on health care. Every patient interaction can be used as an opportunity for teaching.

FACT: Adult learners are goal oriented and performance centered. They need and want information that will assist them in managing and improving their health status.

ACTION: Review the information that you provide to patients and determine whether it is nice to know or necessary to know. Select subject matter that is practical and useful and relates directly to the patient's needs.

FACT: The more information that is presented, the more the patient is likely to forget. Approximately half the information presented to the patient will be forgotten in the first 5 minutes after giving it.

ACTION: Use the following pointers when teaching to help patients learn and retain information:

Keep it short and be specific.
Speak in terms the patient can understand.
Focus on "how" rather than "why."
Repeat and reinforce important information.
Give practical examples and provide ample time for patient practice.

Ask for feedback from the patient to determine whether he or she understands the information.
Provide the patient with written information.

FACT: Each individual has a distinct style of learning and learns best when using his or her preferred learning style. The three main learning styles include reading, listening, and doing. Often, individuals use more than one style for learning.

ACTION: Use a variety of teaching strategies to provide for the different learning styles of patients. Examples of teaching strategies include explanations, printed handouts, audiovisual aids, demonstrations, and discussions.

FACT: Only two thirds of all patients comply with the health care instructions prescribed by the physician. Factors that influence patient compliance include patient adaptation to illness, motivation to change, physical capability, and available support systems.

ACTION: The following help increase patient compliance with prescribed treatment:

Address the patient by name. (Keep in mind that many patients object to being called by their first name by strangers.)
Encourage the patient to take an active role in personal health care.
Help the patient set goals and objectives for change.
Encourage care and support from family members.
Make the patient aware of available outside resources.
Give positive reinforcement when the patient makes needed changes.

4

The medical assistant should explain the purpose of the examination and offer to answer any questions. Patient apprehension and embarrassment can be reduced by addressing the patient by his or her name of choice, by adopting a friendly and supportive attitude, and by speaking clearly, distinctly, and slowly. This also facilitates the physical examination of the patient.

The patient should be asked if he or she needs to empty the bladder before the examination. An empty bladder makes the examination easier and is more comfortable for the patient. If a urine specimen is needed, the patient is requested to void.

Instructions to the patient on disrobing for the examination should be specific, so that he or she understands what items of clothing to remove and where to place the clothing. The disrobing facility should be comfortable and provide privacy. It is helpful to have a place for the patient to sit to make it easier to remove clothing and shoes. The facility should also be equipped with hooks for hanging clothing. Instructions for putting on the examination gown and for locating the gown opening help reduce patient confusion. If the medical assistant senses that the patient will have trouble undressing, assistance should be offered.

The medical assistant is responsible for making the patient's medical record available for review and use by the physician. It is suggested that the medical record be placed outside the examining room; the medical record contains medical terms, which, if seen by the patient, may cause confusion and apprehension. The physician will explain the contents of the medical record, using terms that the patient can understand.

The physical examination is performed with the patient positioned on an examination table, which is specially constructed to facilitate the examination. For safety purposes, it is advisable to help the patient on and off the examining table.

MEASURING WEIGHT AND HEIGHT

☐ The medical assistant routinely measures weight and height on many different types of patients. The process of measuring the patient is known as **mensuration.** A

TABLE 4-2	USDA/DHHS Height and Weight Guidelines	
	Height*	**Range of Weight in Pounds† (Male and Female)**
	5'0"	97–128
	5'1"	101–132
	5'2"	104–137
	5'3"	107–141
	5'4"	111–146
	5'5"	114–150
	5'6"	118–155
	5'7"	121–160
	5'8"	125–164
	5'9"	129–169
	5'10"	132–174
	5'11"	136–179
	6'0"	140–184
	6'1"	144–189
	6'2"	148–195
	6'3"	152–200
	6'4"	156–205
	6'5"	160–211
	6'6"	164–216

*Measured without shoes.
†Measured without clothing.
From: *Dietary guidelines for Americans, 1995* (4th ed.). Washington, DC: U.S. Department of Health and Human Services.

change in weight may be significant in the diagnosis of a patient's condition and in evaluating the course of treatment. Underweight and overweight patients who follow a diet therapy program should be weighed at intervals to determine their progress. Prenatal patients are weighed during each prenatal visit. A sudden gain in weight may indicate edema.

The weight of an adult patient is usually measured during each office visit, whereas adult height is typically measured only during the first visit or when a complete physical examination of the patient is requested. Children are weighed and measured during each office visit to observe their pattern of growth and to calculate medication dosage.

The weight can be compared against a standardized chart that serves as a general guide to determine whether the patient's weight falls within normal limits (Table 4-2).

Text continued on page 133

Guidelines for Measuring Weight and Height

The following guidelines should be followed when using an upright balance scale to measure weight and height.

WEIGHT

1. **Locate the scale to provide for patient privacy.** Place the scale on a hard, level surface in a private location. Many patients are self-conscious about having their weight measured and prefer that it be done in privacy. Be careful not to make weight-sensitive comments during the procedure. This is especially important for patients with weight control problems such as obesity or eating disorders.

2. **Balance the scale before measuring weight.** If the scale is not balanced, the weight measurement will be inaccurate. The scale is balanced when the upper and lower weights are on zero and the indicator point comes to a rest at the center of the balance area.

3. **Assist the patient.** Make sure to assist the patient on and off the scale platform. The scale platform moves slightly and, therefore, may cause the patient to become unsteady.

4. **Obtain an accurate estimation of the patient's weight.** The patient's weight should be measured in normal clothing. The patient should be asked to remove any heavy outer clothing, such as a sweater or a jacket. The patient should always be asked to remove his or her shoes.

5. **Interpret the calibration markings accurately.** The lower calibration bar is divided into 50-pound increments (see Fig. 4–2A). The upper calibration bar is divided into pounds and quarter pounds. The longer calibration lines indicate pound increments and the shorter calibration lines indicate quarter-pound and half-pound increments. (Fig. 4–2B).

6. **Determine the patient's weight correctly.** The patient's weight is determined by adding the measurement on the lower scale to the measurement on the upper scale. The results should be determined to the nearest quarter pound. Occasionally, the patient's

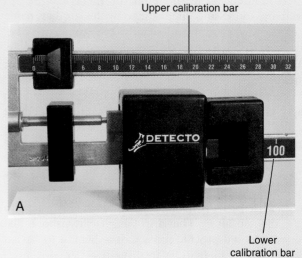

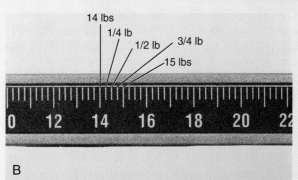

■ **FIGURE 4–2.** Calibration markings for measuring weight on an upright balance scale. *A,* The upper calibration bar is divided into pounds and quarter pounds. *B,* The longer calibration lines indicate pound increments, and the shorter calibration lines indicate quarter-pound and half-pound increments.

weight may need to be converted to kilograms; for example, when determining medication dosage. Refer to the following box for the method used to convert weight from one system to the other.

Weight and Height Conversion

WEIGHT CONVERSION:

Converting pounds to kilograms:
Divide the number of pounds by 2.2

Converting kilograms to pounds:
Multiply the number of kilograms by 2.2

HEIGHT

1. **Provide for the patient's safety.** The medical assistant must be very careful to follow the proper procedure when measuring the patient's height. An example of errors in technique that could result in a

HEIGHT CONVERSION:

To convert inches to centimeters:
Multiply the number of inches by 2.5

To convert centimeters to inches:
Divide the number of centimeters by 2.5

facial injury are as follows: The patient is placed on the scale in a forward position, and the measuring bar is opened up into the patient's face.

Guidelines for Measuring Weight and Height *Continued*

2. **Determine the calibration markings accurately.** Depending on the brand of scale, the calibration markings are divided into either (1) inches or (2) feet and inches (Fig. 4–3). The calibration rod is also calibrated into centimeters, although this unit of measurement is not typically used to measure height.

3. **Read the measurement correctly.** For most patients, the height measurement is read at the junction of the of the stationary calibration rod and the moveable calibration rod (Fig 4–4A). However, if the patient's height is less than the top value of the stationary calibration rod, the measurement is read directly on the stationary rod. For example, (on most scales,) the highest calibration on the stationary rod is 50 inches; therefore, patients with a height of 50 inches or less will have their height read directly off of the stationary rod (Fig. 4–4B).

4. **Record the height measurement correctly.** The height measurement should be recorded in feet and inches. If the scale is calibrated in inches, the reading must be converted to feet and inches by dividing the number of inches by 12. For example, a height measurement of 60 inches is recorded as 5 feet (60 inches divided by 12 equals 5). If the patient's height measurement is 64 inches, the results would be recorded as 5 feet, 4 inches.

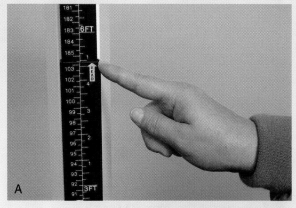

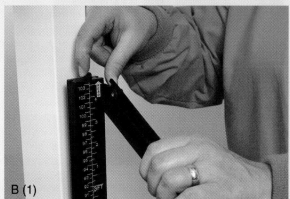

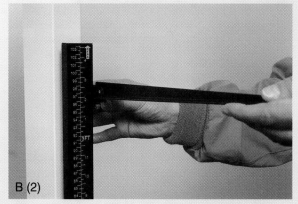

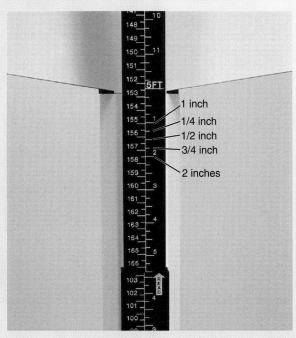

■ FIGURE 4–3. Calibration markings for measuring height on an upright balance scale.

■ FIGURE 4–4. *A,* Reading a height measurement at the junction of the stationary calibration rod and the moveable calibration rod. The height measurement in this illustration is 6 feet and 1 inch. *B(1),* Reading a height measurement on the stationary calibration rod. *Note:* The measuring bar must first be released and moved down to the stationary bar to measure the patient's height. *B(2),* The height is then read at the junction of the bar and the rod. The height measurement in this illustration is 3 feet and 2 inches.

PROCEDURE

4–1

Measuring Weight and Height

EQUIPMENT/SUPPLIES: **Upright balance scale**

WEIGHT

1. **Procedural Step.** Wash the hands.
2. **Procedural Step.** Check the scale to make sure it is balanced as follows:
   a. Make sure the upper and lower weights are on zero. When the weights are on zero, they will be all the way to the left side of the calibration bars.
   b. Look at the indicator point. If the scale is balanced, the indicator point will be resting in the center of the balance area.
   c. If the indicator point rests below the center, adjust the screw on the balance knob by turning it in a clockwise direction (to the right) until the indicator point rests in the center of the balance area.
   d. If the indicator point rests above the center, adjust the screw on the balance knob by turning it

in a counterclockwise direction (to the left) until the indicator point rests in the center of the balance area.
Principle. If the scale is not balanced, the weight measurement will be inaccurate.
3. **Procedural Step.** Greet and identify the patient.
4. **Procedural Step.** Introduce yourself and explain to the patient that you will be measuring his or her height and weight.
5. **Procedural Step.** Instruct the patient to remove his or her shoes and any heavy outer clothing such as a jacket or sweater. A good medical aseptic practice is to place a paper towel on the platform of the scale to protect the patient's feet.
Principle. Removing heavy clothing and shoes provides a more accurate estimation of the patient's weight.

4

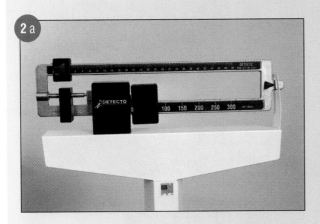

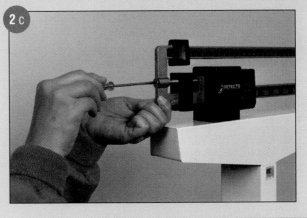

6. **Procedural Step.** Assist the patient onto the scale, and instruct the patient not to move.
   Principle. It is not possible to balance the scale if the patient is moving.

7. **Procedural Step.** Balance the scale as follows:
   a. Move the lower weight to the 50-pound notched groove that does not cause the indicator point to drop to the bottom of the calibration area. Make sure the lower weight is seated firmly in its groove.
   b. Slide the upper weight slowly along its calibration bar by tapping it gently until the indicator point comes to a rest at the center of the balance area.
   Principle. Not seating the lower weight firmly in its groove results in an inaccurate reading.

8. **Procedural Step.** Read the results to the nearest quarter pound by adding the measurement on the lower scale to the measurement on the upper scale.

9. **Procedural Step.** Assist the patient off of the scale platform.

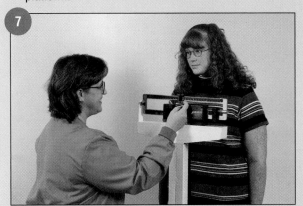

HEIGHT

1. **Procedural Step.** Slide the moveable calibration rod upward until the measuring bar is well above the patient's apparent height. Open the measuring bar to its horizontal position.

2. **Procedural Step.** Instruct the patient to step onto the scale platform with his or her back to the scale. Provide assistance if needed. Instruct the patient to stand erect and to look straight ahead.

   Principle. Asking the patient to look straight ahead ensures an accurate measurement.

3. **Procedural Step.** Carefully lower the measuring bar (while keeping it horizontal) until it rests gently on top of the patient's head.

4. **Procedural Step.** While still keeping the measuring bar in a horizontal position, instruct the patient to step down and put on his or her shoes. Be sure to hold the bar in a horizontal position until the patient has stepped off the scale.

4

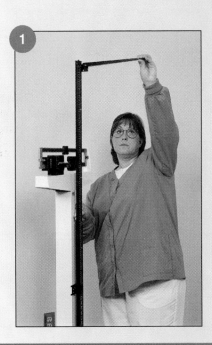

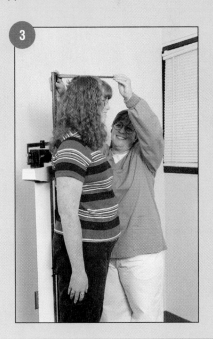

Continued

5. Procedural Step. Read the height measurement to the nearest quarter inch, marking at the junction of the stationary calibration rod and the movable cali-

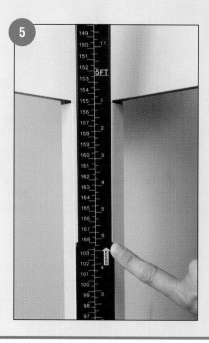

bration rod. (Note: If the patient's height is less than the top value of the stationary rod, the measurement is read directly on the stationary calibration rod.)

6. Procedural Step. Chart the weight and height measurements. The weight should be charted in pounds to the nearest quarter pound and the height should be charted in feet and inches to the nearest quarter inch.

7. Procedural Step. Return the weights to zero. Return the measuring bar to its vertical (resting) position, and slide the movable calibration rod to its lowest position.

CHARTING EXAMPLE

Date	
11/5/2002	10:15 a.m. Wt: 155. Ht: 5' 6¼" ————
	——————————————— J. Smith, CMA

4

Highlight on Interpreting Body Weight

There are various ways used to interpret body weight. The methods used are described in this box.

HEIGHT AND WEIGHT TABLES

One way to interpret body weight is through the use of standardized height and weight tables. In 1959, the Metropolitan Life Insurance Company (MET) issued a set of height and weight tables indicating desirable weight ranges for men and women. In 1983, MET issued revised height and weight tables that listed desirable weight for men and women that were higher than those shown in the 1959 table. Many health experts believe that the desirable weight ranges of the revised tables are too high and, therefore, do not accurately represent healthy body weight.

In 1995, the United States Department of Agriculture (USDA) and the Department of Health and Human Services (DHHS) issued a set of weight guidelines (refer to Table 4–2), that are lower than those of the MET tables. The USDA/DHHS guidelines do not distinguish between weights of men and women, and therefore, must be interpreted by each individual as follows. Women usually have smaller bones and less muscle than men, so they should use the lower end of the range. Men and large-boned muscular women should use the higher end of the weight range to find their healthy body weights.

BODY MASS INDEX (BMI)

Another method for interpreting body weight is the body mass index, or BMI. The BMI expresses the relationship between a individual's weight relative to his or her height. Except for trained athletes, the BMI strongly correlates with total body fat content in adults. This, in turn, provides an indication of the risk of developing chronic health conditions associated with obesity. Many health experts believe that the BMI is a more accurate standard for interpreting body weight than height and weight tables.

Highlight on Interpreting Body Weight *Continued*

Method for Calculating BMI

Use the following steps to calculate your BMI:

Step 1. Multiply your weight in pounds (without clothes or shoes) by 703.

Example for an individual with a weight of 135 pounds:

$$135 \times 703 = 94,905$$

Step 2. Divide this number by your height in inches.
Example for an individual with a height of 66 inches:

$$94,905 \div 66 \text{ inches} = 1438$$

Step 3. Divide this amount again by your height in inches and round off to the nearest whole number:

$$1438 \div 66 = 21.79 \text{ or } 22$$

The BMI of this individual is 22.

Interpretation of the BMI

In June 1998, the National Heart, Lung, and Blood Institute (NHLBI), a federal health agency, issued a set of guidelines for the identification of healthy body weight, overweight, and obesity in adults. One of these guidelines relates to the interpretation of the BMI as is outlined next.

BMI	Interpretation	Health Risk
24 or less	Healthy Weight	Minimal Health Risk
25 to 29.9	Overweight	Low to Moderate Health Risk
30 or more	Obesity	High Health Risk

According to the above NHLBI interpretation, an estimated 97 million adults, or 55 percent of the population, in the United States are overweight or obese. Obesity is associated with higher death rates and, after smoking, is the second leading cause of preventable death in the United States today.

It has been determined that as the BMI rises above normal, there is an increased risk of developing certain diseases associated with overweight and obesity including:

Hypertension
Cardiovascular disease
Dyslipidemia (high blood cholesterol levels and/or high blood triglyceride levels, or both)
Type II diabetes
Sleep apnea
Osteoarthritis
Female infertility

The NHLBI recommends that the BMI be determined in all adults. People of normal weight should have their BMI reassessed every 2 years.

4

POSITIONING AND DRAPING

☐ Correct positioning of the patient facilitates the examination by permitting better access to the part being examined or treated. The basic positions commonly used in the medical office are the supine, prone, dorsal recumbent, lithotomy, Sims, knee-chest and Fowler's.

The position used depends on the type of examination or procedure to be performed. More than one position may be used to examine the same body part during the physical examination. For example, the sitting and supine positions are both used to examine the chest. It is important to know the correct position for each examination or treatment. When positioning a patient, the medical assistant should explain the position to the patient and assist the patient in attaining it.

It is important to take the patient's endurance and degree of wellness into consideration when positioning a patient. Patients who are weak or ill may not be able to assume a position or may require special assistance in attaining it. Some of the positions, such as the lithotomy and knee-chest, are embarrassing and uncomfortable. Therefore, a patient should not be kept in this position any longer than necessary. Some patients (especially elderly ones) become dizzy after being in certain positions such as knee-chest. These patients should be allowed to rest before getting off the examining table.

The patient is draped during positioning to provide for modesty, comfort, and warmth. The part to be examined is the only part that should be exposed. Patient gowns and drapes used in the medical office are usually made of paper but may also be made of cloth.

The procedures for positioning and draping the patient are presented on the following pages.

Text continued on page 143

PROCEDURE

4-2

Sitting Position

Purpose: The sitting position is used to examine the head, neck, chest, and upper extremities and to measure vital signs.

EQUIPMENT/SUPPLIES:	**Examining table** **Patient gown** **Patient drape**

1. **Procedural Step.** Wash hands. Greet and identify the patient. Introduce yourself.
2. **Procedural Step.** Explain to the patient what type of examination or procedure will be performed.
3. **Procedural Step.** Provide the patient with a patient gown. Instruct the patient to remove clothing appropriate for the type of examination being performed and to put on the patient gown with the opening in front. The disrobing facility should provide privacy, a place to sit, and a place for hanging clothing.

4. **Procedural Step.** Pull out the footrest of the examining table, and assist the patient into a sitting position. The patient's buttocks and thighs should be firmly supported on the edge of the table.
5. **Procedural Step.** Place a drape over the patient's thighs and legs to provide warmth and modesty.
6. **Procedural Step.** After completion of the examination, assist the patient down from the table. Instruct the patient to get dressed. Return the footrest to its normal position.

4

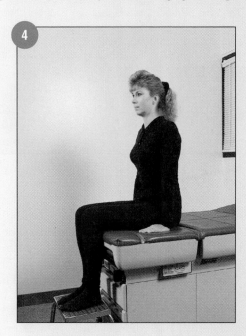

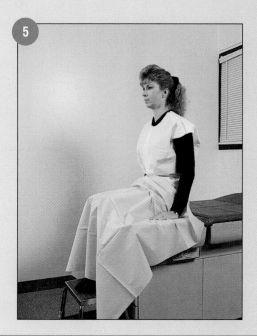

4–3

Supine Position

Purpose: The supine position is used to examine the head, chest, abdomen, and extremities.

EQUIPMENT/SUPPLIES: **Examining table**   **Patient drape**
Patient gown

1. **Procedural Step.** Wash hands. Greet and identify the patient. Introduce yourself.
2. **Procedural Step.** Explain to the patient what type of examination or procedure will be performed.
3. **Procedural Step.** Provide the patient with a patient gown. Instruct the patient to remove clothing appropriate for the type of examination being performed and to put on the patient gown with the opening in front. The disrobing facility should provide privacy, a place to sit, and a place for hanging clothing.
4. **Procedural Step.** Pull out the footrest of the examining table, and assist the patient into a sitting position.
5. **Procedural Step.** Ask the patient to move back on the table. As the patient is doing this, pull out the table extension while supporting the patient's lower legs.

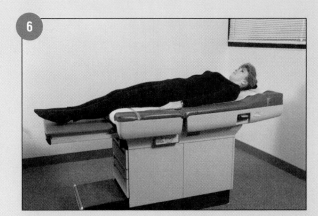

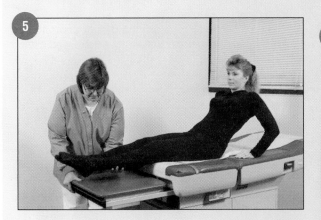

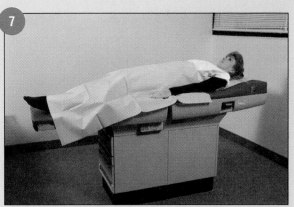

6. **Procedural Step.** Ask the patient to lie down on his or her back with the legs together. Provide assistance if needed. The arms may be placed above the head or alongside the body.
7. **Procedural Step.** Place a drape over the patient to provide warmth and modesty. As the physician examines the patient, move the drape according to the body parts being examined.

8. **Procedural Step.** After completion of the examination, assist the patient back into a sitting position. Slide the table extension back into place while supporting the patient's lower legs.
9. **Procedural Step.** Assist the patient down from the table. Instruct the patient to get dressed. Return the footrest to its normal position.

PROCEDURE

4–4

Prone Position

Purpose: The prone position is used to examine the back and to assess extension of the hip joint.

EQUIPMENT/SUPPLIES: **Examining table**   **Patient drape**
Patient gown

1. **Procedural Step.** Wash hands. Greet and identify the patient. Introduce yourself.
2. **Procedural Step.** Explain to the patient what type of examination or procedure will be performed.
3. **Procedural Step.** Provide the patient with a patient gown. Instruct the patient to remove clothing appropriate for the type of examination being performed and to put on the patient gown with the opening in back. The disrobing facility should provide privacy, a place to sit, and a place for hanging clothing.
4. **Procedural Step.** Pull out the footrest of the examining table, and assist the patient into a sitting position.
5. **Procedural Step.** Ask the patient to move back on the table. As the patient is doing this, pull out the table extension while supporting the patient's lower legs.
6. **Procedural Step.** Ask the patient to lie down on his or her back. Provide assistance, if needed.

7. **Procedural Step.** Ask the patient to turn his or her body over and lie on the abdomen with the legs together and the head turned to one side. Provide assistance for this step. The arms can be placed above the head or alongside the body.
   Principle. Assistance should be provided to prevent the patient from accidentally rolling off the table.
8. **Procedural Step.** Place a drape over the patient to provide warmth and modesty. As the physician examines the patient, move the drape according to the body parts being examined.
9. **Procedural Step.** After completion of the examination, assist the patient back into a supine position and then into a sitting position. Slide the table extension back into place while supporting the patient's lower legs.
10. **Procedural Step.** Assist the patient down from the table. Instruct the patient to get dressed. Return the footrest to its normal position.

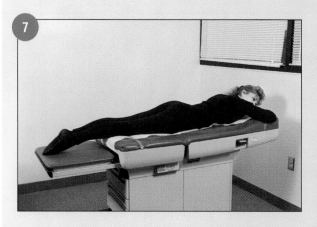

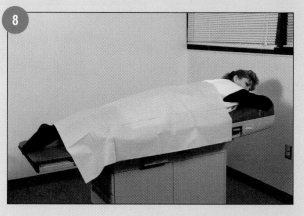

PROCEDURE

Dorsal Recumbent Position

Purpose: The dorsal recumbent position is used for vaginal or rectal examinations, for the insertion of a catheter, and to examine the head, neck, chest, and extremities in patients who have difficulty maintaining the supine position. The supine position is not a comfortable position for patients with respiratory problems, a back injury, or low back pain. Bending the legs (rather than lying flat) is more comfortable for these patients and is easier to maintain.

EQUIPMENT/SUPPLIES:	**Examining table**	**Patient drape**
	Patient gown	

1. **Procedural Step.** Wash hands. Greet and identify the patient. Introduce yourself.
2. **Procedural Step.** Explain what type of examination or procedure will be performed.
3. **Procedural Step.** Provide the patient with a patient gown. Instruct the patient to remove clothing appropriate for the type of examination being performed and to put on the patient gown with the opening in front. The disrobing facility should provide privacy, a place to sit, and a place for hanging clothing.
4. **Procedural Step.** Pull out the footrest of the examining table, and assist the patient into a sitting position.
5. **Procedural Step.** Ask the patient to move back on the table. As the patient is doing this, pull out the table extension while supporting the patient's lower legs.
6. **Procedural Step.** Ask the patient to lie down on his or her back. Provide assistance if needed. The arms can be placed above the head or alongside the body.
7. **Procedural Step.** Place a drape over the patient to provide warmth and modesty. The drape should

be positioned diagonally, with one corner over the patient's chest and the opposite corner over the pubic area.

8. **Procedural Step.** Ask the patient to bend the knees and place each foot at the edge of the examining table with the soles of the feet flat on the table. Provide assistance during this step. Push in the table extension and the footrest.
9. **Procedural Step.** When the physician is ready to examine the genital area, the center corner of the drape is folded back over the abdomen.

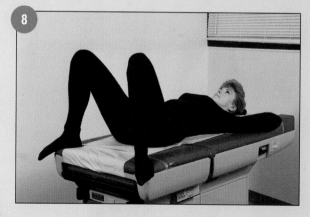

10. **Procedural Step.** After completion of the examination, pull out the footrest and the table extension. Assist the patient back into a supine position and then into a sitting position. Slide the table extension back into place while supporting the patient's lower legs.
11. **Procedural Step.** Assist the patient down from the table. Instruct the patient to get dressed. Return the footrest to its normal position.

4

PROCEDURE

4-6

Lithotomy Position

Purpose: The lithotomy position is used for vaginal, pelvic, or rectal examinations. The lithotomy position is the same as the dorsal recumbent position except that the patient's feet are placed in stirrups. The lithotomy position provides maximum exposure to the genital area and facilitates insertion of a vaginal speculum.

EQUIPMENT/SUPPLIES: **Examining table**   **Patient drape**
Patient gown

1. **Procedural Step.** Wash hands. Greet and identify the patient. Introduce yourself.
2. **Procedural Step.** Explain what type of examination or procedure will be performed.
3. **Procedural Step.** Provide the patient with a patient gown. Instruct the patient to remove clothing appropriate for the type of examination being performed and to put on the patient gown with the opening in front. The disrobing facility should provide privacy, a place to sit, and a place for hanging clothing.
4. **Procedural Step.** Pull out the footrest of the examining table, and assist the patient into a sitting position.
5. **Procedural Step.** Ask the patient to move back on the table. As the patient is doing this, pull out the table extension while supporting the patient's lower legs.
6. **Procedural Step.** Ask the patient to lie down on the back. Provide assistance if needed. The arms can be placed above the head or alongside the body.

7. **Procedural Step.** Place a drape over the patient to provide warmth and modesty. The drape should be positioned diagonally with one corner over the patient's chest and the opposite corner over the pubic area.
8. **Procedural Step.** Ask the patient to bend the knees and place each foot at the edge of the examining table, with the soles of the feet flat on the table. Provide assistance during this step. Push in the table extension and the footrest.
9. **Procedural Step.** Position the stirrups so that they are level with the examining table and pulled out approximately 1 foot from the edge of the table.
10. **Procedural Step.** Ask the patient to move the feet into the stirrups. Provide assistance during this step.
11. **Procedural Step.** Instruct the patient to slide the buttocks to the edge of the examining table and to rotate the thighs outward as far as is comfortable.

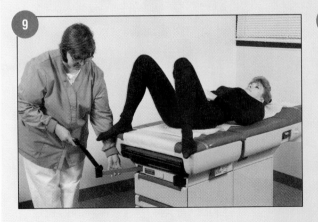

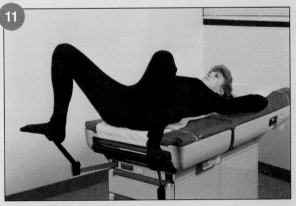

PROCEDURE 4–6

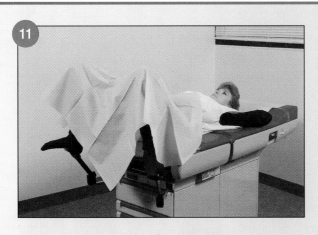

11

12. Procedural Step. When the physician is ready to examine the genital area, the center corner of the drape is folded back over the abdomen.

13. Procedural Step. After completion of the examination, ask the patient to slide the buttocks back from the end of the table. Pull out the footrest and table extension. Lift the patient's legs out of the stirrups at the same time, and place them on the table extension (supine position). Return the stirrups to their normal position. Assist the patient into a sitting position. Slide the table extension back into place while supporting the patient's lower legs.
Principle. When assisting the patient out of the stirrups, both the patient's legs should be lifted at the same time to avoid strain on the back and abdominal muscles.

14. Procedural Step. Assist the patient down from the table. Instruct the patient to get dressed. Return the footrest to its normal position.

PROCEDURE

4–7

Sims Position

Purpose: Sims position, also known as the left lateral position, is used to examine the vagina or rectum, to measure rectal temperature, to perform a flexible sigmoidoscopy, or to administer an enema.

4

EQUIPMENT/SUPPLIES:	**Examining table**	**Patient drape**
	Patient gown	

1. Procedural Step. Wash hands. Greet and identify the patient. Introduce yourself.

2. Procedural Step. Explain what type of examination or procedure will be performed.

3. Procedural Step. Provide the patient with a patient gown. Instruct the patient to remove clothing from the waist down and to put on the patient gown with the opening in back. The disrobing facility should provide privacy, a place to sit, and a place for hanging clothing.

4. Procedural Step. Pull out the footrest of the examining table, and assist the patient into a sitting position.

5. Procedural Step. Ask the patient to move back on the table. As the patient is doing this, pull out the table extension while supporting the patient's lower legs.

6. Procedural Step. Ask the patient to lie down on his or her back. Provide assistance, if needed.

7. Procedural Step. Place a drape over the patient to provide warmth and modesty.

Continued

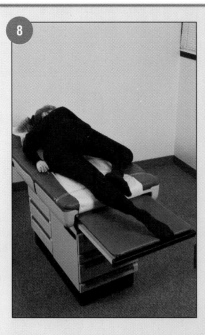

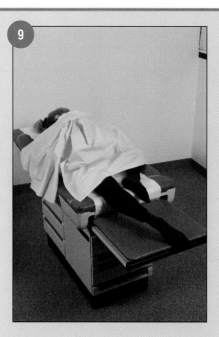

8. **Procedural Step.** Ask the patient to turn on his or her left side. Provide assistance during this step to prevent the patient from accidentally rolling off the table. The left arm should be positioned behind the body and the right arm forward with the elbow bent. Assist the patient in flexing the legs. The right leg is flexed sharply and the left leg is flexed slightly.

9. **Procedural Step.** Adjust the drape as needed. When the physician is ready to examine the patient, a small portion of the drape is folded back to expose the anal area.

10. **Procedural Step.** After completion of the examination, assist the patient back into a supine position and then into a sitting position. Slide the table extension back into place while supporting the patient's lower legs.

11. **Procedural Step.** Assist the patient down from the table. Instruct the patient to get dressed. Return the footrest to its normal position.

4

4-8

Knee-Chest Position

Purpose: The knee-chest position is used to examine the rectum or to perform a proctoscopic examination because it provides maximal exposure to the rectal area. This is a difficult position to maintain; therefore, the patient should not be put into this position until just before the examination.

EQUIPMENT/SUPPLIES:	Examining table Patient drape
	Patient gown

1. **Procedural Step.** Wash hands. Greet and identify the patient. Introduce yourself.

2. **Procedural Step.** Explain what type of examination or procedure will be performed.

3. **Procedural Step.** Provide the patient with a patient gown. Instruct the patient to remove clothing from the waist down and to put on the patient gown with the opening in back. The disrobing facility

PROCEDURE 4–8

should provide privacy, a place to sit, and a place for hanging clothing.

4. **Procedural Step.** Pull out the footrest of the examining table, and assist the patient into a sitting position.

5. **Procedural Step.** Ask the patient to move back on the table. As the patient is doing this, pull out the table extension while supporting the patient's lower legs.

6. **Procedural Step.** Assist the patient into the supine position and then into the prone position. Place a drape over the patient to provide warmth and modesty.

7. **Procedural Step.** Ask the patient to bend the arms at the elbows and rest them alongside of the head. Next ask the patient to elevate the buttocks while keeping the back straight. The patient's head should be turned to one side, and the weight of the body should be supported by the chest. A pillow can be used under the chest for additional support and to promote relaxation. The knees and lower legs are separated approximately 12 inches.

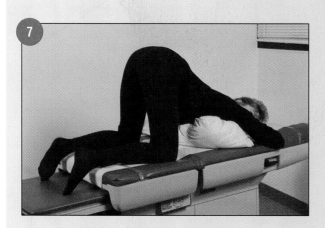

8. **Procedural Step.** Position the drape diagonally with one corner over the patient's back and the opposite corner over the buttocks. When the physician is ready to examine the patient, a small portion of the drape is folded back to expose the anal area.

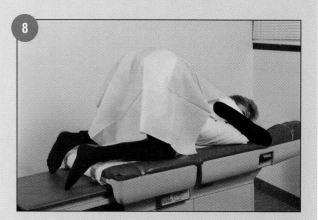

9. **Procedural Step.** After completion of the examination, assist the patient back into a prone position and then into a supine position. Allow the patient to rest in the supine position before sitting up. **Principle.** Patients (especially elderly ones) frequently become dizzy after being in the knee-chest position and should be allowed to rest before sitting up.

10. **Procedural Step.** Assist the patient into a sitting position. Slide the table extension back into place while supporting the patient's lower legs.

11. **Procedural Step.** Assist the patient down from the table. Instruct the patient to get dressed. Return the footrest to its normal position.

4

PROCEDURE

4–9

Fowler's Position

Purpose: Fowler's position is used to examine the upper body on patients with cardiovascular and respiratory problems. These patients find it easier to breathe in this position as compared with a sitting or supine position. This position is also used to draw blood from patients who are likely to faint.

EQUIPMENT/SUPPLIES: Examining table   Patient drape
Patient gown

1. **Procedural Step.** Wash hands. Greet and identify the patient. Introduce yourself.
2. **Procedural Step.** Explain what type of examination or procedure will be performed.
3. **Procedural Step.** Provide the patient with a patient gown. Instruct the patient to remove clothing appropriate for the type of examination being performed and to put on the patient gown with the opening in front. The disrobing facility should provide privacy, a place to sit, and a place for hanging clothing.
4. **Procedural Step.** Position the head of the table as follows:
   a. For a semi-Fowler's position, the table should be positioned at a 45-degree angle.
   b. For a full Fowler's position, the table should be positioned at a 90-degree angle.
5. **Procedural Step.** Pull out the footrest of the examining table, and assist the patient into a sitting position.
6. **Procedural Step.** Pull out the table extension while supporting the patient's lower legs. Ask the patient to lean back against the table head. Provide assistance during this step.
7. **Procedural Step.** Place a drape over the patient to provide warmth and modesty. As the physician examines the patient, move the drape according to the body parts being examined.
8. **Procedural Step.** After completion of the examination, assist the patient back into a sitting position. Slide the table extension back into place while supporting the patient's lower legs.
9. **Procedural Step.** Assist the patient down from the table. Instruct the patient to get dressed. Return the head of the table and the footrest to their normal positions.

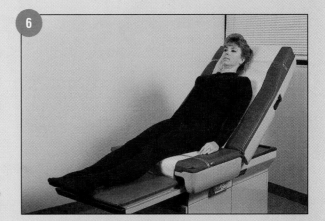

6

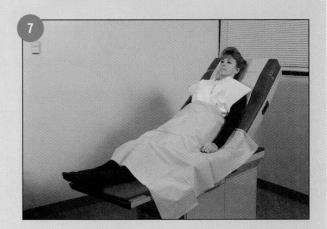

7

4

MEMORIES *from* EXTERNSHIP

HOPE FAUBER. *During my externship at a student health center at a four-year college, I was responsible for working up patients for gynecologic examinations. The drapes were two piece with the top opening in the front and the bottom opening in the back. After explaining this to an Asian student who spoke very little English, I noticed that she had the openings opposite of what I had explained. I explained again, with words and motions, that she needed to reverse the openings. To my surprise, she stood up, turned around in a circle, and sat down!*

ASSESSMENT OF THE PATIENT

☐ The extent of patient assessment during the physical examination depends on the purpose of the examina-

tion and the patient's condition. A complete physical examination involves a thorough assessment of all the body systems. Table 4–3 outlines the specific assessments included in a complete physical examination. In performing a physical examination, the physician uses an organized and systematic approach, starting with a examination of the patient's head and proceeding toward the feet. Using this type of approach facilitates the examination process and requires the fewest number of position changes by the patient.

The results of the physical examination are charted by the physician in the patient's medical record. Figure 4–5 is an example of a preprinted form used for this purpose.

Patients exhibiting symptoms of illness usually require only selected portions of the complete physical examination. For example, a patient who comes to the medical office with the symptoms of bronchitis usually will not require a complete physical examination; rather, the physician examines the body system most at risk for being abnormal.

Four assessment techniques are used to obtain information during the physical examination: inspection, palpation, percussion, and auscultation.

INSPECTION

Inspection involves observation of the patient for any signs of disease and, of the four assessment techniques, is the one most frequently used. Good lighting, either natural or artificial, is important for effective observa-

Text continued on page 148

4

TABLE 4–3

Patient Assessment During the Physical Examination

Body Structure	Assessment	Normal Findings	Abnormal Findings
General Appearance	Observation of body build, posture, and gait	Good posture and balance Steady gait	Poor posture or balance Unsteady, irregular, or staggering gait
	Determination of weight and height	Weight within ideal range	Patient is overweight or underweight
	Observation of hygiene and grooming	Good hygiene and grooming	Poor hygiene and grooming
	Observation for signs of illness	No signs of illness	Obvious signs of illness
	Observation of attitude, emotional state, and mood	Patient speaks clearly and is cooperative	Patients is uncooperative, withdrawn, incoherent, negative, or hostile
Skin	Inspection of the skin for color, vascularity, lesions	Smooth, supple, free of blemishes	Blisters, wounds, lesions, rashes, swelling
	Palpation of the temperature, moisture, turgor, and texture	Warm to the touch No unusual color	Rough, dry, flaky skin Unusual skin color such as flushing, cyanosis, jaundice, or pallor Poor skin turgor

Continued

TABLE 4–3

Patient Assessment During the Physical Examination *Continued*

Body Structure	Assessment	Normal Findings	Abnormal Findings
Arms and Hands	Inspection of the hands and arms for general appearance		Muscle weakness, lack of control or coordination
	Palpation of arm muscles	Firm, strong muscles	Restricted range of motion
	Palpation for tenderness or lumps	Normal range of motion in joints	Tenderness or lumps of the hands or arms
		Good muscle control and coordination	
	Inspection of the fingernails	Colorless nail plate with a convex curve	Indentation, infection, brittleness, thickening, or angulation of the nails
		Smooth nail texture	Cyanosis or pallor of the nails
Head and Neck	Inspection of the size, shape, and contour of the head	Round head with prominences in the front and back	Head is asymmetric or of unusual size
	Inspection of the hair and scalp	Hair is resilient, evenly distributed, and not excessively dry or oily	Loss of hair
	Palpation of the head and neck		Scaliness or dryness of the scalp
			Presence of lice or other parasites
	Palpation of the trachea		Lumps, swelling, tenderness, lesions of the head or neck
Eyes	Evaluation of visual acuity and color vision	Good visual ability with or without glasses or contact lenses	Poor visual acuity or blindness
		Appropriate color perception	Color blindness
	Evaluation of visual field	No visual field loss	Gaps in field of vision
	Inspection of the eyelids and eyeballs	Eyes are bright	Dull or glossy eyes
	Inspection of the conjunctiva	Pink mucous membranes	Inflamed mucous membranes
	Inspection of eye movements	Eyes move equally in all directions	Excessive tearing
	Tests for pupillary reaction using a penlight	Pupils are black, are equal in size, and react appropriately to light	Drainage from the eyes
	Inspection of the internal eye structures using an ophthalmoscope	Reddish pink retina, even caliber, and intact retinal blood vessels	Drooping eyelids
			Uncoordinated eye movements
			Dilated, constricted, or unequal pupils
			Cloudy lens or narrowed blood vessels
Ears	Test for hearing using a tuning fork or audiometer	Good hearing ability	Limited hearing or deafness
	Inspection of the size, shape, and symmetry of the ears	Ears are symmetric and proportionate to the head	Lesions, redness, or swelling of the external ear canal
	Inspection of the external ear canal and tympanic membrane using an otoscope	Cerumen is soft and easily removed	Drainage from the ear
		No drainage or discomfort	Pain when the ear is moved
		Skin of the ear canal is intact, pink, warm, and slightly moist	Impacted cerumen
		Tympanic membrane is pearly gray and semitransparent	Tympanic membrane is red, bulging, or perforated
Nose	Inspection of size, shape, and symmetry of the nose	Nose is symmetric, straight, nontender	Nose is asymmetric, deformed, flaring, or tender
	Inspection of the nostrils using a nasal speculum	Septum is intact and midline	Deviation or perforation of septum
	Test for the sense of smell	Nasal mucosa is moist and pink	Redness, swelling, polyps, or discharge
		Correct or very few incorrect responses to odors	

4

TABLE 4-3

Patient Assessment During the Physical Examination *Continued*

Body Structure	Assessment	Normal Findings	Abnormal Findings
Nose			Nostrils are obstructed Absent, decreased, exaggerated, or unequal responses to the test substances
Mouth and Pharynx	Inspection of the lips for contour, color, and texture Inspection of the mucosa Inspection of the gums and palate Inspection of the teeth Inspection of the tongue Inspection of the pharynx	Pink, moist, soft, smooth lips Pink, moist mucous membranes Smooth, pink, moist, firm gums Hard palate is firm and white Soft palate is pink and cushiony Smooth, white enamel; regularly spaced teeth or well-fitting dentures Moist, pink, slightly rough-surfaced tongue Pink and smooth pharynx Tonsils are pink and normal in size Gag reflex is present	Pallor, cyanosis, blisters, swelling, cracking, excessive dryness of lips Pale or dry mucosa with ulcers or abrasions Missing or loose teeth, dental caries, poor-fitting dentures Gums are red, bleeding, swollen, tender, spongy, or receding Tongue is dry, furry, smooth, red, or ulcerated Pharynx is red, swollen, or ulcerated Tonsils are red or swollen Absent gag reflex
Chest and Lungs	Inspection of the size and shape of the chest Inspection of the respiratory movements Assessment of respiratory rate, rhythm, and depth Percussion of the chest Auscultation of breath sounds Palpation of the ribs	Chest is symmetric Normal respiratory rate, rhythm, and depth Normal breath sounds No cough Ribs slope downward	Abnormal chest contour Labored, slow, rapid, or irregular respirations Flat or dull lung sounds Noisy breath sounds Productive or nonproductive cough Tenderness of the ribs
Heart	Auscultation of heart sounds Auscultation of apical pulse, rate, rhythm, and volume Palpation of peripheral pulses Auscultation of blood pressure Assessment of peripheral vascular perfusion Electrocardiogram to assess heart function	Normal heart sounds Regular, strong heart beats Blood pressure within normal range for age Palpable peripheral pulses Skin is pink, resilient, and moist Immediate return of color to nailbeds Normal heart function	Irregular heart beats or murmur Rates slower or more rapid than normal Weak or absent peripheral pulses Low or high blood pressure Cyanosis, pallor, edema Poor capillary filling in nailbeds Abnormal electrocardiogram
Breasts	Inspection of size, symmetry, and contour Inspection of the nipple Palpation of the breasts Palpation of axillary lymph nodes	Breasts are round, smooth, and symmetric Nipples are round and equal in size, are similar in color, and appear soft and smooth Areola is round and pink	Retraction, dimpling, redness, or swelling of the breasts Bleeding, cracking, discharge, or inversion of the nipples Lumps or tenderness of the breasts or axillary lymph nodes

4

Continued

TABLE 4 – 3

Patient Assessment During the Physical Examination *Continued*

Body Structure	Assessment	Normal Findings	Abnormal Findings
Abdomen	Inspection of contour, symmetry, skin condition, and integrity Auscultation of bowel sounds Percussion to assess underlying organs Palpation of underlying organs, tenderness, and lumps	Symmetric contour Unblemished skin Soft abdomen Active bowel sounds present Normal position and size of the liver and spleen	Asymmetric contour Rash or other skin lesions Abdominal distention Increased, diminished, or absent bowel sounds Tenderness or lumps Enlarged liver or spleen
Genitalia and Rectum	**Male:** Inspection of the penis and urethra Inspection of the scrotum and palpation of the testes Palpation of the rectum and prostate gland Stool specimen to test for occult blood	Penis is smooth Testicles are smooth, firm, and movable within the scrotal sac Scrotum is symmetric Increased pigmentation in the anal area Good anal sphincter tone	Ulceration or discharge from the penis Lumps or tenderness of the scrotum, testes, or prostate gland Enlarged prostate gland Hemorrhoids or relaxed anal sphincter Occult blood in the stool
	Female: Inspection of the external genitalia Inspection of the vagina and cervix using a vaginal speculum Specimen collection from the vagina and cervix for the Pap test Bimanual pelvic examination Palpation of the rectum Stool specimen to test for occult blood	External genitalia are smooth and without lesions Vaginal mucosa is pink and moist Cervix is pink and smooth Increased pigmentation in the anal area Good anal spincter tone	Ulceration or redness or swelling of the external genitalia Lacerations, tenderness, redness, or discharge from the vagina or cervix Tenderness or lumps of the uterus and ovaries Hemorrhoids or relaxed anal sphincter Occult blood in the stool
Lower Extremities	Inspection of the legs for general appearance Palpation of the legs Inspection of the toenails	Firm, strong muscles Normal range of motion in joints Smooth nail texture	Muscle weakness, lack of control or coordination Restricted range of motion Tenderness or lumps Limp or foot dragging during walking Indentation, infection, brittleness, thickening, or angulation of the nails
Neurologic	Determination of mental status and level of consciousness Determination of the sense of pain and touch Use of a percussion hammer to test reflexes	Alert and responds appropriately Oriented to person, place, and time Normal response to pain and touch Normal reflexes	Disoriented Responds inappropriately Diminished or absent response to stimuli Abnormal or absent reflexes

4

PHYSICAL EXAMINATION

INSTRUCTIONS:
(WNL) Within Normal Limits
(POS) Positive findings (X) Omitted

1. GENERAL

a. Posture _____
b. Gait _____
c. Speech _____
d. Appearance _____
e. Emotion _____

2. HEAD

a. Hair _____
b. Masses _____
c. Shape _____
d. Bruits _____
e. Tenderness _____
f. Sinus _____
g. Articulations _____

3. EYES

a. Lids   R ___ L ___   f. Pupils R ___ L ___
b. Sclera   R ___ L ___   g. Fundi   R ___ L ___
c. Conjunctiva R ___ L ___   h. Light   R ___ L ___
d. Muscles   R ___ L ___   i. Bruit   R ___ L ___
e. Cornea   R ___ L ___
               j. Accommodation R ___ L ___

4. EARS

a. Pinna R ___ L ___
b. Canal R ___ L ___
c. Drum   R ___ L ___
d. Weber _____
e. Rinne _____

5. NOSE

a. Septum _____
b. Mucosa R ___ L ___
c. Obstruction ___

6. MOUTH/THROAT

a. Lips _____   f. Teeth _____
b. Breath _____   g. Dentures _____
c. Tongue _____   h. Caries _____
d. Pharynx _____   i. Larynx _____
e. Tonsils _____   j. Floor _____

7. NECK

a. Thyroid _____   d. Nodes R ___ L ___
b. Trachea _____   e. Bruits R ___ L ___
c. Veins _____   f. Carotid R ___ L ___

8. LUNGS

a. Chest _____   e. Bruit _____
b. Symmetry _____   f. Sounds _____
c. Diaphragm _____ g. Fremitus _____
d. Rubs _____

9. HEART

a. PMI _____   e. Rub _____
b. Rate _____   f. Murmur _____
c. Rhythm _____   g. Palpation _____
d. Thrill _____

10. BREASTS

a. Nodes   R ___ L ___
b. Nipple R ___ L ___
c. Areolar R ___ L ___
d. Symmetry _____
e. Discharge _____

11. ABDOMEN

a. Sounds _____   e. Hernia   R ___ L ___
b. Masses _____   f. Bruit   R ___ L ___
c. Tenderness _____ g. Femoral   R ___ L ___
d. Organs _____   h. Ing. Nodes R ___ L ___

12. MUSCULOSKELETAL

a. Cervical _____
b. Thoracic _____
c. Lumbar _____
d. Sacral _____
e. Pelvic _____
f. Rib Cage _____

13. FEMALE GENITALS

a. Labia _____   e. Cervix _____
b. Bartholin _____   f. Uterus _____
   gland   g. Adnexa _____
c. Urethra _____   R ___ L ___
d. Vagina _____   h. Pap smear
                        done _____

14. MALE GENITALS

a. Penis _____   e. Scars _____
b. Scrotum _____   f. Meatus _____
c. Testicles _____ g. Epididymis _____
d. Discharge _____

15. RECTAL

a. Masses _____   f. Fissure _____
b. Anus _____   g. Hemorrhoids _____
c. Sphincter _____ h. Sigmoid _____
d. Prostate _____   _____ cm.
e. Pilonidal _____ i. Mucosa _____
                    j. Other _____

16. SKIN

a. Scars _____
b. Marks _____
c. Texture _____
d. Sweat _____
e. Color _____
f. Ulcers _____

17. NEUROLOGICAL

	Strength*	Reflex**
a. Biceps	R ___ L ___	R ___ L ___
b. Triceps	R ___ L ___	R ___ L ___
c. Knee	R ___ L ___	R ___ L ___
d. Ankle	R ___ L ___	R ___ L ___

e. Romberg _____   i. Coordination _____
f. Babinsky _____ j. Tremor _____
g. Cranial N _____ k. Vibratory _____
h. Sensory _____

*When testing strength use grades:
  Weak (W); Normal (N); Strong (S)

**When testing reflexes use:
  Absent (A); Present (P); Brisk (B)

18. EXTREMITIES

a. Range of Motion
   Shoulder _____   Knee _____
   Elbow _____   Ankle _____
   Wrist _____   Hand _____
   Hip _____   Foot _____
                    Phalanges _____

b. General   UR ___ UL ___ LR ___ LL ___
c. Muscular   UR ___ UL ___ LR ___ LL ___
d. Bruits   UR ___ UL ___ LR ___ LL ___
e. Edema   UR ___ UL ___ LR ___ LL ___
f. Varicosities UR ___ UL ___ LR ___ LL ___

Signature _____

FIGURE 4–5. Example of a preprinted form for recording the results of the physical examination.

4

tion. The patient's color, speech, deformities, skin condition (rashes, scars, warts), body contour and symmetry, orientation to the surroundings, body movements, and anxiety level are assessed through inspection. The medical assistant should develop a high level of detailed observational skills to assist the physician in assessing physical characteristics.

PALPATION

Palpation is the examination of the body using the sense of touch (Fig. 4–6). The physician uses palpation to determine the placement and size of organs, the presence of any lumps, or the existence of pain, swelling, or tenderness. Examining the breasts and taking the pulse are performed by palpation. Palpation often helps verify data obtained during inspection. The patient's verbal and facial expressions are also observed during palpation to assist in the detection of abnormalities.

There are two types of palpation, categorized by the amount of pressure applied: light and deep. **Light palpation** of structures is performed to determine areas of tenderness. The fingertips are placed on the part to be examined and are gently depressed approximately one half inch. **Deep palpation** is used to examine the condition of organs such as those in the abdomen. Two hands are used for deep palpation. One hand is used to support the body from below and the other hand is used to press over the area to be palpated. For example, deep palpation is used by the physician to perform a bimanual pelvic examination.

PERCUSSION

Percussion involves tapping the patient with the fingers and listening to the sounds produced to determine the

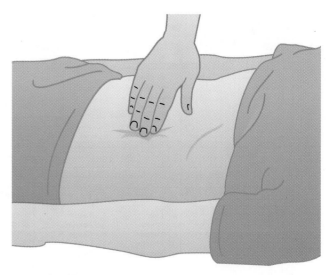

■ **FIGURE 4–6.** Palpation is the examination of the body using the sense of touch.

size, density, and location of underlying organs. This technique is often used to examine the lungs and abdomen.

The fingertips are used to produce a sound vibration similar to that of tapping a drumstick on a drum. The nondominant hand is placed directly on the area to be assessed, with the fingers slightly separated. The dominant hand is used to strike the joint of the middle finger placed on the patient to produce the sound vibration (Fig. 4–7). Structures that are dense, such as the liver, produce a dull sound. Empty or air-filled structures, such as the lungs, produce a hollow sound. Any condition that changes the density of an organ or tissue, such as fluid in the lungs, will cause a change in the quality of the sound.

■ **FIGURE 4–7.** Percussion involves tapping the patient with the fingers. *A,* The nondominant hand is placed directly on the area to be assessed, with the fingers slightly separated. *B,* The fingers of the dominant hand are used to strike the joint of the middle finger to produce a sound vibration.

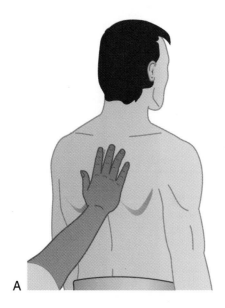

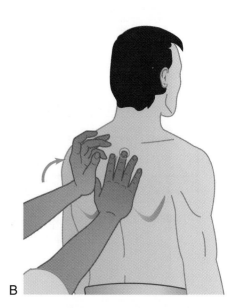

A   B

AUSCULTATION

Auscultation is an examination technique that involves listening with a stethoscope to the sounds produced within the body. This technique is used to listen to the heart and lungs or to measure blood pressure. Environmental noise interferes with effective auscultation of body sounds and, therefore, should be minimized as much as possible. The diaphragm of the stethoscope chestpiece is used to assess high-pitched sounds such as lung and bowel sounds; the bell of the stethoscope chestpiece is used to assess low-pitched sounds such as those produced by the heart or vascular system. The chestpiece should be warmed with the hand before placing it to avoid chilling the patient.

ASSISTING THE PHYSICIAN

☐ During the patient assessment, the medical assistant should assist the physician as required. This includes helping the patient change positions for examination by the physician of the different body systems, handing the physician instruments and supplies, and reassuring the patient to reduce apprehension. Once the examination is completed, the medical assistant should assist the patient off the examining table and provide any additional information needed, such as scheduling a return visit or patient education to promote wellness. The procedure for assisting with the physical examination is presented on the following pages.

PUTTING IT ALL *into* PRACTICE

▶ **HOPE FAUBER:** *I once worked in a private office with a small waiting room and narrow hall. One of my regular patients was a young man who was confined to a wheelchair by spinal injuries. He had great difficulty maneuvering his motorized chair in tight spaces, and he felt uncomfortable and conspicuous sitting in the middle of the waiting room. I began bringing him through the larger back door into the doctor's office, directly into an exam room. Talking about things we had in common, like an interest in sports and cars, made him feel more at ease. By making the situation as easy as possible for him, he was able to keep his dignity and not draw attention to his special needs.*

4

4-10

Assisting with the Physical Examination

EQUIPMENT/SUPPLIES: Examining table
Equipment for the type of examination to be performed
Patient examination gown
Drapes

1. **Procedural Step.** Prepare the examining room. Make sure the room is clean, free of clutter, and well lit, and that the room temperature is comfortable for the patient.
2. **Procedural Step.** Wash the hands.
3. **Procedural Step.** Assemble the equipment according to the type of examination to be performed and physician preference. Arrange the instruments and supplies in a neat and orderly manner on a table or tray. Do not allow one article to lie on top of another.

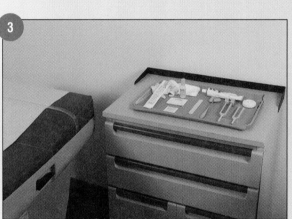

4. **Procedural Step.** Obtain the patient's medical record. Go to the waiting room and ask the patient to come back.
5. **Procedural Step.** Escort the patient to the examining room.
6. **Procedural Step.** Ask the patient to be seated. Greet and identify the patient. Introduce yourself to the patient. Use a calm and friendly manner. **Principle.** Using a calm and friendly manner assists in putting the patient at ease.
7. **Procedural Step.** Seat yourself so that you face the patient at a distance of 3 to 4 feet.
8. **Procedural Step.** Obtain and record the patient's symptoms following the procedure outlined in Chapter 2: Obtaining and Recording Patient Symptoms (Procedure 2-4).

9. **Procedural Step.** Measure the patient's vital signs, and chart the results.
10. **Procedural Step.** Measure the weight and height of the patient, and chart the results.

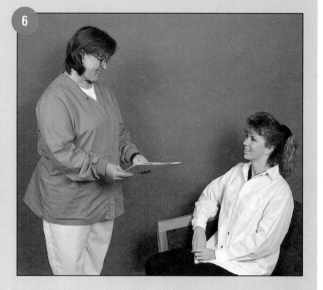

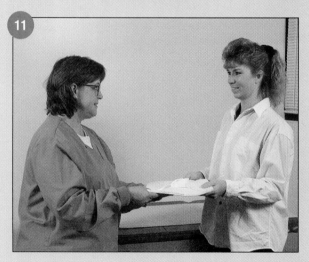

PROCEDURE 4–10

11. Procedural Step. Instruct and prepare the patient for the examination as follows:

a. Ask the patient if he or she needs to empty the bladder before the examination. If a urine specimen is needed, the patient will be required to void into a urine container.

b. Provide the patient with a patient gown. Instruct the patient to remove all clothing and to put on the patient gown with the opening in front. The disrobing facility should provide privacy, a place to sit, and a place for hanging clothing.

c. Ask the patient to have a seat and inform the patient that the physician will be with him or her soon.

Principle. An empty bladder makes the examination easier and is more comfortable for the patient.

12. Procedural Step. Inform the physician that the patient is ready, and make the medical record available to the physician.

13. Procedural Step. Assist the physician with the examination of the body systems as follows:

a. Place the patient in a sitting position on the examining table so that the physician can examine the patient's head, eyes, ears, nose, mouth and pharynx, neck, chest, lungs, and heart.

b. Assist the physician by handing the ophthalmoscope, otoscope, and tongue depressor.

c. Dim the light when the physician is ready to use the ophthalmoscope. The dim light will help dilate the patient's pupils, thus providing the physician with better visualization of the interior of the eye.

d. The tongue depressor should be transferred by holding it at the center to prevent contact with the patient's secretions, which may contain pathogens.

e. Offer reassurance to the patient to help reduce apprehension.

14. Procedural Step. Position the patient as required for examination of the remaining body systems. The medical assistant should place and drape the patient in the proper position for examination of a particular part of the body.

15. Procedural Step. Assist and instruct the patient as follows:

a. Assist the patient off the examining table to prevent falls. Elderly patients frequently become dizzy after being positioned on the examining table.

b. Instruct the patient to get dressed.

c. Provide the patient with any additional instructions, such as patient education, payment of fees, and scheduling a return visit. Instructions given by the medical assistant involving medical care should be explained in terms the patient can understand; medical terms should not be used.

d. Chart any instructions given to the patient in his or her medical record.

e. Escort the patient to the reception area.

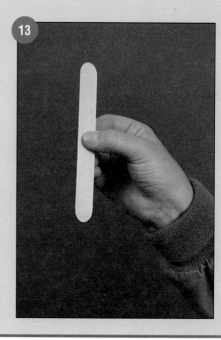

4

Continued

PROCEDURE 4–10

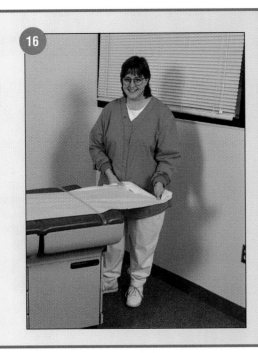

16. Procedural Step. Clean the examining room in preparation for the next patient as follows:
a. Discard the paper on the examining table, and unroll a fresh length of paper on the table.
b. Discard all disposable supplies into an appropriate waste container.
c. Check to make sure that there is an ample supply of clean gowns and drapes and other supplies.
d. Remove reusable equipment to a work area for sanitization, sterilization, or disinfection, as required by the medical office policy.

4

MEDICAL PRACTICE AND THE LAW

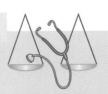

Activities involved in the physical exam can be sensitive for the patient. Information obtained during the patient history is confidential; revealing this information to anyone else is unethical and illegal. A good rapport is essential for obtaining complete information, especially when asking sensitive questions. Complete information is necessary for an accurate diagnosis and treatment.

Preparing the patient for a physical examination can be embarrassing for the patient. Keep in mind your duty to "do good" and "do no harm" to the patient. This involves proper knowledge and techniques, as well as a professional, caring, and helpful attitude. Draping the patient correctly allows a minimum of exposure. Incorrect draping or positioning that is unnecessarily uncomfortable could become a legal issue. Keep in mind that patients who are young, very old, or weak should never be left alone on an examining table. A fall from a table often results in harm and a lawsuit.

Finally, while assisting the physician, be supportive of the patient as much as you are able. While the physician concentrates on the examination, you should continually assess the patient and provide for any needs, including assistance, encouragement, and physical comfort. Be sure to be patient, polite, and professional in all directions given to the patient. You may have done this many times before, but this could be the first time for a frightened, ill patient.

CERTIFICATION REVIEW

- ☐ A patient examination consists of three parts: the health history, the physical examination, and laboratory and diagnostic tests. The results are used by the physician to determine the patient's general state of health, to arrive at a diagnosis and prescribe treatment, and to observe any change in a patient's illness after treatment has been instituted.

- ☐ Diagnosis refers to the scientific method of determining and identifying a patient's condition through the evaluation of the health history, the physical examination, and laboratory tests and diagnostic procedures.

- ☐ The clinical diagnosis is obtained through the evaluation of the health history and the physical examination without the benefit of laboratory or diagnostic tests. The prognosis is the probable course and outcome of a patient's condition.

- ☐ The medical assistant should have the equipment and supplies ready for the examination. They should be arranged for easy access by the physician. The equipment and supplies needed for the physical examination vary according to the type of examination and the physician's preference.

- ☐ The weight of an adult patient is usually measured during each office visit, whereas adult height is typically measured only during the first visit or when a complete physical examination of the patient is requested. Children are weighed and measured during each office visit to observe their pattern of growth and to calculate medication dosage.

- ☐ The scale must be balanced before measuring a patient's weight to ensure an accurate weight measurement. The weight measurement should be recorded in pounds to the nearest quarter of a pound. The height measurement should be recorded in feet and inches to the nearest quarter of an inch.

- ☐ Correct patient positioning facilitates the examination by permitting better access to the part being examined or treated. The positions commonly used in the medical office are the supine, prone, dorsal recumbent, lithotomy, Sims', knee-chest and Fowler's. The position used depends on the type of examination or procedure to be performed.

- ☐ The patient is draped during positioning to provide for modesty, comfort, and warmth. The part to be examined is the only part that should be exposed.

- ☐ A physical examination is performed using an organized and systematic approach starting with a examination of the patient's head and proceeding toward the feet.

- ☐ Assessment techniques used to obtain information during the physical examination include inspection, palpation, percussion, and auscultation.

- ☐ Inspection involves observation of the patient for any signs of disease. Palpation is the examination of the body using the sense of touch. Percussion involves tapping the patient with the fingers and listening to the sounds produced to determine the size, density, and location of underlying organs. Auscultation involves listening with a stethoscope to the sounds produced within the body.

4

RESOURCES

ON THE WEB

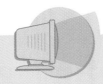

For Information on Nutrition:

American Dietetic Association
www.eatright.org

Ask the Dietitian
www.dietitian.com

CyberDiet
www.cyberdiet.com

For Information on Weight Control and Fitness:

Weight Watchers
www.weightwatchers.com

The Calorie Control Council
www.caloriecontrol.org

Shape Up America
www.shapeup.com

Fitness Link
www.fitnesslink.com

Fitness Partner Connection
primusweb.com/fitnesspartner

For Information on Accessing Health Information:

InteliHealth
www.intelihealth.com

Virtual Hospital
www.vh.org

Mayo Clinic
www.mayo.edu

U.S. Department of Health and Human Services
200 Independence Avenue, SW
Washington, DC 20201
www.os.dhhs.gov

4

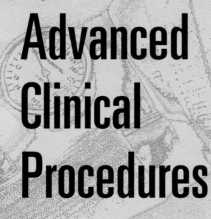

Advanced Clinical Procedures

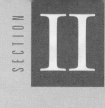

AAMA/CAAHEP COMPETENCES INCLUDED IN THIS SECTION:

CLINICAL COMPETENCIES

Fundamental Principles
- Wrap items for autoclaving
- Perform sterilization techniques

Patient Care
- Prepare patient for and assist with procedures, treatments, and minor office surgery
- Apply pharmacology principles to prepare and administer oral and parenteral medications

TRANSDISCIPLINARY COMPETENCIES

Legal Concepts
- Identify and respond to issues of confidentiality
- Perform within legal and ethical boundaries

Kara Van Dyke, *and I am a Certified Medical Assistant. I am a 1983 graduate of an accredited medical assisting program and have worked for two physicians in a family practice medical office for 10 years. My main interest is the clinical area.*

I started college before graduating from high school, and I always knew that I wanted to work in a health-care field. I find the opportunities to work with patients and help them on a one-on-one basis to be very fulfilling. Medical assisting brings out a caring, nurturing nature in people.

Sterilization and Disinfection

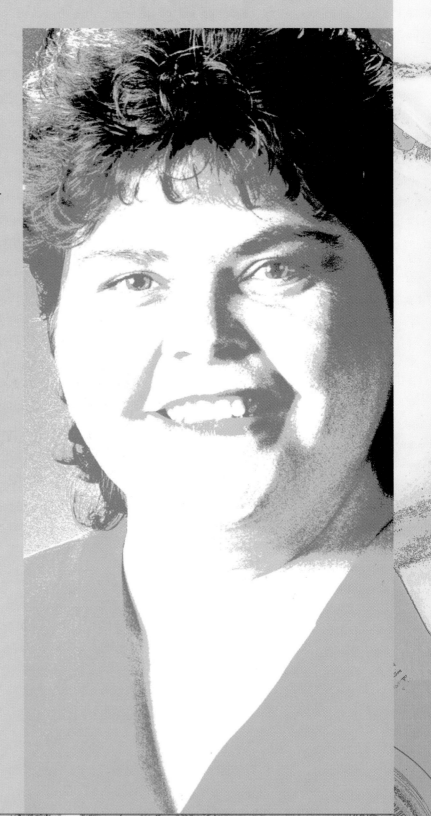

CHAPTER OUTLINE

Definition of Terms
Hazard Communications Standard
  Hazard Communications
    Program
  Inventory of Hazardous
    Chemicals
  Labeling of Hazardous
    Chemicals
  Material Safety Data Sheets
  Employee Information and
    Training
Sanitization
  Sanitizing Instruments
  Guidelines for Sanitizing
    Instruments
Disinfection
  Levels of Disinfection
  Types of Disinfectants
  Guidelines for Disinfection
Sterilization
  Autoclave
  Monitoring Program
  Sterilization Indicators
  Wrapping Articles
  Operating the Autoclave
  Guidelines for Autoclave
    Operation
  Storage
  Maintenance
Other Sterilization Methods
  Dry Heat Oven
  Ethylene Oxide Gas
    Sterilization
  Cold Sterilization
  Radiation

OUTCOMES

After completing this chapter, you should be able to demonstrate the proper procedure to perform the following:

1. Sanitize instruments.
2. Chemically disinfect articles.
3. Wrap articles to be autoclaved.
4. Sterilize articles in the autoclave.
5. Maintain the autoclave.

EDUCATIONAL OBJECTIVES

After completing this chapter, you should be able to do the following:

1. Define the terms listed in the Key Terminology.
2. Explain the purpose of the Hazard Communications Standard.
3. List and describe the information that must be included on the container label of a hazardous chemical.
4. List and describe the information that must be included in a material safety data sheet (MSDS).
5. State the purpose of sanitization.
6. State the advantages of using an ultrasonic cleaner to clean instruments.
7. List and describe the guidelines that should be followed when sanitizing instruments.
8. State the use of the three levels of disinfection: high-level disinfection, intermediate-level disinfection, and low-level disinfection.
9. Explain the difference among the following: critical item, semi-critical item, and noncritical item.
10. List and describe the guidelines that should be followed when disinfecting articles.
11. List and describe the primary use of the disinfectants used in the medical office.
12. Explain how the autoclave functions to sterilize articles.
13. List the components of a sterilization monitoring program.
14. List and describe types of sterilization indicators.
15. Identify the advantages and disadvantages of the following types of wraps: sterilization paper, sterilization pouches, muslin.
16. List the principles that should be followed when the autoclave is loaded.
17. Identify the sterilization times for each of the following categories: unwrapped articles, wrapped articles, liquids, large wrapped packs.
18. Describe the method for storing wrapped articles.
19. Describe the daily, weekly, and monthly maintenance of the autoclave.
20. State the primary use of the following types of sterilization methods: dry heat, ethylene oxide gas, chemicals, and radiation.

KEY TERMINOLOGY

antiseptic (an-Tĭ-sep-tik): A substance that kills disease-producing microorganisms but not their spores. An antiseptic is usually applied to living tissue.

autoclave (au-To-klâv): An apparatus for the sterilization of materials, using steam under pressure.

contaminate (kon-tam-i-nat): To soil, stain, or pollute; to make impure.

critical item: An item that comes in contact with sterile tissue or the vascular system.

detergent (det-ter-jent): An agent that cleanses by emulsifying dirt and oil.

disinfectant (dis-IN-fek-tant): A substance used to destroy disease-producing microorganisms but not necessarily their spores. Disinfectants are usually applied to inanimate objects.

incubate (in-Kû-bât): To provide proper conditions for growth and development.

load: The articles that are being sterilized.

material safety data sheet (MSDS): A sheet that provides information regarding a chemical, its hazards, and measures to take to avoid injury and illness when handling the chemical.

noncritical item: An item that comes into contact with intact skin but not mucous membranes.

sanitization: A cleaning process to reduce the number of microorganisms to a safe level as determined by public health requirements.

semi-critical item: An item that comes into contact with intact mucous membranes.

spore: A hard, thick-walled capsule formed by some bacteria that contains only the essential parts of the protoplasm of the bacterial cell.

sterilization: The process of destroying all forms of microbial life, including bacterial spores.

thermolabile (ther-Mô-lâ-bill): Easily affected or changed by heat.

INTRODUCTION

5

☐ The air and all objects around us contain microorganisms. The medical assistant is responsible for helping to reduce and eliminate microorganisms to prevent the spread of disease. This can be accomplished by practicing good techniques of medical and surgical asepsis (refer to Chapters 1 and 6).

Physical and chemical agents are used to destroy microorganisms in the medical office. The agent to be used depends on the intended use of the article. For example, articles that penetrate sterile tissue or the vascular system, such as surgical instruments, must be sterilized. Articles that come in contact with the skin or mucous membranes should be disinfected, for example, mercury glass thermometers, stethoscopes, and ear specula.

Sanitization, disinfection, and sterilization involve the use of hazardous chemicals. Therefore, it is essential for the medical assistant to acquire a knowledge of the precautions that are required when working with hazardous chemicals.

DEFINITION OF TERMS

Terms that aid in understanding this chapter are listed and defined here.

Sanitization	Sanitization is a cleansing process that lowers the number of microorganisms to a safe level as determined by public health requirements. Sanitization removes all organic material such as blood, body fluids, and tissue from an article. For articles that are used in examinations, treatments, or office surgery to be properly sterilized or disinfected, they must first be sanitized.
Detergent	A detergent is an agent that cleanses by emulsifying dirt and oil.
Disinfection	Disinfection is the process of destroying microorganisms that produce disease; however, it does not necessarily kill the resistant bacterial spores. Disinfectants are generally applied to inanimate objects.
Spore	A spore is a hard, thick-walled capsule that some bacteria form by losing moisture and condensing their contents to contain only the essential parts of the protoplasm of the cell. Spores represent a resting and protective stage of the bacterial cell and are more resistant to drying, sunlight, heat, and disinfectants than is the vegetative form of the bacterium. Favorable conditions cause the spore to germinate into a vegetative bacterium again, capable of reproducing. Two examples of species of bacteria that

Sterilization   form spores are *Clostridium botulinum*, which causes botulism, and *Clostridium tetani*, which causes tetanus.

Sterilization   Sterilization is the process of destroying all forms of microbial life. An object that is **sterile** is free of all living microorganisms and spores. There can be no relative degrees of sterility—an object is classified as either sterile or not sterile. The device most commonly used to sterilize articles in the medical office is the autoclave.

HAZARD COMMUNICATIONS STANDARD

☐ The Hazard Communications Standard (HCS) is a requirement of the Occupational Safety and Health Administration (OSHA). The purpose of the Hazardous Communications Standard is to ensure that employees are informed of the hazards associated with chemicals in their workplaces. A **hazardous chemical** is any chemical that presents a potential threat to the health and safety of an individual coming into contact with it. Examples of hazardous chemicals are those that are corrosive, toxic, flammable, or reactive.

The HCS is based on the concept that employees have a "right to know" about the hazardous chemicals in their workplace as well as the precautions to take to protect themselves when working with hazardous chemicals. In the medical office, sanitization, disinfection, and sterilization procedures involve the use of hazardous chemicals; therefore, the medical assistant must have a thorough knowledge of the HCS.

The HCS consists of the following components:

- Development of a Hazardous Communications Program
- Inventory of Hazardous Chemicals
- Labeling Requirements
- Material Safety Data Sheet Requirements
- Employee Information and Training

Each of these areas is discussed next.

HAZARD COMMUNICATIONS PROGRAM

As part of the HCS, employers are required to develop a Hazard Communications Program (HCP). The HCP consists of a written plan that describes what the facility is doing to meet the requirements of the HCS. The information in the HCP must be made available and communicated to all employees who work with hazardous chemicals.

INVENTORY OF HAZARDOUS CHEMICALS

The employer must develop and maintain a list of hazardous chemicals that are used and stored in the workplace. The list should include the name of the chemical, the name of the manufacturer, the hazardous ingredients, and health and safety ratings of the chemical. The list must be updated as new chemicals are introduced into the workplace. In the medical office, hazardous chemicals often include the following:

- Chemicals used in the back office (e.g., alcohol, laboratory reagents)
- Products used for sanitization, disinfection, and sterilization
- Pharmaceutical products such as local anesthetics (e.g., Xylocaine)
- Front office products (e.g., toner for copying machine)
- Cleaning products

LABELING OF HAZARDOUS CHEMICALS

The HCS requires that each container of a hazardous chemical be labeled by the manufacturer with a warning label to alert the user that the chemical is dangerous (Fig. 5–1). The label must include the possible hazards of the chemical and the steps that can be taken to protect against those risks. The hazard warnings can use words, pictures, or symbols to provide the user with an understanding of the physical and health haz-

5

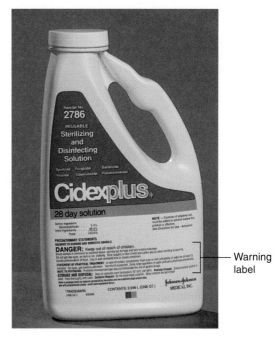

Warning label

■ **FIGURE 5–1.** Hazardous chemical container label.

ards of the chemical. If a label falls off of a product or is damaged, a replacement label must be applied. If a chemical is transferred to a new container, a label with all the required information must be present.

Container Label Requirements

The HCS requires that manufacturers of hazardous chemicals include the following information on container labels:

1. **Name of the chemical.**
2. **Manufacturer information.** The name, address, and emergency phone number of the company that manufacturers the chemical must be stated on the label.
3. **Physical hazards of the chemical.** Examples of physical hazards include the potential of the chemical to catch on fire, explode, or react with other chemicals or materials.
4. **Health hazards of the chemical.** Examples of health hazards include the potential of the chemical to produce irritation to tissue, cancer, a sensitivity reaction, or a toxic or corrosive reaction.
5. **Safety precautions.** The protective clothing, equipment, and procedures that are recommended when working with the chemical must be stated on the label.
6. **Storing and handling the chemical.** Information on how the chemical should be stored and handled must be stated on the label.

MATERIAL SAFETY DATA SHEETS

A material data safety sheet (MSDS) provides information regarding the chemical, its hazards, and measures to take to avoid injury and illness when handling the chemical (Fig. 5–2). An MSDS must be kept on file for each hazardous chemical used or stored in the workplace. MSDSs must be readily accessible to employees and provided to them on request. It is important that the medical assistant review the MSDS before working with a hazardous chemical.

Companies that manufacture and distribute hazardous chemicals must provide an MSDS with each product. A hazardous chemical should never be used unless an MSDS is available. In the event of an accidental exposure, information on the MSDS must be readily available as a reference for emergency treatment. If an MSDS is missing, the supplier or the manufacture of that chemical should be contacted for a replacement.

MSDS Requirements

The HCS requires that manufacturers of hazardous chemicals include the following information on MSDSs (Refer to Fig. 5–2):

1. **Identification.** This section provides information used to identify the chemical and must include the name of the chemical as it appears on the container label, the name and address and emergency phone number of the manufacturer, chemical identification information, common names for the chemical, and the date the MSDS was prepared.
2. **Hazardous ingredients.** This section must provide a list of the hazardous ingredients of the chemical.
3. **Physical and chemical characteristics.** The following physical and chemical characteristics of the chemical must be listed in this section:
   - Appearance and odor
   - Boiling point
   - Vapor pressure
   - Vapor density
   - Water solubility
   - Melting point
   - Freezing point
   - Specific gravity
   - Evaporation rate
   - pH
   - Odor threshold
4. **Fire and explosion data.** Some hazardous chemicals may cause a fire or explosion if used improperly. This section indicates under what circumstances this may occur and what to do if it does occur.
5. **Reactivity data.** Some chemicals react when combined with other chemicals or materials. The reactivity data lists the substances and conditions that the chemical should be kept away from to prevent a dangerous reaction. This information helps in determining where and how to store the chemical.
6. **Health hazard data.** This section is one of the most important areas for health workers. This section includes the following information:
   - Route of entry (e.g., inhalation, ingestion, skin contact, eye contact)
   - Signs and symptoms of exposure (e.g., eye irritation, nausea, dizziness, skin rashes, headache)
   - Emergency first-aid procedures to take if exposed to the chemical (e.g., in case of eye contact, immediately flush eyes with water for 15 minutes)
   - Health hazards that could result from exposure (e.g., permanent eye damage, bronchitis, cancer)

MATERIAL SAFETY DATA SHEET

SECTION 1   IDENTIFICATION

MANUFACTURER'S NAME: Corelis Corporation
ADDRESS: P.O. Box 93
                        Camden, NJ 08106

EMERGENCY TELEPHONE NUMBER: 1 (800) 733-8690

TELEPHONE NUMBER FOR INFORMATION: 1 (800) 331-0766

ISSUED: 10/99

IDENTITY: 2% Aqueous Glutaraldehyde Solution

PREPARED BY: Regulatory Affairs

PRODUCT CODE: 3345

TRADE NAME: Aldecyde

SYNONYMS: None

CHEMICAL FAMILY: Aldehydes

MOLECULAR FORMULA: $OHCC_3H_6CHO$ (Active)

RTECS #: MA 2450000 (Active)

MOLECULAR WEIGHT: 100

HAZARD RATING – HEALTH: 3 (Serious Hazard)   FLAMMABILITY: 0   REACTIVITY: 0   SPECIFIC: NONE

SECTION 2   HAZARDOUS INGREDIENTS/IDENTITY INFORMATION

COMPONENTS (SPECIFIC CHEMICAL IDENTITY)	CAS #	%	OSHA PEL	ACGIH TLV	OSHA 1910.1200
Glutaraldehyde (active)	111-30-8	2	0.2ppm, C	0.2ppm, C	n/a
Inert buffer salts	n/a		None	None	Nonhazardous
Water	7732-18-5	98	None	None	Nonhazardous

SECTION 3   PHYSICAL/CHEMICAL CHARACTERISTICS

APPEARANCE AND ODOR: 2 components: colorless fluid and liquid salts; turns green when activated. Sharp odor masked with peppermint fragrance.

BOILING POINT: 212°F

SPECIFIC GRAVITY (H_2O=1): 1.003 g/cc

VAPOR PRESSURE (mm Hg): same as water

MELTING POINT: n/a

VAPOR DENSITY (AIR=1): same as water

EVAPORATION RATE (H_2O=1): 0.98

SOLUBILITY IN WATER: complete

pH: 8

FREEZING POINT: same as water

ODOR THRESHOLD: .04 ppm, detectable. (ACGIH)

SECTION 4   FIRE AND EXPLOSION HAZARD DATA

FLASH POINT (METHOD USED): None   FLAMMABLE LIMITS – LEL: nd   UEL: nd

EXTINGUISHING MEDIA: If water is evaporated, material can burn. Use carbon dioxide or dry chemical for small fires. Use foam (alcohol, polymer or ordinary) or water fog for large fires.

SPECIAL FIRE FIGHTING PROCEDURES: Self-contained breathing apparatus and protective clothing should be available to fireman.

UNUSUAL FIRE AND EXPLOSION HAZARDS: None

TOXIC GASES PRODUCED: None

SECTION 5   REACTIVITY DATA

STABILITY: 212°F

CONDITIONS TO AVOID: None

INCOMPATIBILITY (MATERIALS TO AVOID): None

HAZARDOUS DECOMPOSITION OR BYPRODUCTS: None

HAZARDOUS POLYMERIZATION: Will not occur

■ **FIGURE 5–2.** Material safety data sheet (MSDS).

5

MATERIAL SAFETY DATA SHEET	MSDS NO. 396
	PAGE 2

SECTION 6 HEALTH HAZARD DATA

ROUTE(S) OF ENTRY – INHALATION: yes   SKIN: yes   INGESTION: yes   EYE: yes

SIGNS AND SYMPTOMS OF EXPOSURE:

EYES: Contact with eyes causes damage.

SKIN: Can cause skin sensitization. Avoid skin contact.

INHALATION: Vapors may be irritating and cause headache, chest discomfort, symptoms of bronchitis.

INGESTION: May cause nausea, vomiting and general systemic illness.

EMERGENCY AND FIRST AID PROCEDURE:

EYES: Flush thoroughly with water. Get medical attention.

SKIN: Flush thoroughly with water. If irritation persists, get medical attention.

INHALATION: Remove to fresh air. If symptoms persist, get medical attention.

INGESTION: Do not induce vomiting. Drink copious amount of milk. Get medical attention.

HEALTH HAZARDS (ACUTE AND CHRONIC):
  Acute: As listed above under Signs and Symptoms of Exposure
  Chronic: None known from currently available information.

MEDICAL CONDITIONS GENERALLY AGGRAVATED BY EXPOSURE: None known from currently available information.

LISTED AS CARCINOGEN BY –   NTP: yes   IARC MONOGRAPHS: no   OSHA: no

TOXICITY: ORAL LD50 (Rat)   Toxicity Rating 1: 500-5000 mg/kg.
            OCULAR (Rabbit)   Toxicity Rating 2: Irritating or moderately persisting more than seven days with.
            DERMAL LD50 (Rabbit)   None by dermal route.
            INHALATION LC50 (Rabbit)   Irritating but non-toxic at highest concentration achieved (2.89 ppm).

SECTION 7 PRECAUTIONS FOR SAFE HANDLING AND USE

STEPS TO BE TAKE IN CASE MATERIAL IS RELEASED OR SPILLED: For LARGE spills, use ammonium carbonate to "neutralize" glutaraldehyde odor. Collect liquid and discard it. For SMALL spills, wipe with sponge or mop down area with an equal mixture of household ammonia and water. Flush with large quantities of water.

WASTE DISPOSAL METHOD: Triple rinse empty container with water and dispose in an incinerator or landfill approved for pesticide containers. Discard solution with large quantities of water.

EPA HAZARDOUS WASTE NUMBER: n/a

PRECAUTIONS TO BE TAKEN IN HANDLING AND STORING: Use normal storage and handling requirements.

SECTION 8 TRANSPORTATION DATA AND ADDITIONAL INFORMATION

DOMESTIC (D.O.T.): Aldehydes, N.O.S.	INTERNATIONAL (I.M.O.): Aldehydes, N.O.S.
PROPER SHIPPING NAME: Glutaraldehyde	PROPER SHIPPING NAME: Glutaraldehyde
HAZARD CLASS: None	HAZARD CLASS: None
LABELS: None Needed	LABELS: None Needed
REPORTABLE QUANTITY: None	UN/NA: 1989

■ **FIGURE 5–2** *Continued*

MATERIAL SAFETY DATA SHEET	MSDS NO. 396
	PAGE 3

SECTION 9 CONTROL MEASURES

VENTILATION:
  ROUTINE: Product should be used in a covered container. Use with standard room ventilation (air conditioning); natural draft.
  EMERGENCY: Enhanced ventilation

RESPIRATORY PROTECTION:
  ROUTINE: None required
  EMERGENCY: Organic vapor cartridge, canister mask

EYE PROTECTION:
  ROUTINE: Safety glasses recommended
  EMERGENCY: Safety glasses

SKIN PROTECTION:
  ROUTINE: Impervious gloves
  EMERGENCY: Impervious gloves; Protective clothing; Rubber boots

WORK/HYGIENIC PRACTICES: Avoid contamination of food

SECTION 10 SPECIAL REQUIREMENTS

None

KEY: n/a = Not Applicable
      nd = Not Determined
       C = Ceiling
     PEL = Permissible Exposure Level
   RTECS = Registry of Toxic Effects of Chemical Substances
       * = Trademark

■ **FIGURE 5–2** *Continued*

5

7. **Precautions for safe handling and use.** This section tells what to do for a spill or leak, the method of disposal of the chemical, and how to handle and store the chemical.
8. **Control measures.** This section lists the engineering controls, work practice controls, and personal protective equipment that should be used to protect oneself from the hazardous chemical. Examples of these measures include using gloves and eye protection and working in a well-ventilated area.

EMPLOYEE INFORMATION AND TRAINING

The HCS requires that employees be provided with information and training regarding hazardous chemicals in the workplace. The training session must be offered at the time of an employee's initial assignment to a work area where hazardous chemicals are present and whenever a new hazard is introduced into the work area. The training program must be an ongoing activity, and each training session must be documented. The HCS requires that the following information be relayed to employees who work with hazardous chemicals:

1. The requirements making up the HCS
2. Physical and health hazards associated with exposure to chemicals in the workplace
3. Measures the employees can take to protect themselves from injury or illness from hazardous chemicals
4. Emergency procedures to take in the event of exposure to a hazardous chemical or a chemical spill
5. The meaning of the information on container labels and how to use that information
6. The meaning of the information on MSDSs and how to use that information
7. The location of the following: HCP plan, list of hazardous chemicals used in the workplace, and MSDS for each chemical in the workplace

SANITIZATION

☐ **Sanitization** involves a series of steps designed to remove organic material from an article and to lower the number of microorganisms on the article to a safe level. Organic material present on an article may result in incomplete sterilization or disinfection. This is because the organic material acts as a physical barrier preventing the physical or chemical agent from reaching the surface of the article to kill microorganisms.

SANITIZING INSTRUMENTS

The most frequent items sanitized in the medical office are medical and surgical instruments. Therefore, this section focuses on the theory and procedure for sanitizing instruments.

The general steps in the sanitization procedure of instruments are as follows:

1. **Initial rinse** of the instruments
2. **Clean** the instruments
3. **Thorough** rinse of the instruments
4. **Dry** the instruments
5. **Check the instruments** for defects and working condition
6. **Lubricate** hinged instruments.

5 Cleaning Instruments

There are two methods that can be used to perform the cleaning step (Step 3 in the preceding list) of the sanitization procedure: the manual method and the ultrasound method.

Manual Method

The **manual method** is used most often in the medical office. It involves the manual cleaning of instruments using a cleaning solution and a brush. Manual cleaning is recommended for delicate instruments because vibrations that occur with the ultrasound method may damage these instruments.

Ultrasound Method

The **ultrasound method** uses a machine known as an ultrasonic cleaner (Fig. 5–3). The ultrasound method offers a safety advantage in that instruments do not have to be handled during the cleaning process. This decreases the incidence of an accidental puncture or cut from a sharp instrument. An **ultrasonic cleaner** works by converting sound waves into mechanical energy, which creates small bubbles all over the instru-

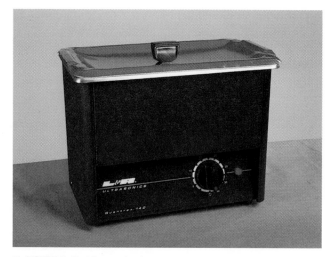

■ **FIGURE 5–3.** Ultrasonic cleaner.

ments. When the bubbles burst, vibrations occur that loosen and remove debris from the instruments. Ultrasonic cleaners are especially good at removing debris from hard to reach areas such as box locks of hemostats and screw locks of scissors.

Before the instruments are placed in the ultrasonic cleaner, they should be separated according to the type of metal making up the instrument (e.g., stainless steel, aluminum, brass). Instruments made of dissimilar metals should not be cleaned together in the ultrasonic cleaner. When different metals are in close contact, the ions from one metal can flow to another. This may

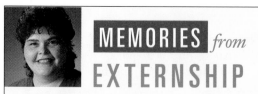

MEMORIES *from* **EXTERNSHIP**

KARA VAN DYKE: *Some of the procedures I performed during externship included the sanitation and sterilization of instruments. I also took patients into the examining room, measured their vital signs, identified the chief complaint, and then prepared them to see the physician. In between patients, I answered the phone, made appointments, and filed charts. I also performed urinalysis, ran electrocardiograms, gave injections, and obtained hematocrit levels. Sometimes all of these things were needed at the same time!*

result in a permanent blue-black stain on an instrument, which can only be removed by having the instrument refinished.

GUIDELINES FOR SANITIZING INSTRUMENTS

The following guidelines should be followed when sanitizing surgical instruments:

1. **Wear gloves during the sanitization process.** Following the OSHA Bloodborne Pathogens Standards, the medical assistant should wear disposable gloves during the entire sanitization procedure. This protects the medical assistant from bloodborne pathogens and other potentially infectious materials. The medical assistant should be especially careful when working with hazardous chemicals and when handling sharp instruments. Heavy-duty utility gloves should be worn over the disposable gloves to provide protection from the irritating effects of chemical agents and accidental punctures or cuts from sharp instruments.

2. **Handle instruments carefully.** Instruments are expensive and delicate, yet durable. They are able to last for many years if properly handled and maintained. Dropping an instrument on the floor or throwing an instrument into a basin may damage it. Instruments should never be piled in a heap, because they will become entangled and may be damaged when separated. Keep sharp instruments separate from the rest of the instruments to prevent damaging or dulling the cutting edge. Also, keep delicate instruments separate to protect them from damage.

3. **Follow instructions on labels of chemical agents.** Before using a chemical agent such as an instrument cleaner or an autoclave cleaner, review the product's MSDS and carefully read the label on the container. Check the label to determine the use, mixing, and storage of the chemical agent. Read and observe precautions listed on the label regarding personal safety such as the use of gloves and eye protection. Also, check the expiration date on the label of the chemical agent. Chemicals have a tendency to lose their potency over time and should not be used past the expiration date.

4. **Use a proper cleaning agent.** A low-sudsing detergent with a neutral pH should be used to clean the instruments. Commercially available instrument cleaners meet these criteria (Fig. 5–4). These cleaners usually come in a concentrated liquid or powder form and must be diluted before use. Never substitute any other type of detergent such as dishwasher detergent or laundry detergent; these detergents may not have the proper pH for sanitizing instru-

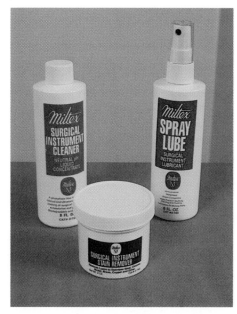

■ **FIGURE 5–4.** Commercially available surgical instrument cleaners. Instrument cleaner *(left)*, stain remover *(center)*, and spray lubricant *(right)*.

ments. If a detergent with an alkaline pH, is used and not completely rinsed off, it could leave a residue on the instrument. This could result in an orange-brown stain on the instrument that resembles rust. Using an acid detergent can also cause staining and permanent corrosion problems.

5. **Use proper cleaning devices.** Proper cleaning devices should be used for the manual cleaning of instruments. A stiff nylon brush should be used to clean the surface of the instrument. A stainless steel wire brush can be used to clean grooves, crevices, or serrations. A stain on an instrument can often be removed using a commercial instrument stain remover (see Fig. 5–4). Never use steel wool or other abrasives to remove stains, because damage could occur to the instrument.

6. **Carefully inspect each instrument for defects and proper working condition.** After cleaning and drying the instrument, it is important to check it for defects and proper working condition as follows:
   a. The blades of an instrument should be straight and not bent.
   b. The tips of an instrument should approximate tightly and evenly when the instrument is closed.
   c. An instrument with a box lock (e.g., hemostatic forceps, needle holders) should move freely but must not be too loose. The pin that holds the box lock together should be flush against the instrument.

d. An instrument with a spring handle (e.g., thumb and tissue forceps) should have sufficient tension to grasp objects tightly.

e. The cutting edge of a sharp instrument should be smooth and devoid of nicks.

f. Scissors should cut cleanly and smoothly. To test for this, the medical assistant should cut into a thin piece of gauze. If they cut all the way to the end of the blade without catching on the gauze, the scissors are in proper working condition.

7. **Lubricate hinged instruments.** Lubricate box locks, screw locks, scissor blades, or any other moving part of each instrument. Use a lubricant that can be penetrated by steam such as a commercial spray lubricant or a lubricant bath (see Fig 5–4). Be sure to lubricate after performing the final rinse; otherwise the lubricant will be rinsed off the instrument. Never use industrial oils or silicon sprays. These substances are not steam penetrable and can build up on the instrument, affecting its working condition.

PROCEDURE

5–1

Sanitization of Instruments

EQUIPMENT/SUPPLIES:

Sink
Disposable gloves
Heavy-duty utility gloves
Contaminated instruments
Instrument container
Instrument cleaning solution

Paper towels
Steam-penetrable lubricant
Stiff nylon brush
Stainless steel wire brush
Ultrasonic cleaner (ultrasound method of cleaning)

5

1. **Procedural Step.** Apply gloves. Remove the contaminated instruments to the cleaning area as soon as possible after use. The instruments should be carried in a covered basin from the examining room to the cleaning area.
   Principle. Disposable gloves act as a barrier to protect the medical assistant from infectious materials. Transporting contaminated instruments in a covered basin promotes infection control.

2. **Procedural Step.** Apply heavy-duty utility gloves over the disposable gloves.
   Principle. Utility gloves help protect the hands from the irritating effects of chemical solutions.

3. **Procedural Step.** Separate sharp instruments and delicate instruments from other instruments.
   Principle. Separating sharp instruments from others prevents damage to or dulling of the cutting edge of these instruments. Delicate instruments should be separated to protect them from damage.

4. **Procedural Step.** Immediately rinse the instruments thoroughly under warm to hot running water (approximately 110°F or 44°C) to remove organic material such as blood, body fluids, and tissue.
   Principle. Rinsing the instruments as soon as possible prevents organic material from drying on the instruments, making it difficult to remove later.

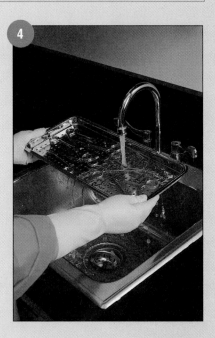

PROCEDURE 5-1

5. Procedural Step. Clean the instruments. The instruments can be cleaned using the manual method or the ultrasound method as follows:

Manual Method for Cleaning Instruments:

a. Check the expiration date of the cleaning agent.

b. Follow the directions on the manufacturer's label for proper use and mixing of the cleaning agent. A low-sudsing detergent with a neutral pH should be used. The detergent may need to be diluted with water. Observe all personal safety precautions listed on the label.

c. Use a stiff nylon brush to clean the surface of the instruments. Be sure to thoroughly scrub all parts of the instrument. Brush delicate instruments carefully to prevent damaging them.

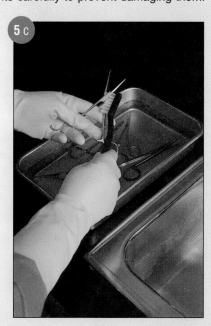

5 c

d. Use a stainless steel wire brush to clean grooves, crevices, or serrations where contaminants such as blood and tissue may collect.

e. If a stain is present on the instrument, attempt to remove it using a damp cloth or sponge to which a commercial stain remover has been applied.

f. Scrub all instruments until they are visibly clean and free from organic material and stains.

g. After cleaning the instruments, dispose of the cleaning solution according to the manufacturer's instructions. It should never be reused.

Principle. A cleaning agent past its expiration date loses its potency and should not be used. A neutral pH detergent should be used to prevent stains from forming on the instruments. Taking appropriate precautions with cleaning agents prevents harm to the medical assistant from hazardous chemicals. All organic material must be removed from the instruments to ensure complete sterilization. Proper disposal of the cleaning solution prevents harm to the environment.

Ultrasound Method for Cleaning Instruments:

a. Prepare the cleaning solution in the ultrasonic cleaner using a cleaning agent recommended by the manufacturer. Observe all personal safety precautions listed on the label.

b. Separate instruments made of dissimilar metals such as stainless steel, aluminum, and bronze.

c. Place the instruments in the ultrasonic cleaner with hinged instruments in an open position.

d. Make sure sharp instruments do not touch other instruments.

e. Make sure all instruments are fully submerged in the cleaning solution.

5

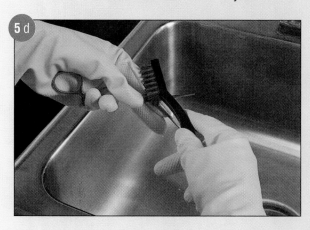

5 d

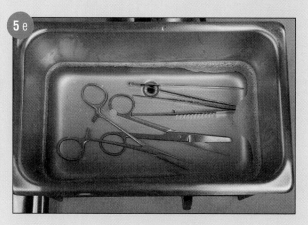

5 e

f. Place the lid on the ultrasonic cleaner.

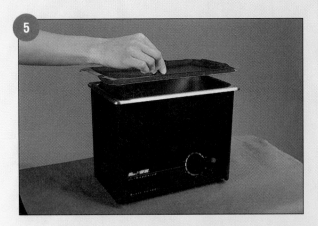

g. Turn on the ultrasonic cleaner and clean the instruments for the length of time recommended by the manufacturer.

h. After completion of the cleaning cycle, remove the instruments from the machine.

i. Change the cleaning solution in the ultrasonic cleaner according to the manufacturer's recommendations.

Principle. Mixing dissimilar metals together could result in permanent stains on the instruments. Instruments must be completely submerged with hinged instruments in an open position so that the solution can reach all parts of the instrument. Taking appropriate precautions with chemical agents prevents harm to the medical assistant from hazardous chemicals.

6. **Procedural Step.** Rinse each instrument thoroughly with warm to hot water (110°F or 44°C) for at least 20 to 30 seconds to remove all traces of the detergent. Open and close hinged instruments to make sure the solution is completely rinsed out of every part of the instrument.

Principle. Detergent residue left on the instrument could cause stains, which could build up and interfere with the proper functioning of the instrument. Using warm to hot water helps to remove the cleaning solution and facilitates the drying process.

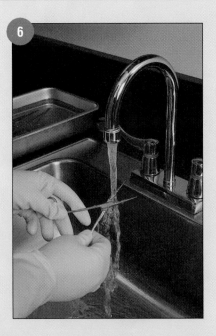

7. **Procedural Step.** Dry each instrument with a paper towel and place the instrument on a dry towel for additional air drying.

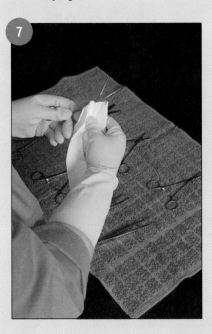

Principle. If the instrument is not completely dry, stains may occur on the instrument.

PROCEDURE 5-1

8. Procedural Step. Check each instrument for defects and proper working condition. If defects are noted or the instrument is not working properly, it must be sent to the manufacturer for repair. However, continue with the sanitization (and sterilization) process so that the instrument is safe to send to the manufacturer.

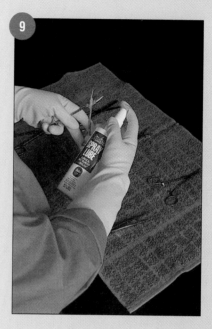

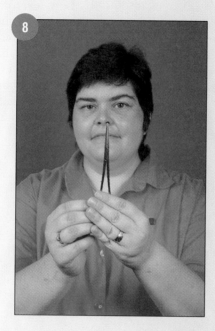

Principle. Instruments that have defects or are not in proper working condition are not safe to use on a patient during a medical or surgical procedure.

9. Procedural Step. Lubricate hinged instruments and any other instrument with moving parts using a steam-penetrable lubricant as follows:

a. Apply the lubricant to a hinged instrument in its open position.

b. Open and close the instrument after applying the lubricant so that it reaches all parts of the hinged area.

c. Place the instrument back on the towel and allow it to drain. Rinsing and wiping are not necessary.

Principle. Lubricating an instrument makes it function better and last longer.

10. Procedural Step. Remove both sets of gloves and wash hands.

11. Procedural Step. Wrap the instruments and sterilize them in the autoclave according to the medical office policy.

5

DISINFECTION

☐ **Disinfection** is the process of destroying pathogenic microorganisms, but it does not necessarily kill bacterial spores. Disinfectants consist of chemical agents that are applied to inanimate objects. In the medical office, most reusable instruments and devices are processed by sterilizing them in an autoclave. Sterilization must be used to process all critical items. A **critical item** is an item that comes in contact with sterile tissue or the vascular system.

Instruments and devices that come into contact with mucous membranes and intact skin can be chemically disinfected (e.g., nasal speculum, vaginal speculum); however, most offices use the autoclave because it is a convenient, efficient, safe, and inexpensive method for destroying microorganisms. Chemical disinfectants, on the other hand, are not only more expensive to use but are also more hazardous and create problems as to their proper disposal.

In some instances, however, medical instruments that are not required to be sterile and that are made of materials damaged by heat must be chemically disinfected. For example, mercury glass thermometers and flexible fiberoptic sigmoidoscopes would be damaged by the heat of an autoclave and must be chemically disinfected.

LEVELS OF DISINFECTION

Disinfection can be classified according to three levels of disinfection based on killing action, as follows:

HIGH-LEVEL DISINFECTION. **High-level disinfection** is a process that destroys all microorganisms with the exception of bacterial spores. High-level disinfection is used to disinfect semi-critical items that are heat-sensitive. A **semi-critical item** is an item that comes in contact with intact mucous membranes such as a flexible fiberoptic sigmoidoscope or a mercury glass thermometer. A frequently used high-level disinfectant is 2 percent glutaraldehyde (Cidex).

INTERMEDIATE-LEVEL DISINFECTION. **Intermediate-level disinfection** is a process that inactivates tubercle bacilli (the causative agent of tuberculosis), vegetative bacteria, most viruses, and most fungi but does not kill bacterial spores. Intermediate-level disinfection is used to disinfect noncritical items. **Noncritical items** are items that come into contact with intact skin but not mucous membranes, such as stethoscopes, blood pressure cuffs, and crutches. An example of a commonly used intermediate-level disinfectant is isopropyl alcohol.

LOW-LEVEL DISINFECTION. **Low-level disinfection** is a process that kills most bacteria, some viruses, and some fungi but cannot be relied on to kill resistant microorganisms such as tubercle bacilli or bacterial spores. Low-level disinfectants are typically used to disinfect surfaces such as examining tables, laboratory countertops, and walls. Low-level disinfectants used in the medical office include sodium hypochlorite (household bleach) and phenolics.

TYPES OF DISINFECTANTS

The disinfectants used most frequently in the medical office are described next. Also refer to Table 5-1 for a list of these disinfectants along with common names and uses for each.

5

TABLE 5-1

Disinfectants Used in the Medical Office

Disinfectant	Common Names	Use in the Medical Office
Glutaraldehyde	Cidex Metricide Procide Omnicide Wavicide	Disinfection of flexible fiberoptic sigmoidoscopes and mercury glass thermometers
Alcohol	Ethyl alcohol Isopropyl alcohol	Disinfection of mercury glass thermometers Disinfection of stethoscopes and percussion hammers; isopropyl alcohol wipes are used to disinfect rubber stoppers of multiple-dose medication vials
Chlorine and chlorine compounds	Sodium hypochlorite (household bleach)	Recommended by OSHA for decontamination of blood spills
Phenolics	Carbolic acid Hydroxybenzene Phenic acid Phenyl hydroxide Phenylic acid	Disinfection of walls, furniture, floors, and laboratory work surfaces
Quaternary ammonium compounds	Benzalkonium chloride	Disinfection of walls, furniture, floors, and laboratory work surfaces

Glutaraldehyde

Glutaraldehyde is categorized as a high-level disinfectant. It has a rapid killing action and is not inactivated by the presence of organic material. Because it does not corrode lenses, metal, or rubber, it is the agent of choice for semi-critical items that cannot be exposed to heat, such as mercury glass thermometers and flexible fiberoptic sigmoidoscopes.

Alcohol

Alcohol is frequently used as a disinfectant in the medical office. The two types that are most commonly used are ethyl and isopropyl alcohol. The disinfecting action of alcohol is increased by the presence of water; therefore, a 70 percent solution of alcohol is recommended. Stronger concentrations (95 to 100 percent) are not as effective. A disadvantage of alcohol is that it tends to dissolve the cement from around the lenses of instruments.

Ethyl alcohol is classified as a high-level disinfectant and can be used for certain types of semi-critical items such as mercury glass thermometers. **Isopropyl alcohol** provides intermediate to low-level disinfection and can be used to disinfect stethoscopes and percussion hammers. Isopropyl alcohol wipes are used to disinfect small surfaces such as rubber stoppers or multiple-dose medication vials.

Chlorine and Chlorine Compounds

Chlorine and chlorine compounds are some of the oldest and most commonly used disinfectants. Their most important use is in the chlorination of water.

In the medical office, chlorine is used in the form of hypochlorites, such as liquid sodium hypochlorite (household bleach). A 10 percent solution of household bleach in water will inactivate hepatitis B virus, human immunodeficiency virus (HIV), and many bacteria in 10 minutes at room temperature. Because of this, household bleach is recommended by OSHA for the decontamination of blood spills. A disadvantage of this disinfectant is that it can be irritating to skin or mucous membranes and is highly corrosive to metal.

Phenolics

Phenolics are used mainly to disinfect walls, furniture, floors, and laboratory work surfaces. This disinfectant is a corrosive poison and tends to be irritating to the eyes and skin. Because of this, eye and skin protective devices should be worn when working with phenolics in the pure form. There are many derivatives of phen-olics that are commonly used and are usually nonirritating, including Lysol and hexachlorophene.

Quaternary Ammonium Compounds

The quaternary ammonium compounds are sometimes used in the medical office for the disinfection of non-critical surfaces such as floors, furniture, and walls.

GUIDELINES FOR DISINFECTION

The following guidelines should be following when disinfecting articles with a chemical agent:

OBSERVE SAFETY PRECAUTIONS. The medical assistant should carefully read the container label and the MSDS before using a chemical disinfectant. All safety precautions should be followed when using the chemical to protect against illness or injury from a hazardous chemical.

SANITIZE THE ARTICLES BEFORE DISINFECTING THEM. The article to be disinfected must first be thoroughly sanitized to remove organic material such as blood, body fluids, and tissue. Organic material prevents the chemical from reaching the surface of the article; therefore, harmful pathogens may not be killed. In addition, with some disinfectants, organic material can absorb the chemical disinfectant and inactivate it. The article should be thoroughly rinsed of the detergent after cleaning because detergent residue may interfere with the disinfecting process. The article must be completely dry before placing it in the disinfectant because water dilutes the chemical and decreases it effectiveness.

PROPERLY PREPARE AND USE THE DISINFECTANT. Products vary substantially among manufacturers; therefore, it is important that the manufacturer's directions on preparation, dilution, and use of the disinfectant be followed very carefully. The disinfectant should be prepared exactly as indicated on the container label. Some disinfectants are used full strength while others require dilution. Some disinfectants (e.g., glutaraldehyde) require the addition of an activator before they can be used. Preparing the disinfectant properly ensures the destruction of microorganisms. A disinfectant must be applied for a certain length of time in order to kill all the pathogens that may be present. The medical assistant must be sure to disinfect for the length of time indicated on the container label.

PROCEDURE

5–2

Chemical Disinfection of Articles

EQUIPMENT/SUPPLIES:

Sink
Disposable gloves
Heavy-duty utility gloves
Contaminated articles

Chemical disinfectant
MSDS
Container to hold the disinfectant
Paper towels

5

1. **Procedural Step.** Review the MSDS for the chemical disinfectant that you will be using.
   Principle. The MSDS provides information regarding the chemical disinfectant, its hazards, and measures to take to avoid injury and illness when handling the disinfectant.

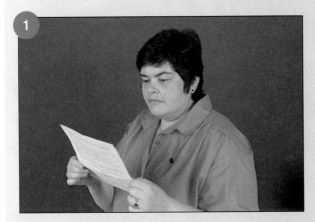

2. **Procedural Step.** Apply gloves. Remove the contaminated articles to a separate work area as soon as possible after use. The articles should be carried in a covered basin from the examining room to the work area with gloved hands.
   Principle. Disposable gloves act as a barrier to protect the medical assistant from infectious materials. Transporting contaminated articles in a covered basin promotes infection control.
3. **Procedural Step.** Apply heavy-duty utility gloves over the disposable gloves.
   Principle. Utility gloves help protect the hands from the irritating effects of chemical solutions.

4. **Procedural Step.** Sanitize the articles by performing the steps outlined in Procedure 5–1, Sanitization of Instruments. The steps include the following:
   Rinse the articles
   Clean the articles
   Thoroughly rinse the articles again
   Dry the articles
   Principle. Sanitizing removes organic matter from the articles. Organic matter left on an article does not allow the disinfectant to reach all parts of the article and may interfere with the proper functioning of the disinfectant. The articles should be thoroughly rinsed of the detergent after cleaning because detergent residue may interfere with the disinfectant process. The articles must be dried completely before immersing them in the disinfectant because water dilutes the chemical, which decreases its effectiveness.
5. **Procedural Step.** Check the expiration date of the chemical disinfectant.
   Principle. A disinfectant past its expiration date loses its potency and should not be used.
6. **Procedural Step.** Follow the directions on the manufacturer's label for proper use and mixing of the disinfectant. The disinfectant may need to be diluted with distilled water. Observe all personal safety precautions listed on the label.
   Principle. Taking appropriate precautions with chemical agents prevents harm to the medical assistant from hazardous chemicals.

PROCEDURE 5–2

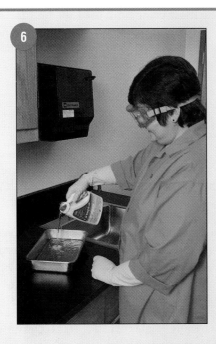

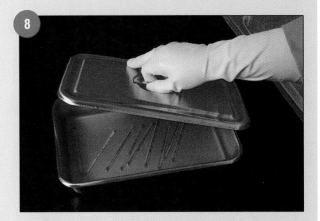

7. **Procedural Step.** Immerse the articles in the chemical disinfectant. Make sure the articles are completely submerged in the disinfectant.

9. **Procedural Step.** Disinfect the articles for the proper length of time as indicated on the label of the container.
   Principle. Proper time requirements must be followed to ensure complete destruction of all microorganisms.

10. **Procedural Step.** Remove the articles from the disinfectant and rinse them thoroughly. Dry the articles with paper towels. Properly dispose of the disinfectant according to the manufacturer's instructions.

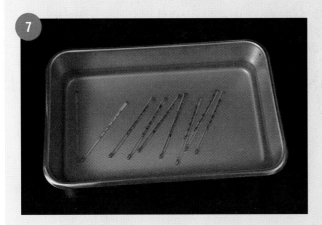

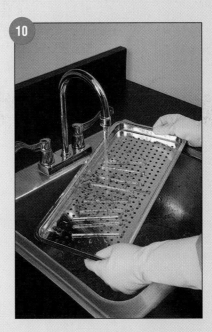

Principle. The articles must be completely submerged to allow the disinfectant to reach all parts of the instrument.

8. **Procedural Step.** Cover the container holding the chemical disinfectant.
   Principle. The container must be kept covered to prevent the escape of toxic fumes and to avoid evaporation of the disinfectant, which could change its potency.

Principle. All traces of the chemical disinfectant must be removed to prevent irritation to the patient's tissues. The disinfectant must be disposed of properly to prevent harm to the environment.

11. **Procedural Step.** Remove both sets of gloves and wash the hands.

12. **Procedural Step.** Store the articles according to the medical office policy.

5

Storage

Chemical disinfectants should be tightly closed and stored under the proper storage conditions recommended by the manufacturer. Chemical disinfectants lose their potency over time; therefore, the medical assistant should strictly adhere to the manufacturer's recommendations for the disinfectant's shelf life, use life, and resuse life. Each of these terms is defined next as it relates to chemical disinfectants.

Shelf life	Shelf life is the length of time a chemical disinfectant may be stored before use and still retain its effectiveness. The shelf life is indicated by an expiration date located on the container. The expiration date should always be checked before using the chemical. Outdated disinfectants should not be used.
Use life	Use life is the period of time a disinfecting solution is effective after it has been activated or prepared for use. For example, Cidex Plus (Johnson & Johnson) is effective for 28 days following activation. At the end of this time, any chemical remaining in the container must be discarded.
Reuse life	Reuse life is the period of time that a disinfecting solution being used and reused remains active. For example, Cidex Plus can be reused for 28 days. At the end of this time, the disinfectant must be discarded.

STERILIZATION

☐ **Sterilization** is the process of destroying all forms of microbial life, including bacterial spores. An item that is **sterile** is free of all living microorganisms and spores. Reusable articles that come in contact with sterile tissue or the vascular system (critical items) must be sterilized before each use.

Sterilization involves the use of either physical or chemical methods. Each method of sterilization has its advantages and disadvantages. The method used to achieve sterility depends primarily upon the nature of the item to be sterilized. The most common physical and chemical sterilization methods include the following:

PHYSICAL METHODS

Steam under pressure (autoclave)
Hot air (dry heat oven)
Radiation

CHEMICAL METHODS

Ethylene oxide gas
Cold sterilization (chemical agents)

The most commonly used method for sterilizing articles in the medical office is steam under pressure using an autoclave. The autoclave is discussed in detail in this chapter, while the other methods of sterilization are briefly described.

AUTOCLAVE

The autoclave is dependable, efficient, and economical and can be used to sterilize items that are not harmed by moisture or high temperature. Refer to the box on this page for a list of heat-resistant items that can be sterilized in the autoclave.

An autoclave consists of an outer jacket surrounding an inner sterilizing chamber. Under pressure, distilled water is converted to steam, which fills the inner sterilizing chamber. The pressure plays no direct part in killing microorganisms; rather, it functions to attain a higher temperature than could be reached by the steam from boiling water (212°F; 100°C). The cooler, drier air already present in the chamber is forced out through an opening known as the air exhaust valve.

It is important that all the air in the chamber be replaced by steam. When air is present, the temperature in the autoclave is reduced and a temperature that is adequate for sterilization is not reached. When all the air has been removed, the air exhaust valve seals off the inner chamber and the temperature in the autoclave begins to rise.

During the sterilization process, the steam penetrates the materials in the sterilizing chamber. The materials are cooler, so the steam condenses into moisture on them, giving up its heat. This heat serves to kill all microorganisms and their spores.

The autoclave is usually operated at approximately 15 pounds of pressure per square inch (psi) at a temperature of 250°F (121°C). While vegetative forms of most microorganisms are killed in a few minutes at temperatures ranging from 130° to 150°F

Items Sterilized in the Autoclave

Surgical instruments
Medical instruments
Linens
Liquids
Brushes
Dressings
Glassware
Treatment trays
Reusable syringes
Utensils

AUTOCLAVE LOG						
Date/Time	Description of the Load	Cycle Time (minutes)	Temperature (F)	Indicator (+/−)	Initial	Comments
7/25/2002 4:00 PM	Surgical instruments	20 min	250° F	−	RR	
7/26/2002 3:00 PM	MOS tray set-ups	30 min	250° F	−	RR	

MAINTENANCE: (Indicate date, vendor name, service, etc)

■ **FIGURE 5–5.** An example of an autoclave log.

(54° to 65° C), certain bacterial spores can withstand a temperature of 240°F (115°C) for more than 3 hours. However, no living thing can survive direct exposure to saturated steam at 250°F (121°C) for 15 minutes or longer.

The sterilization process using the autoclave is discussed in this section (with the exception of sanitization, which was already presented). The sterilization process consists of the following steps:

Monitoring program
Sanitizing articles
Wrapping articles
Operating the autoclave (autoclave cycle)
Storing the packs
Maintaining the autoclave
Each of these is discussed next.

MONITORING PROGRAM

To ensure that instruments and supplies are sterile when used, the Centers for Disease Control and Prevention (CDC) recommends that the medical office establish and maintain a monitoring program of the sterilization process. The monitoring program should consist of the following:

1. Written policies and procedures should exist for each step of the sterilization process.
2. Sterilization indicators should be used to assure that minimum sterilizing conditions have been achieved.
3. Records for each cycle should be maintained in an autoclave log (Fig. 5–5).

The information that should be recorded for each cycle includes the following:

- Date and time of the cycle
- Description of the load
- Exposure time
- Exposure temperature
- Results of the sterilization indicator
- Initials of the operator

Some autoclaves have recorders that automatically print out a portion of this information at the end of the cycle (Fig. 5–6).

STERILIZATION INDICATORS

Materials that are being sterilized must be exposed to steam at a sufficient temperature and for a proper length of time. Sterilization indicators are available to determine the effectiveness of the procedure and to check against improper wrapping of articles, improper loading of the autoclave, or faulty operation of the autoclave.

An article is not considered sterile unless the steam has penetrated to the center of it; therefore, most sterilization indicators are designed to be placed in the center of the article. The medical assistant should thoroughly read the instructions that come with the sterilization indicators. The most reliable indicators check for the attainment of the proper temperature and also indicate the duration of the temperature.

If an indicator does not change properly, a defect may be present in the sterilization technique or in the working condition of the autoclave. The manufacturer's guidelines for proper sterilization techniques should be reviewed and the articles should be resterilized following these guidelines. If the indicator still does not change properly, the autoclave is in need of repair and should not be used until it has been serviced.

Sterilization indicators should be stored in a cool, dry area. Excessive heat or moisture can damage the indicator. The most commonly used sterilization indicators are chemical indicators and biologic indicators, which are described next.

Chemical Indicators

Chemical indicators are impregnated with a thermolabile dye that changes color when exposed to the sterilization process. If the chemical reaction of the indicator does not show the expected results, the item should not be used. Chemical indicators include the following:

AUTOCLAVE TAPE.   Autoclave tape contains a chemical that changes color if it has been exposed to steam. The

READY			
BEGIN			
SET TEMP:	270 F		Temperature
SET TIME:	015	←	Time
RUN #	011	←	Cycle number
DATE			
HEAT UP			
DEG	PSI	MIN	
066	00.0	000	
066	00.0	002	
074	00.0	004	Heat up
164	00.0	006	phase
219	04.1	008	
234	09.4	010	
261	22.6	012	
STERILIZE			
DEG	PSI	MIN	
272	30.2	000	
272	30.7	001	
273	31.3	002	
274	31.0	003	
273	30.7	004	
273	30.4	005	
273	30.1	006	
272	30.0	007	Sterilization
272	30.1	008	phase
272	30.4	009	
272	30.4	010	
272	30.7	011	
273	31.0	012	
273	30.8	013	
274	31.0	014	
273	30.7	015	
VENT			
COMPLETE			

■ **FIGURE 5–6.** An example of a printout of an autoclave cycle.

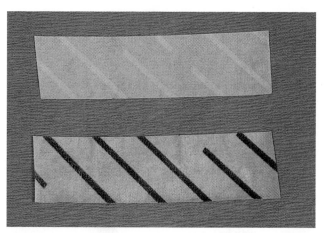

■ **FIGURE 5–7.** Autoclave tape. *Top*: Autoclave tape as it appears before the sterilization process. *Bottom*: Diagonal lines appear on the tape during autoclaving and indicate that the wrapped article has been autoclaved.

tape is available in a variety of colors, can be written on, and is useful for both closing and identifying the wrapped article (Fig. 5–7). Autoclave tape has some definite limitations as an indicator. Since it is placed on the outside of the pack, it cannot assure that steam has penetrated to the center of the pack. Nor does it assure that the item has been sterilized; it merely indicates that an article has been in the autoclave and that a high temperature has been attained.

STERILIZATION STRIPS. Sterilization strips are commercially prepared paper or plastic strips containing a thermolabile dye that change color when exposed to steam under pressure for a certain length of time (Fig. 5–8). Most sterilization strips are designed to change color after being exposed to a temperature of 250°F (121°C) for 15 minutes. The indicator strip should be placed in the center of the wrapped pack with the end containing the dye placed in an area considered to be the hardest for steam to penetrate.

Biologic Indicators

Biologic indicators are the best means available for determining the effectiveness of the sterilization procedure. The CDC recommends that all autoclaves be monitored at least once a week using a biologic indicator.

A biologic indicator is a preparation of living bacterial spores that are commercially available in the form of dry spore strips contained in small glassine envelopes. Biologic monitoring of an autoclave requires the use of a preparation of spores of *Bacillus stearothermophilus*, which is a microorganism having spores that are particularly resistant to moist heat.

Each biologic testing unit includes two spore tests that are sterilized and one spore control that is not

PUTTING IT ALL *into* PRACTICE

▶ KARA VAN DYKE: *As a medical assistant, one of the situations you deal with on an almost daily basis are drug representatives who come to the office to promote their products. Their job is anything but easy. The waiting and the frequent rejections would make most people think twice before applying for the job.*

One winter day, I am sure I made one drug representative really think twice about his career choice. As the representative stopped at our office, he, being a polite young man, let the patient enter the building first with wet snow covered feet. Trying to make a good impression with a new suit and dress shoes, he soon found himself doing a "Spanish fandango" while trying to maintain his balance and eventually crashed to the floor.

Out of compassion, I thought I would help by mopping up the snow tracked floor. What I did not know was the mop had wax on it. Needless to say when he returned with the requested drug samples, we were not able to keep him from falling a second time.

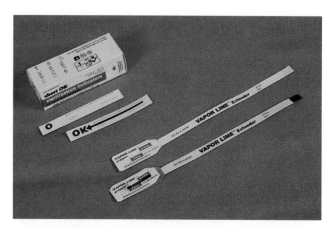

■ **FIGURE 5–8.** Sterilization strips. Sterilization strips contain a thermolabile dye that changes color when exposed to steam under pressure for a certain length of time.

sterilized (Fig. 5–9). The biologic indicator is placed in the center of two different wrapped articles. The articles are placed in areas of the autoclave that are the least accessible to steam penetration, such as on the bottom tray of the autoclave near the front of the autoclave and in the back of the autoclave.

After the indicators have been exposed to sterilization conditions, they must be processed before the results can be obtained. There are two methods for processing results, as follows:

MAIL-IN METHOD. With this method, the processed bacterial spores and the (unprocessed) control are mailed to a processing laboratory. The test is processed by the laboratory and the results are returned to the medical office.

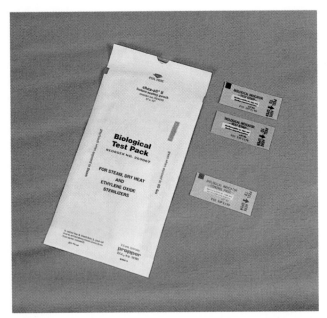

■ **FIGURE 5–9.** Biologic indicator. A biologic indicator includes two spore tests that are sterilized *(top)* and one spore control that is not sterilized *(bottom)*.

IN-HOUSE METHOD. The in-house method involves processing and interpreting the results at the medical office. Following sterilization, the processed spores are incubated for a period of 24 to 48 hours. If sterilization conditions have been met, the processed spores will display a different color or condition as compared to the control. If sterilization conditions have not been met, the processed spores and the unprocessed control will display the same color and condition.

If spores are not killed in routine spore tests, the autoclave should immediately be checked for proper use and function and the spore test repeated. If spore tests remain positive, the autoclave should not be used until it is serviced.

WRAPPING ARTICLES

Articles to be sterilized in the autoclave must first be thoroughly sanitized (see Procedure 5–1). Next, the articles are prepared for autoclaving by wrapping them. The purpose of wrapping articles is to protect them from recontamination during handling and storage.

The wrapping material used should be made of a substance that is not affected by the sterilization process and should allow steam to penetrate while preventing contaminants such as dust, insects, and microorganisms from entering during handling and storage. It should not tear or puncture easily and should allow the sterilized package to be opened without contamination of the contents. A wrapper should not be used if it

is torn or has a hole. Examples of wrapping material used for autoclaving include sterilization paper, sterilization pouches, and muslin. Each of these types of wraps is described next.

Sterilization Paper Wrap

Sterilization paper is a disposable and inexpensive wrapping material. It consists of square sheets of paper of different sizes (Fig. 5–10). The most common sizes are (in inches): 12 × 12, 15 × 15, 18 × 18, 24 × 24, 30 × 30, and 36 × 36. Articles must be wrapped in such a way that they do not become contaminated when the pack is opened. The proper method for wrapping instruments using sterilization paper is outlined in Procedure 5–3. This method of wrapping can be used for all types of instruments and supplies.

The disadvantage of sterilization paper is that it is difficult to spread open for removal of the contents. It has a "memory" and tends to flip back easily and may not open flat to provide a sterile field. (Memory is the ability of a material to retain a specific shape or configuration.) Since sterilization paper is opaque, it is not possible to view the contents of a pack before opening it.

Sterilization Pouches

Sterilization pouches typically consist of a combination of paper and plastic; paper makes up one side of the pouch, and a plastic film makes up the other side (Fig. 5–11). Sterile pouches are available in different sizes; the most common sizes are as follows (in inches): 3 × 9, 5 × 10, and 7 × 12.

Most pouches have a peel-apart seal on one end that is later used to open the pouch for removal of the sterile item. The other end of the pouch is open and is used to insert the item into the pouch. Once inserted,

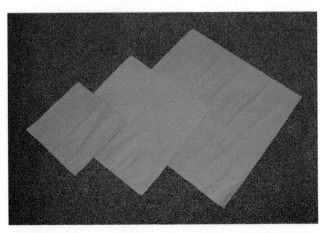

■ **FIGURE 5–10.** Sterilization paper wraps. Sterilization paper consists of square sheets of paper that are available in different sizes.

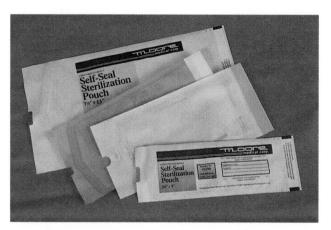

■ **FIGURE 5–11.** Sterilization pouches. Sterilization pouches consist of a combination of paper and plastic, and are available in different sizes.

this end is either heat-sealed or closed with adhesive tape. The proper method for wrapping an instrument using a pouch is outlined in Procedure 5–4.

Sterilization pouches provide good visibility of the contents on the plastic side. Most manufacturers include a sterilization indicator on the outside of the pouch. The medical assistant should check the indicator for proper color change after removing it from the autoclave. If the indicator does not change to the appropriate color (specified by the manufacturer), the contents of the pouch must be resterilized.

Sterilization pouches provide an excellent barrier against microorganisms during storage; most manufacturers indicate contents of their pouches are sterile for up to 1 year when stored under appropriate conditions.

Muslin

Muslin consists of a reusable woven fabric and is available in different sizes. Muslin is flexible and easy to handle and is considered the most economical sterilization wrap because it can be reused. Because of its durability, muslin is frequently used to wrap large packs such as minor office surgery tray set-ups. Muslin is "memory-free" so it will lie flat when opened. A pack wrapped in muslin may be opened on a table so that the wrapper becomes a sterile field. The procedure for wrapping using muslin is the same as that for sterilization paper (see Procedure 5–3).

OPERATING THE AUTOCLAVE

The autoclave must be operated according to the manufacturer's instructions. The medical assistant should carefully read the instruction manual before operating

the autoclave for the first time. Thereafter, the manual should be kept in an accessible location so that it is available if needed as a reference.

The steps that are involved in achieving sterilization using an autoclave are known as the **autoclave cycle.** Accomplishment of each step varies based on whether the autoclave is **manually operated** or **automatically operated.** Figure 5–12 illustrates the autoclave cycle for both manual and automatic autoclave operation.

GUIDELINES FOR AUTOCLAVE OPERATION

General guidelines for operating an autoclave are presented next.

Location of the Autoclave

The autoclave must be placed on a level surface to ensure that the chamber will fill correctly. The front of the autoclave should be located near the front of the support surface so water can be easily drained from the drain tube into a container when flushing out the autoclave.

Filling the Water Reservoir

Use distilled or mineral-free water to fill the water reservoir. Normal tap water contains minerals, such as chlorine, which have corrosive effects on the stainless steel chamber of the autoclave. In addition, using tap water may block the hole of the air exhaust valve. This causes air pockets, which prevent the temperature from rising in the autoclave. Fill the water reservoir to the proper level as indicated in the instruction manual. An autoclave malfunction may occur if the reservoir is overfilled or if there is not enough water in the reservoir.

Loading the Autoclave

For an item to attain sterility, steam must penetrate every fiber and reach every surface of the item at a required temperature and for a specified period of time. To accomplish this, all packs must be positioned in the chamber to allow free circulation and penetration of steam. These guidelines should be followed when loading the autoclave:

1. Small packs are best, because steam penetrates them more easily; it takes longer for steam to reach the center of a large pack to ensure sterilization. A pack should be no larger than 12 × 12 × 20 inches.
2. To allow for proper steam penetration, the materials should be packed as loosely as possible inside the

Text continued on page 184

PROCEDURE

5–3

Wrapping Articles for the Autoclave Using Sterilization Paper or Muslin

EQUIPMENT/SUPPLIES:

Sanitized instrument
Appropriate-sized wrapping material
(sterilization paper or muslin)

Sterilization indicator strip
Autoclave tape
Permanent marker

1. **Procedural Step.** Wash the hands.
2. **Procedural Step.** Assemble the equipment. Select the appropriate-sized wrapping material for the instrument being wrapped. Check the expiration date on the sterilization indicator box. If the sterilization strips are outdated, they should not be used.
   Principle. Instruments are wrapped so that they are protected from recontamination after they have been sterilized. Outdated strip indicators may not provide accurate test results.
3. **Procedural Step.** Place the wrapping material on a clean, flat surface. Turn the wrap in a diagonal position to your body so that it resembles a diamond shape.

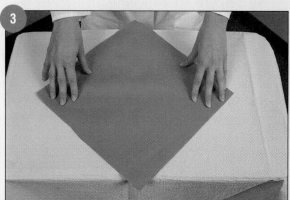

4. **Procedural Step.** Place the instrument in the center of the wrapping material. If the instrument has a movable joint, it should be placed on the wrap in a slightly open position.
   Principle. Instruments with movable joints must be in an open position to allow steam to reach all parts of the instrument. If the instrument is in a closed position, heat exposure could cause the instrument to crack at its weakest part, such as the lock area.

5. **Procedural Step.** Place a sterilization indicator in the center of the pack next to the instrument.

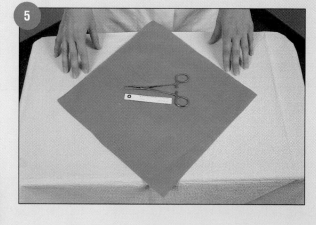

Principle. Sterilization indicators assess the effectiveness of the sterilization process.
6. **Procedural Step.** Fold the wrapping material up from the bottom and double back a small corner.

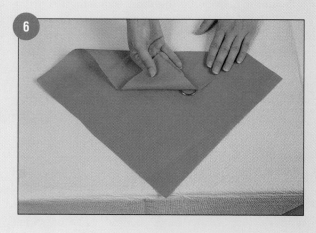

7. **Procedural Step.** Fold over the right edge of the wrapping material and double back the corner.

8. **Procedural Step.** Fold over the left edge of the wrapping material and double back the corner.

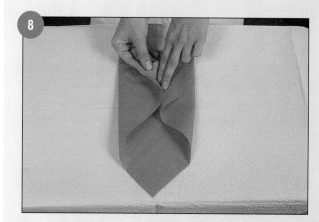

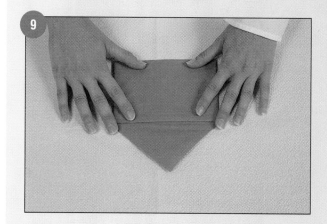

9. **Procedural Step.** Fold the pack up from the bottom and secure it with autoclave tape. Make sure the pack is firm enough for handling but loose enough to permit proper circulation of steam.
   Principle. Instruments must be wrapped properly to permit full penetration of steam and to prevent contaminating them when the wrap is opened. Using autoclave tape will indicate that the pack has been though the autoclave cycle and prevent mix-ups with packs that have not been processed.

10. **Procedural Step.** Label the pack according to its contents. Date the pack with the date of sterilization and your initials.
    Principle. Dating the pack documents its shelf life. After a period of 4 weeks, the contents of the pack are no longer considered sterile and must be resterilized.

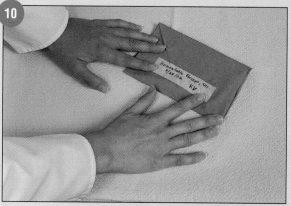

5

PROCEDURE

5–4

Wrapping Instruments for the Autoclave Using a Sterilization Pouch

EQUIPMENT/SUPPLIES: Sanitized instrument   Permanent marker
Appropriate-sized sterilization pouch

1. **Procedural Step.** Wash the hands.
2. **Procedural Step.** Assemble the equipment. Select the appropriate-sized sterilization pouch for the instrument being wrapped. For hinged instruments, make sure to use a bag size wide enough so the instrument can be placed in a slightly open position inside the bag.
   Principle. Instruments are wrapped so that they are protected from recontamination after they have been sterilized.
3. **Procedural Step.** Place the sterilization pouch on a clean, flat surface.
4. **Procedural Step.** Label the pack according to its contents. Date the pack with the date of sterilization and your initials.

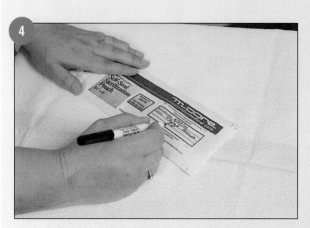

Principle. Dating the pack documents its shelf life. When properly sealed and stored under proper storage conditions, the contents of the pouch are considered sterile for 1 year from the date of sterilization.

5. **Procedural Step.** Insert the instrument to be sterilized into the unsealed, open end of the pouch.

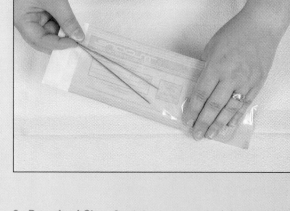

6. **Procedural Step.** Seal the open end of the pouch as follows:
   Adhesive Closure. Peel off the paper strip located above the perforation to expose the adhesive. Fold along the perforation and press firmly to seal the paper to the plastic. Make certain that the seal is secure by running fingers back and forth on both sides of the pouch over the entire sealing area.
   Heat Closure. Seal the pouch using a heat-sealing device.

5

7. **Procedural Step.** Sterilize the pack in the autoclave.

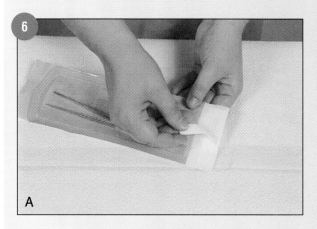
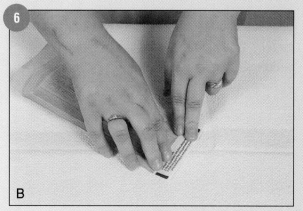

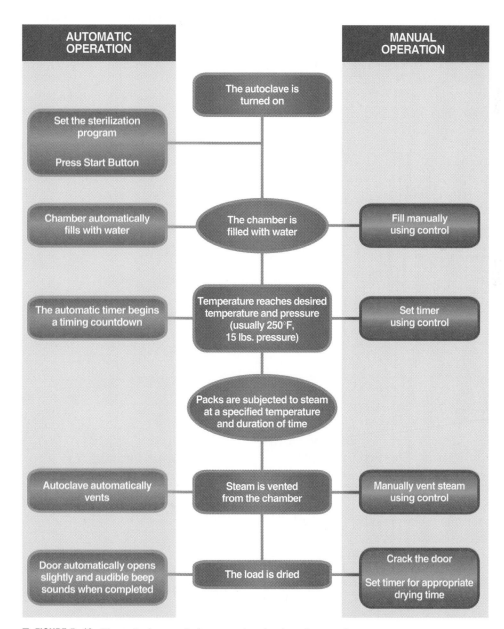

FIGURE 5-12. The autoclave cycle for manual and automatic operation.

■ **FIGURE 5–13.** Arrangement of packs in the autoclave. *A,* Improper arrangement of packs in the autoclave. A large pack (here consisting of four smaller packs held closely together) prevents adequate penetration of steam, resulting in failure to sterilize the portions in the center of the mass. *B,* The large pack has been broken down into four small packs, and these are slightly separated from each other in the autoclave. Steam will now permeate each pack quickly, and in the much shorter period of exposure needed, there will be no oversterilized outer portions. (Courtesy of AMSCO/American Sterilizer Company, Erie, Pennsylvania 16512.)

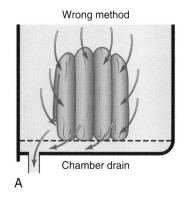

Wrong method

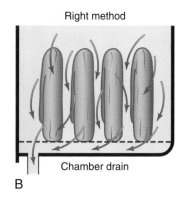

Right method

Chamber drain

A

Chamber drain

B

autoclave, with approximately 1 to 3 inches between small packs and 2 to 4 inches between large packs. Packs should not be allowed to touch surrounding walls, and at least 1 inch should separate the autoclave trays. Placing the articles too close together retards the flow of steam (Fig. 5–13).

3. Jars and glassware should be placed on their sides in the autoclave with their lids removed. If they are placed upright, air may be trapped in them and they will not be properly sterilized. Trapped air must flow out and be replaced by steam during the sterilization process (Fig. 5–14).

4. Packs containing layers of fabric, such as dressings, should be placed in a vertical position. Steam flows from top to bottom, and this method allows the steam to penetrate the layers of fabric.

5. Sterilization pouches should be positioned on their sides to maximize steam circulation and to facilitate the drying process.

Timing the Load

The autoclave is operated at approximately 15 pounds of pressure per square inch with a temperature of 250°F (121°C). The length of time an item is sterilized varies according to what is being sterilized (Table 5–2). For example, steam can easily reach the surfaces of hard, nonporous goods such as unwrapped instruments (e.g., vaginal speculums) to kill microorganisms, requiring less sterilization time. On the other hand, a large minor office surgery pack requires a longer sterilization time because of the time needed for steam to penetrate to the center of the pack. Rubber goods, however, may be damaged by exposure to excessive heat. To prevent this, the medical assistant should make sure to sterilize rubber items for only the prescribed amount of time.

The sterilizing time should not begin until the desired temperature in the autoclave has been reached. Timing the load is accomplished either automatically or manually. Autoclaves with automatic operation begin timing the load automatically once the desired temperature has been reached. With the manual method of operation, the medical assistant must set the timer by hand using a timing control on the front of the autoclave. The medical assistant should not set the timer until the temperature gauge reaches the desired temperature. The articles in the load are not considered sterile unless they have been subjected to steam for the proper length of time.

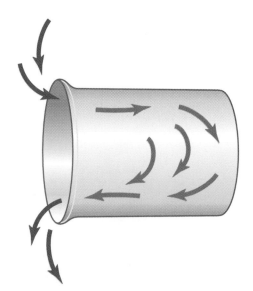

■ **FIGURE 5–14.** Jars and glassware should be placed on their sides in the autoclave with their lids removed. (Courtesy of AMSCO/American Sterilizer Company, Erie, Pennsylvania 16512.)

TABLE 5 – 2

Minimum Sterilizing Times		
Items (Manual Operation)*	Program (Automatic Operation)†	Time (250°F; 121°C)
Unwrapped nonsurgical instruments Open glass or metal canisters Nonsurgical rubber tubing	Unwrapped	15 minutes
Wrapped instruments Fabric or muslin Wrapped trays of loose instruments Rubber tubing	Wrapped	20 minutes
Minor office surgery tray set-up (wrapped)	Packs	30 minutes
Liquids or gels	Liquids	30 minutes

*Manual Operation: The sterilizing time is selected based on the items being sterilized as indicated in this column. The sterilizing time is set using the manual timing control when the autoclave has reached a temperature of 250°F (121°C).

†Automatic Operation: The sterilization program is selected from this column based on what is being autoclaved. The program is selected by pressing the appropriate program button on the front of the autoclave (i.e., Unwrapped, Wrapped, Packs, Liquids). The autoclave automatically begins the proper timing countdown when it reaches 250°F (121°C).

Drying the Load

The sterilized articles are moist and must be allowed to dry before they are removed from the autoclave. This is because microorganisms can move very quickly through the moisture on a wet wrap and onto the sterile article inside, resulting in contamination.

When the load has been subjected to steam for the proper length of time and temperature, the chamber must be vented of steam. Venting the chamber permits the pressure in the autoclave to drop to zero and the chamber to cool, making it safe for the door to be opened. Most autoclaves are designed to vent automatically, which eliminates having to vent them manually.

The door of the autoclave should be opened approximately 1/2 inch but no more than 1 inch. Opening the door more than 1 inch causes cold air from the outside to rush into the autoclave, resulting in condensation of water on the packs. Cracking the door allows the moisture on the articles to change from a liquid to a vapor and thus to escape through the crack. The residual heat in the inner chamber also helps to dry the articles. The load should be allowed to dry for between 15 and 60 minutes, depending on the type of autoclave and the load itself. For example, loads containing large packs require a longer drying time than those with smaller packs. The medical assistant should

follow the manufacturer's recommendations for proper drying times of various loads.

5

STORAGE

Sterilized articles should be stored in clean areas that are free from dust, insects, and other sources of contamination. Articles wrapped in sterilization paper or muslin are considered sterile for 4 weeks. After this time, they should be resterilized. Placing a paper or muslin pack in a sealed airtight plastic bag extends its shelf-life (length of time the article is considered sterile) to 1 year. Plastic bag covers are recommended for low-use items that may not be used within the standard 4-week shelf-life period. The shelf-life of sterilization pouches is typically 1 year from the date of sterilization.

The medical assistant should thoroughly check each sterilized pack at least twice: before storing it and before using it. If the pack is torn or opened or if it is wet, it is no longer sterile and must be rewrapped and resterilized. In addition, the medical assistant should check the sterilization date on each wrapped article before using it to make sure it is still considered sterile.

MAINTENANCE

For the autoclave to work efficiently, it must be properly maintained. The instruction manual that accompanies the autoclave provides specific information for the care and maintenance of that particular type of autoclave.

Safety precautions should be followed when performing maintenance procedures. Before proceeding with preventive maintenance, the autoclave must be cool, the pressure gauge at zero, and the power cord disconnected from the wall socket. Autoclave maintenance is performed on a daily, weekly, and monthly basis as follows:

Daily Maintenance

1. Wipe the outside of the autoclave with a damp cloth and a mild detergent.
2. Wipe the interior of the autoclave and the trays with a damp cloth.
3. Clean the rubber gasket located on the door of the autoclave with a damp cloth.
4. Inspect the rubber door gasket for possible damage that could prevent a good seal.

Weekly Maintenance

1. Wash the inside of the chamber and the trays with a commercial autoclave cleaner according to the manufacturer's instructions. This usually involves the following steps. The water reservoir must first be drained. A soft cloth or a soft brush should be used to clean the chamber, which should be rinsed thoroughly with distilled or demineralized water. Do not use steel wool or a steel brush or other abrasive agents as this can damage the chamber. The chamber must be dried thoroughly and the door left open overnight.
2. The metal shelves should be washed with an autoclave cleaner and rinsed thoroughly with distilled or demineralized water using the same method.

Monthly Maintenance

1. Flush the system to remove any built-up residue, which could cause corrosion of the chamber lines. Carefully follow the manufacturer's directions in the instruction manual to perform this procedure.
2. Check the air trap jet to make sure it is functioning properly. The air trap jet prevents air pockets in the chamber, to ensure adequate sterilization.
3. Check the safety valve to make sure it is functioning properly. The safety valve releases pressure in the chamber if it gets too high.

5

PROCEDURE

5-5

Sterilizing Articles in the Autoclave

EQUIPMENT/SUPPLIES: Autoclave and instruction manual   Wrapped articles
Distilled water   Heat-resistant gloves

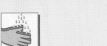

1. **Procedural Step.** Assemble the equipment.
2. **Procedural Step.** Check the level of water in the autoclave and add distilled water, if needed. **Principle.** Water contained in the water reservoir of the autoclave is converted to steam during the

sterilization process. Distilled water is used to prevent corrosion of the stainless steel chamber of the autoclave.

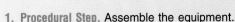

PROCEDURE 5–5

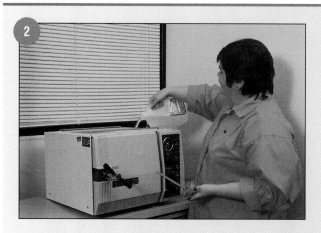

3. **Procedural Step.** Properly load the autoclave following these guidelines:
   a. Do not overload the chamber. Small packs should be placed 1 to 3 inches apart and large packs should be placed 2 to 4 inches apart. The packs should not touch the chamber walls.
   b. At least 1 inch should separate the autoclave trays.
   c. Place jars and glassware on their sides.
   d. Place dressings in a vertical position.
   e. When sterilizing dressings and hard goods together, place dressings on the top shelf and hard goods on the lower shelf.

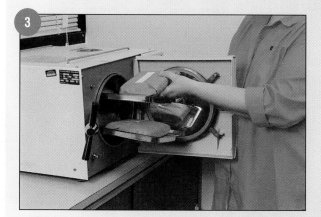

   f. When using sterilization pouches, set the pouches on their sides to maximize steam circulation and to facilitate drying.
   Principle. The autoclave must be loaded properly to assure adequate steam penetration of all articles.
4. **Procedural Step.** Operate the autoclave according to the procedure contained in the instruction manual. A general procedure for both the manual and automatic methods of operation follows.

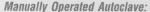

Manually Operated Autoclave:
   a. Determine the sterilizing time for the type of articles being autoclaved (refer to Table 5–2).
   b. Turn on the autoclave.
   c. Fill the chamber with water using the appropriate control.
   d. Securely close and latch the door of the autoclave.
   e. Set the timing control when the temperature on the temperature gauge reaches the desired temperature (usually 250°F or 121°C). At the end of the steam exposure time, an indicator light usually comes on or a beeper sounds.

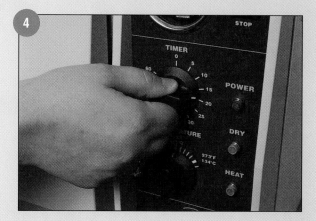

   f. Vent the chamber of steam using the appropriate control if the autoclave does not vent automatically.
   g. Dry the load by cracking open the door approximately 1/2 inch but no more than 1 inch. Set the drying time using the timing control. The drying time will vary between 15 and 60 minutes, depending on the autoclave and the type of load.

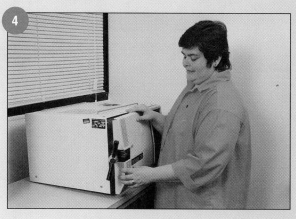

5

5

Principle. The load should not be timed until the proper temperature has been reached to ensure sterilization. The sterility of wrapped packs cannot be ensured unless the wrapped articles are allowed to dry fully. Microorganisms can move through the moisture on a wet wrap and contaminate the sterile article inside.

Automatically Operated Autolave:

   a. Securely close and latch the door of the autoclave.

   b. Turn on the autoclave.

   c. Determine the sterilization program according to what is being autoclaved (refer to Table 5–2). Press the appropriate program button on the front of the autoclave to select the program. Press the start button.

   d. Indicators on the front of the autoclave will tell you what is happening (automatically) in the autoclave.

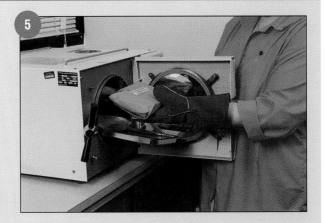

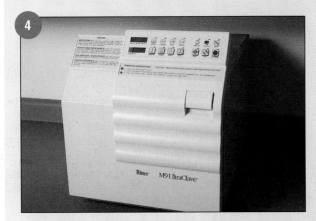

Filling Indicator. Lights up when the chamber is filling with water.

Sterilizing Indicator. Lights up during the heat up and sterilization phase of the cycle.

Temperature Display. Digital display of the temperature in the autoclave.

Time Display. Digital countdown display of the time remaining in the sterilization program.

Drying Indicator. Lights up during the drying phase of the cycle

Complete or Ready Indicator. Illuminates when the autoclave has completed the cycle and sterilized articles can be removed from the autoclave.

5. **Procedural Step.** Turn off the autoclave and remove the load with heat-resistant gloves. Do not touch the inner chamber of the autoclave with your bare hands.

Principle. Heat-resistant gloves protect the medical assistant's hands when the warm packs from the chamber of the autoclave are being removed. The inner chamber of the autoclave is hot and could burn bare hands.

6. **Procedural Step.** Inspect the packs as you take them out of the autoclave. If the packs show any damage such as holes or tears, the articles should be rewrapped and resterilized.

7. **Procedural Step.** Check the sterilization indicators located on the outside of the pack to make sure the proper indicator response has taken place.

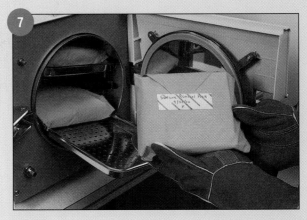

8. **Procedural Step.** Record monitoring information in the autoclave log. Include the date and time of the cycle, a description of the load, the exposure time and temperature, the results of the sterilization indicator, and your initials.

9. **Procedural Step.** Store the articles in a clean, dust-proof area.

10. **Procedural Step.** Maintain appropriate daily care of the autoclave, following the manufacturer's recommendations. The daily care of the autoclave includes the following:
   a. Wipe the outside of the autoclave with a damp cloth and a mild detergent.
   b. Wipe the interior of the autoclave and the trays with a damp cloth.
   c. Clean the rubber gasket located on the door of the autoclave with a damp cloth.
   d. Inspect the rubber door gasket for possible damage that could prevent a good seal.
   Principle. For the autoclave to work efficiently, it must be properly maintained.

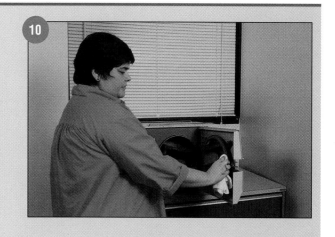

OTHER STERILIZATION METHODS

☐ In addition to the autoclave, other methods can be used to sterilize articles. These methods are not generally used in the medical office and, therefore, are only discussed briefly in this chapter.

DRY HEAT OVEN

Dry heat ovens are used to sterilize articles that either cannot be penetrated by steam or may be damaged by it. For example, dry heat is less corrosive than moist heat for needles and instruments with sharp cutting edges; it does not dull their sharp points or edges. Oil, petroleum jelly, and powder cannot be penetrated by steam and must be sterilized in a dry heat oven. Moist heat sterilization tends to erode the ground glass surfaces of reusable syringes, whereas dry heat does not.

Dry heat ovens operate like an ordinary cooking oven. A longer exposure period is needed with dry heat, because microorganisms and spores are more resistant to dry heat than to moist heat and also because dry heat penetrates more slowly and unevenly than moist heat. The most commonly used temperature for dry heat sterilization is 320°F (160°C) for a duration of 1 to 2 hours, depending on the article being sterilized. The recommended wrapping material for dry heat sterilization is aluminum foil, because it is a good conductor of heat and also protects against recontamination during handling and storage. Dry heat sterilization indicators are available to determine the effectiveness of the sterilization process.

ETHYLENE OXIDE GAS STERILIZATION

Ethylene oxide is a colorless gas that is both toxic and flammable. It is used to sterilize items that are heat sensitive and cannot be sterilized in an autoclave. Once items are sterilized, they must be aerated to remove the toxic reside of the ethylene oxide.

Ethylene oxide sterilization is a more complex and expensive process than steam sterilization. It is frequently used in the medical manufacturing industry for producing prepackaged, presterilized disposable items such as syringes, sutures, catheters, and surgical packs.

COLD STERILIZATION

Cold sterilization involves the use of a chemical agent for an extended length of time. Only those chemicals that are designated as sterilants by the Environmental Protection Agency (EPA) can be used for sterilizing articles. If a chemical agent holds this status, the word "sterilant" will be printed on the front of the container.

The item to be sterilized must be submerged in the chemical for 6 to 24 hours. Over time, prolonged immersion of instruments can damage them. In addition, each time a new instrument is added to the instrument container, the clock must be restarted for the entire amount of time. For these reasons, cold sterilization should only be used when steam, gas, or a dry heat oven are not indicated or are unavailable.

RADIATION

Radiation uses high-energy ionizing radiation to sterilize articles. Radiation is used by medical manufacturers to sterilize prepackaged surgical equipment and for instruments that cannot be sterilized by heat or chemicals.

5

MEDICAL PRACTICE AND THE LAW

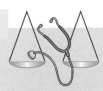

Sterilization and disinfection adversely affect patient outcomes if not performed properly, and can open the medical assistant and office to liability. Meticulous care must be taken to ensure that all procedures are performed correctly and completely.

Sterilization and disinfection procedures include the use of hazardous chemicals. These chemicals must be stored, used, and disposed of in specific ways mandated by law. The autoclave can be a danger-ous machine if it is not used correctly, and it could harm others with hot steam. If you use the autoclave without proper instruction, you could be liable for injuries or accidents resulting from misuse.

Whenever you are dealing with contaminated articles, you have a duty to protect yourself, other employees, patients, and other articles from cross-contamination.

CERTIFICATION REVIEW

☐ The Hazard Communications Standard (HCS) is required by OSHA and its purpose is to ensure that employees are informed of the hazards associated with chemicals in their workplaces and the precautions to take to protect themselves when working with hazardous chemicals.

☐ Employers are required to develop a written Hazard Communications Program describing what their facility is doing to meet the requirements of the HCS.

☐ A hazardous chemical must contain a label that includes the name of the chemical, manufacturer information, physical and health hazards of the chemical, safety precautions, and storing and handling information.

☐ A material safety data sheet (MSDS) provides information regarding the chemical, its hazards, and measures to take to avoid injury and illness when handling the chemical. An MSDS must be kept on file for each hazardous chemical used or stored in the workplace.

☐ The HCS requires that employees be provided with information and training regarding hazardous chemicals in the workplace.

☐ Sanitization is a process that removes organic material from an article and lowers the number of microorganisms to a safe level. The most frequent items sanitized in the medical office are medical and surgical instruments.

☐ Instruments can be cleaned either manually or by using an ultrasonic cleaner. The manual method uses a brush, instrument cleaner, and friction to clean instruments. An ultrasonic cleaner uses a cleaning solution and sound waves to clean the instruments. Items made of dissimilar metals should not be cleaned together to prevent the formation of a permanent stain.

☐ Disinfection is the process of destroying pathogenic microorganisms; it does not necessarily kill bacterial spores. Disinfectants consist of chemical agents that are applied to inanimate objects. The disinfectants used most often in the medical office are glutaraldehyde, alcohol, sodium hypochlorite, phenolics, and quaternary ammonium compounds.

☐ Disinfection can be classified into the following levels: high level, intermediate level, and low level. High-level disinfection is used to disinfect semi-critical items. Intermediate-level disinfection is used for noncritical items, and low-level disinfection is used to disinfect surfaces such as examining tables, countertops, and walls.

☐ Sterilization is the process of destroying all forms of microbial life, including bacterial spores. Sterilization must be used for critical items. Critical items are items that come in contact with sterile tissue or the vascular system.

☐ In the medical office, the autoclave is used most often for sterilization. The autoclave is usually operated at approximately 15 pounds of pressure per square inch at a temperature of 250°F (121°C).

☐ To ensure that instruments and supplies are sterile when used, a monitoring program should be established in the medical office. This program should include sterilization policies and procedures, the use of sterilization indicators, and records for each autoclave cycle.

☐ Sterilization indicators determine the effectiveness of the sterilization process and include chemical indicators and biologic indicators. Chemical indicators use a thermolabile dye that changes color when exposed to the sterilization process. Biologic indicators are the best indicators available and

5

consist of a preparation of heat-resistant bacterial spores.

☐ The purpose of wrapping articles for autoclaving is to protect them from recontamination during handling and storage. Examples of wraps commonly used include sterilization paper, sterilization pouches, and muslin.

☐ The autoclave cycle refers to the steps involved in achieving sterilization. The autoclave must be loaded properly so that steam can easily penetrate the contents of the load. The length of time an item must be sterilized varies according to what is being sterilized. The sterilizing time should not begin until the desired temperature in the autoclave has been reached. To prevent recontamination, articles must be completely dry before removing them from the autoclave.

☐ Sterilized articles should be stored in a clean, dustproof area. Articles wrapped in sterilization paper or muslin are considered sterile for 4 weeks.

☐ The autoclave should be properly maintained following a daily, weekly, and monthly maintenance schedule.

☐ Other methods that can be used to sterilize articles include dry heat, ethylene oxide gas, chemical agents, and radiation. Ethylene oxide and radiation are used by the medical manufacturing industry for producing prepackaged and presterilized disposable items.

ON THE WEB

RESOURCES

For Information on Infection Control in the Health-Care Setting:

Centers for Disease Control and Prevention
www.cdc.gov

Environmental Protection Agency
www.epa.gov

National Institute of Environmental Health Services
www.niehs.nih.gov

Occupational Safety and Health Administration
www.osha.gov

Public Health Service
phs.os.dhhs.gov/phs/ phs.html

5

My name is

Trudy Browning, *and I graduated from an accredited medical assisting program with an associate's degree in Applied Science. I am a Certified Medical Assistant (CMA) and have worked as the office manager of an internal medicine office for the past 3 years. My job includes both front and back office duties, including scheduling appointments, transcription, patient calls, patient work-ups, injections, electrocardiograms, and venipuncture. The most interesting part of my job is dealing with the many different personalities of the patients that I come in contact with daily.*

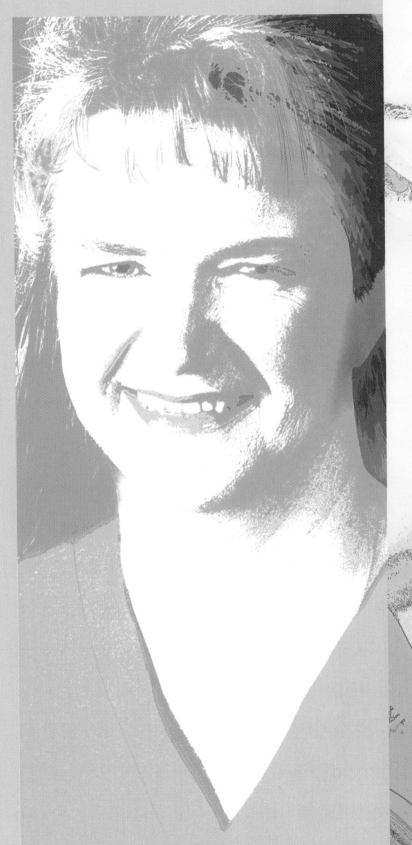

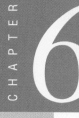
CHAPTER OUTLINE

Surgical Asepsis
Instruments Used in Minor
  Office Surgery
  Care of Surgical Instruments
Commercially Prepared Sterile
  Packages
Wounds
Wound Healing
  Phases of Wound Healing
  Wound Drainage
Sterile Dressing Change
Sutures
  Types of Sutures
  Suture Size and Packaging
  Suture Needles
Insertion of Sutures
Suture Removal
  Surgical Skin Staples
  Adhesive Skin Closures
Assisting with Minor Office
  Surgery
  Tray Set-Up
  Skin Preparation
  Local Anesthetic
  Assisting the Physician
Medical Office Surgical
  Procedures
  Sebaceous Cyst Removal
  Surgical Incision and Drain-
    age of Localized Infections
  Needle Biopsy
  Ingrown Toenail Removal
  Colposcopy
  Cervical Punch Biopsy
  Cryosurgery
Bandaging
  Guidelines for Application
  Types of Bandages
  Bandage Turns
  Tubular Gauze Bandages

OUTCOMES

After completing this chapter, you should be able to demonstrate the proper procedures to perform the following:

1. Apply and remove sterile gloves.
2. Open a sterile package.
3. Add an article to a sterile field.
4. Pour a sterile solution.
5. Change a sterile dressing.
6. Remove sutures.
7. Remove surgical staples.
8. Apply and remove adhesive skin closures.
9. Set up a tray for each of the following surgical procedures: suture insertion, sebaceous cyst removal, incision and drainage of a localized infection, needle biopsy, ingrown toenail removal, colposcopy, cervical punch biopsy, and cryosurgery.
10. Assist the physician with minor office surgery.
11. Apply the following bandage turns: circular, spiral, spiral-reverse, figure-eight, and recurrent.
12. Apply a tubular gauze bandage.

EDUCATIONAL OBJECTIVES

After completing this chapter, you should be able to do the following:

1. Define the terms listed in the Key Terminology.
2. Identify four types of procedure that require the use of surgical asepsis.
3. Describe the medical assistant's responsibilities during a minor surgical procedure.
4. List five guidelines that should be observed during a sterile procedure in order to maintain surgical asepsis.
5. Identify and explain the use and care of instruments commonly used for minor office surgery.
6. Explain the difference between a closed and an open wound, and give an example of one type of closed wound and four types of open wound.
7. List and explain the three phases involved in the healing process.
8. List and describe the different types of wound drainage.
9. List two functions of a dressing.
10. Explain the method used to measure the diameter of suturing material.
11. Describe the two different types of sutures (absorbable and nonabsorbable), and give examples of uses for each.
12. Categorize suturing needles according to their type of point and their shape.
13. Explain the purpose of and procedure for each of the following minor surgical operations: sebaceous cyst removal, incision and drainage of a localized infection, needle biopsy, ingrown toenail removal, colposcopy, cervical punch biopsy, and cryosurgery.
14. State three functions of a bandage, and list four guidelines that should be observed when applying a bandage.
15. Identify the common types of bandages used in the medical office.
16. Explain the use of a tubular gauze bandage.
17. Explain the principles underlying each step in the minor office surgery procedures.

6

KEY TERMINOLOGY

abrasion (Â-brâ-shun): A wound in which the outer layers of the skin are damaged; a scrape.

abscess (AB-sess): A collection of pus in a cavity surrounded by inflamed tissue.

absorbable suture (AB-sorb-a-bl SÛ-chur): Suture material that is gradually digested by tissue enzymes and absorbed by the body.

approximation (a-PROX-i-Mâ-shun): The process of bringing two parts, such as tissue, together, through the use of sutures or other means.

bandage: A strip of woven material used to wrap or cover a part of the body.

biopsy (bî-op-sê): The surgical removal and examination of tissue from the living body. Biopsies are generally performed to determine whether a tumor is benign or malignant.

capillary action (KAP-il-air-ê): That action which causes liquid to rise along a wick, a tube, or a gauze dressing.

colposcope (KUL-pô-skôp): A lighted instrument with a binocular magnifying lens used for the examination of the vagina and cervix.

colposcopy (KUL-pos-kô-pê): The visual examination of the vagina and cervix using a colposcope.

contaminate: As it relates to sterile technique, to cause a sterile object or surface to become unsterile.

contusion (kun-TÛ-shun): An injury to the tissues under the skin causing blood vessels to rupture, allowing blood to seep into the tissues; a bruise.

cryosurgery (KRY-ô-SURG-er-ê): The therapeutic use of freezing temperatures to destroy abnormal tissue.

exudate (X-û-dât): A discharge produced by the body's tissues.

fibroblast (fi-BRÔ-blast): An immature cell from which connective tissue can develop.

forceps (FOR-seps): A two-pronged instrument for grasping and squeezing.

furuncle (fur-UN-kle): A localized staphylococcal infection that originates deep within a hair follicle; also known as a boil.

hemostasis (HÊM-o-STÂ-sis): The arrest of bleeding by natural or artificial means.

incision (IN-sis-shun): A clean cut caused by a cutting instrument.

infection (IN-fek-shun): The condition in which the body or part of it is invaded by a pathogen.

infiltration (IN-fil-TRÂ-shun): The process by which a substance passes into and is deposited within the substance of a cell, tissue, or organ.

inflammation (IN-fla-MÂ-shun): A protective response of the body to trauma and the entrance of foreign matter. The purpose of inflammation is to destroy invading microorganisms and to repair injured tissue.

laceration (LAS-er-Â-shun): A wound in which the tissues are torn apart, leaving ragged and irregular edges.

ligate (LÎ-gât): To tie off and close a structure such as a severed blood vessel.

local anesthetic (LÔ-kul AN-es-THET-ik): A drug that produces a loss of feeling and an inability to perceive pain in only a specific part of the body.

Mayo tray (MÂ-ô TRÂ): A broad, flat metal tray placed on a stand and used to hold sterile instruments and supplies once it has been covered with a sterile towel.

needle biopsy (NÊ-dle BÎ-op-sê): A type of biopsy in which tissue from deep within the body is obtained by the insertion of a biopsy needle through the skin.

nonabsorbable suture (non-AB-sorb-a-bl SÛ-chur): Suture material that is not absorbed by the body and either remains permanently in the body tissue and becomes encapsulated by fibrous tissue or is removed.

postoperative (post-OP-ra-tiv): After a surgical operation.

preoperative (prê-OP-ra-tiv): Preceding a surgical operation.

puncture (punk-SHUR): A wound made by a sharp pointed object piercing the skin.

scalpel (SKAL-pul): A surgical knife used to divide tissues.

scissors: A cutting instrument.

sebaceous cyst (sa-BÂ-shous SIST): A thin, closed sac or capsule containing fatty secretions from a sebaceous gland.

serum (SERE-um): The clear, straw-colored part of the blood that remains after the solid elements have been separated out of it.

sponge: A porous, absorbent pad, such as a 4-inch gauze pad or cotton surrounded by gauze, used to absorb fluids, to apply medication, or to cleanse an area.

sterile: Free from all living microorganisms and bacterial spores.

surgical asepsis (SURG-i-kul Â-SEP-sis): Those practices that keep objects and areas sterile or free from microorganisms.

sutures (SÛ-churs): Material used to approximate tissues with surgical stitches.

swaged needle (SWAGD NÊ-dle): A needle with suturing material permanently attached to the end of the needle.

wound: A break in the continuity of an external or internal surface caused by physical means.

INTRODUCTION

☐ Various types of minor surgical operations may be performed in the medical office, such as insertion of sutures, sebaceous cyst removal, incision and drainage of infections, needle biopsies, cervical biopsies, and ingrown toenail removal. The physician explains the nature of the surgical procedure and any risks to the patient and offers to answer any questions. The medical assistant is responsible for helping reassure the patient and may also be responsible for obtaining the patient's signature on a written consent to treatment form, which grants the physician permission to perform the surgery (Fig. 6–1).

Additional responsibilities of the medical assistant involve preparing the treatment room, preparing the patient, preparing the minor surgery tray, assisting the physician during the procedure, administering postoperative care to the patient, and cleaning the treatment room after the procedure.

The treatment room must be spotlessly clean, and the medical assistant should make sure the physician has adequate lighting for the procedure. The patient is positioned and draped according to the procedure to be performed. Sterile **fenestrated drapes** are often used. They have an opening that is placed directly over the operative area. The skin is prepared as specified by the physician. Hair around the operative site is considered a contaminant and may need to be removed by shaving. The skin is cleansed and an appropriate antiseptic is applied to the area to reduce the number of microorganisms present.

The medical assistant prepares the minor surgery tray using sterile technique. The specific instruments and supplies included in each set-up will vary somewhat, depending on the physician's preference. Therefore, the medical assistant must become familiar with the instruments and supplies required for each surgical procedure performed in the medical office.

During the minor surgery, the medical assistant is present to assist the physician as needed and to lend support to the patient. The medical assistant should become completely familiar with each surgical procedure and learn to anticipate the needs of the physician, to help the procedure proceed quickly and smoothly.

After the minor surgery, the medical assistant should remain with the patient as a safety precaution, to prevent accidental falls or other injuries and to make sure the patient understands the postoperative instructions. The medical assistant then removes and properly cares for all used instruments and supplies and cleans the treatment room in preparation for the next patient.

SURGICAL ASEPSIS

☐ **Surgical asepsis,** also known as sterile technique, refers to those practices that keep objects and areas sterile, or free from all living microorganisms and bacterial spores. Surgical asepsis protects the patient from pathogenic microorganisms that may enter the body and cause disease. It is always employed under the following circumstances: when caring for broken skin, such as open wounds and suture punctures; when a skin surface is being penetrated, as by a surgical incision or the administration of an injection (the needle must remain sterile); or when a body cavity is entered that is normally sterile, such as during the insertion of a urinary cathether. Sterility of instruments and supplies is achieved through the use of disposable sterile items or by sterilizing reusable articles.

A sterile object that touches anything unsterile is automatically considered contaminated and must not be used. A medical assistant in doubt or who has a question concerning the sterility of an article should consider it contaminated and replace it with a sterile article.

Sterility of the hands cannot be attained. Handwashing renders them medically aseptic and must be performed before and after each surgical procedure using proper technique (see Chapter 1). To prevent contamination of sterile articles, sterile gloves must be used to pick up or transfer articles during a sterile procedure.

Specific guidelines must be observed during a sterile procedure to maintain surgical asepsis. These guidelines are presented in a box on page 197.

6

(attach label or complete blanks)

First name: _____   Last name: _____

Date of Birth: _____ Month _____ Day _____ Year

Account Number: _____

Procedure Consent Form

I, _____ ,hereby consent to have

Dr. _____ perform _____ .

I have been fully informed of the following by my physician:

1. The nature of my condition.
2. The nature and purpose of the procedure.
3. An explanation of risks involved with the procedure.
4. Alternative treatments or procedures available.
5. The likely results of the procedure.
6. The risks involved with declining or delaying the procedure.

My physician has offered to answer all questions concerning the proposed procedure.

I am aware that the practice of medicine and surgery is not an exact science, and I acknowledge that no guarantees have been made to me about the results of the procedure.

Patient _____   Date _____
             (or guardian and relationship)

Witnessed _____   Date _____

■ **FIGURE 6–1.** Example of a consent to treatment form.

INSTRUMENTS USED IN MINOR OFFICE SURGERY

☐ A variety of surgical instruments are used for minor office surgery. Most instruments are made from stainless steel and have either a bright, highly polished finish or a dull finish. The medical assistant should become familiar with the name, use, and proper care of the instruments used in the medical office. Some of the more common instruments are described here and are illustrated in Figure 6–2.

Scalpels

A **scalpel** is a small straight surgical knife consisting of a handle and a thin, sharp blade that has a convex edge. It is used to make surgical incisions and can divide tissue with the least possible trauma to the sur-

Guidelines for Surgical Asepsis

1. Take precautions to prevent sterile packages from becoming wet. Wet packages draw microorganisms into the package owing to the capillary action of the liquid, resulting in contamination of the sterile package. If a sterile package that has been prepared at the medical office becomes wet, it must be resterilized; if a disposable sterile package becomes wet, it must be discarded.

2. A 1-inch border around the sterile field is considered contaminated or unsterile, because this area may have become contaminated while the sterile field was being set up.

3. Always face the sterile field. If you must turn your back to it or leave the room, a sterile towel must be placed over the sterile field.

4. Hold all sterile articles above waist level. Anything out of sight may become contaminated. The sterile articles should also be held in front of you and should not be allowed to touch your uniform.

5. To avoid contamination, all sterile items should be placed in the center of the sterile field and not around the edges.

6. Be careful not to spill water or solutions on the sterile field. The area beneath the field is contaminated, and microorganisms will be drawn up onto the field by the capillary action of the liquid, resulting in contamination of the field.

7. Do not talk, cough, or sneeze over a sterile field. Water vapor from the nose, mouth, and lungs will be carried out by the air and contaminate the sterile field.

8. Do not reach over a sterile field. Dust or lint from your clothing may fall onto it or your unsterile clothing may accidentally touch it.

9. Do not pass soiled dressings over the sterile field.

10. Always acknowledge if you have contaminated the sterile field, so that proper steps can be taken to regain sterility.

rounding structures. Both reusable and disposable scalpels are available; scalpels having a reusable handle and a disposable blade are used most frequently.

Scissors

Scissors are cutting instruments that have either straight (str) or curved (cvd) blades. Both blade tips may be sharp (s/s), both may be blunt (b/b), or one tip may be blunt and the other sharp (b/s). The two parts making up a pair of scissors come together at a hinge joint known as a box lock. The type of scissors employed depends on the intended use. The various types of scissors are listed and described next.

- **Operating scissors** have straight delicate blades that have a sharp cutting edge and are used for cutting through tissue. They are available with sharp/sharp, blunt/blunt, or blunt/sharp tips.
- **Suture scissors** are used to remove sutures. The hook on the tip aids in getting under a suture, and the blunt end prevents puncturing of the tissues.
- **Bandage scissors** are inserted beneath a dressing or bandage to cut it for removal. The flat blunt prow can be inserted beneath a dressing without puncturing the skin.
- **Dissecting scissors** have a fine cutting edge used to divide tissue and are available with either straight or curved blades. Both blade tips of dissecting scissors are blunt.

Forceps

Forceps are two-pronged instruments for grasping and squeezing. Some forceps have a spring handle (e.g., thumb, tissue, splinter, and dressing forceps) that provides the proper tension needed for grasping tissue. As you will note from Figure 6–2, some varieties have toothed clasps on the handle, known as ratchets, to hold the tips securely together (e.g., Allis tissue forceps, hemostatic forceps, and sponge forceps). The ratchets are designed to allow closure of the instrument at three or more positions. The various types of forceps are listed and described next.

- **Thumb forceps** have serrated tips and are used to pick up tissue or to hold tissue between adjacent surfaces. Serrations are sawlike teeth that grasp tissue and prevent it from slipping out of the jaws of the instrument.
- **Tissue forceps** have teeth to prevent them from slipping and are used to grasp tissue. Tissue forceps are identified by the number of apposing teeth on each jaw (e.g., 1 × 2, 2 × 3, 3 × 4). The teeth should approximate tightly when the instrument is closed.
- **Splinter forceps** have sharp points that are useful in removing foreign objects, such as splinters, from the tissues.
- **Dressing forceps** are used in the application and removal of dressings. They have a blunt end containing coarse cross striations used for grasping.
- **Hemostatic forceps** have serrated tips, ratchets, and box locks and are available with either straight or curved blades. Hemostats are used to clamp off blood vessels and to establish hemostasis until they can be closed with sutures. The ratchets keep the hemostat tightly shut when it is closed. They should

6

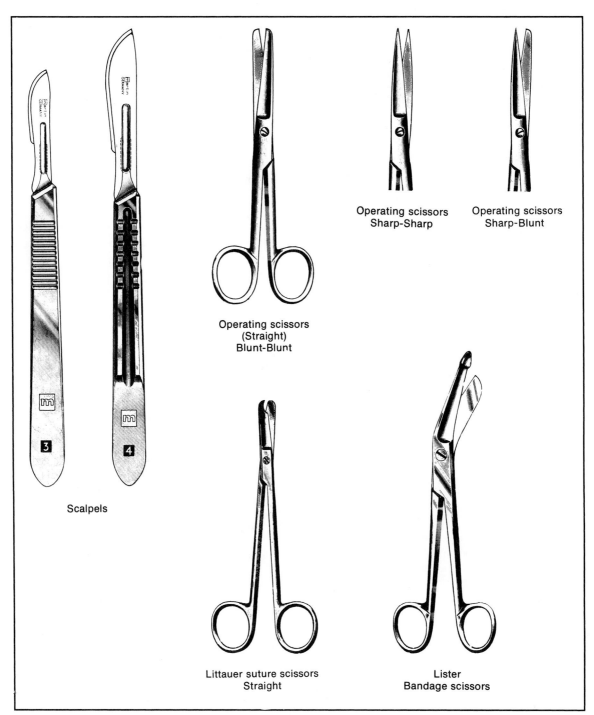

Operating scissors
Sharp-Sharp

Operating scissors
Sharp-Blunt

Operating scissors
(Straight)
Blunt-Blunt

Scalpels

Littauer suture scissors
Straight

Lister
Bandage scissors

■ **FIGURE 6–2.** Instruments used in minor office surgery. (Courtesy of Elmed Incorporated, Addison, Illinois.)

mesh together smoothly when the instrument is closed; if they spring back open, the instrument is in need of repair. The serrations on a hemostat prevent the blood vessel from slipping out of the jaws of the instrument.

■ **Sponge forceps,** as the name implies, have large serrated rings on the tips for holding sponges.

Miscellaneous Instruments

Various types of miscellaneous instruments used in the medical office are listed and described next.

■ **Needle holders** have serrated tips, ratchets, and box locks and are used to grasp a curved needle firmly to insert it through the skin flaps of an incision.

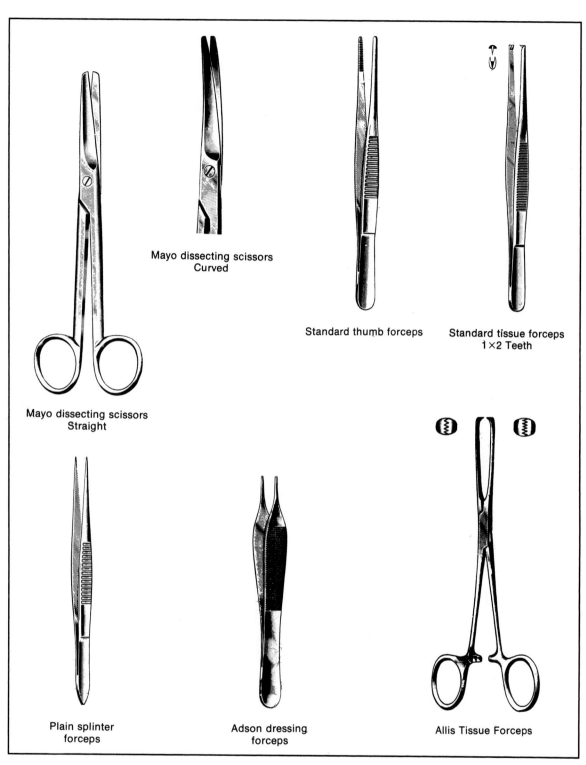

Mayo dissecting scissors
Curved

Standard thumb forceps

Standard tissue forceps
1×2 Teeth

Mayo dissecting scissors
Straight

Plain splinter
forceps

Adson dressing
forceps

Allis Tissue Forceps

■ FIGURE 6–2. *Continued*

Illustration continued on following page

■ **Towel clamps** have two sharp points that are used to hold the edges of a sterile towel in place.

■ **Retractors** are used to hold tissues aside to improve the exposure of the operative area.

■ **Probes** are long slender instruments used to explore wounds or body cavities.

Gynecologic Instruments

Gynecologic surgical procedures are often performed in the medical office; therefore, the medical assistant should be familiar with terms relating to gynecologic instruments. These are listed and described next.

6

6

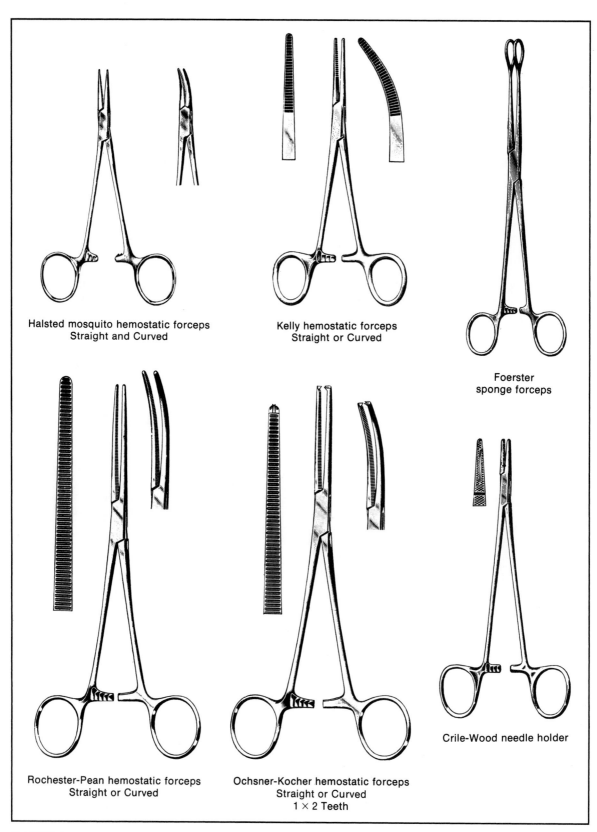

Halsted mosquito hemostatic forceps
Straight and Curved

Kelly hemostatic forceps
Straight or Curved

Foerster
sponge forceps

Rochester-Pean hemostatic forceps
Straight or Curved

Ochsner-Kocher hemostatic forceps
Straight or Curved
1 × 2 Teeth

Crile-Wood needle holder

■ FIGURE 6–2. *Continued*

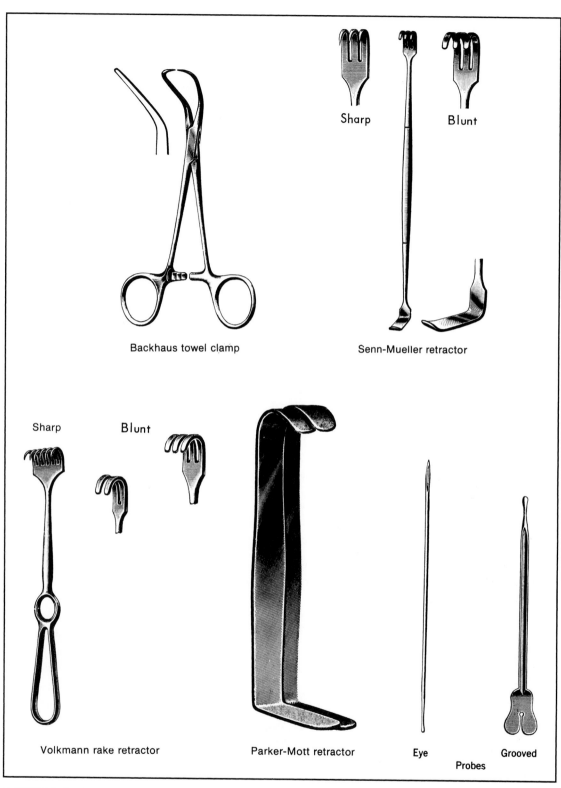

Backhaus towel clamp

Sharp   Blunt

Senn-Mueller retractor

Sharp   Blunt

Volkmann rake retractor

Parker-Mott retractor

Eye   Grooved
Probes

6

■ **FIGURE 6–2.** *Continued*

Illustration continued on following page

GYNECOLOGIC INSTRUMENTS

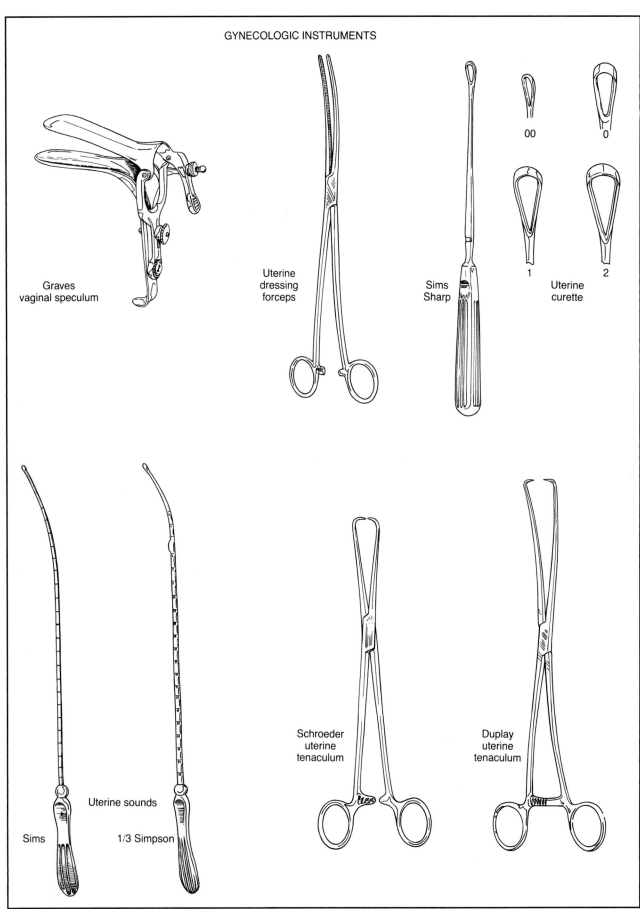

Graves
vaginal speculum

Uterine
dressing
forceps

Sims
Sharp

00   0

1   2

Uterine
curette

6

Uterine sounds

Sims   1/3 Simpson

Schroeder
uterine
tenaculum

Duplay
uterine
tenaculum

■ **FIGURE 6–2.** *Continued*

- A **speculum** is an instrument used to open or distend a body orifice or cavity to permit visual inspection.
- A **tenaculum** is a hooklike instrument used to grasp and hold body parts. For example, a uterine tenaculum is used to grasp and hold the cervix.
- A **sound** is a long slender instrument that is introduced into a body passage or cavity as a means of dilating strictures or to detect the presence of foreign bodies.
- A **curette** is a spoon-shaped instrument used to remove material from the wall of a cavity or other surface.

CARE OF SURGICAL INSTRUMENTS

Surgical instruments are expensive, delicate yet durable, and able to last for many years if properly handled and maintained. The care an instrument receives depends to a large degree on the parts making up the instrument (e.g., box lock, ratchet, cutting edge, serrations). The medical assistant works with instruments while setting up a sterile tray, performing certain procedures such as suture removal or sterile dressing change, and cleaning up after minor office surgery and during the sanitization and sterilization process. During each of these procedures, the following guidelines must be followed to prolong the life span of each instrument and to ensure its proper functioning:

1. Always handle instruments carefully. Dropping an instrument on the floor or throwing an instrument into a basin may damage it.
2. Do not pile instruments in a heap, because they will become entangled and may be damaged when separated.
3. Keep sharp instruments separate from the rest of the instruments to prevent damaging or dulling the cutting edge. Also, keep delicate instruments, such as lensed instruments, separate to protect them from damage.
4. Keep instruments with a ratchet in an open position when not in use, to prolong the proper functioning of the ratchet.
5. Rinse blood and body secretions off an instrument as soon as possible, to prevent them from drying and hardening on the instrument.
6. When performing procedures requiring surgical instruments, one should always use the instrument for the purpose for which it was designed. Substituting one type of instrument for another could damage it.
7. Sanitize and sterilize instruments using proper technique, as outlined in Chapter 5.

Text continued on page 208

6

6–1

PROCEDURE

Applying Sterile Gloves

The medical assistant must wear sterile gloves to perform a sterile procedure, such as a dressing change, or to assist the physician during minor office surgery. The medical assistant must learn to put on the gloves, using the principles of surgical asepsis so as not to contaminate them.

EQUIPMENT/SUPPLIES: **Sterile gloves**

1. **Procedural Step.** Remove all rings; wash the hands.
   Principle. Rings may cause the gloves to tear. The warm, moist environment inside gloves provides ideal growing conditions for the multiplication of transient microorganisms present on the hands. Washing the hands removes these microorganisms and prevents the transmission of pathogens.

2. **Procedural Step.** Place the glove package on a clean flat surface. Open the glove package without touching the inside of the wrapper. The tops of the gloves are turned down to form a cuff.
   Principle. The hands are unsterile and the inside of the wrapper is sterile.

6

3. **Procedural Step.** Pick up the first glove on the inside of the cuff with the fingers of the opposite hand, making sure not to touch the outside of the glove with your ungloved hand.
   Principle. The inside of the cuff will be lying next to your skin and does not remain sterile. Therefore, it is permissible to pick up the glove by the cuff. The outside of the glove is sterile and touching it will contaminate it. If a glove becomes contaminated, a new pair of gloves must be obtained and the procedure repeated, beginning with Procedural Step 2.
4. **Procedural Step.** Pull the glove on. Allow the cuff to remain turned back on itself.
5. **Procedural Step.** Pick up the second glove by slipping your sterile gloved fingers under its cuff.
   Principle. The area under the cuff is sterile and may be touched by the sterile gloved hand.
6. **Procedural Step.** Pull the glove on and turn back the cuff.

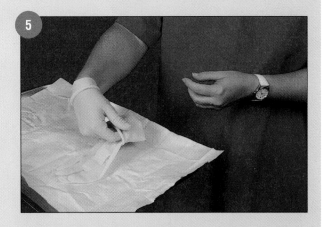

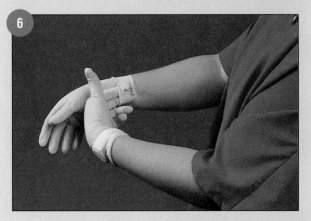

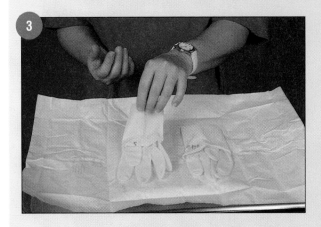

7. **Procedural Step.** Turn back the cuff of the first glove by reaching under the cuff with the other gloved hand. Do not allow the sterile glove to come in contact with the inside of the cuff. Adjust the gloves to a comfortable position. Inspect the gloves for tears.
   Principle. The area under the folded cuff is sterile and may be touched by the sterile gloved hand. The inside of the cuff has previously been touched by your clean hands and is not sterile. If a tear is present, a new pair of gloves must be applied.

6-2

Removing Sterile Gloves

Gloves must be removed in a manner that protects the medical assistant from contaminating the clean hands with possible pathogens that may be present on the outside of the gloves. This is accomplished by not allowing the bare hands to come in contact with the outside of the gloves.

EQUIPMENT/SUPPLIES: Sterile gloves

1. **Procedural Step.** Grasp the outside of the right glove 1 to 2 inches from the top with your gloved left hand. (Note: It does not matter which glove is removed first—you may start with the left glove if you prefer.)
2. **Procedural Step.** Slowly pull the right glove off the hand. It will turn inside out as it is removed from your hand.
3. **Procedural Step.** Pull the right glove free and scrunch it into a ball with your gloved left hand.

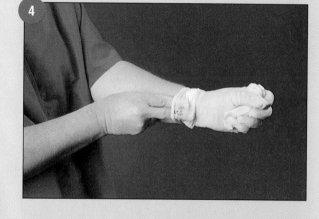

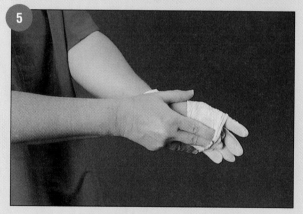

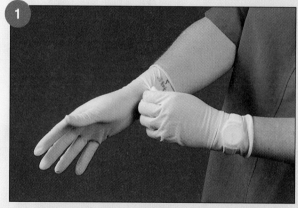

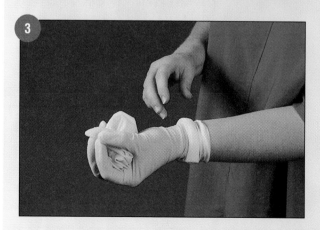

4. **Procedural Step.** Place the index and middle fingers of the right hand on the *inside* of the left glove. Do not allow your clean hand to touch the outside of the glove.
5. **Procedural Step.** Pull the second glove off the left hand. It will turn inside out as it is removed from your hand, enclosing the balled-up right glove. Discard both gloves in an appropriate waste container.
6. **Procedural Step.** Wash hands thoroughly to remove any microorganisms that may have come in contact with your hands.

PROCEDURE

6–3

Opening a Sterile Package

A sterile package that has been wrapped following the procedure for wrapping presented in Chapter 5 is opened using the procedure outlined here. The sterile package may contain an instrument or supplies that need to be transferred to a sterile field, using sterile gloves or by "flipping" the article onto the field using sterile technique. The sterile package may also be in the form of either a commercially prepared disposable package or a pack that has been assembled and sterilized at the medical office; in both cases the inside of the sterile wrapper serves as the sterile field.

EQUIPMENT/SUPPLIES: **Sterile package**

1. **Procedural Step.** Wash the hands.
2. **Procedural Step.** Assemble the equipment.
3. **Procedural Step.** Check the sterilization indicator and expiration date to make sure the wrapped package is sterile.
   Principle. Sterilization indicators are used to determine the effectiveness of the sterilization process. Articles wrapped in muslin or disposable paper are considered sterile for a period of 4 weeks. After this time, they should be resterilized.

4. **Procedural Step.** Place the wrapped package in your hand or on the table so that the top flap of the wrapper will open away from you.
   Principle. Small packages containing an article to be transferred to a sterile field may be opened in your hand.
5. **Procedural Step.** Loosen and remove the fastener on the wrapped package and discard it in a waste container.

6

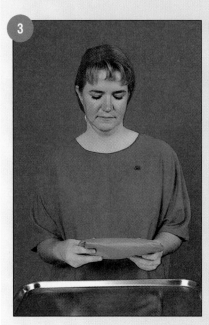

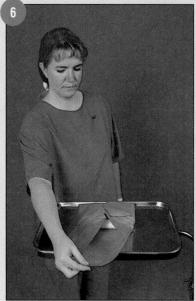

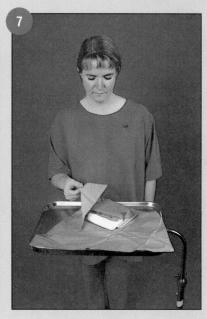

6. **Procedural Step.** Open the first flap away from the body. Handle only the outside of the wrapper.
Principle. The medical assistant should open the sterile package so as not to reach over the sterile contents. Otherwise, dust or lint from unsterile clothing may fall on the contents of the package and cause contamination.

7. **Procedural Step.** Open the left and right flaps without crossing over the sterile field.

8. **Procedural Step.** Open the flap closest to the body by lifting it toward you. Make sure to touch only the outside of the wrapper.

9. **Procedural Step.** Utilize the package as a sterile setup or transfer the contents of the package to the sterile field according to your medical office procedure.

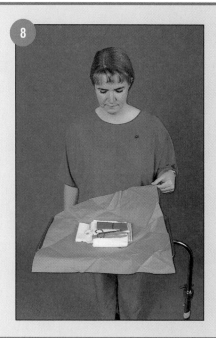

6–4

Pouring a Sterile Solution

The medical assistant may need to pour a sterile solution, such as an antiseptic, into a container located on a sterile field using the principles of surgical asepsis outlined in the following procedure:

EQUIPMENT/SUPPLIES:	Sterile solution Sterile towel Sterile container

1. **Procedural Step.** Read the label to make sure you have the correct solution.

2. **Procedural Step.** Check the expiration date on the solution. An outdated solution should not be used.

3. **Procedural Step.** Palm the label of the bottle.
Principle. Palming the label prevents the solution from dripping on the label and obscuring it.

4. **Procedural Step.** Remove the cap by touching only the outside and place the cap on a flat surface with the open end facing up.

Principle. Handling the cap by the outside prevents contamination of the inside. Placing the cap with the open end facing up prevents contamination of the inside of the cap by the unsterile surface.

5. **Procedural Step.** Rinse the lip of the bottle by pouring a small amount of solution into a separate container.
Principle. Rinsing the lip washes away any microorganisms that may be on it.

Continued

PROCEDURE 6-4

6. **Procedural Step.** Pour the proper amount of solution into the sterile container at a height of approximately 6 inches. Do not allow the neck of the bottle to come in contact with the sterile container, and be careful not to splash any solution onto the sterile field.
Principle. Pouring from a height of approximately 6 inches helps reduce splashing.

7. **Procedural Step.** Replace the cap on the container without contaminating it. Read the label again to make sure you have poured the correct solution.

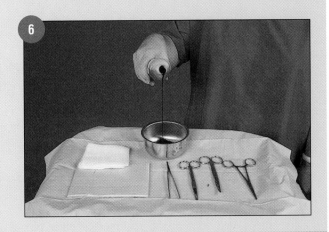

COMMERCIALLY PREPARED STERILE PACKAGES

☐ Commercially prepared disposable packages are frequently utilized and may contain one particular article (such as sterile dressing) or a complete sterile set-up (such as one for the removal of sutures). The directions for opening the package are clearly stated on the outside of the package and should be read carefully to prevent contamination of the sterile contents.

One type of commercially prepared package is the peel-apart package (commonly referred to as a peel-pack). This type of sterile package has an edge with two flaps that can be pulled apart in the following manner: Grasp each unsterile flap between your bent index finger and extended thumb and, using a rolling-outward motion, pull the package apart (Fig. 6–3A). The inside of the wrapper and the contents are sterile and must not be touched with the bare hands, to prevent contamination.

The medical assistant may place the contents of the peel-pack directly on the sterile field by stepping back slightly from the field and then gently ejecting or "flipping" the contents onto it (Fig. 6–3B). Stepping back prevents the unsterile outer wrapper and the medical assistant's hands from crossing over the sterile field, which would result in contamination.

The contents of the package may also be removed with a sterile gloved hand. This technique is useful during minor office surgery in which the physician needs additional supplies such as gauze pads, sutures, and so on. Using a gloved hand, the physician removes the sterile contents from the package, which is being held open by the medical assistant (Fig. 6–3C).

The inside of the package may be used as a sterile field by opening the peel-apart package completely and laying it open flat on a clean dry surface (Fig. 6–3D).

WOUNDS

☐ A **wound** is a break in the continuity of an external or internal surface caused by physical means. Wounds may be accidental or intentional (as when the physician makes an incision during a surgical operation). There are two basic types of wound: closed and open.

A **closed wound** involves an injury to the underlying tissues of the body without a break in the skin surface or mucous membrane; an example is a contusion or bruise. A **contusion** results when the tissues under the skin are injured and is often caused by a blunt object. Blood vessels rupture, allowing blood to seep into the tissues, which results in a bluish discoloration of the skin. After several days, the color of the contusion turns greenish yellow, owing to oxidation of blood pigments. Bruising commonly occurs with injuries such as fractures, sprains, strains, and black eyes.

Open wounds involve a break in the skin surface or mucous membrane that exposes the underlying tissues; examples include incisions, lacerations, punctures, and abrasions.

▪ An **incision** is a clean, smooth cut caused by a sharp cutting instrument such as a knife, razor, or a piece of glass. Deep incisions are accompanied by profuse bleeding; in addition, damage to muscles, tendons, and nerves may occur.

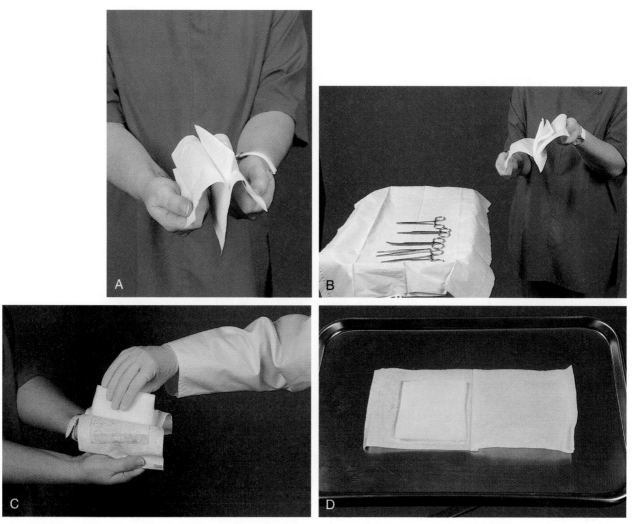

■ **FIGURE 6–3.** Methods for removing the sterile contents of a peel-apart package so that sterility is maintained.

■ A **laceration** is a wound in which the tissues are torn apart, rather than cut, leaving ragged and irregular edges. Lacerations are caused by dull knives, large objects that have been driven into the skin, and heavy machinery. Deep lacerations result in profuse bleeding, and a scar often results from the jagged tearing of the tissues.

■ A **puncture** is a wound made by a sharp-pointed object piercing the skin layers—for example, a nail, splinter, needle, wire, knife, bullet, or animal bite. A puncture wound has a very small external skin opening, and for this reason bleeding is usually minor. A tetanus booster may be administered with this type of wound, because the tetanus bacteria grow best in a warm anaerobic environment as would be found in a puncture.

■ An **abrasion** or scrape is a wound in which the outer layers of the skin are scraped or rubbed off,

resulting in an oozing of blood from ruptured capillaries. Abrasions are caused by falls such as floor burns and include skinned knees and elbows.

Figure 6–4 illustrates the specific wounds just described.

WOUND HEALING

□ The skin acts as a protective barrier for the body and is considered its first line of defense. Once the surface of the skin has been broken, it is easy for microorganisms to enter and cause infection. The body has a natural healing process that works to destroy invading microorganisms and to restore the structure and function of the damaged tissues, as is described next.

6

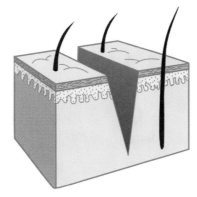

Contusion   Incision   Laceration

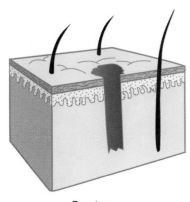

Puncture   Abrasion

■ **FIGURE 6-4.** Types of wounds.

6

PATIENT/TEACHING

WOUND CARE

■ Explain the following to the patient regarding wounds:

The nature of the type of wound that the patient has: incision, laceration, puncture, or abrasion.

The purpose of suturing the wound: to close the skin and protect against further contamination, to facilitate healing, and to leave a smaller scar.

If a tetanus toxoid has been administered, explain the purpose of this immunization: to protect against tetanus (lockjaw).

■ Teach the patient how to care for the wound, as follows:

Keep the dressing clean and dry. If it becomes wet, contact the medical office to schedule a sterile dressing change.

Apply an ice bag for swelling (if prescribed by the physician).

Immediately report any signs that the wound is infected. These include fever, persistent or increased pain, swelling, drainage, red streaks radiating away from the wound.

Return as instructed by the physician for the removal of sutures.

■ Teach the patient the procedure for applying an ice bag (if prescribed by the physician).

■ Provide the patient with written instructions on wound care to refer to at home.

PHASES OF WOUND HEALING

Wound healing takes place in three phases, which are described here and illustrated in Fig. 6–5.

PHASE 1. Phase 1, also called the **inflammatory phase,** begins as soon as the body is injured. This phase lasts approximately 3 to 4 days. During this phase, a fibrin network forms, resulting in a blood clot that "plugs" up the opening of the wound and stops the flow of blood. The blood clot eventually becomes the scab. The inflammatory process also occurs during this phase. **Inflammation** is the protective response of the body to trauma such as cuts and abrasions and to the entrance of foreign matter such as microorganisms. During inflammation, the blood supply to the wound increases, which brings white blood cells and nutrients to the site to assist in the healing process. The four local signs of inflammation are redness, swelling, pain, and warmth. The purpose of inflammation is to destroy invading microorganisms and to remove damaged tissue debris from the area so that proper healing can occur.

PHASE 2. Phase 2 is also called the **granulation phase** and typically lasts from 4 to 20 days. During this phase fibroblasts migrate to the wound and begin to synthesize collagen. Collagen is a white protein that provides strength to the wound. Therefore, as the amount of collagen increases, the wound becomes stronger and the chance that the wound will open decreases. There is also a growth of new capillaries during this phase to provide the damaged tissue with an abundant supply of blood. As the capillary network develops, the tissue becomes a translucent red color. This tissue is known as **granulation tissue.** Granulation tissue consists primarily of collagen and is fragile, shiny, and bleeds easily.

PHASE 3. Phase 3, also known as the **maturation phase,** begins as soon as granulation tissue forms and can last for up to 2 years. During this phase, collagen continues to be synthesized and the granulation tissue eventually hardens to white scar tissue. Scar tissue is not true skin and does not contain nerves or have a blood supply.

The medical assistant should always inspect the wound when providing wound care. The wound should be observed for signs of inflammation and the amount of healing that has taken place. This information should be charted in the patient's record.

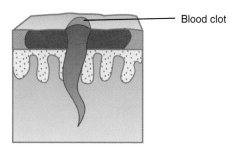

Phase 1: Inflammatory Phase

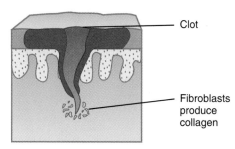

Phase 2: Granulation Phase

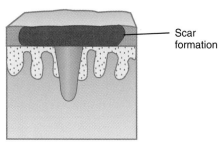

Phase 3: Maturation Phase

■ **FIGURE 6–5.** Phases of the wound healing.

6

WOUND DRAINAGE

The medical term for drainage is exudate. An **exudate** is material, such as fluid and cells, that has escaped from blood vessels during the inflammatory process. The exudate is deposited in tissue or on tissue surfaces and, therefore, is often present in a wound. When providing wound care, the medical assistant should always inspect the wound for the presence of drainage and chart this information in the patient's record. There are three major types of exudates: serous, sanguineous, and purulent. Each is described next.

SEROUS EXUDATE. A serous exudate consists chiefly of serum, which is the clear portion of the blood. Serous drainage is clear and watery. An example of a serous exudate is the fluid in a blister from a burn.

SANGUINEOUS. A sanguineous exudate is red in appearance and consists of red blood cells. This type of drainage results when capillaries are damaged, allowing the escape of red blood cells, and is frequently seen in open wounds. A bright red sanguineous exudate indicates fresh bleeding while a dark exudate indicates older bleeding.

PURULENT. A purulent exudate contains pus, which consists of leukocytes, dead liquefied tissue debris, and dead and living bacteria. Purulent drainage is usually thick and has an unpleasant odor. It is white in color, but may acquire tinges of pink, green, or yellow depending on the type of infecting organism. The process of pus formation is known as **suppuration.**

In addition to the exudates just described, mixed types of exudates are often observed in a wound. A **serosanguineous exudate** consists of clear and blood-tinged drainage and is commonly seen in surgical incisions. A **purosanguineous exudate** consists of pus and blood and is often seen in a new wound that is infected.

STERILE DRESSING CHANGE

☐ Surgical asepsis must be maintained when one is caring for and applying a dry sterile dressing (abbreviated DSD) to an open wound. The medical assistant must take care to prevent infection in clean wounds and to decrease infection in those wounds already infected. The function of a sterile dressing is to protect the wound from contamination and trauma, to absorb drainage, and to restrict motion, which may interfere with proper wound healing. The size, type, and amount of dressing material used during a sterile dressing change depend on the size and location of the wound and the amount of drainage.

Sterile folded **gauze pads** are commonly used in the medical office for a sterile dressing change. This type of dressing functions well in absorbing drainage; however, the gauze has a tendency to stick to the wound when the drainage dries. Gauze pads come in a variety of sizes including 4 × 4, 3 × 3, and 2 × 2; the 4 × 4 size is used most frequently.

Nonadherent pads are also used as a sterile dressing; they have one surface impregnated with agents that prevent the dressing from sticking to the wound. A brand name for this type of dressing material is Telfa pads. The nonadhering side, which is shiny in appearance, is placed next to the wound. Telfa dressings are used when covering burned skin.

The procedure for changing a sterile dressing is presented on the following pages.

PROCEDURE

6

6–5

Changing a Sterile Dressing

EQUIPMENT/SUPPLIES:

SIDE TABLE:
Clean disposable gloves
Antiseptic swabs
Sterile gloves
Waterproof waste bag
Adhesive tape and scissors
Biohazard waste container

STERILE FIELD:
Sterile dressing
Thumb forceps

1. **Procedural Step.** Wash the hands.
2. **Procedural Step.** Assemble the equipment and prepare the sterile field using surgical asepsis. Items are either contained in a prepackaged sterile set-up or placed onto a sterile field. Position the waterproof waste bag in a convenient location for disposal of contaminated items.
3. **Procedural Step.** Greet and identify the patient. Introduce yourself, and explain the procedure.

Instruct the patient not to move during the procedure and not to talk, laugh, sneeze, or cough over the sterile field.
Principle. By moving, the patient may accidentally contaminate the sterile field or touch the wound. Microorganisms are carried in water vapor from the mouth, nose, and lungs and can be transferred onto the sterile field.

PROCEDURE 6–5

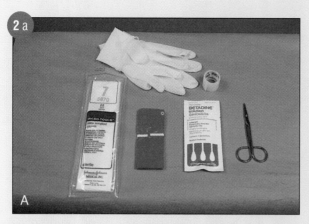

2 a

A

Side Table

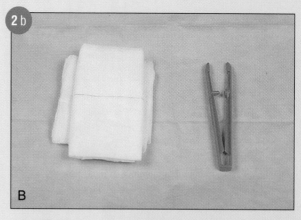

2 b

B

Sterile Field

4. Procedural Step. Apply clean gloves. Loosen the tape on the dressing, and pull it toward the wound. Carefully and gently remove the soiled dressing. If the dressing is stuck to the wound, it can be loosened by moistening it with a normal saline solution. Do not pass the soiled dressing over the sterile field. Place the soiled dressing in the waste bag without allowing the dressing to touch the outside of the bag.
Principle. Gentle tape removal avoids unnecessary stress on the wound. Passing the soiled dressing over the sterile field will contaminate the field.

5. Procedural Step. Inspect the wound and observe for the following: amount of healing, presence of inflammation, presence of drainage, including the amount (scant, moderate, or profuse) and type of drainage.
Principle. Drainage is classified as *serous* (containing serum); *sanguineous* (red and composed of blood); *serosanguineous* (containing serum and blood); *purulent* (containing pus and appearing white with tinges of yellow, pink, or green, depending on the type of infecting microorganism). Purulent drainage is usually thick and has an unpleasant odor.

6. Procedural Step. Remove the gloves, and discard them in the waste bag without contaminating yourself.
Principle. The gloves have touched the unsterile dressing and are considered contaminated.

7. Procedural Step. Open the pouch containing the sterile antiseptic swabs and place in a convenient location such as taping the pouch to the Mayo stand. Open a package of sterile gloves and apply them (refer to Procedure 6–1: Applying Sterile Gloves).

8. Procedural Step. Cleanse the wound using the sterile antiseptic swabs. Cleanse the wound from the top to the bottom, working from the center to the outside of the wound. Use a new swab for each cleansing motion. Discard each contaminated swab in the waste bag after use.

9. Procedural Step. Place the sterile dressing over the wound by dropping it in place using sterile gloves or sterile forceps. Discard the gloves or forceps in the waste bag.
Principle. Dropping the dressing over the wound prevents the possibility of transferring microorganisms from the skin to the center of the wound.

6

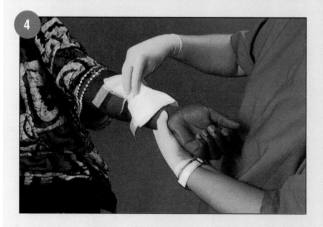

4

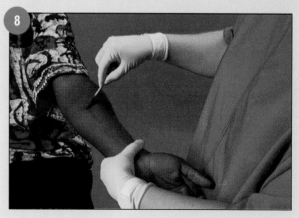

8

Continued

PROCEDURE 6-5

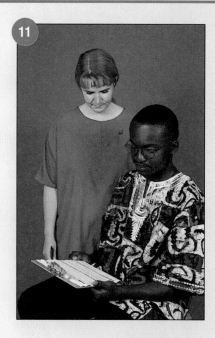

11

d. Witness the patient's signature by signing your name in the appropriate space on the form. Include today's date.

e. Give a signed copy of the wound care instructions to the patient and file a copy in the patient's medical record.

12. **Procedural Step.** Return the equipment. Tightly secure the bag containing the soiled dressing and contaminated articles, and dispose of it in a biohazard waste container.

Principle. Contaminated items must be disposed of properly to prevent the spread of infection.

13. **Procedural Step.** Wash the hands.

14. **Procedural Step.** Chart the procedure. Include the date and time, location of the dressing, condition of the wound, type and amount of drainage, care of the wound, and any problems the patient may have experienced with the wound. Also, chart the instructions given to the patient on wound care.

10. **Procedural Step.** Apply adhesive tape to hold the dressing in place. The tape must be long enough to adhere to the skin but not so long that it will loosen during the patient movement. The strips of tape should be evenly spaced, with strips at each end of the dressing.

11. **Procedural Step.** Instruct the patient in wound care as follows:

a. Provide the patient with written wound care instructions.

b. Explain the wound care instructions and ask the patient if he or she has any questions. The patient should be told to keep the wound clean and dry and to contact the office if signs of inflammation occur.

c. Ask the patient to sign the instruction sheet on the appropriate line.

6

CHARTING EXAMPLE	
Date	
9/20/2002	10:30 a.m. Dressing changed Ⓛ ant forearm. Scant amt of serous drainage noted. Sl redness around incision line. Sutures intact and suture line in good approximation. Incision cleaned c̄ Betadine and DSD applied. No complaints of pain or discomfort. Explained wound care. Written instructions provided. Signed copy filed in chart. To return in 2 days for suture removal. ———— T. Browning, CMA

SUTURES

☐ The insertion and removal of sutures are commonly performed in the medical office. Sutures may be required to close a surgical incision or to repair an accidental wound. They **approximate** or bring together the edges of the wound with surgical stitches and hold them in place until proper healing can occur. Sutures also protect the wound from further contamination and minimize the amount of scar formation. A local anesthetic is necessary to numb the area before the sutures are inserted.

TYPES OF SUTURES

Sutures are available in two different types: absorbable and nonabsorbable.

Absorbable sutures consist of surgical gut or synthetic materials such as polyglycolic acid (Dexon) and polyglactin 910 (Vicryl) (Fig. 6–6A). Surgical gut is made from the submucosa of sheep or beef intestine. This type of suturing material is gradually digested by tissue enzymes and absorbed by the body's tissues from 5 to 20 days after insertion, depending on the kind of surgical gut employed. Plain surgical gut has a rapid

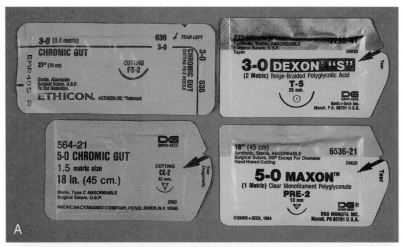

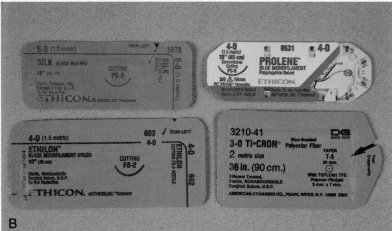

■ **FIGURE 6–6.** Swaged suture packets. *A,* Examples of absorbable sutures. *B,* Examples of nonabsorbable sutures.

absorption time, whereas chromic surgical gut is treated to slow down its rate of absorption in the tissues. Absorbable sutures are frequently used to suture subcutaneous tissue, fascia, intestines, bladder, and peritoneum and to ligate vessels. Since the suturing of this type of tissue is generally done during surgery performed by the physician in a hospital setting with the patient under a general anesthetic, the medical office may not stock absorbable suture material.

Nonabsorbable sutures (Fig. 6–6*B*) are not absorbed by the body and either remain permanently in the body tissues and become encapsulated by fibrous tissue or are removed (e.g., skin sutures). Nonabsorbable sutures are used to suture skin; therefore, this type of suture is frequently used in the medical office.

Nonabsorbable sutures are made from materials that are not affected by tissue enzymes. These materials include silk, cotton, nylon, polyester fiber, polypropylene, stainless steel, and surgical skin staples.

SUTURE SIZE AND PACKAGING

Sutures are measured by their gauge, which refers to the diameter of the suturing material. The size ranges from numbers below 0 (pronounced "aught") to numbers above 0. The diameter of the suture material increases with each number above 0 and decreases with each number below 0. If the size of a particular suture material ranges from 6-0 to 4, the available sizes would include 6-0, 5-0, 4-0, 3-0, 2-0, 0, 1, 2, 3, and 4; 6-0 would be very fine sutures and 4 would be very heavy sutures. For example, size 2-0 (00) sutures have a smaller diameter than size 0 sutures.

Nonabsorbable sutures with a smaller gauge are used for suturing incisions in more delicate tissue such as the face or neck (5-0 to 6-0), whereas heavy sutures are used for firmer tissue such as the chest or abdomen. Finer sutures also leave less scar formation and are used when cosmetic results are desired.

6

Sutures are commercially available in individual packages consisting of an outer peel-apart package and a sterile inner packet. These are labeled according to the type of suture material (e.g., surgical silk), the size (e.g., 4-0), and the length of the suturing material (e.g., 18 inches). The type and size of material used are based on the nature and location of the tissue being sutured and the physician's preference. For example, to repair a laceration of the arm, the physician might use a 4-0 surgical silk suture. The physician informs the medical assistant of the type and size of sutures needed.

SUTURE NEEDLES

Needles used for suturing are categorized according to both their type of point and their shape. A needle with a sharp point is termed a **cutting needle,** and one with a round point is termed a **noncutting needle.** Cutting needles (Fig. 6–7A) are used for durable tissues such as skin; the sharp point helps push the needle through the tissue. Noncutting needles are used to penetrate tissues that offer a small amount of resistance, such as the viscera, subcutaneous tissue, muscle, and peritoneum.

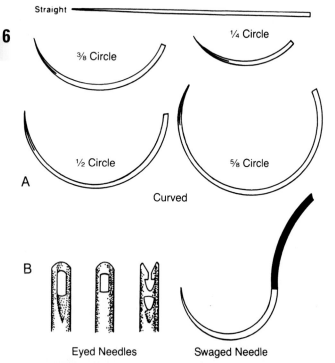

6

■ FIGURE 6–7. Common needle shapes. *A,* Examples of needles with a cutting point. *B,* Examples of eyed needles and a swaged needle. (*A,* from *Perspectives on Sutures,* courtesy of Davis & Geck. *B,* from Nealon, T. F., Jr.: *Fundamental Skills in Surgery,* 3rd ed. Philadelphia, W. B. Saunders Company, 1980.)

The shape of the needle may be either curved or straight (Fig. 6–7A). **Curved needles** permit the physician to dip in and out of the tissue. A needle holder must be used with a curved needle. A **straight needle** is used when the tissue can be displaced sufficiently to permit the needle to be pushed and pulled through the tissue. Straight needles do not require the use of a needle holder.

The needle may have an eye through which the suture material is inserted, or it may be a **swaged needle** (Fig. 6–7B). Swaged means the suture and needle are one continuous unit; in other words, the needle is permanently attached to the end of the suture. Swaged needles are used frequently because they offer several advantages over eyed needles. One advantage is that the suture material does not slip off the needle, as might occur with suture material threaded through the eye of a needle. Another advantage is that tissue trauma is reduced because a swaged needle will have only a single strand of suture that must be pulled through the tissue, compared with a double strand in an eyed needle. Therefore, the swaged needle can be pulled through the tissue with less resulting trauma. Swaged suture packets are labeled to specify the gauge, type, and length of suture material as well as the type of needle point (cutting or noncutting) and the needle shape (curved or straight) (see Fig. 6–6).

INSERTION OF SUTURES

☐ The medical assistant may be responsible for preparing the suture tray and for assisting the physician during the insertion of the sutures. The physician designates the size and type of suture material and needle required. Since sutures, needles, and suture-needle combinations (swaged needles) are contained in peel-apart packages, they can be added to the sterile field by flipping them onto the sterile field or by a sterile gloved hand (Fig. 6–8).

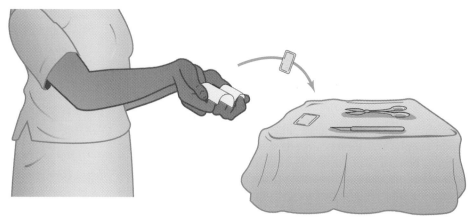

A Flipping sutures onto the sterile field.

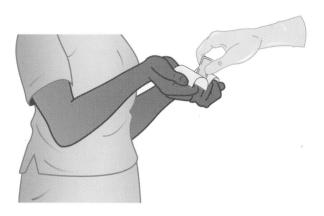

FIGURE 6-8. Adding sutures to a sterile field.

B The physician removing the sutures with a sterile gloved hand.

6

ITEMS PLACED TO THE SIDE OF THE STERILE FIELD
Insertion of Sutures:

- Clean disposable gloves
- Antiseptic solution
- Surgical scrub brush
- Antiseptic swabs
- Sterile gloves
- Local anesthetic
- Alcohol wipe to cleanse the vial
- Tetanus toxoid with needle and syringe
- Biohazard waste container

ITEMS INCLUDED ON THE STERILE FIELD
Insertion of Sutures:

- Fenestrated drape
- Syringe and needle
- Hemostatic forceps
- Thumb forceps
- Tissue forceps
- Dissecting scissors
- Operating scissors
- Needle holder
- Suture
- Sterile 4 × 4 gauze

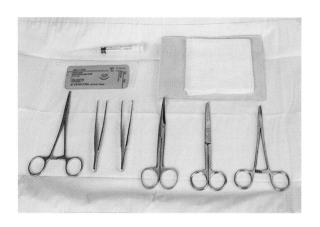

SUTURE REMOVAL

☐ When the wound has healed so that it no longer needs the support of nonabsorbable suture material, the sutures must be removed. The length of time the sutures remain in place depends on their location and the amount of healing that must occur. Some areas of the body, such as the head and neck, have a good blood supply; the sutures do not need to remain there as long, because this area heals more rapidly.

Sutures must always be left in place long enough for proper healing to take place. The physician decides on the length of time, but in general, skin sutures inserted in the head and neck are removed in 3 to 5 days, and sutures inserted in other areas, such as the skin of the arms, legs, and hands, are removed in 7 to 10 days.

The medical assistant is frequently responsible for removing sutures. The procedure for removing sutures is outlined in this section.

SURGICAL SKIN STAPLES

Surgical skin staples are often used to close wounds. Stapling is considered the fastest method of closure of long skin incisions. In addition, trauma to the tissue is reduced because the tissue does not have to be handled very much when inserting the staples.

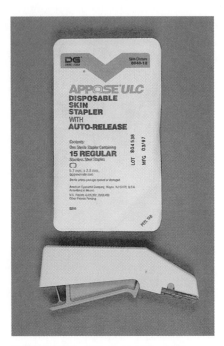

■ **FIGURE 6–9.** Disposable skin stapler.

MEMORIES *from* EXTERNSHIP

TRUDY BROWNING: *Terrified and excited at the same time to be experiencing my first externship, I found myself in a busy pediatric office. After a few days of watching and learning, I prepared to work up a beautiful baby for a well-child examination. Before entering the room I was told by a staff member that the HIV status of the mother of the baby was questionable. Alarmed at first as to how I would feel in this situation, I immediately remembered all the precautions we had talked about in class. As I took the baby from the mother to weigh and measure him, I have to admit many thoughts ran through my mind, but again I was calmed because of all the information we had received in school regarding OSHA precautions. Faced with that situation today, after practicing wisely and safely for 3 years, I would not think twice about it because I know from my education and experience that these types of situations can be handled without alarm.*

Surgical staples consist of stainless steel and are inserted into the skin using a special skin stapler. Skin staplers are available as reusable or disposable devices. The skin stapler holds a cartridge that contains a prescribed number and size of staples (Fig. 6–9).

The physician inserts the staples by gently approximating the tissues with tissue forceps. The skin stapler is then held over the site and the staple is inserted into the skin.

Skin stapling produces excellent cosmetic results and the staples are easily removed with a specially designed staple remover. The procedure for removing skin staples is outlined on the following pages.

PROCEDURE

6-6

Suture and Staple Removal

EQUIPMENT/SUPPLIES:

Antiseptic swabs
Clean disposable gloves
Sterile 4 × 4 gauze
Surgical tape
Biohazard waste container

For Suture Removal:
Suture removal kit, which includes
   Suture scissors
   Thumb forceps
   Sterile 4 × 4 gauze

For Staple Removal:
Staple remover kit, which includes
   Staple remover
   Sterile 4 × 4 gauze

1. **Procedural Step.** Wash the hands and assemble the equipment.
2. **Procedural Step.** Greet and identify the patient. Introduce yourself, and explain the procedure.

3. **Procedural Step.** Position the patient as required. Check to make sure the sutures (or staples) are intact and the incision line is approximated and not gapping. Check the incision line to make sure it is free from infection. If the incision line is not approximated or if redness, swelling, or a discharge is present, do not remove the sutures and notify the physician.

   Principle. The sutures (or staples) should not be removed unless the incision line is approximated and free from infection.

4. **Procedural Step.** Open the suture or staple removal kit, making sure to keep the contents of the kit sterile. Most kits are opened by peeling back a top cover which exposes a plastic tray containing the necessary instruments and supplies.

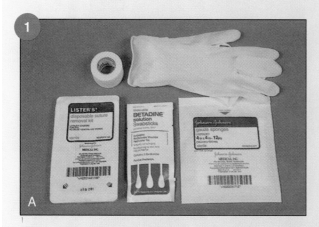

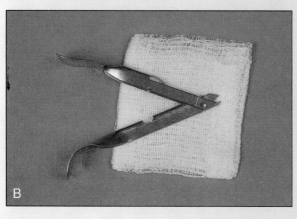

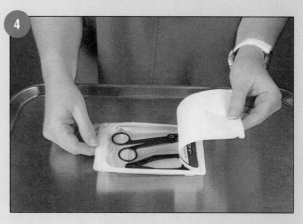

6

Continued

5. **Procedural Step.** Apply clean gloves. Cleanse the incision line with an antiseptic swab to destroy microorganisms and to remove any dried exudate encrusted around the sutures or staples. Clean the wound from the top to the bottom, working from the center to the outside of the wound. Use a new swab for each cleansing motion. Allow the skin to dry.

Principle. Dried exudate must be removed to allow for unimpeded removal of the sutures or staples.

6. **Procedural Step.** Remove the sutures or staples. Tell the patient that he or she will feel a pulling or tugging sensation as each suture (or staple) is removed, but that it will not be painful. Count the number of sutures or staples removed. Refer to the patient's chart to make sure the same number are removed as were inserted by the physician.

To remove sutures:

a. Pick up the knot of the first suture using the sterile thumb forceps provided in the kit.

b. Place the curved tip of the suture scissors under the suture. Cut the suture below the knot on the side of the suture closest to the skin using the sterile suture scissors. Cut the suture as close to the skin as possible.

c. Gently pull the suture out through the outer skin orifice using a smooth, continuous motion. Remove the suture without allowing any portion that was previously outside to be pulled through the skin. Place the suture on the 4 × 4 gauze, included in the suture kit.

d. Continue in this manner until all the sutures have been removed.

Principle. To prevent the risk of infection, the suture must be removed without pulling any portion that has been outside the skin back through the skin.

To remove staples:

a. Gently place the bottom jaws of the staple remover under the staple to be removed.

b. Firmly squeeze the staple handles until they are fully closed.

c. Carefully lift the staple remover upward to remove the staple from the incision line. Place the staple on the 4 × 4 gauze included in the staple kit.

d. Continue in this manner until all the staples have been removed.

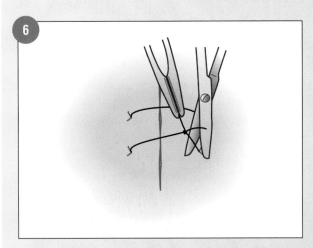

(From Nealon, T. F., Jr.: *Fundamentals in Surgery,* 3rd ed. Philadelphia, W. B. Saunders Company, 1980.)

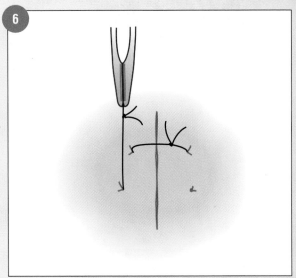

(From Nealon, T. F., Jr.: *Fundamentals in Surgery,* 3rd ed. Philadelphia, W. B. Saunders Company, 1980.)

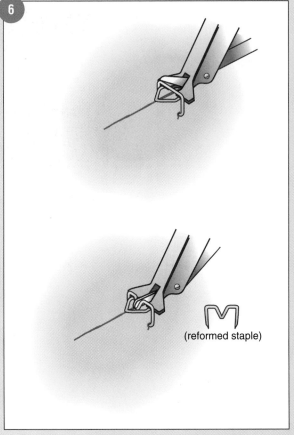

(reformed staple)

(Courtesy of Ethicon Inc., Somerville, NJ.)

7. **Procedural Step.** Cleanse the site with an antiseptic swab. Some physicians may want the medical assistant to apply adhesive skin closures after removing the sutures or staples to provide additional support to the wound as it continues to heal.

8. **Procedural Step.** Apply a dry sterile dressing if indicated by the physician.

9. **Procedural Step.** Properly dispose of all contaminated supplies in a biohazard waste container.

10. **Procedural Step.** Remove the gloves, and wash the hands.

11. **Procedural Step.** Chart the procedure. Include the date and time, the status of the sutures (or staples) and incision line, the number of sutures (or staples) removed, the location of the site, and

care of the wound (i.e., application of an antiseptic or dressing). Chart any instructions given to the patient.

CHARTING EXAMPLE

Date	
9/20/2002	10:30 a.m. Sutures intact and incision line in good approximation. No signs of infection. Sutures x6 removed from ℞ ant forearm. Incision line cleaned c̄ Betadine and DSD applied. Instructions provided on dressing care. ——————— T. Browning, CMA

ADHESIVE SKIN CLOSURES

Adhesive skin closures may be used for wound repair to approximate the edges of a laceration or incision. Skin closures consist of sterile, nonallergenic tape that is commercially available in a variety of widths and lengths and is strong enough to approximate a wound until healing takes place. Brand names for adhesive skin closures are Steri-Strip (3M Corporation) and Proxi-Strips (Johnson and Johnson) (Fig. 6–10).

Adhesive skin closures may be used when not much tension exists on the skin edges. The strips of tape are applied transversely across the line of incision to approximate the skin edges. The advantages of using adhesive skin closures are that they eliminate the need for skin sutures and a local anesthetic, they are easy to apply and remove, and they result in less scarring than skin sutures.

The medical assistant is frequently responsible for applying and removing adhesive skin closures. These procedures are outlined on the following pages.

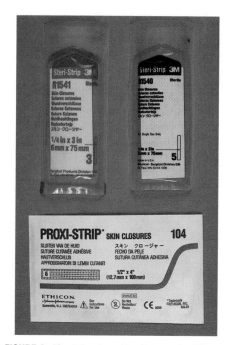

■ **FIGURE 6–10.** Adhesive skin closures in different sizes.

PROCEDURE

6–7

Application and Removal of Adhesive Skin Closures

EQUIPMENT/SUPPLIES:

Box of clean disposable gloves
Sterile gloves
Antiseptic solution
Surgical scrub brush
Antiseptic swabs
Tincture of benzoin

Sterile cotton-tipped applicator
Adhesive skin closure strips
Sterile 4 × 4 gauze pads
Surgical tape
Biohazard waste container

Application of Adhesive Skin Closures:

1. **Procedural Step.** Wash the hands, and assemble the equipment.
2. **Procedural Step.** Greet and identify the patient.
3. **Procedural Step.** Introduce yourself, and explain the procedure.
4. **Procedural Step.** Position the patient as required. Apply clean gloves. Inspect the appearance of the wound for signs of redness, swelling, and drainage. (Note: This information is charted in the patient's record at the end of the procedure.)
5. **Procedural Step.** Gently scrub the wound using an antiseptic solution (e.g., Betadine solution) and a sterile gauze pad or a surgical scrub brush. Clean at least 3 inches around the wound, making sure to remove all debris, skin oil, and exudates. Allow the skin to dry or pat dry with gauze squares. (Note: Change gloves as needed to maintain cleanliness.)

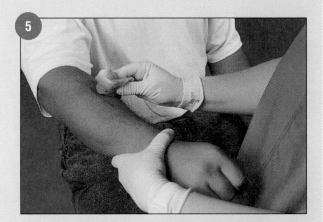

6. **Procedural Step.** Cleanse the site using antiseptic swabs such as Betadine or alcohol swabs. Clean the wound from the top to the bottom, working from the center to the outside of the wound. Use a new swab for each cleansing motion. Allow the skin to dry.

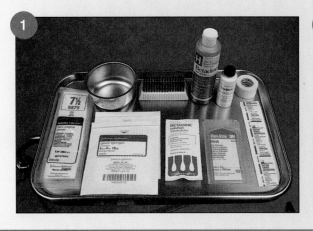

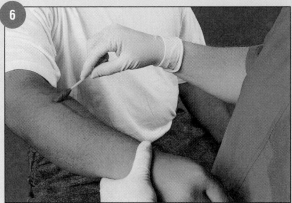

PROCEDURE 6–7

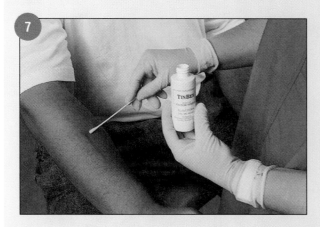

7. Procedural Step. If dictated by the medical office policy, apply a thin coat of tincture of benzoin to the skin parallel to the wound using a sterile cotton-tipped applicator. Do not allow the tincture of benzoin to touch the wound. Allow the skin to dry. Remove gloves and wash the hands.
Principle. Tincture of benzoin facilitates adhesion of the strips to the skin.

8. Procedural Step. Open the plastic peel-apart package of strips using sterile technique as follows:
a. Grasp each flap of the package between the thumbs and pull the package apart.
b. Peel back the package until it is completely open.
c. Lay the opened package flat on a clean dry surface. The inside of the package serves as the sterile field.

9. Procedural Step. Apply sterile gloves. Fold the card of strips along its perforated tab and tear off the tab, which exposes the ends of the strips, making them easier to grasp. Peel a strip of tape off the card at a 45-degree angle to the card.

10. Procedural Step. Check to make sure the skin surface is dry. Position the first strip over the center of the wound as follows:
a. Secure one end of the strip of tape to the skin on one side of the wound by pressing down firmly on the tape.
b. Stretch the strip transversely across the line of the incision until the edges of the wound are approximated exactly. If necessary, use your gloved hand to assist in bringing the edges of the wound together.
c. Secure the strip on the skin on the other side of the wound by pressing down firmly on the tape.

Principle. Approximating the wound exactly provides for good healing and less scar formation.

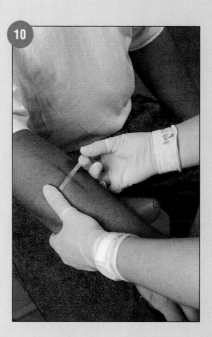

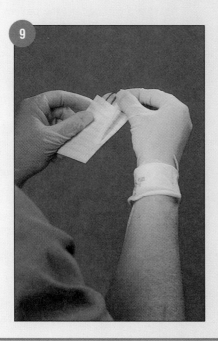

6

Continued

PROCEDURE 6–7

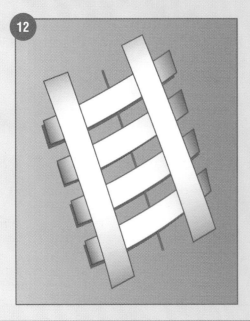

11

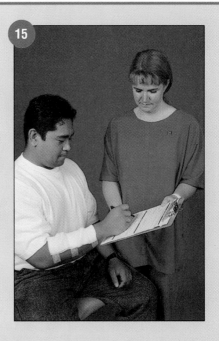

15

6

11. Procedural Step. Apply the next strip midway between the middle (first) strip and one end of the wound. Apply a third strip between the middle strip and the other end of the wound. Continue applying the strips at 1/8-inch intervals until the edges of the wound are approximated. If at any time the skin surfaces become moist with perspiration, blood, or serum, wipe the area dry with a sterile gauze pad before applying the next strip.
Principle. Applying the strips in this manner facilitates good approximation of the wound. Spacing the strips at 1/8-inch intervals allows for proper drainage of the wound.

12

12. Procedural Step. Apply two closures approximately 1/2 inch from the ends of the strips and parallel to the wound (ladder fashion).
Principle. Applying a strip along each edge redistributes the tension and assists in holding the strips firmly in place.

13. Procedural Step. Apply a dry sterile dressing over the strips if indicated by the physician (Refer to Procedure 6–5).

14. Procedural Step. Remove the gloves, and wash the hands.

15. Procedural Step. Instruct the patient in wound care as follows:
a. Provide the patient with written wound care instructions.
b. Explain the wound care instructions and ask the patient if he or she has any questions.
c. Ask the patient to sign the instruction sheet on the appropriate line.
d. Witness the patient's signature by signing your name in the appropriate space on the form. Include today's date.
e. Give a signed copy of the wound care instructions to the patient and file a copy in the patient's medical record.
Principle. An instruction sheet signed by the patient provides legal documentation that wound care instructions were provided to the patient.

16. Procedural Step. Chart the procedure. Include the date and time, the appearance of the wound, wound preparation, the number of strips applied, the location of the wound, and care of the wound. Chart instructions given to the patient about wound care.

PROCEDURE 6-7

CHARTING EXAMPLE

Date	
9/20/2002	10:30 a.m. Incision approx 5 cm long located on ®️ post forearm. Redness noted on edge of wound. Sl amt of serous drainage noted. Wound scrubbed c̄ Betadine sol and Betadine antiseptic applied. Applied Steri-Strips x5. Incision in good approximation. Applied DSD. Explained wound care. Written instructions provided. Signed copy filed in chart. To return in 5 days for removal of strips. ————
	———————————— T. Browning, CMA

Removal of Adhesive Skin Closures

1. **Procedural Step.** Wash the hands. Greet and identify the patient. Introduce yourself, and explain the procedure.

2. **Procedural Step.** Position the patient as required. Check to made sure the skin closures are intact and the incision line is approximated and not gapping. Check the incision line to make sure it is free from infection. If the incision line is not approximated or if redness, swelling, or a discharge is present, do not remove the skin closures and notify the physician.

3. **Procedural Step.** Position a 4 × 4 gauze pad in a convenient location. Apply clean gloves.

4. **Procedural Step.** Remove the skin closures as follows:
   a. Peel off each half of the strip of tape from the outside toward the wound margin. Never pull the strips away from the wound, because tension on the wound site may disrupt the healing process.
   b. Gently lift the strip away from the wound surface. Place the strip on a 4 × 4 gauze.
   c. Continue in this manner until all the skin closures have been removed.

5. **Procedural Step.** Cleanse the site with an antiseptic swab. Apply a dry sterile dressing if indicated by the physician. (Refer to Procedure 6–5.)

6. **Procedural Step.** Properly dispose of all contaminated supplies. Remove the gloves, and wash the hands.

7. **Procedural Step.** Chart the procedure. Include the date and time, the status of the skin closures, the number of skin closures removed, the location of the site, and care of the wound. Chart any instructions given to the patient.

CHARTING EXAMPLE

Date	
9/20/2002	10:30 a.m. Skin closures intact and in good approximation. No signs of infection. Strips x 4 removed from ®️ post forearm. Incision line cleaned c̄ Betadine and DSD applied. Instructions provided on dressing care.
	———————————— T. Browning, CMA

6

ASSISTING WITH MINOR OFFICE SURGERY

TRAY SET-UP

Assisting with minor office surgery requires a thorough knowledge of the instruments and supplies for each tray set-up and the type of assistance required by the physician during the surgery. The medical assistant must be able to work quickly and efficiently and to anticipate the physician's needs.

The instruments and supplies for the surgery must be set up on a sterile field. Many offices maintain index cards indicating the appropriate instruments and supplies for each minor office surgery tray set-up. The card may also indicate information regarding the type of skin preparation, the position of the patient, the physician's glove size, the type of suture material, preoperative instructions, and postoperative instructions. The index cards are generally kept in a file box and are filed alphabetically by the type of surgery. The medical assistant should pull the card before setting up for the minor office surgery and use it as a guide to make sure all the required articles are placed on the sterile field. The medical assistant may set up the sterile tray either before or after preparing the patient's skin. The sterile tray set-up must not be permitted to become contaminated. If the medical assistant must turn away from the sterile tray or leave the room after setting up, a sterile towel must be placed over the tray to maintain sterility.

Methods Used to Set Up a Sterile Tray

A common method used to set up a sterile tray is to use prepackaged sterile set-ups wrapped in disposable sterilization paper or muslin that are prepared by the medical office through autoclave sterilization. These set-ups are labeled according to their specific use (e.g., suture pack, cyst removal pack) and contain most of the instruments and supplies required for the minor office surgery indicated on the label. The medical assistant opens the wrapped package on a flat surface, such as a Mayo stand; the inside of the wrapper is sterile and serves as the sterile field. Several additional articles not contained in the prepackaged set-up (e.g., an antiseptic, sterile 4 × 4 gauze pads, disposable syringes and needles, and sutures) may need to be added to the sterile field once the package is opened. The antiseptic is added to the sterile field according to the procedure previously outlined in this chapter. Items in peel-apart packages are added by flipping them onto the sterile field or by using sterile transfer forceps.

Another method used to set up a sterile tray is to place all the necessary articles on the sterile field by flipping them onto the sterile field from peel-apart packages. In using this method, the sterile field is prepared by placing a sterile towel over a tray such as a Mayo stand or other flat surface. The sterile towel must be handled by the corners only so as not to contaminate it. It must not be fanned through the air but laid down gently and slowly to prevent airborne contamination.

Side Table

Some articles required for minor office surgery are not placed on the sterile field but are set up off to the side on an adjacent table or stand. These articles, such as the label required for a specimen container, may be medically aseptic and therefore should not be placed on the sterile field, or they may be sterile but enclosed in a medically aseptic package or container. The local anesthetic, which is a sterile solution, is in a vial that is medically aseptic and therefore must not be placed on the sterile field. The physician needs to apply gloves to perform the surgery. Although the gloves are sterile, the outside wrapper is not; therefore, the package of gloves must not be placed on the sterile field. In addition, it is easier for the physician to apply gloves from a side table or stand. The medical assistant opens the outside wrapper for the physician, to facilitate applying the gloves.

SKIN PREPARATION

The patient's skin must be prepared prior to the minor office surgery, because the skin contains an abundance

of microorganisms. If these microorganisms were to enter the body, a wound infection could develop. It is not possible to sterilize skin, because chemical agents required to kill all living microorganisms are too strong to be placed on the skin surfaces. Therefore, the operative site and an area surrounding it must be cleaned and prepared in such a way as to remove as many microorganisms as possible to reduce the risk of surgical wound contamination.

Shaving the Site

Hair supports the growth of microorganisms, and the physician may therefore want the medical assistant to shave the skin at and around the operative site. Disposable shave prep trays are commercially available and include several gauze sponges, a measured amount of antiseptic soap, a container for soapy water, and a disposable safety razor. The skin should be pulled taut as it is shaved, and the medical assistant must be careful to prevent nicks. Once all the hair has been removed, the shaved area should be rinsed and dried thoroughly.

Cleansing the Site

The site must next be cleaned with an antiseptic solution such as Betadine solution (povidone-iodine) or Hibiclens (chlorhexidine) (Fig. 6–11). The medical assistant should scrub the area with a surgical scrub brush using a firm circular motion, moving from the inside outward. The area is then rinsed using gauze pads saturated with water and is blotted dry with sterile gauze.

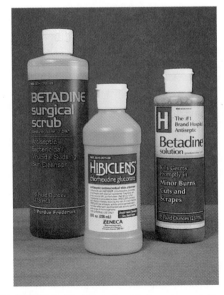

■ **FIGURE 6–11.** Examples of cleansing solutions.

Antiseptic Application

Once the patient's skin has been shaved (if required) and cleansed, an antiseptic is applied to the operative area, followed by the application of a sterile drape. The antiseptic decreases the number of microorganisms on the patient's skin; an example of a commonly used antiseptic is Betadine (povidone-iodine). A disposable sterile **fenestrated drape** is most commonly used; it will cover a wide area of skin around the operative area, leaving only the operative site exposed. The drape provides a sterile area around the operative site and thereby decreases contamination of the patient's surgical wound.

LOCAL ANESTHETIC

Minor office surgeries often require the use of a local anesthetic; examples of local anesthetics frequently used in the medical office include lidocaine hydrochloride (Xylocaine) and procaine hydrochloride (Novocain). The physician injects the local anesthetic into the tissue surrounding the operative site, a process termed **infiltration,** to produce a loss of sensation in that area and thereby prevent the patient from feeling pain during the surgery. Local anesthetics begin working in 5 to 15 minutes and have a duration of action of from 1 to 3 hours, depending on the type of anesthetic used.

Some physicians may prefer to use a local anesthetic containing **epinephrine,** a vasoconstrictor that prolongs the local effect of the anesthetic and decreases the rate of systemic absorption of the local anesthetic by constricting blood vessels at the operative site. The physician will inform the medical assistant as to the type, strength, and amount of the local anesthetic needed for the minor office surgery. For example, Xylocaine is available in 0.5, 1.0, 1.5, and 2.0 percent solutions. The physician may order 1 ml of Xylocaine

6

Highlight on the History of Surgery

Surgery evolved from very primitive beginnings. The first record of a surgical operation dates back to 350,000 B.C. Primitive humans believed that headaches were caused by demons that had gained entrance into the head and were unable to get out. To release the demons, a hole was chiseled through the patient's skull with a sharp flint. Early operating instruments consisted of sharpened flints and crude hammers. Sharpened animal teeth were used for blood-letting and drainage of abscesses. Ancient records show that suturing materials consisted of dried gut, dried tendon, strips of hide, horsehair, and fibers from tree bark. To help form a clot, bleeding wounds were covered with materials such as rabbit fur, shredded tree bark, egg yolk, and cobwebs.

As late as the early 1800s, surgical instruments were still almost nonexistent. Kitchen knives and penknives doubled as scalpels, and table forks were used as retractors. Physicians would use household pincushions to hold their suturing needles. The same sponges were used for every patient to wipe away blood and other secretions. Because of this, the most trivial operations were likely to be followed by infection, and death occurred in up to half of all surgical operations. Joseph Lister, an English surgeon, was one of the first individuals to advocate the use of antiseptics during surgery. Lister insisted on the use of antiseptics on the hands of his surgical team, instruments, wounds, and dressings. Lister's ideas were ridiculed by many surgeons, but in 1879 his antiseptic principles were, at long last, formally adopted by the medical profession. Today Joseph Lister is known as the father of modern surgery.

Anesthetic agents, such as ether and chloroform, were discovered in the mid-1800s. Before this time, various methods were used to subdue and restrain patients during surgery, such as having the patient consume alcohol before the operation and strapping the patient to the operating table. With the advent of anesthetics, new surgical procedures never before considered possible came into existence. This resulted in new demands for surgical instruments, as well as the necessity for smaller and more delicate instruments.

The late 1800s and early 1900s saw dramatic advances in surgical operations and techniques. The most notable of these included the invention of the steam sterilizer, which permitted sterilization of surgical instruments and supplies; the use of surgical gowns, caps, masks, and gloves during surgery; the monitoring of a patient's condition while under anesthesia; the development of stainless steel, which provided a superior material for manufacturing surgical instruments; and the establishment of standards for manufacturing and packaging sutures. Other discoveries important to surgery during this same time period included the discovery of x-rays by Wilhelm Roentgen, the discovery of penicillin by Alexander Fleming, the discovery by William Halsted that cocaine could be used as a local anesthetic, and the development of endoscopic instruments such as the laryngoscope, bronchoscope, and sigmoidoscope for viewing internal structures of the body.

The breakthroughs in surgical technology established through the ages laid the foundation for our present-day complex surgical procedures such as laser surgery, open-heart surgery, and microsurgery. It is incredible indeed to think that it all started with a sharpened flint!

2.0 percent with epinephrine to suture a laceration of the forearm.

Preparing the Anesthetic

The local anesthetic is drawn up into the syringe using the information presented in Chapter 7 (Procedure 7–3: Preparing the Injection). The vial must first be cleansed using an alcohol wipe. The correct amount of anesthetic solution is then withdrawn into the syringe. This may be performed by either the medical assistant or the physician. The medical assistant withdraws the anesthetic into the syringe and hands it to the physician, who has not yet applied gloves. The physician injects the anesthetic into the patient's tissues and then applies gloves to begin the surgery.

The physician may prefer to draw the anesthetic solution into the syringe after he or she has applied gloves. The medical assistant should first show the label of the vial to the physician and then hold the vial securely while the physician withdraws the medication (Fig. 6–12). The medical assistant must hold the vial, because the outside of the vial is medically aseptic and cannot be touched by the physician's sterile gloved hand.

If the medical assistant prepares the anesthetic injection, the needle and syringe are not placed on the sterile field but are assembled off to the side, using aseptic technique. If the physician withdraws the anesthetic, the needle and syringe are placed on the sterile field.

ASSISTING THE PHYSICIAN

The type of assistance required by the physician during minor office surgery is based on the type of surgery performed and physician's preference.

Some physicians want the medical assistant to apply sterile gloves and assist directly by handing instruments and supplies from the sterile field. An instrument should be handed to the physician in a firm, confident manner and should be placed in the physician's hand in its functional position, that is, the position in which it is to be used (Fig. 6–13). If the instrument is handed correctly, the physician should not have to reposition the instrument to use it.

The medical assistant is responsible for adding any instruments or supplies to the sterile field that are required by the physician after the surgery has begun, such as another hemostat, additional 4 × 4 gauze pads, or sutures. This is generally accomplished using peel-apart packages and either flipping the contents onto the sterile field or holding the package open and allowing the physician to remove the contents with a gloved hand. In assisting with minor office surgery, it is essen-

6

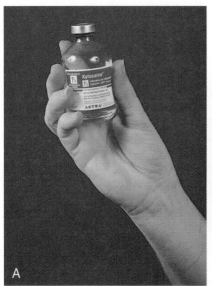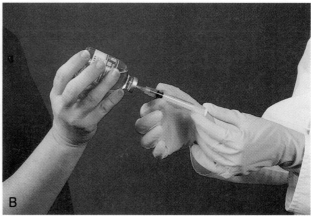

■ **FIGURE 6–12.** Drawing up the local anesthetic. *A,* Trudy holds up the vial so that the physician can verify the name and strength of the local anesthetic. *B,* Trudy holds the vial securely while the physician withdraws the medication.

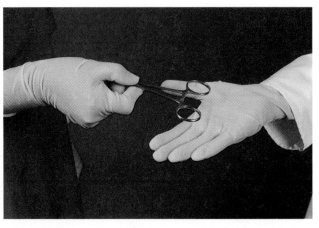

■ **FIGURE 6–13.** Trudy hands a hemostat to the physician in its functional position.

tial to know all steps in the procedure so that the physician's needs are anticipated and the surgery proceeds smoothly and efficiently.

The physician may obtain a tissue specimen that is sent to the laboratory for histologic examination. The specimen must be placed in an appropriate-sized container with a preservative. The medical assistant is responsible for labeling the specimen container with the patient's name, the date, and the type of specimen. The medical assistant must also complete a laboratory requisition to accompany the specimen; this is known as a biopsy requisition (Fig. 6–14).

Once the minor office surgery is completed, the physician may want the medical assistant to place a dry sterile dressing over the surgical wound to protect it from contamination or injury or to absorb drainage. The medical assistant is also responsible for assisting the patient and cleaning the examining room.

A general procedure for assisting with minor office surgery is outlined in the following pages. Specific instruments and supplies required for the minor office surgery depend on the type of surgery being performed and the physician's preference. Knowing the name and function of each of the surgical instruments presented in Figure 6–2 enables the medical assistant to set up for each type of minor surgery performed in the medical office. If the medical office utilizes prepackaged sterile set-ups, the medical assistant will have already assembled the instruments and supplies in the package during the sanitization and sterilization process; however, the instruments and supplies should be rechecked after the pack is opened to make sure all the sterile articles are included.

6

DIAGNOSTIC PATHOLOGY ASSOCIATES, INC

HISTOPATHOLOGY/CYTOPATHOLOGY REQUISITION

BILL TO: ☐ ACCOUNT ☐ MEDICARE ☐ BLUE SHIELD ☐ PATIENT ☐ MEDICAID ☐ OTHER	PATIENT NAME (LAST, FIRST, MIDDLE INITIAL)	PATIENT ID	ROOM NO.

SEX	BIRTHDATE / /	DATE COLLECTED	TIME COLLECTED A.M. P.M.	REQUESTING PHYSICIAN	SPECIAL INSTRUCTIONS

RESPONSIBLE PARTY NAME	RESPONSIBLE PARTY ADDRESS	CITY, STATE, ZIP

PHONE	MEDICAID ID NUMBER	MEDICARE HIC NUMBER	INSURANCE COMPANY NAME

INSURANCE COMPANY ADDRESS	GROUP NUMBER	CONTRACT NUMBER	COVERAGE CODE	PATIENT/INSURED RELATIONSHIP ☐ SELF ☐ SPOUSE ☐ DEPEND.

PATIENT AUTHORIZATION: I AUTHORIZE THE RELEASE OF ANY MEDICAL INFORMATION NECESSARY TO PROCESS A CLAIM. I PERMIT A COPY OF THIS AUTHORIZATION TO BE USED IN PLACE OF THE ORIGINAL AND REQUEST PAYMENT OF ANY MEDICAL INSURANCE BENEFITS EITHER TO ME OR TO THE PARTY WHO ACCEPTS ASSIGNMENT.   SIGNED X_____   DATE _____

TISSUE EXAM: ☐ GROSS & MICROSCOPIC ☐ GROSS ONLY **SPECIMEN TYPE:** ☐ BIOPSY ☐ SCRAPING ☐ BRUSHING ☐ WASHING ☐ FLUIDS ☐ FINE NEEDLE ☐ OTHER _____	**SOURCE OF SPECIMEN:** ☐ PHONE REPORT (NEXT WORKING DAY) COPIES TO: _____	CLINICAL DIAGNOSIS: PATIENT HISTORY:

■ **FIGURE 6–14.** Biopsy requisition. (Courtesy of Diagnostic Pathology Associates, Inc., Columbus, Ohio.)

PROCEDURE

6–8

Assisting with Minor Office Surgery

EQUIPMENT/SUPPLIES: Instruments and supplies for the type of surgery to be performed

Preparing the Tray

1. **Procedural Step.** Determine the type of minor office surgery to be performed. The physician instructs the medical assistant as to the type of surgery as well as any additional information needed to set up for the surgery, such as the appropriate anesthetic and suture material. If the medical office maintains a minor office surgery filing system, pull the file card indicating the instruments and supplies that are required for the type of surgery to be performed.

2. **Procedural Step.** Prepare the examining room. Make sure the room is spotlessly clean and well lighted.

3. **Procedural Step.** Wash the hands.

4. **Procedural Step.** Set up any medically aseptic articles required on a side stand or table.
   Principle. Articles that are medically aseptic cannot be placed on the sterile field because they would contaminate it.

5. **Procedural Step.** Wash the hands and set up the minor office surgery tray on a clean, dry, flat sur-

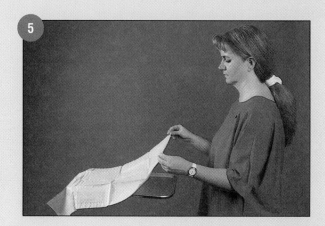

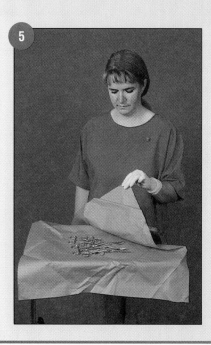

face, using the principles of surgical asepsis. The sterile tray can be set up as follows:

Prepackaged Set-Up.
Use a prepackaged sterile set-up. Select the appropriate package from the supply shelf and place it on a Mayo stand or other flat surface. Open the set-up using the inside of the wrapper as the sterile field. Add any other articles to the sterile field that are needed for the surgery but not contained in the sterile package.

Transferring Articles to a Sterile Field.
Place a sterile towel on a Mayo stand or other flat surface to provide a sterile field and transfer instruments and supplies to it from wrapped or peel-apart packages. Pick up the folded sterile towel by two corner ends and allow it to unfold; make sure it does not touch an unsterile surface. Lay the sterile towel down gently and slowly over the Mayo stand, making sure it does not brush against an unsterile surface such as your uniform. Do not allow your arms to pass over the towel as you lay it down, because this would result in contamination of the sterile field.
Principle. The principles of surgical asepsis must be followed to prevent contamination of the sterile field.

6

6. Procedural Step. Arrange the articles neatly on the sterile field using sterile gloves. Do not allow one article to lie on top of another. Recheck to make sure all the instruments and supplies required for the surgery are available on the sterile field.
Principle. Instruments and supplies can be located quickly and efficiently on a neat and orderly sterile field. Sterile gloves must be used to prevent contamination of the sterile articles.

7. Procedural Step. Cover the tray set-up with a sterile towel by picking up the towel by two corner ends and placing it gently and slowly over the set-up. Do not allow your arms to pass over the sterile field as you lay it down.
Principle. The towel prevents the sterile tray from becoming contaminated. The towel must be picked up by the corner ends to prevent contaminating it and should be moved slowly and not fanned through the air to prevent airborne contamination. Passing the arms over the sterile field results in contamination of the field.

Preparing the Patient

8. Procedural Step. Greet and identify the patient. Introduce yourself. Explain the procedure, and prepare the patient for the minor office surgery. Help allay patient fears. Ask the patient if he or she needs to void before the surgery. Provide instructions to the patient on any clothing that must be removed and putting on an examination gown, if required. Enough clothing must be removed to completely expose the operative area. Instruct the patient not to move during the procedure and not to talk, laugh, sneeze, or cough over the sterile field.

Principle. Minor office surgery is often a frightening experience for the patient, and reassurance should be offered to help reduce apprehension. The amount of clothing that must be removed will depend on the type of minor office surgery being performed. By moving, the patient may accidentally contaminate the sterile field or touch the operative site. Microorganisms are carried in water vapor from the mouth, nose, and lungs and can be transferred onto the sterile field.

9. Procedural Step. Position the patient. The type of position is determined by the type of minor office surgery to be performed. The patient is positioned in such a way as to provide the best possible exposure and accessibility to the operative site. *Note:* If a difficult position must be maintained, such as the knee-chest position, the patient should not be positioned until the physician is ready to begin the minor office surgery.

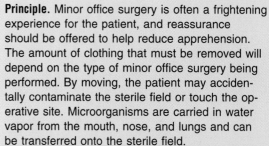

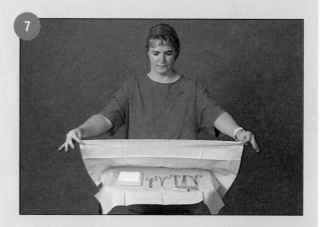

6

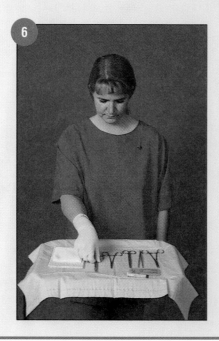

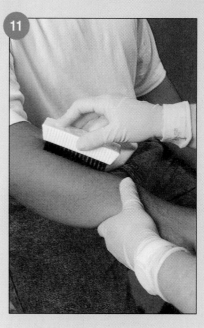

Continued

6

10. **Procedural Step.** Adjust the light so that it is focused on the operative site.

11. **Procedural Step.** Apply clean disposable gloves. Prepare the patient's skin as specified by the physician. The skin at and around the operative site may need to be shaved. The skin should be pulled taut as it is shaved. The area is then rinsed and dried thoroughly.

    Cleanse the patient's skin with an antiseptic solution and a surgical scrub brush using a firm, circular motion and moving from the inside outward. Do not return to an area just cleansed. The area is then rinsed using gauze pads saturated with water and blotted dry with a sterile gauze pad.

    Cleanse the site using antiseptic swabs such as Betadine or alcohol swabs. Allow the skin to dry. Remove the gloves and wash hands.

12. **Procedural Step.** Check to make sure everything is prepared for the minor office surgery and inform the physician that the patient is ready.

Assisting the Physician

13. **Procedural Step.** Assist the physician as required during the minor office surgery, following the principles of surgical asepsis. The physician will inject the local anesthetic, drape the patient, and perform the surgery.

    The responsibilities of the medical assistant may include:

    a. Uncovering the sterile tray set-up by picking up the sterile towel covering it. The towel should be picked up by two corner ends and removed slowly and gently without allowing the arms to pass over the sterile field.

    b. Withdrawing the local anesthetic into a syringe and handing it to the physician or holding the vial while the physician withdraws the local anesthetic.

    c. Opening the outer glove wrapper for the physician to facilitate the application of sterile gloves.

    d. Adjusting the light as needed by the physician for good visualization of the operative site.

    e. Restraining patients such as children.

    f. Relaxing and reassuring the patient during the minor office surgery.

    g. Handing instruments and supplies to the physician. (Sterile gloves required.)

    h. Keeping the sterile field neat and orderly. (Sterile gloves required.)

    i. Holding a basin in which the physician can deposit soiled instruments and supplies, such as hemostats and gauze sponges. (Clean gloves required.)

    j. Retracting tissue from an area to allow the physician better access and visibility of the operative site. (Sterile gloves required.)

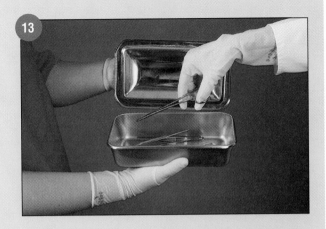

    k. Sponging blood from the operative site. (Sterile gloves required.)

    l. Adding instruments and supplies to the sterile field as required by the physician.

    m. Holding the specimen container to accept a specimen received from the physician. (Clean gloves required.) Do not touch the inside of the container because it is sterile. Label the specimen container with the patient's name, the date, and the type of specimen.

14. **Procedural Step.** Apply a sterile dressing to the surgical wound, if ordered by the physician (refer to Procedure 6–5: Changing a Sterile Dressing). **Principle.** The sterile dressing protects the wound from contamination and injury and helps absorb drainage.

15. **Procedural Step.** Stay with the patient as a safety precaution and to assist and instruct the patient. The patient may need to rest before getting off the examining table. Help the patient off the table to

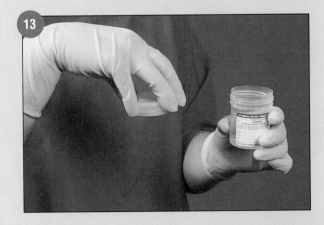

PROCEDURE 6-8

prevent falls. Instruct the patient to dress, offering assistance if needed. Make sure postoperative instructions regarding any type of medical care to be administered at home are understood. Relay information regarding the return visit for postoperative care, such as the removal of sutures or a dressing change. If the patient has a wound or if sutures have been inserted, he or she should be told to keep the area clean and dry and to report any signs of inflammation such as redness, swelling, discharge, or increase in pain. Any instructions given must be charted in the patient's medical record.

Principle. The patient (especially an elderly one) may become dizzy after the minor office surgery and should be allowed to rest before getting off the examining table. Patient instructions must be charted to protect the physician legally, in the event that the patient fails to follow instructions and causes harm or damage to the operative site.

16. **Procedural Step.** If a specimen was collected, it must be transferred to the laboratory in a tightly closed, properly labeled specimen container. Complete a biopsy request form to accompany the specimen. Record information in the patient's

chart, including the date the specimen was picked up or sent to the laboratory, as well as the name of the laboratory.

Principle. Recording information regarding the specimen transport documents that the specimen was sent to the laboratory.

17. **Procedural Step.** Clean the examining room. Handle the instruments carefully so as not to damage them. Be especially careful with sharp instruments to prevent cutting yourself. Blood and body secretions should be rinsed off the instruments immediately, to prevent them from drying and hardening. The instruments must then be sanitized and sterilized, when it is convenient to do so, following the procedures presented in Chapter 5. Discard disposable articles contaminated with blood or other potentially infectious materials in a biohazard waste container.

Principle. Surgical instruments are expensive and must be handled carefully to prolong their life span. Hardened blood and secretions on an instrument are difficult to remove. Disposable articles must be discarded in an appropriate manner to prevent the spread of infection.

6

MEDICAL OFFICE SURGICAL PROCEDURES

☐ The most common surgical procedures performed in the medical office are presented on the following pages. A discussion of the procedure and the items required for each tray set-up are included. The medical assistant should take into account, however, that the instruments and supplies may vary slightly from those listed here, based on the physician's preference.

SEBACEOUS CYST REMOVAL

A **sebaceous cyst** is a thin, closed sac or capsule containing secretions from a sebaceous or oil gland. It forms when the outlet of the gland becomes obstructed. The built-up secretion of sebum from the gland causes swelling, and the lining of the cyst consists of the stretched sebaceous gland. Sebaceous cysts

are soft to firm in consistency and are generally elevated and filled with an odorous cheesy material. This type of cyst may occur anywhere on the body except on the palms and the soles—these areas do not contain sebaceous glands. Sebaceous cysts tend to occur most frequently on the scalp, face, ears, neck, and back.

A sebaceous cyst is usually painless and nontender, although it may become infected; to avoid this, the cyst should be excised by the physician. If it is already infected, the physician does not excise the cyst but drains it and performs the removal at a later time. A sebaceous cyst is removed as follows:

1. A local anesthetic is used to numb the area.
2. The physician makes an incision, removes the cyst, and sutures the surgical incision (Fig. 6–15).
3. The cyst is placed in the specimen container with a preservative and sent to the laboratory for examination by a pathologist.
4. A sterile dressing is then applied to the operative site.

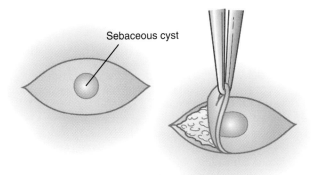

Sebaceous cyst

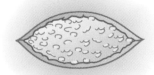

■ **FIGURE 6–15.** Sebaceous cyst removal. The physician makes an incision, removes the cyst, and sutures the surgical incision. (From Nealon, T. F., Jr.: *Fundamentals in Surgery,* 3rd ed. Philadelphia, W. B. Saunders Company, 1980.)

ITEMS PLACED TO THE SIDE OF THE STERILE FIELD
Sebaceous Cyst Removal:
- Clean disposable gloves
- Antiseptic solution
- Surgical scrub brush
- Antiseptic swabs
- Sterile gloves
- Local anesthetic
- Alcohol wipe to cleanse the vial
- Specimen container with preservative and label
- Laboratory request form
- Surgical tape
- Biohazard waste container

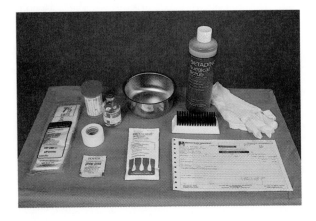

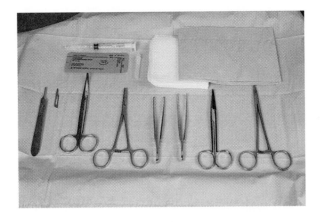

ITEMS INCLUDED ON THE STERILE FIELD
Sebaceous Cyst Removal:
- Fenestrated drape
- Needle and syringe for drawing up the local anesthetic
- Scalpel and blade
- Dissecting scissors
- Hemostatic forceps
- Tissue forceps
- Thumb forceps
- Operating scissors
- Needle holder
- Sutures
- Sterile 4 × 4 gauze

SURGICAL INCISION AND DRAINAGE OF LOCALIZED INFECTIONS

An **abscess** is a collection of pus in a cavity surrounded by inflamed tissue (Fig. 6–16). It is caused by a pathogen that invades the tissues, usually by way of a break in the skin. An abscess serves as a defense mechanism of the body to keep an infection localized by walling off the microorganisms, preventing them from spreading through the body. A **furuncle,** also known as a boil, is a localized staphylococcal infection that originates deep within a hair follicle. Furuncles produce pain and itching. The skin initially becomes red and then turns white and necrotic over the top of the furuncle. Erythema and induration usually surround it.

Localized infections, such as abscesses, furuncles, and infected sebaceous cysts that do not rupture and drain naturally, may need to be incised and drained by the physician as follows:

1. A local anesthetic is generally used for the procedure.
2. A scalpel is used to make the incision. Then either a rubber Penrose drainage tube or a gauze wick is inserted into the wound to keep the edges of the tissues apart, which facilitates drainage of the exudate. The exudate contains pathogenic microorga-

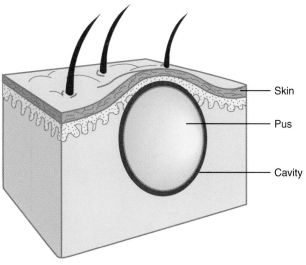

Skin

Pus

Cavity

■ **FIGURE 6–16.** An abscess is a collection of pus in a cavity surrounded by inflamed tissue. (From Nealon, T. F., Jr.: *Fundamentals in Surgery,* 3rd ed. Philadelphia, W. B. Saunders Company, 1980.)

nisms; therefore, the medical assistant should be careful to avoid contact with the exudate while assisting with the minor surgery.

3. A sterile dressing of several thicknesses is applied over the operative site to absorb the drainage.
4. The patient may be instructed to apply warm moist compresses at home to promote healing.

ITEMS PLACED TO THE SIDE OF THE STERILE FIELD

Incision and Drainage:

- Clean disposable gloves
- Antiseptic solution
- Surgical scrub brush
- Antiseptic swabs
- Sterile gloves
- Local anesthetic
- Alcohol wipe to cleanse the vial
- Rubber Penrose drain or gauze wick
- Iodoform packing material
- Surgical tape
- Biohazard waste container

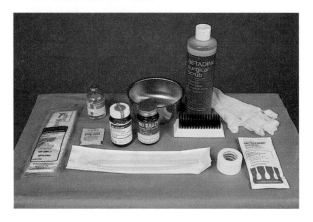

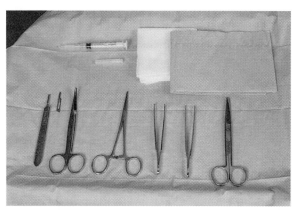

ITEMS INCLUDED ON THE STERILE FIELD

Incision and Drainage:

- Fenestrated drape
- Needle or syringe for drawing up the anesthetic
- Scalpel and blade
- Dissecting scissors
- Hemostatic forceps
- Tissue forceps
- Thumb forceps
- Operating scissors
- Sterile 4 × 4 gauze

PUTTING IT ALL *into* PRACTICE

▶ **TRUDY BROWNING:** *Working in an internal medicine office where a majority of the patients are elderly, I occasionally come across individuals who are not very cooperative and are "set in their ways." One 90-year-old lady, in particular, had a reputation in the office of being cantankerous and difficult to work with. One day when the physician ordered lab work on her, I prepared to draw blood from her tiny, frail body, praying that everything would go smoothly. As I helped her up after a successful "stick," she, of all people, reached to give me a hug and said to me, "I like you. That didn't even hurt"! She continued to hold my hand and talk to me as I walked her out of the office. This turned out to be the last time I would see her as she moved out of town, but not out of my heart, leaving a lasting impression on my life.*

6

NEEDLE BIOPSY

A **biopsy** is the removal and examination of tissue from the living body. The tissue is usually examined under a microscope. Biopsies are most often performed to determine whether a tumor is malignant or benign; however, a biopsy may also be used as a diagnostic aid for other conditions, such as infections. A **needle biopsy** is a type of biopsy in which tissue from deep within the body is obtained by the insertion of a biopsy needle through the skin. A biopsy needle consists of an outer needle for making the puncture and a forked inner needle for obtaining the tissue specimen (Fig. 6–17A). The inner needle detaches tissue from a part of the body and brings it to the surface through its lumen (Fig. 6–17B).

The advantage of a needle biopsy is that a sample of tissue can be obtained that might otherwise require a major surgical operation. The procedure is performed under a local anesthetic, and, since an incision is not required, the patient does not have to undergo the discomfort and inconvenience of an operative recovery. The tissue specimen is placed in a container with a preservative and sent to the laboratory for examination by a pathologist. A small dressing, placed over the needle puncture site, is usually sufficient to protect the operative site and promote healing. After the procedure, the patient should be observed for any evidence of complications related to the procedure.

Needle Biopsy Set-Up

The items required for a needle biopsy are listed here.

ITEMS PLACED TO THE SIDE OF THE STERILE FIELD
Needle Biopsy:
- Clean disposable gloves
- Antiseptic solution
- Surgical scrub brush
- Antiseptic swabs
- Sterile gloves
- Local anesthetic
- Alcohol wipe to cleanse the vial
- Specimen container with preservative and label
- Laboratory request form
- Surgical tape
- Biohazard waste container

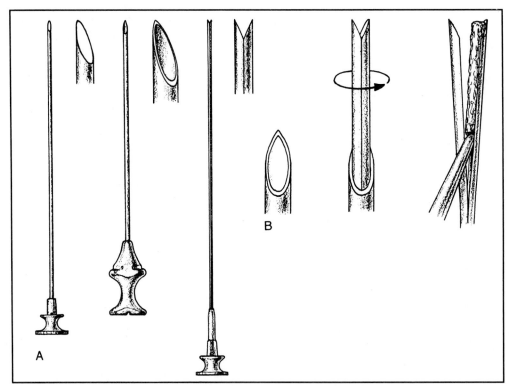

■ **FIGURE 6–17.** Biopsy needle. *A,* A biopsy needle consists of an outer needle for making the puncture and a forked inner needle for obtaining the specimen. *B,* The inner needle detaches tissue from a part of the body and brings it to the surface through its lumen. (From Nealon, T. F., Jr.: *Fundamentals in Surgery,* 3rd ed. Philadelphia, W. B. Saunders Company, 1980.)

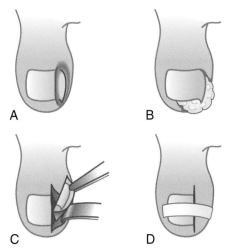

■ **FIGURE 6–18.** Ingrown toenail. *A,* The edge of the toenail grows deeply into the nail groove. *B,* In mild cases, treatment consists of inserting a small piece of cotton packing under the toenail. *C,* In severe and recurring cases, a wedge of the nail is surgically removed, and *D,* a strip of surgical tape is applied over the area. (From Nealon, T. F., Jr.: *Fundamentals in Surgery,* 3rd ed. Philadelphia, W. B. Saunders Company, 1980.)

ITEMS INCLUDED ON THE STERILE FIELD

Needle Biopsy:

- Fenestrated drape
- Needle and syringe for drawing up the local anesthetic
- Biopsy needle
- Sterile 4 × 4 gauze

INGROWN TOENAIL REMOVAL

An ingrown toenail occurs when the edge of the toenail grows deeply into the nail groove and penetrates the surrounding skin, resulting in pain and discomfort to the patient (Fig. 6–18*A*). Ingrown toenails are caused by external pressure, such as from tight shoes or hose, or from trauma, improper nail trimming, or infection. The protruding nail acts as a foreign body, usually resulting in secondary infection and inflammation. In mild cases, this condition is treated by inserting a small piece of cotton packing under the toenail to raise the nail edge away from the tissue of the nail groove (Fig. 6–18*B*). In severe and recurring cases, part of the nail must be surgically removed, which relieves pain by decreasing the nail pressure on the soft tissues.

Ingrown Toenail Removal Set-up

The items required for the removal of an ingrown toenail are listed here.

ITEMS PLACED TO THE SIDE OF THE STERILE FIELD

Ingrown Toenail Removal:

- Clean disposable gloves
- Antiseptic solution
- Surgical scrub brush
- Antiseptic swabs
- Sterile gloves
- Local anesthetic
- Alcohol wipe to cleanse the vial
- Surgical tape
- Biohazard waste container

ITEMS INCLUDED ON THE STERILE FIELD

Ingrown Toenail Removal:

- Fenestrated drape
- Needle and syringe for drawing up the local anesthetic
- Surgical toenail scissors
- Hemostatic forceps
- Operating scissors
- Sterile 4 × 4 gauze

Procedure

An ingrown toenail is removed as follows:

1. Before the surgical procedure is performed, the affected foot must first be soaked in tepid water containing an antibacterial skin solution for 10 to 15 minutes to soften the nail plate and decrease the possibility of bacterial infection.
2. The patient is placed in a reclining position with the foot adequately supported, and the toe is shaved to remove hair, which would act as a contaminant.
3. An antiseptic is applied to the affected toe, which is then numbed using a local anesthetic.
4. The physician surgically removes a wedge of the nail using surgical toenail scissors (Fig. 6–18*C*).
5. A sterile gauze dressing or a strip of surgical tape is applied over the area to protect the operative site and to promote healing (Fig. 6–18*D*).

COLPOSCOPY

Colposcopy is the visual examination of the vagina and cervix by means of a lighted instrument with a binocular magnifying lens, known as a **colposcope.** (Fig. 6–19). The purpose of colposcopy is to examine the vagina and cervix to determine areas of abnormal tissue growth. Colposcopy is performed following an abnormal cytology report from a Papanicolaou (Pap) smear, to evaluate a vaginal or cervical lesion observed during a pelvic examination, or after treatment for cancer of the cervix. The lens of the colposcope magnifies tissue, thereby facilitating the inspection of cervical cells and the obtaining of a biopsy. For a routine col-

6

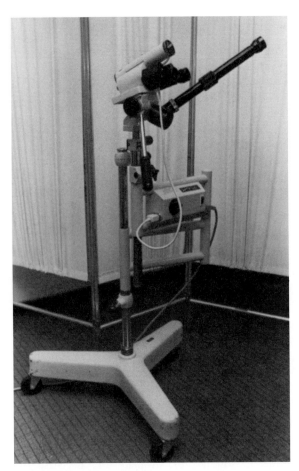

■ **FIGURE 6–19.** Colposcope

6

poscopic examination, a magnification of × 16 is generally used. The colposcope may be placed on an adjustable stand or attached to the side of the examining table and swung out prior to use.

Colposcopy Set-Up

The items required for colposcopy are listed here.

ITEMS PLACED TO THE SIDE OF THE STERILE FIELD
Colposcopy:

- Colposcope
- Sterile gloves
- Monsel's solution
- Specimen container with preservative and label
- Laboratory request form
- Biohazard waste container

ITEMS INCLUDED ON THE STERILE FIELD
Colposcopy:

- Vaginal speculum
- Normal saline
- Acetic acid (3 percent)
- Staining solution (Lugol's solution or Gram's iodine)
- Long, sterile cotton-tipped applicators
- Cervical punch biopsy forceps
- Uterine tenaculum
- Uterine dressing forceps

Procedure

Colposcopy is performed as follows:

1. The patient is placed in a lithotomy position and prepared as for the pelvic examination.
2. The physician inserts a warmed, unlubricated vaginal speculum into the vagina.
3. A long, cotton-tipped applicator moistened with saline is used to wipe the cervix to remove the mucus film that normally covers it. The saline also provides better visualization of the cervical epithelium, because dry cervical epithelium is not transparent and therefore does not allow satisfactory viewing of the vascular pattern of the cervix.
4. The colposcope is focused on the cervix, and the physician inspects the saline-moistened cervix.
5. The cervix is swabbed with acetic acid, using a long, cotton-tipped applicator. The acetic acid helps in dissolving cervical mucus and other secretions; furthermore, the acetic acid provides the best contrast between normal and abnormal tissue, allowing for easier visualization of dysplastic and neoplastic epithelium.
6. The cervical epithelium may also be stained with a solution such as Lugol's solution or Gram's iodine, using a long, cotton-tipped applicator. The stain is another means to identify unhealthy epithelium. The healthy epithelium of the cervix contains glycogen, which is able to absorb these stains. Conversely, abnormal epithelium, such as would constitute a malignancy, does not contain glycogen and therefore is unable to absorb the stain.
7. If an abnormal area is observed, the physician will obtain a cervical biopsy using punch biopsy forceps.

CERVICAL PUNCH BIOPSY

A cervical biopsy is usually performed in combination with colposcopy to remove a cervical tissue specimen for examination by a pathologist. The purpose of the biopsy is to determine whether the specimen is benign or malignant. Cervical biopsies are often performed after an abnormal Pap smear cytology report. The procedure is usually performed a week after the end of the menstrual period, when the cervix is the least vascular.

Cervical Punch Biopsy Set-Up

The items required for a cervical punch biopsy are listed here.

ITEMS PLACED TO THE SIDE OF THE STERILE FIELD
Cervical Punch Biopsy:

- Sterile gloves
- Monsel's solution
- Specimen container with preservative and label
- Laboratory request form
- Tampons
- Colposcope (if required)
- Biohazard waste container

ITEMS INCLUDED ON THE STERILE FIELD
Cervical Punch Biopsy:

- Vaginal speculum
- Staining solution (Lugol's solution or Gram's iodine)
- Long, sterile cotton-tipped applicators
- Cervial punch biopsy forceps
- Uterine dressing forceps
- Uterine tenaculum
- Sterile 4 × 4 gauze

Procedure

A cervical biopsy is performed as follows:

1. The patient is positioned and draped in a lithotomy position. An anesthetic is not needed; because the cervix has few pain receptors, the patient experiences little discomfort from the procedure.
2. The physician inserts a vaginal speculum into the vagina for proper visualization of the cervix.
3. To assist in obtaining the specimen, the physician may stain the cervix with Lugol's solution or Gram's iodine.
4. If a colposcope is being used, it is focused on the cervix and utilized according to the information discussed on page 238.
5. The physician obtains several tissue specimens (Fig. 6–20A) from the abnormal cervical epithelium, using cervical biopsy punch forceps (Fig. 6–20B).
6. The specimen is placed in a container with a preservative and is sent to the laboratory for examination by a pathologist.
7. If bleeding occurs, the physician controls it with gauze packing, a hemostatic solution (e.g., Monsel's solution), or electrocautery.

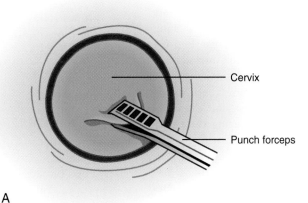

A

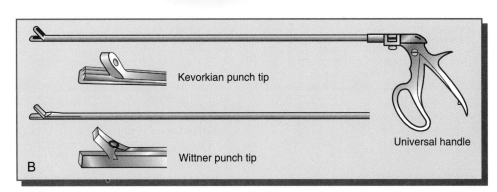

B

■ **FIGURE 6–20.** Cervical punch biopsy. *A,* Obtaining a tissue specimen from the cervix using cervical biopsy punch forceps. *B,* Cervical biopsy punch forceps. (Courtesy of Elmed Incorporated, Addison, Illinois.)

8. A vaginal tampon is inserted after the procedure is finished to absorb drainage and should be left in place usually for 8 to 24 hours.

9. The patient should be instructed not to insert another tampon unless directed to do so by the physician as it may irritate the cervix and could cause bleeding.

10. The patient should be informed that a minimum amount of bleeding may follow the procedure; however, the patient should be instructed to contact the physician if bleeding is heavier than normal menstrual bleeding.

11. A foul-smelling gray-green vaginal discharge may occur several days after the procedure and continue for a period of up to 3 weeks. The patient should be informed that this discharge results from normal healing of cervical tissue and will gradually diminish as the healing progresses.

CRYOSURGERY

Cervical

Cervial cryosurgery, also known as **cryotherapy,** is often used to treat chronic cervicitis and cervical erosion through the use of freezing temperatures. The procedure can be performed without an anesthetic, although occasionally a mild analgesia is necessary immediately afterward. The cryosurgery unit consists of a long metal probe attached to a cooling-agent tank (Fig. 6–21). The principal cooling agents available include liquid nitrogen, nitrous oxide, and carbon dioxide gas; of these, liquid nitrogen is used most often. The probe is placed in contact with the infected area, and the cooling agent flows through the probe, freezing the cervical tissue to $-40°$ to $-80°C$. This causes the cells to die and slough off so that the cervical covering can eventually be replaced with new, healthy epithelial tissue. The regeneration of the new cervical tissue occurs within approximately 4 to 6 weeks after the procedure.

Cryosurgery Set-Up

The items required for cryosurgery are listed here.

ITEMS PLACED TO THE SIDE OF THE STERILE FIELD
Cryosurgery:
- Cryosurgery unit
- Sanitary pads
- Biohazard waste container

ITEMS INCLUDED ON THE STERILE FIELD
Cryosurgery:
- Vaginal speculum
- Acid-saline solution
- Long, cotton-tipped applicators

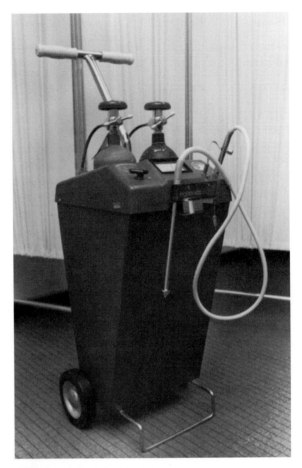

■ **FIGURE 6–21.** Cryosurgery unit.

Procedure

Cryosurgery is performed as follows:

1. The patient is draped and placed in the lithotomy position.

2. The physician inserts a vaginal speculum for proper visualization of the cervix.

3. The cervix is swabbed with an acid-saline solution to remove mucus and other contaminants.

4. The metal probe is placed in contact with the affected area, and the cryosurgery unit is turned on.

5. The cooling agent is permitted to flow over the cervical area for approximately 3 minutes. During the procedure, the patient may experience some pain resembling menstrual cramping that usually lasts about 30 minutes.

6. Once the procedure has been completed, the medical assistant should assist the patient as necessary and observe for any signs of discomfort or vertigo.

7. The patient is given a sanitary pad at the office following the procedure to absorb any discharge.

8. On the first postoperative day following the procedure, the patient will develop a heavy, clear, watery

vaginal discharge, which usually reaches its maximum by the sixth day.

9. The patient should be told to use sanitary pads at home rather than tampons. In addition, a vaginal cream may be prescribed to promote wound healing and the formation of new epithelial tissue.

10. The patient should be told that continuation of the discharge for approximately 4 weeks is normal, but that the development of a foul odor should be reported to the physician.

11. The patient should be informed that the next menstrual period will be heavier than normal and may involve some cramping.

12. The patient is usually instructed to abstain from intercourse for 4 weeks following the procedure and to douche with a solution of dilute vinegar and water.

13. The patient will be required to schedule a return visit 6 weeks following the procedure to make sure proper wound healing has taken place.

Skin Lesions

In the medical office, cryosurgery may also be used to remove benign skin lesions, such as common warts. Only a small amount of cooling agent is required for skin lesions, therefore the cryosurgery unit is considerably smaller than the one just described for cervical cryosurgery. Most physicians use liquid nitrogen contained in a small, pressurized stainless steel canister with an attached probe. The physician applies the liquid nitrogen to the skin lesion until it turns white, which indicates that freezing of the tissue has taken place. During the procedure, the patient will feel a slight burning or stinging sensation as the cooling agent is applied. Following cryosurgery, a blister develops and dries to a scab in a week to 10 days and eventually sloughs off. The patient should be told to keep the area clean and dry until the scab has sloughed off. In some cases, the treatment may not result in complete destruction of the lesion; two or more treatments may be required to remove the lesion.

BANDAGING

☐ A bandage is a strip of woven material used to wrap or cover a part of the body. The function of the bandage may be to apply pressure to control bleeding; to protect a wound from contamination; to hold a dressing in place; or to protect, support, or immobilize an injured part of the body.

GUIDELINES FOR APPLICATION

The bandage should be applied so that it feels comfortable to the patient, and it must be fastened securely with adhesive tape, metal clips, or safety pins. Guidelines for applying a bandage follow.

1. Observe the principles of medical asepsis during the application of a bandage.

2. Be sure that the area to which a bandage is applied is clean and dry.

3. Do not apply a bandage directly over an open wound. Rather, a sterile dressing should first be applied, and then the bandage. The dressing should be covered with the bandage by at least 2 inches (5 cm) beyond the edge of the dressing, to prevent contamination of the wound.

4. To prevent irritation, do not allow the skin surfaces of two body parts (for example, two fingers) to touch. In addition, the patient's perspiration provides a moist environment that encourages the growth of microorganisms. A piece of gauze should be inserted between the two body parts.

5. Be sure that joints and prominent parts of bones are padded to prevent the bandage from rubbing the skin and causing irritation.

6. Bandage the body part in its normal position with joints slightly flexed to avoid muscle strain.

7. Apply the bandage from the distal to the proximal part of the body to aid in the venous return of blood to the heart.

8. As you apply the bandage, ask the patient if it feels comfortable. The bandage should fit snugly enough so it does not fall off but not so tightly that it impedes circulation. If possible, the fingers and toes should be exposed when bandaging an extremity. This provides the opportunity to check them for signs of an impairment in circulation. Signs indicating that the bandage is too tight include coldness, pallor, numbness, cyanosis of the nailbeds, swelling, pain, or tingling sensations. If any of these signs occur, the medical assistant should loosen the bandage immediately.

9. If a bandage roll is dropped during the procedure, obtain a new bandage and begin again.

TYPES OF BANDAGES

Three basic types of bandages are utilized in the medical office. A **roller bandage** is a long strip of soft material wound on itself to form a roll. It ranges from 1/2 to 6 inches (1.3 to 15.2 cm) in width and from 2 to 5 yards (1.83 to 4.57 m) in length. The width used depends on the part being bandaged. Roller bandages are usually made of sterilized gauze. Gauze is porous and light in weight, molds easily to a body part, and is

6

relatively inexpensive and easily disposed of. However, since it is made of loosely woven cotton, it may slip and fray easily. **Kling gauze** is a special type of gauze that stretches; this allows it to cling, and, as a result, it molds and conforms better to the body part than does regular gauze.

Elastic bandages are made of woven cotton containing elastic fibers. One brand name for this bandage is the Ace bandage. Although elastic bandages are expensive, they can be washed and used again. The medical assistant must be extremely careful when applying an elastic bandage because it is easy to apply it too tightly and impede circulation, owing to its elastic nature. Elastic adhesive bandages may also be utilized; these have an adhesive backing to provide a secure fit.

BANDAGE TURNS

Five basic bandage turns are used, alone or in combination with one another. The type of turn used depends on which body part is to be bandaged and whether the bandage is used for support or immobilization or for holding a dressing in place.

The **circular turn** is applied to a part of uniform width, such as toes, fingers, or the head. Each turn completely overlaps the previous turn. Two circular turns are used to anchor a bandage at the beginning and end of a spiral, spiral-reverse, figure-eight, or recurrent turn (Fig. 6–22).

The **spiral turn** is applied to a part of uniform circumference, such as the fingers, upper arm, upper leg, chest, or abdomen. Each spiral turn is carried upward at a slight angle and should overlap the previous turn by one half to two thirds the width of the bandage (Fig. 6–23).

The **spiral-reverse turn** is useful for bandaging a part that varies in width, such as the forearm or lower leg. Reversing each spiral turn allows for a smoother fit and prevents gaping due to the variation in the contour of the limb. The thumb is used to make the reverse halfway through each spiral turn. The bandage is then directed downward and folded on itself while it is kept parallel to the lower edge of the previous turn. Each turn should overlap the previous one by two thirds of

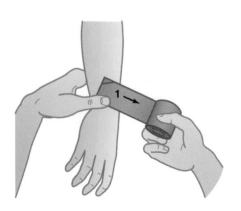

1. Place the end of the bandage on a slant.

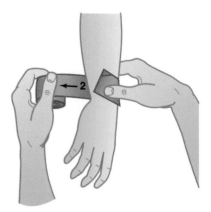

2. Encircle the part while allowing the corner of the bandage to extend.

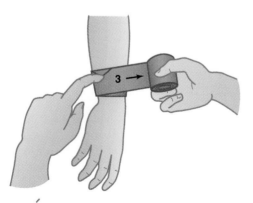

3. Turn down the corner of the bandage.

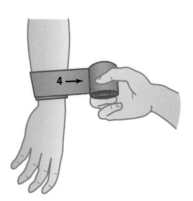

4. Make another circular turn around the part.

■ **FIGURE 6–22.** The procedure for anchoring a bandage.

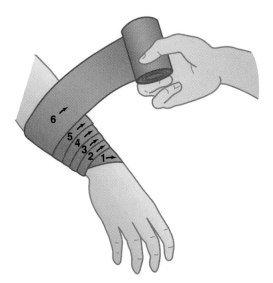

■ **FIGURE 6–23.** The procedure for making the spiral turn.

the width of the bandage. The reverse turns are utilized as often as is necessary to provide a uniform fit (Fig. 6–24).

The **figure-eight turn** is generally used to hold a dressing in place or to support and immobilize an injured joint, such as the ankle, knee, elbow, or wrist. The figure-eight consists of slanting turns that alternately ascend and descend around the part and cross over one another in the middle, resembling the figure 8. Each turn overlaps the previous one by two thirds of the width of the bandage (Fig. 6–25).

The **recurrent turn** is a series of back-and-forth turns used to bandage the tips of fingers or toes, the stump of an amputated extremity, or the head. The bandage is anchored by using two circular turns and then is passed back and forth over the tip of the part to be bandaged, first on one side and then on the other side of the first center turn. Each turn should overlap the previous turn by two thirds of the width of the bandage (Fig. 6–26).

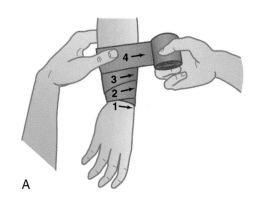

A

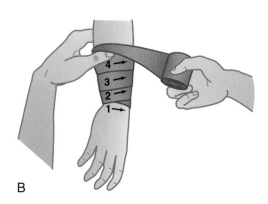

B

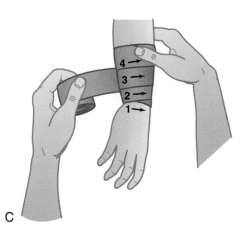

C

■ **FIGURE 6–24.** The procedure for making the spiral-reverse turn. A. Encircle the part while keeping the bandage at a slant. B. Reverse the spiral turn using the thumb and direct the bandage downward and fold it on itself. C. Keep the bandage parallel to the lower edge of the previous turn.

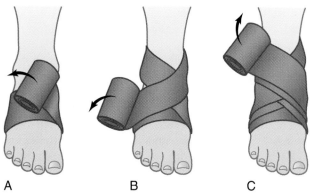

■ FIGURE 6–25. The procedure for applying an elastic bandage around the ankle using a figure-eight turn. (From Leake, M. J.: *A Manual of Simple Nursing Procedures.* Philadelphia, W. B. Saunders Company, 1971.)

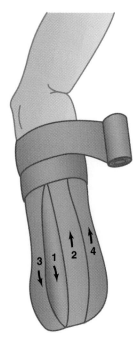

■ FIGURE 6–26. The procedure for using the recurrent turn to bandage the end of a stump.

TUBULAR GAUZE BANDAGE

A tubular gauze bandage consists of seamless elasticized gauze fabric dispensed in a roll. It is used to cover round body parts such as fingers, toes, arms, and legs and resembles a sleeve in fit. This type of bandage is easier to apply than a roller bandage, and it also adheres more securely to the body part. Tubular gauze is not sterile and therefore should not be applied over open wounds; however, it can be applied over a sterile dressing to hold it in place. The gauze is available in varying widths; selection of the width is based upon the body part to be bandaged. Refer to Table 6–1 for a list of tubular gauze widths and the body parts each size can be used to bandage.

The gauze is applied by means of a plastic or metal framelike applicator, which comes in different sizes. The applicator selected must be somewhat larger than the part to be bandaged to allow the gauze to slide easily over the body part. To assist in selecting the proper gauze width, each applicator is marked with a size number that corresponds to the size number on the tubular gauze bandage box.

The procedure for applying a tubular gauze bandage to a finger is outlined on the following pages.

TABLE 6 – 1

Tubular Gauze Bandage Widths and Recommended Application Sites

Width	Recommended Application Sites
⅝ inch	Fingers and toes of infants
	Small fingers and toes of adults
1 inch	Hands and feet of infants
	Fingers and toes of adults
	Over bulky dressings
1½ inches	Arms and legs of infants
	Arms and feet of children
	Small hands, arms, and feet of adults
2⅝ inches	Legs, thighs and heads of children
	Arms and lower legs of adults
	Small thighs, small heads of adults
3⅝ inches	Legs, thighs, lower legs, shoulders, arms, heads of adults
	Trunks of infants
5 inches	Large heads, small trunks of adults
7 inches	Trunks of adults

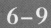

PROCEDURE

6-9

Applying a Tubular Gauze Bandage

EQUIPMENT/SUPPLIES: Applicator Adhesive tape
Roll of tubular gauze Bandage scissors

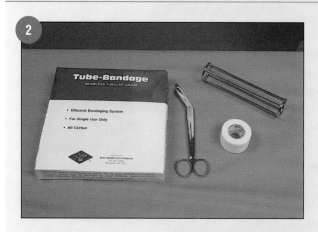

3. **Procedural Step.** Place the gauze bandage on the applicator as follows:
   a. Pull a sufficient length of gauze from the dispensing box roll.
   b. Spread apart the open end of the gauze, using your fingers.
   c. Slide the gauze over one end of the applicator. Continue loading the applicator by gathering enough gauze on the applicator to complete the bandage.
   d. Cut the roll of gauze near the opening of the box.
4. **Procedural Step.** Place the applicator over the proximal end of the patient's finger.

1. **Procedural Step.** Wash the hands. Greet and identify the patient. Introduce yourself and explain the procedure.
2. **Procedural Step.** Assemble the equipment. The applicator selected should be somewhat larger than the part to be bandaged. The proper gauze width must be used to ensure a secure fit.
   Principle. The applicator should be larger than the body part to allow the gauze to slide easily over the body part.

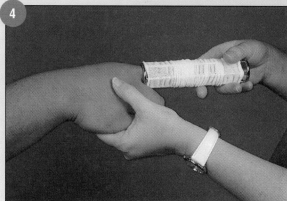

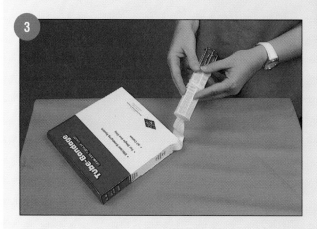

5. **Procedural Step.** Move the applicator from the proximal end to the distal end of the patient's finger, while leaving the bandage on the length of the finger. The bandage should be held in place at the base of the patient's fingers with your fingers.
   Principle. The bandage should be held in place to prevent it from sliding, which would not ensure complete coverage of the affected part.

6

PROCEDURE 6–9

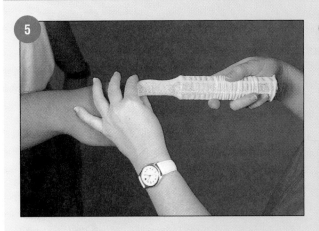

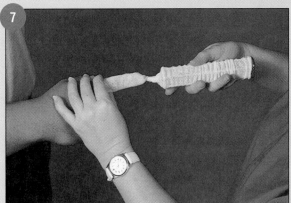

6. **Procedural Step.** Pull the applicator 1 to 2 inches past the end of the patient's finger. Continue to hold the bandage in place with your fingers.
Principle. The bandage must extend beyond the length of the patient's finger in order to secure it at the distal end.
7. **Procedural Step.** Rotate the applicator one full turn to anchor the bandage.
Principle. Anchoring the bandage holds it securely in place.
8. **Procedural Step.** Move the applicator forward again toward the proximal end of the patient's finger.
Principle. Moving the applicator forward applies a second layer of bandaging material to the patient's finger.
9. **Procedural Step.** Move the applicator forward approximately 1 inch past the original starting point of the bandage and anchor it using another rotating motion.
Principle. Anchoring the bandage holds it securely in place.
10. **Procedural Step.** Repeat this procedure for the number of layers desired. Finish the last layer at

the proximal end. Cut any unused gauze from the applicator and remove the applicator.
11. **Procedural Step.** Apply adhesive tape at the base of the finger to secure the bandage.
12. **Procedural Step.** Wash the hands and record the procedure. Include the date and time and location of the bandage application.

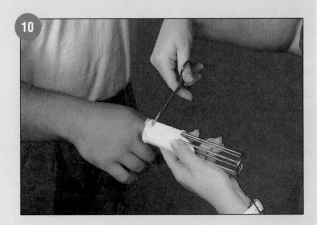

6

MEDICAL PRACTICE AND THE LAW

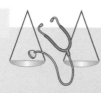

Surgical procedures are invasive and painful, and they have the potential for harmful complications, and therefore, lawsuits.

Before having a surgical procedure performed, the patient must sign a consent to treatment form. It is the medical assistant's responsibility to witness the patient's signature, but it is the physician's responsibility to inform the patient of the procedure to be performed, and its risks, alternative procedures, and benefits. The physician may delegate some or all of these tasks to the medical assistant, but *do not* accept this responsibility. Patients cannot sign for themselves if they are minors, or are impaired by drugs or disease such as Alzheimer's. In these cases, consent must be obtained from the legal guardian or next of kin. Before asking a patient to sign a consent to treatment form, ask if he or she has any questions. If so, make sure the information is given before the consent is signed. Make sure you know what procedures require informed consent in your office. Refer to Chapter 2 (The Medical Record) for specific guidelines to follow in obtaining the patient's consent.

During the procedure, your duty is to assist the physician and maintain surgical asepsis. If this is broken, you must inform the physician and remedy the situation. There is no such thing as "almost sterile."

After the surgical procedure, the medical assistant must give the patient home-care instructions. These must be performed exactly to assure proper healing. Instructions should be given verbally, demonstrated, and given in writing. Written instructions must be in the correct language, and at the patient's reading level. Pictures included in the written instructions can help clarify difficult points. Many offices purchase preprinted instructions for common surgical procedures. Make sure the signs of infection are listed on these sheets, along with instructions to call the physician if they occur, or if any other problems or questions arise.

CERTIFICATION REVIEW

6

☐ Surgical asepsis refers to those practices that keep objects and areas sterile or free from all living microorganisms. It is always employed when caring for broken skin, when a skin surface is being penetrated, or when a body cavity is entered that is normally sterile.

☐ Specific guidelines must be followed during a sterile procedure. Do not allow sterile packages to become wet. A 1-inch border around the sterile field is considered contaminated. Always face the sterile field. Hold all sterile articles above waist level. All sterile items should be placed in the center of the sterile field. Do not spill water or solutions on the sterile field. Do not talk, cough, or sneeze over a sterile field. Do not reach over a sterile field. Do not pass soiled dressings over a sterile field. Always acknowledge if you have contaminated the sterile field.

☐ A wound is a break in the continuity of an external or internal surface caused by physical means. The two basic types of wounds are closed and open. A closed wound involves an injury to the underlying tissue without a break in the skin surface, such as a contusion. An open wound involves a break in the skin surface that exposes the underlying tissues; examples include incisions, lacerations, punctures, and abrasions.

☐ The body has a natural healing process that works to destroy invading microorganisms and to restore the structure and function of the damaged tissue. Wound healing takes places in three phases: the inflammatory phase, the granulation phase, and the maturation phase.

☐ The function of a sterile dressing is to protect a wound from contamination and trauma, to absorb drainage, and to restrict motion, which may interfere with proper wound healing.

☐ Sutures are available in two different types: absorbable and nonabsorbable. Absorbable sutures consist of surgical gut or synthetic materials that are gradually digested by tissue enzymes and absorbed by the body's tissues. Nonabsorbable sutures are not absorbed by the body and either remain permanently in the body tissues or are removed. They are made from silk, cotton, nylon, polyester fiber, polypropylene, stainless steel and surgical skin staples.

Continued

□ Needles for suturing are categorized as cutting needles (having a sharp point) or noncutting needles (having a round point). Cutting needles are used for skin, and noncutting needles are used to penetrate tissues that offer a small amount of resistance, such as the viscera, subcutaneous tissue, muscle, and peritoneum. A swaged needle is one in which the suture and needle are one continuous unit.

□ Surgical skin staples are often used to close wounds. Stapling is considered the fastest method of closing of long skin incisions. In addition, trauma to the tissue is reduced because the tissue does not have to be handled very much when inserting the staples.

□ Adhesive skin closures may be used for wound repair to approximate the edges of a laceration or incision. They are used when not much tension exists on the skin edges. The advantages of adhesive skin closures are that they eliminate the need for skin sutures and a local anesthetic, they are easy to apply and remove, and they result in less scarring than skin sutures.

□ The instruments and supplies for a minor office surgery depend upon the surgery to be performed. Many offices maintain index cards indicating the appropriate instruments and supplies for each minor office surgery tray set-up.

□ The patient's skin must be prepared prior to the minor office surgery, because the skin contains an abundance of microorganisms. Skin preparation involves shaving the site, scrubbing the site with an antiseptic cleansing solution, and applying an antiseptic.

□ The use of a local anesthetic, such as Xylocaine, is often required for minor office surgery. Xylocaine with epinephrine contains a vasoconstrictor that prolongs the local effect of the anesthetic and decreases the rate of systemic absorption by constricting blood vessels at the operative site.

□ A sebaceous cyst is a thin, closed sac or capsule containing secretions from a sebaceous or oil gland. It forms when the outlet of the gland becomes obstructed. A sebaceous cyst is usually painless and nontender, although it may become infected; to avoid this, the cyst should be excised by the physician.

□ An abscess is a collection of pus in a cavity surrounded by inflamed tissue. An abscess serves as a defense mechanism of the body to keep an infection localized by walling off the microorganisms, preventing them from spreading through the body. A furuncle (boil) is a localized staphylococcal infection that originates deep within a hair follicle.

□ A biopsy is the removal and examination of tissue from the living body. It is most often performed to determine whether a tumor is malignant or benign. A needle biopsy is a type of biopsy in which tissue from deep within the body is obtained by the insertion of a biopsy needle through the skin. The advantage of a needle biopsy is that a sample of tissue can be obtained that might otherwise require a major surgical operation.

□ An ingrown toenail occurs when the edge of the toenail grows deeply into the nail groove and penetrates the surrounding skin, resulting in pain and discomfort to the patient. The protruding nail acts as a foreign body, usually resulting in secondary infection and inflammation.

□ Colposcopy is the visual examination of the vagina and cervix by means of a lighted instrument with a binocular magnifying lens, known as a colposcope. The purpose of colposcopy is to examine the vagina and cervix to determine areas of abnormal tissue growth. Colposcopy is performed following an abnormal cytology report from a Pap smear, to evaluate a vaginal or cervical lesion observed during a pelvic examination, or after treatment for cancer of the cervix.

□ A cervical punch biopsy is usually performed in combination with colposcopy to remove a cervical tissue specimen to determine if it is benign or malignant. Cervical biopsies are often performed after an abnormal Pap smear cytology report.

□ Cervical cryosurgery is often used to treat chronic cervicitis and cervical erosion through the use of freezing temperatures. A cooling agent is applied to the infected area, which causes the cells to die and slough off so that the cervical covering can eventually be replaced with new, healthy epithelial tissue.

□ A bandage is a strip of woven material used to wrap or cover a part of the body. The function of the bandage may be to apply pressure to control bleeding, to protect a wound from contamination, to hold a dressing in place, or to protect, support, or immobilize an injured part of the body.

6

RESOURCES

ON THE WEB

For information on surgery and emergency medicine:

The American College of
  Surgeons
www.facs.org

American Red Cross
www.crossnet.org

Ethicon Incorporated
www.ethiconinc.com

Federal Emergency Manage-
  ment Agency
www.fema.gov

Global Emergency Medical
  Services
www.globalmed.com

LSU Trauma Center
www.trauma.lsumc.edu

6

Theresa Cline, *and I am a Certified Medical Assistant. I graduated from an accredited medical assistant program and have an associate's degree in Applied Science. I work for two physicians in a family practice medical office. I have worked there ever since I graduated from college in 1983. My primary job responsibilities include those of being a receptionist and a billing and insurance manager. However, I do perform clinical duties when the need arises. The reason that I prefer the administrative aspect of being a medical assistant is that I find it very rewarding to be able to help people with their insurance difficulties, especially the elderly, who sometimes find such matters overwhelming and very confusing. Dealing with insurance companies in this day and age is a constant challenge. Things are changing all the time, and the need to keep abreast of these changes is very important to the flow of the medical office.*

Administration of Medication

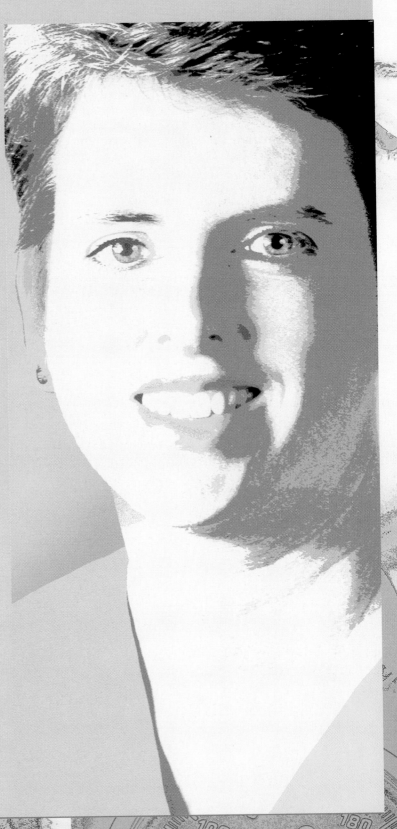

OUTCOMES

After completing this chapter, you should be able to demonstrate the proper procedures to perform the following:

1. Convert between the metric, apothecary, and household systems of measurement.
2. Prepare and administer oral medication.
3. Reconstitute a powdered drug for parenteral administration.
4. Withdraw medication from a vial.
5. Withdraw medication from an ampule.
6. Prepare and administer a subcutaneous injection.
7. Locate the following intramuscular injection sites: dorsogluteal, deltoid, vastus lateralis, and ventrogluteal.
8. Prepare and administer an intramuscular injection.
9. Administer an injection using the Z-track method.
10. Prepare and administer an intradermal injection.
11. Administer a tine test and read the test results.

EDUCATIONAL OBJECTIVES

After completing this chapter, you should be able to do the following:

1. Define the terms listed in the Key Terminology.
2. List eight routes for administration of medication.
3. Explain the difference between administering, prescribing, and dispensing medication.
4. List and define the four names of drugs.
5. Classify drugs according to preparation.
6. Classify drugs according to the action they have on the body.
7. List the guidelines that should be followed in writing metric and apothecary notations.
8. List and explain the different parts of a prescription.
9. Identify four factors that affect the action of drugs in the body.
10. List the guidelines that should be followed when preparing and administering medication.
11. State the advantages and disadvantages of using the parenteral route of administration.
12. Explain which tissue layers of the body are used for an intradermal, a subcutaneous, and an intramuscular injection.
13. Identify the parts of a needle and syringe and explain their function. Read correctly the calibrations on the syringe.
14. Explain the purpose for using the Z-track method to administer medication.
15. Explain the purpose of tuberculin skin testing.
16. Explain the significance of a positive reaction to a tuberculin skin test and list the diagnostic procedures that will be performed as a result of a positive reaction.
17. Explain the principle underlying each step in the procedures for administering oral and parenteral medication and for performing a tine test.
18. Explain the purpose and method of performing each of the following types of allergy tests: patch testing, scratch testing, intradermal skin testing, and RAST testing.

KEY TERMINOLOGY

allergen (AL-er-gen): A substance that is capable of causing an allergic reaction.

allergy: An abnormal hypersensitivity of the body to substances that are ordinarily harmless.

ampule (AM-pûl): A small sealed glass container containing a single dose of medication.

aspirate (AS-pir-âte): To remove by suction.

avoirdupois (av-er-DÛ-poys): A system of weight used in English-speaking countries for weighing heavy articles. This system is not used to weigh drugs and precious stones and metals.

conversion: Changing from one unit of measurement to another.

cubic centimeter: The amount of space occupied by 1 milliliter (1 ml = 1 cc).

dermis (DUR-mis): The true skin; the main thickness of the skin, with an active blood supply.

dose: The quantity of a drug to be administered at one time.

epidermis (EP-a-derm-is): The outermost, nonvascular layer of the skin.

induration (in-DUR-Â-shun): An area of hardened tissue.

inhalation administration (in-HAL-Â-shun ad-MIN-is-trâ-shun): The administration of medication by way of air or other vapor being drawn into the lungs.

intradermal injection (in-TRA-derm-al in-JEK-shun): Introducing medication into the dermal layer of the skin.

intramuscular injection (in-TRA-mus-kû-lar in-JEK-shun): Introducing medication into the muscular layer of the body.

intravenous injection (in-TRA-vên-us in-JEK-shun): Introducing medication into the bloodstream directly through a vein.

length: A unit of linear measurement used to measure length or distance.

oral administration: Administration of medication by mouth.

prescription (prê-SKRIP-shun): Order for a drug or other therapy written by a physician.

subcutaneous injection (sub-CÛ-tane-ê-us in-JEK-shun): Introducing medication beneath the skin, into the subcutaneous or fatty layer of the body.

sublingual administration (sub-lêng-wul ad-MIN-is-TRÂ-shun): Administration of medication by placing it under the tongue, where it dissolves and is absorbed through the mucous membrane.

topical administration: Applying a drug to a particular spot, usually for a local action.

vesiculation (VES-ik-û-LÂ-shun): The formation of vesicles (fluid-containing lesions of the skin).

vial: A closed glass container with a rubber stopper.

volume: The amount of space occupied by a substance.

weight: The measure of heaviness of a substance.

wheal (WHÊL): A small raised area of the skin.

INTRODUCTION

☐ The study of drugs is known as **pharmacology.** This discipline includes the preparation, use, and action of drugs. A **drug** is a chemical that is used for the treatment, prevention, or diagnosis of disease. Most drugs are produced synthetically, but they may also be obtained from other sources such as animals, plants, and minerals.

In the medical office, medication may be administered, prescribed, or dispensed. Medication that is **administered** is actually given to the patient at the office. Medication is **prescribed** when a physician provides the patient with a written prescription for a drug to be filled at a pharmacy. Prescriptions may also be telephoned to the pharmacy by the physician, depending on the preference of the patient. **Dispensed** medication is either given or sold to the patient at the office, to be taken at home.

An important responsibility of the medical assistant is the administration of medication. (However, one should first check the laws of the state to make sure that it is legally permissible for the medical assistant to administer medication.) Common routes of administration are oral, sublingual, inhalation, rectal, urethral, vaginal, topical, intradermal, subcutaneous, intramuscular, and intravenous. The route of administration used depends on the type of drug being given, the intended action, and the rapidity of response desired. The routes by which medication is most commonly given in the medical office are the oral and the parenteral routes. **Parenteral** refers to sites outside the gastrointestinal tract; this term is most commonly used to indicate the administration of medication by injection.

The medical assistant is obligated to become familiar with the drugs that are most frequently used in his or her office. It is essential to have a knowledge of their indications, precautions, common side effects, adverse reactions, route of administration, dosage, and storage. With each drug, the manufacturer includes a package insert that contains valuable information regarding the drug. In addition, many drug references are available. The *Physician's Desk Reference* is frequently used in the medical office.

The medical assistant should administer and dispense medication only under the instructions of the physician. It is unlawful to act without his or her consent.

DRUG NOMENCLATURE

☐ Each drug has four names: the chemical, generic, official, and brand, or trade, name. The **chemical name** provides a precise description of the drug's chemical composition; drug manufacturers and pharmacists are most concerned with the chemical make-up of a drug.

The **generic name** is assigned by the pharmaceutical manufacturer who first develops the drug, before it receives official approval by the Food and Drug Administration (FDA). The generic name is often a shortened derivative of the chemical name.

The **official name** is the name under which the drug is listed in official publications such as the *United States Pharmacopeia (USP)* and the *National Formulary (NF)*. Official publications set specific standards to regulate the strength, purity, packaging, safety, labeling, and dosage form for each drug. The generic name is frequently used for the official name.

The **brand name** is the name under which a pharmaceutical manufacturer markets a drug. Because a drug may be manufactured by more than one pharmaceutical company, it may have several brand names. For example, the generic name of a commonly used analgesic is acetaminophen; brand names for this drug include Tylenol, Aceta, Exdol, Tempra, and Panadol.

The medical assistant should be familiar with the generic and brand names of the medications prescribed and administered in the medical office. (*Note:* For a current list of the most frequently prescribed drugs in the US, refer to the following Internet site: RxList: The Internet Drug Index; www.rxlist.com).

CLASSIFICATION OF DRUGS BASED ON PREPARATION

☐ Drugs are available in two basic forms: liquid and solid. The same medication may be available in both a liquid and solid form, which permits it to be administered by different routes. For example, a liquid preparation of an antibiotic is administered to young children, whereas the solid preparation (e.g., tablets, capsules) of the same medication is administered to older children and adults. The following list includes the common categories of drugs based on preparation.

LIQUID PREPARATIONS

Aerosol	A pressurized dosage form in which solid or liquid drug particles are suspended in a gas to be dispensed in a cloud or mist. Example: Proventil Inhalation Aerosol.
Elixir	A drug that is dissolved in a solution of alcohol and water. Elixirs are sweetened and flavored and are taken orally. Example: Tylenol Elixir.
Emulsion	A mixture of fats or oils in water. Example: cod liver oil emulsion.
Liniment	A drug combined with oil, soap, alcohol, or water. Liniments are applied externally, using friction, to produce a feeling of heat or warmth. Example: camphor liniment.
Lotion	An aqueous preparation that contains suspended ingredients. Lotions are used to treat external skin conditions. They work to soothe, protect, and moisten the skin and or to destroy harmful bacteria. Example: Nutraderm Lotion.
Solution	A liquid preparation containing one or more completely dissolved substances. The dissolved substance is known as the solute, and the liquid in which it is dissolved is known as the solvent. Example: Adrenalin Chloride solution.
Spirit	A drug combined with an alcoholic solution that is volatile (a substance that is volatile evaporates readily). Example: aromatic spirit of ammonia.
Spray	A fine stream of medicated vapor, usually used to treat nose and throat conditions. Example: Dristan nasal spray.
Suspension	A drug containing solid insoluble drug particles in a liquid; the preparation must be shaken before administration. Example: Amoxicillin Oral Suspension.
Syrup	A drug dissolved in a solution of sugar, water, and a flavoring that may be added to disguise an unpleasant taste. Example: Robitussin Cough Syrup.

Tincture   A drug dissolved in a solution of alcohol or alcohol and water. Example: tincture of iodine.

SOLID PREPARATIONS

Capsule   A drug contained in a gelatin capsule that is water soluble and functions to prevent the patient from tasting the drug. Example: Benadryl Capsules.
Sustained-release capsules contain granules that dissolve at different rates to provide a gradual and continuous release of medication. This reduces the number of doses that must be administered. Example: Contac 12-Hour Sustained-Release Capsules.

Cream   Drug combined in base that is generally nongreasy, resulting in a semisolid preparation. Creams are applied externally to the skin. Example: Aristocort Topical Cream.

Lozenge   A drug contained in a candy-like base. Lozenges have a circular shape and are designed to dissolve on the tongue. Example: Cēpacol Throat Lozenges.

Ointment   A drug combined with an oil base, resulting in a semisolid preparation. Ointments are applied externally to the skin and are usually greasy in nature. Example: Polysporin Ointment.

Suppository   A drug mixed with a firm base, such as cocoa butter, that is designed to melt at body temperature. A suppository is shaped into a cylinder or a cone for easy insertion into a body cavity, such as the rectum or vagina. Example: Nupercainal Suppositories.

Tablet   Powdered drugs that have been pressed into discs. Some tablets are **scored,** meaning they are marked with an indentation so they can be broken into halves or quarters for proper dosage. Example: aspirin tablets.
Tablets and capsules may be **enteric-coated,** meaning that they are coated with a substance that prevents them from dissolving until they reach the intestines. The purpose of this is to protect the drug from being destroyed by gastric juices or to prevent it from irritating the stomach lining. Enteric-coated tablets must not be crushed or chewed to prevent the active ingredients from being released prematurely in the stomach. Example: Ecotrin Enteric-Coated Aspirin.

Transdermal Patch   A patch with an adhesive backing containing a drug that is applied to the skin. The drug enters the circulation after being absorbed through the skin. Example: nitroglycerin patches (Nitro-Dur).

CLASSIFICATION OF DRUGS BASED ON ACTION

☐ Drugs can also be classified according to the action they have on the body. The medical assistant should know in which category a particular drug belongs. Table 7–1 presents a classification of common categories of drugs based on action, along with an example of each.

SYSTEMS OF MEASUREMENT USED TO ADMINISTER MEDICATION

☐ Three systems of measurement are used in the United States for prescribing and administering medication: the metric system, the apothecary system, and the household system. The metric system is the most common, because it is more accurate and easier to use. However, some physicians originally trained in the apothecary system may still use it to order medication. Therefore, it is important for the medical assistant to be familiar with both of these systems. The third, the household system, is the least accurate and is generally used only when a patient takes liquid medication at home.

Systems of measurement have units of weight, volume, and length. **Weight** refers to the heaviness of an item, whereas **volume** refers to the amount of space occupied by a substance. **Length** is a unit of linear measurement used to measure the distance from one point to another. Although length is not used to administer medication, it is used in other aspects of the medical office. For example, the head circumference of infants is measured in centimeters (cm), a metric unit of linear measurement.

To prepare and administer medication properly and to avoid medication errors, the medical assistant must

TABLE 7–1

Common Drug Classifications, Therapeutic Effects, and Examples

Drug Classification and Major Therapeutic Effects	Example
α-Adrenergic blocking agents Prevent vasoconstriction normally caused by the catecholamines epinephrine and norepinephrine	Phentolamine (Regitine)
Analgesic Relieves pain	Acetaminophen (Tylenol)
Antacids Neutralize gastric acid	Magnesium hydroxide (Milk of Magnesia)
Antianginals Increase blood supply to myocardial tissue primarily through vasodilation	Isosorbide dinitrate (Sorbitrate)
Antiarrhythmics Promote normal cardiac rate and rhythm	Procainamide (Pronestyl)
Anticholinergics Block the effects of acetylcholine at muscarinic receptor sites in the autonomic nervous system	Atropine sulfate
Anticoagulants Prevent the formation and/or extension of clots	Coumadin
Anticonvulsants Control seizures	Phenytoin (Dilantin)
Antidepressants Elevate the mood by promoting accumulation of neutrotransmitters (norepinephrine and serotonin) at CNS synapses	Amitriptyline (Elavil)
Antidiabetic agents Reduce blood sugar levels	Insulin (regular or NPH)
Antidiarrheals Promote defecation of normally formed stools	Loperamide (Imodium)
Antiemetics Prevent nausea and vomiting	Prochlorperazine (Compazine)
Antifungals Kill or inhibit growth of susceptible fungi	Fluconazole (Diflucan)
Antigout agents Control symptoms of gout	Allopurinol (Zyloprim)
Antihistamines Block the effects of histamine to help relieve allergic symptoms	Diphenhydramine (Benadryl)
Antihyperlipidemic agents Decrease blood lipid levels	Clofibrate (Atromid-S)
Antihypertensive agents Reduce blood pressure	Enalapril (Vasotec)
Anti-infectives Kill or inhibit growth of susceptible bacteria	Penicillin
Antimanic agents Treat and prevent recurrence of manic episodes	Lithium
Antineoplastics Treat and control symptoms of malignant neoplasms	Cisplatin (Platinol-AQ)
Antiparkinson agents Treat symptoms of Parkinson's disease by restoring balance between acetylcholine and dopamine in the basal ganglia of the brain	Benztropine (Cogentin)
Antiplatelets Interfere with the ability of platelets to adhere to each other	Dipyridamole (Persantine)

7

Continued

TABLE 7–1

Common Drug Classifications, Therapeutic Effects, and Examples *Continued*

Drug Classification and Major Therapeutic Effects	Example
Antipsychotics Alleviate psychotic symptoms by blocking dopamine receptors in the brain	Chlorpromazine (Thorazine)
Antipyretics Lower body temperature	Acetaminophen (Tylenol)
Antithyroid agents Inhibit thyroid hormone synthesis, thereby reducing basal metabolic rate	Propylthiouracil
Antituberculars Kill or inhibit growth of mycobacteria	Isoniazid (INH)
Antitussives Suppress cough reflex	Codeine
Antivirals Inhibit viral growth	Acyclovir (Zovirax)
β-Adrenergic blocking agents Block the effects of the catecholamines epinephrine and norepinephrine on β-adrenergic receptors in the automatic nervous system	Propranolol (Inderal)
Bronchodilators Relieve bronchospasm through bronchodilation	Theophylline
Calcium channel blockers Treat angina pectoris, hypertension, and coronary artery spasm by vasodilation	Verapamil (Calan)
Central nervous system stimulants Increase levels of catecholamines in the central nervous system	Amphetamine
Cholinergics Prolong the action of acetylcholine at receptor sites in the body	Bethanechol (Urecholine)
Diuretics Increase urine output by the kidney	Furosemide (Lasix)
Expectorants Decrease viscosity of bronchial secretions	Guaifenesin and alcohol (Robitussin)
Glucocorticoids Affect carbohydrate, fat, and protein metabolism; depress the immune response; exhibit anti-inflammatory effects	Prednisone
Hematologic agents Increase blood-forming components of the circulatory system	Ferrous sulfate (Feosol)
Histamine (H_1) antagonists Inhibit gastric acid secretion by blocking H_1 receptors	Cimetidine (Tagamet)
Immunosuppressants Inhibit cell-mediated immune responses in the body	Cyclosporine (Sandimmune)
Inotropic agents Increase strength and force of myocardial contractility	Digoxin (Lanoxin)
Laxatives Promote defecation of normal, soft stool, thus relieving constipation	Psyllium (Metamucil)
Narcotic analgesics Relieve moderate or severe pain	Morphine
Neuromuscular blocking agents Block transmission of nerve impulses at the neuromuscular junction in the peripheral nervous system	Succinylcholine (Anectine)
Nonnarcotic analgesics Relieve mild to moderate pain	Aspirin

TABLE 7-1

Common Drug Classifications, Therapeutic Effects, and Examples *Continued*	
Drug Classification and Major Therapeutic Effects	*Example*

Nonsteroidal anti-inflammatory drugs
   Relieve mild to moderate pain, fever, and inflammation through
   inhibition of prostaglandin synthesis
	Ibuprofen (Motrin)

Sedatives and hypnotics Reduce anxiety, promote sleep	Phenobarbital (Luminal)
Skeletal muscle relaxants Decrease skeletal muscle spasm	Baclofen (Lioresal)
Thrombolytic agents Dissolve existing blood clots	Alteplase (Activase)

Thyroid hormones
   Increase basal metabolic rate through replacement of deficient
   thyroid levels
	Levothyroxine (Synthroid)

Vasopressors
   Increase blood pressure, cardiac output, and urinary output by
   affecting vasoconstriction
	Dopamine (Intropin)

From Leahy JM, Kizilay PE: *Foundation of Nursing Practice: A Nursing Process Approach.* Philadelphia, W. B. Saunders, 1998.

have a thorough knowledge of the specific units of measurement for each of these three systems and must be able to convert within each, as well as from one system to another. A basic discussion of the metric, apothecary, and household systems is presented next. A more thorough study of these systems, including conversion of units and dose calculation, is included in the *Student Manual* (Chapter 7: Drug Dosage Calculation).

METRIC SYSTEM

The metric system was developed in France in the latter part of the eighteenth century in an effort to simplify measurement. Most European countries are required by law to use this system for the measurement of weight, volume, and length. Overall, the metric system is used for most scientific and medical measurements. Pharmaceutical companies use the metric system for labeling medications.

The metric system employs a uniform decimal scale and is based upon units of 10, making it very flexible and logical. The basic metric units of measurement are the gram, liter, and meter. The **gram** is a unit of weight used to measure solids. The **liter** is a unit of volume used to measure liquids, and the **meter** is a linear unit used to measure length or distance. The metric units used most often in the administration of medication in the medical office are the milligram, gram, milliliter, and cubic centimeter. Because a

cubic centimeter (cc) is the amount of space occupied by 1 milliliter (ml), these two units can be used interchangeably (i.e., 1 ml = 1 cc).

Prefixes added to the words gram, liter, and meter designate smaller or larger units of measurement in the metric system. The same prefixes are used with all three units. For example, *milli-* is used as follows: *milli*gram, *milli*liter, and *milli*meter. Each prefix changes the value of the basic unit of measurement by the same amount. The prefix milli- denotes a unit that is 1/1000 of the basic unit. Therefore, 1 gram is equal to 1000 milligrams, 1 liter is equal to 1000 milliliters, and 1 meter is equal to 1000 millimeters. Table 7-2 lists the units of measurement in the metric system and equivalent values between the units.

TABLE 7-2

Metric System: Conversion of Equivalent Values	
Weight	
1000 micrograms	= 1 milligram
1000 milligrams	= 1 gram
1000 grams	= 1 kilogram
Volume	
1000 milliliters	= 1 liter
1000 liters	= 1 kiloliter
1 milliliter	= 1 cubic centimeter

Metric Notation Guidelines

Specific guidelines are used in the medical notation of metric units of measurement and dose quantity. To read prescriptions and medication orders, to record medication administration, and, most important, to avoid medication errors, the medical assistant must be familiar with and be able to use these guidelines.

1. The units of metric measurement are written using the following abbreviations:

Weight	microgram: μg (formerly mcg)
	milligram: mg
	gram: g
	kilogram: kg
Volume	milliliter: ml
	cubic centimeter: cc
	liter: L

2. A period should not be used with the abbreviation of the units of measurement.

   Example   Correct: mg
   ml
   Incorrect: mg.
   ml.

3. Arabic numerals (1, 2, 3, 4) are used to express the quantity of the dose.

   Example   Correct: 4 mg
   Incorrect: īv mg

4. The numeral expressing the quantity of the dose is placed in front of the abbreviation. To make it easier to read, a (single) space should be left between the quantity and abbreviation.

   Example   Correct: 5 ml
   Incorrect: ml 5 and 5ml

5. A fraction of a dose is written as a decimal.

   Example   Correct: 0.5 g
   Incorrect: ½ g

6. If the dose is a fraction of a gram, a zero must be placed before the decimal as a means of focusing on the fractional dose. This reduces the possibility of misreading the dose as a whole number.

   Example   Correct: 0.5 g (this reduces the possibility of not seeing the decimal point and reading the dose as 5 grams)
   Incorrect: .5 g

7. A decimal point and a zero should not be placed after a whole number. The decimal point may be overlooked, resulting in a tenfold overdose error.

   Example   Correct: 1 ml (this reduces the possibility of not seeing the decimal point and reading the dose as 10 ml)
   Incorrect: 1.0 ml

APOTHECARY SYSTEM

The apothecary system is older and less accurate than the metric system. It was brought to the United States from England during the eighteenth century. Pharmacists used this system during the colonial period to compound and measure medications. This system is gradually being phased out in preference to the metric system. Until that process is completed, however, the medical assistant must be familiar with this system and be able to use it to administer medication.

The basic unit of weight in the apothecary system is the grain, derived from the weight of a large grain of wheat, which was used to balance the material being weighed. The next largest unit of measurement is the scruple; however, this unit is not used to administer medication. The remaining units, in order of increasing weight, are the dram, ounce, and pound. The pound is not generally used in the administration of medication. The medical assistant should note, however, that in the apothecary system the pound is equal to 12 ounces, in contrast to the more familiar *avoirdupois* pound used to measure body weight, which is equal to 16 ounces.

Measures of liquid volume in the apothecary system correlate closely with measures of dry weight in the same system. The smallest unit of measurement is the minim, meaning "the least." A minim is approximately equivalent to a volume of water weighing 1 grain. A minim glass or a syringe calibrated in minims must be used to measure with this unit. The remaining units of liquid volume in the apothecary system, in order of increasing volume, are the fluidram, fluidounce, pint, quart, and gallon. The basic unit of linear measurement is the inch, followed by the foot, yard, and mile. Most Americans are familiar with apothecary units of measurement because of their frequent use in everyday life. For example, milk is available in pints, quarts, and gallons, and height is measured in feet and inches.

Table 7–3 lists the units of measurement in the apothecary system and equivalent values between units.

Apothecary Notation Guidelines

The following guidelines are used in the medical notation of apothecary units of measurement and dose quantity.

1. The units of apothecary measurement are usually written using abbreviations and symbols as follows:

Weight	grain: gr
	dram: ʒ
	ounce: ℥

TABLE 7 – 3

Apothecary System: Conversion of Equivalent Values

Weight

60 grains	= 1 dram
8 drams	= 1 ounce
12 ounces	= 1 pound

Volume

60 minims	= 1 fluidram
8 fluidrams	= 1 fluidounce
16 fluidounces	= 1 pint
2 pints	= 1 quart
4 quarts	= 1 gallon

Volume   minim: ℳ
fluidram: f ℨ
fluidounce: f ℥
pint: pt
quart: qt
gallon: gal

2. When symbols and abbreviations are used to express apothecary units, lower case roman numerals must be used to express the dose quantity.

   Example   Correct: ℥ vi (6 ounces)
   Incorrect: 6 ℥; ℥ 6

3. The roman numeral expressing dose quantity must *follow* the symbol or abbreviation.

   Example   Correct: ℨ ii (2 drams); gr v (5 grains)
   Incorrect: ii ℨ; v gr

4. A line may be placed over the roman numerals. Dots are placed above the line for emphasis as a safeguard against error.

   Example   Correct: f ℨ iii (3 fluidrams)
   Incorrect: f ℨ 111

5. The symbol ss is used to designate one half of a dose and must follow the apothecary symbol or abbreviation.

   Example   Correct: gr ss
   Incorrect: gr ½

6. Fractions (other than ½) are written in arabic numerals and must follow the apothecary symbol or abbreviation.

   Example   Correct: gr ¼
   Incorrect: gr 0.25; ¼ gr

   (*Note:* If abbreviations and symbols are *not* used to express apothecary units of measurement, arabic numerals must be used to express dose quantity and are placed before the unit of measurement.)

Example   Correct: 5 grains; ½ ounce
Incorrect: grains 5; ounce ½ or ounce ss

HOUSEHOLD SYSTEM

The household system is more complicated and less accurate for administering liquid medication than either the metric or apothecary system. Nevertheless, most individuals are familiar with this system because of its frequent use in the United States. Thus, this system of measurement may be the only one the patient can fully relate to and therefore safely use to administer liquid medication at home. For example, most patients are more comfortable measuring medication in drops and teaspoons, rather than minims and milliliters. In addition, the patient is more likely to have household measuring devices on hand than to have metric measuring devices. If a precise measurement is needed, however, the metric system must be used, and the medical assistant should instruct the patient in the use of the metric measuring device.

Volume is the only household unit of measurement used to administer medication. The basic unit of liquid volume in the household system is the drop (gtt), which is approximately equal to 0.6 ml in the metric system and 1 minim in the apothecary system. These units cannot be considered exact equivalents, because the size of the drop varies based upon temperature, the viscosity of the liquid, and the size of the dropper. The remaining units, in order of increasing volume, are the teaspoon, tablespoon, ounce (fluidounce), cup, and glass. Table 7–4 lists the units of liquid volume measurement in the household system and equivalent values between units.

TABLE 7 – 4

Household System: Conversion of Equivalent Values

Abbreviations

drop: gtt
teaspoon: t or tsp
tablespoon: T or tbs
ounce: oz
cup: c

Volume

60 drops	= 1 teaspoon
3 teaspoons	= 1 tablespoon
6 teaspoons	= 1 ounce
2 tablespoons	= 1 ounce
6 ounces	= 1 teacup
8 ounces	= 1 glass

CONVERSION BETWEEN UNITS OF MEASUREMENT

☐ Changing from one unit of measurement to another is known as **conversion.** Conversion is required when medication is ordered in one unit of measurement and the medication label expresses the drug strength in a different unit. The dose quantity must be mathematically translated or converted to the unit of measurement of the medication on hand. For example, if the physician orders 5 grams of an oral solid medication and the medication label expresses the drug strength in milligrams, the medical assistant would need to convert the grams into milligrams to know how much medication to administer. Converting units of measurement can be classified into the following categories: (1) conversion of units within a measurement system and (2) conversion of units from one measurement system to another.

Converting units within a measurement system allows a quantity to be expressed in a different, but equal, unit of measurement within the *same* system. An example of converting between units of weight within the metric system is as follows: 1 gram is equal to 1000 milligrams. Converting from one measurement system to another allows a quantity to be expressed in a unit of measurement from *another* system. An example of a conversion between the apothecary and metric systems is as follows: 1 grain (apothecary system) is equivalent to 60 milligrams (metric system).

Conversion requires the use of a conversion table to indicate the equivalent values between various units of measurement. Conversion tables of equivalent values used to convert within each of the three measurement systems have previously been discussed and are included in these tables.

- Metric Conversion—Table 7–2
- Apothecary Conversion—Table 7–3
- Household Conversion—Table 7–4

Tables used to convert between systems consist of approximate equivalents, rather than exact equivalents, and a 10 percent error usually occurs in making these conversions. Conversion tables used to convert from one system to another are presented in Tables 7–5 and 7–6.

TABLE 7 – 5

Conversion Chart for Metric and Apothecary Systems (Commonly Used Approximate Equivalents)

Metric System to Apothecary System		Apothecary System to Metric System		
Weight		**Weight**		
60 mg	= 1 grain	15 grains =	1000	mg (1 g)
1 g	= 15 grains	10 grains =	600	mg
4 g	= 1 dram	7½ grains =	500	mg
30 mg	= 1 ounce	5 grains =	300	mg
1 kg	= 2.2 pounds	3 grains =	200	mg
		1½ grains =	100	mg
Volume		1 grain =	60	mg
0.06 ml	= 1 minim	¾ grain =	50	mg
1 ml (cc)	= 15 minims	½ grain =	30	mg
4 ml	= 1 fluidram	¼ grain =	15	mg
30 ml	= 1 fluidounce	⅙ grain =	10	mg
500 ml	= 1 pint	⅛ grain =	8.0	mg
1000 ml (1 L)	= 1 quart	1/12 grain =	5.0	mg
		1/15 grain =	4.0	mg
		1/20 grain =	3.0	mg
		1/30 grain =	2.0	mg
		1/40 grain =	1.5	mg
		1/50 grain =	1.2	mg
		1/60 grain =	1.0	mg
		1/100 grain =	0.6	mg
		1/120 grain =	0.5	mg
		1/150 grain =	0.4	mg
		1/200 grain =	0.3	mg
		1/300 grain =	0.2	mg
		1/600 grain =	0.1	mg

TABLE 7 – 6

Conversion Chart for Apothecary and Metric Equivalents of Household Measures (Volume)

Household	Apothecary	Metric
1 drop	= 1 minim	= 0.06 milliliter
15 drops	= 15 minims	= 1 milliliter (1 cc)
1 teaspoon	= 1 fluidram	= 5 (4) milliliters*
1 tablespoon	= 4 fluidrams	= 15 milliliters
2 tablespoons	= 1 fluidounce	= 30 milliliters
1 ounce	= 1 fluidounce	= 30 milliliters
1 teacup	= 6 fluidounces	= 180 milliliters
1 glass	= 8 fluidounces	= 240 milliliters

*The American standard teaspoon is accepted as 5 ml; however, 4 ml can be used as the equivalent to provide a more accurate conversion.

TABLE 7 – 7

Abbreviations and Symbols Commonly Used in the Medical Office

Abbreviation or Symbol	Meaning	Abbreviation or Symbol	Meaning
aa	of each	ml	milliliter
ac	before meals	non rep	do not repeat
AD	right ear	NPO	nothing by mouth
ad lib	as desired	OD	right eye
aq	water	OS	left eye
AS	left ear	OU	in each eye
AU	in each ear	ʒ or oz	ounce
bid	twice a day	pc	after meals
c̄	with	po	by mouth
caps	capsules	prn	as needed
cc	cubic centimeter	pt	patient
dil	dilute	qd	every day
ʒ	dram	qh	every hour
EENT	eye, ear, nose, and throat	q (2, 3, 4) h	every (2, 3, 4) hours
elix	elixir	qid	four times a day
g	gram	qod	every other day
GI	gastrointestinal	qs	of sufficient quantity
gr	grain	Rx	take
gtt (s)	drop (drops)	s̄	without
GU	genitourinary	SC	subcutaneous
h	hour	sol	solution
hs	at bedtime	SOS	if necessary
ID	intradermal	ss	one half
IM	intramuscular	stat	at once
IV	intravenous	tab	tablet
kg	kilogram	tbs	tablespoon
L	liter	tid	three times a day
liq	liquid	tr	tincture
♏	minim	tsp	teaspoon
mg	milligram	ung	ointment

7

The medical assistant must be careful when using conversion tables to avoid errors in interpolation. The numbers on conversion tables are small and close together; therefore, it is possible to misread the chart from one column to the other. To reduce the possibility, a straight edge should be used when obtaining a value from a conversion table.

THE PRESCRIPTION

☐ A **prescription** is an order written by a physician for the dispensing of drugs (or other forms of therapy). Abbreviations and symbols are used to write a prescription. They are also used when recording in the patient's chart. A list of the common abbreviations used in the medical office is included in Table 7–7. A more extensive list of medical abbreviations is included in Appendix A. The prescription is written on a specially designed form. It includes directions to the pharmacist for filling the prescription and instructions to the patient for taking the medication (Fig. 7–1). The specific information that the prescription must include is

1. The patient's name and address.
2. The date.
3. The **superscription,** which consists of the symbol ℞. This symbol comes from the Latin word *recipe* and means "take."
4. The **inscription,** which states the name of the drug, the dosage form, and the amount per dose. Drug dosage is stated in either metric or apothecary units of measurement.
5. The **subscription,** which gives directions to the pharmacist. At present, it is generally used to designate the number of doses to be dispensed.

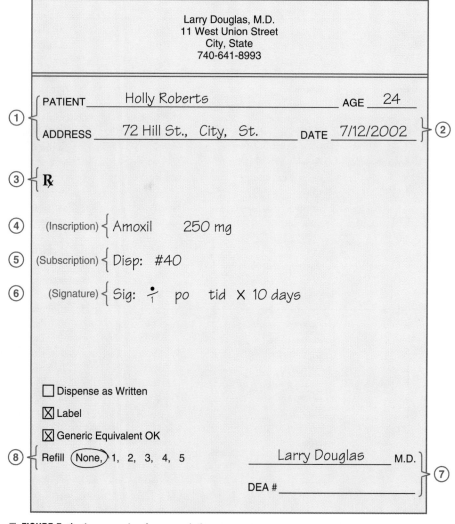

FIGURE 7–1. An example of a prescription.

TABLE 7–8 Classification of Controlled Substances

Classification	Description	Examples
Schedule I	Drugs having a high potential for abuse and no accepted medical use. (The drug container is marked C-I.)	Heroin LSD Marihuana Peyote
Schedule II	Drugs having a high potential for abuse but with accepted medical use. Abuse may lead to severe psychologic or physical dependence. (The drug container is marked C-II.)	Amobarbital Amphetamine Cocaine Codeine Meperidine hydrochloride (Demerol) Methadone Morphine
Schedule III	Drugs have an accepted medical use with moderate or low potential for physical dependence and high potential for psychologic dependence. (The containers are marked C-III.)	Codeine-containing medications Thiopental sodium Glutethimide
Schedule IV	Drugs having accepted medical use and that may cause mild physical or psychologic dependence. (The container is marked C-IV.)	Chloral hydrate (Noctec) Diazepam (Valium) Meprobamate (Equanil) Phenobarbital
Schedule V	Drugs having accepted medical use and that have limited potential for causing physical or psychologic dependence. (The container is marked C-V.)	Drug mixtures containing small quantities of narcotics such as cough syrups containing codeine (e.g., Robitussin A-C) Diphenoxylate and atropine preparations (e.g., Lomotil)

6. The **signature** (abbreviated S or Sig), which indicates the information to be included on the medication label. It consists of directions to the patient for taking the medication. Most physicians also prefer that the name of the drug be included on the label, because this helps the patient identify the medication.

7. The physician's signature, address, and telephone number. The Drug Enforcement Agency (DEA) number must be included if a narcotic is being prescribed.

8. Instructions indicating the number of times the prescription may be refilled.

The medical assistant should make sure that all prescription pads are kept in a safe place and out of reach of individuals who may want to obtain drugs illegally. The stock supply of prescription pads should be locked in a drawer.

CONTROLLED DRUGS

By means of federal and state legislation, restrictions are placed on drugs that have potential for abuse. These medications are known as **controlled drugs** and are classified into five categories, called schedules, which are based on their abuse potential. Refer to Table 7–8 for a list and description of the schedules for controlled drugs.

To prescribe or dispense controlled drugs, the physician must register each year with the DEA. The physician is assigned a registration number known as the **DEA number.** Each time a prescription for a controlled drug is written, the DEA number must be indicated in the appropriate space on the prescription blank (see Fig. 7–1).

GENERIC PRESCRIBING

Generic prescribing means that the physician has written the prescription using the generic name, rather than the brand name, of the drug. Because a number of pharmaceutical manufacturers may produce the same generic drug (but by a different brand name), price competition often results. If the physician prescribes a drug using its generic name (rather than the brand name), the pharmacist is permitted to fill it with the drug offering the best savings to the patient. In addition, some states allow the pharmacist the option of filling the prescription with a generically equivalent drug, even if the prescription has been prescribed by brand name. In this case, if the physician desires the prescription to be filled with a specific brand of drug, instructions must be indicated on the prescription form, such as "Dispense as Written (DAW)," or words of a similar meaning (see Fig. 7–1).

FACTORS AFFECTING DRUG ACTION

THERAPEUTIC EFFECT

Each drug has an intended therapeutic effect, which is the desired effect of the medication, in other words, the reason why the patient takes the medication. Certain factors affect the therapeutic action of drugs in the body, causing patients to respond differently to the same drug. Because of this, the drug therapy may need to be adjusted to meet these individual variations, which include the following:

AGE. Children and elderly people tend to respond more strongly to drugs than do young and middle-aged adults. The physician may calculate smaller doses for these very young and old patients.

ROUTE OF ADMINISTRATION. Medications administered by different routes will be absorbed at different rates. Drugs administered orally will be absorbed slowly, because they must first be digested. Parenterally administered drugs are usually absorbed more quickly than orally administered drugs because they are injected directly into the body.

BODY SIZE. The body size of a patient has an effect on drug action. A thin person may require a smaller quantity of a drug, whereas an obese person may require more.

TIME OF ADMINISTRATION. A drug administered through the oral route will be absorbed more rapidly when the stomach is empty than when food is present. A drug may not produce the desired effect or may be absorbed too slowly if it is taken when food is present. However, some drugs are irritating to the stomach lining and must therefore be taken with food. The medical assistant should check the drug insert or a drug reference to make sure that the drug is being administered at the proper time.

TOLERANCE. A patient taking a certain drug over a period of time may develop a tolerance to it. This means that the same dose of a drug no longer produces the desired effect after prolonged administration. The physician should be notified to determine whether a change of drug or alteration of dosage is needed.

PATIENT/TEACHING

PRESCRIPTION MEDICATIONS

■ Teach patients the proper guidelines for taking prescription medication to avoid adverse reactions, which include the following:

Take your medication exactly as prescribed, at the right times and in the right amounts. The medication may not work properly unless it is taken as directed. If the dose is too small, the drug may not produce its intended therapeutic effect; exceeding the recommended dosage could result in a toxic effect that could be harmful.

Inform the physician if any new symptoms or adverse effects develop when taking the medication. The physician may need to change your dosage or prescribe a different medication. There are usually a number of alternative medications that the physician can prescribe to treat your condition.

Take the medication for the prescribed duration of time, even after you begin to feel better. If you don't complete the entire course of drug therapy, your condition may recur. For example, not taking all of a prescribed antibiotic may cause an infection to return and it may be worse than the first infection.

Be sure to tell the physician if you decide not to take your medication. The physician may otherwise think your medication is not working. Not taking a medication prescribed by the physician could be serious because it may allow your condition to get worse.

Do not take additional medications, including over-the-counter (OTC) medications, without first checking with the physician. All drugs, including OTC medications, are designed to have an effect on the body. Sometimes various combinations of drugs can cause serious reactions. In other cases, one drug may cancel the effects of another and not allow it to work at all.

Never take a prescription medication that was prescribed for someone else. Physicians prescribe medication based on an individual's age, weight, sex, and condition. Taking a medication prescribed for someone else can have serious results.

Store your medications in a safe place, away from the reach of children. Accidental drug poisoning in children is a common and preventable problem. Also, do not take your medication in front of small children, because they may want to mimic your example.

Discard unused portions of prescription medications and outdated OTC medications. Medications should be discarded by flushing them down the toilet. Medications that are past their expiration date may produce adverse effects in the body.

ADVERSE REACTIONS

A drug may cause unintended adverse reactions, which may occur immediately or be delayed hours or even days following administration of the medication. These include the following.

Drug Interactions

When certain medications are used at the same time, drug interactions may produce undesirable effects. The medical assistant should inquire about other medications the patient is taking and record this information in the patient's chart for review by the physician.

Allergic Drug Reaction

The patient may exhibit an allergic reaction to a drug after administration. The reaction is often mild and may take the form of a rash, rhinitis, or pruritus. However, occasionally it may be a severe allergic reaction and occur suddenly and immediately. It is then known as an **anaphylactic reaction.**

An anaphylactic reaction is the least common type of allergic reaction but the most serious. Symptoms begin with sneezing, hives, itching, angioedema, erythema, and disorientation. The symptoms quickly increase in severity and progress to dyspnea, cyanosis, and shock. Blood pressure decreases, and the pulse becomes weak and thready. Convulsions, loss of consciousness, and death may occur if treatment is not initiated promptly.

To aid in preventing an allergic reaction from a drug or to reduce its danger, the medical assistant should stay with the patient after administration of the medication. The medical assistant should be especially alert for signs of an anaphylactic reaction after administering allergy skin tests or a penicillin or allergy injection. If a reaction occurs, the physician should be notified immediately to begin treatment, which generally consists of one or more injections of epinephrine, depending on the severity of the reaction. Epinephrine goes to work immediately to reverse the life-threatening symptoms of an anaphylactic reaction. Once the patient is stabilized, he or she is usually given an injection of an antihistimine. The antihistamine takes longer to begin working but helps alleviate some of the symptoms of the reaction such as hives, itching, angioedema, and erythema. The medical assistant must make sure that an ample supply of epinephrine is kept on hand at all times. Many offices maintain emergency carts for this purpose.

Side Effects

The majority of drugs produce side effects, which are secondary effects that occur along with the therapeutic effect of the drug. Side effects may be harmless and, therefore, tolerated in order to obtain the therapeutic effect of the drug. For example, most patients are willing to tolerate the dry mouth and drowsiness that may accompany an antihistamine in order to obtain its therapeutic effect. Other side effects may be harmful to the patient and warrant discontinuing the medication, such as a drop in blood pressure or an allergic reaction.

Idiosyncratic Reactions

An idiosyncratic reaction is an abnormal or peculiar response to a drug that is unexplained and unpredictable. Elderly patients are most prone to exhibit idiosyncratic reactions to drugs and therefore should be monitored more closely when taking a new medication.

GUIDELINES FOR THE PREPARATION AND ADMINISTRATION OF MEDICATION

□ The medical assistant should follow these guidelines when preparing and administering any drug to prevent medication errors.

1. Work in a quiet, well-lit atmosphere that is free from distractions.
2. Know the drug to be given; be sure to give the correct drug at the proper dose. The term **dose** refers to the quantity of a drug to be administered at one time. Each medication will have a certain **dosage range,** or range of quantities of the drug, that can produce therapeutic effects. It is important to administer the exact dose of the drug. If the dose is too small, it will not produce a therapeutic effect, whereas a dose that is too large could be harmful or even fatal to the patient.
3. Read the label of the medication as it is taken from its storage location, before pouring the medication, and before replacing the medication into its storage location. Do not use a drug if the label is missing or is difficult to read.
4. Do not use a drug if the color has changed, if a precipitate has formed, or if it has an unusual odor.
5. Check the expiration date before pouring the drug.

7

6. Check the patient's records or question the patient to make sure that he or she is not allergic to the medication before administering it.

7. Choose an appropriate site at which to administer an injection; the proper location is dictated by the type of injection being given. The site must be intact and free from abrasions, lesions, bruises, and edema.

8. Make sure you give the drug to the intended patient.

9. Stay with the patient after giving the medication.

10. Record information properly in the patient's chart immediately after administering the drug. Make sure the recording is clear and written in legible handwriting to avoid confusion by individuals reading it. Include the date and time, the name of the medication, the dose given, the route of administration, the site of administration, and any unusual observations or patient reactions. If you administer a medication that contains a fraction of a gram, place a 0 before the decimal point (e.g., 0.5 mg) so that the dosage is not misread as 5 mg. An example of a medication recording is as follows:

CHARTING EXAMPLE	
Date	
9/15/2002	10:30 a.m. DPT, 0.5 ml, IM, (L) vastus lateralis.
	——————————— T. Cline, CMA

11. Follow the six "rights" of preparing and administering medication:

Right drug	Right time
Right dose	Right patient
Right route	Right technique

ORAL ADMINISTRATION

☐ The oral route is the most convenient and the most widely used method of administering medication. Oral means that the drug is given by mouth in either a solid form (such as a tablet or capsule) or in a liquid form (such as a solution or syrup). Absorption of most oral medication takes place in the small intestine, although some may be absorbed in the mouth and stomach.

Many patients find it easier to swallow a tablet or capsule with half a glass of water. However, water should not be offered after the patient has received a cough syrup, because the water would dilute its beneficial effects. Unless the patient has a malabsorption problem or is unable to swallow, the oral route is considered the safest and most desirable route for administering medication.

PARENTERAL ADMINISTRATION

☐ There are several advantages to using the parenteral route of administration (subcutaneous, intramuscular, intravenous). Medications are absorbed more rapidly and completely than through the oral route. In some cases, the parenteral route is the only way a drug can be given. For example, if the patient is unconscious or has a gastric disturbance such as nausea or vomiting, the parenteral route would be used. If the state laws permit, the medical assistant is usually responsible for administering subcutaneous, intramuscular, and intradermal injections. Intravenous injections are given when an immediate effect is needed; in the medical office, they are usually administered by the physician in an emergency situation.

There are also disadvantages with the parenteral route, such as pain and the chance that infection may result, owing to the break in the skin. The medical assistant can help reduce pain by inserting and withdrawing the needle quickly and smoothly, and by withdrawing the needle using the angle of insertion.

If injections are given repeatedly (e.g., allergy injections), the sites should be rotated to prevent the overuse of one particular site, which may result in irritation and tissue damage. Rotating sites also allows for better absorption of the drug. When recording the procedure in the patient's chart, the medical assistant must be sure to include the site of the injection (e.g., right upper arm, left dorsogluteal). This assists in proper site rotation for patients requiring more than one injection. In addition, the information provides a reference point should a problem arise with the injection site.

Medical asepsis must be used when parenteral medications are administered. In addition, the needle, the inside of the syringe, and the outside of the lower end of the plunger should remain sterile. This reduces the danger of microorganisms entering the patient's body. The medical assistant must be sure to follow the OSHA Standard when administering medication as a means of protecting oneself from bloodborne pathogens. Refer to Chapter 1 to review medical asepsis and the OSHA Standard and to Chapter 6 to review sterile technique.

PROCEDURE

7–1

Administering Oral Medication

EQUIPMENT/SUPPLIES: Medication ordered by the physician   Medication tray
Medicine cup

1. **Procedural Step.** Wash the hands.
2. **Procedural Step.** Assemble the equipment.
3. **Procedural Step.** Work in a quiet, well-lit atmosphere.
   Principle. Good lighting aids the medical assistant in reading the medication label.
4. **Procedural Step.** Select the correct medication from the shelf, and check the expiration date. Compare the medication with the physician's instructions. The drug label must be checked three times: before removing the medication from the shelf, while pouring the medication, and before returning it to its proper place.

5. **Procedural Step.** Calculate the correct dose to be given, if necessary.
6. **Procedural Step.** Remove the bottle cap touching the outside of the lid only.
   Principle. Touching the inside of the lid will contaminate it.
7. **Procedural Step.** Check the drug label and pour the medication.
   Solid Medications. Pour the correct number of capsules or tablets into the bottle cap. Transfer the medication to a medicine cup, being careful not to touch the inside of the cup.

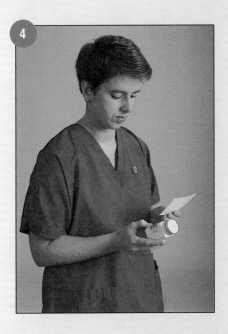

Principle. If the medication is outdated, consult the physician, because it may produce undesirable effects for which the medical assistant could be held responsible. The medication should be carefully compared with the physician's instructions to prevent a drug error.

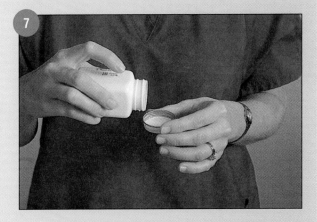

Principle. Pouring the medication into the lid prevents contamination of the medication and lid.
Liquid Medication. Place the lid of the bottle upside down on a flat surface with the open end facing up. Palm the surface of the label. With the opposite hand, place the thumbnail at the proper calibration on the medicine cup, and hold the cup at eye level. Pour the medication and read the dose at the lowest level of the meniscus. (The meniscus is the curved surface of the liquid in a container. When a liquid is poured into a medicine cup, capillary action will cause the liquid in contact with the cup to be drawn upward, resulting in a curved surface in the middle.)

Continued

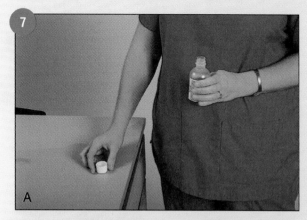

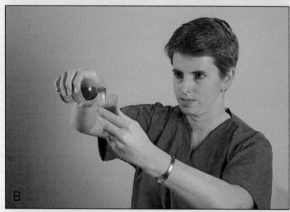

Principle. Placing the bottle cap with the open end facing up prevents contamination of the inside of the cap. Palming the medication label prevents

the medication from dripping on the label and obscuring it.

8. **Procedural Step.** Check the drug label and return the medication to the shelf.

9. **Procedural Step.** Greet and identify the patient. Introduce yourself and explain the procedure. Explain the purpose of administering the medication.
   Principle. It is crucial that no error be made in patient identity.

10. **Procedural Step.** Hand the medicine cup containing the medication to the patient, along with a glass of water. (Water should not be offered if the medication is a cough syrup.)
    Principle. Water helps the patient swallow the medication.

11. **Procedural Step.** Remain with the patient until the medication is swallowed. If the patient experiences any unusual reaction, notify the physician.

12. **Procedural Step.** Wash the hands.

13. **Procedural Step.** Chart the procedure. Include the date and time, the name of the medication, the dosage given, the route of administration, and any significant observations or patient reactions. The Latin abbreviation *po* can be used to indicate the route of administration. This abbreviation means *by mouth.*

CHARTING EXAMPLE

Date	
2/12/2002	*9:30 a.m. Acetaminophen, 650 mg, po.*
	———————————————— T. Cline, CMA

PARTS OF A NEEDLE AND SYRINGE

Needle

The needle consists of several parts (Fig. 7–2). The **hub** of the needle fits onto the top of the syringe. The **shaft,** also known as the cannula, is inserted into the body tissue. The opening in the shaft of the needle, known as the **lumen,** is continuous with the needle hub. Medication flows from the syringe and through the lumen of the needle. The **point** of the needle is located at the end of the needle shaft. The point is sharp so that it can penetrate the body tissues easily. The top of the needle is slanted and is called the

bevel. The bevel is designed to make a narrow, slitlike opening in the skin that heals quickly.

Each needle has a certain **gauge;** needle gauges for administering medication range between 18 and 27. The gauge of a needle is determined by the diameter of the lumen: As the size of the gauge increases, the diameter of the lumen decreases. Thus, a needle with a gauge of 23 has a smaller lumen diameter than a needle with a gauge of 21. Thick or oily preparations must be given with a large lumen because they are too thick to pass through a smaller one. A needle with a larger lumen causes a larger needle track to be made in the tissues. To help reduce pain and tissue damage, a

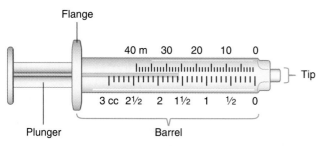

■ **FIGURE 7-2.** Diagram of a needle and a 3-cc syringe, with parts identified.

needle with the smallest gauge appropriate for the solution and route of administration is always chosen. The **length** of the needle ranges between ⅜ and 3 inches; the length used will be based on the type of injection being given. For instance, the needle used to give an intramuscular injection must be longer than

one used for a subcutaneous injection so that it penetrates deeply enough to reach the muscle tissue.

Syringe

The syringe is used for inserting fluids into the body and usually is made of plastic. Plastic syringes must be disposed of after one use. Plastic syringes are available individually packaged for sterility in a paper or cellophane wrapper or a rigid plastic container. The medical assistant needs to attach a needle to the syringe, which is available individually wrapped. Individually packaged syringes are also available with the needle already attached. Information regarding the syringe capacity and the length and gauge of the needle is found on the wrapper of the syringe and/or needle (Fig. 7–3).

The parts of a syringe are the barrel, flange, and plunger (see Fig. 7–2). The **barrel** of the syringe holds the medication and contains calibrated markings to measure the proper amount of medication. Most syringes are calibrated in both cubic centimeters (cc) and minims; cubic centimeters are used most often in administering medication. The medical assistant should become familiar with reading the graduated scales on syringes. At the end of the barrel is a rim known as

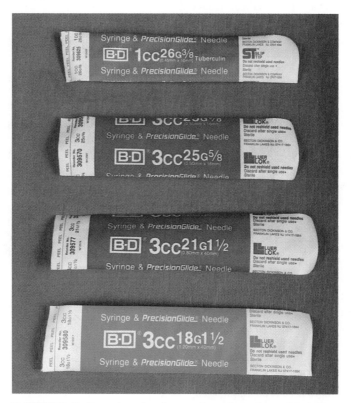

■ **FIGURE 7-3.** Examples of syringe and needle packages labeled according to contents.

the **flange,** which helps in injecting the medication. The flange also prevents the syringe from rolling when it is placed on a flat surface. The **plunger** is a movable cylinder that slides back and forth within the barrel. It is used to draw substances into and out of the barrel.

Various types of syringes are available to administer injections. The choice is based on the type of injection (e.g., allergy skin test, insulin, antibiotic) and the amount of medication being administered. The types used most often in the medical office include hypodermic, insulin, and tuberculin (Fig. 7–4). **Hypodermic syringes** are available in 2-, 2.5-, 3-, and 5-cc sizes and have two sets of calibrations—cc and minims. They are commonly used to administer intramuscular injections.

The **insulin syringe** is designed especially for the administration of an insulin injection, and the barrel is calibrated in units. The most commonly used type is the U-100 syringe, which is calibrated into 100 units and divided into increments of 2 units.

Tuberculin syringes are employed when a very small dose of medication is to be administered, such as in the tuberculin skin test. The tuberculin syringe has a capacity of 1 cc, and the calibrations are divided into tenths (0.1) and hundredths (0.01) of a cubic centimeter.

Syringes are also available with capacities of 10, 20, and 50 cc; however, they are not used for administering medication but rather for medical treatments such as irrigating wounds and draining fluid from cysts.

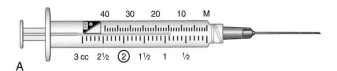

A

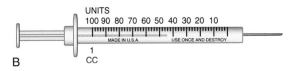

B

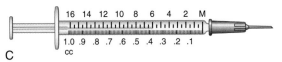

C

■ **FIGURE 7–4.** Various types of syringes used to administer injections. *A,* Hypodermic. *B,* Insulin (U-100). *C,* Tuberculin.

MEMORIES *from* EXTERNSHIP

THERESA CLINE: *I had a very bad first experience performing venipuncture at my third and final externship site. I had, of course, performed venipuncture in the classroom and felt fairly confident in doing it. However, my first two externship sites did not do in-office venipunctures. They sent all of their patients that needed blood work to an ancillary facility.*

I was working with the phlebotomist at my externship site, and a pleasant young man came in as our first patient. He was very willing to be a "guinea pig" and let me draw his blood. I was somewhat nervous but reassured that he seemed confident enough to let me practice on him. I put the tourniquet on his arm, found a good vein with no problem, and drew his blood. However, after I pulled out the needle and laid down the tube of blood, I turned around and immediately realized that I had forgotten to take the tourniquet off of his arm because he had a huge hematoma at the draw site. I was horrified and so was the patient but my supervisor removed the tourniquet and reassured both of us that it would be fine. I felt so bad because this man had been nice enough to let me draw his blood even though I was a student and it was his option whether he wanted me to perform the procedure or not. He wasn't nearly as upset as I was, but I did learn a valuable lesson and have made sure that the same mistake did not happen again.

PREPARATION OF PARENTERAL MEDICATION

Medication used for injections is available in different types of dispensing units: vials, ampules, and prefilled syringes and cartridges.

Vials

A **vial** is a closed glass container with a rubber stopper; a soft metal cap protects the rubber stopper and must be removed the first time the medication is used. Single-dose and multiple-dose vials are available (Fig. 7–5).

Some vials may require mixing before the medication can be withdrawn (e.g., reconstituting a powdered drug or mixing a vial that separates upon standing). Vials requiring mixing should be rolled between the hands rather than shaken, because shaking will cause the medication to foam, thus creating air bubbles that may enter the syringe when the medication is withdrawn. To remove medication, an amount of air exactly equal to the amount of liquid to be removed is injected into the vial. The air should be inserted above the fluid level to avoid creating bubbles in the medication. If air is not injected first, a partial vacuum will be created and it will be difficult to remove the medication. During the withdrawal of medication, the needle opening should be inserted below the fluid level to prevent the entrance of air bubbles. Air bubbles can be removed by tapping the barrel of the syringe with the fingertips. If they are allowed to remain, they take up space that the medication should occupy.

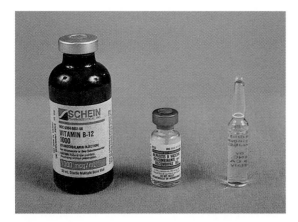

■ **FIGURE 7–5.** The multiple-dose vial (*left*) and the single-dose vial (*middle*) consist of a closed glass container with a rubber stopper. The ampule (*right*) consists of a small, sealed glass container that holds a single dose of medication.

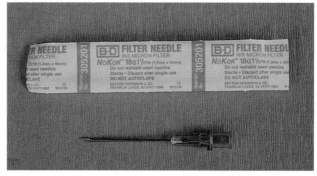

■ **FIGURE 7–6.** Filter needle used to withdraw medication from an ampule.

Ampules

An **ampule** is a small, sealed glass container that holds a single dose of medication (Fig. 7–5). An ampule has a constriction in the stem, known as the neck, that helps in opening it. Before opening, make sure that there is no medication in the stem by tapping it lightly.

A colored ring around the neck indicates where the ampule is prescored for easy opening. The ampule is opened by holding it firmly with gauze and breaking off the stem using moderate pressure.

A potential hazard with medication in ampules is the presence of small glass particles in the ampule after the container is broken. When the medication is withdrawn into the syringe, the glass particles may also be withdrawn. To prevent this problem, a needle with a filter should be used that filters out any small glass particles (Fig. 7–6).

The needle opening is inserted into the base of the ampule below the fluid level to withdraw medication. To prevent contamination, the needle should not touch the edge of the ampule. Air should never be injected into the ampule, because this may force out some of the medication.

If a filter needle has been used to withdraw the medication, the filter needle must be recapped, removed from the syringe, and discarded in a biohazard sharps container. The appropriate size and gauge needle for administering the medication must then be applied to the syringe.

Prefilled Syringes and Cartridges

Some drugs come in **prefilled disposable syringes,** or **cartridges.** Using this type of dispensing unit does not require drawing up the medication. The name of the

TUBEX® Injector
NOTE: The TUBEX® Injector is reusable: do not discard.

DIRECTIONS FOR USE:

Ribbed Collar

TUBEX® Sterile Cartridge-Needle Unit

Plunger Rod   Plunger

To administer
Method of administration is the same as with conventional syringe. Remove needle cover by grasping it securely; twist and pull. Introduce needle into patient, aspirate by pulling back slightly on the plunger, and inject.

To load a TUBEX® Sterile Cartridge-Needle Unit into the TUBEX® Injector

CLOSE   OPEN

1. Turn the ribbed collar to the "OPEN" position until it stops.

CLOSE

2. Hold the Injector with the open end up and fully insert the TUBEX® Sterile Cartridge-Needle Unit. Firmly tighten the ribbed collar in the direction of the "CLOSE" arrow.

3. Thread the plunger rod into the plunger of the TUBEX® Sterile Cartridge-Needle Unit until slight resistance is felt.
The Injector is now ready for use in the usual manner.

To load an E.S.I. DOSETTE® Sterile Cartridge-Needle Unit into the TUBEX® Injector

Ribbed Collar

E.S.I. DOSETTE® Sterile Cartridge-Needle Unit

Plunger Rod   Plunger

To administer
Method of administration is the same as with conventional syringe. Remove needle cover by grasping it securely; twist and pull. Introduce needle into patient, aspirate by pulling back slightly on the plunger, and inject.

CLOSE

1. Turn the ribbed collar to the "OPEN" position until it stops.

CLOSE

2. Hold the Injector with the open end up and fully insert the E.S.I. DOSETTE® Sterile Cartridge-Needle Unit. Firmly tighten the ribbed collar in the direction of the "CLOSE" arrow.

3. Thread the plunger rod into the plunger of the E.S.I. DOSETTE® Sterile Cartridge-Needle Unit until slight resistance is felt.

4. Engage the needle-cap assembly by pulling the cap down over the silver cartridge hub. The needle is fully engaged when the silver hub is completely covered.

The injector is now ready for use in the usual manner.

To remove the empty TUBEX® or DOSETTE® Cartridge-Needle Unit and dispose into a biohazard sharps container:

OPEN

1. Do not recap the needle. Disengage the plunger rod.

2. Hold the Injector, needle down, over a biohazard container and loosen the ribbed collar. TUBEX® or DOSETTE® Cartridge-NeedleUnit will drop into the container.

BIOHAZARD

3. Discard the needle cover.

The TUBEX® Injector is reusable and should not be discarded.

Used TUBEX® or DOSETTE® Cartridge-Needle Units should not be employed for successive injections or as multiple-dose containers. They are intended to be used only once and discarded.

NOTE: Any graduated markings on TUBEX® or DOSETTE® Cartridge-Needle Units are to be used only as a guide in mixing, withdrawing, or administering measured doses.

A

■ **FIGURE 7–8.** Procedure for administering an injection using a Tubex Injector. (*A,* Courtesy of ESI Lederle, Division of American Home Products Corporation, St. Davids, PA.)

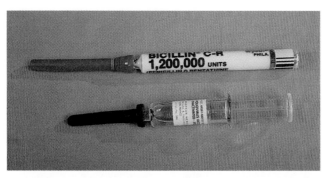

■ FIGURE 7–7. *Top,* An example of a prefilled disposable cartridge containing medication. Disposable cartridges must be inserted into a specially designed syringe for administration of the injection. *Bottom,* An example of a prefilled disposable syringe.

tions are prepared and stored in a powdered form and require the addition of a liquid before administration. Examples include the measles, mumps, and rubella (MMR) immunization (Fig. 7–9) and potassium penicillin G. The process of adding a liquid to a powdered drug is known as **reconstitution.** The liquid used is usually sterile water or sterile normal saline. The powdered drug is contained in a single-dose or multiple-dose vial and is accompanied by specific instructions for reconstitution. A general procedure for reconstituting powdered drugs is outlined in Procedure 7–2.

drug, the dose, and the expiration date are included on the syringe or cartridge (Fig. 7–7). An example is the Tubex Injector, consisting of a reusable syringe that holds a Tubex sterile cartridge-needle unit. The procedure for administering an injection using the Tubex Injector is presented in Figure 7–8.

STORAGE

The medical assistant should always read the drug package insert to determine the proper method for storing each parenteral medication, because improper storage may alter the effectiveness of the medication.

RECONSTITUTION OF POWDERED DRUGS

Some parenteral medications are stable for only a short period of time in liquid form; therefore, these medica-

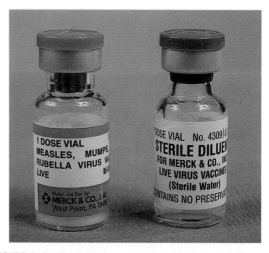

■ FIGURE 7–9. The measles, mumps, and rubella (MMR) vaccine is an example of a parenteral medication that requires reconstitution before administration. The vial on the left contains the medication in powdered form, and the vial on the right contains the sterile diluent.

7

7–2

Reconstituting Powdered Drugs

1. **Procedural Step.** From the vial containing the powdered drug, withdraw an amount of air equal to the amount of liquid to be injected into the vial.
2. **Procedural Step.** Add the appropriate amount of reconstituting liquid to the powdered drug.
3. **Procedural Step.** Roll the vial between the hands to mix the powdered drug and liquid.

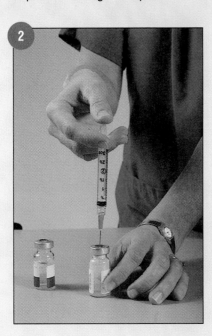

4. **Procedural Step.** Label multiple-dose vials with the name of the medication, the date of preparation, and your initials.

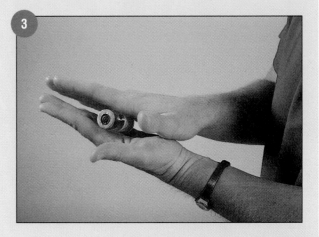

5. **Procedural Step.** Store multiple-dose vials as indicated by the manufacturer's instructions. Because reconstituted drugs are stable for a short period of time, be sure to check carefully the date of preparation on the multiple-dose vial before administering it.

7–3

Preparing the Injection

EQUIPMENT/SUPPLIES:	Medication ordered by the physician	Antiseptic wipe
	Appropriate needle and syringe	Medication tray

1. **Procedural Step.** Wash the hands.
2. **Procedural Step.** Assemble the equipment.
3. **Procedural Step.** Work in a quiet, well-lit atmosphere.
   Principle. Good lighting aids the medical assistant in reading the medication label.
4. **Procedural Step.** Select the proper medication, and check the expiration date. Compare the medication with the physician's instructions. The drug label must be checked three times: while removing the medication from its storage location, before withdrawing the medication into the syringe, and before returning it to its proper place.
   Principle. If the medication is outdated, consult the physician, it may produce undesirable effects and the medical assistant could be held responsible. The medication should be carefully compared with the physician's instructions to prevent a drug error.
5. **Procedural Step.** Calculate the correct dose to be given, if necessary.
6. **Procedural Step.** Open the antiseptic; wipe and cleanse the vial or ampule.
   Principle. Cleansing the vial or ampule removes dust and bacteria.
7. **Procedural Step.** Open the syringe and needle package. Assemble the needle and syringe if necessary.
   Principle. Disposable needles and syringes may come together in a package, already assembled or in separate packages, requiring assembly of the needle and syringe.
8. **Procedural Step.** Remove the needle guard and check to make sure that the needle is attached firmly to the syringe by grasping the needle at the hub and turning it clockwise.

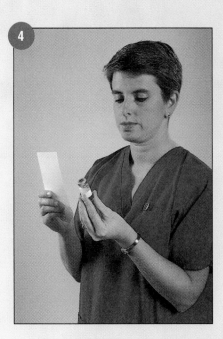

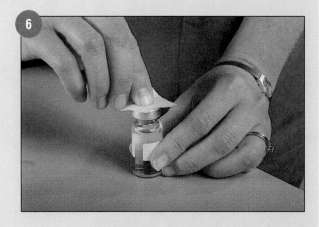

9. **Procedural Step.** Check the drug label, and withdraw the proper amount of medication from the vial or ampule as follows:

9.A. Vial
   a. Pull back on the plunger to draw an amount of air into the syringe equal to the amount of medication to be withdrawn from the vial. Air must first be injected into the vial to prevent the formation of a partial vacuum in the vial, making it difficult to remove medication.
   b. Using moderate pressure, insert the needle through the center of the rubber stopper, until it reaches the empty space between the stopper and fluid level.
   c. Push down on the plunger to inject the air into the vial, making sure to keep the needle opening above the fluid level. The air must be inserted above the fluid level to avoid creating air bubbles in the medication.
   d. Invert the vial while holding onto the syringe and plunger.
   e. Hold the syringe at eye level, and withdraw the proper amount of medication. Keep the needle opening below the fluid level to prevent the entrance of air bubbles into the syringe.
   f. Remove any air bubbles in the syringe by holding the syringe in a vertical position and tapping the barrel with the fingertips until they disappear. Air bubbles take up space the medication should occupy.
   g. Remove any air remaining at the top of the syringe by slowly depressing the plunger and allowing the air to flow back into the vial.
   h. Carefully remove the needle from the rubber stopper.

9.B. Ampule
   a. Tap the stem of the ampule lightly to remove any medication in the neck of the ampule.
   b. Place a piece of gauze around the neck of the ampule.

Continued

7

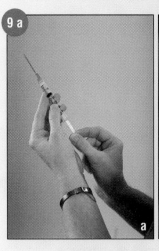

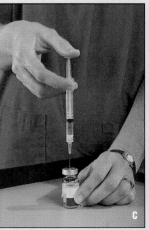

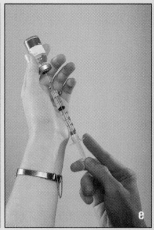

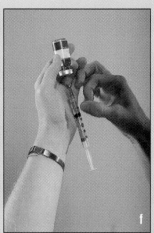

c. Using both hands, hold the ampule firmly between the fingers.

d. Break off the stem by snapping it quickly and firmly away from the body.

e. Insert the needle opening below the fluid level. (Note: It is recommended that a filter needle be used to withdraw the medication. A filter needle prevents glass particles from being withdrawn into the syringe.)

f. Withdraw the proper amount of medication by pulling back on the plunger. Be sure to keep the needle opening below the fluid level to prevent the entrance of air bubbles into the syringe. Air bubbles take up space the medication should occupy resulting in an inaccurate measurement of medication.

g. Remove the needle from the ampule without allowing the needle to touch the edge of the ampule.

h. If air bubbles are in the syringe hold the syringe in a vertical position and tap the barrel with the fingertips until they disappear. Draw back slightly on the plunger and slowly push the plunger forward to eject the air. Do not eject the fluid.

10. **Procedural Step.** Replace the needle guard. If a filter needle has been used to withdraw the medi-

cation, remove it from the syringe and discard it in a biohazard sharps container. Replace it with the appropriate size and gauge needle for administering the medication.

Principle. The needle must remain sterile. The needle guard prevents the needle from becoming contaminated.

11. **Procedural Step.** Check the drug label and return the medication to its proper storage compartment.

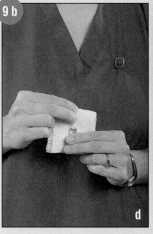

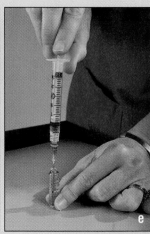

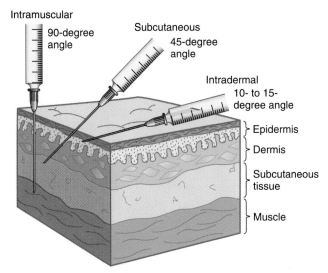

■ **FIGURE 7–10.** Angle of insertion for intradermal, subcutaneous, and intramuscular injections.

SUBCUTANEOUS INJECTIONS

A subcutaneous injection is made into the subcutaneous tissue, which is located just under the skin (see Fig. 7–10). This consists of adipose (fat) tissue. Subcutaneous tissue is located all over the body; however, certain sites are more commonly used in which bones and blood vessels are not near the surface of the skin. These include the upper lateral part of the arms, the anterior thigh, the upper back, and the abdomen (Fig. 7–11). Absorption of medication from a subcutaneous injection occurs mainly through capillaries, resulting in a slower absorption rate than with intramuscular injections. To ensure proper absorption, tissue that is grossly adipose, hardened, inflamed, or edematous should not be used as an injection site.

The needle length varies from ½ to ⅝ inch, and the gauge ranges from 23 to 25. Elderly and dehydrated patients tend to have less subcutaneous tissue, whereas obese patients have more. The length of the needle should be adjusted accordingly, to make sure the injec-

tion is given into the subcutaneous tissue and not into muscle tissue.

Subcutaneous tissue is sensitive to irritating solutions and large volumes of medications; therefore, drugs given subcutaneously must be isotonic, nonirritating, nonviscous, and water soluble. The amount of medication injected through the subcutaneous route should not exceed 1 cc. More than this amount results in pressure on sensory nerve endings, causing discomfort and pain.

Medications commonly administered through the subcutaneous route include epinephrine, insulin, and allergy injections. Patients receiving an allergy injection must wait in the medical office for 15 to 20 minutes following the injection to be observed for the occurrence of any unusual reactions.

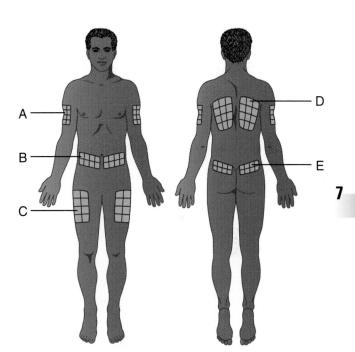

■ **FIGURE 7–11.** Common sites for subcutaneous injections. *A*, Upper outer arm; *B*, lower abdomen; *C*, upper outer thigh; *D*, upper back; *E*, flank region.

7

PROCEDURE

7–4

Administering a Subcutaneous Injection

EQUIPMENT/SUPPLIES: Medication ordered by the physician
Appropriate needle and syringe
Antiseptic wipe

Disposable gloves
Biohazard sharps container

1. **Procedural Step.** Greet and identify the patient. Introduce yourself and explain the procedure and purpose of the injection.
   Principle. It is crucial that no error be made in patient identity. An apprehensive patient may need reassurance.

2. **Procedural Step.** Select an appropriate injection site. The upper arm, thigh, back, and abdomen are recommended sites for a subcutaneous injection. Refer to Figure 7–11.
   Principle. The entire area should be exposed to ensure a safe and comfortable injection.

3. **Procedural Step.** Prepare the injection site. Cleanse the area with an antiseptic wipe. Using a circular motion start with the injection site and move outward. Do not touch the site after cleansing it.
   Principle. Using a circular motion carries contaminants away from the injection site. Touching the site after cleansing will contaminate it, and the cleansing process will need to be repeated.

4. **Procedural Step.** Allow the area to dry completely.
   Principle. If the area is not permitted to dry, the antiseptic may enter the tissues when the skin is pierced, resulting in irritation and patient discomfort.

5. **Procedural Step.** Apply gloves, and remove the needle guard. Position your nondominant hand on the area surrounding the injection site. The skin may be held taut, or the area surrounding the injection site may be grasped and held in a cushion fashion.
   Principle. Gloves provide a barrier precaution against bloodborne pathogens. In normal adults, the needle will enter the subcutaneous tissue when the skin is held taut. Grasping the area around the injection site is recommended for a thin or dehydrated patient. It will ensure that the subcutaneous tissue, and not muscle tissue, is entered.

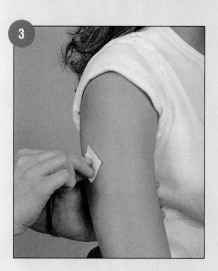

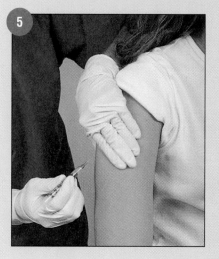

6. **Procedural Step.** Insert the needle quickly and smoothly at a 45-degree or 90-degree angle, depending on the length of the needle. The barrel of the syringe should be held between the thumb and the index finger. Insert the needle to the hub.

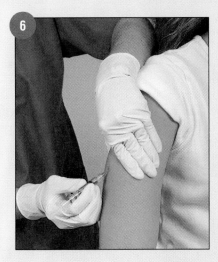

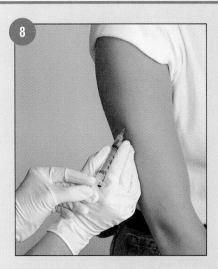

Principle. Inserting the needle quickly and smoothly minimizes tissue trauma and pain. Needle length determines the angle of insertion to ensure placement of the medication in subcutaneous tissue. With a ½-inch needle, a 90-degree angle should be used; with a ⅝-inch needle, a 45-degree angle should be used.

7. **Procedural Step.** Remove your hand from the skin.
Principle. Medication injected into compressed tissue causes pressure against nerve fibers and is uncomfortable for the patient.

8. **Procedural Step.** Hold the syringe steady and pull back gently on the plunger to determine whether the needle is in a blood vessel, in which case blood will appear in the syringe. If blood appears, withdraw the needle, prepare a new injection, and begin again.
Principle. Moving the syringe once the needle has entered the tissue causes patient discomfort. Drugs intended for subcutaneous administration but injected into a blood vessel are absorbed too quickly, and undesirable results may occur.

9. **Procedural Step.** Inject the medication slowly and steadily by depressing the plunger.
Principle. Rapid injection creates pressure and destroys tissue, which are uncomfortable for the patient.

10. **Procedural Step.** Place the antiseptic wipe gently over the injection site and quickly remove the needle, keeping it at the same angle as for insertion.
Principle. Withdrawing the needle quickly and at the same angle as for insertion reduces patient

discomfort. The antiseptic wipe placed over the injection site helps prevent tissue movement as the needle is withdrawn, reducing patient discomfort.

11. **Procedural Step.** Gently massage the injection site with an antiseptic wipe.
Principle. Massaging helps distribute the medication so that it is more completely absorbed.

12. **Procedural Step.** Properly dispose of the needle and syringe in a biohazard sharps container.
Principle. Proper disposal is required by the OSHA Standard to prevent accidental needlestick injuries.

13. **Procedural Step.** Remove the gloves, and wash the hands.

14. **Procedural Step.** Chart the procedure. Include the date and time, the name of the medication, the dosage given, the route of administration, the injection site used, and any significant observations or patient reactions.

15. **Procedural Step.** Stay with the patient to make sure he or she is not experiencing any unusual reactions. (*Note:* If an allergy injection has been given, the patient should remain at the medical office for at least 15 minutes to make sure that a reaction does not occur.) If the patient experiences an unusual reaction, notify the physician.

CHARTING EXAMPLE

Date	
2/17/2002	3:30 p.m. Ragweed allergy inj, 0.20 cc, SC Ⓡ upper arm. Arm checked 15 minutes following administration. No reaction noted. ———— ———————————— T. Cline, CMA

7

INTRAMUSCULAR INJECTIONS

Intramuscular injections are made into the muscular layer of the body, which lies below the skin and subcutaneous layers (see Figure 7–10). The amount of medication injected into muscle tissue may be larger than the amount injected into subcutaneous tissue. An amount of up to 3 cc may be injected into the gluteal or vastus lateralis muscles, although older adults and very thin adults are able to tolerate only 2 cc or less in these sites.

Absorption is more rapid by this route than by the subcutaneous route, because there are more blood vessels in muscle tissue. Medication that is irritating to subcutaneous tissue is often given intramuscularly, because there are fewer nerve endings in deep muscle tissue. Most parenteral medications administered in the medical office are given through the intramuscular route; examples include antibiotics, immunizations, vitamin B$_{12}$, and corticosteroids.

The length of the needle varies from 1 to 3 inches; a 1.5-inch needle is typically used for an average-sized adult. The gauge of the needle ranges from 18 to 23, depending on the viscosity of the medication.

The sites chosen for intramuscular injections are away from large nerves and blood vessels. The medical assistant should practice locating these sites to become familiar with them. The area should always be fully exposed to permit clear visualization of the injection site. Intramuscular injection sites are described in the following sections.

Dorsogluteal Site

The dorsogluteal site is often used to administer intramuscular injections. In adults and children older than 3 years of age, the gluteal muscles are well developed and can absorb a large amount of medication. The patient should lie on the abdomen with the toes pointed inward, which aids in relaxation of the gluteus muscles. The injection is made into the upper outer quadrant of the gluteal area, in the area located above and outside a diagonal line drawn from the greater trochanter to the posterior superior iliac spine. These landmarks should be identified through palpation. The medical assistant must be *extremely* careful to maintain the proper boundary lines to avoid injection into the sciatic nerve or superior gluteal artery (Fig. 7–12).

Deltoid Site

The deltoid area is easily accessible and can be used when the patient is in a sitting or lying position (see Fig. 7–12). This area forms a rectangle, bounded on top by the lower edge of the acromion process and on the bottom by the lateral side of the arm, opposite the axilla. The side boundaries of the rectangle are parallel to the arm. They are located one third and two thirds of the way around the site of the arm. The medication is injected into the deltoid muscle. This site is small, because major nerves and blood vessels surround it, and large amounts of medication (no more than 1 cc) and repeated injections should not be given in this area.

The medical assistant should make sure that the entire arm is exposed by having the patient's sleeve completely pulled up or by removing the sleeve from the arm if it cannot be pulled up. A tight sleeve constricts the arm and causes unnecessary bleeding from the puncture site.

Vastus Lateralis Site

The vastus lateralis is now used more frequently, because it is away from major nerves and blood vessels and is a relatively thick muscle (see Fig. 7–12). This site is particularly desirable for infants and children younger than 3 years of age whose gluteal muscles are not yet well developed. The area is bounded by the midanterior thigh on the front of the leg and the midlateral thigh on the side. The proximal boundary is a hand's breadth below the greater trochanter, and the distal boundary is a hand's breadth above the knee. It is easier to give an injection in the vastus lateralis if the patient is lying down, but a sitting position may also be used.

Ventrogluteal Site

Also growing in acceptability is the ventrogluteal site. The subcutaneous layer is relatively small, and the muscle layer is thick. The site is located away from major nerves and blood vessels. Through palpation, the greater trochanter of the femur, the anterior superior iliac spine, and the iliac crest can be located. If the injection is being made into the left side of the patient, the palm of the right hand is placed on the greater trochanter, and the index finger is placed on the anterior superior iliac spine. The middle finger is spread posteriorly as far as possible away from the index finger, to touch the iliac crest. The hand position is reversed if the injection is being made into the right side of the patient. The triangle formed by the fingers is the area into which the injection is given. An injection into the ventrogluteal site can be administered when the patient is lying prone or on one side (see Fig. 7–12).

7

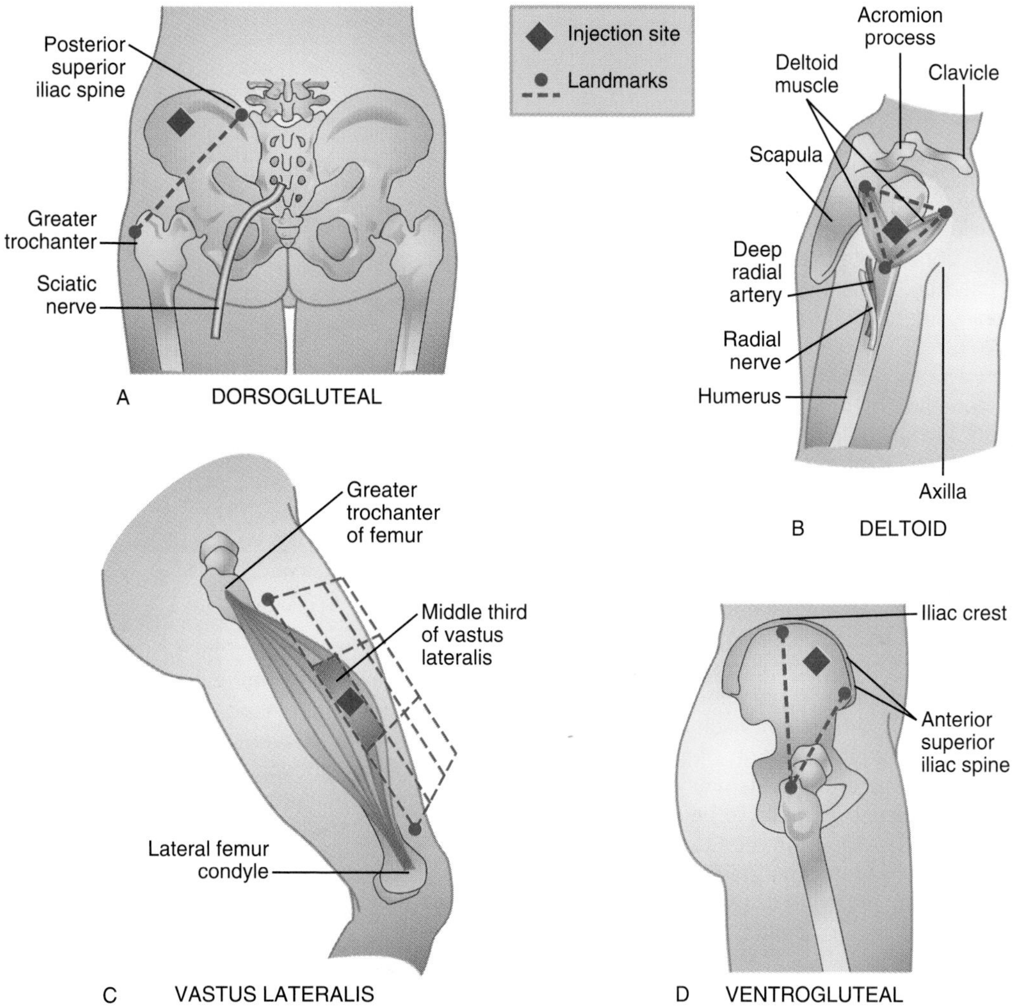

FIGURE 7-12. Sites of intramuscular injections. *A,* Dorsogluteal muscle; *B,* deltoid muscle; *C,* vastus lateralis; *D,* ventrogluteal muscle. (From Leahy, J. M., Kizilay, P. E.: *Foundations of Nursing Practice: A Nursing Process Approach.* Philadelphia, W. B. Saunders, 1998.)

PROCEDURE

7–5

Administering an Intramuscular Injection

EQUIPMENT/SUPPLIES: Medication ordered by the physician   Disposable gloves
Appropriate needle and syringe   Biohazard sharps container
Antiseptic wipe

1. **Procedural Step.** Greet and identify the patient. Introduce yourself and explain the procedure.
Principle. Make sure that you are giving the medication to the right patient. Explain the purpose of the injection. Assistance may be needed for restraining infants and children.

2. **Procedural Step.** Select an appropriate injection site. Refer to Figure 7–12 for the recommended intramuscular injection sites. Remove the patient's clothing as necessary to make sure the entire area is exposed.
Principle. Major nerves and blood vessels may lie in close proximity to the intramuscular injection sites. The medical assistant should develop skill and accuracy in locating the proper sites.

3. **Procedural Step.** Prepare the injection site. Cleanse the area with an antiseptic wipe. Using a circular motion, start with the injection site and move outward. Do not touch the site after cleansing it.
Principle. Using a circular motion carries contaminants away from the injection site. Touching the site after cleansing will contaminate it, and the cleansing process will need to be repeated.

4. **Procedural Step.** Allow the area to dry completely.
Principle. If the area is not permitted to dry the antiseptic may enter the tissues when the skin is pierced, resulting in irritation and patient discomfort.

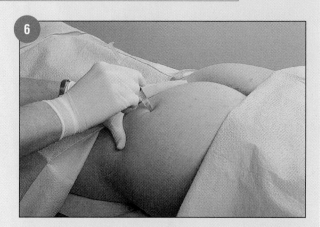

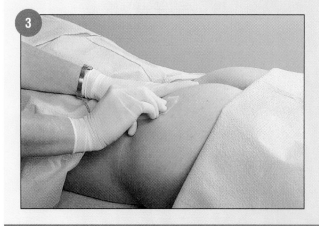

5. **Procedural Step.** Apply gloves and remove the needle guard. Stretch the skin taut over the injection site using the thumb and first two fingers of the nondominant hand.
Principle. Gloves provide a barrier precaution against bloodborne pathogens. Stretching the skin taut permits easier insertion of the needle and helps ensure that the needle enters muscle tissue.

6. **Procedural Step.** Hold the barrel of the syringe like a dart and insert the needle quickly and smoothly at a 90-degree angle to the patient's skin with a firm motion. Insert the needle to the hub.
Principle. The needle is inserted at a 90-degree angle to ensure that it reaches muscle tissue. Inserting the needle quickly and smoothly minimizes tissue trauma and pain.

7. **Procedural Step.** Hold the syringe steady, and pull back gently on the plunger to determine whether the needle is in a blood vessel. If blood appears, withdraw the needle, prepare a new injection, and begin again.
Principle. Moving the syringe once the needle has penetrated the tissue causes patient discomfort. If drugs that are intended for intramuscular administration are injected into a blood vessel, the result is faster absorption of the medication. This may produce undesirable results.

7

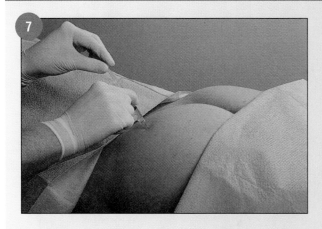

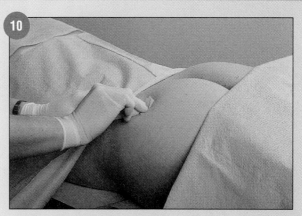

8. **Procedural Step.** Inject the medication slowly and steadily by depressing the plunger.
   Principle. Rapid injection creates pressure and destroys tissue, thus causing discomfort for the patient.

9. **Procedural Step.** Place the antiseptic wipe gently over the injection site and remove the needle quickly keeping it at the same angle as for insertion.
   Principle. Withdrawing the needle quickly and at the same angle as for insertion reduces patient discomfort. Placing the antiseptic wipe over the injection site helps prevent tissue movement as the needle is withdrawn, also reducing patient discomfort.

10. **Procedural Step.** Gently massage the injection site with an antiseptic wipe.
    Principle. Massaging helps distribute the medication so that it is absorbed by the muscle tissue.

11. **Procedural Step.** Properly dispose of the needle and syringe in a biohazard sharps container.
    Principle. Proper disposal is required by the OSHA Standard to prevent accidental needlestick injuries.

12. **Procedural Step.** Remove the gloves, and wash the hands.

13. **Procedural Step.** Chart the procedure. Include the date and time, the name of the medication, the dosage given, the route of administration, the injection site used, and any significant observations or patient reactions.

14. **Procedural Step.** Stay with the patient to make sure he or she is not experiencing any unusual reactions.
    Principle. If the patient experiences an unusual reaction, notify the physician.

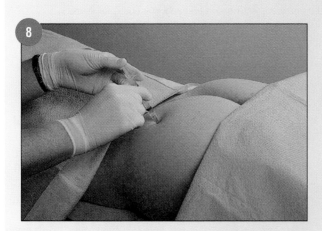

7

CHARTING EXAMPLE

Date	
2/20/2002	9:30 a.m. Penicillin G benzathine, 900,000 units, IM, (L) dorsogluteal. Tolerated injection well. ——————————————— T. Cline, CMA

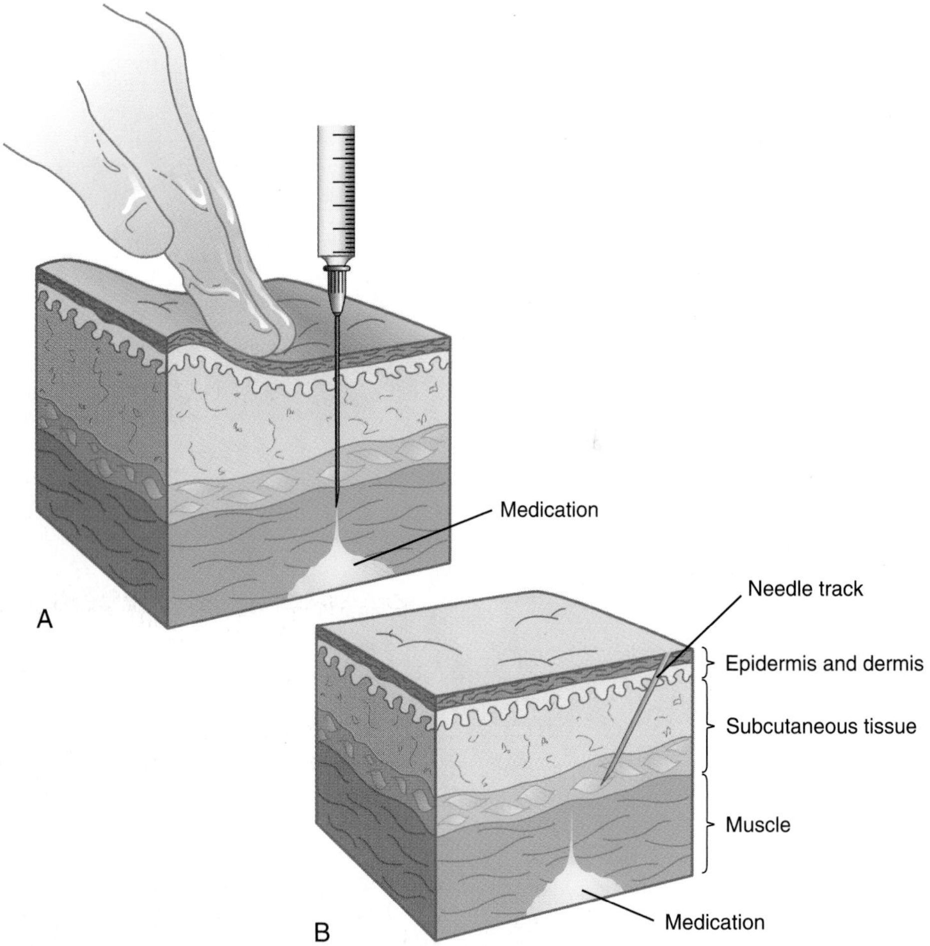

■ **FIGURE 7–13.** The Z-track intramuscular injection method. *A,* The skin and subcutaneous tissue are pulled to the side before the needle is inserted. *B,* This causes a zigzag path through the tissue once the skin is released, which seals off the needle track.

Z-TRACK METHOD

Medications that are irritating to subcutaneous and skin tissue or that discolor the skin must be given intramuscularly using the Z-track method; an example of a medication that is administered by this method is iron dextran. The dorsogluteal, ventrogluteal, and vastus lateralis sites can all be used as areas to administer a Z-track injection.

The Z-track method is very similar to the intramuscular injection procedure, except that the skin and subcutaneous tissue at the injection site are pulled to the side before the needle is inserted. This causes a zigzag path through the tissues once the skin is released, preventing the medication from reaching the subcutaneous layer or skin surface by sealing off the needle track (Fig. 7–13). The procedure for administering medication using the Z-track method uses concepts previously presented in the discussion of the intramuscular injection procedure.

INTRADERMAL INJECTIONS

An intradermal injection is given into the dermal layer of the skin, at an angle almost parallel to the skin (see Fig. 7–10). Absorption is slow; therefore, only a small amount of medication may be injected (0.01 to 0.2 cc). The sites most often used for an intradermal injection are areas where the skin is thin, such as the anterior forearm and the middle of the back.

The needle used is short, usually ⅜ to ⅝ inch long, and the lumen has a small diameter, usually 25 to 27 gauge. A tuberculin syringe is often used for administering the injection. The capacity of the syringe is small (1 cc), and the calibrations are divided into tenths and hundredths of a cubic centimeter. The fine calibrations allow for a very small amount of medication to be administered, which is required with an intradermal injection.

The most frequent use of intradermal injections is to administer a skin test such as an allergy skin test or

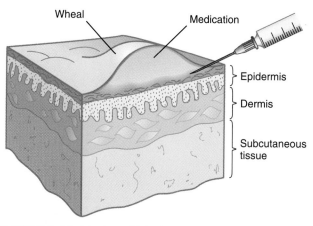

■ FIGURE 7–14. Intradermal injections are used to administer skin tests. Enough medication must be deposited in the skin layers to form a wheal.

a tuberculin skin test. The medication for the appropriate test is placed into the skin layers, and a small raised area known as a wheal is produced at the injection site, owing to distention of the skin (Fig. 7–14). At a time dictated by the type of test being administered, the results are read and interpreted. For example, the majority of allergy skin tests may be read and interpreted at the medical office within a short period of time (usually 15 to 20 minutes) after administration of the test, whereas tuberculin skin testing requires 48 hours before the test results may be read.

The skin testing medication interacts with the body tissues; if no reaction occurs, the wheal disappears within a short period of time, and the only visible sign left is the puncture site. If a reaction to the skin test occurs, induration results, indicating a positive reaction. Erythema may also be present at the test site; however, for most skin tests, the extent of induration is the only criterion used to assess a positive reaction.

PROCEDURE

7–6

Z-Track Intramuscular Injection Technique

7

1. **Procedural Step.** Follow Steps 1 to 4 of the intramuscular injection procedure. Procedure 7–5.
2. **Procedural Step.** Apply gloves, and remove the needle guard. With the nondominant hand, pull the skin away laterally from the injection site approximately 1 to 1½ inches.
3. **Procedural Step.** Insert the needle quickly and smoothly at a 90-degree angle.
4. **Procedural Step.** Aspirate to determine whether the needle is in a blood vessel (refer to Step 7 of the intramuscular injection procedure.)
5. **Procedural Step.** Inject the medication slowly and steadily.
6. **Procedural Step.** After injecting the medication, wait 10 seconds before withdrawing the needle to allow initial absorption of the medication.
7. **Procedural Step.** Withdraw the needle quickly at the same angle of insertion.
8. **Procedural Step.** Release the traction on the skin in order to seal off the needle track; doing so pre-

vents the medication from reaching the subcutaneous tissue and skin surface. Properly dispose of the needle and syringe.
9. **Procedural Step.** Do not massage the site; massaging may cause the medication to seep out. If bleeding occurs at the injection site, apply gentle pressure with a sterile gauze pad.
10. **Procedural Step.** Complete the procedure by following Steps 12 to 14 of the intramuscular injection procedure.

CHARTING EXAMPLE

Date	
2/20/2002	10:30 a.m. Iron dextran, 100 mg, IM, Z-track into Ⓡ dorsogluteal. No complaints of discomfort. ———————— T. Cline, CMA

7-7

Administering an Intradermal Injection

EQUIPMENT/SUPPLIES: Medication ordered by the physician
Appropriate needle and syringe
Antiseptic wipe

Disposable gloves
Biohazard sharps container

1. **Procedural Step.** Greet and identify the patient. Introduce yourself and explain the procedure.
   Principle. It is crucial that no error be made in patient identity. Explain the purpose of the injection to help reassure an apprehensive patient.
2. **Procedural Step.** Select an appropriate injection site. The anterior forearm and the middle of the back are recommended sites for an intradermal injection.
   Principle. The entire area should be exposed to ensure a safe and comfortable injection.
3. **Procedural Step.** Prepare the injection site. Cleanse the area with an antiseptic wipe. Using a circular motion, start with the injection site and move outward. Do not touch the site after cleansing it.
   Principle. Using a circular motions will carry material away from the injection site. Touching the site after cleansing will contaminate it, and the cleansing process will need to be repeated.
4. **Procedural Step.** Allow the area to dry completely.
   Principle. If the area is not permitted to dry the antiseptic may enter the tissue when the skin is pierced, resulting in irritation and patient discomfort. In addition, the antiseptic may cause a reaction that could be mistaken for a positive test response.
5. **Procedural Step.** Apply gloves, and remove the needle guard. With the nondominant hand, stretch the skin taut at the proposed site of administra-

tion. Insert the needle at a 10- to 15-degree angle, with the bevel upward. The needle should be inserted about one eighth of an inch until the bevel of the needle just penetrates the skin. No aspiration is needed.
   Principle. Gloves provide a barrier precaution against bloodborne pathogens. Stretching the patient's skin taut will permit easier insertion of the needle. The needle should be inserted at an angle almost parallel to the skin, to ensure penetration within the dermal layer of the skin. The needle must be inserted with the bevel facing upward to allow for proper wheal formation. If the needle is inserted with the bevel facing downward the medication will be absorbed and a wheal will not form.
6. **Procedural Step.** Hold the syringe steady, and inject the medication slowly and steadily by depressing the plunger until a tense, white wheal forms (approximately 6 mm in diameter). Expect to feel a certain amount of resistance as you inject the medication; this helps in indicating that the needle is properly located in the superficial skin layers rather than in the deeper subcutaneous tissue.
   Principle. Moving the syringe once the needle has entered the skin causes patient discomfort.
7. **Procedural Step.** Place the antiseptic wipe gently over the injection site; remove the needle quickly and at the same angle as for insertion.

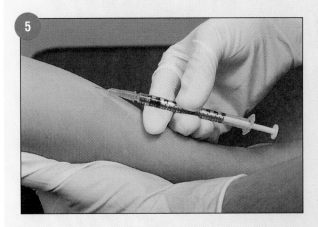

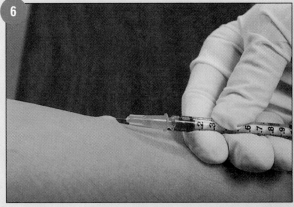

PROCEDURE 7-7

Principle. Withdrawing the needle quickly and at the angle of insertion reduces patient discomfort. The antiseptic wipe placed over the injection site helps prevent tissue movement as the needle is withdrawn, also reducing patient discomfort.

8. **Procedural Step.** Do not massage the injection site. The wheal will be quickly absorbed and no adhesive bandage is needed.

   Principle. Massaging is not needed because the medication is not intended to be distributed into the tissues. In addition, massaging may cause leakage of the testing solution through the needle puncture site, which could interfere with the test results.

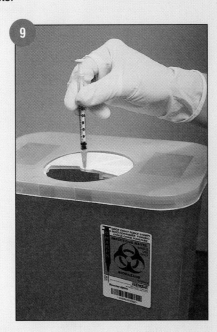

9. **Procedural Step.** Properly dispose of the needle and syringe in a biohazard sharps container.

   Principle. Proper disposal of the needle and syringe is required by the OSHA Standard to prevent accidental needlestick injuries.

10. **Procedural Step.** Remove the gloves, and wash the hands.

11. **Procedural Step.** Stay with the patient to make sure that he or she is not experiencing any unusual reactions. Perform *one* of the following, based on the type of skin test being administered, the length of time required for the body tissues to react to the test, and the medical office policy.
    a. Read the test results, using inspection and palpation at the site of the injection to assess the presence of and/or to determine the amount of induration.

    or
    b. Inform the patient of a date and time to return to the medical office to have the results read.

    or
    c. Instruct the patient in the proper procedure for reading and interpreting the results at home and reporting them to the medical office.

    In all cases, the results must be read and interpreted according to the manufacturer's instructions that accompany the test. (*Note:* The medical assistant should be especially careful and alert for any sign of a patient reaction when administering allergy skin tests.) If the patient experiences an unusual reaction, notify the physician immediately.

12. **Procedural Step.** Chart the procedure. Include the date and time, the name of the medication, the dosage given, the route of administration, the injection site used, the skin test results, and any significant observations or patient reactions. (*Note:* If the skin test results are to be recorded at a later date, the test results will not be recorded at this time.)

7

CHARTING EXAMPLE	
Date	
2/15/2002	2:30 p.m. Mantoux tuberculin test, 0.10 ml, ID, ⓡ ant forearm. Instructed patient to return on 2/17 to have results read.
	———————————— T. Cline, CMA

TUBERCULIN SKIN TESTING

TUBERCULOSIS

Tuberculosis is an infectious disease that usually attacks the lungs, although it may occur in almost any other part of the body, particularly the brain and kidney. The causative agent of tuberculosis is the tubercle bacillus (*Mycobacterium tuberculosis*), which is a rod-shaped bacterium. The symptoms of active pulmonary tuberculosis include fatigue, weakness, weight loss, low-grade fever, night sweats, a cough that produces mucopurulent sputum, and occasional hemoptysis (coughing up blood) and chest pain.

PURPOSE OF TUBERCULIN SKIN TESTING

The purpose of tuberculin skin testing is to detect the presence of a tuberculin infection. The test is often performed as a screening measure to assist in the early detection of unsuspected cases of tuberculosis before the patient becomes symptomatic. In this way, appropriate therapeutic measures can be instituted, leading to early treatment, which also helps prevent the spread of the disease. Tuberculin skin testing is usually included as part of a regular health screen, or it may be required as a prerequisite for employment, college entrance, entrance into the military service, and so on. The medical assistant is responsible for administering the tuberculin skin test and for interpreting the test results. Although tuberculin skin testing is relatively easy to perform, the procedure must be followed exactly to ensure accurate results. A patient with a tuberculous infection may fail to react to the test if it is performed inaccurately.

SKIN TEST REACTIONS

The substance used in the skin test is tuberculin, which consists of a purified protein derivative (PPD) extracted from a culture of tubercle bacilli (the causative agent of tuberculosis), to test for sensitivity to the microorganism. When introduced into the skin of an individual with an active or dormant case of tuberculosis, tuberculin will cause a localized thickening of the skin, resulting in an abnormally hard spot termed **induration.** Induration is caused by an accumulation of small sensitized lymphocytes and occurs in the area in which the tuberculin was injected into the skin. Tuberculin skin test reactions are based on the amount of induration present and are interpreted according to the manufacturer's instructions that accompany the test.

POSITIVE REACTION

A positive reaction to a tuberculin skin test indicates the presence of a tuberculous infection; however, it does not differentiate between the active and dormant states of the infection. This means that the individual had or now has a tuberculous infection but does not necessarily mean that the patient has the active tuberculosis disease. Therefore, a positive reaction will warrant further diagnostic procedures before the physician can make a final diagnosis. Additional procedures used to detect the presence of an active tuberculous infection include an x-ray study of the patient's chest and microbiologic examination of the patient's sputum for the presence of tubercle bacilli.

METHODS FOR TUBERCULIN SKIN TESTING

Several methods are used for tuberculin skin testing; the most commonly used methods are the **Mantoux**

PUTTING IT ALL *into* PRACTICE

▶ **THERESA CLINE:** *There was one experience that I will* never *forget relating to the administration of an injection because it taught our entire office staff a very valuable lesson. It involved a woman who came to our office because she had lacerated her wrist while using a butcher knife. After the wound was sutured, I proceeded to give her a tetanus injection because she was past due for one. Shortly thereafter, she became very nauseated and dizzy, and I made her lie down on the examining table. She asked me to get her a cold drink of water and I left the room to do so. Apparently, while I was gone she must have tried to sit up or turn over because she rolled off the table and struck the back of her head on the floor. She sustained a laceration to her scalp which also had to be sutured. Owing to her persistent symptoms of severe nausea, vomiting, and headache, it was decided that she should be admitted to the hospital for neurologic observation and x-ray studies.*

The vitally important lesson that this experience taught everyone in our office was that you must never leave a patient alone, not even for a minute to get something if there is the slightest indication that they are not feeling perfectly fine. Another staff member should be called to obtain whatever is needed, and from that point on, this has always been our office policy and procedure.

test and the **tine test.** The Mantoux test is administered using an intradermal needle and syringe, whereas the tine test uses a sterile plastic unit containing four stainless steel tines for puncturing the skin. The Mantoux test and the tine test have similar guidelines for administering and reading the tests, which are presented next. Procedures specific to each test are presented following these general guidelines.

ADMINISTERING THE TUBERCULIN SKIN TEST

1. The anterior forearm, approximately 4 inches below the bend in the elbow, should be used as the site of administration of the test; hairy areas of the skin, scar tissue, and areas without adequate subcutaneous tissue should be avoided.
2. The skin must be cleansed thoroughly and allowed to dry completely before the test is administered. Commonly used cleansing agents include alcohol and acetone.
3. The tuberculin must be deposited in the superficial layers of the skin. If blood appears at the puncture site once the test has been administered, it is not significant and will not interfere with the test.
4. Once the test has been administered, it must be read within 48 to 72 hours. The patient may be instructed to return to the medical office to have it read, or the medical assistant may need to instruct the patient in the proper procedure for reading the test at home.

READING THE TUBERCULIN TEST RESULTS

1. The test results must be read in good lighting (within 48 to 72 hours).
2. The medical assistant must instruct the patient to flex the arm at the elbow.
3. The test results are read using both inspection and palpation. If induration is present, the medical assistant should rub the finger lightly from the area of normal skin (without induration) to the indurated area to assess its size. The area of induration is then measured in millimeters. The extent of induration present is the only criterion used in determining a positive reaction. If erythema is present without induration, the results are interpreted as negative.

MANTOUX TEST

The Mantoux test is administered through an intradermal injection using a tuberculin syringe with a capacity of 1.0 ml and a short (⅜ to ½ inch) needle with a gauge of 26 to 27. The amount of solution that is injected is 0.1 ml, which is drawn into the syringe from a multiple-dose vial containing the Mantoux tuberculin solution.

It is important that the medical assistant draw up the proper amount of tuberculin solution. Injecting too much of the solution might elicit a reaction not caused by a tuberculous infection, whereas injecting too little of the solution results in not enough solution being injected into the skin to elicit a reaction. This will invalidate the test, because if no reaction occurs, it cannot be accepted as a negative reaction. Procedure 7–3, Preparing the Injection, and Procedure 7–7, Ad-

ministering an Intradermal Injection, should be followed to prepare and administer the Mantoux test.

The medical assistant must make sure to inject the solution into the superficial skin layers to form a wheal. If the injection is made into the subcutaneous layer, a wheal will not form and the test will yield a false-negative result, whereas a too-shallow injection may cause leakage of the tuberculin solution onto the skin. In either case, the medical assistant must repeat the test again at another site at least 2 inches away.

The medical assistant should not massage the site after injecting the solution because the solution is not intended to be absorbed into the tissues. In addition, massaging may cause leakage of the tuberculin solution out through the needle puncture site.

The test results must be read in good lighting within 48 to 72 hours. The diameter of induration should be measured transversely to the long axis of the forearm, and the results should be recorded in millimeters. Results should never be recorded as positive or negative. Mantoux tuberculin skin test results are interpreted as follows:

Positive Induration of 10 mm or more constitutes a positive reaction and warrants further diagnostic procedures to determine whether active tuberculosis is present. (*Note:* An induration of 5 mm or even smaller should be interpreted as a positive reaction for HIV-infected persons and close contacts of a person with infectious tuberculosis).

Doubtful Induration measuring 5 to 9 mm means that retesting is recommended, using a different site of injection.

Negative Induration of less than 5 mm constitutes a negative reaction.

TINE TEST

The tine test, a multiple puncture test, is convenient and easy to administer; therefore, it is especially useful for tuberculin screening. A sterile disposable intradermal test device is used that consists of a stainless steel disc attached to a plastic handle. Four triangular prongs or tines, approximately 2 mm long, project from the disc; these tines have been impregnated with tuberculin. The patient is inoculated intradermally to a depth of 1 to 2 mm by simple pressure on the skin, and the tuberculin on the tines is deposited into the skin layers.

The medical assistant frequently administers the tine test in the medical office and is also responsible for reading the test results in the office or instructing the patient in reading the results at home and reporting them to the office. If the tine test reaction is positive, most physicians confirm the positive reaction by performing the Mantoux test. The procedure for administering and reading a tine test follows in Procedure 7–8.

Highlight on Tuberculosis

For the first time since 1953, the incidence of tuberculosis (TB) in the United States appears to be rising. Until now, public health officials considered TB a disease that had been conquered. Ten million people are infected with tuberculosis, and 4 to 5 percent of new cases remain undiagnosed until death. In addition, outbreaks of drug-resistant strains of TB have appeared in patients in hospitals, prisons, and community health clinics across the country.

Although any part of the body can be infected, the TB organism prefers body tissues with high oxygen concentrations, such as the lungs. That is why approximately 85 percent of individuals with TB have pulmonary tuberculosis. TB is not highly contagious, and prolonged contact with an infected individual is usually required before the disease develops. This is because the natural defense mechanisms in the upper respiratory tract prevent most inhaled TB organisms from reaching the lungs.

Individuals at greatest risk for contracting tuberculosis from infected patients are young children whose immune systems are not fully developed, the elderly whose immune systems are diminished, and individuals with immune deficiency diseases such as AIDS. There has also been an increase in environments conducive to the transmission of tuberculosis, which include long-term care facilities such as nursing homes and prisons.

The tuberculin skin test is used to identify individuals infected with the TB organism. A positive reaction occurs in 2 to 10 weeks after an individual becomes infected with tuberculosis. Most authorities believe that the Mantoux tuberculin test is more specific and accurate than the tine test. This is because the Mantoux test uses a known amount of tuberculin (0.10 ml of PPD), compared with the tine test in which the tuberculin cannot be as precisely controlled. Because of this, authorities recommend that the tine test be used only for screening individuals at low risk for tuberculosis infection.

Fortunately, TB can be treated. Antibiotics have been available since the 1940s to cure TB and thereby help prevent its spread. Unless antibiotic drug resistance occurs, most patients are able to leave the hospital shortly after beginning drug therapy. Discharge, however, does not mean that the patient is completely cured. Compared with most other infectious diseases, treatment for TB is lengthy, typically lasting 6 months to a year. After 2 to 4 weeks of drug therapy, the disease is no longer contagious to others and the patient can resume a normal lifestyle. If the patient does not comply with the drug therapy regimen, however, some of the TB organisms will survive and the patient will be at risk for a recurrence of the disease.

TB is a reportable disease; therefore, physicians must notify the local health department of cases of tuberculosis. The physician is also required to keep public health officials informed of the patient's compliance with the drug therapy regimen. To help prevent the spread of tuberculosis, public health officials conduct investigations in an attempt to locate anyone who may have become infected from each known case.

7

PROCEDURE

7–8

Administering a Tine Test

EQUIPMENT/SUPPLIES:	Tine test	Disposable gloves
	Antiseptic wipe	Biohazard sharps container

1. **Procedural Step.** Wash the hands.
2. **Procedural Step.** Greet and identify the patient. Introduce yourself and explain the procedure.
3. **Procedural Step.** Select an appropriate site to administer the tine test. The anterior surface of the forearm, approximately 4 inches below the bend of the elbow, is recommended. Hairy areas of the skin, areas with blemishes, scar tissue, and areas without adequate subcutaneous tissue should be avoided.
   Principle. Hairy areas of the skin and areas with blemishes make it difficult to read the test results.

4. **Procedural Step.** Prepare the site. Cleanse the area with an antiseptic wipe. Allow the area to dry completely. Do not touch the site once it has been cleansed.

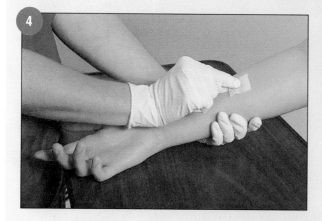

Principle. Touching the site after cleansing contaminates it, and the cleansing process will need to be repeated.

5. **Procedural Step.** Apply gloves. Expose the four tuberculin-coated tines using the following technique: Hold the protective plastic cap with one hand and, with the other hand, use a twisting pulling motion on the cap covering the tines, thereby removing the cap and exposing the tines.
Principle. Gloves provide a barrier precaution against bloodborne pathogens.

6. **Procedural Step.** Grasp the forearm with the nondominant hand immediately behind the proposed

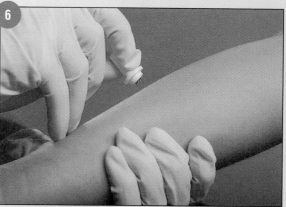

site of administration of the test, and stretch the skin of the forearm tightly to prevent the patient's arm from jerking during administration.
Principle. If the patient jerked the arm during administration of the test, it could result in a scratch on the arm. Stretching the skin will permit easier insertion of the tines.

7. **Procedural Step.** Hold the tine test device in the dominant hand, place the plastic disc (with the four tines) on the patient's skin, and hold for at least 1 second (between 1 and 2 seconds is recommended) to allow the tines to pierce the skin. Sufficient pressure should be exerted so that the four puncture sites and the circular depression from the plastic base are visible on the patient's skin.
Principle. The tines penetrate the skin, thereby introducing the tuberculin on the tines into the patient's skin.

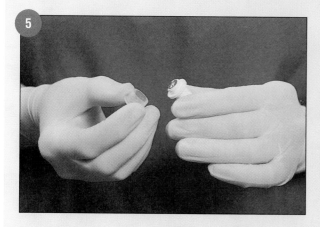

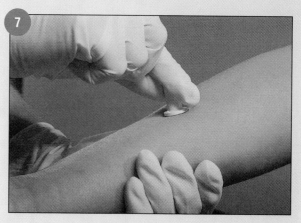

Continued

8. **Procedural Step.** Release the tension from the grasp on the patient's forearm, and withdraw the tine test unit. Do *not* massage or rub the test site after application of the tines.

Principle. The incidence of bleeding at the test site is reduced if the tension on the forearm is released before the tines are withdrawn. The test site should not be massaged because the tuberculin is intended to be deposited into the skin layers and not absorbed into the tissues.

9. **Procedural Step.** Discard the plastic disc in a biohazard sharps container. Local care of the skin is not necessary. Some minor bleeding may occur, but this does not interfere with the test results.

Principle. Once used, the tine test unit is contaminated and should never be reused.

10. **Procedural Step.** Remove gloves, and wash the hands.

11. **Procedural Step.** Instruct the patient to return for a reading of the test in 48 to 72 hours, or instruct the patient in reading the test at home and reporting results.

Principle. The response to the tuberculin deposited in the patient's skin occurs within 24 to 72 hours; therefore, the skin test results must be read within 48 to 72 hours.

12. **Procedural Step.** Chart the procedure. Include the date and time, the name of the test administered (tine test), the site of administration, and any unusual patient reactions.

Principle. Recording the site of administration facilitates locating the test site if the patient will be returning to the medical office to have the test read.

CHARTING EXAMPLE

Date	
2/21/2002	1:15 p.m. Tine test admin to the ⓡ ant forearm. Instructed patient to return on 2/23 to have results read. ———— T. Cline, CMA

7–9

Reading the Tine Test Results

EQUIPMENT/SUPPLIES: **Millimeter ruler**
Disposable gloves

1. **Procedural Step.** Greet and identify the patient. Introduce yourself and explain the procedure.
2. **Procedural Step.** Work in a quiet well-lit atmosphere.
3. **Procedural Step.** Wash the hands and apply gloves.
4. **Procedural Step.** Ask the patient to flex the arm at the elbow.
5. **Procedural Step.** Locate the application site by inspecting the patient's arm for the presence of the four-point pattern.
6. **Procedural Step.** Read the test results. Gently rub your finger over the test site to palpate for the presence of induration. If induration is present, the area should be lightly rubbed from the area of normal skin (without induration) to the indurated area

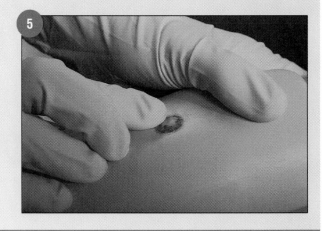

to assess the size of the area of induration present. Measure the diameter of the largest single reaction around one of the puncture sites with a millimeter ruler (supplied by the manufacturer). The results of the tine test are interpreted as follows:

A. Positive Reactions

a. Vesiculation: **Vesiculation** is the formation of vesicles, which are fluid-containing lesions of the skin. If vesiculation is present, the test is interpreted as positive and will warrant further diagnostic procedures to determine whether active tuberculosis is present.

b. Induration 2 mm or greater is interpreted as a positive reaction. Most physicians confirm the positive reaction by performing the Mantoux test (before performing further diagnostic procedures).

B. Negative Reaction: Induration less than 2 mm constitutes a negative reaction.

Principle. Vesiculation or induration 2 mm or greater is the only criterion used to determine a positive reaction. Erythema without the presence of vesicles or induration constitutes a negative reaction.

7. **Procedural Step.** Wash the hands.

8. **Procedural Step.** Chart the results. Include the date and time, the name of the test (tine test), and the test results (recorded in millimeters).

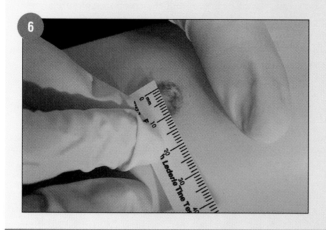

CHARTING EXAMPLE

Date	
2/23/2002	2:00 p.m. Tine test: 9 mm induration.
	No vesicles present. ———— T. Cline, CMA

ALLERGY TESTING

ALLERGY

An allergy is an abnormal hypersensitivity of the body to substances that are ordinarily harmless; these substances are known as **allergens.** Allergens enter the body by being inhaled, by being swallowed, by being injected, or by contact with the skin. Almost any substance in the environment can be an allergen. Common examples of allergens include plant pollens, molds, house dust, animal danders, feather pillows, dyes, soaps, detergents, cosmetics, certain foods and medications, and insect stings.

The exact cause of allergies is not fully understood. In many cases, the tendency to develop allergies seems to be inherited because children of allergic parents tend to exhibit more allergic symptoms than children of nonallergic parents do. Although allergies can develop at any age, children are more apt to develop allergies than are older individuals.

ALLERGIC REACTION

When an allergen enters the body of an allergic person for the first time, it stimulates the body to produce antibodies to that allergen. These antibodies are usually of a type known as IgE antibodies. After the initial sensitization, allergic antibodies combine with the allergen in the body, resulting in an allergen-antibody reaction. When such a reaction occurs, histamine is released in significant amounts, causing allergic symptoms. Allergen-antibody reactions may involve any system of the body; however, the ones most frequently affected are the respiratory and the integumentary systems. Allergic symptoms can range from mild to very severe, as is the case with the potentially fatal anaphylactic reaction.

Depending on the allergen and the body system affected, allergies appear in different forms in an individual. Table 7–9 lists the common clinical forms and symptoms of allergies.

TABLE 7-9

Clinical Forms of Allergies

Allergic Rhinitis	An inflammation of the mucous membrane of the nose caused by allergies. Symptoms include nasal congestion, sneezing, and a runny nose. An individual may have seasonal allergic rhinitis, meaning that the nasal mucosa is inflamed only during certain seasons of the year, as typically occurs with hay fever. On the other hand, an individual may have perennial rhinitis in which the nasal mucosa is inflamed year-round. This type of allergic rhinitis is commonly caused by allergens that are always present in the environment, such as house dust and animal danders.
Hay Fever	Caused by an allergy to molds or the pollen of trees, grasses, or weeds. The term *hay fever* is completely misleading, because hay fever is not caused by hay nor does it result in a fever. The term was first used in the early 1800s by English physicians treating patients with allergies to grass pollens. The symptoms of hay fever and the common cold are almost identical. Sufferers of both experience episodes of sneezing, itching and watery eyes, runny and stuffy nose, and a burning sensation of the palate and throat. Hay fever is seasonal in nature, occurring when there is pollen in the air. Depending on the geographic location, hay fever may occur in the spring, summer, or fall and last until the first frost.
Asthma	A condition characterized by wheezing, coughing, and dyspnea. During an asthmatic attack, the bronchioles constrict and become clogged with mucus, which accounts for many of the symptoms of asthma. Asthma may occur at any age but is more common in children and young adults and, if not treated, can lead to serious complications such as permanent lung damage. It is frequently, but not always, associated with a family history of allergy. Any of the common allergens such as house dust, pollens, molds, or animal danders may trigger an asthmatic attack. Asthmatic attacks also may be caused by nonspecific factors such as air pollutants, tobacco smoke, chemical fumes, vigorous exercise, respiratory infections, exposure to cold, and emotional stress.
Urticaria	Urticaria, or hives, is an outbreak on the skin of welts of varying size that are redder or paler than the surrounding skin and are accompanied by intense itching. When the swellings are large and invade deeper tissues, the condition is known as angioedema. Hives may develop on the face or lips or even internally. Allergies to food or drugs (especially penicillin and aspirin) and insect bites often cause hives to occur, but they may also result from an underlying disease state or occur after exercise. In many cases, the exact cause of the urticaria cannot be determined.
Contact Dermatitis	A rash caused by direct contact with the skin of an allergen such as cosmetics, perfumes, deodorants, rubber, plastics, and clothing treated with certain preservatives or dyes. Symptoms include swelling, blistering, oozing, and scaling. The rash usually occurs only on the area of the body that has come into contact with the allergen. The most common cause of contact dermatitis is poison ivy, poison oak, and sumac.
Eczema	A noncontagious rash accompanied by redness, itching, vesicles, oozing, crusting, and scaling. Eczema is a common allergic reaction in children, but it may also occur in adults, usually in a more severe form. The rash commonly appears on the face, neck, and folds of the elbows and knees. Eczema is frequently associated with allergies, and substances to which a person is allergic may aggravate it. Foods may be important areas of this problem, particularly milk, fish, or eggs. Allergens that are inhaled, such as dust and pollen, rarely cause eczema.

7

DIAGNOSIS AND TREATMENT

The best means of preventing allergic symptoms is to identify and avoid the offending allergen or allergens. The first and most important step in this process involves the completion of a very careful and detailed medical history by the physician. Of particular importance to the diagnosis of an allergy are the patient's home and work environment, diet, and living habits. The physician also performs a thorough physical exam-ination to detect conditions resulting from allergies, such as nasal polyps, wheezing, skin rashes, and urti-caria.

Once the medical history and physical examination have been completed, the physician may order diagnos-tic allergy tests. Allergy testing is performed to confirm information obtained through the medical history and physical examination. The most common type of al-lergy tests ordered include direct skin testing and the

Highlight on Allergens

HOUSE DUST

There are many components in house dust to which an individual may be allergic—the most significant of these is the house dust mite. Dust mites thrive in warm humid conditions and feed on scales shed from human skin; therefore they are commonly found in mattresses, carpets, stuffed animals, and upholstered furniture. It is the waste products of these dust mites to which an individual reacts who is allergic to house dust.

There is no shortage of food for the dust mite, since one person sheds up to 1 gram of scales per day, which is enough to feed thousands of mites for months. *Dermatophagoides pteronyssinus* and *Dermatophagoides farinae* are the most common house dust mites and are present in varying numbers in virtually every home. Mites occur in greatest numbers in bedding, particularly in mattresses; there may be up to 5,000 mites in each gram of dust from a mattress. Sufferers will often notice that symptoms become much worse when the bedding is disturbed and allergenic material becomes airborne. Practices that eliminate dust also reduce the number of dust mites in a household.

INSECT STINGS

It is estimated that one of every 125 Americans is allergic to insect stings. Approximately 40 people in the United States die each year from a severe allergic reaction to insect stings. The incidence of deaths is low because most people know they need to obtain medical attention immediately if an allergic reaction begins to occur.

Almost all the insects whose venom can cause allergic reactions belong to a group called Hymenoptera, which includes honeybees and bumblebees, wasps, yellow jackets, and hornets. When a honeybee stings, its stinger remains imbedded in the skin of the victim, causing the bee to die as it tries to tear itself away. Wasps, yellow jackets, and hornets are more aggressive than bees and can sting repeatedly. Hornets are the most aggressive of the group and may sting even when not provoked. Yellow jackets are close behind in aggressiveness, whereas wasps usually sting only if someone interferes with them near their nest.

If an insect sting does not cause an allergic reaction within 30 minutes, chances are excellent that no problem will occur. A normal reaction to an insect sting includes localized pain, redness, swelling, and itching lasting 1 to 2 days. Any generalized reaction not arising directly from the area of the sting is almost certain to be an anaphylatic reaction, which begins with such symptoms as sneezing, hives, itching, angioedema, erythema, and disorientation and progresses to difficulty in breathing, dizziness, faintness, and loss of consciousness. Medical care should be sought immediately because most fatalities occur within the first 2 hours after the sting. Because time is a factor, individuals who are known to have a severe allergy to insect stings are provided with an anaphylactic emergency treatment kit containing epinephrine in a prefilled syringe and oral antihistamines. In this way, treatment for a severe allergic reaction can be started as soon as possible.

PENICILLIN

Penicillin is one of the most common causes of allergic drug reactions. Approximately 2 to 5 percent of individuals are allergic to penicillin. The reaction may be mild and completely overlooked or confused with the symptoms of the disease being treated with the drug, or it can be more serious and take the form of severe dermatitis or an anaphylactic reaction. Death due to a severe anaphylactic reaction is rare, occurring only in 0.01 percent of patients being treated with penicillin.

Penicillin was discovered in 1929 by Sir Alexander Fleming but was not used as a therapeutic drug until 1940. By 1944, it was evident that some of the side effects of penicillin were allergic in nature; the first recorded death due to an anaphylactic reaction occurred in 1945.

Oral administration of penicillin is safer than a penicillin injection because it has a lower frequency of severe allergic reactions. There have been only six reported deaths from oral administration of penicillin.

Approximately 95 percent of serious reactions occur within 1 hour following a penicillin injection. The best preventive measure, therefore, is to keep the patient under direct observation for at least 30 minutes after administration of the injection.

radioallergosorbent assay (RAST) test, which are described in more detail in the following section.

The general treatment of allergies includes avoidance of the allergen (if possible); alleviation of the symptoms through drug therapy, such as antihistamines, decongestants, bronchodilators, and inhaled steroids; and decreasing the sensitivity of the body to the allergen by the administration of allergy injections, or desensitization injections.

TYPES OF ALLERGY TESTS

The purpose of allergy testing is to determine the specific substances or allergens that are causing the patient's allergic symptoms. The two main categories of allergy tests are the direct skin tests and the RAST test. The medical assistant is often responsible for performing direct skin testing in the medical office. The RAST test is performed by an outside laboratory on a blood specimen. The medical assistant may be responsible for performing a venipuncture to obtain the blood specimen.

Direct Skin Testing

Direct skin testing involves applying extracts of common allergens to the skin and observing the body's reaction to them. The extract is applied either topically to the skin (patch testing) or into the superficial skin layers (skin-prick and intradermal testing). The advantage of direct skin testing is that test results are obtained immediately. This in vivo administration of allergens, however, has the potential to cause adverse reactions, the least common but most serious being an anaphylactic reaction. The medical assistant should have a thorough knowledge of the symptoms of an anaphylactic reaction and alert the physician immediately if they begin in the patient.

Regardless of the specific type of skin test (patch, skin-prick, or intradermal), some general guidelines should be followed:

1. The patient should be instructed to discontinue the use of antihistamines for 3 days before the skin testing; otherwise false-negative results may occur.
2. The area of application should be free from hair, scar tissue, and dermatitis, and it should be lightly pigmented to permit good visualization and palpation of test reactions. Recommended sites include the anterior forearm and the middle of the back. The back is usually used for patch and skin-prick testing, whereas the forearm is typically used for intradermal skin testing.
3. The area of application should be cleansed thoroughly with an antiseptic wipe and allowed to dry completely.
4. Gloves should be worn when the allergy testing involves puncture of the skin which includes both skin-prick testing and intradermal skin testing. Gloves protect the medical assistant from exposure to bloodborne pathogens, as required by the OSHA Standard.
5. The allergen extracts should be spaced approximately 2 inches apart to provide enough surface area for a sizeable reaction to take place. If not enough surface area is available; large adjacent reactions may run together, making it difficult to read test results.
6. The test sites should be labeled so that the site of application of each allergen extract can be later identified when reading results.
7. The skin testing may cause a mild allergic reaction, such as a runny nose, sneezing, and mild wheezing 8 to 24 hours following skin-prick and intradermal skin testing. The patient should be made aware of

this reaction and told to contact the physician if a more severe reaction than this occurs.

Patch Testing

Patch testing is primarily used to identify allergens causing contact dermatitis. Patch testing involves the topical application of each allergen to the skin, using a "patch." A patch consists of a small piece of gauze or filter paper impregnated with the allergen, which is applied to the skin and taped in place with hypoallergenic tape (Fig. 7–15). Allergens commonly applied include plants, topical drugs, resins, metals, cosmetics, dyes, and chemicals. The patient should be instructed to leave the patches in place, keep them dry, and return to the medical office in 48 hours to have the results read. When the patient returns to the office, the patches are carefully removed and the results are read 20 minutes later. The delayed reading time allows for lessening of any redness that may occur from the tape removal.

Test results are recorded as positive or negative. Positive reactions are characterized by itching, erythema, and induration, often accompanied by vesiculation. In strongly positive responses, the reaction may extend beyond the margin of the patch. Positive results are further graded on a quantitative 1+ to 3+ scoring system according to the type of reaction (Table 7–10).

Skin-Prick Testing

Skin-prick testing is usually performed to diagnose allergies to common allergens, particularly those that are inhaled, such as house dust, pollens, and molds. Skin-prick testing involves the application of a number of allergen extracts to the skin, followed by pricking each with a sterile needle or other sharp instrument (Fig. 7–16). The number of allergen extracts applied during one office visit usually ranges between 20 and 30. Pricking the skin deposits the allergens in the outer

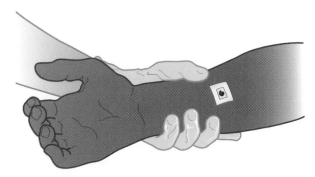

■ **FIGURE 7–15.** Patch testing. A patch consists of a small piece of gauze or filter paper impregnated with the allergen, which is applied to the skin and taped in place.

Guidelines for Recording Direct Skin Test Results

Patch Test

—	No reaction
+1	Presence of erythema and edema, possibly papules
+2	Presence of erythema, edema, and vesicles, possibly papules
+3	Erythema, vesicles, and severe edema

Skin-Prick Testing and Intradermal Testing

—	No reaction
±1	Induration of 1 mm or less
+1	Induration greater than 1 mm and up to 5 mm in diameter
+2	Induration greater than 5 mm and up to 10 mm in diameter
+3	Induration greater than 10 mm and up to 15 mm in diameter
+4	Induration greater than 15 mm in diameter

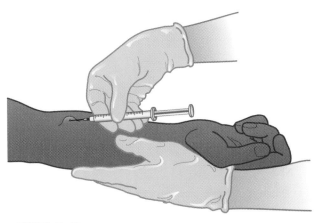

■ **FIGURE 7–17.** Intradermal skin testing. Intradermal testing involves the injection of a small amount of allergen extract into the superficial skin layers through the intradermal route of administration.

layers of the skin to allow each to react with the body tissues.

The following guidelines should be followed for skin-prick testing: The extracts should be placed on the skin in rows in a specific pattern. This, along with labeling the test sites with a felt-tipped pen, helps keep track of the location of each extract. Only a single drop of extract should be placed on the skin; more than this amount may cause the extracts to diffuse and run together. A sterile needle should be passed through

the drop, and the point should lightly lift the top layer of skin without causing bleeding. It is important to wipe the needle dry with a sterile swab between each prick to prevent one extract from mixing with the next, leading to inaccurate test results.

The maximum reaction is usually seen between 15 and 20 minutes. During this time, the test sites should be left uncovered and the patient should be instructed not to touch them. The area should not be wiped, because this removes the allergen extract, resulting in false-negative results. The results are read (after 15 to 20 minutes) using a millimeter ruler.

Positive reactions are characterized by an area of induration surrounded by redness and itching. Positive results are recorded by measuring the size of the induration in millimeters and converting it to a numerical scale based on the extent of the induration present (refer to Table 7–10). Any redness should be ignored. Refer to Figure 7–18 for an illustration of skin test results. If only a mild reaction occurs, the physician may perform more specific intradermal skin testing.

Intradermal Skin Testing

Intradermal skin testing is similar to skin-prick testing but it is more specific. The number of skin tests performed during one office visit ranges from 5 to 30. Because there is a greater chance of adverse allergic reactions occurring with intradermal skin testing, the physician often starts with skin-prick testing in individuals who are suspected of being highly allergic as determined by the medical history and the results of the physical examination.

Intradermal skin testing involves the injection of a small amount of allergen extract into the superficial skin layers (0.02 to 0.05 ml) through the intradermal route of administration (Fig. 7–17). A tuberculin sy-

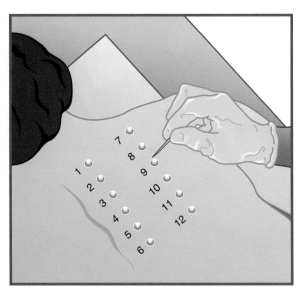

■ **FIGURE 7–16.** Skin-prick testing. Skin-prick testing involves the application of a number of allergen extracts to the skin, followed by the pricking of each with a sterile needle.

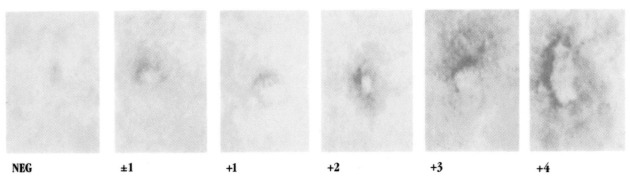

| NEG | ±1 | +1 | +2 | +3 | +4 |

■ **FIGURE 7–18.** Skin-prick and intradermal skin test results. (Copyright and courtesy of Hollister-Stier.)

ringe is used to administer the test, and the allergen extract is injected until a wheal forms following the procedure for administering an intradermal injection (Procedure 7–7). After 15 to 20 minutes, the test sites are observed for reactions. Positive reactions are characterized by an area of induration surrounded by redness and itching. As with skin-prick testing, positive results are recorded by measuring the size of the induration in millimeters and converting it to a numeric scale based on the amount of induration present (refer to Fig. 7–18 and Table 7–10).

RAST Testing

The RAST (radioallergosorbent test) measures the amount of IgE antibodies in the blood to common allergens. A sample of the patient's blood is sent to an outside laboratory, where it is exposed to radioactively tagged allergens. A radiation detection device is then used to measure the amount of IgE antibodies to the allergens. The advantages of the RAST test over direct skin testing are as follows: The results are not affected by medications (such as antihistamines); there is no danger of adverse allergic reactions occurring because the test is performed in vitro, meaning outside the body; and RAST testing can be performed on patients who have skin eruptions and are unable to undergo direct skin testing because of a lack of an intact skin surface area. On the other hand, RAST testing is expensive and does not provide immediate test results as does direct skin testing.

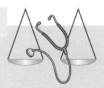

MEDICAL PRACTICE AND THE LAW

Medications have the potential to do great good and also to do great harm. One of the most common sources of lawsuits is medication related, so the medical assistant has a tremendous responsibility to follow all procedures in order to avoid doing harm.

Many patients are prescribed multiple medications from various physicians. When performing a medication evaluation, it is best to ask the patient to bring in all medications they are currently taking. Be sure to include over-the-counter medications such as vitamins, aspirin, or nutritional supplements.

When administering medications, first check a

current medication reference to determine potential adverse effects. Refer to the *Physician's Desk Reference* or package insert for this information. This information may also be available on a computer program. Next, check for patient allergies. Check the chart, then ask the patient this question before administering the medication. Be sure the patient is informed why the drug is being given, its name, and common side effects. Watch the patient take the drug if given orally. If given parenterally, be sure to use proper technique to prevent injury. Follow the six "rights" of medication administration and make sure to check the medication label three times before

administering any medication. This all may seem cumbersome, but if any steps are omitted and the patient has an adverse reaction, you could be held liable.

Controlled drugs have specific laws that regulate their ordering, storing, and dispensing. Failure to adhere to these regulations could cause the physician to lose his or her license. Be aware of drug-seeking behavior of patients, as well as physical symptoms of addiction. You also have a duty to be aware of coworkers' behavior, and report to the physician any individual who appears chemically impaired, or you suspect of diverting medications for themselves.

CERTIFICATION REVIEW

- A drug is a chemical that is used for the treatment, prevention, or diagnosis of disease. Medication that is administered is given to the patient at the office. Medication is prescribed when a physician provides the patient with a written prescription for a drug to be filled at a pharmacy. Dispensed medication is either given or sold to the patient at the office to be taken at home.
- The chemical name of a drug provides a precise description of a drug's chemical composition. The generic name is assigned by the pharmaceutical manufacturer who first develops the drug. The official name is the name under which the drug is listed in official publications. The brand name is the name under which a pharmaceutical manufacturer markets a drug.
- Three systems of measurement are used in the United States for prescribing and administering medication: the metric system, the apothecary system, and the household system. The metric system is the most common because it is more accurate and easier to use.
- A prescription is an order written by a physician for the dispensing of drugs. The prescription includes directions to the pharmacist for filling the prescription and instructions to the patient for taking the medication.
- Controlled drugs are drugs that have potential for abuse. They are classified into five categories based on their abuse potential. To prescribe or dispense controlled drugs, the physician must register each year with the DEA.
- A patient may experience an allergic reaction to a drug after administration. The reaction is usually mild and may take the form of a rash, rhinitis, or

pruritus. Occasionally, it may be a severe allergic reaction and occur suddenly and immediately. This reaction is known as an anaphylactic reaction.
- The majority of drugs produce side effects. They may be harmless and tolerated in order to obtain the therapeutic effect of the drug. Other side effects may be harmful to the patient and warrant discontinuing the medication.
- The oral route is the most convenient and most widely used method of administering medication. Absorption of most oral medication takes place in the small intestine, although some may be absorbed in the mouth and stomach.
- The parenteral route of administration includes subcutaneous, intramuscular, and intravenous administration of medication. With parenteral administration, medications are absorbed more rapidly and completely. In some cases, the parenteral route is the only way a drug can be given, such as when a patient is unconscious.
- The syringe is used for inserting fluids into the body. Various types of syringes are available to administer injections. The types used most often in the medical office include hypodermic, insulin, and tuberculin. Each needle has a certain gauge; needle gauges for administering medication range between 18 and 27. As the size of the gauge increases, the diameter of the lumen decreases. The length of the needle ranges between 3/8 inch and 3 inches; the length used will be based on the type of injection being given.
- A vial is a closed glass container with a rubber stopper; single-dose and multiple-dose vials are available. An ampule is a small, sealed glass con-

Continued

7

CERTIFICATION REVIEW *Continued*

tainer that holds a single dose of medication. A prefilled disposable syringe or cartridge holds a single dose of medication and does not require drawing up the medication.

☐ A subcutaneous injection is made into the subcutaneous tissue consisting of adipose tissue. The needle length varies from 1/2 to 5/8 inch, and the gauge ranges from 23 to 25. The amount of medication injected through the subcutaneous route should not exceed 1 cc.

☐ Intramuscular injections are made into the muscular layer of the body. An amount of up to 3 cc may be given through the intramuscular route. The length of the needle varies from 1 to 3 inches, and the gauge ranges from 18 to 23, depending on the viscosity of the medication. Intramuscular injection sites include the following: dorsogluteal, deltoid, vastus lateralis, and ventrogluteal.

☐ An intradermal injection is given into the dermal layer of the skin. The size of the needle ranges from 3/8 to 5/8 inch, and the lumen ranges from 25 to 27. The most frequent use of intradermal injections is to administer a skin test such as an allergy skin test of a tuberculin skin test (Mantoux text).

☐ TB is an infectious disease that usually attacks the lungs. The purpose of tuberculin skin testing is to detect the presence of a tuberculin infection. A positive reaction to a tuberculin skin test indicates the presence of a TB infection; however, it does not differentiate between the active and dormant states of the infection; a positive reaction warrants further diagnostic procedures before a final diagnosis can be made.

☐ Allergy skin testing determines the specific allergens that are causing the patient's allergic symptoms. Direct skin testing involves applying extracts of common allergens to the skin then observing the body's reaction to them. Direct skin testing includes patch testing, skin-prick testing, and intradermal skin testing. The RAST test is performed by an outside laboratory on a blood specimen and measures the amount of antibodies in the blood to common allergens.

7

RESOURCES

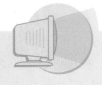

ON THE WEB

For information on pharmacology:

Food and Drug Administration
www.fda.gov

Pharm Info Net
www.pharminfo.com

Drug Enforcement Agency
www.usdoj.gov/dea

RxList: The Internet Drug Index
www.rxlist.com

WWW Virtual Pharmacy
www.cpb.uokhsc.edu/pharmacy/pharmint.html

Pharm Web
www.pharmweb.net

Merck and Company
www.merck.com

For information on allergies:

American Academy of Allergy, Asthma, and Immunology
www.aaaai.org

National Institute of Allergy and Infectious Diseases (NIAID)
www.niaid.nih.gov

For information on alcohol abuse:

Alcoholics Anonymous (AA)
www.alcoholics-anonymous.org

National Institute on Alcohol Abuse and Alcoholism (NIAAA)
www.niaaa.nih.gov

National Council on Alcoholism and Drug Dependency (NCADD)
www.ncadd.org

National Clearinghouse for Alcohol and Drug Information
www.health.org

Al-Anon/Alateen
www.Al-Anon-Alateen.org

Mothers Against Drunk Drivers (MADD)
www.madd.org

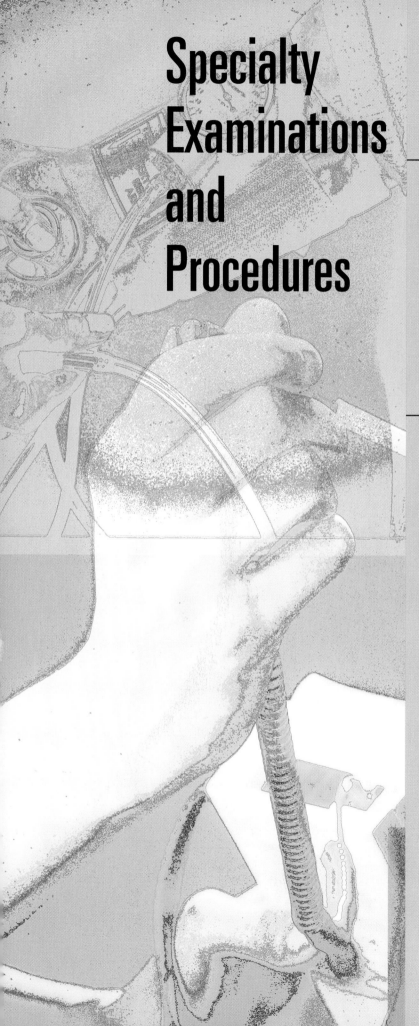

Specialty Examinations and Procedures

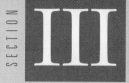
AAMA/CAAHEP COMPETENCIES INCLUDED IN THIS SECTION:

Clinical Competencies

Patient Care

- Obtain vital signs.
- Obtain and record patient history.
- Prepare and maintain examination and treatment areas.
- Prepare patient for and assist with routine and specialty examinations.
- Prepare patient for and assist with procedures, treatments, and minor office surgery.
- Apply pharmacology principles to prepare and administer oral and parenteral medications.
- Maintain medication and immunization records.

Transdisciplinary Competencies

Communicate

- Respond to and initiate written communications.
- Recognize and respond to verbal communications.
- Recognize and respond to nonverbal communications.

Patient Instruction

- Instruct individuals according to their needs.
- Provide instruction for health maintenance and disease prevention.

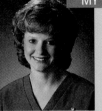

MY NAME IS

Cammie Lindner. *I graduated from an accredited medical assisting program and received an associate's degree in Applied Science. I am a Certified Medical Assistant. In addition, I have completed a course in Otorhinolaryngic Allergies, focusing on allergy testing techniques and treatments.*

I have worked for 10 years for an ear, nose, and throat surgeon. There are administrative responsibilities in my job; however, the focus is mainly on the clinical aspects, including vital signs measurement, allergy testing, immunotherapy, and assisting with office surgeries, such as biopsies, excision of skin lesions, and tympanostomy tube insertions.

I have found my career to be quite rewarding. In particular, I enjoy the allergy practice. The nearly 2 hours of testing allows me the opportunity to learn more about my patients, their interests, and their families.

I went straight from high school to college and always knew that I wanted to work in the health care field.

Eye and Ear Assessment and Procedures

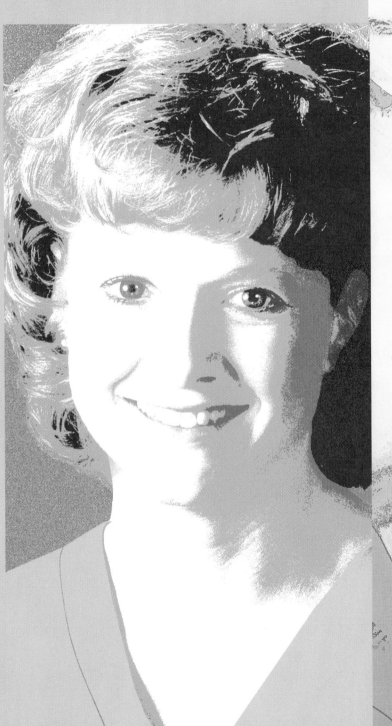

CHAPTER OUTLINE

The Eye
Structure of the Eye
Visual Acuity
  Assessment of Distance Visual
  Acuity
  Assessment of Near Visual
  Acuity
Assessment of Color Vision
  The Ishihara Test
Eye Irrigation
Eye Instillation

The Ear
Structure of the Ear
Assessment of Hearing Acuity
  Types of Hearing Loss
  Hearing Acuity Tests
Ear Irrigation
Ear Instillation

OUTCOMES

After completing this chapter,
you should be able to demonstrate the proper procedures to
perform the following:

1. Assess distance visual acuity.
2. Assess near visual acuity.
3. Assess color vision.
4. Perform an eye irrigation.
5. Perform an eye instillation.
6. Perform an ear irrigation.
7. Perform an ear instillation.

EDUCATIONAL OBJECTIVES

After completing this chapter,
you should be able to do the following:

1. List four tests or procedures
   that are performed on the
   eye and ear in the medical
   office.
2. Define the terms listed in
   the Key Terminology.
3. Identify the structures that
   constitute the eye, and explain the function of each.
4. Define visual acuity.
5. State the causes of myopia,
   hyperopia, and presbyopia,
   and indicate what visual difficulty is present with each.
6. Explain the differences
   among an ophthalmologist,
   an optometrist, and an optician.
7. Explain the significance of
   the top and bottom numbers
   next to each line of letters
   on the Snellen eye chart.
8. Explain the difference between congenital and acquired color vision defects.
9. State three reasons each for
   performing an eye irrigation
   and an eye instillation.
10. Explain the principles underlying the steps in each eye
    procedure.
11. Identify the structures making up the external, middle,
    and outer ear and explain
    the function of each.
12. Identify conditions that may
    cause conductive and sensorineural hearing loss.
13. List and describe three ways
    hearing acuity may be tested.
14. State three reasons each for
    performing an ear irrigation
    and an ear instillation.
15. Explain the principles underlying the steps in each ear
    procedure.

CHAPTER 8

303

8

KEY TERMINOLOGY

audiometer: An instrument used to measure hearing acuity quantitatively for the various frequencies of sound waves.

canthus (KAN-thus): The junction of the eyelids at either corner of the eye.

cerumen: Ear wax.

hyperopia (hî-PER-op-êa): Farsightedness.

impacted: Being wedged firmly together so as to be immovable.

instillation: The dropping of a liquid into a body cavity.

irrigation: The washing of a body canal with a flowing solution.

myopia: Nearsightedness.

ophthalmologist (OP-tha-mall-ô-gist): A medical doctor who specializes in diagnosing and treating disorders of the eye.

optician (OP-tish-in): A professional who interprets and fills ophthalmic prescriptions.

optometrist (OP-tom-i-trist): A licensed practitioner who is skilled in measuring visual acuity and is qualified to prescribe corrective lenses.

otoscope: An instrument for examining the external ear canal and tympanic membrane.

presbyopia (pres-BÊ-ôp-êa): A decrease in the elasticity of the lens due to aging, resulting in a decreased ability to focus on close objects.

refraction (rê-FRAK-shun): The deflection or bending of light rays by a lens.

tympanic membrane: A thin, semi-transparent membrane located between the external ear canal and middle ear that receives and transmits sound waves. (Also known as the eardrum.)

INTRODUCTION

☐ The medical assistant is responsible for performing a variety of assessments and procedures involving the eye and the ear. An understanding of the structure and function of the eye and the ear is essential in mastering skill in these areas.

A distance and near visual acuity test is usually included as part of the routine physical examination. This test is used as a screening device to detect deficiencies in vision.

The medical assistant may be responsible for assessing color vision with the use of specially prepared colored plates. As a result of this testing, color blindness can be detected. Color blindness is an inability to distinguish certain colors; the most common problem is with the colors red and green. This is particularly significant if the patient is involved in an activity or employment that relies upon the ability to distinguish colors, such as electronics, interior decorating, flying a plane, and art.

Hearing tests may also be included as part of the routine physical examination. During contact with the patient, the medical assistant should be alert to any signs that may indicate the patient is having difficulty hearing what is being said. A whispered voice or a ticking watch held next to the patient's ear can be used as a screening test for hearing acuity. The use of tuning forks or an audiometer provides for a more accurate determination of hearing acuity. An **audiometer** is an instrument that emits sound waves at various frequencies. The patient is instructed to indicate when a sound at a given frequency can be heard.

Performing or teaching the patient to perform eye and ear irrigations and instillations is a frequent responsibility of the medical assistant. **Irrigation** is washing a body canal with a flowing solution. **Instillation** is dropping a liquid into a body cavity. Eye and ear irrigations and instillations should be performed using the important principles of medical asepsis outlined in Chapter 1.

The Eye

STRUCTURE OF THE EYE

☐ Three different layers make up the eye (Fig. 8–1). The outer layer is the **sclera,** which is composed of tough, white fibrous connective tissue. The front part of the sclera is modified to form a transparent covering over the colored part of the eye; this covering is known as the **cornea.**

The middle layer of the eye is the **choroid.** It is composed of many blood vessels and is highly pigmented. The blood vessels nourish the other layers of the eye, whereas the pigment works to absorb stray light rays. The front part of the choroid is specialized into the ciliary body, the suspensory ligaments, and the iris. The **ciliary body** contains muscles that control the shape of the lens. The function of the **suspensory ligaments** is to suspend the lens in place. The **lens** itself is responsible for focusing the light rays on the retina. The colored part of the eye is the **iris,** which controls the size of the pupil. The **pupil** is the opening in the eye that permits the entrance of light rays.

The third and innermost layer of the eye is the **retina.** Light rays come to a focus on the retina and

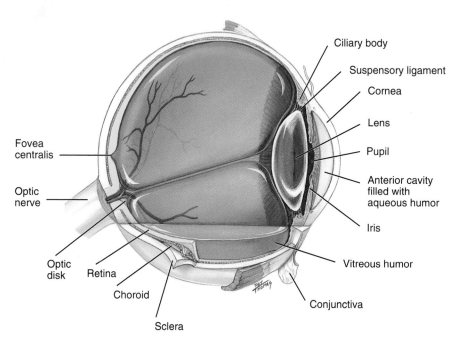

■ **FIGURE 8–1.** The internal structure of the eye. (From Applegate, E. J.: *The Anatomy and Physiology Learning System.* Philadelphia, W. B. Saunders, 1995, p. 191.)

Ciliary body
Suspensory ligament
Cornea
Lens
Pupil
Anterior cavity filled with aqueous humor
Iris
Vitreous humor
Conjunctiva

Fovea centralis
Optic nerve
Optic disk
Retina
Choroid
Sclera

are subsequently transmitted to the brain, by way of the optic nerve, to be interpreted.

The **anterior chamber** is the area between the cornea and iris, and the **posterior chamber** is the area between the iris and lens. Both chambers are filled with a substance known as the **aqueous humor.** Between the lens and the retina is a transparent, jelly-like material filling the eyeball, known as the **vitreous humor.** Its function is to help maintain the shape of the eyeball.

The **conjunctiva** is a membrane that lines the eyelids and covers the front of the eye, except for the cornea. The conjunctiva covering the sclera is transparent except for some capillaries, which allows the white sclera to show through.

VISUAL ACUITY

☐ Visual acuity refers to acuteness or sharpness of vision. A person with normal visual acuity can see clearly and is able to distinguish fine details both close up and at some distance.

Errors of refraction are the most common causes of defects in visual acuity. **Refraction** refers to the ability of the eye to bend the parallel light rays coming into it so they can be focused on the retina. An error of refraction means that the light rays are not being refracted or bent properly and therefore are not adequately focused on the retina. A defect in the shape of the eyeball can cause a refractive error. Errors of refraction can be improved with the use of corrective lenses.

A person who is nearsighted has a condition termed **myopia.** The eyeball is too long from front to back, causing the light rays to be brought to a focus in front of the retina. The myopic person has difficulty seeing objects at a distance and may squint and have headaches as a result of eye strain (Fig. 8–2). A concave lens is used to correct this condition by causing the light rays to come to a focus on the retina.

A person who is farsighted has a condition known as **hyperopia.** The eyeball is too short from front to back, resulting in a different type of refractive error, in which the light rays are brought to a focus behind the retina. This person has difficulty viewing objects at a reading or working distance (Fig. 8–3). A convex lens is used to correct this condition by causing the light rays to come to a focus on the retina.

In most people, a decrease in the elasticity of the lens of the eye begins to occur after age 40 years. This condition is known as **presbyopia,** and it results in a decreased ability to focus clearly on objects close up.

If a defect in visual acuity is detected, the patient is referred to an eye specialist for further evaluation. Several types of specialists are involved in the care of the eyes. An **ophthalmologist** is a medical doctor who specializes in diagnosing and treating disorders of the eye. An ophthalmologist is qualified to prescribe drugs and corrective lenses and to perform eye surgery. An **optometrist** is a licensed practitioner who is skilled in measuring visual acuity. The optometrist is qualified to prescribe corrective lenses for the treatment of refractive errors. This professional is not a physician and therefore is not permitted to diagnose or treat other eye disorders or to perform eye surgery. An **optician** is

8

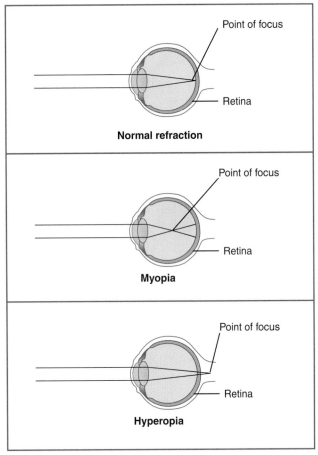

Errors of Refraction

■ **FIGURE 8–2.** Diagram of normal refraction as compared with myopia (nearsightedness) and hyperopia (farsightedness), which are errors of refraction that cause visual defects.

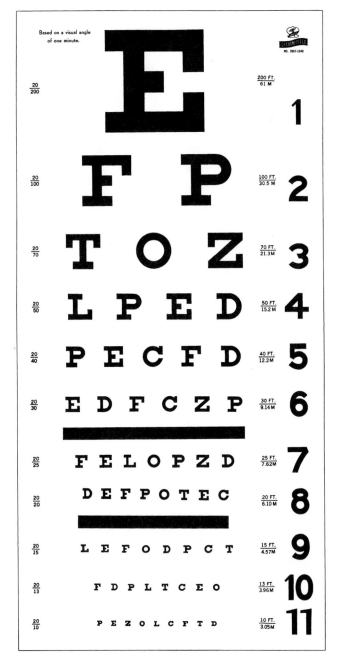

■ **FIGURE 8–3.** A Snellen eye chart consisting of letters in decreasing sizes, which is used to measure distance visual acuity.

a professional who interprets and fills prescriptions for eyeglasses or contact lenses.

ASSESSMENT OF DISTANCE VISUAL ACUITY

Myopia can be diagnosed (in combination with other tests) by a distance visual acuity test. In the medical office, the Snellen eye chart is most often used. There are two types of charts (Figs. 8–3 and 8–4): one type, used for school-aged children and adults, consists of a chart of letters in decreasing sizes. The other type, used for preschool children, non–English-speaking people, and nonreaders, is composed of the capital letter E in decreasing sizes and arranged in different directions. Visual acuity charts with pictures of common objects are also available for use with preschoolers. These charts tend to be less accurate than the Snellen charts. Some children are unable to identify the objects because of lack of recognition rather than a defect in

visual acuity. It is suggested that the Snellen Big E chart be used with preschoolers.

Conducting a Snellen Test

The visual acuity test should be performed in a well-lit room that is free from distractions. The test is usually performed at a distance of 20 feet; this can be conveniently marked off in the medical office with paint or a

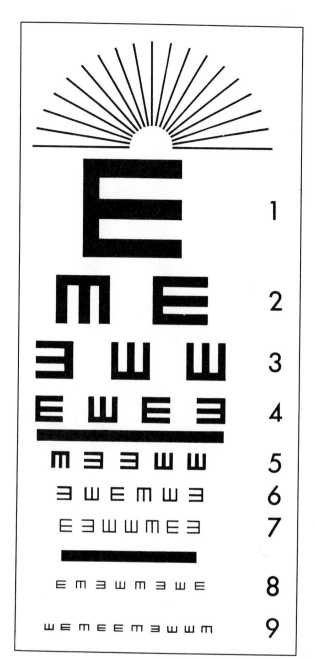

FIGURE 8–4. A Snellen Big E eye chart consisting of the capital letter E in decreasing sizes and arranged in different directions, which is used to measure distance visual acuity.

Highlight on Eye Assessment

It is recommended that individuals under the age of 40 years have a complete eye examination every 3 to 5 years. Individuals from ages 40 to 65 years should have an eye examination every 2 to 4 years. Individuals over age 65 years should have yearly eye examinations.

Individuals who have risk factors for eye disorders should have an eye examination each year. Examples of risk factors include diabetes and hypertension.

Visual acuity is considered normal for the various age groups if it falls within the following values:

Infant	20/200
Child (18 months to 4 years)	20/50
(4 to 8 years)	20/30
(9 years to adult)	20/20
Adult	20/20

Legal blindness is defined as a visual acuity measurement of 20/200 or less in both eyes with the use of corrective lenses.

The term "color blind" is not an accurate term to describe an individual with abnormal color vision, because the inability to distinguish any colors at all is extremely rare. Most individuals with a color vision abnormality are unable to distinguish certain hues of color, such as red and green. Therefore, a better term to use is "color vision defect."

Defective color vision is usually congenital. It is found in 8 percent of men and 5 percent of women.

Studies have shown that there is no significant correlation between defective color vision and increased automobile accidents. The majority of drivers who have a color vision defect are able to distinguish traffic light by the different light intensities and by the position of the light on the traffic signal itself.

piece of tape so that it does not have to be remeasured each time the test is given.

At the side of each row of letters on the chart are two numbers, separated by a line. The number above the line represents the distance (in feet) at which the test is conducted. It is usually 20, as most eye tests are conducted at this distance. The number below the line represents the distance from which a person with normal visual acuity can read the row of letters. The line marked 20/20 indicates normal distance visual acuity, or 20/20 vision. This means a person could read what he or she was supposed to read at a distance of 20 feet.

A visual acuity reading of 20/30 means this was the smallest line that the individual could read at a distance of 20 feet. People with normal acuity would be able to read this line at a distance of 30 feet.

A visual acuity reading of 20/15 means this was the smallest line that the individual could read at a distance of 20 feet. It indicates above-average acuity for distance vision. People with normal acuity would be able to read this line at 15 feet.

The acuity should be measured in each eye separately, traditionally beginning with the right eye. Most physicians prefer that the patient keep contact lenses or glasses on during the test, except for reading glasses;

PROCEDURE

8–1

Assessing Distance Visual Acuity–Snellen Chart

EQUIPMENT/SUPPLIES: Snellen eye chart   Eye occluder

1. **Procedural Step.** Wash the hands.
2. **Procedural Step.** Assemble the equipment. Perform the test in a well-lit room that is free from distractions.
3. **Procedural Step.** Greet and identify the patient. Introduce yourself and explain the procedure. The patient should be told that he or she will be asked to read several lines of letters. The patient should not have an opportunity to study or memorize the letters before beginning the test. The patient should be instructed not to squint during the test, as squinting temporarily improves vision.
4. **Procedural Step.** Determine whether the patient wears contact lenses or glasses (other than reading glasses). If the patient wears such aids, he or she should be told to keep them on during the test.
5. **Procedural Step.** Place the patient in a comfortable position 20 feet from the chart. The patient may sit or stand. (It is helpful to have the distance permanently marked off to prevent having to measure each time the test is performed.)
6. **Procedural Step.** Position the center of the Snellen chart at the patient's eye level. The medical assistant stands next to the chart during the test to indicate to the patient the line to be identified.
   Principle. Make sure the chart is at the patient's eye level rather than your eye level, to provide the most accurate results.
7. **Procedural Step.** Ask the patient to cover the left eye with the eye occluder. Instruct the patient to keep the left eye open. During the test, the medical assistant should check to make sure the patient is keeping the left eye open.
   Principle. Keeping the left eye open prevents squinting of the right eye.
8. **Procedural Step.** Measure the visual acuity of the right eye first. Ask the patient to identify orally one line at a time on the Snellen chart, starting with the 20/70 line (or a line that is several lines above the 20/20 line).

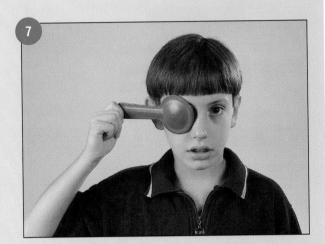

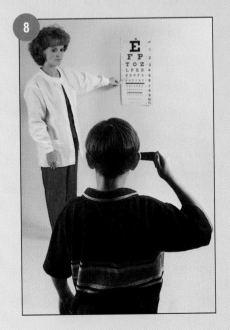

PROCEDURE 8–1

Principle. It is best to start at a line that is above the 20/20 line to give the patient a chance to gain confidence and to become familiar with the test procedure. The medical assistant should establish a pattern of beginning with the same eye each time the test is performed (traditionally the right eye). This helps to reduce errors during the recording of results.

9. **Procedural Step.** If the patient is able to read the 20/70 line, proceed down the chart until the smallest line of letters the patient can read is reached. If the patient is unable to read the 20/70 line, proceed up the chart until the smallest line of letters the patient can read is reached.

10. **Procedural Step.** Observe the patient for any unusual symptoms while he or she is reading the letters, such as squinting, tilting of the head, or watering of the eyes.

    Principle. These symptoms may indicate that the patient is having difficulty identifying the letters.

11. **Procedural Step.** Ask the patient to cover the right eye with the eye occluder and to keep the right eye open. Measure the visual acuity in the left eye as described in Steps 8 through 10.

    During the test the medical assistant should check to make sure the patient is keeping the right eye open.

    Principle. Keeping the right eye open prevents squinting of the left eye.

12. **Procedural Step.** Chart the procedure. Include the date and time, the name of the test (Snellen Test), the visual acuity results, and any unusual symptoms the patient may have exhibited during the test. Also chart whether or not the patient was wearing corrective lenses during the test. Use the following abbreviations.

    $\overline{s}c$—without correction
    $\overline{c}c$—with correction

    To chart the visual acuity results, observe the numbers to the side of the smallest line of letters that the patient was able to read. If one or two letters were missed, the visual acuity is recorded with a minus sign next to the bottom number, along with the number of letters missed. (If more than two letters are missed, the previous line should be recorded.) Latin abbreviations are used to record the visual acuity in each eye. The abbreviations for the right eye is OD and the abbreviation for the left eye is OS.

CHARTING EXAMPLE	
Date	
11/5/2002	3:30 p.m. Snellen Test: OD 20/20-1.
	OS 20/25, $\overline{s}$c. Exhibited squinting while reading
	20/20 line, OD. ————— C. Lindner, CMA

8

---

the medical assistant should record in the patient's chart that corrective lenses were worn by the patient during the test. An eye occluder should be held over the eye not being tested. The patient's hands should not be used to cover the eye, as this may encourage peeking through the fingers, especially in the case of children. The patient should be instructed to leave open the eye not being tested, since closing it causes squinting of the eye that is being tested.

Assessing Distance Visual Acuity in Preschoolers

With minor variations, Procedure 8–1: Assessing Distance Visual Acuity can be used to test distance visual acuity in preschoolers. The Snellen Big E chart is utilized for this purpose.

A child needs a complete and thorough explanation of what is expected of him or her before beginning the test. Tell the child you will be playing a pointing game. Do not force the child to play the game, because the results would then tend to be inaccurate. Draw the capital letter E on an index card, and teach the child to point in the direction of the open part of the E by turning the card in different directions (up, down, to the right, and to the left). Using such phrases as the "fingers" or the "legs of the table" to describe the open part of the E helps the child understand what is expected (Fig. 8–5). Allow the child to practice the pointing game with the index card until you are sure this level of skill has been mastered. Be sure to praise the child when the correct response is given.

The child may need help in holding the eye occluder in place. The aid of another person such as the parent would then be required.

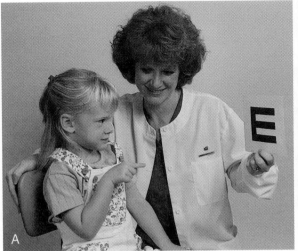
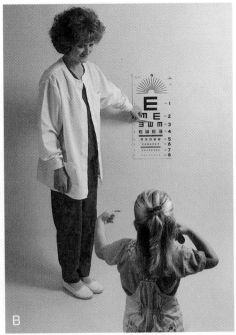

■ **FIGURE 8–5.** *A,* Cammie teaches a preschooler to point in the direction of the open part of the capital letter E. *B,* Cammie performs the Snellen Big E visual acuity test.

No. 1.
.37M

    In the second century of the Christian era, the empire of Rome comprehended the fairest part of the earth, and the most civilized portion of mankind. The frontiers of that extensive monarchy were guarded by ancient renown and disciplined valor. The gentle but powerful influence of laws and manners had gradually cemented the union of the provinces. Their peaceful inhabitants enjoyed and abused the advantages of wealth.

No. 2.
.50M

fourscore years, the public administration was conducted by the virtue and abilities of Nerva, Trajan, Hadrian, and the two Antonines. It is the design of this, and of the two succeeding chapters, to describe the prosperous condition of their empire; and afterwards, from the death of Marcus Antoninus, to deduce the most important circumstances of its decline and fall; a revolution which will ever be remembered, and is still felt by

No. 3.
.62M

the nations of the earth. The principal conquests of the Romans were achieved under the republic; and the emperors, for the most part, were satisfied with preserving those dominions which had been acquired by the policy of the senate, the active emulations of the consuls, and the martial enthusiasm of the people. The seven first centuries were filled with a rapid succession of triumphs; but it was

No. 4.
.75M

reserved for Augustus to relinquish the ambitious design of subduing the whole earth, and to introduce a spirit of moderation into the public councils. Inclined to peace by his temper and situation, it was very easy for him to discover that Rome, in her present exalted situation, had much less to hope than to fear from the chance of arms; and that, in the prosecution of

No. 5.
1.00M

the undertaking became every day more difficult, the event more doubtful, and the possession more precarious, and less beneficial. The experience of Augustus added weight to these salutary reflections, and effectually convinced him that, by the prudent vigor of

No. 6.
1.25M

his counsels, it would be easy to secure every concession which the safety or the dignity of Rome might require from the most formidable barbarians. Instead of exposing his person or his legions to the arrows of the Parthians, he obtained, by an honor-

No. 7.
1.50M

able treaty, the restitution of the standards and prisoners which had been taken in the defeat of Crassus. His generals, in the early part of his reign, attempted the reduction of Ethiopia and Arabia Felix. They marched near a thou-

No. 8.
1.75M

sand miles to the south of the tropic; but the heat of the climate soon repelled the invaders, and protected the unwarlike natives of those sequestered regions

No. 9.
2.00M

The northern countries of Europe scarcely deserved the expense and labor of conquest. The forests and morasses of Germany were

No. 10.
2.25M

filled with a hardy race of barbarians who despised life when it was separated from freedom; and though, on the first

No. 11.
2.50M

attack, they seemed to yield to the weight of the Roman power, they soon, by a signal

■ **FIGURE 8–6.** Example of a near visual acuity card.

ASSESSMENT OF NEAR VISUAL ACUITY

Near visual acuity testing assesses the patient's ability to read objects close up (i.e., at a reading or working distance); the test results are used to detect patients with hyperopia and presbyopia.

The test is conducted with a card similar to the Snellen eye chart, except for the size of the type, which ranges from the size of newspaper headlines down to considerably smaller print such as would be found in a telephone directory (Fig. 8–6). The test card is available in a variety of forms such as printed paragraphs, printed words, pictures, and Es.

The test should be performed in a well-lit room free from distractions. It is conducted with the patient holding the test card at a distance between 14 and 16 inches. The acuity should be measured in each eye separately, traditionally beginning with the right eye. The eye not being tested should be kept closed. If the patient wears reading glasses, they should be worn during the test.

The patient is asked to identify orally each line or paragraph of type. During the test, the patient should be observed for any unusual symptoms such as squinting, tilting the head, or watering of the eyes, which may indicate that the patient is having difficulty reading the card. The patient continues until reaching the smallest type that can be read.

The results are recorded as the smallest type that the patient could comfortably read with each eye at the distance at which the card is held (i.e., 14 to 16 inches). The recording will be based upon the type of test card used to conduct the test. For example, one type of card utilizes a recording method similar to that used with the Snellen eye test. For this type of near visual acuity card, the results would be recorded as 14/14 for a patient with normal near visual acuity. This means the patient read what was supposed to be read at a distance of 14 inches. Using the Jaeger system, a recording for a patient with normal visual acuity would be J2. Also included in the recording should be the date and time, corrective lenses worn, and any unusual symptoms exhibited by the patient.

ASSESSMENT OF COLOR VISION

☐ Defects in color vision may be classified as congenital or acquired. **Congenital defects** are the most common type and refer to a color vision deficiency that is inherited and therefore is present at birth. Congenital color vision deficiencies most often affect males. **Acquired defects** refer to a color vision deficiency that is acquired after birth, resulting from such factors as an

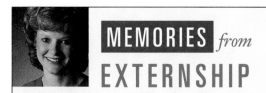

MEMORIES *from* **EXTERNSHIP**

CAMMIE LINDNER: *There is one characteristic that is shared by all patients. I first noticed this during my externships, and it does not seem to matter what type of practice it is. Patients like to feel special and to be treated that way. They like consistency in their doctor and in the office staff, in seeing familiar faces. This is especially hard during externship. The time spent is too short to truly get to know the patients, but it is a great learning experience.*

It is important to observe the staff and patient communication and interaction skills. By doing this, you can decide which ones you admire and those that you do not wish to copy. The following are just a few of the guidelines that have helped me. (1) Call patients by name, and be sure that they know your name. (2) Follow through with what you have told a patient you will do, and keep them updated if circumstances change. (3) Smile and do not let one patient's negative attitude interfere with your care of others. (4) Take time to listen.

When you do begin your career, it does not take long to get into a routine and to start knowing your patients. When patients see a familiar face, they are more willing to share information that can contribute to improved communication.

eye injury, disease, or certain drugs. Color vision tests, such as the Ishihara test (Fig. 8–7), detect color vision disturbances of congenital origin and are commonly performed as a screening measure in the medical office. A very rough screening for color vision can be performed by asking the patient to identify the red and green colored lines present on most Snellen charts.

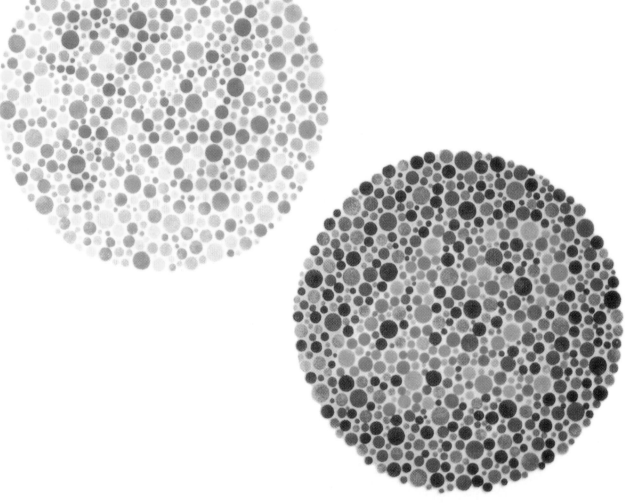

■ FIGURE 8–7. Ishihara color plates. Polychromatic plates. In the upper figure the normal person reads 74, whereas the red-green color blind person reads 21. In the lower figure, the red-blind person (protanope) reads 2, whereas the green-blind person (deuteranope) reads 4. The normal-vision person reads 42. (From Ishihara J.: *Tests for Color Blindness.* Tokyo, Kanehara and Co., 1920. Note that reproduced plates are not good for the test for color deficiency.)

THE ISHIHARA TEST

The Ishihara test for color blindness is a convenient and accurate method used to detect total color blindness and red-green blindness of congenital origin by assessing an individual's ability to perceive primary colors and shades of color.

The Ishihara book contains a series of polychromatic plates consisting of primary colored dots arranged to form a numeral against a background of similar dots of contrasting colors (Fig. 8–7). Patients with normal color vision are able to read the appropriate numeral; however, patients with color vision defects read the dots as either not forming a number at all or as forming a completely different number than the one

identified by the individual with normal color vision. The first plate in the Ishihara book is designed to be read correctly by all individuals (those with normal vision and those exhibiting color vision deficiencies) and should be used to explain the procedure to the patient. Plates are also included in the book with winding colored lines for patients who are unable to read numbers, such as preschoolers and non–English-speaking individuals. The patient is asked to trace the line formed by the colored dots.

The Ishihara test should be conducted in a quiet room illuminated by natural daylight. If this is not possible, a room lit with electric light may be used; however, the light should be adjusted to resemble the effect of natural daylight as much as possible. Using

PROCEDURE

8-2

Assessing Color Vision—Ishihara Test

EQUIPMENT/SUPPLIES: **Ishihara book**

1. **Procedural Step.** Wash hands. Assemble the equipment.
2. **Procedural Step.** Conduct the test in a quiet room illuminated by natural daylight.
   Principle. Using unnatural light may change the appearance of the shades of color on the plates, leading to inaccurate test results.
3. **Procedural Step.** Greet and identify the patient. Introduce yourself and explain the procedure. Using the first (practice) plate as an example, instruct the patient to orally identify numbers formed by colored dots. The patient should be told that 3 seconds will be given to identify each plate.
   Principle. The first plate is designed to be read correctly by all individuals and is used to explain the procedure to the patient.
4. **Procedural Step.** Hold the first color plate 30 inches (75 cm) from the patient. The plate should be held at a right angle to the patient's line of vision. Both eyes should be kept open during the test.
5. **Procedural Step.** Ask the patient to identify the number on the plate. Record results after each plate. Continue until the patient has viewed all the plates.

   To record the color vision results, use the plate identification number and the number given by the patient. If the patient is unable to identify a number, the mark X should be recorded to indicate that the plate could not be read by the patient. Examples:

   Plate 5: 21 (This means the patient read the number 21 on Plate 5.)

   Plate 6: X (This means the patient could not identify a number on Plate 6.)

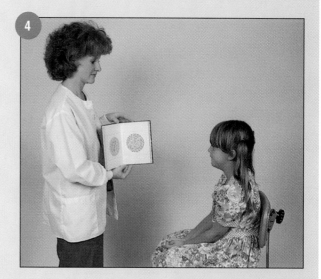

6. **Procedural Step.** Chart the procedure. Include the date and time, the name of the test (Ishihara test), the color vision results, and any unusual symptoms that the patient may have exhibited during the test, such as squinting or rubbing the eyes.
7. **Procedural Step.** Return the Ishihara book to its proper place. The book of color plates must be stored in a closed position to protect it from light.
   Principle. Exposing the plates to excessive and unnecessary light results in fading of the color.

8

light other than just described, such as bright sunlight, may change the appearance of shades of color on the plates, leading to inaccurate test results.

The medical assistant is responsible for performing the color vision test and recording results in the patient's chart. The physician will assess the results to determine whether the patient has a deficiency in color vision.

The Ishihara test consists of 14 color plates. Plates 1 through 11 are used to conduct the basic test, whereas Plates 12, 13, and 14 are used to further assess patients exhibiting a red-green color deficiency. Therefore, it is not necessary to include these plates (12, 13, and 14) in the test for those patients exhibiting normal color vision. In interpreting the results, if 10 or more plates are read normally, the patient's color vision is considered normal. If only 7 (or fewer than 7) of the 11 Ishihara plates are read correctly, the patient is identified as having a color vision deficiency. It would be unusual for the medical assistant to obtain results in which the patient read 8 or 9 plates correctly. The test is structured so that a patient with a color vision defect generally does not read 8 or 9 plates correctly and the rest incorrectly.

If a defect in color vision is detected, the patient is referred to an ophthalmologist or optometrist for additional assessment of color vision, using more precise color vision tests. The procedure for assessing color vision using the Ishihara color plates is outlined in Procedure 8–2.

EYE IRRIGATION

☐ An eye irrigation involves washing the eye with a flowing solution. Eye irrigations are performed for the following purposes: to cleanse the eye by washing away foreign particles, ocular discharges, or harmful chemicals; to relieve inflammation through the application of heat; or to apply an antiseptic solution.

PROCEDURE

8–3

Performing an Eye Irrigation

EQUIPMENT/SUPPLIES:
Disposable gloves
Sterile irrigating solution
Sterile container to hold the solution
Sterile rubber bulb syringe

Basin for the returned solution
Moisture-resistant towel
Sterile gauze pads

1. **Procedural Step.** Wash the hands.
2. **Procedural Step.** Assemble the equipment. Normal saline is generally used to irrigate the eye. Check the irrigating solution carefully with the physician's instructions to make sure you have obtained the correct solution. Check the expiration date of the solution. Check the solution label three times: while removing the solution from the shelf, while pouring the solution, and before returning it to its proper place. Warm the irrigating solution to body temperature (98.6°F, or 37°C).
   Principle. The solution should be carefully compared with the physician's instructions to prevent an error. If the solution is outdated, consult the physician; it may produce undesirable effects, and the medical assistant could be held responsible. If the solution is too cold or too warm, it will be uncomfortable for the patient.
3. **Procedural Step.** Greet and identify the patient. Introduce yourself and explain the procedure.
   Principle. Explain the purpose of the irrigation to the patient.
4. **Procedural Step.** Apply gloves. Position the patient.

The patient may be placed in a sitting or lying position with the head turned in the direction of the affected eye. A basin should be positioned tightly against the patient's cheek under the affected eye to catch the irrigating solution. A moisture-resistant towel should be placed on the patient's shoulder to protect the patient's clothing. If both eyes are to be irrigated, two separate sets of equipment must be used to prevent cross-infection from one eye to the other.
   Principle. The patient is positioned so the solution will flow away from the unaffected eye to prevent cross-infection.
5. **Procedural Step.** Note the diagram of the external structures of the eye. Cleanse the eyelids from inner to outer canthus with a moistened gauze pad to remove any discharge or debris on the lids. The inner canthus is the inner junction of the eyelids next to the nose. The outer canthus is the junction of the eyelids farthest from the nose. Normal saline or the solution ordered for the irrigation may be used. Discard the gauze pad after each wipe.

PROCEDURE 8-3

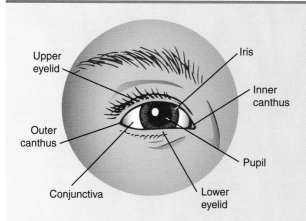

Upper eyelid
Iris
Inner canthus
Outer canthus
Pupil
Conjunctiva
Lower eyelid

Principle. The eyelids should be clean to prevent any foreign particles from entering the eye during the irrigation. Cleansing from inner to outer canthus prevents cross-infection.

6. **Procedural Step.** Fill the irrigating syringe with the solution by squeezing the bulb and slowly releasing it until the desired amount of solution enters the bulb.

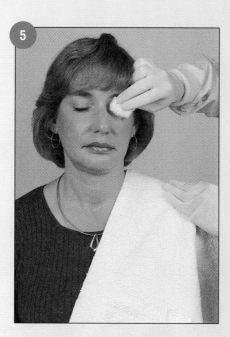

7. **Procedural Step.** Separate the eyelids with the index finger and thumb to expose the lower conjunctiva and to hold the upper eyelid open.
Principle. The medical assistant must hold the eye open during the procedure, because the patient will have a tendency to close it.

8. **Procedural Step.** Hold the tip of the syringe approximately 1 inch above the eye. Gently release the solution onto the eye at the inner canthus. This allows the solution to flow over the eye at a moderate rate from the inner to the outer canthus.

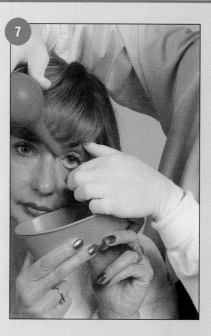

Direct the solution to the lower conjunctiva. To prevent injury, do not allow the syringe to touch the eye.
Principle. The solution flows away from the unaffected eye to prevent cross-infection. The cornea is sensitive and can be harmed easily. Therefore, the irrigating solution must be directed to the lower conjunctiva to prevent injury to the cornea.

9. **Procedural Step.** Refill the syringe and continue irrigating until the desired results have been obtained or all the solution is used, depending on the purpose of the irrigation.

10. **Procedural Step.** Dry the eyelids from inner to outer canthus with a gauze pad.

11. **Procedural Step.** Remove the gloves and wash the hands.

12. **Procedural Step.** Chart the procedure. Include the following: the date and time; which eye was irrigated; the type, strength, and amount of solution used; and any significant observations and patient reactions. Use one of these abbreviations to indicate which eye was irrigated:

OU Both eyes
OD Right eye
OS Left eye

13. **Procedural Step.** Return the equipment.

8

CHARTING EXAMPLE	
Date	
11/5/2002	10:30 a.m. OS irrigated c̄ sterile normal saline, 98.6° F. No complaints of discomfort.
	———————————— C. Lindner, CMA

EYE INSTILLATION

☐ Eye instillations are performed to treat eye infections (with medication), to soothe an irritated eye, to dilate the pupil, or to anesthetize the eye during an eye examination or treatment. Medication to be instilled in the eye may come in a liquid form, as ophthalmic drops, or as an ophthalmic ointment. The eye drops may be dispensed in a bottle with an eye dropper or in a flexible plastic container with an attached tip for administering the eye drops. Eye ointment is dispensed in a small metal tube with a small tip for applying the medication.

PROCEDURE

8-4

Performing an Eye Instillation

EQUIPMENT/SUPPLIES:
Disposable gloves
Ophthalmic drops with a sterile eye dropper or ophthalmic ointment ordered by the physician

Sterile tissues
Sterile gauze pads

1. **Procedural Step.** Wash the hands.
2. **Procedural Step.** Assemble the equipment. Check the medication carefully against the physician's instructions to make sure you have obtained the correct medication. The medication should bear the word *ophthalmic.* Check the expiration date. Check the drug label three times: while removing the medication from the shelf, before removing the cap or withdrawing the medication into the dropper, and before instilling the medication.
   Principle. The medication should be carefully compared with the physician's instructions to prevent a drug error. Medication not bearing the word *ophthalmic* should never be placed in the eye because it could result in an injury to the eye. If the medication is outdated, consult the physician; it may produce undesirable effects, and the medical assistant could be held responsible.
3. **Procedural Step.** Greet and identify the patient. Introduce yourself and explain the procedure.
   Principle. Explain the purpose of the instillation to the patient.
4. **Procedural Step.** Place the patient in a sitting or supine position.
5. **Procedural Step.** Apply gloves. Prepare the medication. *Eye drops:* Withdraw the medication into the dropper. *Eye ointment:* Remove the cap from the tip of the tube.
6. **Procedural Step.** Ask the patient to look up to the ceiling, and expose the lower conjunctival sac by using the fingers of the nondominant hand placed

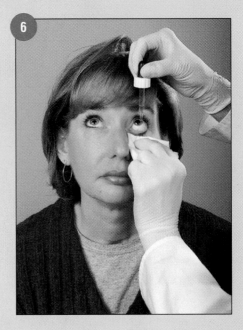

over a tissue. The fingers should be placed on the patient's cheekbone just below the eye, and the skin of the cheek should be drawn downward gently.
Principle. Looking up helps keep the dropper from touching the cornea. It also helps keep the patient from blinking when the drops are instilled.

7. **Procedural Step.** Insert the medication. *Eye drops:* Place the correct number of eye drops in the center of the lower conjunctival sac. The tip of the dropper should be held approximately ½ inch above the eye sac. Do not allow the dropper to touch the eye. *Eye ointment:* Place a thin ribbon of ointment along the length of the lower conjunctival sac from inner to outer canthus. Be careful not to touch the tip of the ointment tube to the eye. Discontinue the ribbon by twisting the tube.
Principle. The medication must be placed in the conjunctival sac, rather than directly on the eyeball itself, as the medication may harm the cornea. Touching the dropper or tube to the eye results in contamination of these items.

8. **Procedural Step.** Discard any unused solution from the eye dropper. Do not touch the dropper to the outside of the bottle when returning it to the bottle.
Principle. Touching the dropper to the outside of the bottle contaminates the dropper. Unused solution should not be returned to the bottle because it will contaminate the medication remaining in the bottle.

9. **Procedural Step.** Ask the patient to close his or her eyes gently and move the eyeballs. Tell the patient that the instillation may blur the vision temporarily.

Principle. Moving the eyeballs helps distribute the medication over the entire eye. If the eyes are shut tightly, the drops or ointment is pushed out.

10. **Procedural Step.** Dry the eyelid from inner to outer canthus with a gauze pad to remove any excess medication.

11. **Procedural Step.** Remove the gloves, and wash the hands.

12. **Procedural Step.** Chart the procedure. Include the date and time, the name and strength of the medication, number of drops or amount of ointment, which eye received the instillation, any observations made by the medical assistant, and the patient's reaction.

CHARTING EXAMPLE

Date	
11/5/2002	2:30 p.m. Atropine sulfate, 1% , gtts ii
	instilled OU. Pt states a temporary blurring
	of vision. ——————— C. Lindner, CMA

PATIENT/TEACHING

CONJUNCTIVITIS

■ Answer questions patients have about conjunctivitis.

What is Pinkeye?

Pinkeye is medically referred to as conjunctivitis. It occurs when the conjunctiva, the lining of the eye, becomes infected with a bacterium or virus. Other causes of conjunctivitis include allergies and irritation from wind, dust, and smoke. Pinkeye is almost always harmless and will clear up by itself within 2 weeks. If it is caused by bacteria, the physician may prescribe antibiotic eye drops or ointment.

What Are the Symptoms of Pinkeye?

Most types of pinkeye are relatively painless. The eye is red or pink due to irritation, and there is a feeling of sandiness or grittiness in the eye. A discharge is commonly present, which may cause the eyelids to be stuck together in the morning. Other symptoms include tearing and itching of the eye and sensitivity to light.

Is Pinkeye Contagious?

Pinkeye caused by a virus or bacteria is highly contagious. It can be spread easily from one eye to another and throughout a family or classroom in a matter of days.

What Can Be Done to Prevent Spreading Pinkeye?

The following measures help prevent the spread of pinkeye:

Avoid touching or rubbing the infected eye, which can spread the infection to the other eye or other people

Wash the hands frequently with soap, particularly after touching the eyes or face

Do not share washcloths, towels, or pillows with family members

Do not use contact lenses or eye make-up until the pinkeye is completely gone

■ Encourage the patient to practice techniques that prevent the spread of pinkeye.

■ If the physician has prescribed eye medication, teach the patient (or parent) the proper procedure for performing an eye instillation.

■ Provide the patient with educational materials on conjunctivitis.

The Ear

STRUCTURE OF THE EAR

☐ The ear has functions in hearing and in maintaining equilibrium. It consists of three divisions: the **external ear,** the **middle ear,** and the **inner ear.** The structures in the ear are illustrated in Figure 8–8 and described next.

The external ear is composed of the auricle (or pinna) and the external auditory canal, also known as the external ear canal. The opening into this canal is the **external auditory meatus.**

The **auricle** is a flap of cartilage covered with skin that projects from the side of the head. Its function is to receive and collect sound waves and to direct them toward the external auditory canal.

The **external auditory canal** is approximately 1 inch long in an adult and extends from the auricle to the tympanic membrane. It is lined with skin containing fine hairs, nerve endings, and glands. The glands secrete ear wax or cerumen, which lubricates and protects the ear canal. The canal has an S-shaped curve as it leads inward. During either an examination with the otoscope or an ear instillation or irrigation, the canal must be straightened.

The **tympanic membrane** is at the end of the external auditory canal. It is a pearly gray semi-transparent membrane that functions in receiving sound waves.

The middle ear is an air-filled cavity that contains three small bones, or **ossicles:** the malleus, the incus, and the stapes. The **eustachian tube** connects the middle ear to the nasopharynx. Air pressure between the external atmosphere and the middle ear is stabilized through the eustachian tube.

The inner ear contains the **cochlea,** which is the essential organ of hearing. The **semicircular canals** are also located in the inner ear and function in maintaining equilibrium.

ASSESSMENT OF HEARING ACUITY

☐ The assessment of hearing acuity is considered an integral part of a complete physical examination. It is quite possible for an individual to have a hearing loss and yet not be aware of it. Early detection and treatment of hearing problems help prevent permanent hearing loss.

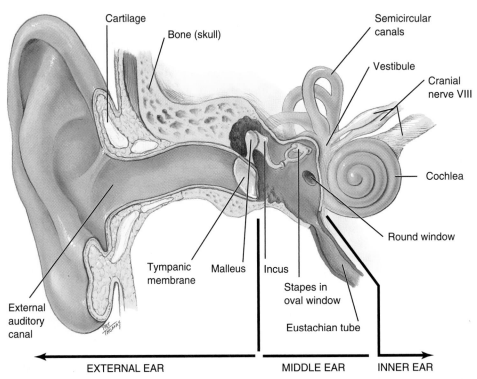

■ **FIGURE 8–8.** Structure of the ear. (From Applegate, E. J.: *The Anatomy and Physiology Learning System.* Philadelphia, W. B. Saunders, 1995, p. 196.)

OTITIS MEDIA

■ Answer questions patients have about otitis media.

What Is a Middle Ear Infection?

A middle ear infection is medically referred to as otitis media. It is an inflammation of the middle ear caused by an infection and can occur in one or both ears. It is very common in young children between the ages of 3 months and 3 years but unusual in adults. A middle ear infection is not serious if treated promptly and effectively. If not treated, middle ear infections can cause permanent hearing loss and other types of complications.

What Causes a Middle Ear Infection?

It is believed that a middle ear infection is caused by a blocked eustachian tube. The blockage causes fluid to build up in the middle ear. This fluid is an ideal place for bacteria to grow, which results in infection.

What Are the Symptoms of a Middle Ear Infection?

The most common symptoms are considerable pain and a feeling of fullness in the ear, fever, and temporary hearing loss. Other symptoms may include nasal congestion, dizziness, and nausea and vomiting.

How Does the Physician Know Whether a Middle Ear Infection is Present?

The physician examines the ears with an otoscope. If a middle ear infection is present, the eardrum will be red, caused by irritation from the infection, and there will be fluid behind the eardrum.

How Is It Treated?

To fight the infection, a middle ear infection is treated with an antibiotic for a period of 7 to 10 days. It is important to take all the antibiotic prescribed; otherwise the ear infection may recur. A decongestant may also be recommended by the physician to help open the blocked eustachian tube.

Why Are Middle Ear Infections so Common in Children?

In children, the eustachian tube is positioned horizontally and is shorter and narrower than in adults. Hence, when a child has an upper respiratory infection, bacteria can travel easily to the middle ear. In addition, swelling from the respiratory infection can block this narrow tube, which causes fluid to build up in the middle ear.

■ Encourage the patient to complete the entire prescribed course of antibiotics.

■ If the physician has prescribed ear drops, teach the patient (or parent) the proper procedure for performing an ear instillation.

■ Encourage early treatment of upper respiratory infections.

■ Provide the patient with educational materials on otitis media.

An individual with normal hearing should be able to hear the frequencies of normal speech, which range from 500 to 3000 hertz (Hz) (cycles per second) at a normal sound intensity (25 decibels). Patients who exhibit hearing loss are referred to an otolaryngologist or an audiologist for further evaluation.

TYPES OF HEARING LOSS

There are three types of hearing loss: conductive, sensorineural, and mixed. **Conductive loss** is the most common and results when there is a physical interference with the normal conduction of sound waves through the external and middle ear. Because of the interference, the amount of sound reaching the inner ear is less than normal, resulting in hearing impairment. Conductive loss in the external ear may be due to an obstruction in the external ear canal, such as impacted cerumen, swelling from external otitis media, foreign bodies, or benign growths such as polyps. If the conductive loss is in the middle ear, it may be due to fluid or infection in the middle ear, a perforated tympanic membrane, or otosclerosis. The cause of conductive hearing loss often can be detected by examining the external ear canal with an otoscope. Hearing is frequently restored by removing the obstruction (e.g., impacted cerumen) or treating the disorder (e.g., otitis media).

Sensorineural hearing loss results from damage to the inner ear or auditory nerve. With this type of hearing loss, the sound is conducted normally through the outer and middle ear structures but, because of a problem with the perception of sound waves, a hearing deficit occurs. Specific causes of sensorineural loss include hereditary factors; infectious diseases such as measles, mumps, and meningitis; ototoxicity caused by certain medications; intense noise; tumors; and degenerative changes from the normal aging process.

Mixed loss is a combination of both conductive and sensorineural loss.

HEARING ACUITY TESTS

A number of tests can be used to assess hearing acuity. They range from the very simple gross screening test to qualitative tests using a tuning fork to highly specific quantitative tests using an audiometer. It is important to test only one ear at a time because a hearing deficit may exist in one ear only. The ear not being tested should be blocked by an ear plug or masked. **Masking** involves the presentation of sound (usually noise) to the ear not being tested so that the patient's response is based only on hearing in the ear being tested.

8

Gross Screening Test

The gross hearing test is a simple and quick screening test used to identify a very large hearing impairment. It is performed by the physician during the physical examination. Hearing is assessed by asking the patient to repeat a simple word or series of numbers whispered from a distance of 1 to 2 feet from the ear. A gross hearing test may also be conducted by determining whether the patient can hear the ticking of a watch at a distance of 4 to 6 inches from the ear. When a hearing loss is found, a tuning fork or audiometer is used for a more precise assessment of hearing.

Tuning Fork Tests

Tuning fork tests provide a general assessment of hearing acuity and may be included as part of the physical examination. A tuning fork with a frequency of 512 or 1024 Hz is generally used, because these frequencies fall within the range of normal speech. The Weber and Rinne tests are the tuning fork tests most commonly performed by the physician; they are used to identify conductive and sensorineural hearing loss.

The Weber test is a useful assessment of hearing loss when one ear hears better than the other. The tuning fork is set in vibration and the base of the fork is placed on the center of the patient's head. The patient is then asked to indicate where the sound is heard best. A patient with normal hearing will hear the sound equally in both ears or in the center of the head. Figure 8–9 illustrates the Weber test and describes the interpretation of results.

The Rinne test compares the duration of sound perception by air conduction with bone conduction. An individual with normal hearing is able to hear sound that is conducted through air longer than sound that is conducted through bone. The tuning fork is set in vibration and the prongs of the fork are placed in the air about an inch away from the opening of the patient's ear canal, just long enough for the patient to hear the sound. The base of the fork is then placed against the bone of the mastoid process. The physician continues to alternate the tuning fork back and forth

Highlight on Hearing Impairment

The number of individuals with a hearing impairment has gradually increased over the past 20 years. Factors contributing to this increase include an aging population and a noisier environment.

It is estimated that approximately 28 million people in the United States suffer from a hearing loss severe enough to interfere with their daily activities, while another 2 million individuals are profoundly deaf.

Precise screening of preschoolers for hearing loss is difficult. This is because tuning fork tests and audiometry require the ability to signal in response to sound, and children up to the age of 4 or 5 years have trouble mastering this skill.

Most state, county, and local school systems require hearing screening as a prerequisite for entrance into school and again at periodic intervals, usually during the first, third, fifth, and seventh grades.

Risk factors for hearing impairment in children include family history of deafness, rubella during pregnancy, premature birth, low birth weight, measles, mumps, high fevers, meningitis, and recurrent or chronic ear infections.

Signs of hearing impairment in children are poor attentiveness, delayed speech development, and persistent problems with articulation. Signs of hearing impairment in adults include frequent requests for words or statements to be repeated, leaning toward the speaker, turning the head, cupping the ears, and speaking in a loud or unvaried tone of voice.

The most common cause of conductive hearing loss in children is the presence of fluid in the middle ear, which prevents the tympanic membrane from vibrating freely. In adults, the most common cause of conductive loss is otosclerosis, a condition in which the stapes becomes fixed because of calcium deposits and less able to pass on vibrations when sound enters the ear.

Permanent sensorineural hearing loss can result when the ear is repeatedly bombarded with loud sound. The loudness of sound is measured in units called **decibels.** Sounds of less than 75 decibels, even after long exposure, are unlikely to cause hearing loss. Normal conversation is approximately 60 to 70 decibels, while the humming of a refrigerator is 40 decibels and city traffic can reach 80 decibels.

Sounds above 75 decibels, especially when prolonged, are known to damage the tiny hair cells of the organ of Corti, a structure in the inner ear responsible for converting sound waves into nerve impulses for transmission to the brain. This type of sensorineural hearing loss, known as noise-induced hearing loss (NIHL), is most often seen in individuals who frequently listen to loud music, fire guns without the use of ear protection, or are exposed to loud noise as part of their jobs. For example, motorcycles, fire crackers, and small arms all emit sounds from 120 to 140 decibels.

The individual who benefits most from a hearing aid is one with a mild-to-moderate conductive hearing loss. An individual with a sensorineural or mixed loss has more trouble finding a suitable hearing aid and often gets less satisfactory results.

8

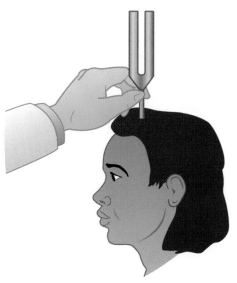

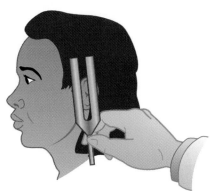

Air conduction

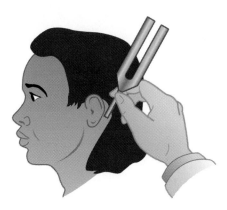

Bone conduction

■ **FIGURE 8–9.** The Weber test. Normal hearing: The patient hears the sound equally in both ears or in the center of the head. If a conductive loss is present, the patient will hear the sound better in the problem ear. If a sensorineural loss is present, the patient will not hear the sound as well in the problem ear.

■ **FIGURE 8–10.** The Rinne test. Normal hearing: The patient will hear the sound at least twice as long through air conduction as through bone conduction. If a conductive loss is present, the patient will hear the sound longer by bone conduction than by air conduction.

PUTTING IT ALL *into* PRACTICE

▶ **CAMMIE LINDNER:** *Over the past 10 years in an ENT practice, there have been many challenging and rewarding situations. A recent incident was one that certainly fell into the rewards category.*

A young girl came into the office from the emergency department for repair of a facial laceration. It had been quite a day for her, so it was understandable that she was a bit nervous and upset. As the suturing was performed, she grasped her mother's hand as I tried to discuss interests and school with her. She did fine and was very relieved when the last suture was done.

On her return visit for the suture removal her mother could not accompany her. As I was showing her to the examination room, she quietly asked if I would be in the room. I said, "If you would like, I certainly will." She anxiously nodded yes. The sutures were removed as she squeezed my hand tighter and tighter. After all of them were out, she first checked her appearance in the mirror, then turned before going out the door giving me a big hug and a "Thank you."

It is days like this one that truly are great rewards and make you feel you really can make a difference in someone's care.

until it stops vibrating. The patient is asked to indicate which sound is heard for a longer duration of time. Figure 8–10 illustrates the Rinne test and describes the interpretation of results.

Audiometry

Audiometry is the measurement of the hearing acuity for the various frequencies of sound waves. It is a more specific hearing acuity test because it provides informa-

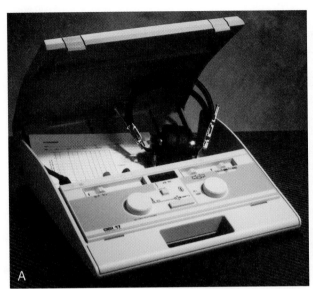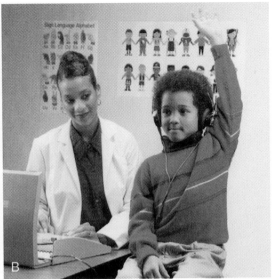

■ **FIGURE 8–11.** *A,* Audiometer. *B,* The patient signals when he hears a sound. (Courtesy of GSI [Grayson-Stadler], Milford, NH.)

8

tion on how extensive a hearing loss a patient has and which frequencies are involved. It is important that audiometry be conducted in a quiet room, because outside noise may affect the test results, especially in the lower frequencies. The patient wears headphones placed snugly over the ears (Fig. 8–11). The audiometer delivers a single frequency at a time at specific intensities, starting with low-frequency tones of 250 or 500 Hz and going up to very high frequencies of 6000 or 8000 Hz. The patient is asked to signal when he or she hears a sound, so that the patient's hearing threshold for each frequency can be determined. The hearing acuity in each ear is assessed separately, and the results are plotted on a graph known as an **audiogram.** The medical assistant may be responsible for performing audiometry in the medical office. Before operating an audiometer, however, the medical assistant must be provided with extensive on-site training by an audiologist to ensure that proper technique is used in conducting the test.

Tympanometry

Tympanometry is not a hearing test, but it does help determine the cause of hearing loss; so it is presented in this section. The tympanometer consists of an earpiece attached to an electronic device (Fig. 8–12). The earpiece is placed snugly in the patient's ear, and low-frequency sound waves are directed against the eardrum while pressure is applied in the ear canal. With a normal ear, the eardrum will exhibit mobility in response to the pressure, as indicated on a graphic readout known as a **tympanogram.** If there is fluid in the

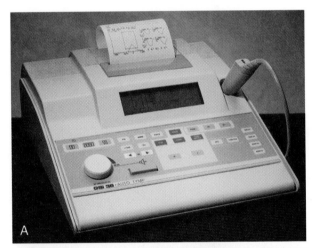

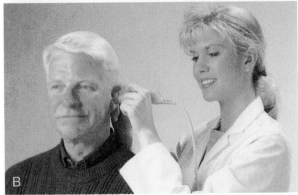

■ **FIGURE 8–12.** *A,* Tympanometer. *B,* The earpiece is placed snugly in the patient's ear. (Courtesy of GSI [Grayson-Stadler], Milford, NH.)

middle ear, the eardrum will not move but remain stiff, as indicated on the tympanogram. Hence tympanometry is useful in diagnosing serous otitis media (fluid in the middle ear), which is a common cause of hearing loss in children.

EAR IRRIGATION

☐ An ear irrigation is the washing of the external auditory canal with a flowing solution. Ear irrigations are performed for the following purposes: to cleanse the external auditory canal to remove cerumen, discharge, or a foreign body; to relieve inflammation by applying an antiseptic solution; or to apply heat to the ear. Impacted cerumen must first be softened by instilling warm mineral oil or hydrogen peroxide for 10 to 15 minutes before irrigating.

An ear irrigation should not be performed if the tympanic membrane is perforated, because this could result in a severe irritation or infection of the middle ear.

PROCEDURE 8–5

Performing an Ear Irrigation

EQUIPMENT/SUPPLIES:

Disposable gloves
Irrigating solution
Container to hold the solution
Irrigating syringe

Ear basin for the returned solution
Moisture-resistant towel
Cotton balls

1. **Procedural Step.** Wash the hands.
2. **Procedural Step.** Assemble the equipment. Check the irrigating solution carefully against the physician's instructions to make sure you have obtained the correct solution. Check the expiration date of the solution. Check the label of the irrigating solution three times: while removing the solution from the shelf, while pouring the solution, and before returning it to its proper place. Warm the irrigating solution to body temperature (98.6°F, or 37°C).
   Principle. The solution should be carefully compared with the physician's instructions to prevent an error. If the solution is outdated, consult the physician; it may produce undesirable effects, and the medical assistant could be held responsible. If the solution is too cold or too warm, the patient will become dizzy due to stimulation of the inner ear.
3. **Procedural Step.** Greet and identify the patient. Introduce yourself, and explain the procedure. Explain the purpose of performing the irrigation—for

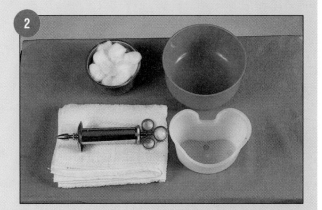

example to remove cerumen. Tell the patient the procedure is not painful; however, he or she may feel a minimal amount of discomfort and occasional dizziness, fullness, and warmth as the ear solution comes in contact with the tympanic membrane.

Continued

8

4. Procedural Step. Place the patient in a sitting position with the head tilted toward the affected ear. A moisture-resistant towel should be placed on the patient's shoulder under the ear to be irrigated, to protect clothing and to prevent water from running down the neck. Instruct the patient to hold the ear basin against the head under the affected ear to catch the irrigating solution.
Principle. The patient is positioned so gravity aids the flow of the solution out of the ear and into the basin.

5. Procedural Step. Apply gloves. Cleanse the outer ear with a moistened cotton ball to remove any discharge or debris present. Normal saline or the solution ordered for the irrigation may be used.
Principle. The outer ear should be clean to prevent any foreign particle from entering the ear canal during the irrigation.

6. Procedural Step. Fill the syringe with the irrigating solution (approximately 50 ml). Expel air from the syringe.
Principle. Air forced into the ear is uncomfortable for the patient.

7. Procedural Step. Straighten the external ear canal. The canal is straightened by gently pulling the ear upward and backward for adults and children over 3 years old and downward and backward for children 3 years of age and younger.
Principle. Straightening the canal permits the irrigating solution to reach all areas of the canal.

8. Procedural Step. Insert the syringe tip into the ear and inject the irrigating solution toward the roof of the ear canal. It is important that the solution be injected toward the roof of the canal to prevent it from being injected directly onto the tympanic membrane. Do not insert the tip of the syringe too deeply.
Principle. The tip of the syringe should be directed at the roof of the canal to prevent injury to the tympanic membrane and to aid in the removal of foreign particles by allowing the solution to flow down the length of the canal and out of the bottom. In addition, severe patient discomfort and dizziness may occur from the solution's being injected directly onto the tympanic membrane. Inserting the tip of the syringe too deeply causes discomfort for the patient.

9. Procedural Step. Refill the syringe and continue irrigating until the desired results have been obtained or all the solution is used, depending on the purpose of the irrigation. Make sure the tip of the syringe does not obstruct the canal opening so that the solution can flow freely out of the canal. Observe the returning solution to note the material present (e.g., cerumen, discharge, or a foreign object) and the amount (small, moderate, large).

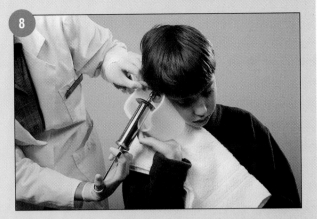

Principle. Obstruction of the canal opening causes pressure that results in patient discomfort and possible injury to the tympanic membrane.

10. Procedural Step. Dry the outside of the ear with a cotton ball. Have the patient lie on the affected side on the treatment table. Tell the patient that the ear will feel sensitive for a short period of time. Place a cotton wick loosely in the ear canal for 15 minutes if instructed to do so by the physician.
Principle. Any remaining solution in the ear canal should be allowed to drain out. A cotton wick will help make the patient's ear feel less sensitive after the irrigation.

11. Procedural Step. Remove the gloves and wash the hands.

12. Procedural Step. Chart the procedure. Include the following: the date and time; which ear was irrigated; the type, strength, and amount of solution used; the amount and type of material returned in the irrigating solution; any significant observations; and patient reactions. Use one of these abbreviations to indicate which ear was irrigated:

AU Both ears
AD Right ear
AS Left ear

13. Procedural Step. Return the equipment.

CHARTING EXAMPLE

Date	
11/15/2002	2:15 p.m. Irrigated AD c̄ normal saline, 200 ml @ 98.6° F. Mod amt of cerumen present in returned solution. Cotton wick placed in ear canal for 15 minutes. No complaints of discomfort or dizziness. ————————— C. Lindner, CMA

EAR INSTILLATION

☐ An ear instillation involves the dropping of a liquid into the external auditory canal. Ear instillations are performed to soften impacted cerumen, to combat infection with the use of antibiotic ear drops, or to relieve pain.

PROCEDURE

8-6

Performing an Ear Instillation

EQUIPMENT/SUPPLIES: Disposable gloves   Cotton balls
Otic drops with a sterile dropper

1. **Procedural Step.** Wash the hands.
2. **Procedural Step.** Assemble the equipment. Check the medication carefully against the physician's instructions to make sure you have obtained the correct medication. The medication should bear the word *otic*. Check the expiration date. Check the drug label three times: while removing the medication from the shelf, before withdrawing the medication into the dropper, and before instilling the medication.
   Principle. The medication should be carefully compared with the physician's instructions to prevent a drug error. Medication not bearing the word *otic* should not be placed in the ear because it could result in an injury to the ear. If the medication is outdated, consult the physician; it may produce undesirable effects, and the medical assistant could be held responsible.
3. **Procedural Step.** Greet and identify the patient. Introduce yourself, and explain the procedure.
   Principle. Explain the purpose of the instillation to the patient.
4. **Procedural Step.** Place the patient in a sitting position with the head tilted in the direction of the unaffected ear.
   Principle. Gravity aids in the flow of the medication into the ear canal.
5. **Procedural Step.** Apply gloves. Withdraw the medication into the dropper.
6. **Procedural Step.** Straighten the external auditory canal. The canal is straightened by pulling the ear

upward and backward for adults and children over 3 years old and downward and backward for children 3 years of age and younger.

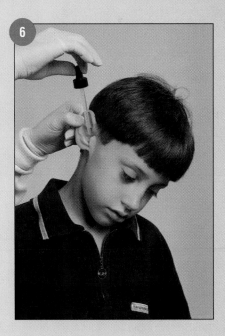

Principle. Straightening the canal permits the medication to reach all areas of the canal.

Continued

PROCEDURE 8–6

7. Procedural Step. Place the tip of the dropper in the ear canal, and insert the proper amount of medication by squeezing the rubber bulb and instilling the correct number of drops along the side of the canal.

8. Procedural Step. Instruct the patient to lie on the unaffected side for 2 to 3 minutes.
Principle. Lying on the unaffected side prevents the medication from running out and allows complete distribution of the medication.

9. Procedural Step. Place a moistened cotton wick loosely in the ear canal for 15 minutes if instructed to do so by the physician.
Principle. The cotton wick prevents the medication from running out when the patient is up. Moistening the wick will prevent the medication from being absorbed by the cotton.

10. Procedural Step. Remove the gloves and wash the hands.

11. Procedural Step. Chart the procedure. Include the date and time, the name and strength of the medication, number of drops, which ear(s) received the instillation, any significant observations, and the patient's reaction.

12. Procedural Step. Replace the equipment.

CHARTING EXAMPLE

Date	
11/20/2002	9:30 a.m. Auralgan, gtts ii instilled, AD. No discharge present. Pt states a relief of pain.
	———————————— C. Lindner, CMA

MEDICAL PRACTICE AND THE LAW

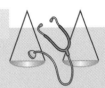

Eye and ear assessment issues are similar to those of any assessment. Accurate assessments done properly are necessary for accurate diagnoses and treatment and to prevent injuries to these structures.

Patient Rights

Patients entering the office have six major rights, which are based on values and enforced by laws.

1. The right to have the physician and medical assistant **do good** for them. Failure results in malpractice.
2. The right to **be treated fairly.** This is enforced by discrimination and employment laws.
3. The right to **be free.** This is exercised by giving informed consent and advance directives.
4. The right **not to be harmed.** Licensure protects patients by assuring a minimal level of skill.
5. The right of fidelity, or **being true.** This includes confidentiality, telling the truth, and loyalty to the patient.
6. The right to **life.** This appears with cases of abortion, assisted suicide, and euthanasia.

If any of these rights are violated, the patient has the right to sue.

8

CERTIFICATION REVIEW

☐ Visual acuity refers to acuteness or sharpness of vision. A person with normal visual acuity can see clearly and is able to distinguish fine details both close up and at some distance.

☐ Errors of refraction are the most common cause of defects in visual acuity. A person who is nearsighted has a condition termed myopia and has difficulty seeing objects at a distance. A person who is farsighted has a condition known as hyperopia and has difficulty viewing objects at a reading or working distance. A decrease in the elasticity of the lens due to aging is known as presbyopia and results in a decreased ability to focus clearly on objects close up.

CERTIFICATION REVIEW *Continued*

- ☐ An ophthalmologist is a medical doctor who specializes in diagnosing and treating disorders of the eye. An optometrist is a licensed practitioner who is skilled in measuring visual acuity. An optician is a professional who interprets and fills prescriptions for eyeglasses or contact lenses.

- ☐ A distance visual acuity test assesses an individual's ability to see objects at a distance. The Snellen test is generally used in the medical office as a screening test for distance visual acuity. A reading of 20/20 indicates normal distance visual acuity.

- ☐ Near visual acuity testing assesses an individual's ability to read objects close up. The test results are used to detect patients with hyperopia and presbyopia. The results are recorded as the smallest type the patient can comfortably read.

- ☐ Congenital color defects are inherited and refer to a color vision deficiency that is inherited and therefore is present at birth. Acquired defects refer to a color vision deficiency that is acquired after birth. Color vision tests, such as the Ishihara test, detect color vision disturbances of congenital origin.

- ☐ An eye irrigation involves washing the eye with a flowing solution. Eye irrigations are performed to cleanse the eye of ocular discharges or harmful chemicals; to relieve inflammation through the application of heat; or to apply an antiseptic solution.

- ☐ Eye instillations are performed to treat eye infections, to soothe an irritated eye, or to dilate the pupil or anesthetize the eye during an eye examination or treatment. Eye medications come in the form of ophthalmic drops or as an ophthalmic ointment.

- ☐ There are three types of hearing loss: conductive, sensorineural, and mixed. A conductive loss results from an interference with the conduction of sound waves through the external and middle ear. Sensorineural loss results from damage to the inner ear or auditory nerve. Mixed loss is a combination of both conductive and sensoineural loss.

- ☐ Tests that can be used to assess hearing acuity include the following: gross screening test, tuning fork tests, audiometry, and tympanometry. Of these, audiometry is the most specific hearing acuity test because it provides information on how extensive a hearing loss a patient has and which frequencies are involved.

- ☐ An ear irrigation is the washing of the external auditory canal with a flowing solution. Ear irrigations are performed to remove cerumen, discharge, or a foreign body; to relieve inflammation by applying an antiseptic solution; or to apply heat to the ear.

- ☐ An ear instillation involves the dropping of a liquid into the external auditory canal. Ear instillations are performed to soften impacted cerumen, to combat infection with the use of antibiotic drops, or to relieve pain.

8

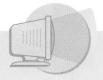

ON THE WEB

RESOURCES

For Information on the eye:

American Optometric Association
www.aoanet.org

Eyenet
www.eyenet.org

National Eye Institute
www.nei.nih.gov

Prevent Blindness America
www.prevent-blindness.org

For information on the ear:

American Academy of Audiology (AAA)
www.audiology.com

American Academy of Otolaryngology
www.entnet.org

Deaf World Web
www.deafworldweb.org

National Institute on Deafness and Other Communication Disorders (NIDCD)
www.nih.gov/nidcd

Marlyne Cooper, *and I am a Certified Medical Assistant. I graduated from an accredited medical assisting program and have an associate's degree in Applied Science. I work in a community health center and have worked as a medical assistant for 5 years. My primary responsibilities are to take patients back to the examination rooms and to prepare them for procedures and treatments. I take the patient's chief complaint, along with the health history. I greet each patient in a kind and calm way. This helps put the patient at ease before the physician goes into the examining room.*

Physical Agents to Promote Tissue Healing

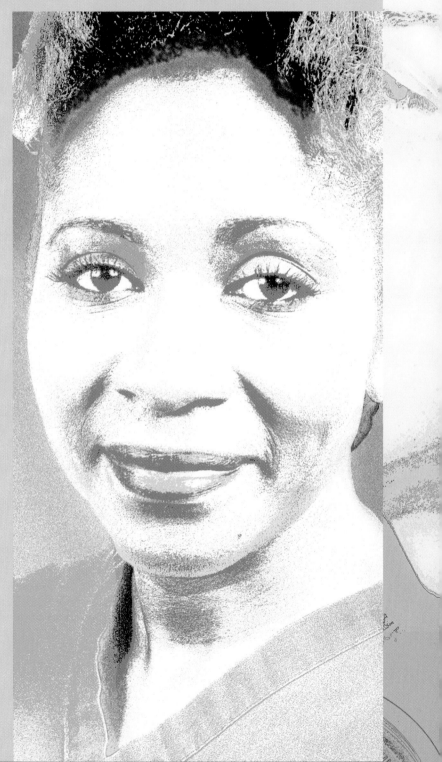

OUTCOMES

After completing this chapter, you should be able to demonstrate the proper procedure to perform the following:

1. Apply the following heat treatments: hot water bag, heating pad, hot soak, and hot compress.
2. Apply the following cold treatments: ice bag, cold compress, and chemical cold pack.
3. Administer an ultrasound treatment.
4. Instruct an individual in the proper guidelines for cast care.
5. Measure an individual for axillary crutches.
6. Instruct an individual in the proper guidelines for the use of crutches.
7. Instruct an individual in the proper procedure for each of the following crutch gaits: four-point, two-point, three-point, swing-to, and swing-through.
8. Instruct an individual in the proper procedure for using a cane.
9. Instruct an individual in the proper procedure for using a walker.

EDUCATIONAL OBJECTIVES

After completing this chapter, you should be able to do the following:

1. Define the terms listed in the Key Terminology.
2. Give examples of moist and dry applications of heat and cold.
3. List the effects that occur from the local application of heat, and state three reasons for applying heat.
4. List the effects that occur from the local application of cold, and state three reasons for applying cold.
5. State three factors that should be taken into considerations when applying heat and cold.
6. Describe the general use of therapeutic ultrasound.
7. Explain the purpose of the ultrasound coupling agent.
8. List three reasons for applying a cast.
9. Identify the advantages and disadvantages of synthetic casts.
10. Describe the cast application procedure.
11. List four factors that are taken into consideration when ambulatory aids are prescribed.
12. Explain the difference between an axillary crutch and a Lofstrand crutch.
13. State three conditions that may result when axillary crutches are not fitted properly.
14. List the guidelines that should be followed by the patient to ensure safety during crutch use.
15. State the use of each of the following crutch gaits: four-point gait, two-point gait, three-point gait, swing-to-gait, and swing-through gait.
16. List and describe the three types of canes.
17. Identify the patient conditions that warrant the use of a cane or walker.

KEY TERMINOLOGY

ambulation (AM-bû-LÂ-shun): The ability to walk as opposed to being confined to bed.

compress: A soft, moist, absorbent cloth that is folded in several layers and applied to a part of the body in the local application of heat or cold.

edema (a-DÊÊM-a): The retention of fluid in the tissues, resulting in swelling.

erythema (a-RITH-mê-a): Redness of the skin caused by congestion of capillaries in the lower layers of skin.

exudate (X-Û-dâte): A discharge produced by the body tissues.

inflammation (in-FLA-mâ-shun): The protective response of the tissues to injury or destruction. Local symptoms occurring at the site of the inflammation include pain, swelling, redness, and warmth.

long arm cast: A cast that extends from the axilla to the fingers of the hand, usually with a bend in the elbow.

long leg cast: A cast that extends from the midthigh to the toes.

orthopedist (orth-Ô-pêd-ist): A physician who deals with the prevention and correction of disorders of the locomotor structures of the body.

short arm cast: A cast that extends from below the elbow to the fingers.

short leg cast: A cast that begins just below the knee and extends to the toes.

soak: The direct immersion of a body part in water or a medicated solution.

sprain: Trauma to a joint that causes injury to the ligaments.

strain: An overstretching of a muscle due to trauma.

suppuration (SUPP-er-Â-shun): The process of pus formation.

toxin (ToX-in): A poisonous or noxious substance.

INTRODUCTION

9 ☐ Physical agents are often employed in the medical office to promote tissue healing for individuals who experience a disability following an injury, disease, or loss of a body part. Physical agents are used therapeutically to improve circulation, provide support, and promote the return of motion so that the individual can perform the activities of daily living. Physical agents frequently used in the medical office include heat and cold applied locally, therapeutic ultrasound, casts, and ambulatory aids such crutches, canes, and walkers.

LOCAL APPLICATION OF HEAT AND COLD

☐ The application of heat and cold is used therapeutically to treat pathologic conditions such as infection and trauma. The medical assistant may be responsible for applying various forms of heat and cold at the medical office or for instructing patients in the proper procedure for applying heat or cold at home. Therefore, the medical assistant should have a basic understanding of the physiologic effects of heat and cold on the body and any adverse reactions that may occur if they are not administered correctly.

Heat and cold can be applied in either moist or dry forms. Examples of moist and dry applications of heat and cold commonly used are

1. Dry heat: hot water bag, heating pad
2. Moist heat: hot soak, hot compress
3. Dry cold: ice bag, chemical cold pack
4. Moist cold: cold compress

Heat and cold are applied for short periods of time (generally 15 to 30 minutes) to produce desired therapeutic results. The application may be repeated at time intervals specified by the physician. Prolonged application of heat or cold is not recommended, as it can result in adverse secondary effects. The type of heat or cold application used for a particular condition depends on the purpose of the application, the location and condition of the affected area, and the age and general health of the patient. The physician will instruct the medical assistant to apply a heat or cold treatment based upon these factors.

Heat and cold receptors located in the skin readily adapt to changes in temperature, eventually resulting in diminished heat or cold sensations. The temperature actually remains the same and is providing the intended therapeutic effects. However, the patient, not perceiving the same degree of temperature, may want to increase the intensity of the application without realizing the inherent dangers involved. Excessive heat or cold could result in tissue damage. The medical assistant should fully explain to the patient the necessity of maintaining a safe temperature range during the application.

HEAT

Local Effects of Heat

The local effects of applying moderate heat to the body for a short period of time (approximately 15 to 30 minutes) include dilatation, or an increase in diameter, of the blood vessels in the area as the body tries to rid itself of excess heat from the blood to the environment (Fig. 9–1). This results in an increased blood supply to the area, and tissue metabolism increases. Nutrients and oxygen are provided to the cells at a faster rate, and wastes and toxins are carried away faster. The skin in the area becomes warm and exhibits

erythema. **Erythema** is the redness of the skin caused by congestion of capillaries in the lower layers of the skin.

These physiologic effects of moderate heat applied to a localized area promote healing. However, prolonged application of heat (more than 1 hour) produces secondary effects that reverse this healing process. Blood vessels constrict, and blood supply to the area decreases. The medical assistant must be careful to apply heat for the length of time specified by the physician.

Purpose of Applying Heat

Heat functions in relieving pain, congestion, muscle spasms, and inflammation. Heat promotes muscle relaxation and, therefore, is often used for the relief of pain due to the excessive contraction of muscle fibers.

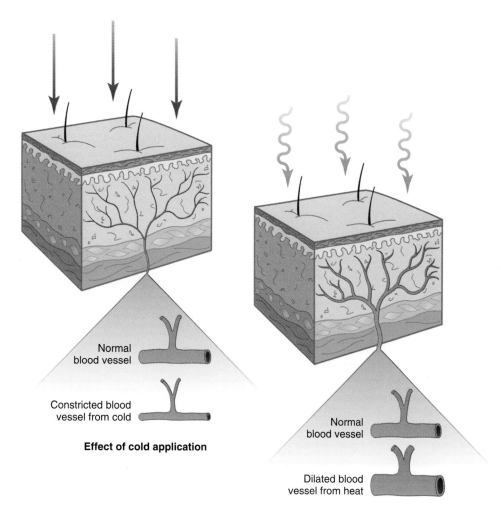

Normal blood vessel

Constricted blood vessel from cold

Effect of cold application

Normal blood vessel

Dilated blood vessel from heat

Effect of heat application

■ **FIGURE 9–1.** Effects of the local application of heat and cold. (From Wood, L. A., Rambo, B. J.: *Nursing Skills for Allied Health Services,* Vol 2. Philadelphia, W. B. Saunders, 1980.)

Edema or swelling already present in the tissues can be reduced through the application of heat, because the increased blood supply functions to increase the absorption of fluid from the tissues through the lymphatic system.

Heat, usually in the form of a moist compress, can be used to soften exudates. An **exudate** is a discharge produced by the body's tissues. At times, exudates may form a hard crust over an area and require removal. Heat also increases **suppuration,** or the process of pus formation, to help in the relief of inflammation by breaking down infected tissues. However, heat is not recommended for the initial treatment of acute inflammation or trauma.

Examples of conditions for which the local application of heat is often prescribed are low back pain, arthritis, menstrual cramping, and localized abscesses.

COLD

Local Effects of Cold

The application of moderate cold to a localized area produces constriction, or a decrease in diameter, of blood vessels in the area as the body attempts to prevent heat loss from the blood to the environment (see Fig. 9–1). This leads to decreased blood supply to the area. Tissue metabolism decreases, less oxygen is used, and fewer wastes accumulate. The skin becomes cool and pale. Prolonged application of cold (more than 1 hour) has a reverse secondary effect. Blood vessels dilate, and there is an increase in tissue metabolism. The medical assistant must apply cold for the recommended length of time only, to prevent secondary effects.

Purpose of Applying Cold

The application of moderate cold for a short period of time is used to prevent edema or swelling. Cold may be applied immediately after an individual has suffered direct trauma such as a bruise, sprain, muscle strain, joint injury, or fracture. The cold limits the accumulation of fluid in the body tissues by constricting blood vessels and reducing the leakage of fluid into the tissues. Through the constriction of peripheral blood vessels, cold can be used to control bleeding. Cold temporarily relieves pain because of its anesthetic, or numbing, effect, which reduces stimulation of the nerve receptors. Cold also slows the movement of blood and tissue fluids in the affected area, resulting in less pressure against nerve receptors and, therefore, less pain. In the early stages of an infection, the local application of cold will function to inhibit the activity of microorganisms. In this way, suppuration is decreased

and inflammation is reduced. Cold applications should always be placed in a protective covering, because applying cold directly to the skin could result in a skin burn.

FACTORS AFFECTING THE APPLICATION OF HEAT AND COLD

Before the application of heat or cold, certain factors must be taken into consideration to prevent unfavorable reactions such as tissue necrosis. The temperature may need to be adjusted based on the following conditions:

1. **The age of the patient.** Young children and elderly patients tend to be more sensitive to the application of heat or cold.
2. **Location of the application.** Certain areas of the body are more sensitive to the application of heat or cold, especially thin areas of the skin and areas that are usually covered by clothing, such as the chest, back, and abdomen. The skin of the hands and face is not as sensitive and is better able to tolerate temperature change. Broken skin, such as is found with an open wound, is more sensitive to heat and cold as well as being more prone to tissue damage.
3. **Impaired circulation.** Patients with impaired circulation tend to be more sensitive to heat or cold. This impairment may be at the site of the application or may be a systemic problem involving the entire body due to conditions such as peripheral vascular disease, diabetes mellitus, or congestive heart failure.
4. **Impaired sensation.** Patients with impaired sensation must be watched very carefully, because tissue damage may occur from the application of heat or cold without the patient's awareness.
5. **Individual tolerance to change in temperature.** Some individuals cannot tolerate temperature change as easily as others. The medical assistant should observe the area to which the heat or cold has been applied before, during, and after the treatment for signs indicating that a modification in temperature is needed. Prolonged erythema or paleness, pain, swelling, or blisters should be reported to the physician. The medical assistant should also ask the patient if the application feels comfortable, or if it is too hot or too cold.

Procedures for the local application of heat and cold are presented on the following pages; heat application procedures (hot water bag, heating pad, hot soak, and hot compress) are presented first, followed by cold application procedures (ice bag, cold compress, and chemical packs).

Text continued on page 341

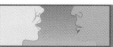

LOW BACK PAIN

■ Answer questions patients have about low back pain.

What causes low back pain?

Low back pain is one of the most common health problems in the United States. Between 50 and 80 percent of individuals are affected by low back pain at some time during their life. The most frequent cause of low back pain is poor posture and poor body mechanics, which strain the muscles and ligaments supporting the back. Other causes include physical inactivity, excessive body weight, disc damage, osteoarthritis, and congenital deformities.

How might the physician treat low back pain?

To treat low back pain caused by strain, the physician might prescribe bed rest, local application of heat, massage, medications, back manipulation, the use of back-supporting devices, deep-heating treatments such as ultrasound, and back exercises to strengthen the supporting structures of the back and prevent the back pain from becoming recurrent or chronic.

What can be done to prevent low back pain?

Most cases of low back pain can be prevented by practicing good posture and body mechanics.

■ Encourage patients to follow practices that prevent strain to the lower back.

■ Teach the patient the procedure for the local application of heat as prescribed by the physician.

■ Provide the patient with a sheet illustrating the back exercises prescribed by the physician.

■ Provide the patient with educational materials on low back pain.

BODY MECHANICS

■ Teach patients the essentials of good posture and body mechanics as follows:

Standing and walking.

Stand and walk with the chin tucked in, head up, back flattened, and the pelvis held straight. Wear comfortable low-heeled shoes that offer good support.

Lifting.

To lift an object, always bend the body at the knees and hips. Never bend from the waist. Lift the object with the leg muscles and hold it close to the body at waist level. Never lift anything heavier than you can easily manage or higher than waist level.

Sitting.

Sit in a chair with a firm back. The feet should be flat on the floor with the knees level with the hips. Sit firmly against the back of the chair; avoid slumping. Using a pillow in the small of the back, or a footstool to raise the knees, also helps reduce strain on the back.

Driving.

Make sure the car seat is not too far back. Stretching for the pedals places strain on the back. The car seat should be positioned so that the driver's back is straight and the knees are raised.

Sleeping.

Sleep on a firm, comfortable mattress that supports the back and does not allow it to sag. Sleep on the side with knees bent or on the back with a pillow under the knees. Do not sleep on the stomach, because this causes the body to sag into the mattress, resulting in strain on the back, neck, and shoulders.

9

9–1

Applying a Hot Water Bag

EQUIPMENT/SUPPLIES:	Hot water bag with a protective covering	Pitcher to hold water
	Bath thermometer	

1. **Procedural Step.** Wash the hands.
2. **Procedural Step.** Assemble the equipment.
3. **Procedural Step.** Greet and identify the patient.

Introduce yourself, and explain the procedure. Explain the purpose of applying the hot water bag—for example, to relieve pain.

Continued

333

9

4. **Procedural Step.** Fill the pitcher with hot tap water. Test the temperature of the water with a bath thermometer. It should range between 115 and 125°F (46 and 52°C) for adults and older children and between 105 and 115°F (41 and 46°C) for infants, children under 2 years of age, and elderly patients.

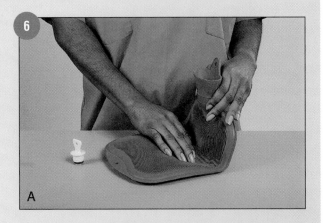

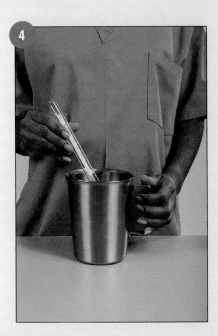

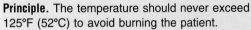

Principle. The temperature should never exceed 125°F (52°C) to avoid burning the patient.

5. **Procedural Step.** Fill the hot water bag one third to one half full of water.
Principle. A hot water bag that is not completely full is lighter in weight and easier to mold to the body area.

6. **Procedural Step.** Expel the excess air from the bag by resting the bag on the table and flattening it while holding the neck upright until the water reaches the neck. Air can also be expelled by holding the bag upright and squeezing the unfilled part until the water reaches the neck. Screw in the stopper or fasten the top with special closure tabs.
Principle. Air is a poor conductor of heat and also makes it difficult to mold the hot water bag to the body area.

7. **Procedural Step.** Dry the outside of the bag and test for leakage by holding the bag upside down.
Principle. Leaking water will get the patient wet and may burn the patient.

8. **Procedural Step.** Place the bag in the protective covering.

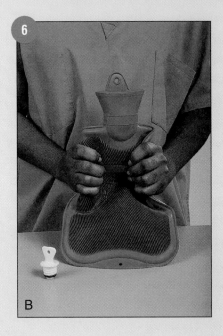

Principle. The cover helps absorb perspiration and lessens the danger of burning the patient.

9. **Procedural Step.** Place the bag on the patient's affected body area. Ask the patient how the temperature feels. The hot water bag should feel warm but not uncomfortable.
Principle. Individuals vary in their ability to tolerate heat.

10. **Procedural Step.** Administer the treatment for the proper length of time, as designated by the physician. Check the patient's skin periodically for signs of an increase or decrease in redness or swelling and ask the patient whether the site is painful.

11. **Procedural Step.** Refill the bag with hot water as needed to maintain the proper temperature making sure to remove an equal amount of the cooler water.

PROCEDURE 9–1

12. **Procedural Step.** Wash the hands and chart the procedure. Include the date and time, method of heat application (hot water bag), temperature of the hot water, location and duration of the application, appearance of the application site, and the patient's reaction.

13. **Procedural Step.** Properly care for the hot water bag. Dispose of or launder the protective covering. Cleanse the hot water bag with a warm detergent solution, rinse thoroughly, and dry by hanging the bag upside down with the top removed. Store the bag by screwing on the stopper, leaving air inside to prevent the sides from sticking together.

CHARTING EXAMPLE

Date	
12/5/2002	2:30 p.m. Hot water bag @ 110°F applied to Ⓡ ant thigh x 20 minutes. Area appears pink following application. Pt states a relief of muscle spasm. Provided instructions for the application of a hot water bag at home.
	———————————— M. Cooper, CMA

9–2

PROCEDURE

Applying a Heating Pad

The electric heating pad consists of a network of wires that function to convert electric energy into heat to provide a constant and even heat application. The wires must not be bent or crushed. This could damage the pad, resulting in overheating of parts of the pad and leading to burns or fire. Pins must not be inserted in the pad as a means of securing it, because if a pin comes in contact with a wire, an electric shock could result. To prevent electric hazards, heating pads should not be used over areas containing moisture such as wet dressings.

EQUIPMENT/SUPPLIES: **Heating pad with a protective covering**

1. **Procedural Step.** Wash the hands.
2. **Procedural Step.** Assemble the equipment.
3. **Procedural Step.** Greet and identify the patient. Introduce yourself, and explain the procedure. Patients should be instructed not to lie on the heating pad.
   Principle. Lying on the pad causes heat to accumulate and burn the patient.
4. **Procedural Step.** Place the heating pad in the protective covering.
   Principle. The protective covering provides more comfort for the patient and functions to absorb perspiration.
5. **Procedural Step.** Connect the plug to an electric outlet. Set the selector switch at the proper setting, as designated by the physician (usually low or medium).
6. **Procedural Step.** Place the heating pad on the patient's affected body area. Ask the patient how the temperature feels. The heating pad should feel warm but not uncomfortable.

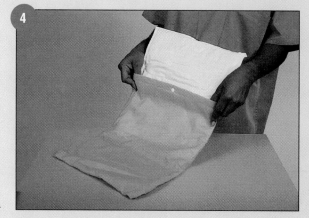

7. **Procedural Step.** Instruct the patient not to turn the control higher, so as to prevent a burn that may be caused by excessive heat.
   Principle. The patient's heat receptors eventually become adjusted to the temperature change, result-

Continued

9

ing in a decreased heat sensation, and the patient may be tempted to increase the temperature.

8. **Procedural Step.** Administer the treatment for the proper length of time as designated by the physician. Check the patient periodically for signs of an increase or decrease in redness or swelling, and ask the patient if the site is painful.

9. **Procedural Step.** Wash hands and chart the procedure. Include the date and time, method of heat application (heating pad), temperature setting of the pad, location and duration of the application, appearance of the application site, and the patient's reaction.

10. **Procedural Step.** Return equipment.

CHARTING EXAMPLE

Date	
12/10/2002	10:15 a.m. Heating pad on medium setting applied to lower back x 20 minutes. Area appears pink following application. Pt states a relief of pain and better mobility Provided instructions on the application of a heating pad at home. ———— M. Cooper, CMA

9–3

Applying a Hot Soak

A **soak** is the direct immersion of a body part in water or a medicated solution. A soak can be applied to an extremity or a part of the torso. Hot soaks function to cleanse open wounds, to increase suppuration, to increase the blood supply to an area to hasten the healing process, or to apply a medicated solution to an area. Applying a soak to an open wound requires the use of sterile technique.

EQUIPMENT/SUPPLIES:	Soaking solution ordered by the physician	Basin
	Bath thermometer	Bath towels

1. **Procedural Step.** Wash the hands.
2. **Procedural Step.** Assemble the equipment.
3. **Procedural Step.** Greet and identify the patient. Introduce yourself, and explain the procedure.
4. **Procedural Step.** Fill the basin half full with the warmed soaking solution.
5. **Procedural Step.** Check the temperature of the solution with a bath thermometer. The temperature for an adult should range between 105 and 110°F (41 and 44°C).
6. **Procedural Step.** Place the patient in a comfortable position to avoid fatigue and muscle strain. Pad the side of the basin with a towel to provide for patient comfort.
7. **Procedural Step.** Slowly and gradually immerse the patient's affected body part in the solution. Ask the patient how the temperature feels.
Principle. The affected body part should be allowed to become accustomed to the change in temperature gradually.

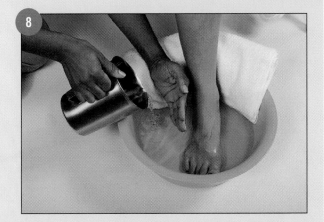

8. **Procedural Step.** Test the temperature of the solution frequently. Remove cooler fluid every 5 minutes to keep the solution at a constant temperature. Pour the hot water in near the edge of the

PROCEDURE 9-3

basin by placing your hand between the patient and water. Stir the water as you pour.

Principle. Water should be added away from the patient's body part to prevent splashing hot water on the patient. Stirring in the water helps distribute the heat and keep the temperature constant.

9. **Procedural Step.** Apply the hot soak for the proper length of time as designated by the physician (usually 15 to 20 minutes). Check the patient's skin periodically for signs of an increase or decrease in redness or swelling, and ask the patient whether the site is painful.

10. **Procedural Step.** Completely and gently dry the affected part.

11. **Procedural Step.** Wash the hands and chart the procedure. Include the date and time, method of heat application (hot soak), name and strength of

the solution, the temperature of the soak, location and duration of the application, the appearance of the application site, and the patient's reaction.

12. **Procedural Step.** Return and properly care for the equipment.

CHARTING EXAMPLE

Date	
12/12/2002	1:15 p.m. Normal saline hot soak @ 105°F applied to (R) ankle x 20 minutes. Area appears pink following application. Pt states less stiffness in ankle. —— M. Cooper, CMA

PROCEDURE

9-4

Applying a Hot Compress

A **compress** is a soft, moist, absorbent cloth, such as a washcloth, applied to a body part. Hot compresses are used to increase suppuration, to improve circulation to a body part to aid in healing, and to promote drainage from infection. Applying a hot compress to an open wound requires the use of sterile technique.

EQUIPMENT/SUPPLIES: Solution ordered by the physician   Basin
Bath thermometer   Washcloths

1. **Procedural Step.** Wash the hands.
2. **Procedural Step.** Assemble the equipment.
3. **Procedural Step.** Greet and identify the patient. Introduce yourself, and explain the procedure.
4. **Procedural Step.** Fill the basin half full with warmed solution. Check the temperature of the solution with the bath thermometer. The temperature for an adult should range between 105 and 110°F (41 and 44°C).
5. **Procedural Step.** Completely immerse the compress in the solution. Wring out the compress to rid it of excess moisture. The compress should be wet but not dripping. Apply it lightly at first to the affected site to allow the patient gradually to become used to the heat. The medical assistant may want to

cover the compress with a waterproof cover to help hold the heat in. Ask the patient how the temperature feels. The compress should be applied as hot as the patient can comfortably tolerate.

Principle. The waterproof cover prevents cool air currents from coming in contact with the compress and reduces the number of times the compress needs to be changed.

6. **Procedural Step.** Place additional compresses in the solution so they are ready for use.
7. **Procedural Step.** Repeat the application of the compress every 2 to 3 minutes for the duration of time specified by the physician (usually 15 to 20 minutes). Check the patient's skin periodically for signs of an increase or decrease in redness or

9

Continued

PROCEDURE 9–4

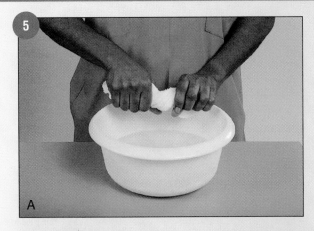

A

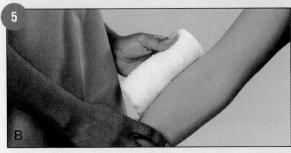

B

swelling and ask the patient whether the site is painful.

8. **Procedural Step.** Check the temperature of the water periodically. Add more hot water if needed.

9. **Procedural Step.** Thoroughly and gently dry the affected part.

10. **Procedural Step.** Wash hands and chart the procedure. Include the date and time, method of heat application (hot compress), name and strength of the solution, temperature of the solution, location and duration of the application, appearance of the application site, and the patient's reaction.

11. **Procedural Step.** Return and properly care for the equipment.

CHARTING EXAMPLE

Date	
12/20/2002	10:30 a.m. Normal saline hot compress @ 110°F applied to Ⓡ forearm x 20 minutes. Abscess appears to be coming to a head. No complaints of discomfort.— M. Cooper, CMA

9–5

PROCEDURE

Applying an Ice Bag

EQUIPMENT/SUPPLIES: Ice bag with a protective covering
Small pieces of ice (ice chips or crushed ice)

1. **Procedural Step.** Wash the hands.
2. **Procedural Step.** Assemble the equipment.
3. **Procedural Step.** Greet and identify the patient. Introduce yourself, and explain the procedure. Explain the purpose of applying the ice bag—for example, to prevent swelling.
4. **Procedural Step.** Check the ice bag for leakage.
   Principle. A leaking bag will get the patient wet and cause chilling.
5. **Procedural Step.** Fill the bag one half to two thirds full with small pieces of ice.

Principle. Small pieces of ice work better than larger pieces because they reduce the amount of air spaces in the bag, resulting in better conduction of cold. In addition, small pieces of ice allow the bag to mold better to the body area.

6. **Procedural Step.** Expel air from the bag by squeezing the empty top half of the bag together and screwing on the stopper.
   Principle. Air is a poor conductor of cold and also makes it difficult to mold the ice bag to the body area.

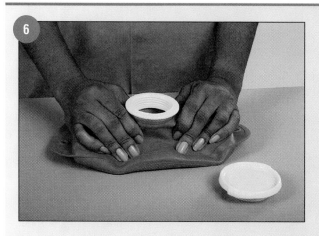

6

7. Procedural Step. Thoroughly dry the bag and place it in the protective covering.
Principle. The protective covering provides for patient comfort and absorbs the moisture that condenses on the outside of the bag.

8. Procedural Step. Place the bag on the patient's affected body area. Ask the patient how the temperature feels. The application of ice is usually uncomfortable, but most patients tolerate it if they know how much benefit may be derived from it.
Principle. Individuals vary in their ability to tolerate cold.

9. Procedural Step. Administer the treatment for the proper length of time, as designated by the physician (*usually until the area feels numb,* approximately 20 to 30 minutes). Check the patient's skin periodically for signs of an increase or decrease in redness or swelling and ask the patient whether

the site is painful. If extreme paleness and numbness or a mottled blue appearance occur at the application site, remove the bag and notify the physician.

10. Procedural Step. Refill the bag with ice as necessary, and change the protective covering if needed.

11. Procedural Step. Wash the hands, and chart the procedure. Include the date and time, method of cold application (ice bag), location and duration of the application, appearance of the application site, and the patient's reaction.

12. Procedural Step. Properly care for the ice bag. Dispose of or launder the protective covering as required. Cleanse the ice bag with a warm detergent, solution, rinse thoroughly and dry by hanging the bag upside down with the top removed. Store the bag by screwing on the stopper, leaving air inside to prevent the sides from sticking together.

CHARTING EXAMPLE

Date	
12/22/2002	11:30 a.m. Icebag applied to (R) knee x 20 minutes. Pt complained of slight discomfort during the application. Area appears less swollen following application. Provided instructions on the application of an ice bag at home. ———————— M. Cooper, CMA

9

9–6

Applying a Cold Compress

Cold compresses are used to relieve pain and inflammation and to treat conditions such as headaches, injury to the eyes, and pain after tooth extraction.

EQUIPMENT/SUPPLIES:	Ice cubes Washcloths
	Basin

1. Procedural Step. Wash the hands.
2. Procedural Step. Assemble the equipment.

3. Procedural Step. Greet and identify the patient. Introduce yourself, and explain the procedure.

Continued

PROCEDURE 9–6

4. **Procedural Step.** Prepare the water by placing large ice cubes in the basin and adding a small amount of water.

Principle. Using larger pieces of ice prevents them from sticking to the compress and slows the rate at which they melt in the water.

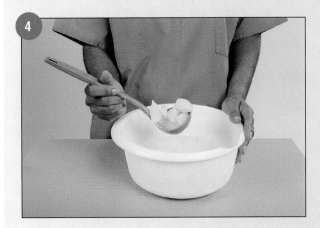

5. **Procedural Step.** Completely immerse the compress in the solution. Wring out the compress to rid it of excess moisture. The compress should be wet but not dripping. Apply it lightly at first to the affected site to allow the patient gradually to become used to the cold. The medical assistant may want to cover the compress with an ice bag to help keep it cold and to reduce the number of times it needs

to be changed. Ask the patient how the temperature feels.

6. **Procedural Step.** Place additional compresses in the solution to be ready for use.

7. **Procedural Step.** Repeat the application of the compress every 2 to 3 minutes for the duration of time specified by the physician (usually 15 to 20 minutes). Check the patient's skin periodically for signs of an increase or decrease in redness or swelling and ask the patient whether the site is painful.

8. **Procedural Step.** Add ice if needed to keep the water cold.

9. **Procedural Step.** Thoroughly dry the affected part.

10. **Procedural Step.** Wash hands and chart the procedure. Include the date and time, method of cold application (cold compress), location and duration of the application, appearance of the application site, and the patient's reaction.

11. **Procedural Step.** Return and properly care for the equipment.

CHARTING EXAMPLE

Date	
12/27/2002	9:15 a.m. Cold compress applied to bridge of nose x 15 minutes. Nose appears less swollen following application. Tolerated application well. ——————— M. Cooper, CMA

9–7

PROCEDURE

Applying a Chemical Cold and Hot Pack

Chemical Cold Pack

Chemical cold packs are available in a variety of sizes and shapes. Once activated, they provide a specific degree of coldness for a specific period of time (usually 30 to 60 minutes), as indicated on the package label. Most cold packs consist of a vinyl bag containing ammonium nitrate crystals. Enclosed within this bag is a smaller vinyl bag containing water. The cold pack is activated by applying pressure until the inner bag ruptures. This releases the water into the larger bag, and a chemical reaction occurs between the crystals and water, producing coldness. These packs are disposable and once the coldness diminishes they should be discarded in an appropriate receptacle. Chemical cold packs should be stored at room temperature and are used as an alternative to ice bags for the local application of cold.

PROCEDURE 9–7

Chemical Hot Pack

A chemical hot pack is similar to a chemical cold pack except that heat is generated once the bag is activated. The vinyl bag contains calcium chloride crystals, and the smaller bag (encased within the vinyl bag) contains water. Pressure is applied to break the inner bag. The water in the inner bag combines with the calcium chloride crystals to produce heat. After using the pack, it should be discarded in an appropriate receptacle.

The procedure for applying a chemical cold or hot pack is as follows:

1. **Procedural Step.** Shake the crystals to the bottom of the bag.
2. **Procedural Step.** Squeeze the bag firmly to break the inner water bag.
3. **Procedural Step.** Shake the bag vigorously to mix the contents.
4. **Procedural Step.** Apply the bag to the affected area.
5. **Procedural Step.** Administer the treatment for the proper length of time.
6. **Procedural Step.** Discard the bag in an appropriate receptacle.

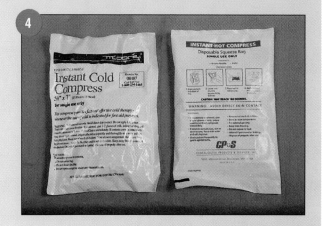

THERAPEUTIC ULTRASOUND

☐ Therapeutic ultrasound uses high-frequency sound waves as a penetrating, deep-heating agent for the soft tissues of the body, such as tendons and muscles. Many physicians use ultrasound in the medical office for the local application of heat to treat musculoskeletal disorders.

The beneficial physiologic effects of ultrasound are primarily due to the deep heat produced in the tissues and include reduction of edema, breakup of exudates and precipitates, increased cellular metabolism, relief of pain, and micromassage. The physician may order ultrasound to treat such musculoskeletal conditions as sprains, joint contractures, neuritis, arthritis, edema, synovitis, scar tissue, bursitis, fibrositis, strains, and dislocations. Therapeutic ultrasound must *not* be used over the eyeball, over malignant tumors, directly over the spinal cord, over the heart or brain, over reproductive organs or a pregnant uterus, or over areas of impaired sensation or inadequate circulation.

The medical assistant is responsible for performing the ultrasound treatment, which includes preparing the patient, operating the machine, and administering the treatment.

PARTS OF THE ULTRASOUND MACHINE

The ultrasound machine consists of two main parts: the generator and the transducer. The generator is located within the main unit of the machine, which also contains the controls to operate the machine. The transducer consists of a crystal inserted between two electrodes; it is located in a device termed the applicator head or sound head. The applicator head is a lightweight, hand-held device attached to the ultrasound machine by a connector cord (Fig. 9–2). The generator produces a high-frequency electric current that causes the crystal (located in the transducer) to vibrate and generate sound waves. The frequency of the sound waves produced by the transducer is above the frequency of sound waves audible to the human ear; therefore, no sound is heard when the machine is in operation.

The controls on the ultrasound machine include a timing control and an intensity control; additional controls may be present, depending on the type of machine in use. The **timing control** measures time in minutes; the time limit of most machines ranges from 0 to 15 minutes, which is sufficient because the majority of treatments rarely exceed 10 minutes. The **intensity control** governs the intensity of the sound waves, which are measured in watts; therapeutic ultrasound intensity usually ranges from 1 to 4 watts. A digital display screen indicates the intensity at which the machine has been set.

The medical assistant must be able to operate each control; for example, if the physician orders an ultrasound treatment at 4 watts for a duration of 5 minutes, the medical assistant first sets the timing control at 5 (minutes) and then sets the intensity control until the display screen indicates that the intensity is at 4 watts.

9

Timing control

Density control

Applicator head

Connector card

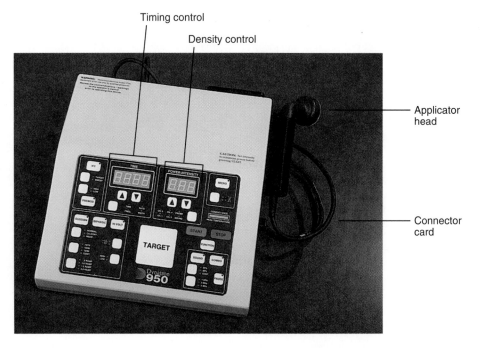

■ **FIGURE 9–2.** The parts of an ultrasound machine.

MEMORIES *from* EXTERNSHIP

MARLYNE COOPER: *At my first externship site, I was scared to death about having to give injections to small children. I didn't want to hurt them. A 6-month-old baby came to the office for her immunizations. My externship supervisor wanted me to give the injections. The baby was so small, and she was crying before I even gave her the first injection. I knew that when I gave the injection, she was going to cry even more, and that made me feel bad. My supervisor was there with me, and she talked me through it. It turned out that it wasn't as bad as I thought it would be. My supervisor was very helpful in keeping me calm. After that first experience, I felt much more comfortable when I had to give an injection to a small child.*

Coupling Agents

Air is a poor conductor of sound; therefore, a coupling agent must be used with ultrasound treatments to increase conductivity, thereby providing a good transmission of the sound waves to the patient's tissues. The coupling agent produces an air-free contact between the applicator head and the patient's skin and is available in the form of a commercially available lotion or gel.

The coupling agent must be at room temperature and must be applied liberally to the treatment area of the patient's skin. Water may also be used as a coupling agent because it is a good conductor of sound. In this method, both the patient's skin surface to be treated and the applicator head are completely submerged under water. The applicator head is held ½ to 1 inch away from the patient's skin and is slowly and steadily moved, using a circular motion. The underwater method is advocated when the patient's skin is sensitive and cannot tolerate the direct pressure of the applicator head or when the body surface to be treated is uneven, as are the hands or feet, where it would be difficult to obtain a good contact between the patient's skin and the applicator head.

ADMINISTERING ULTRASOUND THERAPY

The applicator head is firmly placed on the patient's skin surface and is slowly and steadily moved over the treatment area, which allows the sound waves to penetrate the patient's soft tissues. As the sound waves travel through the tissues, part of the waves are absorbed by the tissues and transformed into heat. This produces a vigorous deep heating in the soft tissues of the body. A micromassage effect is also produced owing to the mechanical vibration of the sound waves as they pass through the tissues, massaging them.

The applicator head must be moved continuously during the treatment in either a back-and-forth stroking motion or in a circular motion at a rate of 1 to 2 inches per second. The method used depends in large part on the area of the body to which the treatment is being applied. It is usually easier to use the stroking motion over larger body areas such as the back, and the circular motion over smaller areas such as the ankle. Moving the applicator head ensures a uniform distribution of heat in the tissues and prevents the occurrence of hot spots. A hot spot is a very small area in which the temperature rises rapidly if the applicator head is allowed to remain stationary. This could cause burns to the patient's tissues.

Ultrasound dosage is expressed in watt-minutes. Watt refers to the intensity of the sound waves ordered by the physician, and minutes refers to the duration of the treatment. The dosage ordered by the physician depends on the area of the body that is receiving the treatment and the patient's condition. An acute condition requires a lower intensity treatment, whereas a chronic condition warrants a higher intensity treatment. The underwater method also requires a higher intensity because some of the sound waves are absorbed and reflected by the water.

Ultrasound therapy is generally administered in a series of 6 to 12 treatments; the frequency of the treatment varies from once daily to three times per week. The duration of administration of the treatment usually progresses from 5 minutes at the beginning of the series to 8 to 10 minutes near the end of the treatments. An ultrasound treatment should never exceed 20 minutes.

During the treatment, the patient normally should not feel the ultrasound waves. If the patient indicates a feeling of burning or pain, the medical assistant should stop the treatment immediately and inform the physician. Any pain or discomfort usually indicates that the treatment dosage is too intense. Other causes of pain or discomfort include application of an insufficient amount of coupling medium to the treatment area and keeping the applicator head on one area too long.

9

PROCEDURE

9–8

Administering an Ultrasound Treatment

EQUIPMENT/SUPPLIES: **Ultrasound machine**   **Paper towels**
Coupling agent

1. **Procedural Step.** Wash the hands.
2. **Procedural Step.** Assemble the equipment.
3. **Procedural Step.** Greet and identify the patient. Introduce yourself, and explain the procedure. Tell the patient that the treatment will not take long and that any pain or discomfort experienced during the treatment should be reported immediately.
   Principle. Pain or discomfort during the treatment may indicate that the intensity of the treatment dosage is too high.

4. **Procedural Step.** Ask the patient to remove appropriate clothing to expose the treatment area. Position the patient and prepare the skin. Make sure the coupling agent is at room temperature, and apply it liberally to the treatment area. Tell the patient that the coupling agent will feel cold. Use the applicator head to spread the coupling agent evenly over the treatment area. The coupling agent should completely cover, but should not flood, the area. Do not place the coupling agent on the ultrasound machine.

Continued

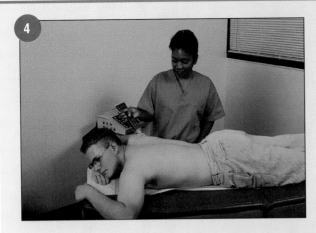

7. Procedural Step. Move the applicator head in a back-and-forth stroking motion or in a circular motion. If the stroking method is employed, use short strokes (approximately 1 inch in length), and gradually move the applicator head so that each stroke overlaps the previous stroke by one half. Move the applicator head continually at a rate of 1 to 2 inches per second.

Principle. Moving the applicator head continually ensures a uniform distribution of heat in the tissues and prevents overheating of the tissue in a small area (hot spot).

Principle. The coupling agent permits a good transmission of the sound waves to the patient's tissues. The coupling agent should be applied at room temperature so as not to be too uncomfortable for the patient.

5. Procedural Step. Set the intensity control at the minimum position, and set the timer to the amount of time stipulated for the ultrasound treatment as specified by the physician. Once the timer has activated the machine check to make sure the intensity is at 0 watts.

6. Procedural Step. Advance the intensity control to the treatment level (measured in watts) specified by the physician. Tell the patient that the applicator head will feel cold. Hold the applicator at a right angle to the patient's skin, and using a firm pressure, place the application head into the coupling agent in the treatment area.

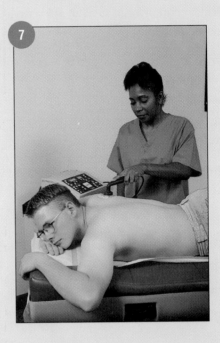

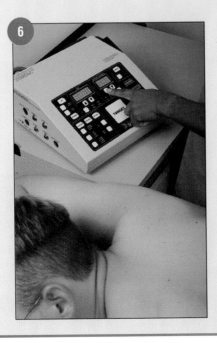

8. Procedural Step. Continue the ultrasound treatment until the timer goes off. During the treatment, perform the following:
   a. Move the applicator head continually.
   b. Do not remove the applicator head from the patient's skin and hold it up in the air.
   c. Stop the treatment immediately and notify the physician if the patient complains of any pain or discomfort.

Principle. Holding the applicator head in the air causes it to become hot and it may burn the patient when it is placed back on the skin. The excessive heat may also damage the crystal in the applicator head.

9. Procedural Step. When the treatment time is completed, the timer automatically shuts off the machine. Remove the applicator head from the patient's skin.

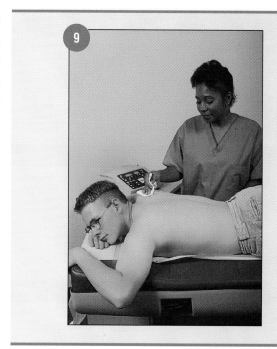

10. **Procedural Step.** Wipe the excess coupling medium from the patient's skin and applicator head with a paper towel. Instruct the patient to get dressed.

11. **Procedural Step.** Wash the hands, and chart the procedure. Include the date and time, the location of the treatment, the duration (in minutes) and the intensity used (in watts), and the patient's reaction.

CHARTING EXAMPLE

Date	
12/10/2002	10:45 a.m. Ultrasound applied to the Ⓡ
	upper back @ 2 watts x 5 minutes. No
	complaints of discomfort. Pt states a relief
	of pain and feeling of relaxed muscles. ——
	—— M. Cooper, CMA

CASTS

☐ A cast is a stiff cylindrical casing that is used to immobilize a body part. Casts are applied most often when an individual sustains a fracture. The cast keeps the fractured bones aligned until proper healing takes place. Other uses of a cast are to support and stabilize weak or dislocated joints; to promote healing after a surgical correction, such as knee surgery; and to aid in the nonsurgical correction of deformities such as congenital dislocation of the hip.

Casts are usually applied by an **orthopedist,** a specialist who deals with the prevention and correction of disorders of the locomotor structures of the body. The role of the medical assistant in cast application is to assemble the equipment and supplies, prepare the patient for the procedure, assist the physician during the application, provide or reinforce cast care instructions, and clean the examining room following the application.

One of the most important goals of cast management is the prevention of pressure areas, which are most apt to occur over bony prominences. A **pressure area** occurs when the cast presses or rubs against the patient's skin, resulting in inadequate circulation to the area. If permitted to continue, a pressure area can cause the skin to break down, which is then susceptible to infection by invading organisms.

CAST MATERIALS

Casts are categorized as either plaster casts or synthetic casts according to the materials they consist of. Plaster casts are preferred for acute, complicated fractures, whereas synthetic casts are often used for simple, uncomplicated fractures.

PLASTER CASTS. The traditional plaster cast consists of powdered calcium sulfate crystals formed into a bandage that must be soaked in tepid water to activate the crystals. When wet, the plaster bandage becomes pliable and self-adhering, allowing it to be molded to the body part. Plaster bandages are available in individual rolls of various widths ranging from 2 to 6 inches. The width used depends on the body part to be casted: the smaller widths are used for the arms and the larger widths for the legs and trunk.

SYNTHETIC CASTS. Synthetic casts consist of tape made of fiberglass, polyester and cotton, or plastic. The tape is impregnated with polyurethane resin that is activated when it is soaked in water. Of the three types of synthetic materials, fiberglass is the one most commonly used. Synthetic tape comes in individual rolls of varying widths ranging from 2 to 5 inches.

9

The advantages of synthetic casts as compared with plaster casts are

■ Synthetic casts dry and set much more quickly than plaster casts. Because of this, they are able to bear weight within a short period of time following application.

■ Synthetic casts are less likely to become indented because of their fast drying time. Indentations can result in pressure areas.

■ Synthetic casts weigh less than plaster casts and, therefore, are less restrictive, which allows the patient greater activity and mobility.

■ Synthetic casts are less bulky than plaster casts; therefore, patients usually can wear regular clothing over them.

■ The material making up synthetic casts is moisture resistant. If a nonabsorbent lining has been used in applying the cast, the physician may allow the patient to immerse the cast in water. After immersion, the cast must be thoroughly dried as soon as possible to avoid skin problems. The outside of the cast should first be blotted with an absorbent towel. This should be followed by the application of a blow dryer on a cool setting using a sweeping motion over the entire cast until it is completely dry. Because this procedure takes about an hour, some patients who could otherwise do so choose not to get their cast wet.

Disadvantages of synthetic casts as compared with plaster casts include

■ Synthetic casts cannot be molded to the body part as easily as plaster casts, so they are less effective for immobilizing severely displaced bones or unstable fractures.

■ Because of the cost of the materials making them up, synthetic casts are more expensive than plaster casts.

■ The surface of a synthetic cast is rougher than that of a plaster cast; therefore, there is an increased chance of snagging clothes, scratching furniture, and causing abrasions on other parts of the body with the cast.

CAST APPLICATION

The physician applies the cast so that it fits snugly but still allows for adequate circulation necessary for proper healing. A period of 4 to 6 weeks is usually required for complete healing to take place.

Casts are classified according to the body part they cover. The types of casts most frequently applied in the medical office are illustrated and described in Figure 9–3. The type of cast applied depends on the nature of the patient's injury or condition. For exam-

Short arm cast

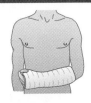

Extends from below the elbow to the fingers.

Long arm cast

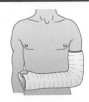

Extends from the axilla to the fingers, usually with a bend in the elbow.

Short leg cast

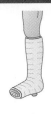

Begins just below the knee and extends to the toes; a walking heel is usually attached to a lower extremity cast so that the patient is able to ambulate.

Long leg cast

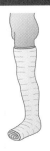

Extends from the midthigh to the toes.

■ **FIGURE 9–3.** Types of casts.

ple, a short arm cast is used for a dislocated wrist, and a long arm cast is used for a fracture of the humerus.

Regardless of the casting material used (plaster or synthetic), the following steps are performed in applying a cast:

1. **Inspection of the Skin**
   The area to which the cast will be applied should be clean and dry. The patient's skin should be inspected for redness, bruises, or open areas. This information should be recorded in the patient's chart, which may assist in evaluating patient complaints after the cast has been applied.

2. **Application of the Stockinette**
   Before applying the cast, the physician covers the body part with a stockinette (Fig. 9–4). Stockinette consists of a soft, tubular, knitted cotton material

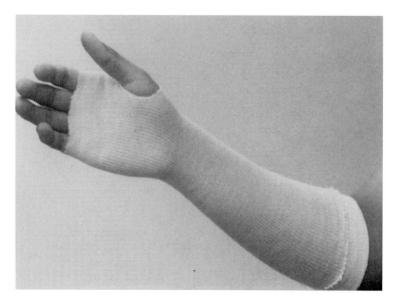

■ **FIGURE 9–4.** Application of stockinette. (Courtesy of 3M Health Care, St. Paul, MN.)

that stretches up to three times its normal width to accommodate the diameter of the body part. It is applied like putting on a stocking. The purpose of the stockinette is to provide for patient comfort and to cover the rough edges at the ends of the cast.

Stockinette comes in widths ranging from 2 to 12 inches; the width used depends on the diameter of the part to be covered. Typically, a 3-inch width is used for arm casts, while a 4-inch width is used for leg casts and a 10- to 12-inch width is used for body casts.

3. **Application of Cast Padding**
   Cast padding consists of a soft cotton material that comes in a roll of widths ranging from 2 to 4 inches. The purpose of cast padding is to prevent pressure areas and to shield the patient's skin when the cast is removed. Between two and three layers are applied directly over the stockinette, using a spiral turn. Each turn overlaps the preceding one by half of the width of the roll. Extra layers of padding are applied over bony prominences (Fig. 9–5).

4. **Application of the Cast Bandage or Tape**
   The plaster cast bandage or synthetic tape is applied over the cast padding. The number of rolls used depends on the desired strength of the finished cast. Usually, between 4 and 6 layers are applied for a plaster cast and between 3 and 5 layers are applied for a synthetic cast.

   The physician wears rubber gloves during the procedure to protect the hands from the casting material. Following application, the cast must be allowed to dry: The time varies based on the type of casting material used. Because of their porous nature, plaster casts require a longer drying period

than synthetic casts. Only when a cast is completely dry does it become hard and inflexible and able to bear weight. The physician usually prescribes a supportive device, such as a sling or crutches, to prevent unnecessary strain and to minimize swelling during the healing process. Specific information on applying plaster casts and synthetic casts is presented next.

Plaster Cast

To activate the plaster, the bandage roll must be completely immersed in tepid water (70 to 95°F;

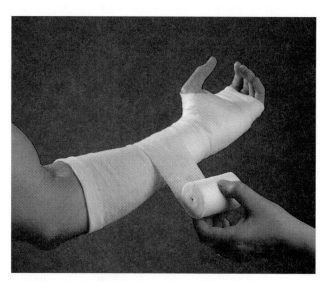

■ **FIGURE 9–5.** Application of cast padding. (Courtesy of 3M Health Care, St. Paul, MN.)

21 to 35°C) until bubbles no longer rise from the roll. The edges of the roll are then gently squeezed (but not wrung) toward the center to remove excess water. A properly squeezed roll should be fully saturated with water, but not dripping.

The physician wraps the body part with the plaster bandage, using a spiral turn, until the desired number of layers have been applied. The stockinette is folded over the edges of the cast and anchored with the cast bandage to produce a smooth, comfortable edge on the cast. The physician molds and smooths the plaster to conform to the contours of the body part until the cast is firmly set. Finally, the physician trims the ends of the cast with a cast knife to remove rough edges and to provide freedom of movement for the uninvolved part of the extremity such as the thumb, fingers, or toes.

As the plaster begins to harden, a chemical reaction occurs that releases heat. Because of this, the patient may feel warmth during and after the application. Most patients find that the warmth has a soothing effect. The patient should not put any weight on the cast until it is completely dry; otherwise, the cast may break down. It takes approximately 24 to 48 hours for the standard plaster cast to dry completely.

Synthetic Cast

9

A synthetic cast is applied in a similar manner to that for a plaster cast. The roll of synthetic tape is fully immersed in cool water for a period of time recommended by the manufacturer (Fig. 9–6). For example, fiberglass tape is immersed for 10 to 15 seconds. The tape is then wrapped over the body part, using a spiral turn, until the desired number of layers have been applied (Fig. 9–7). To help smooth the rough exterior surface associated with a synthetic cast, a silicone cream is rubbed over the surface of the cast. The cast is then allowed to dry for a period of time specified by the manufacturer; for example, a fiberglass cast dries in 30 minutes.

PRECAUTIONS

The following precautions should be observed during and after cast application:

- Do not cover a wet cast with a towel, plastic, or any other material. Covers prevent heat from escaping, which could result in a burn to the patient's skin.
- Take precautions to prevent indentations, particularly with a plaster cast, which could lead to pressure areas. This is accomplished by not allowing the

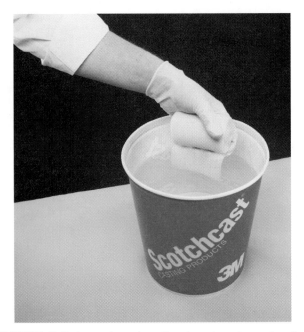

■ **FIGURE 9–6.** Immersion of a fiberglass tape in cool water. (Courtesy of 3M Health Care, St. Paul, MN.)

cast to come in contact with a hard surface while it is drying and by handling a wet cast with the palms of the hands rather than the fingertips.

- Remove any crumbs of plaster from the patient's skin, using a cloth dampened with warm water. Remove synthetic casting material with a swab moistened with alcohol or acetone. If cast particles are not removed, they may work their way into the cast and result in irritation and infection.
- Before the patient leaves the medical office, the physician will check the circulation, sensation, and

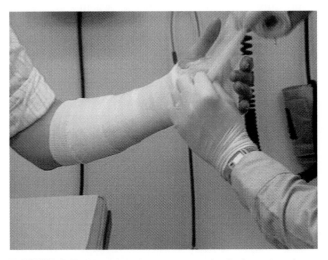

■ **FIGURE 9–7.** Wrapping the tape over the body part, using a spiral turn. (Courtesy of 3M Health Care, St. Paul, MN.)

movement of the extremities to make sure the cast is not too tight. The physician will also make sure that all joints excluded from the cast are free to move.

GUIDELINES FOR CAST CARE

The medical assistant is often responsible for explaining or reinforcing the guidelines that should be followed by a patient with a cast. These guidelines are often presented on an instruction sheet that is signed by the patient, with a copy filed in the patient's chart. Guidelines for cast care include the following:

- Wait at least 24 hours before putting any pressure or weight on a plaster cast. Synthetic casts can bear weight 1 hour following application.
- Elevate the cast above heart level for the first 24 hours to decrease swelling and pain.
- Move toes or fingers to help prevent swelling. Do this often if it does not cause pain.
- Take precautions to prevent dirt, sand, and other foreign particles from becoming trapped under the cast. These may cause irritation to the skin and lead to infection.
- Do not use any object to scratch the skin under the cast. Inserting anything into the cast, such as a pencil, coat hanger, or knitting needle, may cause a break in the skin, which could then become infected. Also, the object may become lost in the cast.
- Keep plaster casts dry at all times. If a plaster cast becomes wet, it loses its shape and may break down. Waterproof cast protectors are available to keep the cast dry during showering or bathing.
- Report the following symptoms *immediately* to the physician, which may indicate that the cast is too tight or an infection is developing: increased pain or swelling; coldness, paleness, or blueness of the fingers or toes; foul odor or drainage coming from the cast; tingling of, numbness of, or inability to move the fingers or toes; and chills, fever, nausea, or vomiting.

CAST REMOVAL

The easiest and safest way to remove a cast is to bivalve it—this means cutting the cast into two halves, resulting in an anterior and a posterior shell. To bivalve a cast, the physician cuts the entire length of the cast on two opposite sides down to the level of the cast padding. The cuts are made with a cast cutter, which is a hand-held electric saw with a circular blade that oscillates (Fig. 9–8). The medical assistant should reassure the patient that, although the saw is noisy, only a

PATIENT/TEACHING

CAST CARE

Teach the patient the important guidelines of cast care.

Emphasize the importance of contacting the physician immediately if any signs of circulatory impairment or infection occur.

If cold has been prescribed by the physician to reduce swelling, teach the patient the procedure for applying an ice bag to the casted extremity.

Emphasize the importance of returning to have the cast checked by the physician.

If isometric exercises to help maintain the muscle tone of the affected extremity are prescribed by the physician, provide the patient with a sheet illustrating the exercises.

Provide the patient with printed materials on cast care.

tickling sensation and some heat will be felt from the saw's vibration. After cutting the cast, the physician pries it apart with a cast spreader. Next, the physician uses bandage scissors to cut through the cast padding and stockinette. The cast is then carefully removed from the patient's extremity.

The skin of the affected extremity will appear yellow and scaly. The extremity will also appear thinner, and the muscles will be flabby. The medical assistant should explain to the patient that this is considered normal because of lack of use of the extremity. The physician may recommend exercises or physical therapy or both to help the patient regain strength and function of the body part.

AMBULATORY AIDS

☐ Mechanical assistive devices are used by individuals requiring aid in ambulation. The term **ambulation** refers to walking; patients who are ambulatory are able to walk as opposed to being confined to a wheelchair or bed. Examples of ambulatory aids include crutches, canes, and walkers. The type of device used depends on factors such as the type and severity of the disability, the amount of support required, and the patient's age and degree of muscular coordination. The ambulatory aid may be prescribed for a temporary condition, such as a fracture or a sprain to a lower extremity, or for disability following orthopedic surgery. It may also be prescribed for a more permanent condition, such as paralysis, deformity, or permanent weakness of the lower extremities.

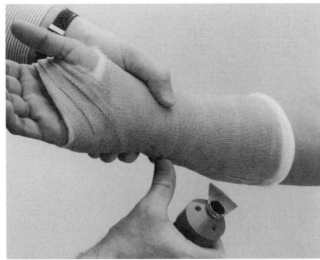

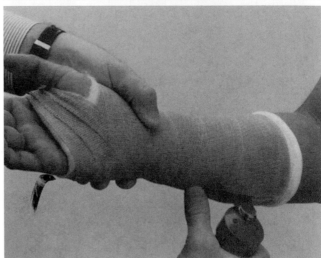

■ **FIGURE 9–8.** Cast removal using a cast cutter. (Courtesy of 3M Health Care, St. Paul, MN.)

9

CRUTCHES

Crutches are artificial supports consisting of wood or tubular aluminum. They are used for patients requiring assistance in walking as a result of disease, injury, or birth defects of the lower extremities. Crutches function by removing weight from the legs and transferring it to the arms.

The two main types of crutch are the axillary crutch and the Lofstrand crutch (Fig. 9–9). The **axillary crutch** is used most frequently and is made of wood or tubular aluminum. This type of crutch has a shoulder rest and handgrips and extends from the ground almost to the patient's axilla. The **Lofstrand crutch** consists of a single adjustable tube of aluminum that extends only to the forearm. A metal cuff, attached to the crutch, fits securely around the patient's forearm, while a handgrip covered with rubber extends from the crutch for weight bearing. The metal cuff and the handgrip function in stabilizing the patient's wrists to make walking safer and easier. One advantge of the Lofstrand crutch is that the individual can release the handgrip, enabling use of the hand, while the metal cuff holds the crutch in place. The Lofstrand crutch is most often used by individuals who are paraplegic or have cerebral palsy. Both the axillary and Lofstrand crutch require tips, which are generally

Highlight on Ambulatory Aids

Many people who could benefit from ambulatory aids are not using them. The primary reason for this is because they do not know how to use them correctly, become discouraged, and then quit using them.

Other types of aids available to assist individuals with physical disabilities include raised toilet seats, carrying devices, tub seats, overbed tables, and swivel cushions for assistance in getting into and out of cars.

If an individual with a physical disability needs help in driving, the local bureau of vocational rehabilitation or the state motor vehicle department can provide information on qualified instruction available in the community.

Walking with an ambulatory aid is a physiologic stressor to the body since energy expenditure is increased compared with normal walking. Because of this, individuals need to rest frequently when using an ambulatory aid.

Many people need to have their crutches lengthened after they have had them for a while. This is because their posture improves as they gain confidence in walking with them. Children and teenagers who use crutches for a long period of time also need frequent adjustments as they grow.

A cane can provide security to the individual using it; however, it can be more trouble than it is worth if it is the incorrect size. It is estimated that two thirds of people who buy canes select one that is too long.

Some walkers are designed to fit over chairs and toilets, allowing the user additional support when rising or sitting. Folding walkers are available, which helps in storing and transporting them.

PATIENT/TEACHING

CRUTCHES

Teach patients the guidelines for the proper use of crutches.

Provide the patient with an exercise sheet illustrating exercises for strengthening arm muscles before beginning crutch walking.

Teach the patient the crutch gait or gaits prescribed by the physician.

Provide the patient with a list of local vendors who provide crutch services such as repairs and crutch supplies (rubber tips, crutch pads, and so on).

Provide the patient with printed educational materials on the use of crutches and crutch gaits.

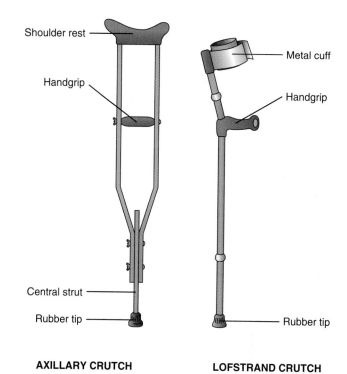

■ FIGURE 9–9. Types of crutches. (Courtesy of 3M Health Care, St. Paul, MN.)

made of rubber. The tips increase the surface tension to help prevent the crutches from slipping on the floor.

Axillary Crutch Measurement

The patient must be measured for axillary crutches to ensure the correct crutch length and the proper placement of the handgrip. Incorrectly fitted crutches increase the patient's risk of developing back pain, nerve damage, and injuries to the axilla and palms of the hands, as follows: If the crutch is too long, the shoulder rest exerts pressure on the patient's axilla. This can injure the radial nerve in the brachial plexus, which eventually may lead to **crutch palsy,** a condition of muscular weakness in the forearm, wrist, and hand. In addition, crutches that are too long cause the patient's shoulders to be forced forward, preventing the patient from pushing his or her body off the ground. Crutches that are too short force the patient to be bent over and uncomfortable, also making them awkward to use. If the handgrips are too low, pressure results on the patient's axilla, whereas handgrips that are too high are awkward. Crutches are designed using bolts and wing nuts, which allow for proper adjustment of both the length and handgrip level.

PUTTING IT ALL *into* PRACTICE

▶ **MARLYNE COOPER:** *One of my most rewarding experiences was when a young woman came into the office with severe chest pains. I immediately got up from my desk and helped her back to an examining room. I then ran an electrocardiogram (ECG) as ordered by the physician. After the physician read the ECG, he indicated the results did not look good and that the patient would have to be transported to the hospital. I went into the patient's room to comfort her. She asked me if she was going to have to go to the hospital. I replied, "Possibly." She immediately said, "No." Then I began to explain to her that it was important to have more tests. She finally agreed to go. After being taken to the hospital by an ambulance, she was later transferred to another hospital for a heart catheterization. A few weeks passed and she came into the office. She hugged me and thanked me for possibly saving her life. It felt so good that I could help make a difference in a patient's life.*

Crutch Guidelines

It is important that the patient be provided with specific guidelines to ensure safety while using crutches, to prevent injuries or falls. The medical assistant is responsible for instructing the patient in these guidelines, as outlined:

1. The weight of the body should be supported by the hands on the handgrips and the axillary pads pressing against the sides of the rib cage. The body weight should not be supported by the axilla, because pressure on the axilla may result in crutch palsy.
2. Tingling or numbness in the upper body should be reported to the physician. It may indicate that the crutches are being used incorrectly or that the crutches are the wrong size.
3. The patient should practice correct posture to prevent strain on muscles and joints and to maintain proper body balance.
4. The shoulder rests of axillary crutches can be slightly padded for comfort, but the padding must press against not the axilla but rather against the lateral rib cage. The handgrips can also be padded for increased patient comfort.
5. The crutches should be moved forward to the side, to prevent obstruction of the pathway for the feet.
6. Each step taken with crutches should be at a safe and comfortable distance, preferably 6 inches. When first learning to use the crutches, the patient should take small steps, rather than large ones. The crutches should not be moved forward more than 12 to 15 inches with each step. A distance greater than this may cause the crutches to slide forward.
7. The crutch tips should be securely attached and inspected on a regular basis. If the crutch tips are worn down, they should be replaced with tips of the proper size.
8. Crutch tips should be kept dry to maintain their surface friction. If they become wet, the patient should dry them well before use.
9. The wing nuts holding the central strut and handgrips in place periodically should be checked for tightness.
10. Well-fitting flat shoes with firm, nonskid soles should be worn to provide good traction and stability.
11. The patient should look ahead when walking rather than down at his or her feet.
12. The surface the patient is walking on must be clean, flat, dry, and well lighted. Throw rugs and objects serving as obstacles should temporarily be removed from the patient's environment.

Crutch Gaits

The type of crutch gait used depends upon the amount of weight the patient is able to support with one or both legs, the patient's physical condition, and muscular coordination. The patient should learn both a fast and a slow gait. The faster gait is used for making speed in open areas, and the slower one is used in crowded places. In addition, learning more than one gait reduces patient fatigue, because a different combination of muscles is used for each gait.

Text continued on page 357

PROCEDURE

9–9

Measuring for Axillary Crutches

Determining Crutch Length

To determine crutch length correctly the patient must wear shoes while being measured. The measurement can be taken with the patient in a standing position.

1. **Procedural Step.** Ask the patient to stand erect.
2. **Procedural Step.** Position the crutches with the crutch tips at a distance of 2 inches (5 cm) in front of and 4 to 6 inches (15 cm) to the side of each foot. (The large dots in the figure represent crutch tips.)

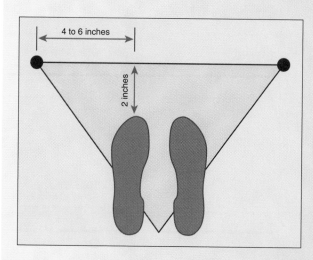

3. **Procedural Step.** Adjust the crutch length so that the shoulder rests are approximately 1½ to 2 inches (about 2 finger-widths) below the axilla. The length of the crutch is adjusted by removing the bolt and wing nut and sliding the central strut (support piece) at the bottom either upward or downward, as necessary, to attain the proper length. The strut is then secured by replacing the bolt and securely fastening the wing nut.

Handgrip Positioning

Once the crutch length measurement procedure has been completed, the correct placement of the handgrips must be determined.

1. **Procedural Step.** Ask the patient to stand erect with a crutch under each arm and to support his or her weight by the handgrips.
2. **Procedural Step.** Adjust the handgrips on the crutches so that the patient's elbow is flexed to an angle of approximately 30 degrees. The handgrip level is adjusted by removing the bolt and wing nut and sliding the handgrip upward or downward, as required. The handgrip is then secured by replacing the bolt and tightly fastening the wing nut. The angle of elbow flexion can be verified using a measuring device known as a **goniometer.**
3. **Procedural Step.** Check the fit of the crutches. If the crutches are measured correctly, the medical assistant should be able to insert two fingers between the top of the crutch and the axilla, when the patient is standing erect with the crutches under the arms.

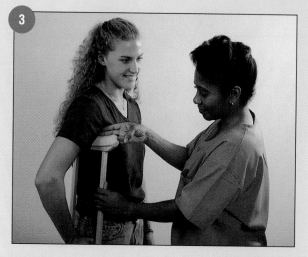

9

PROCEDURE

9–10

Instructing the Patient in Crutch Gaits

Tripod Position

The tripod position is the basic crutch stance used before crutch walking. It provides a wide base of support and enhances stability and balance.

Instruct the patient in the tripod position as outlined below.

1. **Procedural Step.** Stand erect, and face straight ahead.
2. **Procedural Step.** Place the tips of the crutches 4 to 6 inches (15 cm) in front of the feet and 4 to 6 inches (15 cm) to the side of each foot. (The large dots in the figure represent crutch tips.)

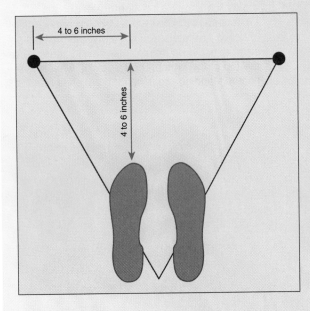

Four-Point Gait

The four-point gait is a very basic and slow gait. In order to use this gait, the patient must be able to bear considerable weight on both legs. The four-point gait is the most stable and safest of the crutch gaits, because it provides at least three points of support at all times. It is most often used with patients who have leg muscle weakness or spasticity, poor muscular coordination or balance, or degenerative leg joint disease. Instruct the patient in the procedure for the four-point gait following the steps in the figure.

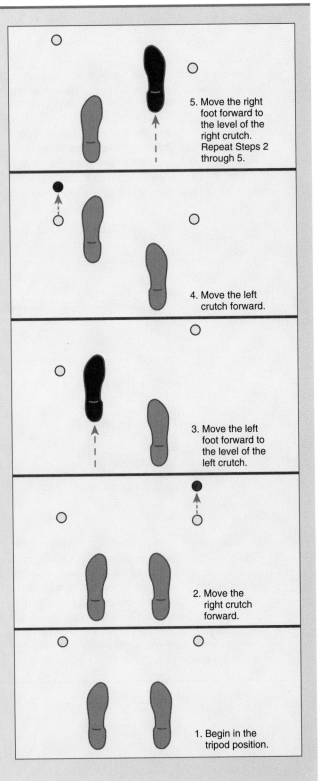

5. Move the right foot forward to the level of the right crutch. Repeat Steps 2 through 5.

4. Move the left crutch forward.

3. Move the left foot forward to the level of the left crutch.

2. Move the right crutch forward.

1. Begin in the tripod position.

9

PROCEDURE 9-10

Two Point Gait

The two-point gait is similar to, but faster than, the four-point gait. This gait requires more balance because only two points support the body at one time. The two-point gait is used when the patient is capable of partial weight bearing on each foot and has good muscular coordination. Instruct the patient in the procedure for the two-point gait following the steps in the figure.

Three Point Gait

The three-point gait is used for the patient who cannot bear weight on one leg. The patient must be able to support his or her full weight on the unaffected leg. With this gait, the crutches and the unaffected leg alternatively bear the patient's weight. This gait is used most often for amputees without a prosthesis, patients with musculoskeletal or soft tissue trauma to a lower extremity (e.g., fracture, sprain), patients with acute leg inflammation, or patients who have had recent leg surgery. To use this gait, the patient must have good muscular coordination and arm strength. Instruct the patient in the procedure for the three-point gait, following the steps in the figure.

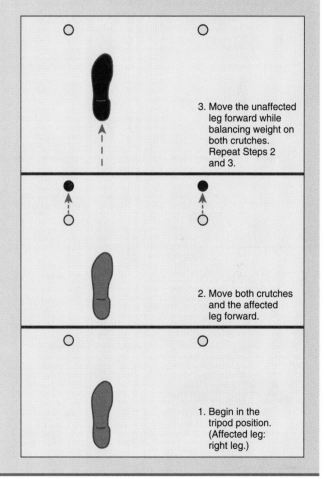

3. Move the right crutch and left foot forward at the same time. Repeat Steps 2 and 3.

2. Move the left crutch and right foot forward at the same time.

1. Begin in the tripod position.

3. Move the unaffected leg forward while balancing weight on both crutches. Repeat Steps 2 and 3.

2. Move both crutches and the affected leg forward.

1. Begin in the tripod position. (Affected leg: right leg.)

9

Swing Gaits

The swing gaits include the swing-to gait and the swing-through gait and are used by patients with severe lower extremity disabilities such as paralysis and by patients wearing supporting braces on their legs.

Instruct the patient in the procedure for the swing-to crutch gait, following the steps in the figure.

Instruct the patient in the procedure for the swing-through crutch gait, following the steps in the figure.

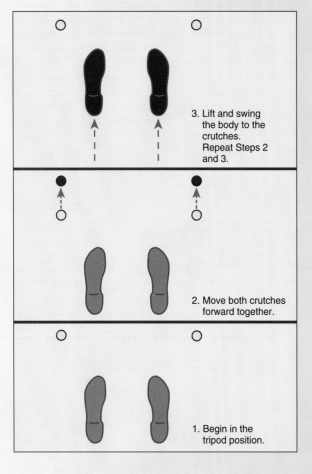

SWING-TO GAIT

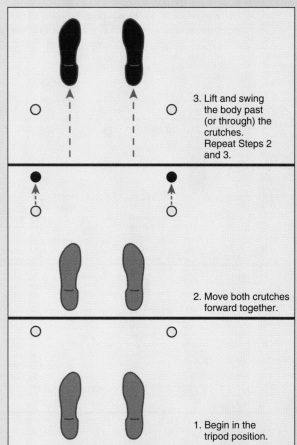

SWING-THROUGH GAIT

9–11

Instructing the Patient in Use of a Cane

Instruct the patient in the use of a cane as outlined below:

1. **Procedural Step.** Hold the cane on the strong side of the body (i.e., in the hand opposite the affected extremity).
2. **Procedural Step.** The tip of the cane should be placed 4 to 6 inches to the side of the foot.
3. **Procedural Step.** Move the cane forward approximately 12 inches (1 foot).
4. **Procedural Step.** Move the affected leg forward to the level of the cane.
5. **Procedural Step.** Move the strong leg forward and ahead of the cane and weak leg.
6. **Procedural Step.** Repeat Steps 3 through 5.

Note: The cane and affected leg can be moved forward simultaneously (Steps 3 and 4); however, the patient has less support with this method.

PROCEDURE

9–12

Instructing the Patient in Use of a Walker

Instruct the patient in the use of a walker as outlined below:

1. **Procedural Step.** Pick up the walker, and move it forward approximately 6 inches.
2. **Procedural Step.** Move the right foot and then the left foot up to the walker.
3. **Procedural Step.** Repeat Steps 1 and 2.

CANES

A cane is a lightweight, easily movable device, made of wood or aluminum with rubber tips, used to help provide balance and support. Canes are generally used by patients who have weakness on one side of the body, such as those with hemiparesis, joint disabilities, or defects of the neuromuscular system. The three main types of canes are the **standard cane,** the **tripod cane,** and the **quad cane** (Fig. 9–10). The standard cane provides the least amount of support and is used by patients requiring only slight assistance in walking. The tripod and quad canes have three and four legs, respectively, a bent shaft, and a T-shaped handle with grips. They are easier to hold and provide greater stability than the standard cane because of the wider base of support. In addition, multilegged canes are able to stand alone, which frees the arms when the patient is getting up from a chair. The disadvantage of the multilegged cane is that it is bulkier and therefore more difficult to move.

The cane length must be properly adjusted to ensure optimum stability. The cane handle should be approximately level with the greater trochanter, and the elbow should be flexed at 25- to 30-degree angle. The patient should be instructed to stand erect and not lean on the cane to ensure good balance.

WALKERS

A walker is an ambulatory aid consisting of an aluminum frame with handgrips and four widely placed legs with rubber suction tips and one open side (Fig. 9–11). A walker is light and, therefore, easily movable.

9

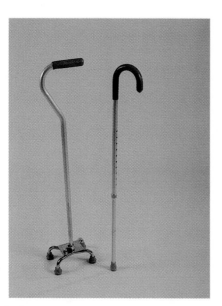

■ **FIGURE 9–10.** Examples of a standard cane (*right*) and a quad cane (*left*). (Courtesy of 3M Health Care, St. Paul, MN.)

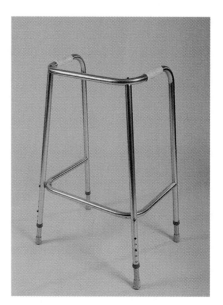

■ **FIGURE 9–11.** A walker.

For proper ambulation, the walker should extend from the ground to approximately the level of the patient's hip joint.

Walkers are most often used by geriatric patients with weakness or balance problems. Because of its wide-base support, a walker provides the patient with a great amount of stability and security. Disadvantages of a walker include a slow pace and difficulty in maneuvering the walker in a small room.

MEDICAL PRACTICE AND THE LAW

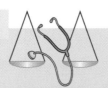

The activities described in this chapter deal with the goal of returning full function to an injured area. Sometimes, despite correct treatment, full function may not return. This problem can become a legal issue if the patient believes he or she should have healed fully or cannot return to work. To protect yourself, follow each procedure to the letter, and record the patient's progress (or lack of progress) carefully in the medical record. Sometimes, the patient is involved in an insurance fraud and falsely complains of pain or impaired function to continue receiving disability benefits. If you suspect this is the case, objectively document the functions you have seen the patient perform, and notify the physician to avoid implication in possible fraud.

The application of heat and cold must be performed precisely in order to maximize effectiveness of the treatment without injury to the patient. Failure to follow procedures correctly or to obtain the correct temperature could leave you legally liable.

The ultrasound machine, if used incorrectly, can burn the patient. To protect yourself and benefit the patient, keep the applicator head moving at all times and keep adequate coupling agent on the skin at all times.

Ambulatory aids used correctly can assist the patient with regaining mobility. If crutches are improperly used, the patient could fall or develop nerve or other injuries. When instructing about ambulation aid use, be sure to allow enough time for the patient to give a return demonstration, and send home written instructions to consult if he or she forgets what was taught.

9

CERTIFICATION REVIEW

☐ The application of heat or cold is used to treat pathologic conditions such as infection and trauma. Heat and cold are applied for short periods of time, usually ranging from 15 to 30 minutes. The type of heat or cold application used depends upon the purpose of the application, the location and condition of the affected area, and the age and general health of the patient.

☐ The local effects of applying heat to the body include dilation of the blood vessels in the area. Nutrients and oxygen are provided to the cells at a faster rate, and wastes are carried away faster. Erythema is the redness of the skin caused by congestion of capillaries in the lower layers of the skin. Heat functions in relieving pain, congestion, muscle spasms, and inflammation.

☐ The local application of cold produces constriction of blood vessels. Because of this factor, tissue metabolism decreases, less oxygen is used, and fewer wastes accumulate. The local application of cold is used to prevent edema and may be applied immediately after an individual has suffered direct trauma such as a bruise, sprain, muscle strain, joint injury, or fracture.

☐ Factors that affect the local application of heat and cold include the age of the patient, the location of the application, impaired circulation and sensation, and individual tolerance to change in temperature.

☐ Therapeutic ultrasound uses high-frequency sound waves as a deep-heating agent for the soft tissues of the body. Ultrasound may be ordered to treat the following conditions: sprains, joint contractures, neuritis, arthritis, edema, synovitis, scar tissue, bursitis, fibrositis, strains, and dislocations. Ultrasound must not be used over the eyeball, over malignant tumors, directly over the spinal cord, over the heart or brain, over reproductive organs or a pregnant uterus, or over areas of impaired sensation or inadequate circulation.

CERTIFICATION REVIEW *Continued*

☐ A cast is a stiff cylindrical casing that is used to immobilize a body part. Casts are applied most often when an individual sustains a fracture. Other uses of a cast are to support and stabilize weak or dislocated joints; to promote healing after a surgical correction; and to aid in the nonsurgical correction of deformities.

☐ An orthopedist is a specialist who deals with the prevention and correction of disorders of the locomotor structures of the body. Plaster casts are preferred for acute, complicated fractures, whereas synthetic casts are often used for simple, uncomplicated fractures.

☐ Casts are classified according to the body part they cover. The types of cast most frequently applied include: short arm cast, long arm cast, short leg cast, and long leg cast. The type of cast applied depends on the nature of the patient's injury or condition.

☐ Mechanical assistive devices are used by individuals requiring aid in ambulation. Examples of ambulatory aids include crutches, canes, and walkers. The type of device used depends on factors such as the type and severity of the disability, the amount of support required, and the patient's age and degree of muscular coordination.

☐ Crutches are artificial supports consisting of wood or tubular aluminum. They are used for patients requiring assistance in walking as a result of disease, injury, or birth defects of the lower extremities. Crutches function by removing weight from the legs and transferring it to the arms.

☐ The type of crutch gait used depends on the amount of weight the patient is able to support with one or both legs, the patient's physical condition, and muscular coordination. Types of crutch gaits include the four-point gait, the two-point gait, the three-point gait, and the swing gaits.

☐ A cane is a lightweight, easily movable device used to help provide balance and support. Canes are generally used by patients who have weakness on one side of the body. A walker is an ambulatory aid that is most often used by geriatric patients with weakness or balance problems.

9

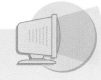

O N   T H E   W E B

RESOURCES

For information on rehabilitation and disability:

National Rehabilitation Information Center (NARIC)
www.naric.com

Cure Paralysis Now (CPN)
www.cureparalysis.org

The National Stroke Association (NSA)
www.stroke.org

Arthritis Foundation
www.arthritis.org

Alzheimer's Association
www.alz.org

MY NAME IS

Michele Parsons, *and I am a Certified Medical Assistant. I graduated from an accredited program and have an associate's degree in Applied Science. I have worked in the field of medical assisting for 13 years, and at present I work with five physicians in a college student health clinic.*

My primary job responsibilities include documenting patient histories and complaints, taking vital signs, and assisting physicians with patient examinations and procedures. Some examples include gynecologic examinations, cleaning and packing of pilonidal cysts, and cleaning and dressing of wounds and burns.

What I find most interesting about my job are the different types of illnesses and injuries I see. Because I work in an outpatient ambulatory care clinic for college students, I see patients with a lot of different conditions. I also enjoy working with this age group of patients.

I went straight into a medical assisting program after graduating from high school. I prefer working in a health care setting in a practice rather than a hospital. I feel there is more continuity to my job and a better chance to get to know my patients. And, working in a college clinic gives me the added benefits of having spring and winter breaks off as well!

The Gynecologic Examination and Prenatal Care

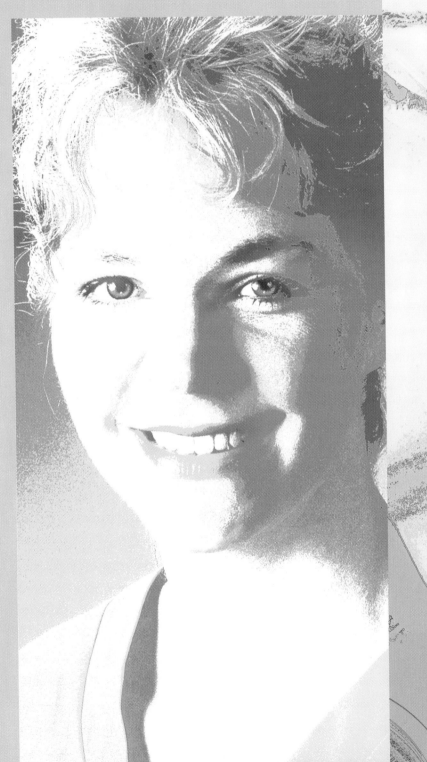

OUTCOMES

After completing this chapter, you should be able to demonstrate the proper procedures to perform the following:

1. Instruct an individual in the procedure for a breast self-examination.
2. Prepare a patient for a gynecologic examination.
3. Assist the physician with a gynecologic examination.
4. Complete a cytology requisition for a Papanicolaou test.
5. Complete a prenatal health history.
6. Assist with an initial prenatal examination.
7. Assist with a return prenatal examination.
8. Assist with a 6-weeks-postpartum examination.

EDUCATIONAL OBJECTIVES

After completing this unit, you should be able to do the following:

1. Define the terms listed in the Key Terminology.
2. List the parts of the gynecologic examination.
3. Explain the purpose of performing each of the following: breast examination; inspection of the external genitalia, vagina, and cervix; Papanicolaou test; bimanual pelvic examination; and rectal-vaginal examination.
4. Explain how the results of the Pap test are reported.
5. Explain the methods used to identify each of the following vaginal infections and the supplies required for the collection and evaluation of each: trichomoniasis, candidiasis, gonorrhea, and chlamydia.
6. Explain the purpose of prenatal care.
7. Explain the purpose of each of the following four components of the first prenatal visit: prenatal record, initial prenatal examination, patient education, and laboratory tests.
8. Record the patient's pregnancy in terms of gravidity and parity.
9. Calculate the expected date of delivery (EDD) using Nägele's rule and a gestation calculator.
10. List and explain the purpose of each procedure included in the initial prenatal examination.
11. List and explain the purpose of each laboratory test included in the prenatal laboratory work-up.
12. Explain the purpose of return prenatal visits. List and explain the purpose of each of the procedures included in the return prenatal examination.
13. Describe the purpose of each of the following special tests and procedures: alpha-fetoprotein analysis, obstetric ultrasound scanning, amniocentesis, and fetal heart rate monitoring.
14. Explain the purpose of the 6-weeks-postpartum visit.
15. List and explain the purpose of each of the procedures included in the 6-weeks-postpartum examination.

KEY TERMINOLOGY

abortion: The loss of a pregnancy before the stage of viability.

adnexal (ad-NEX-al): Ajacent.

atypical: Deviation from the normal.

Braxton Hicks contractions: Intermittent and irregular painless uterine contractions that occur throughout pregnancy. They occur more frequently toward the end of pregnancy and are sometimes mistaken for true labor pains.

cytology (SÎ-TOL-ô-gê): The science that deals with the study of cells, including their origin, structure, function, and pathology.

dilation (of the cervix) (dî-LÂ-shun): The stretching of the external os from an opening a few millimeters in size to an opening large enough to allow the passage of an infant (approximately 10 cm).

EDD: Expected date of delivery, or due date.

effacement (ê-FÂS-Ment): The thinning and shortening of the cervical canal from its normal length of 1 to 2 cm to a structure with paper-thin edges in which there is no canal at all. Effacement occurs late in pregnancy or during labor, or both. The purpose of effacement along with dilation is to permit the passage of the infant into the birth canal.

endocervix (in-DÔ-serv-ix): The mucous membrane lining the cervical canal.

engagement: The entrance of the fetal head or the presenting part into the pelvic inlet.

exfoliated cells (X-FOL-ê-ât-ed SELLS): Cells that have been sloughed off from the surface of tissues into the secretions bathing those tissues.

external os (X-tern-al os): The opening of the cervical canal of the uterus into the vagina.

fetal heart rate: The number of times the fetal heart beats per minute.

fetal heart tones: The heart beat of the fetus as heard through the mother's abdominal wall.

fetus (FÊ-tus): The child in utero, from the third month after conception to birth; during the first 2 months of development, it is called an embryo.

fundus (FUN-dus): The dome-shaped upper portion of the uterus between the fallopian tubes.

gestation (Jes-tâ-shun): The period of intrauterine development from conception to birth; the period of pregnancy. The average pregnancy lasts about 280 days or 40 weeks from the date of conception to childbirth.

gravid (GRAV-id): Pregnant.

gravida (GRAV-id-a): A woman who is or has been pregnant.

gravidity (GRAV-id-i-tê): The total number of pregnancies a woman has had regardless of duration, including a current pregnancy.

gynecology (GÎN-e-KUL-ô-jê): The branch of medicine that deals with the diseases of the reproductive organs of women.

high-risk: Having an increased possibility of suffering harm, damage, or death.

infant: A child from birth to 1 year of age.

internal os (in-TERN-al os): The internal opening of the cervical canal into the uterus.

lochia (LOK-ê-a): A discharge from the uterus after delivery, consisting of blood, tissue, white blood cells, and some bacteria.

multigravida (mul-TÊ-GRAV-i-da): A woman who has been pregnant more than once.

multipara (mul-TÊ-pare-a): A woman who has completed two or more pregnancies to the age of viability regardless of whether they ended in live infants or stillbirths.

nullipara (nul-Ê-pare-a): A woman who has not carried a pregnancy to the point of viability (20 weeks of gestation).

obstetrics (OB-stet-riks): That branch of medicine concerned with the care of the woman during pregnancy, childbirth, and the postpartal period.

para: A term used to refer to past pregnancies that reached viability (20 weeks of gestation), regardless of whether the infant was stillborn or alive at birth.

parity (PARE-it-ê): The condition of having borne offspring who had attained the age of viability (20 weeks of gestation), regardless of whether they were live infants or stillbirths.

pelvimetry (PELV-iM-it-rê): Measurement of the capacity and diameter of the maternal pelvis, which helps determine whether it will be possible to deliver the infant through the vaginal route.

perineum (PER-in-ê-UM): The external region between the vaginal orifice and the anus in a female and between the scrotum and the anus in a male.

position: The relation of the presenting part of the fetus to the maternal pelvis.

postpartum (POST-par-tuM): Occuring after childbirth.

pre-eclampsia (PRÊ-ê-KLAMP-sê-a): A major complication of pregnancy of unknown cause, characterized by increasing hypertension, albuminuria, and

10

edema. If this condition is neglected or not treated properly, it may develop into eclampsia, which could cause maternal convulsions and coma. Pre-eclampsia generally occurs between the twentieth week of pregnancy and the end of the first week postpartum.

prenatal (PRÊ-nâ-TUL): Before birth.

presentation: The part of the fetus that is closest to the cervix and will be delivered first. A cephalic presentation is a delivery in which the fetal head is presenting against the cervix. A breech presentation is a delivery in which the buttocks or feet are presented instead of the head.

primigravida (PRÎM-i-GRAV-id-a): A woman who is pregnant for the first time (gravida I).

primipara (PRÎM-ip-a-ra): A woman who has carried a pregnancy to viability (20 weeks of gestation) for the first time, regardless of whether the infant was stillborn or alive at birth (para I).

puerperium (PURE-per-ê-uM): The period of time (usually 4 to 6 weeks) in which the uterus and the body systems are returning to normal following delivery.

quickening: The first movements of the fetus in utero as felt by the mother, which usually occurs between the sixteenth and twentieth weeks of gestation and is felt consistently thereafter.

toxemia (TOX-êM-ê-a): A pathologic condition occurring in pregnant women that includes pre-eclampsia and eclampsia. If pre-eclampsia goes undiagnosed or is not satisfactorily controlled, it could develop into eclampsia, characterized by convulsions and coma.

trimester: Three months, or one-third, of the gestational period of pregnancy.

vulva (VUL-va): The region of the external genital organs in the female.

INTRODUCTION

☐ The medical assistant should have a knowledge of gynecology and obstetrics to assist in examinations and treatments in these specialty areas. Gynecologic examinations are frequently and routinely performed in the medical office. Prenatal care consists of a series of scheduled medical office visits for the promotion of the health of the mother and fetus during the pregnancy. Obtaining the patient's cooperation helps make the gynecologic or prenatal examination proceed more smoothly and, as a result, makes the patient feel more comfortable. The medical assistant can help by explaining the purpose of the procedure to the patient. If the individual understands the beneficial results to be derived from the examination, she is more likely to participate as required. This chapter presents a discussion of both the gynecologic examination and prenatal care, as well as the procedures involved with each.

The Gynecologic Examination

GYNECOLOGY

☐ **Gynecology** is the branch of medicine that deals with diseases of the reproductive organs of women. Gynecologic examinations are frequently and routinely performed in the medical office and generally include a breast and pelvic examination. The gynecologic exami-

nation may be included as part of the physical examination or may be performed by itself.

The purpose of the gynecologic examination is to assess the health of the female reproductive organs in order to detect early signs of disease, leading to early diagnosis and treatment. Although assisting with the gynecologic examination is a routine procedure for the medical assistant, the patient may not consider it a routine examination. The medical assistant should fully explain the procedure and offer to answer any questions to reduce the patient's possible apprehension or embarrassment.

THE BREAST EXAMINATION

☐ The physician generally begins with the breast examination. The medical assistant helps the patient into the supine position. The physician inspects the breasts for any localized redness or inflammation and any dimpling scaling, or puckering of the skin. The nipples are checked for abnormalities such as bleeding or discharge, and the breasts and axillary lymph nodes are palpated for lumps.

The patient should know how to examine her breasts at home for the presence of lumps by learning to perform a **breast self-examination (BSE).** Most breast cancers are first discovered by women themselves. The medical assistant may be responsible for instructing the patient in this procedure. The American Cancer Society recommends that women 20 years and older examine their breasts monthly, approximately

10

Highlight on Breast Cancer

Breast cancer is one of the most common types of cancer among American women. The American Cancer Society estimates that one of every nine women in the United States will develop breast cancer at some point in her lifetime. Each year, more than 175,000 women learn they have breast cancer. Two thirds of them will be more than 50 years old, but breast cancer does occur in younger women.

The 5-year survival rate from the time of diagnosis for all stages of malignant breast tumors is 75 percent. For small, localized tumors, the survival rate can approach 90 percent. These encouraging statistics are due to advances in early detection of breast cancer, improved surgical procedures, hormonal therapy, and chemotherapy.

A three-point program is recommended by the American Cancer Society and the National Cancer Institute for the early detection of breast cancer: a monthly breast self-examination, a periodic clinical breast examination by a physician, and screening mammography.

Breast cancer results from the abnormal growth of cells in breast tissue. It occurs more often in the left breast than in the right, and more often in the upper outer quadrant of the breast. It is not known what causes this abnormal growth to occur; therefore every woman should consider herself at risk for breast cancer. Certain risk factors, however, appear to place a woman at higher than normal risk for breast cancer. These include the following:

- Age (the risk of breast cancer increases as women get older)
- A family history of breast cancer, particularly in a first-degree relative (i.e., mother, sister, or daughter)
- Beginning menstrual periods early (before age 12 years)
- Late menopause (after age 55 years)
- No children, or first birth after age 30 years.
- Exposure to low-level ionizing radiation
- Obesity
- The consumption of a diet high in fat

The warning signs of possible breast cancer include a lump or thickening in the breast or armpit, a change in breast skin color or texture, dimpling or puckering, nipple discharge, changes in the size or shape of the breast, and an enlargement of the lymph nodes.

A biopsy is the only conclusive method of determining whether a breast lump or suspicious area seen on a mammogram is benign or malignant. A biopsy involves the surgical removal and analysis of all or part of the lump. There are several biopsy methods, including needle biopsy, incisional biopsy (removal of a portion of the lump), excisional biopsy (removal of the entire lump), and mammographic localization with biopsy. The physician may recommend one or more of these procedures to evaluate a lump or other change in the breast.

Fortunately, 80 percent of all breast lumps are benign; hence a lump or suspicious area is often the result of a benign breast condition such as normal hormonal changes, fibrocystic breast disease, or a fibroadenoma.

---

1 week after the menstrual period, when the breasts are usually not tender or swollen. After menopause, the breast self-examination should be performed on the same day each month.

Figure 10–1 demonstrates the procedure for performing a breast self-examination. If a lump or discharge is discovered, the woman should schedule an appointment with her physician as soon as possible. Most breast lumps are not cancerous, but the physician is the one to make that diagnosis.

THE PELVIC EXAMINATION

☐ The purpose of the pelvic examination is to assess the size, shape, and location of the reproductive organs and to detect the presence of disease. The pelvic examination consists of the following components:

1. Inspection of the external genitalia, vagina, and cervix.
2. Collection of a specimen for a Pap test.
3. Bimanual pelvic examination.
4. Rectal-vaginal examination

The most common position for the pelvic examination is the lithotomy position. The patient should lie on the table on her back, with her feet in the stirrups and her buttocks at the bottom edge of the table. The stirrups should be level with the examining table and pulled out approximately 1 foot from the edge of the table. The patient's knees should be bent and relaxed, and her thighs should be rotated outward as far as is comfortable. This position helps relax the vulva and perineum and facilitates insertion of the vaginal speculum. The patient should be properly draped to reduce exposure and to provide warmth. The lithotomy position is difficult to maintain, and the patient should not be placed in this position until the physician is ready to begin the examination.

The medical assistant can help the patient relax during the examination by telling her to breathe deeply, slowly, and evenly through the mouth. If the patient is relaxed, it is easier for the physician to insert the vagi-

1

Before a mirror:

Inspect your breasts with arms at your sides. Next, raise your arms high overhead. Look for any changes in shape or contour of each breast, a swelling, dimpling of skin or changes in the nipple.

   Then, rest palms on hips and press down firmly to flex your chest muscles. Left and right breast will not exactly match — few women's do. Gently squeeze the nipple and look for a discharge.

   Regular inspection shows what is normal for you and will give you confidence in your examination.

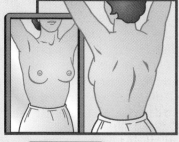

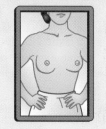

2

Lying down:

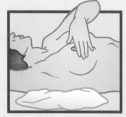

Lie down. Flatten your right breast by placing a pillow under your right shoulder. Fingers flat, use the sensitive pads of the middle three fingers on your left hand. Feel for lumps or changes using a rubbing motion. Press firmly enough to feel the different breast tissues. Completely feel all of the breast and chest area from your collarbone to the base of a properly fitted bra; and from your breast bone to the underarm. Pay special attention to the area between the breast and the underarm, including the underarm itself. Allow enough time for a complete exam.

   The diagrams show the three patterns preferred by women and their doctors; the circular, clock or oval pattern, the vertical strip, and the wedge. Choose the method easiest for you and use the same pattern to feel every part of the breast tissue.

   After you have completely examined your right breast, then examine your left breast using the same method. Compare what you have felt in one breast with the other.

3

In the shower:

Examine your breasts during bath or shower; hands glide easier over wet skin. Fingers flat, move gently over every part of each breast. Check for any lump, hard knot or thickening.

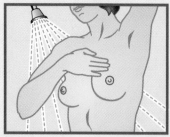

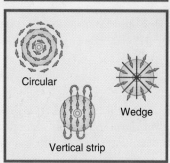

Circular

Wedge

Vertical strip

This diagram shows the three patterns preferred by women and their doctors: 1) the circular, clock or oval pattern, 2) the vertical strip and 3) the wedge. Choose the method easiest for you. Use the same pattern to feel every part of the breast tissue.

10

■ **FIGURE 10–1.** Breast self-examination.

nal speculum and to perform the bimanual pelvic examination; it is also more comfortable for the patient. It is recommended that the medical assistant remain in the room during the pelvic examination to provide legal protection for the physician, to reassure the patient, and to assist the physician.

INSPECTION OF THE EXTERNAL GENITALIA, VAGINA, AND CERVIX

The physician begins the examination with inspection of the external genitalia. The vulva is inspected for swelling, ulceration, or redness.

Next, the physician inserts a vaginal speculum into the vagina. Specula are available in two forms—metal and plastic. Metal specula are reusable and therefore must be sanitized and sterilized after each use. Plastic specula are disposable and are designed for one use

only. Vaginal specula come in three sizes: small, medium, and large. The physician determines the size required based on the physical and sexual maturity of the patient. The function of the speculum is to hold the walls of the vagina apart to allow visual inspection of the vagina and cervix (Fig. 10–2).

If a Papanicolaou (Pap) smear or a specimen for microbiologic examination is to be obtained, the speculum should not be lubricated because this would interfere with the test results. It should be warmed before use by moistening it with warm water, by placing it on a heating pad, or by storing it in an examining table that has a warming drawer. Moistening the speculum helps lubricate it, which allows easier insertion when a lubricant cannot be used.

The physician inspects the vagina and cervix for color, lacerations, ulcerations, tenderness, nodules, or discharge. If an abnormal discharge is present, the physician obtains a specimen for microbiologic examina-

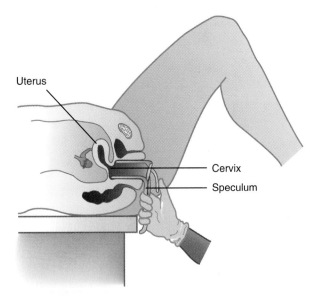

Uterus

Cervix

Speculum

■ **FIGURE 10–2.** Insertion of the vaginal speculum for visualization of the vagina and cervix.

tion. Examples of pathologic conditions producing a discharge include vaginal infections such as *trichomoniasis*, *candidiasis*, *gonorrhea*, and *chlamydia*, which are discussed in detail later in this chapter.

THE PAPANICOLAOU TEST

Purpose

A Pap test is usually included as part of the pelvic examination. It is a simple and painless cytologic screening test named after its developer, Dr. George Papanicolaou (1883–1962). It is used for early detection of precancerous or cancerous conditions of the cervix and endometrium and makes early treatment possible, which may lead to a cure.

Currently the American Cancer Society recommends an annual Pap test and pelvic examination for all women starting at the onset of sexual activity or at age 18 years, whichever is earlier. The guidelines further state that after a woman has tested negative for three or more consecutive examinations, the Pap test may be performed less frequently at the discretion of the physician. Women who are at high risk for cancer or who have had a positive test result should have Pap smears more often.

Patient Instructions

Women should be instructed not to douche or insert vaginal medications for 48 hours before having a Pap smear taken. Douching reduces the number of cells

available for analysis, and vaginal medications change the pH of the vagina, making the specimen nonrepresentative or invalid. The patient should be told to abstain from sexual intercourse for 48 hours before the collection of a Pap smear. Recent sexual intercourse can produce inflammatory changes that can obscure visualization of abnormal cells. In addition, a Pap smear must not be taken from a woman during her menstrual period, because the red blood cells obscure the smear and interfere with an accurate reading. The ideal time is at the midpoint of the patient's menstrual cycle.

Specimen Collection

The Pap test is based on the fact that tissues, including malignant uterine tumors, slough off cells into the surrounding cervical and vaginal mucus; these are known as **exfoliated cells.** A scraping of mucus containing these exfoliated cells may be taken from the vagina, cervix, and endocervical canal. The mucus is thinly spread on a glass slide having a frosted edge; smears should always be made on the slide surface that carries the frosted edge. The medical assistant must label each slide on its frosted edge with a lead pencil according to the source of the specimen as follows: **V** (vaginal), **C** (cervical), and **E** (endocervical). (Note: Slides are also available on which all three specimens can be placed. The slide is divided into thirds and prelabeled with a V, C, and E.)

VAGINAL SPECIMEN. The physician obtains the vaginal specimen from the vaginal pool in the posterior fornix of the vagina (just below the cervix), using the spatula end of the cervical scraper and thinly spreading the mucus on the appropriate slide (Fig. 10–3*A*). The vaginal specimen is also used in the determination of the maturation index.

CERVICAL SPECIMEN. The physician obtains the cervical specimen by placing the S-shaped end of the cervical scraper just inside the cervical canal at the external os and then rotating the blade 360 degrees over the surface of the cervix at the squamocolumnar junction, where cervical cancer is most often found (Fig. 10–3*B*). The physician then thinly spreads the mucus specimen on the appropriate slide.

ENDOCERVICAL SPECIMEN. The physician collects the endocervical specimen from the endocervical canal. This is accomplished using a moistened cotton-tipped applicator or a cytology brush, inserting it into the endocervical canal, and then rotating the applicator or brush. The physician then thinly rolls the specimen over the surface of the appropriate slide (Fig. 10–3*C*).

A. Vaginal Specimen

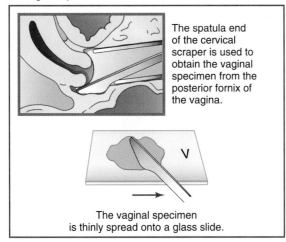

The spatula end of the cervical scraper is used to obtain the vaginal specimen from the posterior fornix of the vagina.

The vaginal specimen is thinly spread onto a glass slide.

B. Cervical Specimen

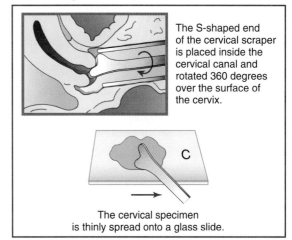

The S-shaped end of the cervical scraper is placed inside the cervical canal and rotated 360 degrees over the surface of the cervix.

The cervical specimen is thinly spread onto a glass slide.

C. Endocervical Specimen

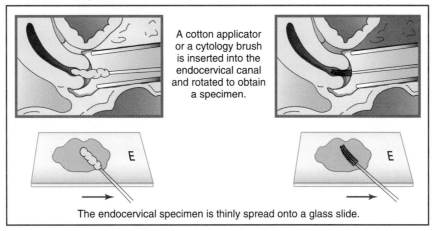

A cotton applicator or a cytology brush is inserted into the endocervical canal and rotated to obtain a specimen.

The endocervical specimen is thinly spread onto a glass slide.

■ **FIGURE 10–3.** Obtaining the Pap smear.

Fixing the Smear

The smears must be fixed immediately by flooding the slides with 95 percent ethyl alcohol or by lightly spraying the slides with a commercial cytology spray fixative. The slides must be fixed before they dry to avoid inaccurate results. The purpose of the fixative is to maintain the normal appearance of the cells, to protect the slides from contaminants in the air such as dust and bacteria, and to attach the smear to the slide firmly. The cytology fixative must be allowed to dry thoroughly; the slides are then ready for transport to a cytology laboratory for evaluation.

Cytology Request

A cytology request must accompany all Pap smears. It should include the physician's name and address; the date; the source of the specimen; the patient's name,

address, age, and date of last menstrual period (abbreviated LMP); and history, including any previous abnormal Pap smears, hormone therapy, treatment for cancer, and abnormal vaginal bleeding or discharge. Refer to Figure 10–4 for an example of a cytology request form. If the results of the Pap smear are abnormal, the physician may want to repeat the test. On repeat smears, the previous laboratory number and date must also be included on the request form.

Maturation Index

The maturation index (MI) provides the physician with an endocrine evaluation of the patient, which can assist in evaluating the cause of infertility, menopausal or postmenopausal bleeding, or amenorrhea and can help assess the results of treatment with hormones. The maturation index refers to the percentage of parabasal, intermediate, and superficial cells present in the smear.

10

Please Print or Type
NAME OF
PATIENT _____

| DO NOT WRITE HERE | Last | First | Date of Birth | Age |

_____

Number and Street　　City　　State　　Zip

TYPE OF SPECIMEN
☐ Vaginal　☐ Maturation Index
☐ Cervical　☐ Other

Last Menstrual Period

_____

Month　　Day　　Year

Physicians Name and Address

☐ Abnormal Vaginal Bleeding
☐ Abnormal Vaginal Discharge
☐ Previous Pelvic Surgery (Type) _____
☐ Radiation Therapy Date _____ ☐ Previous Cytology _____
Clinical Diagnosis and Remarks _____

☐ Hormone Therapy
☐ Pregnancy

BILLING INFORMATION:
☐ Bill Patient　☐ Bill Physician　☐ Bill Medicare #
☐ Bill Welfare # _____
Case Name _____ Pt. 2 Digit # _____
Other _____

CYTOPATHOLOGY CONSULTATION REQUEST　　Date _____

■ **FIGURE 10–4.** Cytology request form.

If the physician orders a maturation index along with the Pap test, the medical assistant must be sure to indicate this on the cytology request by checking the appropriate square labeled Maturation Index (see Fig. 10–4). Numerous factors may affect the results of the maturation index; therefore, it is important to indicate on the cytology request the presence of abnormal bleeding, hormone treatment, or treatment with digitalis, corticosteroids, or thyroid medication.

Analysis of the Pap Smear

To protect the slides during transport to a cytology laboratory, they must be carefully placed in a slide container designed especially for this purpose and bearing a label indicating that the contents include a medical specimen. The smears are then mailed to a cytology laboratory where they are stained and manually studied under a microscope by a cytopathologist for evidence of infection, abnormal cells (dysplasia), or cancerous cells. The cytologic findings are recorded on a cytologic report form and returned to the medical office.

A recent development in the examination of Pap slides is the use of computer technology. An abnormal slide may contain only a few abnormal cells among thousands of normal cells and the manual method may result in missing these abnormal cells. If the manual inspection determines that the slide is negative, an au-

tomated cytology analyzer can be used to reexamine the slide. The analyzer is able to examine every cell on the smear and select and display those cells that appear "most abnormal." The cytopathologist can then review these cells before issuing a negative report.

Results of the Pap Test

The terminology employed in reporting cytologic findings seen on a Pap smear has undergone several modifications over the years. Dr. Papanicolaou originally categorized findings into classes I through V, with class I as normal and class V practically conclusive for malignancy. More recently, Pap smears have been classified according to the **Bethesda system.** The Bethesda system was developed in 1988 by the National Cancer Institute in Bethesda, Maryland. This system separates the cytology report (Fig. 10–5) into three main categories:

1. A statement of the adequacy of the specimen (e.g., specimen is satisfactory for evaluation).
2. A general categorization of the specimen as normal or abnormal (e.g., within normal limits).
3. A descriptive diagnosis by which the cytopathologist elaborates on any abnormal findings. This part of the report provides the physician with a detailed description of any infection, dysplasia, or cancerous cells observed on the slide by the cytopathologist.

RIVERVIEW HOSPITAL
DEPARTMENT OF PATHOLOGY
2501 GRANT AVENUE
ST. LOUIS, MO 63146
(314) 883-3443

PATIENT: HEATHER JONES
PT NO: 45876
SEX: FEMALE
AGE: 32 YEARS
SUBMITTING: T. WOODSIDE, MD

ACCESSION DATE: 6/30/2002   ACCESSION: GY-33-8903

GYN CYTOLOGY REPORT

CLINICAL INFORMATION

LMP: 6/18/2002

Previous cytology: 7/2000 WNL

SPECIMEN ADEQUACY

Specimen is satisfactory for evaluation.

DIAGNOSIS

**ABNORMAL CYTOLOGY/INFECTION
FEATURES CONSISTENT WITH CANDIDA SPECIES**

■ **FIGURE 10–5.** Cytology report form (Bethesda system).

The Bethesda system has been adopted by the American College of Pathology and the American College of Obstetricians and Gynecologists and is now considered the standard for reporting cervical cytology on Pap smears. Because this system provides a detailed cytologic description rather than a numerical result (as with the previous class I through V system), it is considered a more effective means of communciating the results of the Pap test to the physician.

Abnormal cytologic findings on the Pap smear indicate that further tests should be conducted. Examples of additional procedures that may be performed include colposcopy, cervical biopsy, and endocervical curettage.

BIMANUAL PELVIC EXAMINATION

After obtaining the smear for the Pap test, the physician withdraws the speculum and performs a bimanual pelvic examination. The physician inserts the index and middle fingers of a lubricated gloved hand into the vagina. The fingers of the other hand are placed on the patient's lower abdomen. Between the two hands, the physician can palpate the size, shape, and position of the uterus and ovaries and detect tenderness or lumps (Fig. 10–6).

RECTAL-VAGINAL EXAMINATION

The last part of the pelvic examination is a rectal-vaginal examination. The physician inserts one gloved finger into the vagina and another gloved finger into the rectum to gain information about the tone and alignment of the pelvic organs and the adnexal region (the ovaries, fallopian tubes, and ligaments of the uterus). The presence of hemorrhoids, fistulas, and fissures can also be noted during the examination.

10

MEMORIES *from* EXTERNSHIP

MICHELE PARSONS: *Orthopedics was my third externship site, and I remember thinking, "Good, another speciality." My initial duties were administrative. I made appointments, billed insurance providers, and processed patients. I preferred clinical duties, but I did not mind the administrative duties.*

Finally, my chance for clinical work arrived. I assisted with cast applications, helped apply splints, and processed x-rays. I was so excited to be able to do this work. One day, a young boy came into the office. He had a cast in place on his arm. After reviewing his history, none of the staff could believe what had happened. The patient had a fracture to the elbow region and pins were in place. The pins should have been removed approximately 1 to 2 weeks after placement, but the patient had come to the office approximately 2 months later instead.

I assisted the physician in cast removal but found myself having to leave the room because of the overwhelming odor—infection! I remember being so embarrassed. The office staff were very understanding, however, and made me feel much better about having had to leave the examination room. The patient was scheduled for immediate surgery because of the risk of gangrene infection. Following surgery, the patient was fine, and everything turned out all right.

VAGINAL INFECTIONS

☐ The vagina provides a warm, moist environment, which tends to encourage the growth of various organisms, resulting in a vaginal infection, or **vaginitis.** If an unusual vaginal discharge is present, suggesting a vaginal infection, a specimen is obtained for culture or microscopic examination to identify the invading organism. A specimen of the discharge is collected at the medical office and is either evaluated there or placed on a culture or transport medium that is picked up or sent to an outside medical laboratory for evaluation. The patient should be instructed not to douche before coming to the medical office, because the physician will be unable to observe the discharge or to obtain a specimen for microbiologic analysis.

The medical assistant is responsible for assembling the appropriate supplies for the collection and evaluation of the suspected invading organism. She or he must be sure to label all specimens with the patient's name, the date, and the source of the specimen. If it will be transported to an outside medical laboratory for evaluation, a laboratory request form must be completed, including the source of the specimen, the physician's clinical diagnosis, the microbiologic examination requested, and any other pertinent information such as medications the patient is taking. The physician's clinical assessment of the patient's signs and symptoms, along with the results of the laboratory evaluation of the specimen, are used to diagnose the presence of a vaginal infection.

Medical assistants should take precautions to protect themselves from being infected with a pathogen while

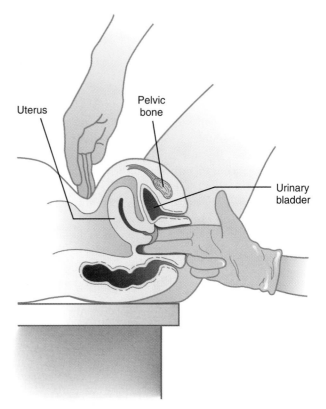

■ **FIGURE 10–6.** The bimanual pelvic examination.

PROCEDURE

10–1

Assisting with a Gynecologic Examination

The following procedure describes the medical assistant's role in assisting with a gynecologic examination consisting of a breast and pelvic examination, including a Pap smear.

EQUIPMENT/SUPPLIES:	
Disposable gloves	Glass slides with a frosted edge
Examining gown and drape	Cytology fixative
Vaginal speculum	Lubricant
Cervical scraper	Tissues
Cotton-tipped applicator or cytology brush	Biohazard waste container

1. **Procedural Step.** Wash the hands.
2. **Procedural Step.** Assemble the equipment. Using a lead pencil, identify the slides on the frosted edge with the patient's name, the date, and the source of the specimen. Use a **V** to identify the slide of the smear taken from the vagina, a **C** to identify the slide of the smear taken from the cervix, and an **E** to identify the slide of the smear taken from the endocervical canal. Place the equipment and supplies within easy reaching distance of the physician.

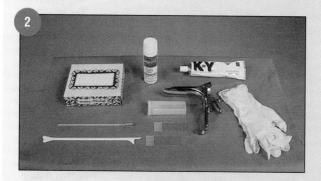

3. **Procedural Step.** Complete the cytology request form, making sure to include all essential information required by the cytology laboratory.
4. **Procedural Step.** Greet and identify the patient. Introduce yourself, and explain the procedure. Ask the patient if she needs to empty her bladder before the examination. If a urine specimen is needed, she is requested to void into a specimen container.

Principle. An empty bladder makes the pelvic examination easier and is more comfortable for the patient.

5. **Procedural Step.** Prepare and instruct the patient for the examination. Measure the patient's vital signs and height and weight and chart the results. Instruct the patient to undress completely and wear the examining gown with the opening positioned in front.
6. **Procedural Step.** Assist the patient onto the examining table. Position and drape her in a supine position for the breast examination. Refer to Chapter 4: Procedure 4–3 for the procedure for placing a patient in the supine position.
7. **Procedural Step.** Assist the patient into the lithotomy position for the pelvic examination. Properly drape the patient. Refer to Chapter 4: Procedure 4–6 for the procedure for placing a patient in the lithotomy position. Adjust and focus the light for the physician. Reassure the patient and help her relax the abdominal muscles during the examination by telling her to breathe deeply, slowly, and evenly through the mouth.

Principle. Visualization of the vagina and cervix requires direct light. If the patient is relaxed, the examination proceeds more smoothly and is more comfortable for the patient.

8. **Procedural Step.** Assist the physician as follows for the pelvic examination:
   a. Warm the vaginal speculum by moistening it with warm water, by placing it on a heating pad, or by storing it in a warming drawer. Inserting a cold speculum into the vagina causes the patient discomfort and results in contraction of the vaginal muscles, making it difficult for the physician to insert the speculum.

10

Continued

PROCEDURE 10–1

8. **b.** Assist the physician with the application of the gloves.

c. Apply gloves and fix the Pap slides by flooding them with 95 percent ethyl alcohol or with a cytology spray fixative, following the directions on the spray container. The smears must be fixed immediately (within 10 seconds after collection) to maintain the normal appearance of the cells and to prevent the smears from being exposed to contaminants in the air. The medical assistant must be sure to hold the nozzle of the spray fixative the recommended distance from the slides (usually 5 to 6 inches). Holding the spray nozzle too close may result in blowing the cells off the slides. The slides should be sprayed lightly with a continuous motion from left to right, then right to left, and allowed to dry thoroughly, usually for 5 to 10 minutes.

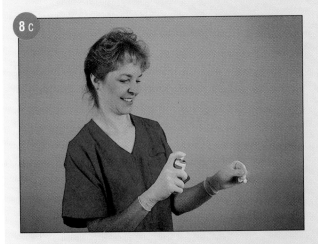

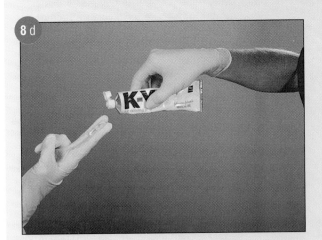

d. Apply lubricant to the physician's glove for the bimanual and rectal-vaginal examinations. Be careful not to allow the tube of lubricant to touch the physician's fingers to prevent contamination of the contents of the tube.

9. **Procedural Step.** After the examination, have the patient move back on the table (assist the patient if needed). Pull out the footrest and table extension and remove both legs from the stirrups simultaneously and place them on the table extension. Allow the patient to rest for a minute in the supine position. Return the stirrups to their normal position. Offer the patient tissues to remove excess lubricating jelly from the perineum. Help the patient into a sitting position, push in the table extension while supporting the patient's lower legs. Assist the patient off the examining table, so no falls will occur. Instruct the patient to get dressed. Inform the patient of the method used by the medical office to relay test results.

Principle. Patients (especially elderly ones) frequently become dizzy after being on the examining table and should be allowed to rest before sitting up.

10. **Procedural Step.** Prepare the Pap slides for transportation to the laboratory by placing them in a protective slide container. Be sure to include the completed cytology request form. Chart the transport of the Pap smear to an outside laboratory.

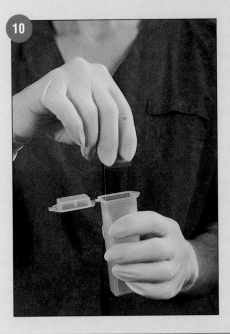

PROCEDURE 10-1

11. Procedural Step. Clean the examining room in preparation for the next patient. Rinse the vaginal speculum in cold water to remove secretions or they will dry and be more difficult to remove later on. Then sanitize and sterilize the speculum when it is convenient to do so, according to the medical office policy.

CHARTING EXAMPLE	
Date	
9/7/2002	10:00 a.m. Pap smear sent to Medical Center Laboratory for cytology.——M. Parsons, CMA

assisting with the collection and evaluation of the specimen by practicing good techniques of medical asepsis. Methods used to identify the invading organism and the supplies required for the collection and evaluation of organisms causing common vaginal infections are presented in the following paragraphs.

TRICHOMONIASIS

Trichomonas vaginalis, the causative agent of trichomoniasis (trich), is a pear-shaped protozoan possessing four flagella, which allows for the motility of the organism (Fig. 10-7). Trichomoniasis is most commonly spread through sexual intercourse. Symptoms of this infection include a profuse, frothy vaginal discharge that is usually yellowish green in color, itching and irritation of the vulva and vagina, and dysuria. The cervix may exhibit red spots, a condition known as "strawberry cervix."

Trichomonas may be identified at the medical office by the preparation of a wet mount, which involves placing a small amount of the discharge on a microscope slide using a sterile swab, adding a drop of isotonic saline to it, and then placing a coverslip over the mixture to protect it (Fig. 10-8). The slide is then examined under the microscope and observed for the

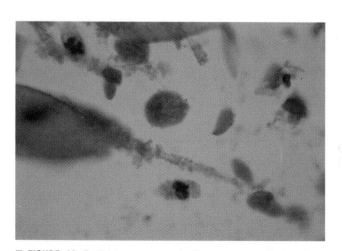

■ **FIGURE 10-7.** *Trichomonas vaginalis* as seen under a microscope. (From Mahon, C., Manuselis G.: *Diagnostic Microbiology.* Philadelphia, W. B. Saunders, 1995, p. 746.)

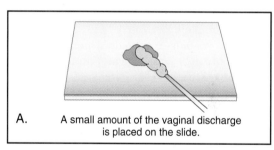

A. A small amount of the vaginal discharge is placed on the slide.

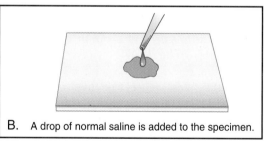

B. A drop of normal saline is added to the specimen.

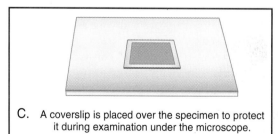

C. A coverslip is placed over the specimen to protect it during examination under the microscope.

■ **FIGURE 10-8.** Preparation of a wet mount for the identification of *Trichomonas vaginalis*.

10

presence of the lashing movements of the flagella and the motility of the organism.

If the physician prefers to have an outside laboratory evaluate the specimen, it must be placed in a sterile culture tube containing isotonic saline; a brand name of a commercially available form is the Culturette. It is important that the specimen be transported as soon as possible to prevent it from dying, which would impede visualization of the motility of the organism.

The treatment of trichomoniasis involves the oral administration of metronidazole (Flagyl). Both the woman and her sexual partner must be treated at the same time to prevent reinfection, because the partner may harbor the organism without displaying noticeable symptoms.

CANDIDIASIS

Candida albicans is a yeastlike fungus normally found in the intestinal tract and is therefore a frequent contaminant of the vagina; however, it usually does not produce symptoms indicating a vaginal infection. Conditions such as pregnancy, diabetes mellitus, and prolonged antibiotic therapy produce changes within the vagina that may precipitate a candidal infection of the vagina, commonly referred to as a yeast infection. Symptoms of candidiasis include white patches on the mucous membrane of the vagina along with a thick, odorless cottage cheese–like discharge. The discharge is extremely irritating and usually results in burning and intense itching. The patient generally experiences severe vulval irritation and dysuria.

Candida may be identified microscopically in the medical office by placing a specimen of the vaginal discharge on a slide using a sterile swab and adding a drop of a 10 to 20 percent solution of potassium hydroxide (KOH). The KOH dissolves cellular debris present in the smear and allows for better visualization of yeast buds, spores, or hyphae (fungus filaments), indicating the presence of *Candida albicans* (Fig. 10–9).

If the specimen is to be transported to a medical laboratory for identification, it must be placed on a transport medium to prevent drying and death; a commonly used medium is the Culturette.

The treatment of candidiasis consists of the application of vaginal ointments or suppositories such as miconazole (Monistat), clotrimazole (Gyne-Lotrimin), and nystatin (Mycostatin). Candidiasis has a tendency to recur; therefore, the woman should be instructed to contact the medical office if the symptoms of the yeast infection reappear.

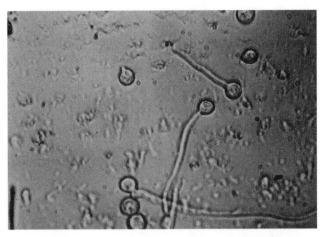

■ **FIGURE 10–9.** *Candida albicans* as seen under a microscope. (From Mahon, C., Manuselis G.: *Diagnostic Microbiology*. Philadelphia, W.B. Saunders, 1995, p. 721.)

GONORRHEA

Neisseria gonorrhoeae, a gram-negative diplococcus, is the causative agent of gonorrhea, the most common venereal disease. Gonorrhea is an infection of the genitourinary tract that is transmitted through sexual intercourse.

Women who have contracted gonorrhea may be asymptomatic or may exhibit a purulent vaginal discharge. As the disease progresses, it may spread to the lining of the uterus, resulting in pelvic inflammatory disease (PID) with the symptoms of lower abdominal pain, fever, nausea, and vomiting. If gonorrhea is left undiagnosed or untreated, it could result in sterility.

Neisseria gonorrhoeae is a **fastidious organism,** meaning it is difficult to grow and requires specialized growth conditions; therefore, special precautions must be followed when culturing the organism to prevent it from dying.

The growing conditions for *Neisseria gonorrhoeae* must include an atmosphere of carbon dioxide (devoid of oxygen) as well as a specially enriched blood medium known as chocolate agar. Thayer-Martin medium contains chocolate agar, which should be kept refrigerated and then warmed to room temperature just before using to provide the proper temperature growth requirement. Using a cold medium results in the death of any gonococci present in the specimen. The physician inoculates the Thayer-Martin medium and then places it in an atmosphere of carbon dioxide.

The Jambec collection system is a commercially available chocolate agar culture medium (see Fig. 10–10). This collection system is frequently used in the medical office to culture gonorrhea in females. The physician collects the specimen from the endocervical canal using a sterile swab. Specimens from the vagina and rectum may also be collected. The specimen must be inoculated on the culture medium immediately after collection to prevent death of the organism. The medical assistant is responsible for removing the lid and holding the plate while the physician inoculates it, using a Z pattern. The lid must be removed during inoculation only; unnecessary removal results in contamination of the specimen with extraneous microorganisms.

To provide an atmosphere devoid of oxygen using the Jambec system, a carbon dioxide-generating tablet packed in a foil pouch is unwrapped and placed in a circle in front of the plate (Fig. 10–10). The plate is then turned upside down and placed in a gas-impermeable plastic bag, which is sealed tightly to maintain the carbon dioxide atmosphere, allowing for proper growth of the gonococci, and to prevent air from entering and killing the gonococci. The inoculated plate is either stored at room temperature or placed in an incubator in its carbon dioxide environment until transport to the laboratory.

In men, gonorrhea usually can be identified with a gram-stained smear. The physician collects a specimen of the purulent urethral exudate and spreads the material on a slide. The slide should be allowed to air dry; a fixative should not be used. The laboratory stains the smear and then examines it for the presence of gram-negative intracellular diplococci, which indicate the presence of the gonococcus. A smear is not considered an accurate method of identification of *Neisseria gonorrhoeae* for women because other strains of gram-negative diplococci reside in the vagina that are not indicative of *Neisseria gonorrhoeae*, thereby confusing the diagnosis. Men who have contracted gonorrhea exhibit more symptoms than do women, including urethritis, dysuria, and a profuse yellow purulent discharge.

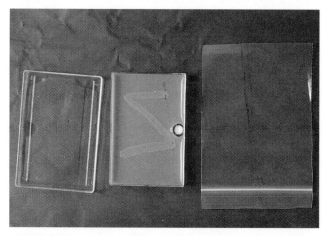

FIGURE 10–10. The Jambec collection system. (From Mahon, C., Manuselis, G.: *Diagnostic Microbiology*. Philadelphia, W. B. Saunders, 1995, p. 397.)

Gonorrhea is one of the infectious diseases that must be reported to the local Department of Health, so that all sexual partners can be followed up and treated.

CHLAMYDIA

Chlamydia is a gram-negative intracellular bacterium, meaning it grows and multiplies in the cytoplasm of the host cell. The name of the species affecting humans is *Chlamydia trachomatis*. Chlamydia is transmitted through sexual intercourse, and in the past decade it has become one of the most prevalent sexually transmitted diseases in the United States. Chlamydia often occurs in association with gonorrhea; approximately 25 to 50 percent of patients with gonorrhea also have chlamydia.

Individuals with chlamydia may be asymptomatic, and therefore the patient may not be aware of having the condition. Because of this, the patient may not seek medical care until serious complications have occurred. Women with symptoms have itching and burning in the genital area, an odorless, thick, yellow-white vaginal discharge, dull abdominal pain, and bleeding between menstrual periods. The genital site most commonly affected in women is the cervix; chlamydial cervicitis can extend into the fallopian tubes, resulting in salpingitis. Chlamydia is also thought to be a cause of PID, an inflammation of the cervix, uterus, fallopian tubes, and ovaries.

If left untreated, a chlamydial infection in a woman can lead to scarring in the fallopian tubes, infertility, and tubal pregnancy. In men, symptoms of a chlamydial infection include dysuria and a watery discharge from the penis. A chlamydial infection in a man is often described as **nongonococcal urethritis** and, if left untreated, can lead to epididymitis and sterility.

Chlamydia can be diagnosed through cell culture isolation and examination of a stained smear, serum-antibody detection, and direct-antigen detection. The equipment and supplies needed for the tray set-up depend upon the method used to diagnose chlamydia. The cell culture isolation and direct antigen detection involve the collection of a specimen from the endocervix in women and the urethra in men, using a sterile swab. The specimen must be placed in a tube containing a transport medium to preserve the specimen until it reaches the laboratory. The patient should be instructed not to void for 1 hour before the collection of the specimen to prevent any chlamydia organisms from being washed away. The serum antibody detection of chlamydia requires the collection of a blood specimen from the patient.

10

Prenatal Care

OBSTETRICS

☐ **Obstetrics** is the branch of medicine dealing with the supervision of women during pregnancy, childbirth, and the puerperium. **Prenatal** or **antepartal care** refers to the care of the pregnant woman before delivery of the infant. Prenatal care consists of a series of scheduled medical office visits for the promotion of the health of the mother and fetus through the prevention of disease and the provision of early detection, diagnosis, and treatment of problems common to pregnancy (e.g., anemia, urinary tract infection, and pre-eclampsia). Early detection of medical problems helps prevent serious complications in the mother and fetus.

The medical office visits for providing prenatal and postpartal care to the pregnant woman can be grouped into three major categories as follows:

1. First prenatal visit.
2. Return prenatal visits.
3. Six-weeks-postpartum visit.

Each of these categories and the responsibilities of the medical assistant during each are presented in this section.

THE FIRST PRENATAL VISIT

☐ The first prenatal visit generally occurs after the woman has missed her second menstrual period; if problems exist, the woman is seen after missing her first menstrual period. The first visit is often a stressful experience, and the medical assistant plays an important role in helping relax the patient and relieve her anxiety.

The first prenatal visit requires more time than the subsequent or return prenatal visits; therefore, sufficient time should be scheduled to allow for a complete and accurate initial assessment of the pregnant woman. The components of the first prenatal visit vary, depending on the medical office, but they generally include the following:

1. Completion of a prenatal record form.
2. Initial prenatal examination, consisting of a complete physical examination. Of particular importance are the breast, abdominal, and pelvic examinations. Pelvic measurements may be taken at this time or during a return prenatal visit.
3. Prenatal patient education.
4. Laboratory tests.

Each component of the first prenatal visit is described in more detail in the following pages.

THE PRENATAL RECORD

☐ The prenatal record provides information regarding the past and present health status of the patient and also serves as a data base and flow sheet for subsequent prenatal visits. The prenatal record is essential in helping identify high-risk patients. The medical assistant is usually responsible for collecting a portion of the information required for the prenatal record. Many different types of printed prenatal record forms are available (see Fig. 10–11 for one example). The form utilized in your medical office will be based on physician preference and the method used for conducting the prenatal examination.

Obtaining and recording information in the prenatal record provides an opportunity for the medical assistant to develop a rapport with the patient. It is also an excellent time to relay information to her regarding various aspects of the prenatal and postnatal period, such as an explanation of the changes taking place within her body, information relating to the Lamaze method of childbirth, the signs and symptoms of oncoming labor, nutrition of the infant (breast feeding and bottle feeding), and care of the newborn infant. Providing a quiet setting free from distractions allows the patient the confidence to discuss areas of concern openly; this helps assure a complete and accurate prenatal history.

During the first prenatal visit, the medical assistant should relay his or her name and position to the patient to help build a supportive relationship with her as well as to allow her to ask for the medical assistant by name when contacting the medical office.

The prenatal record is similar to and contains much of the same information as the health history described in Chapter 2. Particular attention is given to factors that may influence the course of pregnancy, as will be described in the following paragraphs.

PAST MEDICAL HISTORY

The past medical history focuses on those conditions that could affect the health of the mother and fetus such as kidney disease, heart disease, hypertension, venereal disease, phlebitis, diabetes, tuberculosis, endocrine disorders, drug allergies, alcohol and tobacco intake, drug addiction, and so on. In addition, the medical assistant solicits information from the patient regarding past immunizations and childhood diseases to provide the physician with the information needed to assess her antibody protection against such diseases.

Prenatal Health History Summary   Date:

Patient's name _____

_____

Age_____ Race_____ Religion_____ Marital status_____ Years married_____ Education_____ Occupation_____

Home address_____ Home tel._____ Work tel._____

Nearest relative_____ Relative's employer_____ Work tel._____

Referring physician_____ Attending physician_____

PAST MEDICAL HISTORY	Patient	Family
1. Congenital anomalies		
2. Genetic diseases		
3. Multiple births		
4. Diabetes mellitus		
5. Malignancies		
6. Hypertension		
7. Heart disease		
8. Rheumatic fever		
9. Pulmonary disease		
10. GI problems		
11. Renal disease		
12. Other urinary tract problems		
13. Genitourinary anomalies		
14. Abnormal uterine bleeding		
15. Infertility		
16. Venereal disease		
17. Phlebitis, varicosities		
18. Nervous/mental disorders		
19. Convulsive disorders		
20. Metabol./endocrine disorders		
21. Anemia/hemoglobinopathy		
22. Blood dyscrasias		
23. Drug addiction		
24. Smoking/alcohol		
25. Infectious diseases		
26. Operations/accidents		
27. Blood transfusions		
28. Other hospitalizations		
29. **No known disease**		

Check and detail positive findings including date and place of treatment. Precede findings by reference number.

Menstrual History Onset _____ age   Cycle _____ q.   _____ days   Length _____ days   Amount _____   Last contraceptive   ☐ None   Type _____   Last used _____

PAST OBSTETRICAL HISTORY   Grav   Para   Pret   Abort   Live

No.	Month/year	Sex	Weight at birth	Wks. gest.	Hrs. in labor	Type of delivery	Details of delivery: include anesthesia and maternal or newborn complications. Use Risk Guide numbers where applicable
1							
2							
3							
4							
5							
6							
7							
8							

Sensitivities (detail positive findings)
30. ☐ **None known**
31. ☐ Antibiotics
32. ☐ Analgesics
33. ☐ Sedatives
34. ☐ Anesthesia
35. ☐ Other

Preexisting Risk Guide
Indicates pregnancy/outcome at risk
36. ☐ Age < 15 or > 35
37. ☐ < 8th grade education
38. ☐ Cardiac disease (class I or II)
39. ☐ Tuberculosis, active
40. ☐ Chronic pulmonary disease
41. ☐ Thrombophlebitis
42. ☐ Endocrinopathy
43. ☐ Epilepsy (on medication)
44. ☐ Infertility (treated)
45. ☐ 2 abortions (spontaneous/induced)
46. ☐ ≥ 7 deliveries
47. ☐ Previous preterm or SGA infants
48. ☐ Infants ≥ 4,000 gms
49. ☐ Iosimmunization (ABO, etc.)
50. ☐ Hemorrhage during previous preg.
51. ☐ Previous preeclampsia
52. ☐ Surgically scarred uterus
53. ☐ _____

Indicates pregnancy/outcome at **high** risk
54. ☐ Age ≥ 40
55. ☐ Diabetes mellitus
56. ☐ Hypertension
57. ☐ Cardiac disease (class III or IV)
58. ☐ Chronic renal disease
59. ☐ Congenital/chromosomal anomalies
60. ☐ Hemoglobinopathies
61. ☐ Isoimmunization (Rh)
62. ☐ Drug addiction/alcoholism
63. ☐ Habitual abortions
64. ☐ Incompetent cervix
65. ☐ Prior fetal or neonatal death
66. ☐ Prior neurologically damaged infant
67. ☐ _____

Initial Risk Assessment
68. ☐ No risk factors noted
69. ☐ At risk
70. ☐ At high risk

Signature

10

■ **FIGURE 10–11.** Example of a prenatal record form.

INTERVAL PRENATAL HISTORY

Flow Chart Date	Weight this visit	Year Pregravid Blood pressure	Urine Protein	Sugar	Est. weeks gestation (dates/sizes)	Fundal height	Fetal heart rate	Edema	PROGRESS NOTES	See Add Prog Note

10

Risk Guide for Pregnancy and Outcome

Risk Guide for Pregnancy and Outcome

☐ (0) No risk factors noted _____

☐ (1) At risk _____

☐ (2) **High risk** _____

Continuing Risk Guide

Mo/day	Potential risk factors	Mo/day	High risk factors
/	3. Preg. without familial support	/	18. Diabetes mellitis
/	4. Second pregnancy in 12 months	/	19. Hypertension
/	5. Smoking (≥ 1 pack per day)	/	20. Thrombophlebitis
/	6. Rh negative (nonsensitized)	/	21. Herpes (type 2)
/	7. Uterine/cervical malformation	/	22. Rh sensitization
/	8. Inadequate pelvis	/	23. Uterine bleeding
/	9. Venereal disease	/	24. Hydramnois
/	10. Anemia (Hct < 30%:Hgb < 10%)	/	25. Severe preeclampsia
/	11. Acute pyelonephritis	/	26. Fetal growth retardation
/	12. Failure to gain weight	/	27. Premature rupt. membranes
/	13. Multiple pregnancy (term)	/	28. Multiple pregnancy (preterm)
/	14. Abnormal presentation	/	29. Low/failing estriols
/	15. Postterm pregnancy	/	30. Significant social problems
/	16.	/	31. Alcohol and drug abuse
/	17.	/	32.

Comments:

■ **FIGURE 10–11.** *Continued*

PRESENT PREGNANCY HISTORY

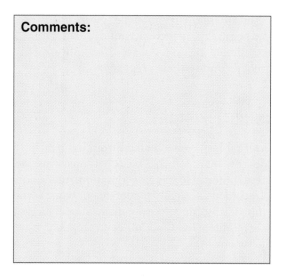

Comments:

History Since LMP	Patient
1. Headaches	
2. Nausea/vomiting	
3. Abdominal pain	
4. Urinary complaints	
5. Vaginal discharge	
6. Vaginal bleeding	
7. Edema (specify area)	
8. Febrile episode	
9. Rubella exposure	
10. Other viral exposure	
11. Drug exposure	
12. Radiation exposure	
13. Other	

```
L
M
P        date     quality
E
D
C
```

16.   Medications Since LMP

(Rx, non-Rx, vitamins)   ☐ None

Describe: _____

_____

_____

_____

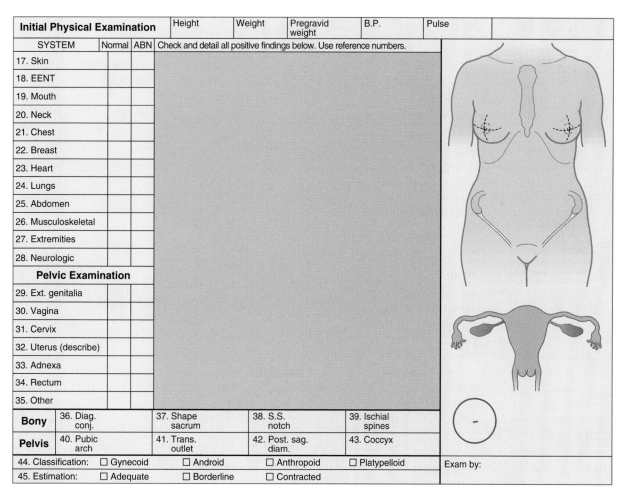

Initial Physical Examination		Height	Weight	Pregravid weight	B.P.	Pulse	
SYSTEM	Normal	ABN	Check and detail all positive findings below. Use reference numbers.				
17. Skin							
18. EENT							
19. Mouth							
20. Neck							
21. Chest							
22. Breast							
23. Heart							
24. Lungs							
25. Abdomen							
26. Musculoskeletal							
27. Extremities							
28. Neurologic							

Pelvic Examination

	Normal	ABN	
29. Ext. genitalia			
30. Vagina			
31. Cervix			
32. Uterus (describe)			
33. Adnexa			
34. Rectum			
35. Other			

Bony	36. Diag. conj.	37. Shape sacrum	38. S.S. notch	39. Ischial spines
Pelvis	40. Pubic arch	41. Trans. outlet	42. Post. sag. diam.	43. Coccyx

44. Classification:	☐ Gynecoid	☐ Android	☐ Anthropoid	☐ Platypelloid	Exam by:
45. Estimation:	☐ Adequate	☐ Borderline	☐ Contracted		

■ **FIGURE 10–11.** *Continued*

Rubella, if contracted during pregnancy, can be dangerous to the developing fetus; the earlier in pregnancy the infection occurs, the greater is the chance of birth defects. The infant may be born with heart defects, cataracts, mental retardation, and deafness. Patients who do not have antibody protection against rubella are given a rubella immunization within 6 weeks after delivery. The rubella vaccination is made from a live virus and therefore cannot be given to a pregnant woman because it may be harmful to the fetus. These patients should be told to avoid exposure to children with rubella during their pregnancy.

MENSTRUAL HISTORY

A menstrual history is obtained from the patient, which includes the date of the onset of menstruation, the menstrual interval cycle, the duration, the amount of flow (recorded as small, moderate, or large), and any gynecologic disorders. The patient should be asked if she was using a method of contraception when she became pregnant.

PAST OBSTETRIC HISTORY

A thorough past obstetric history is also included as a component of the prenatal record and provides the opportunity to obtain information from the patient relating to previous pregnancies. Information that is obtained and explored includes gravidity, parity, premature births, multiple births, abortions, stillbirths, and any problems relating to infertility.

Gravidity and parity provide data with respect to the pregnancy, and the medical assistant should develop skill in recording this information. **Gravidity** refers to the total number of times a woman has been pregnant, regardless of the duration of the pregnancy and including the current pregnancy. **Parity** refers to the number of children the patient has delivered that reached the age of viability, regardless of whether the child was born alive or stillborn. An infant is considered viable after 20 weeks of gestation. Both these terms (gravidity and parity) refer to the pregnancy rather than the fetus; for example, multiple births (twins, triplets) count as only one pregnancy (gravida) and one delivery (para). **Abortion** (ab) refers to a fetus that did not reach the age of viability, or 20 weeks of gestation.

For example, if a woman is pregnant for the first time, the medical assistant would record the information as follows: gravida I, para 0. After delivery, regardless of whether the infant is born alive or stillborn (as long as it was carried to the point of viability or 20 weeks of gestation.), she becomes gravida I, para I. If she delivers twins from this pregnancy, the recording is still gravida I, para I, remembering that multiple births count as only one delivery. If she becomes pregnant again and loses the fetus before the age of viability (abortion), the medical assistant would record the information as follows: gravida II, para I, ab I.

If a woman is a multigravida, information is obtained relating to each previous pregnancy, including length of pregnancy, hours of labor, type of delivery

(vaginal or cesarean section), and maternal or infant complications. The obstetric history assists in identifying areas that may need to be further investigated or monitored during the prenatal period.

PRESENT PREGNANCY HISTORY

The present pregnancy history establishes a baseline for the present health status of the prenatal patient. In addition, the patient is queried regarding any warning signs that may be present, such as persistent headaches, visual disturbances, abdominal pain, vaginal bleeding, or discharge that may place the mother or fetus in jeopardy. The patient is also asked if she has experienced any of the early signs of pregnancy such as nausea, vomiting, fatigue, or breast changes.

Any prescribed or over-the-counter medications being taken by the patient must also be recorded. Certain medications cross the placental barrier and could be harmful to the developing fetus. Therefore, the patient should not take any medications while pregnant without first checking with the physician.

In the space provided under the present pregnancy history, the medical assistant will also need to record the first day of the patient's last menstrual period (LMP). The LMP is used to calculate due date, or **expected date of delivery** (EDD), by using **Nägele's rule:** Add 7 days to the first day of the LMP, subtract 3 months, and add 1 year (EDD = LMP + 7 days − 3 months + 1 year). For example, if the first day of the patient's LMP was June 10, 2000, the EDD is March 17, 2001. The problem is set up as follows:

$$\frac{\begin{array}{ccc} 6 & 10 & 2000 \\ -3 + & 7 + & 1 \end{array}}{\begin{array}{ccc} 3 - & 17 - & 2001 \end{array}} \quad \begin{array}{l} \text{(LMP)} \\ \text{(Applying Nägele's rule)} \\ \text{(Delivery date)} \end{array}$$

Using Nägele's rule, approximately 4 percent of patients deliver spontaneously on the EDD and the majority of patients deliver during the period extending 7 days before to 7 days after the EDD.

Gestation calculators are commercially available that may also be used to determine the delivery date by lining up an arrow adjacent to the date of the LMP, using a movable inner cardboard wheel (Fig. 10–12). These calculators require less time to determine the EDD than using Nägele's rule, and they provide information on the probable size (length and weight) of the fetus on any given date. The accuracy of gestation calculators is comparable to that of Nägele's rule. If the patient is unsure of the date of her LMP, the physician estimates the length of gestation by using other methods such as fundal height measurement or sonography.

10

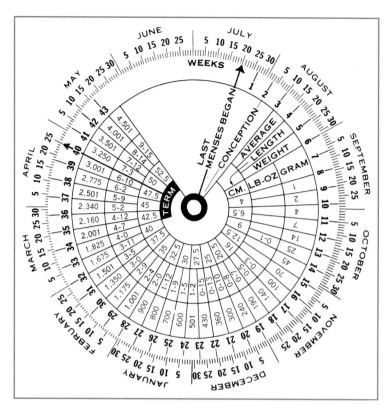

■ **FIGURE 10–12.** Gestation calculator. The last menstrual period is July 20 and the estimated date of delivery is April 25.

INTERVAL PRENATAL HISTORY

The interval prenatal history is also included in the prenatal record form; its purpose is to update the record at each return visit. Essential data are collected and recorded in this section during each return visit, including the weight, blood pressure, urine testing results, fundal height measurement, and fetal heart rate. A general inquiry is made regarding the occurrence of any additional signs of pregnancy such as quickening or Braxton Hicks contractions, as well as a general inquiry as to how the patient is feeling or the presence of any concerns or symptoms since the last prenatal visit.

This information is recorded and assists the medical staff in planning, implementing, and evaluating individual needs. Particular attention is focused on risk factors such as hypertension, thrombophlebitis, and uterine bleeding, which could influence the course of the pregnancy.

INITIAL PRENATAL EXAMINATION

PURPOSE

The initial prenatal examination is of particular importance because it results in confirmation of the pregnancy and establishes a baseline for the woman's state of health. It includes a thorough gynecologic examination (breast and pelvic examinations) and a general physical examination of the other body systems, although the latter may be performed during a subsequent prenatal visit, depending on the medical office routine.

Women often have little or no medical supervision during their child-bearing years; therefore, the physical examination is of particular importance in establishing a baseline for the woman's general state of health and in helping identify high-risk prenatal patients. Conditions such as obesity, hypertension, severe varicosities, and uterine size inappropriate for the due date can be diagnosed by the physician, and necessary treatment or monitoring can be instituted to help prevent complications.

PREPARATION OF THE PATIENT

Once the patient arrives at the medical office and the prenatal record form has been completed, the medical assistant is responsible for taking and recording the patient's vital signs, height, and weight to provide a data base for subsequent prenatal visits. The patient is then asked to disrobe completely and put on an examining gown with the opening in front. The medical assistant must make sure to give complete and thorough instructions so the patient knows exactly what is expected. The patient should be asked if she needs to

10

empty her bladder because an empty bladder facilitates the examination and is more comfortable for her. If the office policy is such that a specimen is needed for urine testing at the initial prenatal visit, the patient will be required to void.

Special precautions should be taken in assisting the prenatal patient onto and off of the examination table. The footstool should be placed in a convenient position next to the table, and the medical assistant should help the patient onto and off of the table to assure her safety and comfort. This is especially important as the pregnancy progresses and the patient becomes more awkward and off-balance.

The medical assistant is responsible for setting up the tray required for the examination. The set-up includes the equipment and supplies required for each procedure included. During the prenatal examination, the medical assistant is responsible for positioning the patient as required for each aspect of the examination as well as assisting the physician as necessary. Table 10-1 lists the procedures commonly included in the prenatal examination and the purpose, implications, and (when applicable) the patient position for each. Most of the procedures included in the initial prenatal examination are presented elsewhere in the text; the number of the chapter that contains the step-by-step procedure is included in Table 10-1.

PATIENT EDUCATION

At the conclusion of the initial prenatal examination and after the patient is dressed, the physician talks with her regarding instructions on diet, weight gain, rest, sleep, clothing, employment, exercise, travel, intercourse, bowel function, dental care, smoking, alcohol, and drugs. Many offices have a prenatal guidebook designed especially for this purpose that is given to each patient to use as a reference. Some offices also utilize a series of teaching films that the patient views during the return prenatal visit while waiting to see the physician. The physician usually prescribes a daily vitamin supplement to be taken during the prenatal period to help ensure that the mother and fetus obtain an adequate supply of vitamins and minerals.

TEST REQUIREMENTS

During the first visit, the patient is also given a laboratory request to have the required specimens collected and tested at an outside medical laboratory. Some offices collect blood and urine specimens; these are then picked up or mailed to an outside laboratory for testing. However, most offices find it more convenient to have the specimens collected at an outside laboratory. The prenatal laboratory tests, generally referred to as the prenatal profile, are discussed in more detail on the following pages.

FOLLOW-UP

When the physician is finished talking with the patient, the medical assistant is responsible for scheduling the next prenatal visit and for making sure the patient understands the instructions for maintaining health and preventing disease during the pregnancy. The medical assistant should tell the patient to report the occurrence of any of the warning signs of problems in the pregnancy and not to take any medications without first checking with the physician. The patient should also be encouraged to contact the medical office should any questions or problems arise.

LABORATORY TESTS

A number of laboratory tests are ordered by the physician to assist in the overall initial assessment of the state of health of the prenatal patient and to detect problems that may put the pregnancy at risk. The physician gives the patient a laboratory request at the first prenatal visit for tests that will be collected and evaluated at an outside laboratory. Several of the tests, such as the Pap smear and gonorrhea culture, require the physician to collect the specimens at the medical office and then have them transported to an outside laboratory for evaluation. The blood specimen required for the hematologic tests must be obtained through a venipuncture to provide sufficient quantity for the number of tests ordered.

The medical assistant should stress to the patient the importance of having these tests completed as soon as possible to provide the physician with the test results by the time of the next scheduled prenatal visit. Based on the results of the prenatal examination and the laboratory tests, the physician may order further tests, if needed, to assess the patient's condition. The following tests are generally included in the prenatal laboratory work-up.

Urine Tests

URINALYSIS.　A complete urinalysis is performed, including a physical, chemical, and microscopic analysis of the urine; a clean-catch midstream urine specimen is generally required for the test. If bacteria are found in the urine specimen, the physician usually requests a urine culture and sensitivity test to determine the pos-

TABLE 10–1

Elements of the Initial Prenatal Examination

Procedure	Purpose and Implications
Vital signs (Chapter 3) Temperature Pulse Respiration Blood pressure	To provide a baseline for subsequent prenatal visits. The blood pressure drops slightly during the first and second trimesters and returns to normal or slightly above normal during the last trimester. An elevation in the blood pressure during the pregnancy is used in conjunction with other patient signs and symptoms to assess the presence of a possible pathologic condition. An elevation in the blood pressure may be indicative of possible pre-eclampsia or other hypertensive disorders.
Weight (Chapter 4)	To provide a baseline weight measurement for comparison with all future weight measurements at subsequent prenatal visits. The medical assistant will be plotting the patient's weight on a graph or flow sheet at each prenatal visit, and any deviations from expected progressions will be evaluated by the physician. Measuring and recording the maternal weight gain or loss are helpful in assessing fetal development and to some extent the mother's nutrition and state of health. A sudden unexplained weight gain may be indicative of possible pre-eclampsia of pregnancy.
Physical examination (Chapter 4)	To establish a baseline for the woman's general state of health to be certain the patient is entering pregnancy in the best possible physical condition. The physical examination includes an examination of the patient's eyes, ears, nose, and throat; chest, lungs, and heart; breasts; abdomen; reproductive organs; rectum; and extremities. Of particular importance are the breast, abdominal, and pelvic examinations, which are outlined in a separate category.
Breast examination (Chapter 10)	To check for cysts or lumps and the breast changes that take place during pregnancy, such as tenderness and fullness and darkening of the nipple and areola. Patient position: supine.
Abdominal examination (Chapter 10)	To detect any masses or lumps other than the developing fetus. The abdomen is inspected for scars or striations, and the initial measurement of the fundal height is generally made to provide a baseline for future fundal height measurements. Patient position: supine.
Pelvic examination (Chapter 10)	To provide data to confirm the pregnancy and to determine the length of gestation. To identify pelvic characteristics and any abnormalities that may result in complications during the pregnancy or delivery. The pelvic examination generally includes the following: a. Inspection of the external genitalia b. Speculum examination of the vagina and cervix c. Pap smear d. Specimen for gonorrhea culture e. Vaginal specimen if an infection is suspected f. Bimanual examination Patient position: lithotomy.
Rectal-vaginal examination (Chapter 10)	To assess the strength and irregularity of the posterior vaginal wall and the posterior cervix. The anus is inspected for hemorrhoids and fissures, and the rectum is inspected for any herniation and masses. Patient position: lithotomy.
Pelvic measurements (Chapter 10)	To assure that the size and shape of the pelvis are within normal limits to allow the full-term fetus to pass safely through the pelvic inlet in the normal vaginal route of delivery; if not, a cesarean section will be required. Some physicians delay taking the pelvic measurements until later in the pregnancy. At that time, the prenatal patient's perineal muscles are more relaxed, allowing the pelvic measurements to be taken with less patient discomfort and more accuracy. The pelvic measurements are taken using the hands and an instrument specifically designed for this purpose, known as a *pelvimeter*. The process of measuring the capacity and diameter of the maternal pelvis is known as *pelvimetry*. Patient position: supine and lateral (side).

10

sible presence of a urinary tract infection. A pregnancy test may also be performed on the urine specimen, if ordered by the physician.

Smears and Cultures

PAPANICOLAOU SMEAR. A Pap smear is prepared for the detection of abnormalities of cell growth to diagnose precancerous or cancerous conditions of the cervix and uterus. This test can also be used for hormonal assessment and to assist in the detection of vaginal infections.

GONORRHEA AND CHLAMYDIA. These specimens are taken from the endocervical canal to rule out gonorrhea and chlamydia. If a gonorrheal infection is present at the time of delivery, the *Neisseria gonorrhoeae* organism could infect the infant's eyes and cause **ophthalmia neonatorum,** which could result in blindness. A chlamydial infection may cause the infant to develop neonatal conjunctivitis and pneumonia following delivery. A patient who has contracted gonorrhea or chlamydia requires treatment with an appropriate antibiotic. A gonorrhea culture on prenatal patients is generally mandated by state law.

TRICHOMONIASIS AND CANDIDIASIS. If an excessive irritating vaginal discharge is present, the physician usually obtains a specimen to rule out trichomoniasis and candidiasis. It is important to control candidiasis before delivery to prevent the development of a yeastlike infection of the mucous membrane of the mouth or throat of the infant, known as thrush.

Blood Tests

COMPLETE BLOOD COUNT (CBC). The CBC is a basic screening test used to assist in assessing the patient's state of health. It includes a hemoglobin, hematocrit, white blood count, red blood count, differential white cell count, and red blood cell indices; of particular importance with respect to the prenatal patient are the hemoglobin and hematocrit evaluations, which are described here.

HEMOGLOBIN AND HEMATOCRIT. Low hemoglobin or hematocrit values are seen in cases of anemia. Prenatal patients have a tendency to develop anemia because there is an increased demand for and correlating increased production of red blood cells during pregnancy; therefore, the physician carefully reviews the results of these tests. If the hemoglobin or hematocrit value is low, further hematologic evaluation is usually required. If necessary, therapy is instituted, which usually consists of an iron supplement and nutritional counseling. The hemoglobin and hematocrit values are

checked again at approximately 32 weeks of gestation as a precaution against anemia before delivery.

Rh FACTOR AND ABO BLOOD TYPE. These tests are performed to anticipate any ABO or Rh incompatibilities. If the patient is Rh−, the father's blood type must also be evaluated. If the father's blood type is Rh+, the possibility of an Rh incompatibility may exist. This warrants the performance of an Rh antibody titer test as well as repeat antibody titers throughout the pregnancy to determine whether the mother's antibody level is increasing. An increased Rh antibody level could be dangerous to the developing fetus.

GLUCOSE TOLERANCE TEST. A 1-hour glucose tolerance test is performed between 24 and 28 weeks of gestation to screen for gestational diabetes, since approximately 30 percent of women develop this condition during pregnancy. The patient is instructed to fast for 12 hours before the test. During the test, a flavored glucose solution is given to the patient to drink, and 1 hour later the patient's blood is drawn and measured for the glucose level. Patients exhibiting elevated results are further evaluated to determine whether gestational diabetes is present.

SEROLOGY TEST FOR SYPHILIS. The microorganism that causes syphilis, *Treponema pallidum*, is able to cross the placental barrier and infect the fetus; this could result in intrauterine death or could cause the fetus to be born with congenital syphilis. Children with congenital syphilis are often born with deformities and may become blind, deaf, paralyzed, or insane. The tests most commonly employed to screen for the presence of syphilis are the Venereal Disease Research Laboratories (VDRL) test and the rapid plasma reagin (RPR) test. The test results are reported as nonreactive, weakly reactive, or reactive. Because these tests are screening tests, a weakly reactive or reactive test result warrants more specific testing to arrive at a diagnosis for syphilis. Examples of these tests are the FTA-ABS (fluorescent treponemal antibody absorption) test and the MHA-TIP (microhemagglutination-treponema pallidum) test.

A prenatal serology test for syphilis is usually mandated by state law and should be performed early in the pregnancy, before fetal damage occurs. A patient who has contracted syphilis requires treatment with an appropriate antibiotic.

RUBELLA TITER. This test assesses the level of antibody against rubella (German measles) present in the patient's blood and is used to determine whether or not the woman has immunity to rubella. If the mother contracts rubella during pregnancy, serious congenital abnormalities can occur in the fetus. Those patients

10

who lack immunity should be immunized against rubella within 6 weeks following delivery.

Rh ANTIBODY TITER (ON Rh– BLOOD SPECIMENS). This test detects the amount of circulating Rh antibodies against red blood cells. These antibodies can occur in a pregnant woman who is Rh– and is carrying an Rh+ fetus; therefore, an Rh antibody titer is performed in all Rh– blood specimens. Repeat antibody titer levels are also performed during the pregnancy to determine whether the woman's antibody level is increasing. As

previously indicated, an increased Rh antibody level could be dangerous to the developing fetus.

HEPATITIS B AND HIV. The Centers for Disease Control and Prevention recommends that pregnant women have a blood test to screen for exposure to the hepatitis B virus. Women who have positive test results have an increased risk of spontaneous abortion or preterm labor. In addition, the mother may transmit hepatitis B to the infant, particularly during delivery or in the first few days of life. This risk can be greatly reduced by administering hepatitis immunoglobin and the hepatitis B vaccine to the newborn infants of women who have tested positive for hepatitis B. It is also recommended that testing for HIV (the AIDS virus) be offered to pregnant women who are at risk for contracting AIDS. Babies born to women who are HIV-positive have a high risk of developing the disease.

PUTTING IT ALL *into* PRACTICE

▶ **MICHELE PARSONS:** *A patient who had not been to the clinic for a while came in one day. His graduation from college had been delayed because he had developed a pilonidal cyst that needed to be surgically removed. At onset, these cysts can be very painful and usually require daily cleaning and packing. From my past experience with pilonidal cyst care, I knew that 1 to 2 months of treatment are usually required before full recovery is achieved.*

The physician and I prepared for the initial treatment and noticed the surgical site was very large and deep. We knew this treatment would take much longer than usual. Treatment was provided daily for 3 months. Subsequent treatments continued every other day for 2 months. Through our continuous contact, we became good friends with the patient.

Our patient graduated at the end of the spring quarter and moved out of state. He stays in contact with us and is still undergoing treatment. I feel he made a difference in our lives because he always maintained a positive attitude and was very pleasant, therefore making our job easier. We made a difference in his life through the good health care we provided and our continuing friendship.

RETURN PRENATAL VISITS

☐ Return prenatal visits provide the opportunity for a continuous assessment of the state of health of the mother and fetus. During each visit, essential data are collected and recorded in the prenatal record, resulting in an updated record at each visit, as discussed in this section. If signs or symptoms of a pathologic condition are present, the physician performs selected aspects of the physical examination as necessary to diagnose and treat the condition. In addition, diagnostic and laboratory tests may be ordered to assist in diagnosis and treatment.

The return prenatal visit also provides the opportunity for the physician and the medical assistant to lend support to the mother and to provide her with ongoing prenatal education to help reduce apprehension and anxiety and to ensure that the mother is well informed and prepared during her pregnancy, childbirth, and the postpartum period. The medical assistant plays an important role in prenatal education and should take the necessary time with each patient to provide appropriate information and to allow the patient the opportunity to ask questions.

For convenience, the 9 months of pregnancy are divided into three **trimesters,** each consisting of 3 months. During the first 6 months, or first two trimesters, of the pregnancy, the patient is seen once a month at the medical office. The patient is then seen every 2 weeks during the seventh and eighth months and then each week during the ninth month until delivery. The patient exhibiting complications is seen more frequently for closer monitoring.

The patient is asked to collect a first-voided morning urine specimen on the day of each return visit to be brought to the medical office for testing. Some physicians also require that the specimens be a clean-

10

catch midstream collection. A responsibility of the medical assistant is to instruct the patient in the proper collection techniques and care and handling of the specimen until it reaches the office. The medical assistant is responsible for testing the specimen for glucose and protein, using a reagent strip, and for recording results in the prenatal record. A positive reaction to glucose may indicate the development of diabetes mellitus or a prediabetic condition, whereas a positive reaction to protein may indicate pre-eclampsia. Further testing is usually needed to arrive at a final diagnosis and to institute treatment.

During the return visit the physician performs one or more of the following procedures, depending on the stage of the pregnancy: (1) palpation of the woman's abdomen to measure fundal height, (2) measurement of the fetal heart rate, and (3) a vaginal examination. These procedures are discussed in detail in the following paragraphs.

FUNDAL HEIGHT MEASUREMENT

The pregnant uterus rises gradually into the abdominal cavity, and the fundus is palpable between the eighth and thirteenth weeks of the pregnancy. The first fundal height measurement, which is usually performed during the first prenatal visit, is used as a guideline for all subsequent measurements. The physician measures the fundal height by placing one end of a flexible, nonstretchable centimeter tape measure on the superior aspect of the symphysis pubis and measuring to the crest or top of the uterine fundus (Fig. 10–13). The measurement is then recorded on a graph or flow chart in the patient's prenatal record. By 20 weeks the fundus reaches the lower border of the umbilicus, and between 36 and 37 weeks it reaches the tip of the sternum. During the first and second trimesters, measuring the fundal height provides a gross estimate of the duration of the pregnancy; the fundal height measurement is considered accurate to within 4 weeks using McDonald's rule:

Calculation of the duration of the pregnancy using McDonald's rule:

Height of the fundus (in centimeters) $\times 8/7 =$ duration of the pregnancy in weeks.

Example: 21 cm $\times$ 8/7 = 24 weeks

Height of the fundus (in centimeters) $\times 2/7 =$ duration of the pregnancy in lunar months.

Example: 21 cm $\times$ 2/7 = 6 months

Because fetal weights vary considerably during the third trimester, it is difficult to use fundal height measurements as an estimate of the duration of the pregnancy in the last trimester.

In addition to assessing the duration of the pregnancy, the fundal height measurements permit variations from normal to become apparent and are used to assess whether or not fetal development is progressing normally. Growth that is too rapid or too slow must be evaluated further by the physician as a possible indication of high-risk conditions such as multiple pregnan-

10

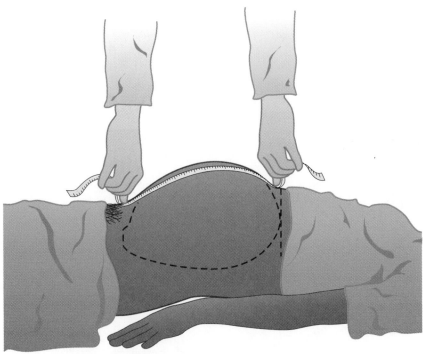

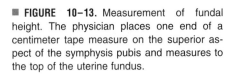

■ **FIGURE 10–13.** Measurement of fundal height. The physician places one end of a centimeter tape measure on the superior aspect of the symphysis pubis and measures to the top of the uterine fundus.

cies, polyhydramnios, ovarian tumor, intrauterine growth retardation (IUGR), intrauterine death, or an error in estimating the fetal progress.

FETAL HEART TONES

The normal fetal heart rate falls between 120 and 160 beats per minute with a regular rhythm. A very slow or rapid fetal heart rate usually indicates fetal distress. The fetal heart tones (FHT) can be heard with a Doppler fetal pulse detector between the tenth and twelfth weeks of gestation. The Doppler fetal pulse detector detects the fetal pulse rate through the conversion of ultrasonic waves into audible sounds of the fetal pulse.

The Doppler device consists of an instrument containing a crystal faceplate at its narrow end. Attached to the instrument by means of a jack is a stethoscope-type headset for listening to sounds (Fig. 10–14A). Because air is a poor conductor of soundwaves, an ultrasound coupling agent must first be spread on the

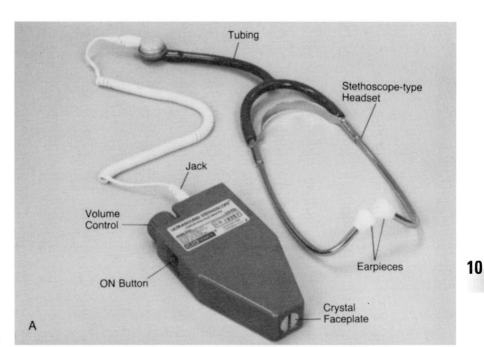

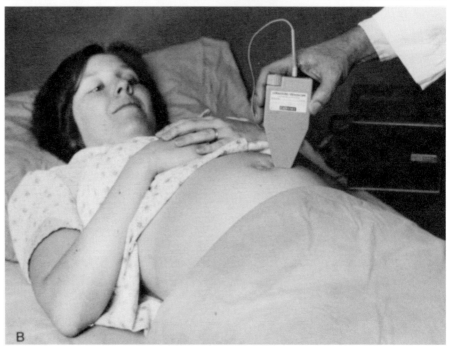

■ **FIGURE 10–14.** *A,* The parts of a Doppler device. *B,* The crystal faceplate of the Doppler device is moved across the abdomen to detect the fetal pulse. (Courtesy of Media Sonics, Mountain View, California.)

10

mother's abdomen in the area to be examined to increase conductivity of the sound waves between the abdomen and the crystal faceplate. The earpieces of the headset are then placed in the examiner's ears and the crystal faceplate is slowly moved across the abdomen to detect the fetal pulse (Fig. 10–14*B*).

VAGINAL EXAMINATION

In the absence of vaginal bleeding, vaginal examinations may be performed at any time during the pregnancy; however, in a normal pregnancy, there is usually no need to perform a vaginal examination until the patient nears term. The vaginal examination is usually begun approximately 2 to 3 weeks from the EDD and is performed to confirm the presenting part and to determine the degree, if any, of cervical dilation and effacement. The purpose of dilation and effacement is to permit the passage of the infant from the uterus into the birth canal (Fig. 10–15).

SPECIAL TESTS AND PROCEDURES

The physician may want to evaluate the pregnancy using one or more of the following procedures: alpha-fetoprotein analysis, obstetric ultrasound scanning, amniocentesis, and fetal heart rate monitoring. These are not considered routine procedures; however, they involve very little risk to the mother or fetus. Because some of these tests may be performed in the obstetric medical office, such as obstetric ultrasound scanning, amniocentesis, and nonstress fetal heart rate monitoring, the medical assistant should have a general knowledge of these procedures.

Alpha-Fetoprotein Analysis

The alpha-fetoprotein (AFP) analysis is a laboratory test performed on the serum of the mother's blood at 15 to 18 weeks of pregnancy. Its purpose is to screen for the presence of certain fetal abnormalities. Alpha-

fetoprotein is a glycoprotein produced by the fetus. During pregnancy, some AFP crosses from the amniotic fluid to the mother's bloodstream. When the neural tube of the fetus is not properly formed, increased amounts of AFP appear in the maternal blood. Hence, elevated test results indicate the possibility that a neural tube defect may be present in the fetus, such as spina bifida or anencephaly. A decreased AFP level, on the other hand, is associated with an increased risk of having a baby with Down's syndrome. Because the AFP analysis is a screening test, abnormal test results require further testing, such as ultrasound or aminocentesis, to determine whether a fetal abnormality actually exists.

Obstetric Ultrasound Scanning

Obstetric ultrasound scanning is a diagnostic imaging technique used to view the fetus in utero. It allows for the continuous viewing of the fetus and also shows fetal movement.

The procedure is performed by a physician or an ultrasonographer using high-frequency sound waves that are directed into the uterus through an **abdominal transducer** (Fig. 10–16). The mother lies on an examining table in a supine position and is draped for modesty with her abdomen exposed. A coupling agent, in the form of a liquid gel, is applied to the mother's abdomen to increase the transmission of the sound waves. When the sound waves reach the uterus, they "bounce" back to the transducer, similar to an echo. These reflected sound waves are then converted into an image or **sonogram** (Fig. 10–17) that is displayed on a viewing screen known as an oscilloscope. The display screen is usually positioned so the mother can observe the image on the screen if she wishes.

Obstetric ultrasound is most frequently performed between 16 and 22 weeks of gestation to determine gestational age and to confirm the due date. This is accomplished by taking various measurements of the fetus on the oscilloscope, such as the biparietal diameter (side-to-side measurement of the fetal head). The

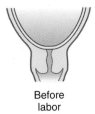 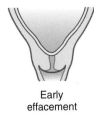 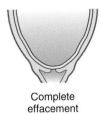 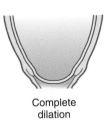

| Before labor | Early effacement | Complete effacement | Complete dilation |

■ **FIGURE 10–15.** Effacement and dilation occur to permit the passage of the infant into the birth canal. The cervical canal will shorten from its normal length of 1 to 2 cm to a structure with paper-thin edges in which there is no canal at all. The cervix will dilate from an opening a few millimeters in size to an opening large enough to allow the passage of the infant (approximately 10 cm).

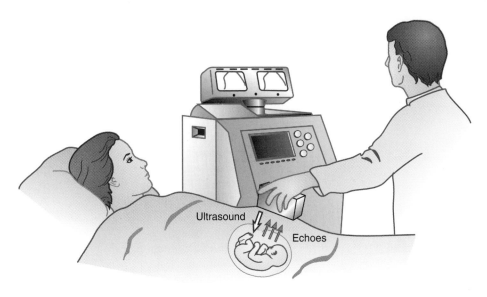

■ **FIGURE 10–16.** Obstetric ultrasound scanning. (From Kremkau, F.: *Diagnostic Ultrasound,* 4th ed. Philadelphia, W. B. Saunders, 1993, p. 2.)

routine examination also includes a thorough review of the fetal anatomy, including the brain, spinal cord, heart, lungs, gastrointestinal tract, kidneys, bladder, bowel, and extremities. Other reasons for performing ultrasound are to

■ Confirm the presence of fetal life
■ Evaluate fetal growth
■ Estimate fetal weight
■ Detect the presence of multiple fetuses
■ Determine the cause of bleeding or spotting
■ Detect congenital abnormalities
■ Determine placental position
■ Detect ectopic pregnancy
■ Determine the baby's position and size late in pregnancy

■ View the fetus, placenta, and amniotic fluid during tests such as amniocentesis or chorionic villus sampling

The patient must have a full bladder for an ultrasound examination that uses an **abdominal transducer.** This is accomplished by instructing the patient to consume 32 ounces of fluid approximately 1 hour before the procedure. A full bladder acts as an "acoustic window" through which the sound waves can travel to provide a clear visualization of the uterus. In addition, a full bladder holds the uterus stable and pushes away any bowel that might interfere with the image.

In the very early stages of the pregnancy (up to 12 weeks), a **vaginal transducer** may be used for the ultrasound examination, instead of an abdominal transducer. The advantage is that a full bladder is not required, thus making the examination more comfortable for the patient.

Vaginal ultrasound provides clearer visualization of the uterus in the beginning of the pregnancy because the probe of the transducer is situated in the vagina, which places it closer to the uterus. As the pregnancy progresses, however, abdominal ultrasound is generally preferred for producing the best image.

Amniocentesis

Amniocentesis is a diagnostic procedure that can be performed as early as the fourteenth to sixteenth week of the pregnancy. Amniocentesis provides for prenatal diagnosis of certain genetically transmitted errors of metabolism, congenital abnormalities, and chromosomal disorders such as Down's syndrome. It is also used to detect fetal jeopardy or distress and, later in the preg-

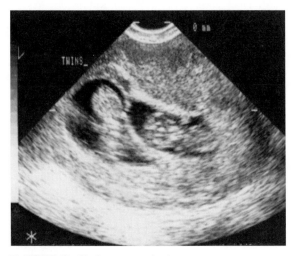

■ **FIGURE 10–17.** Sonogram of twins.

10

10

PATIENT/TEACHING

OBSTETRIC ULTRASOUND SCANNING

Answer questions patients have about obstetric ultrasound scanning:

What Is Ultrasound?

Ultrasound is a technique used to look at the baby in the uterus with the use of sound waves. During the examination, a gel is spread over the mother's abdomen, and a scanning device is moved lightly over the area. The baby's image is displayed on a monitor similar to a television screen. During the examination, Polaroid pictures of the baby will be taken and you will be given a copy for your baby album. If you so choose, you may bring a standard VHS tape for the ultrasonographer to record your baby on videotape for you. The ultrasound examination usually takes no longer than 30 minutes to perform.

Why Is Ultrasound Performed?

Ultrasound scanning is used to determine the age and position of the unborn baby, the location of the placenta, the number of babies present, and overall, to help the physician monitor and manage the pregnancy.

What Preparation Is Needed?

To prepare for an abdominal ultrasound, you will need to drink 32 ounces of fluid 1 hour before the examination. Drink all the water within a 15- to 20-minute time period, and then you should not void until the examination has been completed. You should wear comfortable clothing. A two-piece outfit is recommended so that you do not have to undress completely.

Is Ultrasound Safe?

There are no known side effects or risks to the mother or fetus during an ultrasound examination. Ultrasound does not use x-rays. No long-term risks have been detected. The procedure is painless and should not cause discomfort except that your full bladder may make you feel you need to go to the bathroom. Once the examination is completed, you will have the opportunity to do so.

Can I Learn the Sex of My Baby Through Ultrasound?

Although ultrasound is not performed to determine the sex of the baby, it is sometimes possible to tell whether the baby is a boy or girl, depending on the position of the baby in the uterus. Because not all parents want to know their baby's sex in advance, you will not automatically be told the baby's sex if it is determined, but you will be given the opportunity to make the choice of knowing or not knowing.

- Emphasize the importance of preparing properly for the examination.
- Provide the patient with educational materials on obstetric ultrasound.

nancy, to assess fetal lung maturity. Amniocentesis can also determine whether the baby is a boy or girl.

To perform the procedure, the physician inserts a long, thin needle through the mother's abdomen and into the amniotic sac surrounding the fetus (Fig. 10–18). A sample of fluid is withdrawn, which contains fetal cells. The fluid is then sent to a laboratory for study. Obstetric ultrasound is always performed in conjunction with amniocentesis so that the physician can view the position of the fetus, placenta, and amniotic fluid. This allows the physician to know the exact place to insert the needle.

Although the complication rate for an amniocentesis is extremely low, it is not risk-free. There is a slight risk of bleeding, leakage of fluid, and infection of the amniotic fluid. There is also a remote possibility of miscarriage. Because of these risk factors, amniocentesis is offered only to women whose pregnancies are at risk for fetal abnormalities. These include women who are 35 years or older or who have a previous history of a child with a genetic or neural tube defect; women who have abnormal AFP blood tests results; and when one parent has a chromosomal abnormality or is a carrier for a metabolic disease.

Fetal Heart Rate Monitoring

Fetal heart rate (FHR) monitoring is performed later in the pregnancy to obtain information on the physical condition of the fetus. Specific conditions that may warrant this procedure are fetal growth that is not

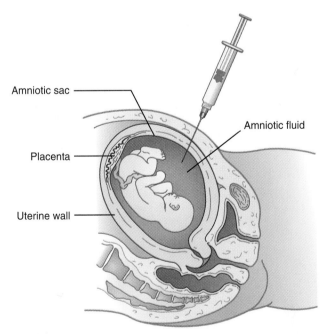

■ **FIGURE 10–18.** Amniocentesis.

progressing well, decreased amniotic fluid, decreased fetal activity, elevation of the mother's blood pressure, gestational diabetes, and an overdue fetus.

To perform the procedure, an electronic microphone is placed on the mother's abdomen, which amplifies the fetal heartbeat. A gel is usually applied under the microphone to make the sounds clearer. The heartbeat can be heard by and is also digitally displayed and recorded by the fetal heart rate monitor.

There are two types of fetal heart rate monitoring procedures: the nonstress test and the contraction stress test. The **nonstress test (NST)** monitors changes in the fetal heart rate in response to the baby's spontaneous movements. The mother is instructed to press a button when she feels the baby move. In a normal test, the baby's heart rate increases when the baby moves. To prepare for the NST, the mother must be instructed to eat a light meal within 2 hours of the procedure, which helps stimulate fetal movement.

If the results of the nonstress test are abnormal, a **contraction stress test (CST)** may be performed. This test is similar to the NST, except that mild contractions of the uterus are stimulated for a short period of time. The CST is used to evaluate the response of

the baby's heart rate to the contractions, to determine whether the baby will be able to withstand the stress of repeated contractions during labor. If the results of the test are abnormal, further evaluation is required to evaluate the well-being of the baby and to determine how and when delivery of the baby should be carried out.

MEDICAL ASSISTING RESPONSIBILITIES

The medical assistant has many important responsibilities in the return prenatal examination, which are outlined on the following pages under the Procedure for Assisting with a Return Prenatal Visit. The medical assistant is responsible for assembling the equipment and supplies required for the examination, for obtaining information to update the prenatal record, for preparing the patient for the examination, and for assisting the physician during the examination. The physician depends on the medical assistant to have the urine test results and certain measurements such as blood pressure and weight completed and recorded in advance to allow him or her the opportunity to review these measurements before examining the patient.

PROCEDURE

10–2

Assisting with a Return Prenatal Examination

10

| EQUIPMENT/SUPPLIES: | Flexible, nonstretchable centimeter tape measure
Doppler fetal pulse detector
Ultrasound coupling agent
Vaginal speculum | Disposable gloves
Lubricant
Examining gown and drape
Biohazard container |

1. **Procedural Step.** Wash the hands.
2. **Procedural Step.** Set up the tray for the prenatal examination. The equipment and supplies needed depend on the procedures included in the examination as follows:
   a. Fundal height measurement
   b. Measurement of fetal heart tones
   c. Examination of the legs, feet, and face for edema and the development of varicosities
   d. Taking a specimen for the diagnosis of a vaginal infection
   e. Vaginal examination

3. **Procedural Step.** Greet and identify the patient. Introduce yourself and explain the procedure. Obtain the urine specimen from the patient, which she has collected at home. Determine whether the patient has taken the necessary precautions to preserve the specimen before bringing it to the medical office. **Principle.** Specimens that have been left standing out produce inaccurate test results.
4. **Procedural Step.** Ask the patient if she has experienced any problems since the last prenatal visit, and record any information in the appropriate section in her prenatal record.

Continued

PROCEDURE 10-2

Principle. The physician further investigates any unusual or abnormal signs or symptoms relayed by the patient.

5. **Procedural Step.** Measure the patient's blood pressure, and chart the results in the prenatal record. If the blood pressure is elevated, allow the patient to relax, then measure the blood pressure again.

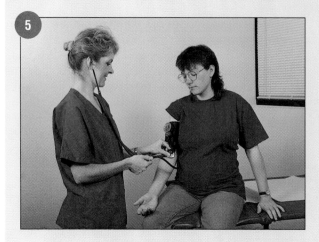

Principle. Taking an elevated blood pressure again gives the opportunity to determine whether the elevation was due to emotional excitement.

6. **Procedural Step.** Weigh the patient and chart the results in the prenatal record.

10

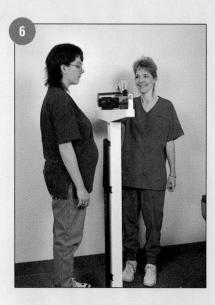

Principle. Maternal weight gain or loss assists in assessing fetal development as well as the mother's nutrition and state of health.

7. **Procedural Step.** Ask the patient if she needs to empty her bladder before the examination.
   Principle. An empty bladder makes the examination easier and more comfortable for the patient.

8. **Procedural Step.** Instruct and prepare the patient for the examination. Have her remove her outer clothing to expose the abdominal area. If the physician will be performing a vaginal examination, the patient must also remove her panties; otherwise she may leave them on.

9. **Procedural Step.** Test the urine specimen for glucose and protein using a reagent strip, and chart the results. *Note:* The urine specimen may be tested at any time before the physician examines the patient; however, a convenient time to test the specimen is while the patient is disrobing.
   Principle. The prenatal patient's urine must be tested at each visit to assist in the early detection and prevention of disease.

10. **Procedural Step.** Place the footstool close to the examining table. Assist the patient onto the table. Place her in a supine position and properly drape her. Provide support and reassurance to the patient to help her relax during the examination.
    Principle. The medical assistant should make sure to provide for the safety of the prenatal patient while she is getting onto and off of the examining table. The patient should be properly draped to provide for warmth and comfort.

11. **Procedural Step.** Place the patient's chart in a convenient location for review by the physician. Inform the physician that the patient is ready to be examined.
    Principle. The physician will first want to review the measurements taken by the medical assistant and compare them with his or her findings during the prenatal examination.

12. **Procedural Step.** Assist the physician as required for the prenatal examination. The medical assistant may be responsible for the following:
    a. Handing the physician the tape measure for the determination of the fundal height and recording the measurement in the patient's prenatal record.
    b. Handing the physician the Doppler fetal pulse detector for measurement of the fetal heart tones. The medical assistant may also be responsible for spreading the ultrasound coupling agent on the patient's abdomen.
    c. Assisting the patient into the lithotomy position if a vaginal specimen is to be taken for the detection of a vaginal infection. The medical assistant will also need to hold the appropriate medium or slide (labeled with the patient's name, the date, and the source of the specimen) so that the physician can place the specimen on it. In addition, the medical assistant is

usually responsible for completing the laboratory request if the specimen will be transported to an outside medical laboratory for evaluation. If the specimen is to be examined at the medical office, the medical assistant needs to prepare it as necessary for identification of the

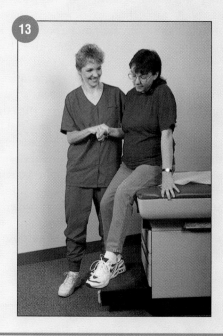

invading organism. Make sure to follow the OSHA Standard during specimen collection to prevent infection with a pathogen.

d. Assisting the patient into the lithotomy position if a vaginal examination is performed and assisting the physician with the application of the glove and the application of lubricant to the glove for the examination. Be careful not to allow the tube of lubricant to touch the physician's fingers, to prevent contamination of the contents of the tube.

13. **Procedural Step.** After the examination, assist the patient into a sitting position and allow her the opportunity to rest for a moment. If a vaginal examination was performed, offer the patient tissues to remove excess lubricating jelly from the perineum. Assist her off the examining table, using the footstool to prevent falls. Instruct the patient to get dressed.
Principle. The patient may become dizzy after being on the examining table and should be allowed to rest before getting off.

14. **Procedural Step.** Provide prenatal patient teaching and further explanation of the physician's instructions as required to meet individual patient needs.

15. **Procedural Step.** Clean the examining room in preparation for the next patient and, if necessary, prepare specimens for transport to an outside medical laboratory, including the completed laboratory request.

10

SIX-WEEKS-POSTPARTUM VISIT

☐ The **puerperium** includes the period of time in which the body systems are returning to their prepregnant or nearly prepregnant state, which usually extends for 4 to 6 weeks after delivery. During this time period, numerous changes take place within the woman's body. The involution of the uterus (i.e., the process by which it returns to its normal size and state) occurs; this includes healing of any injuries sustained to the birth canal during delivery.

During the puerperium, the patient experiences a vaginal discharge shed from the lining of the uterus, known as **lochia.** Lochia consists of blood, tissue, white blood cells, mucus, and some bacteria. The color of the lochia is an indication of the progress of the healing of the uterus. For the first 3 days after delivery, the lochia consists almost entirely of blood and because of its red color is termed **lochia rubra.** By

approximately the fourth day postpartum, the amount of blood decreases and the discharge becomes pink or brownish in color and is known as **lochia serosa.** By the tenth day postpartum, the amount of flow should decrease and the lochia should become yellowish-white; this is known as **lochia alba.** Lochia usually continues in consistently decreasing amounts (from moderate to scant to occasional spotting) and becomes more pale in color until the third week following delivery, when it usually disappears altogether. However, it would not be considered unusual for the discharge to last the entire 6 weeks.

The patient should be instructed to contact the medical office under the following circumstances: if the amount of discharge increases rather than decreases; if the discharge is absent within the first 2 weeks after delivery; if it changes to red after having been yellowish white, which indicates bleeding; or if it takes on a foul odor, which indicates infection. Menstruation usually begins approximately 2 months after delivery in the non-nursing mother and 3 to 6 months after delivery in the nursing mother.

During the puerperium, the patient should be encouraged to avoid fatigue, to avoid lifting heavy objects, and to consume a nutritious, well-balanced diet that helps maintain health and promote healing during this period.

The physician will want to see the patient at the medical office at the end of the 6-week period. The purpose of the 6-weeks-postpartum visit is to evaluate the general physical condition of the patient, to make sure there are no residual problems from childbearing, and to provide the patient with education regarding methods of birth control and infant care. The patient is queried during this visit regarding the presence of any problems or abnormalities relating to vaginal discharge, urinary or bowel function, or breast feeding in the nursing mother. This information is recorded in the patient's chart. The postpartum visit provides an excellent opportunity for the medical assistant to instruct the patient in the technique for performing a breast self-examination and to educate her in the importance of returning to the medical office periodically for a Pap test.

During the postpartal examination, the physician evaluates the patient's general appearance, performs breast and pelvic examinations, and checks to determine whether the muscle tone has returned to the muscles of the abdominal wall. During the puerperium, atypical cells may be sloughed off into the cervical and vaginal mucus as part of the normal healing process. Because of this, the Pap test is not included in the postpartum visit. If the patient has problems with hemorrhoids or varicosities, the physician discusses any further treatment required. If the patient does not have antibody protection to rubella, as has been evidenced through the prenatal laboratory tests, she receives rubella immunization at this time (if it has not previously been administered in the hospital). In addition, hemoglobin and hematocrit determinations are usually performed on the postpartum patient to screen for anemia due to blood loss during delivery and the puerperium.

The responsibilities of the medical assistant during the postpartum visit include measuring and recording the patient's vital signs and weight, and preparing the patient for the examination. The patient is required to disrobe completely for this examination and to put on an examining gown with the opening in front. Table 10–2 lists the procedures commonly included in the 6-weeks-postpartum visit and the purpose of each.

TABLE 10–2

Six-Weeks-Postpartum Examination

Procedure	Purpose
Vital signs (Chapter 3) Temperature Pulse Respiration Blood pressure	To make sure the vital signs fall within normal limits and that the blood pressure has returned to its normal prepregnant level. Elevated blood pressure may indicate essential hypertension or renal disease.
Weight (Chapter 4)	To determine whether the patient's weight has returned to its prepregnant measurement. If not, nutritional counseling may be indicated.
Breast examination (Chapter 10)	To make sure the breasts are not sore or tender and no cysts or masses are present. In the non-nursing mother, the breasts will be examined to determine whether they have returned to their prepregnant size. In the nursing mother, the nipples will be examined for cracks, redness, soreness, and fissures.
Pelvic examination (Chapter 10)	To make sure involution of the uterus is complete and to determine whether the cervix has healed. To make sure the episotomy and any injuries sustained by the birth canal have healed. To make sure no abnormal vaginal discharge is present.
Rectal-vaginal examination (Chapter 10)	To make sure the pelvic floor has regained its muscle tone. To determine whether hemorrhoids are present.
Evaluation of the patient's general physical condition (Chapter 4)	To make sure the body systems have returned to their prepregnant state.

MEDICAL PRACTICE AND THE LAW

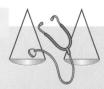

Gynecologic and prenatal examinations are very intimate and can be embarrassing to the patient. Give clear instructions for disrobing, positioning, and draping to maximize patient comfort and coverage. Some offices have a policy of having a female staff member present when a male physician examines a female patient. Make sure your presence is documented in the chart. The prenatal period is one of tremendous change, and for a first pregnancy, much patient teaching is needed. Often, preprinted information is available for each trimester. If you work in a obstetric office, know that lawsuits involving damage to newborns are among the highest monetary amounts awarded.

CERTIFICATION REVIEW

- ☐ Gynecology is the branch of medicine that deals with diseases of the reproductive organs of women. Gynecologic examinations include a breast and pelvic examination. The purpose of the examination is to assess the health status of the female reproductive organs and to detect early signs of disease, leading to early diagnosis and treatment.

- ☐ During the breast examination, the physician inspects the breasts for localized redness or inflammation and any dimpling, scaling, or puckering of the skin. The nipples are checked for abnormalities and the breasts and axial lymph nodes are palpated for lumps. Women should perform a breast self-examination at home each month, approximately 1 week after the menstrual period.

- ☐ The purpose of the pelvic examination is to assess the size, shape, and location of the reproductive organs and to detect the presence of disease. The pelvic examination consists of an inspection of the external genitalia, vagina, and cervix; collection of a specimen for a Pap test; bimanual pelvic examination; and a rectal-vaginal examination.

- ☐ The purpose of the Pap test is to provide for the early detection of precancerous or cancerous conditions of the cervix and endometrium, making early treatment possible. Abnormal cytologic findings on the Pap smear indicate that further tests should be conducted such as colposcopy, cervical biopsy, and endocervical curettage.

- ☐ The purpose of the bimanual pelvic examination is to determine the size, shape, and position of the uterus and ovaries and detect tenderness or lumps. The purpose of the rectal-vaginal examination is to obtain information about the tone and alignment of the pelvic organs and the adnexal region. The presence of hemorrhoids, fistulas, and fissures can also be noted during this examination.

- ☐ Trichomoniasis is a vaginal infection caused by a protozoan and is most commonly spread through sexual intercourse. Symptoms include a profuse, frothy yellowish green vaginal discharge, itching and irritation of the vulva and vagina, and dysuria. The cervix may exhibit red spots; this is known as "strawberry cervix."

- ☐ Candidiasis is a vaginal infection caused by a yeastlike fungus. Conditions such as pregnancy, diabetes mellitus, and prolonged antibiotic therapy may precipitate a candidal infection of the vagina, commonly referred to as a yeast infection. Symptoms of candidiasis include white patches on the mucous membrane of the vagina along with a thick, odorless cottage cheese–like discharge that causes severe vulval irritation and dysuria.

- ☐ Gonorrhea is the most common venereal disease. It is an infection of the genitourinary tract and is caused by a bacterium that is transmitted through sexual intercourse. Women who have contracted gonorrhea may be asymptomatic or may exhibit a purulent vaginal discharge. As the disease progresses, it may spread to the lining of the uterus, resulting in pelvic inflammatory disease (PID).

- ☐ Chlamydia is caused by a bacterium that is transmitted through sexual intercourse. Individuals with

Continued

chlamydia may be asymptomatic. Women with symptoms have itching and burning in the genital area; an odorless thick, yellowish-white vaginal discharge; dull abdominal pain; and bleeding between menstrual periods.

☐ Obstetrics is the branch of medicine dealing with the supervision of women during pregnancy, childbirth, and the puerperium. Prenatal refers to the care of the pregnant woman before delivery of the infant to promote health of the mother and fetus through the prevention of disease and the provision of early detection, diagnosis, and treatment of problems common to pregnancy.

☐ The first prenatal examination consists of the completion of a prenatal record form, an initial prenatal examination, prenatal patient education, and laboratory tests.

☐ The prenatal record provides information regarding the past and present health status of the patient and also serves as a data base and flow sheet for subsequent prenatal visits.

☐ Gravidity refers to the total number of times a woman has been pregnant, regardless of the duration of the pregnancy and including the current pregnancy. Parity refers to the number of children the patient has delivered that reached the age of viability (20 weeks of gestation), regardless of whether the child was born alive or stillborn. Abortion refers to a fetus that did not reach the age of viability.

☐ The expected date of delivery (EDD) can be determined using Nägele's rule and a gestation calculator. Using these methods to calculate the EDD, approximately 4 percent of patients deliver spontaneously on the EDD and the majority of patients deliver during the period extending 7 days before to 7 days after the EDD.

☐ The purpose of the initial prenatal examination is to confirm the pregnancy and to establish a baseline for the woman's state of health. It includes a thorough gynecologic examination (breast and pelvic) and a general physical examination of the other body systems.

☐ A number of laboratory tests are ordered on the prenatal patient to assist in the overall initial assessment of the state of health of the prenatal patient and to detect problems that may put the pregnancy at risk. Tests that may be included in the prenatal laboratory work-up include: a complete urinalysis, Pap smear, gonorrhea and chlamydia, trichomoniasis and candidiasis (if warranted), complete blood count, hemoglobin and hematocrit, Rh factor and ABO blood type, glucose tolerance test, serology test for syphilis, rubella titer, Rh antibody titer, hepatitis B, and HIV.

☐ Return prenatal visits provide the opportunity for a continuous assessment of the state of health of the mother and fetus. During the return visit the physician performs one or more of the following procedures: palpation of the woman's abdomen to measure fundal height, measurement of the fetal heart rate, and a vaginal examination. The 9 months of pregnancy are divided into three trimesters, each consisting of 3 months.

☐ The alfa-fetoprotein (AFP) analysis is a laboratory test performed to screen for the presence of certain fetal abnormalities. Abnormal test results may indicate the possibility of a neural tube defect such as spina bifida, anencephaly, or Down's syndrome.

☐ Obstetric ultrasound scanning is used to view the fetus in utero. It is used most frequently to determine gestational age and to confirm the due date. Other reasons for performing ultrasound are to confirm the presence of fetal life, evaluate fetal growth, estimate fetal weight, detect the presence of multiple fetuses, determine the cause of bleeding or spotting, detect congenital abnormalities, determine placental position, detect ectopic pregnancy, determine the baby's position and size late in pregnancy, or to view the fetus, placenta, and amniotic fluid during tests such as amniocentesis or chorionic villlus sampling.

☐ Amniocentesis is performed to diagnose certain genetically transmitted errors of metabolism, congenital abnormalities, and chromosomal disorders such as Down's syndrome. Fetal heart rate monitoring is performed to obtain information on the physical condition of the fetus.

☐ The puerperium includes the period of time in which the body systems are returning to the prepregnant or nearly prepregnant state, which usually extends for 4 to 6 weeks after delivery. The physician will want to see the patient at the medical office at the end of the 6-week period. The purpose of this postpartum visit is to evaluate the general physical condition of the patient, to make sure there are no residual problems from childbearing, and to provide the patient with education regarding methods of birth control and infant care.

10

RESOURCES

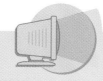

ON THE WEB

For information on gynecology and obstetrics:

American Society for Reproductive Medicine (ASRM)
www.asrm.com

The North American Menopause Society (NAMS)
www.menopause.org

Obstetric Ultrasound
www.ob-ultrasound.net

Planned Parenthood Federation of American
www.plannedparenthood.org

For information on sexually transmitted diseases:

COHIS STDs
web.bu.edu/COHIS/std/aboutstd.htm

International Herpes Management Forum (IHMF)
www.ihmf.org

10

Traci Powell, *and I am a Certified Medical Assistant with an associate's degree in Applied Science. I graduated from an accredited medical assisting program, and I have been a CMA for 13 years. I work in the pediatrics department of a large multispecialty clinic. My job responsibilities are mostly clinical; however, I do assist in the front office when needed. I love working with the children and have enjoyed watching them grow over the years.*

A coworker and I recently organized a local AAMA (American Association of Medical Assistants) chapter. Our chapter provides AAMA continuing education units (CEUs). Our members attend both state and national conventions each year, and they also hold state and national leadership positions. It is my goal to see the medical assisting profession continue to grow and advance in the health care field. With advanced training for CMAs being developed by the AAMA and the great increase in managed care, opportunities for Certified Medical Assistants are growing tremendously.

The Pediatric Examination

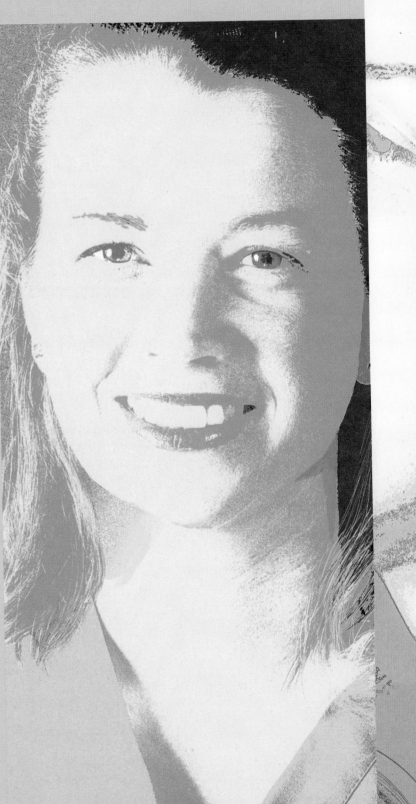

OUTCOMES

After completing this chapter, you should be able to demonstrate the proper procedures to perform the following:

1. Carry an infant, using the following positions: cradle and upright.
2. Measure the weight and length of an infant.
3. Measure the head and chest circumference of an infant.
4. Plot pediatric growth values on a growth chart.
5. Collect a urine specimen from an infant, using a pediatric urine collector bag.
6. Administer an intramuscular injection to an infant.
7. Collect a specimen for a phenylketonuria (PKU) screening test.

EDUCATIONAL OBJECTIVES

After completing this unit, you should be able to do the following:

1. Define the terms listed in the Key Terminology.
2. List the two categories of pediatric patient office visits and what functions are performed during each.
3. Explain why it is important to develop a rapport with the pediatric patient.
4. State the importance of measuring the child's weight, height (or length), and head circumference during each office visit.
5. Locate the following pediatric intramuscular injection sites and explain the use of each in regard to the age of the pediatric patient: dorsogluteal, vastus lateralis, and deltoid.
6. Describe the schedule for immunization of infants and children recommended by the American Academy of Pediatrics.
7. Explain the purpose of performing a PKU screening test.

CHAPTER 11

KEY TERMINOLOGY

immunity (IM-ûn-it-ê): The resistance of the body to the effects of a harmful agent such as a pathogenic microorganism or its toxins.

immunization (active, artificial) (IM-ûn-i-zâ-shun): The process of becoming immune or of rendering an individual immune through the use of a vaccine or toxoid.

infant: A child from birth to 1 year of age.

length (recumbent): The measurement from the vertex of the head to the heel of the foot in a supine position.

pediatrician: A medical doctor who specializes in the care and development of children and the diagnosis and treatment of diseases of children.

pediatrics: The branch of medicine dealing with the care and development of children and the diagnosis and treatment of diseases of children.

stature: The height of the body in a standing position.

toxoid (Tox-ôid): A toxin (poisonous substance produced by a bacterium) that has been treated by heat or chemicals to destroy its harmful properties. It is administered to an individual to prevent an infectious disease by stimulating the production of antibodies in that individual.

vaccine (VAK-sên): A suspension of attenuated (weakened) or killed microorganisms administered to an individual to prevent an infectious disease by stimulating the production of antibodies in that individual.

vertex (VER-tex): The summit, or top, especially the top of the head.

INTRODUCTION

☐ **Pediatrics** is the branch of medicine dealing with the care and development of children and the diagnosis and treatment of diseases in children. A **pediatrician** is a medical doctor who specializes in pediatrics. Many physicians involved in general practice also handle pediatric patients. It is essential that the medical assistant develop the skills needed to assist the physician in the care and treatment of children.

PEDIATRIC OFFICE VISITS

☐ There are two broad categories of pediatric patient office visits. The first is the **health maintenance visit,** in which the physician progressively evaluates the growth and development of the child. A physical examination is performed during each health maintenance visit and is directed toward discovering any abnormal conditions commonly associated with the stage of development reached by the child. Refer to Table 11–1 for an outline of normal development during infancy. The child will also receive any necessary immunizations during these visits.

Another important component of the health maintenance visit is anticipatory guidance. **Anticipatory guidance** is the process of providing parents with information to prepare them for anticipated developmental events and to assist them in promoting their children's well-being (Table 11–2). Topics that are commonly included are safety, nutrition, sleep, play, exercise, development, and discipline. Refer to Table 11–3 for a presentation of child safety guidelines by age group.

The interval between health maintenance visits depends on the medical office, but it frequently follows this schedule after birth: 1 month, 2 months, 4 months, 6 months, 9 months, 12 months, 15 months, 18 months, 24 months, and yearly thereafter.

The other category is the **sick child visit.** The child is exhibiting the signs and symptoms of disease, and the physician evaluates the patient's condition to arrive at a diagnosis and to prescribe treatment.

During both the health maintenance and sick child visits, the medical assistant utilizes many of the same techniques that have been presented in previous chapters (e.g., temperature and pulse readings, measurement of respiration and blood pressure, measurement of weight and height, measurement of visual acuity, assisting with the physical examination, and others). Techniques relating specifically to the pediatric patient and variations in techniques already presented are discussed in this chapter.

DEVELOPING RAPPORT

☐ The medical assistant must establish a rapport with the pediatric patient. If he or she gains the child's trust and confidence, the child is more likely to cooperate during an examination or procedure. Interacting with

Text continued on page 411

TABLE 11–1

Milestones of Gross and Fine Motor Development in Infancy

Average Age (months)	Gross Motor	Fine Motor
1	Turns head from side to side	Grasping reflex present
2	Holds head at 45-degree angle when prone	Holds rattle briefly
3	Begins rolling over	Grasps rattle or dangling objects
4	Slight head lag when pulled to sitting position	Brings objects to mouth
5	No head wobble when held in sitting position	Transfers objects from hand to hand
6	Sits without support	Manipulates and examines large objects with hands
7	Stands while holding on	Reaches for, grabs, and retains object
8	Pulls self to stand	Grasps objects with thumb and finger
9	Crawls backwards	Begins to show hand preference
10	Creeps on hands and knees	Hits cup with spoon
11	Walks using furniture for support	Picks up small objects with thumb and forefinger (pincer grasp)
12	Stands alone easily	Puts three or more objects into a container
12–16	Walks alone easily	Turns two or three pages in a large cardboard book

From Leahy, J. M., Kizilay, P. E.: *Foundations of Nursing Practice*. Philadelphia, W. B. Saunders, 1998, Table 16–4, p. 289.

TABLE 11–2

Anticipatory Guidance

Anticipatory Guidance in Infancy

Issue	Rationale	Guidance
Thumb sucking or use of pacifier	Sucking is a major pleasure for the infant Benefits such as decreased crying and increased relaxation have been identified by meeting the infant's need for non-nutritive sucking Infants will generally find their fingers or hands to suck on to meet this need without the use of a pacifier As the need for non-nutritive sucking decreases, so does the need for the pacifier or thumb, unless their use is treated as a reinforcement by children's parents to relieve infant distress	Explore parents' feelings regarding the infant's need to use a pacifier If pacifiers are to be used, review safety considerations in their use (e.g., preferably constructed in one piece, have a flange with at least two ventilation holes and be large enough to prevent aspiration, remove from infant when not in use, never secure to infant by tying with a cord around the neck) Thumb sucking is generally abandoned by the age when dental problems may become an issue (when permanent teeth erupt) If a pacifier is used, try removing it around 6 months of age, when the infant is not yet old enough to remember or miss it for long If pacifiers are used beyond the first year, unless you are meticulous about sterilizing them they can be very unhygienic as the child toddles around with them; this is a good reason to discontinue pacifier use

11

Table continued on following page

TABLE 11–2

Anticipatory Guidance in Infancy		
Issue	**Rationale**	**Guidance**
Teething	Teething seldom causes discomfort in an infant younger than 4 months of age At 5 or 6 months, as the first tooth emerges, drooling, chewing on hard objects, and some irritability may accompany the minor inflammation of the gums Most discomfort is felt by the infant with the eruption of the first molars at age 12 to 15 months	Believing that an infant younger than 4 months of age is irritable for long periods due to "teething" may cause a parent to neglect a real illness Medical attention should be sought for any infant experiencing fever, diarrhea, vomiting, or loss of appetite as these are not symptoms of teething Avoid the use of teething gels because they contain anesthetics that may cause untoward effects in the infant if overused Provide something cold to bite on; for example, a frozen gel-filled teething ring
Separation/stranger fear	Around 8 months of age, infants have sufficient capacity to recognize their primary caregivers and find comfort in their presence Because they have not yet developed the task of object permanence, infants experience great displeasure when their caregivers leave them alone or with an unfamiliar substitute This behavior may continue into toddlerhood	Parents (caregivers) should accustom the infant to new persons, especially those that may be called on to babysit in the future (the more frequent the exposure, the less likely the fear) Give infants opportunities to explore strangers at their own pace to allow a "warm-up" period of adjustment Talk to infants when leaving them and greet them when you return. This can aid the development of object permanence and reassure them that you will always return Use a transitional object such as your scarf or a toy to reassure them of your continued presence
Spoiling/limit setting	When infants' needs are not promptly met or are only met after a period of delay, they become anxious, quicker to fuss or cry, and slower to accept comfort; therefore, the less you meet the infants' needs, the more demanding they become As infants become more mobile toward the latter half of the first year, parents need to set limits to provide for their safety; however, there is no substitute for vigilant parental monitoring	Prompt attention to the crying infant often is greeted by the infant's smile and comfort Delaying attention to the crying infant leads to an encounter with a miserably distressed infant who does not settle down easily, has a stomach full of air from excessive crying, and will most likely start crying again before long Limit setting is done with the older infant through consistent and age-appropriate methods A negative voice and stern eye-to-eye contact may be all that is needed A quiet period for the infant in the playpen may be warranted Parents who express concern over discipline in the infant stage should recognize that the earlier it is started, the easier it is to maintain throughout childhood

Injury prevention	Unintentional injury is the second leading cause of death in infancy
	Common risks associated with this developmental stage include
	    Choking or suffocation
	    Falls
	    Motor vehicle crash injuries
	    Burns
		Parents and caregivers should be instructed in the techniques of cardiopulmonary resuscitation (CPR)
		Home and environmental safety check list should be reviewed with parents
		Refer to the prevention guidelines in Table 11–3

TABLE 11-2

Anticipatory Guidance *Continued*

Anticipatory Guidance in Infancy

Issue	Rationale	Guidance
Crying/colic	Periods of crying of up to 2 hours per day are considered normal and part of the infant's temperament Colicky infants are described as those who cry for long periods with legs drawn up, generally for periods in excess of 3 hours daily Colic has no known cause but has been associated with intolerance to cow's milk formula or ingestion of milk products by breast-feeding mothers and passive smoking As infants cry, they swallow more air, distend the abdomen, cry some more, and pass flatus, and the cycle continues	Reassurance should be given to parents that the crying period is a source of energy release for the infant Parents should always initially respond to the infant's cry to determine the cause Continuation of long periods of crying should be reported to the health care provider When no cause for the crying episodes can be identified, time of onset should be noted; immediate response to the infant by chainging position, massaging the abdomen, swaddling in blanket, taking for car ride, or placing the infant in wind-up swing has been successful Avoid smoking near the infant Provide, small frequent feedings; burp during and after feeding; have the infant sit upright for half an hour after feeding

Anticipatory Guidance in Toddlerhood

Issue	Rationale	Guidance
Toilet training	The ability to master control over elimination requires muscular maturation as well as cognitive maturity The toddler needs to understand instructions as well as the purpose for accomplishing this task for which there is no tangible reward other than that of "pleasing" a caregiver Eighty-four percent of 3-year-old children are dry throughout the day, and 66 percent, throughout the night	Most parents initiate toilet training efforts between 20 and 24 months Parents should be informed that "successful" toilet training at a very early age is usually because the *parent* is "trained" to recognize the child's readiness and places the child on the potty at the appropriate time Teach parents to keep a record of the toddler's pattern and signals of elimination for several weeks prior to starting Have parents obtain a sturdy potty chair, if possible, so the child can independently sit and get up, or a sturdy step stool to access toilet with adult supervision Have parents dress child in loose-fitting clothing to aid easy access and prevent accidents Inform parents that when the child signals that a bowel movement or voiding may be on the way, they should casually suggest to the child that he or she may want to sit on the potty Encourage parents not to force the child to sit on the potty or to show disappointment if attempts are unsuccessful Explain to parents that accidents will happen and will need to be taken in stride Nagging and punishing a child for being uncooperative or for having "accidents" will mean certain failure, as the toddler will become overwhelmed and confused about what is expected

11

Table continued on following page

TABLE 11–2

Anticipatory Guidance *Continued*

Anticipatory Guidance in Toddlerhood

Issue	Rationale	Guidance
Temper tantrums	Temper tantrums are commonly seen toward the end of the second year of life Tantrums are the result of excessive frustration; for example, when a child becomes overwhelmed with emotion and feelings of tension, an explosive outburst is a means of release Tantrums often involve screaming, thrashing, and breath-holding spells	Parents should be taught that a temper tantrum is like an "emotional blown fuse," which is not something that the toddler can control Parents need to recognize a balance between a frustration level that their child can tolerate and that is useful for learning and the amount of frustration that will cause the fuse to blow During a tantrum, a parent should be instructed to try to protect child from harm but not to overpower him or her, as this physical restriction may heighten the anger Reassure parents that breath-holding spells, although alarming to watch, do not result in physical harm. The body's natural reflex to breathe will allow the child to take in air before any damage can occur
Stress, anxiety, and fear	Toddlers live on an emotional see-saw, with most of the stress and tears arising from the basic contradiction of wanting independence and the desire to be protected and loved by their caregivers Again they need a balance of autonomy yet protection from separation anxiety A toddler begins to feel anxious whenever his or her own feelings become uncontrollable, leading to crying or temper tantrums	Inform parents to recognize cues from the toddler that indicates an impending problem; for example, excessive clinginess, less adventurous behavior, increased shyness Instruct parents to offer more affection, attention, and protection for several days until the toddler regains a normal sense of independence and adventure
Bedtime struggles	As many as 50 percent of all children between the ages of 1 and 2 years engage in fussing or bedtime struggles lasting for more than an hour Sometimes these struggles are associated with family stress, such as illness or change in normal routines Most times they are caused by continued infancy routines of "being put to sleep" by nursing, rocking, or coddling	Inform parents that they are not alone with this struggle—that it is very common Inform parents that if they continue to coddle, rock, or nurse their toddlers to sleep at this age, it will be harder to institute a different bedtime routine Instruct parents to alter the routine by providing about 20 minutes of sedentary activity, such as quiet conversation or storytelling Have parents keep a night light on if it makes the child more comfortable Tell parents to finish their sedentary time with a pleasant "goodnight," and if child begins to cry and continues for several minutes, they should go back in the room, repeat "goodnight" and leave again; this performance should be repeated every few minutes for as long as it takes toddler to settle down Any sleep problem that persists over several months should be referred to the child's health care provider

TABLE 11–2   **Anticipatory Guidance** *Continued*

Anticipatory Guidance in Toddlerhood

Issue	Rationale	Guidance

Unintentional injuries	Unintentional injury is the leading cause of death and disability in toddlerhood
	Toddlers are especially vulnerable to unintentional injuries due to their activity level, developing motor skills, and inability to perceive dangerous situations
	Common risks associated with this developmental stage include
	    Drowning
	    Burns or scalds
	    Motor vehicle injuries
	    Falls
	    Poisoning
		Parents and caregivers should be instructed in the techniques of CPR
		Home and environmental safety checklist should be reviewed with parents and caregivers
		Refer to the prevention guidelines in Table 11–3
		Reinforce with parents and caregivers the importance of vigilant child monitoring and supervision during this highly vulnerable developmental stage

Play activities	Play is the "work" of the young; it helps children to use their muscles and gain mastery over what they think, see, and do—a form of learning Pretending or imaginative play emerges during this period—the toddler reenacts past experiences through retained mental pictures of things seen or heard; for example, a little boy might dip a sock in the dog's water bowl and use it to clean his toy truck after having observed his father wash the car the previous month	Inform parents that providing a safe place, safe toys or other play equipment, and time is all that is needed to promote healthy play activities in the toddler If the toddler gets frustrated, the toys or activities may be too advanced, or he or she may be asking for some assistance or guidance Boredom will ensue if the play space and the activities are not varied from time to time Inform parents that toys need not be expensive; children at this age are content to play with household objects, such as plastic bowls and wooden spoons Instruct parents to be responsible consumers: when purchasing toys, they should (1) inspect them for small pieces or loose parts that may present a choking hazard, (2) determine if they are age appropriate for their child, and (3) not sacrifice safety and quality for price

Anticipatory Guidance for the Preschool Child

Issue	Rationale	Guidance
Aggression	A hostile act may be intended to hurt somebody or to establish dominance and is usually triggered by the social conflicts that arise in the course of cooperative play during the preschool years Children between 2 and 5 years of age who fight the most tend to be the most sociable and competent In many cases, a decline in physical aggression is often accompanied by an increase in verbal aggression, usually in the form of name calling Even in a normal child, aggression can get out of hand and become dangerous Since the 1950s, research has correlated televised violence with aggressive behavior in children	Parents can often reduce aggressive tendencies by the way they act or react to the situation Teach parents to deal with misbehavior by reasoning with the child, reinforcing good behavior, and being consistent in their approach to discipline Spanking causes a child to suffer frustration, pain, and humiliation, and it is poor role modeling—the child sees hitting as an acceptable solution to a problem Encourage parents to monitor their child's television viewing by limiting total time allowed for viewing and selecting model shows that are educational and prosocial

11

Table continued on following page

TABLE 11-2

Anticipatory Guidance for the Preschool Child

Issue	Rationale	Guidance
Fearfulness	Preschoolers have an inability to distinguish "pretend" from reality as part of normal development Preschoolers have an intense sense of fantasy and are more likely to be frightened by something that looks "scary" than by something that can cause real harm Common fears of this age group include separation from parent, dark, animals, and noises—especially those in the dark Sometimes the anxiety is grounded in reality: for example, a child who was bitten by a dog may fear that the event will happen again	Parents can often reduce fears by instilling a sense of trust and normal caution without being overprotective Teach parents to avoid ridiculing their child but to provide reassurance and encourage open expression of feelings Have parents avoid coercion and logical persuasion, because developmentally, the child is unable to process such statements as "Pet the nice parrot—it won't hurt you," or "Lions are only found in a zoo" Encourage parents to seek out modeling behavior and expose their child to it; by observing fearlessness in other children, their child will gradually overcome the perceived threat

Daycare or preschool	Preschoolers can thrive physically, intellectually, and emotionally in daycare and preschool settings that have small groups, high adult-to-child ratios, and a stable, competent, and involved staff
	
	Preschoolers develop best when they have a balance between structured activities and freedom to explore on their own
	
	Parents may feel less stress knowing that their child is being well cared for while they are earning the income needed or fulfilling personal achievements
		Teach parents strategies for choosing a good program for their child that includes the following:
		  Provides a safe, clean setting
		  Welcomes parents who visit unannounced
		  Has warm and friendly personnel that are responsive to the children
		  Fosters social skills, self-esteem, and respect for others
		  Helps parents improve their parenting skills
		Teach parents to avoid programs that
		  Employ staff members who are not educated, trained in CPR, or experienced in child care or child education
		  Are not licensed by the state
		  Have no written plan for meals or emergencies
		  Have poor ventilation or lighting or no smoke alarms, fire extinguisher, or first-aid kit

Sleep disorders	Approximately one in four preschoolers suffers from either night terrors or nightmares Night terrors are identified by abrupt awakening from deep sleep in a state of panic; the child is not really awake and will quiet down quickly and not remember the incident in the morning Night terrors do not indicate underlying emotional problems and are thought to be an effect of very deep sleep states Nightmares usually come toward the early morning and are vividly remembered by the child Persistent nightmares, especially those that cause fear and anxiety to the child during the day, may indicate excessive stress in the child	Explain to parents that these are common sleep problems in preschoolers Teach parents to enlist a pleasant and relaxed bedtime ritual to share with their child, such as recalling a happy family outing or event Recommend that parents leave a small light on that does not produce shadows on the wall Encourage parents to provide their child with comfort and reassurance each and every time an episode occurs

TABLE 11–2

Anticipatory Guidance *Continued*

Anticipatory Guidance for the Preschool Child

Issue	Rationale	Guidance

Unintentional injuries	Unintentional injury continues to be the leading cause of death and disability in preschool children
	
	Preschoolers are no longer content with their home environment and venture outside of the home, often with less supervision than in previous years
	
	Common risks associated with this developmental stage include
	    Motor vehicle injuries
	    Burns or scalds
	    Drowning
	    Falls
	    Poisoning
		Parents and caregivers should be instructed in the techniques of CPR
		
		Home and environmental safety checklist should be reviewed with parents and caregivers
		
		Reinforce with parents and caregivers the importance of vigilant child monitoring and supervision

Anticipatory Guidance in School-Age Children

Issue	Rationale	Guidance
School anxiety or phobia	Adjusting to grade school is a significant change for a 6-year-old, even if preschool was attended; no longer is the focus play, the sessions are full days, and the expectations are high Major tasks occur in first and second grade as children learn to read and write and have to meet the teacher's expectations Competing with schoolmates for the teacher's attention and approval can cause strain and anxiety Children sometimes resist attending school by becoming physically sick—abdominal pain or complaints of headache last until the child is allowed to stay home for the day	Encourage parents to communicate with the child's teacher on a regular basis to stay well informed on progress and to help identify problems early on Have parents spend time each evening reviewing the child's day and homework assignments and provide guidance and security when indicated Inform parents that school adjustments take place not only in first grade but every time there is a change in grade, teacher, and classmates and when other stressful events are happening around the child If continuous anxiety or other school difficulties persist, suggest that the parent have the child evaluated by a health care provider or refer for counseling
Dental problems	As primary teeth are shed and secondary teeth erupt, the child is at risk for malocclusion, a condition where the upper and lower teeth malalign, predisposing the child to permanent jaw and dental problems	Orthodontic referrals for braces are usually made during early adolescence after all of the primary teeth are shed; however, in the case of malocclusion, prompt referral should be made as soon as the problem is evident

Table continued on following page

11

TABLE 11–2

Anticipatory Guidance *Continued*

Anticipatory Guidance in School-Age Children

Issue	Rationale	Guidance
Dental problems *(Continued)*	Dental caries are a significant health problem in all age groups; however, because school-age children are relied on to independently perform all self-care activities, dental hygiene measures often are neglected Tooth evulsion, or loss due to trauma, occurs commonly in this active age group because children participate in more risky and challenging physical activites than when they were younger, such as contact sports and rollerblading	Stress to parents the importance of dental checkups every 6 months and daily oral hygiene measures to prevent formation of dental caries In addition to brushing and using fluoride supplements, school-age children should floss their teeth on a regular basis; nurses can provide instruction and reinforce teaching in this area Instruct parents and children about what to do if a permanent tooth is traumatically knocked out; tell them to hold the tooth by the crown and avoid touching the root; if dirty, rinse under running water, then insert the root end into the socket and seek medical care immediately Always stress the importance of wearing protective gear, including mouth shields, when playing contact sports and other physical activities to minimize injuries
Sleeptalking or sleepwalking	Approximately one in every six children experiences an episode of sleepwalking during the school-age years, with few who walk persistently Sleepwalking and talking occur during the first 1 to 2 hours after onset of sleep and are associated with neurologic immaturity or anxiety-provoking daytime experiences Almost all children outgrow this behavior and do not develop persistent sleeping problems	Inform parents of the self-limiting nature of this problem and have them focus on maintaining safety for the child who wanders from bed at night by keeping doors securely locked Guiding the sleepwalking child back to bed before ready may result in the child getting up again during the night; remain with the child until he or she returns to bed or awakens from the trance If these behaviors suddenly develop in the child, have parents try to identify a possible stressor or exciting event that the child recently experienced as the potential cause of the sleep problem Instruct parents to prevent their children from watching action-packed television or videos prior to sleep and to encourage more sedentary activities like reading or playing a card game instead

11

TABLE 11-2

Anticipatory Guidance *Continued*

Anticipatory Guidance in School-Age Children

Issue	Rationale	Guidance
Sex education	Ideally, the preteen years are the time when parents need to be available to answer their child's questions regarding sex Many parents are extremely uncomfortable discussing sex with their children because they are ignorant about the topic themselves As they enter puberty, older school-age children have many questions about sex and often have no place to get answers; they turn to misinformed peers for information Nurses are in a good position to educate parents and children about sexuality but only after examining their own beliefs and attitudes about such issues	Introduce the subject of sex education to parents of preteens and assess their knowledge and comfort level with the topic Ask parents if they are willing to introduce the topic of sex to their children, and if not, would they allow you to Approach the topic initially from a physiological perspective, informing them about the outward changes that will occur as they go through puberty; then advance to more social and emotional issues when they are ready A matter-of-fact tone should be used when presenting information to children so they can observe the lack of spirited emotion attached to the subject Reinforce to them that no person has a right to touch them in places that make them feel uncomfortable

From Leahy, J. M., Kizilay, P. E.: *Foundations of Nursing Practice.* Philadelphia, W. B. Saunders, 1998, Table 16–7, pp. 294–311.

TABLE 11-3

Child Safety Guidelines

Age	Common Injury	Prevention Strategies
Infancy	Motor vehicle crash	Use infant car restraints that meet safety standards Infants weighing <20 lb (9.1 kg) face rear in center back seat of car (never in passenger front seat because of danger of airbag deployment) Install restraint and secure infant appropriately according to manufacturer's guidelines
	Falls	Never leave child unattended on bed, changing table, or other high place Keep cribs away from windows; put mattress in lowest position Use safety gates at top and bottom of staircases
	Burns/scalds	Never hold child while handling hot foods, liquids, or cigarettes Keep water heater temperature at 110–120°F (43.3–48.9°C) Test water prior to bathing Use outlet covers; keep electric cords out of reach Use sunscreen with sun protection factor ≥30; expose to sun gradually
	Drowning	Hold on to infant at all times during bath Never leave infant unattended while bathing or near water
	Choking/suffocation	Avoid propping bottles for feeding Keep small objects out of reach Keep plastic bags and balloons out of reach Check all toys for loose parts Avoid tying pacifier around neck Keep cribs away from drapery and dangling cords Learn cardiopulmonary resuscitation (CPR)

11

Table continued on following page

TABLE 11-3

11

Child Safety Guidelines *Continued*

Age	Common Injury	Prevention Strategies
Toddler	Poisoning	Use cabinet latches on all low cabinets
		Keep house plants out of reach
		Keep syrup of ipecac handy
		Post poison control center phone number by the telephone
	Motor vehicle crash	Switch to toddler car restraint when child weighs >20 lb (9.1 kg)
		Avoid placing children <12 years of age in front passenger seat to avoid injuries from airbag deployment
		Hold child's hand when crossing street
		Begin teaching proper street crossing and safety rules
		Set a good example when crossing streets
	Falls	Continue infant guidelines
		Switch to youth bed when child can climb over crib rails or leave the rails down
		Install window guards on windows that open more than 4 inches
	Burns/scalds	Continue infant guidelines
		Avoid placing hot objects within child's reach
		Restrict child from cooking areas
		Cook on back burners of stove and turn pot handles inward
		Avoid using table cloths
		Keep matches/lighters out of reach
		Begin teaching the meaning of "hot"
	Drowning	Supervise continually in bath and near lakes, ocean, rivers, and pools
		Begin teaching water safety and swimming
		Keep away from toilets and buckets of water
	Choking	Continue infant guidelines
		Cut table foods well and instruct not to talk or run while eating
		Avoid feeding hard candies, peanuts, raw vegetable sticks, raisins, and frankfurters
Preschool	Poisoning	Continue infant guidelines
		Use cabinet latches on all high and low cabinets
		Avoid taking pills in child's presence
	Motor vehicle crash	Continue toddler guidelines
		Use regular car safety restraints for children ≥40 lb or 4 years of age
	Falls	Continue toddler guidelines
		Supervise playground activities
		Ensure padded ground in playground areas
		Use approved helmet and knee and elbow pads for bicycling and skating
	Burns/scalds	Continue toddler guidelines
		Teach stop, drop, roll, and cool in event of flame burns
		Practice home fire safety drills
	Choking	Instruct not to talk or run while eating
		Instruct to chew food well
		Learn CPR
School Age	Poisoning	Continue toddler guidelines
	Motor vehicle crash	Continue use of car safety restraints
		Most at risk for pedestrian injury
		Stress street crossing safety guidelines
		Stress bicycling, skating, and motorized vehicle safety
	Falls	Continue preschool guidelines
	Burns/scalds	Continue preschool guidelines
	Drowning	Continue supervision when in and around water
		Teach swimming and proper diving guidelines if not already done
	Choking	Continue preschool guidelines
		Learn CPR

TABLE 11-3

Child Safety Guidelines *Continued*

Age	Common Injury	Prevention Strategies
	Poisoning	Monitor for signs of depression or despondency, which may lead to intentional ingestion
	Firearm injury	Store all guns unloaded and out of reach Install trigger latches on all firearms Have child attend hunting safety classes if appropriate
Adolescence	Motor vehicle crash	Monitor for signs of alcohol use and counsel to avoid drinking and driving Instruct teen to avoid riding with an impaired driver Continue to stress safety restraint use Have teen attend driver education classes
	Falls	Instruct regarding proper use of protective gear to prevent sports-related injuries
	Burns	Instruct regarding dangers of smoking, and smoking in bed
	Drowning	Instruct regarding dangers of diving into unknown (shallow) bodies of water to prevent head injury Stress attending boating/coast guard safety course
	Choking	Continue stressing not talking while eating, especially if alcohol impaired Learn CPR
	Poisoning	Continue school-age guidelines
	Firearm injury	Continue school-age guidelines

From Leahy, J. M., Kizilay, P. E.: *Foundations of Nursing Practice.* Philadelphia, W. B. Saunders, 1998, Table 16–3, pp. 285–286.

children requires special techniques, depending on the age of the child. For example, children in the age group of 2 to 4 years often respond well to making a game of the procedure. Explaining the purpose of an instrument (e.g., the stethoscope) and allowing the child to hold the instrument or even to help during the procedure may also aid in overcome fears (Fig. 11-1).

The medical assistant should always explain the procedure to children who are able to understand. Each child must be approached at his or her level of understanding. In order to do this, the medical assistant

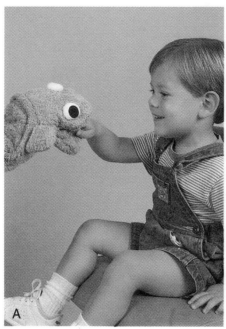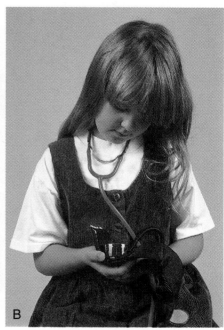

FIGURE 11-1. The medical assistant should develop a rapport with young children to gain their trust and cooperation. Making a game of the procedure (*A*) and explaining the purpose of the stethoscope and allowing the child to hold it (*B*) help the child overcome fears.

should have a knowledge of what to expect from a child at a particular age, in terms of both motor and social development. It should be kept in mind, however, that each child has his or her own rate of development. The descriptions of normal development based on age are meant to serve as a guide only and may have to be modified to meet individual needs. It is also important to realize that it is normal for an ill child to regress to an earlier level of behavior.

CARRYING THE INFANT

☐ The medical assistant needs to lift and carry the infant in order to perform various procedures, such as measurement of length and weight. The infant should be lifted and carried in a manner that is both safe and comfortable. These positions include the cradle and upright positions, which are described here.

CRADLE POSITION. The medical assistant slides the left hand and arm under the infant's back and grasps the baby's upper arm from behind. The thumb and fingers should encircle the infant's upper arm. The infant's head, shoulders, and back are supported by the medical assistant's arm. Next the medical assistant slips the right arm up and under the baby's buttocks. The infant is cradled in the arm with the child's body resting against the medical assistant's chest (Fig. 11–2).

11

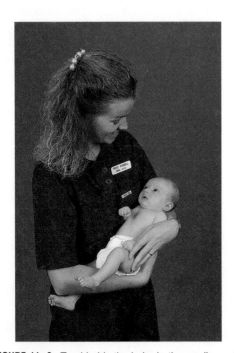

█ **FIGURE 11–2.** Traci holds the baby in the cradle position.

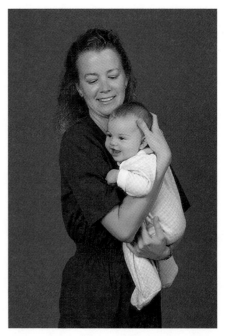

█ **FIGURE 11–3.** Traci holds the infant in the upright position.

UPRIGHT POSITION. The medical assistant slips the right hand under the infant's head and shoulders. The fingers should be spread apart to support the infant's head and neck. The left forearm is then slipped under the infant's buttocks to help support the baby's weight. The infant should be allowed to rest against the medical assistant's chest with the cheek resting on the medical assistant's shoulder (Fig. 11–3).

GROWTH PATTERNS

☐ One of the best methods to evaluate the progress of a child is to measure his or her growth. The weight, height (or length), and head circumference (up to age 3 years) of a child should be measured during each office visit and plotted on a growth chart.

GROWTH MEASUREMENTS

Weight

The weight of a child is often utilized to determine nutritional needs and the proper dosage of a medication to administer to the child. Therefore, the medical assistant should exercise care in measuring weight. Infants are weighed in a recumbent position as is outlined in Procedure 11–1. Older children are weighed

MEMORIES *from* EXTERNSHIP

TRACI POWELL: *I still remember how difficult it was at times as a student. I had been out of high school for over a year, so I had to get back into the routine of studying. I worried about whether I would do well, whether I would be able to find a good job, and if I would like medical assisting. Adding to these concerns was the financial burden of putting myself through school. I took advantage of grants and a student loan. Throughout the last 6 months of my education, I also worked full-time as an aide on the midnight shift at a nursing home while attending school full-time during the day. As if that was not enough, my first child was well on her way into this world as I was finishing up the last quarter of my degree. There were so many times that I was tired, frustrated, and broke, but I kept pushing myself to do my best because I knew this was going to be my lifetime career and I wanted to excel in my profession. My determination paid off. Today, I have a great medical assisting position that I love, with an institution that is one of the best employers in the area.*

Length

Another measure of a child's growth is length or height. Length is measured in children less than 24 months old. The recumbent length is a measurement from the vertex of the head to the heel of the infant in a supine position as is outlined in Procedure 11–2. Two people are needed to accurately determine the length of an infant. The parent's help can be solicited

if the medical assistant gives explicit instructions on what is to be done. Older children have their height measured in a standing position (Fig. 11–4), as presented in Chapter 4 (The Physical Examination).

Head and Chest Circumference

Infancy is a period of rapid brain growth. Because of this, the head circumference measurement is one of the most important parameters to obtain. The head circumference for a newborn ranges between 32 and 38 centimeters or 12.5 and 15 inches. A 4-inch (10-cm) increase in head circumference occurs within the first year of life.

Head circumference should be routinely measured on all children under 3 years of age and plotted on a head circumference growth chart. Measurement of head circumference is an important screening measure for microencephaly and macroencephaly.

At birth, a newborn's head circumference is about 2 centimeters larger than his or her chest circumference. The chest grows at a faster rate than the cranium, and between 6 months and 2 years of age, both measurements are about the same. After age 2, the chest circumference is greater than the head circumference. The measurement of the chest circumference is valuable in a comparison with the head circumference but not necessarily by itself. The chest circumference is not typically measured on a routine basis, but only when there is a suspected heart or lung abnormality.

11

in a standing position, as presented in Chapter 4 (The Physical Examination).

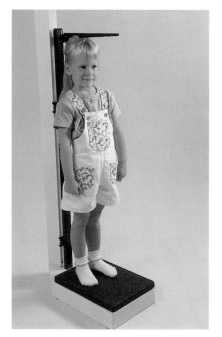

■ **FIGURE 11–4.** Measuring the height of a child.

PROCEDURE

11–1

Measuring the Weight of an Infant

EQUIPMENT: **Pediatric balance scale**

1. **Procedural Step.** Wash the hands.
2. **Procedural Step.** Greet the child's parent, and identify the child. Introduce yourself, and explain the procedure.
3. **Procedural Step.** Unlock the pediatric scale, and place a clean paper protector on it. Check the balance scale for accuracy, making sure to compensate for the weight of the paper.
   Principle. The paper protector prevents cross-contamination and reduces the spread of disease from one patient to another.
4. **Procedural Step.** Remove the infant's clothing, including the diaper.
   Principle. Bulky diapers tend to increase the child's weight considerably. In addition, growth charts for infants and young children generally base their percentiles on the weight of the child without clothing.
5. **Procedural Step.** Gently place the infant on his or her back on the scale. Place one hand slightly above the infant as a safety precaution.
6. **Procedural Step.** Balance the scale as follows:
   a. Move the lower weight to the 10-pound mark on the notched groove that does not cause the indicator point to drop to the bottom of the calibration area. Make sure the lower weight is seated firmly in its groove.
   b. Slowly slide the upper weight along its calibration bar by tapping it gently until the indicator point comes to a rest at the center of the balance area.
   Principle. Not seating the lower weight firmly in its groove results in an inaccurate reading.
7. **Procedural Step.** Read the results in pounds and ounces while the infant is lying still. (*Note:* The result on this scale is 15 pounds and 2 ounces.)
8. **Procedural Step.** Return the balance to its resting position and lock the scale.

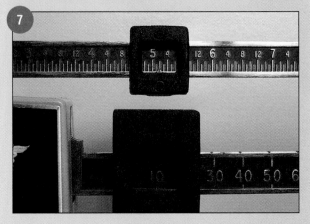

9. **Procedural Step.** Gently remove the infant from the scale and chart the results.
10. **Procedural Step.** Plot the weight on the infant's growth chart.

GROWTH CHARTS

Growth charts should be included in every child's permanent record. They provide a means for assessing the child's rate of growth and for comparing it with that of other children of the same age (Fig. 11–5). The physi-

cian will want to investigate any significant change or rapid rise or drop in the child's growth pattern. The charts can be used to identify children with growth or nutritional abnormalities.

The medical assistant may be responsible for plotting the child's growth measurements on the chart.

PROCEDURE

11–2

Measuring the Length of an Infant

EQUIPMENT: **Pediatric balance scale**

1. **Procedural Step.** Place the infant on his or her back on the examining table. Be careful not to let him or her roll off the table.
2. **Procedural Step.** Place the vertex of the infant's head against the headboard at the zero mark. Ask the parent to hold the infant's head in this position.

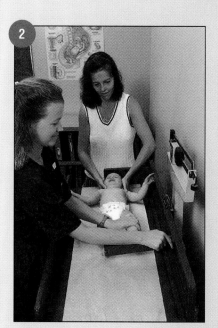

3. **Procedural Step.** Straighten the infant's knees and place the soles of his or her feet firmly against an upright foot board (to create a right angle).

4. **Procedural Step.** Read the infant's length in inches (to the nearest ¼ inch) from the measure and return the footboard to its resting position. (*Note:* The result on this scale is 25½ inches.)

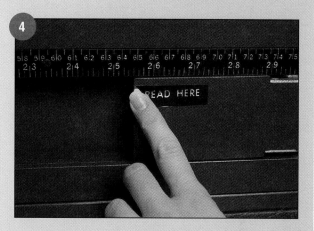

5. **Procedural Step.** Gently remove the infant from the table and chart the results.
6. **Procedural Step.** Plot the length on the infant's growth chart.

CHARTING EXAMPLE

Date	
8/10/2002	9:30 a.m. Wt. 15 lb 2 oz. Ht. 25 ½ in. —————
————————— T. Powell, CMA

11

The procedure for using growth charts is as follows: Locate the growth value in the vertical column under the appropriate category (weight, length or stature, and head circumference). Next, locate the child's age in the horizontal column. Find the site at which the two lines (extending from these values) intersect on the graph. Place an **X** on this site. To determine the percentile in which the child falls in relation to other children of the same age, follow the percentile line upward to read the value located on the side of the chart. (Interpolation is needed if the value does not fall exactly on a percentile line.) Chart the results as instructed by the physician.

Text continued on page 423

PROCEDURE

11–3

Measuring Head and Chest Circumference of an Infant

EQUIPMENT: **Flexible nonstretch tape measure**

Measurement of Head Circumference:

1. **Procedural Step.** Wash the hands, and assemble the equipment. The tape measure should consist of either paper or plastic; a cloth tape should not be used.
   Principle. Cloth tape measures can stretch and give a falsely low reading.
2. **Procedural Step.** Position the infant. The infant should be placed on his or her back on the examining table. An alternative to this is to have the parent hold the child.
3. **Procedural Step.** Position the tape measure around the infant's head at the greatest circumference. This is usually accomplished by placing the tape slightly above the eyebrows and pinna of the ears and around the occipital prominence at the back of the skull.

11

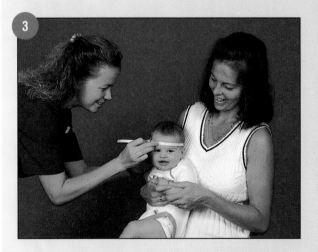

4. **Procedural Step.** Read the results in centimeters (or inches) to the nearest 0.5 cm (or ¼ inch). Chart the results.
5. **Procedural Step.** Plot the head circumference value on the infant's growth chart.

CHARTING EXAMPLE

Date	
8/10/2002	10:00 a.m. Head circumference: 42 ½ cm. —————————————— T. Powell, CMA

Measurement of Chest Circumference:

1. **Procedural Step.** Position the infant on his or her back on the examining table.
2. **Procedural Step.** Encircle the tape around the infant's chest at the nipple line. It should be snug but not so tight that it leaves a mark.

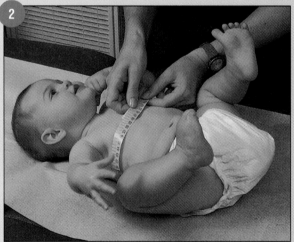

3. **Procedural Step.** Read the results in centimeters (or inches) to the nearest 0.5 cm (or 1/4 inch). Chart the results.

CHARTING EXAMPLE

Date	
8/15/2002	10:00 a.m. Chest circumference: 42 cm. —————————————— T. Powell, CMA

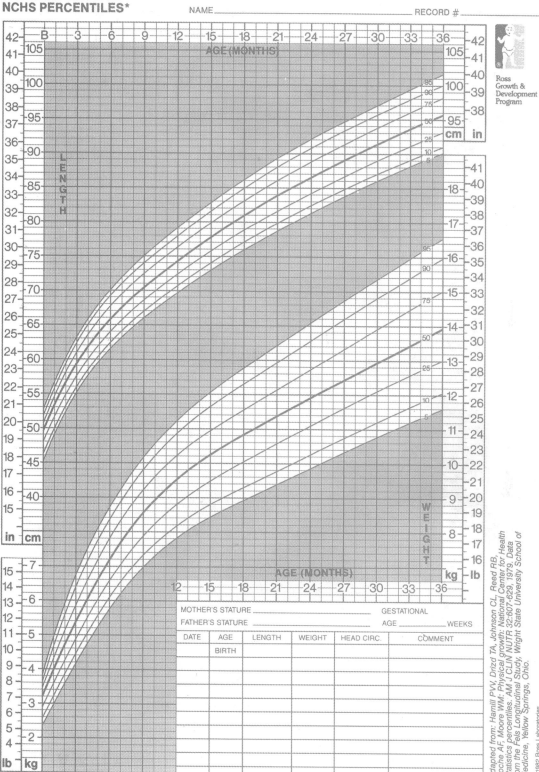

■ **FIGURE 11–5.** Growth charts. *A,* Chart for length and weight of girls, birth to 36 months.

Illustration continued on following page

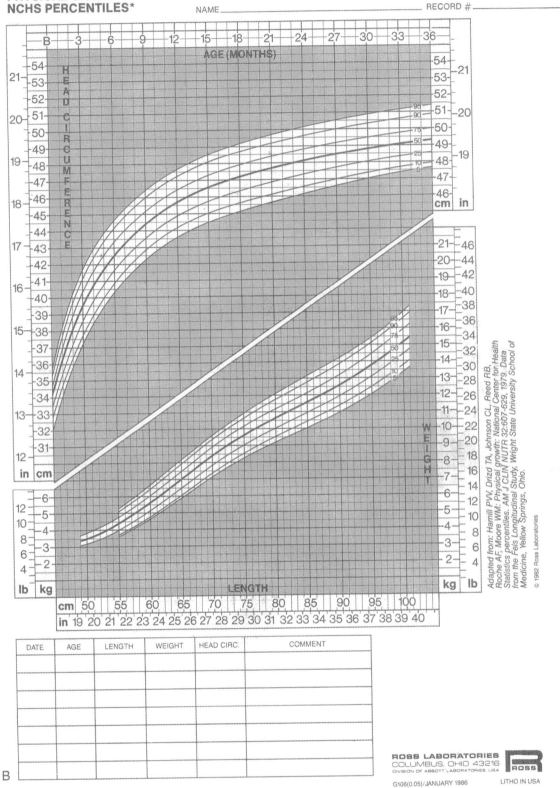

GIRLS: BIRTH TO 36 MONTHS
PHYSICAL GROWTH
NCHS PERCENTILES*

NAME _____   RECORD # _____

Adapted from: Hamill PVV, Drizd TA, Johnson CL, Reed RB, Roche AF, Moore WM: Physical growth: National Center for Health Statistics percentiles. AM J CLIN NUTR 32:607-629, 1979. Data from the Fels Longitudinal Study, Wright State University School of Medicine, Yellow Springs, Ohio.

© 1982 Ross Laboratories

DATE	AGE	LENGTH	WEIGHT	HEAD CIRC.	COMMENT

B

ROSS LABORATORIES
COLUMBUS, OHIO 43216
DIVISION OF ABBOTT LABORATORIES, USA

G106(0.05)/JANUARY 1986   LITHO IN USA

■ **FIGURE 11–5.** *Continued B,* Chart for head circumference of girls, birth to 36 months.

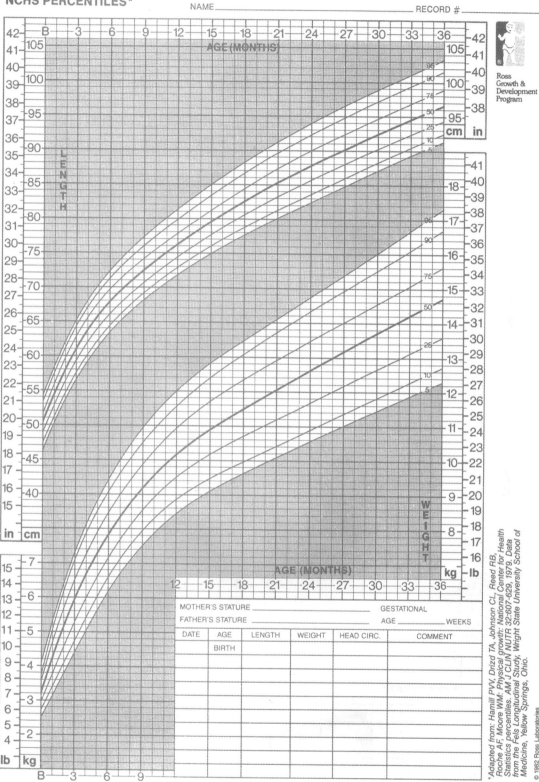

BOYS: BIRTH TO 36 MONTHS
PHYSICAL GROWTH
NCHS PERCENTILES*

NAME _____   RECORD # _____

*Adapted from: Hamill PVV, Drizd TA, Johnson CL, Reed RB, Roche AF, Moore WM: Physical growth: National Center for Health Statistics percentiles. AM J CLIN NUTR 32:607-629, 1979. Data from the Fels Longitudinal Study, Wright State University School of Medicine, Yellow Springs, Ohio.

© 1982 Ross Laboratories

Ross
Growth &
Development
Program

MOTHER'S STATURE _____   GESTATIONAL
FATHER'S STATURE _____   AGE _____ WEEKS

DATE	AGE	LENGTH	WEIGHT	HEAD CIRC.	COMMENT
	BIRTH				

■ **FIGURE 11–5.** *Continued C,* Chart for length and weight of boys, birth to 36 months.

Illustration continued on following page

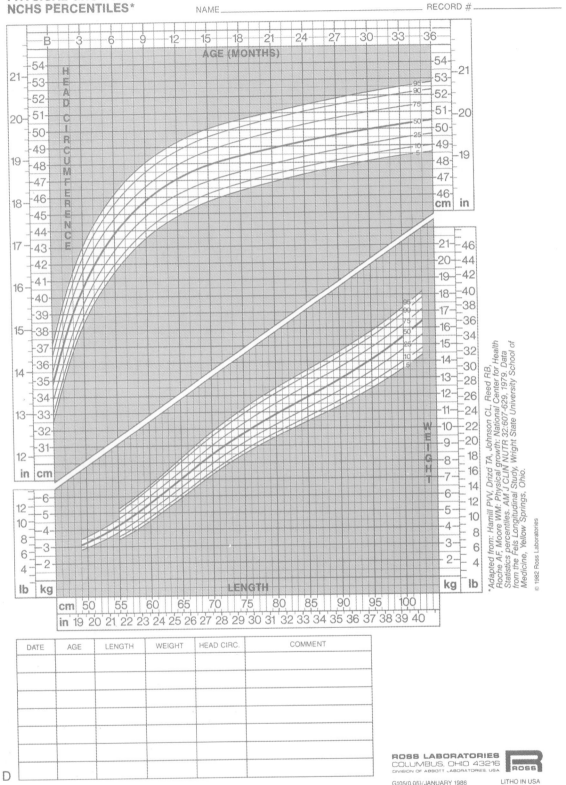

■ **FIGURE 11–5.** *Continued D,* Chart for head circumference of boys, birth to 36 months.

FIGURE 11-5. *Continued E,* Chart for stature and weight of girls, 2 to 18 years.

Illustration continued on following page

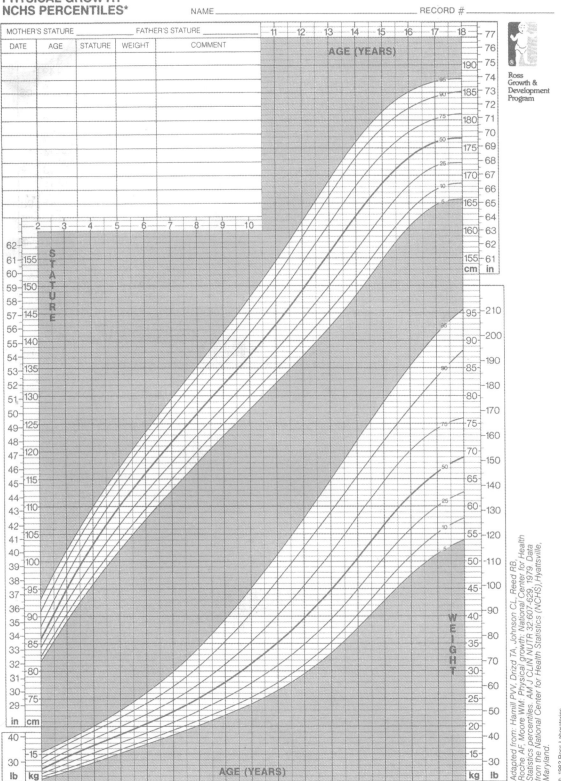

■ **FIGURE 11–5.** *Continued F,* Chart for stature and weight of boys, 2 to 18 years. (Adapted from Hamill PVV, Drizd TA, Johnson CL, Reed RB, Roche AF, Moore WM: Physical growth: National Center for Health Statistics percentiles. *Am J Clin Nutr* 32:607-629, 1979. Data from the National Center for Health Statistics [NCHS], Hyattsville, Maryland.)

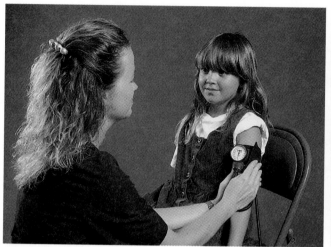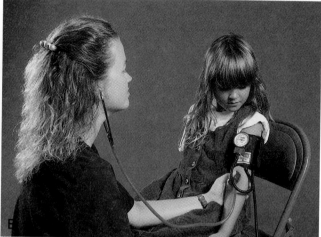

FIGURE 11-6. Traci measures the blood pressure of a pediatric patient.

PEDIATRIC BLOOD PRESSURE MEASUREMENT

☐ The American Academy of Pediatrics recommends that all children 3 years of age and older have their blood pressure measured annually. Measuring pediatric blood pressure helps to identify children at risk for developing hypertension as adults.

The procedure for measuring blood pressure in children is the same as for adults and is presented in Chapter 3: Vital Signs (also refer to Fig. 11-6). The most important criterion in taking pediatric blood pressure is the size of the cuff. The width of the cuff should be 20 percent greater than the diameter of the child's limb. If the cuff is too small, the reading may be falsely high. On the other hand, if the cuff is too large, the reading may be falsely low. The cuff should fit snugly and should be applied so that the center of the inflatable bag is directly over the artery to be compressed.

Another important factor to consider when taking pediatric blood pressure is preparing the child for the procedure. It is important to gain the child's cooperation and to make sure that the child is relaxed. Apprehension can cause the blood pressure to be falsely high. To reduce a child's anxiety level, carefully explain the procedure to the child and allow him or her to handle the equipment before measuring blood pressure.

COLLECTION OF A URINE SPECIMEN

☐ A urine specimen may be required from a pediatric patient as part of a general physical examination, to assist in the diagnosis of a pathologic condition, or to evaluate the effectiveness of therapy.

The collection of a urine specimen in a child exhibiting bladder control is performed using the technique outlined in Chapter 16. Collecting a urine specimen from an infant or young child who cannot urinate voluntarily involves the use of a pediatric urine collector. The urine collector consists of a clear plastic bag containing a soft sponge ring coated with a pressure-sensitive adhesive around the opening. The adhesive firmly attaches the urine collector to the genitalia. Most pediatric urine collectors are designed to be used with both sexes.

PROCEDURE

11–4

Applying a Pediatric Urine Collector

EQUIPMENT/SUPPLIES: Disposable gloves
Personal wipes or gauze squares and an antiseptic solution
Pediatric urine collector bag
Urine specimen container and label
Biohazard waste container

1. **Procedural Step.** Wash the hands.
2. **Procedural Step.** Assemble the equipment.

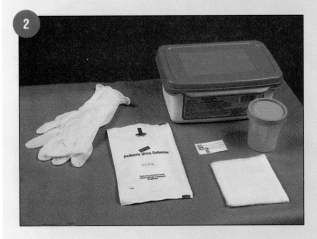

3. **Procedural Step.** Greet the child's parent, and identify the child. Introduce yourself, and explain the procedure.
4. **Procedural Step.** Apply gloves. Position the child. The child should be placed on the back with the legs spread apart. The medical assistant may need another individual to hold the child's legs apart.
   Principle. This position facilitates cleansing of the genitalia and permits proper application of the urine collector bag.
5. **Procedural Step.** Cleanse the child's genitalia.
   Female. Using a front-to-back motion (pubis to anus), cleanse each side of the meatus with a separate wipe or gauze square saturated with an antiseptic solution. With a third wipe or gauze square cleanse directly down the middle (directly

over the urinary meatus). Thoroughly rinse the area and wipe it dry.
   Male. If the child is not circumcised, retract the foreskin of the penis. Cleanse the area around the meatus and the urethral opening (meatal orifice) in a manner similar to that used in the female patient. Be sure to use a separate wipe or gauze square (saturated with an antiseptic solution) for each swipe. Cleanse the scrotum last, using a fresh wipe or gauze square. Rinse the area and thoroughly wipe it dry.
   Principle. The urinary meatus and surrounding area must be cleansed to prevent contaminants such as baby powder, fecal material, and microorganisms from entering the urine specimen, which could affect the test results. A front-to-back motion must be used to prevent drawing microorganisms from the anal area into the area being cleansed. The cleansing agent must be rinsed off to prevent it from entering the urine specimen, which could affect the accuracy of the test results. The area must be wiped dry to assure an airtight adhesion of the collection bag to prevent leakage of urine.
6. **Procedural Step.** Remove the paper backing from the urine collector bag, thereby exposing the adhesive surface. Firmly attach the bag in the following manner:
   Female. The round opening of the bag should be placed so as to cover the upper half of the external genitalia. The opening of the bag should be directly over the urinary meatus.
   Male. The bag should be positioned so the child's penis and scrotum are projected through the opening of the bag.
   Principle. The urine collector bag must be attached securely to prevent leakage.
7. **Procedural Step.** Loosely diaper the child. Check the urine collector bag every 15 minutes until a urine specimen is obtained.

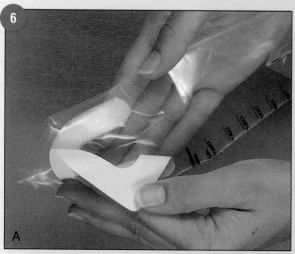

A

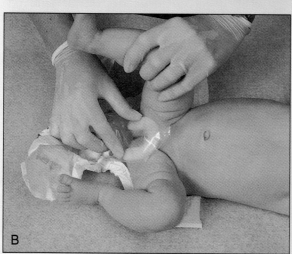

B

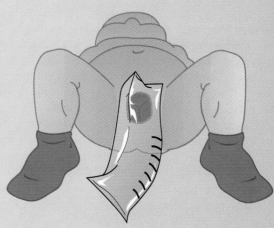

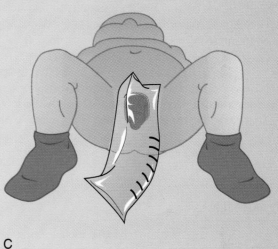

C

11

Principle. The diaper helps hold the urine collector bag in place.

8. **Procedural Step.** Once the child has voided, gently remove the urine collector bag.
   Principle. The bag must be removed gently because pulling the adhesive away too quickly may cause discomfort and irritation of the child's skin.

9. **Procedural Step.** Clean the genital area and rediaper the child.

10. **Procedural Step.** Transfer the urine specimen into a urine specimen container and tightly apply the lid. Label the container with the child's name, the date, the time of collection, and the type of specimen (i.e., urine). Dispose of the collector bag in a biohazard waste container. Based on the medical office routine, test the urine specimen or prepare it for transfer to an outside laboratory, making sure to include a completed laboratory request. If the specimen cannot be tested or transferred immediately, preserve it by placing it in the refrigerator.

Principle. Changes take place in a urine specimen that is left sitting out.

11. **Procedural Step.** Remove the gloves, and wash the hands.

12. **Procedural Step.** Chart the procedure. Include the date, the time of collection, and the type of specimen (i.e., urine). If the specimen is to be transported to an outside laboratory, indicate this information, including the laboratory tests ordered.

CHARTING EXAMPLE	
Date	
8/12/2002	10:15 a.m. Urine specimen collected for culture. Picked up by Medical Center Lab on 8/12/2002. ——————— T. Powell, CMA

PEDIATRIC INTRAMUSCULAR INJECTIONS

□ Administering an intramuscular (IM) injection to a child is an important responsibility. The experience a child has with early injections influences his or her attitude toward later ones. If the child is old enough to understand, the procedure should be explained. The medical assistant should be honest and attempt to gain the child's trust and cooperation. The child should be told the truth about the injection—that it will hurt but only for a short time. It is also advisable to explain that the medicine will help him or her get better. Another person should be present to assist. The assistant can help position the child and can divert or restrain him or her if necessary. If the child struggles and fights excessively, however, the medical assistant should delay the injection and consult the physician.

The administration of IM injections has already been described in Chapter 7. Before undertaking the study of pediatric IM injections, the medical assistant should review that chapter thoroughly, concentrating on the location of injection sites and the procedure for the administration of an injection. The same basic technique used to administer an IM injection to an adult is used for a child. Variations in procedure are explained in the following section.

Type of Needle

The gauge and length of the needle used for the IM injection vary, depending on the consistency of the medication to be administered and the size of the child. Thick or oily preparations require a larger needle lumen, and the needle must be of sufficient length to reach muscle tissue.

Injection Sites

There are variations in pediatric injection sites based on the age of the child. The specific site to be utilized is stated in the package insert accompanying the medication. Until the child is walking, the gluteus muscle is small, not well developed, and covered with a thick layer of fat. Moreover, an injection in the dorsogluteal site may come dangerously close to the sciatic nerve. The danger is increased if the child is squirming or fighting. Because serious trauma can result from incorrect administration of an injection in this area, it is recommended that the dorsogluteal site not be used until the child has been walking for at least a year (Fig. 11–7).

The vastus lateralis muscle site is recommended instead in infants and young children. It is located on the

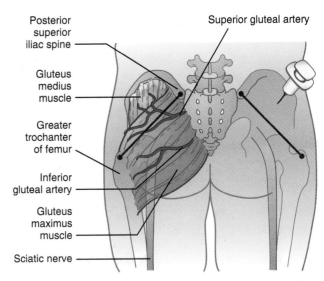

■ **FIGURE 11–7.** Dorsogluteal intramuscular injection site. (Courtesy of Wyeth Laboratories, Philadelphia, PA.)

anterior surface of the midlateral thigh, away from major nerves and blood vessels, and it is large enough to accommodate the injected medication (Fig. 11–8). The length of the needle used depends on the overall size of the thigh. It should be long enough to penetrate the muscle belly for proper absorption to take place. A 1-inch needle is often utilized. To administer the injection, the infant is placed on the back. The thigh is grasped in order to compress the muscle tissue and to stabilize the extremity. The injection is administered following the procedure outlined in Chapter 7 (Procedure 7–5. Administering an Intramuscular Injection).

The deltoid muscle is shallow and can accommodate only a very small amount of medication. In addition,

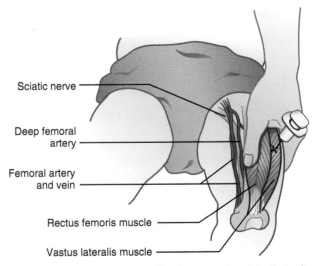

■ **FIGURE 11–8.** Vastus lateralis intramuscular injection site. (Courtesy of Wyeth Laboratories, Philadelphia, PA.)

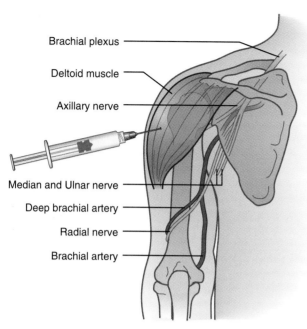

Brachial plexus

Deltoid muscle

Axillary nerve

Median and Ulnar nerve

Deep brachial artery

Radial nerve

Brachial artery

■ **FIGURE 11–9.** Deltoid intramuscular injection site. (Courtesy of Wyeth Laboratories, Philadelphia, PA.)

repeated injections to this site are painful. As during an injection into the vastus lateralis, the muscle mass should be grasped at the injection site and compressed between the thumb and fingers. The needle should be inserted pointing slightly upward toward the shoulder (Fig. 11–9).

After giving the injection, the medical assistant or the child's parent should hold the infant and provide comfort and show approval so that the child associates something other than pain with this procedure.

IMMUNIZATIONS

☐ **Immunity** is the resistance of the body to the effects of harmful agents such as pathogenic microorganisms or their toxins. The process of becoming immune or rendering an individual immune through the use of a vaccine or toxoid is known as active, artificial **immunization.** Immunizations build up the body's defenses and protect an individual from attack by certain infectious diseases.

Common immunizations administered to infants and children include the following: diphtheria and tetanus toxoids combined with acellular pertussis vaccine (DTaP); polio vaccine; measles (rubeola), mumps, and rubella (MMR) combined vaccines; *Haemophilus influenzae* type b (Hib) vaccine; hepatitis B; and chickenpox (varicella). Prevention of disease is one of the most important goals in the care of children.

PUTTING IT ALL *into* PRACTICE

▶ **TRACI POWELL:** *It is interesting how your education, training, and experience all come together, especially in a crisis. Early one morning, when I arrived at work, a mother was waiting with a small child who was approximately 2 years of age. The child was dusky in color, panicky, and having a great deal of trouble breathing. Apparently the child had gotten into some dry beans the previous night and had inhaled one into her lung. None of the physicians were in the building yet, and this child was in respiratory distress. We immediately called a Code Blue, put her on oxygen, and then made arrangements for a squad car to take her to Children's Hospital, where a surgeon was waiting. Fortunately, all went well and she is a very healthy little girl today.*

Looking back, I am grateful for a good, solid medical assisting education, a PALS (Pediatric Advance Life Support) certification, and experience in working with children so that I was able to help that child overcome a life-threatening experience. I firmly believe that no matter how long a person has been in the medical field or what his or her profession is, continuing education is essential to stay current in the ever-changing health care field.

Immunizations should be administered to infants and young children during health maintenance visits according to an immunization schedule. The American Academy of Pediatrics recommends following the schedule outlined in the accompanying box. This schedule is intended as a guide to be used with any modifications needed to meet the requirements of an individual or group.

11

Recommended Childhood Immunization Schedule, United States, January–December 1999

Vaccines[1] are listed under routinely recommended ages. [Bars] indicate range of recommended ages for immunization. Any dose not given at the recommended age should be given as a "catchup" immunization at any subsequent visit when indicated and feasible. (Ovals) indicate vaccines to be given if previously recommended doses were missed or given earlier than the recommended minimum age.

Age ▲ Vaccine ▼	Birth	1 mo	2 mos	4 mos	6 mos	12 mos	15 mos	18 mos	4-6 yrs	11-12 yrs	14-16 yrs
Hepatitis B[2]	Hep B		Hep B		Hep B					(Hep B)	
Diphtheria, Tetanus, Pertussis[3]			DTaP	DTaP	DTaP	P	DTaP[3]		DTaP	Td	
H. influenzae type b[4]			Hib	Hib	Hib	Hib					
Polio[5]			IPV	IPV	Polio				Polio		
Rotavirus[6]			Rv[6]	Rv[6]	Rv[6]						
Measles, Mumps, Rubella[7]						MMR			MMR[7]	(MMR[7])	
Varicella Zoster Virus Vaccine[8]						Var				(Var[8])	

Approved by the Advisory Committee on Immunization Practices (ACIP), the American Academy of Pediatrics (AAP), and the American Academy of Family Physicians (AAFP).

1. This schedule indicates the recommended ages for routine administration of currently licensed childhood vaccines. Combination vaccines may be used whenever any components of the combination are indicated and its other components are not contraindicated. Providers should consult the manufacturers' package inserts for detailed recommendations.

2. *Infants born to HBsAg-negative mothers* should receive the second dose of hepatitis B vaccine at least 1 month after the 1st dose. The third dose should be administered at least 4 months after the first dose and at least 2 months after the second dose but not before 6 months of age for infants.

   Infants born to HBsAg-positive mothers should receive hepatitis B vaccine and 0.5 ml of hepatitis B immune globulin (HBIG) within 12 hours of birth at separate sites. The second dose is recommended at 1 to 2 months of age and the third dose at 6 months of age.

   Infants born to mothers whose HBsAg status is unknown should receive hepatitis B vaccine within 12 hours of birth. Maternal blood should be drawn at the time of delivery to determine the mother's HBsAg status; if the HBsAG test is positive, the infant should receive HBIG as soon as possible (no later than 1 week of age).

   All children and adolescents (through 18 years of age) who have not been immunized against hepatitis B may begin the series during any visit. Special efforts should be made to immunize children who were born in or whose parents were born in areas of the world with moderate or high endemicity of HBV infection.

3. DTaP (diphtheria and tetanus toxoids and acellular pertussis vaccine) is the preferred vaccine for all doses in the immunization series, including completion of the series in children who have received 1 or more doses of whole-cell DTP vaccine. Whole-cell DTP is an acceptable alternative to DTaP. The fourth dose (DTP or DTaP) may be administered as early as 12 months of age, provided 6 months have elapsed since the third dose and if the child is unlikely to return at age 15 to 18 months. Td (tetanus and diphtheria toxoids) is recommended at 11 to 12 years of age if at least 5 years have elapsed since the last dose of DTP, DTaP, or DT. Subsequent routine Td boosters are recommended every 10 years.

4. Three *Haemophilus influenzae* type b (HIB) conjugate vaccines are licensed for infant use. If PRP-OMP (PedvaxHIB and COMVAX [Merck]) is administered at 2 and 4 months of age, a dose at 6 months is not required. Because clinical studies in infants have demonstrated that using some combination products may induce a lower immune response to the HIB vaccine component, DTaP/HIB combination products should not be used for primary immunization in infants at 2, 4, or 6 months of age, unless they are FDA-approved for these ages.

5. Two poliovirus vaccines currently are licensed in the United States: inactivated poliovirus vaccine (IPV) and oral poliovirus vaccine (OPV). The ACIP, AAP, and AAFP now recommend that the first two doses of poliovirus vaccine should be IPV. The ACIP continues to recommend a sequential schedule of two doses of IPV administered at ages 2 and 4 months,

Recommended Childhood Immunization Schedule, United States, January–December 1999 *Continued*

followed by two doses of OPV at 12 to 18 months and 4 to 6 years. Use of IPV for all doses also is acceptable and is recommended for immunocompromised persons and their household contacts. OPV is no longer recommended for the first two doses of the schedule and is acceptable only for special circumstances, such as for children of parents who do not accept the recommended number of injections; late initiation of immunization, which would require an unacceptable number of injections; and imminent travel to polio-endemic areas. OPV remains the vaccine of choice for mass immunization campaigns to control outbreaks due to wild poliovirus.

6. *Rotavirus vaccination:* Clinicians temporarily should suspend administration of rotavirus vaccine to unimmunized and partially immunized children, pending collection and evaluation of additional information.

7. The second dose of measles, mumps, and rubella vaccine (MMR) is recommended routinely at 4 to 6 years of age but may be administered during any visit, provided at least 4 weeks have elapsed since receipt of the first dose and that both doses are administered beginning at or after 12 months of age. Those who have not previously received the second dose should complete the schedule by the visit when the child is 11 to 12 years old.

8. Varicella vaccine is recommended at any visit on or after the first birthday for susceptible children, i.e., those who lack a reliable history of chickenpox (as judged by a health-care provider) and who have not been immunized. Susceptible persons 13 years of age or older should receive two doses, given at least 4 weeks apart.

Text courtesy of The American Academy of Pediatrics, Elk Grove Village, Illinois.

 PATIENT/TEACHING

CHILDHOOD IMMUNIZATIONS

■ Answer questions patients have about childhood immunizations:

What Is Immunity?

Immunity is the resistance of the body to microorganisms that cause disease. When an individual has an infection, the body responds by producing disease-fighting substances known as antibodies. Antibodies usually remain in the body even after the individual has recovered from the disease. This protects the individual from getting the same disease again.

How Do Immunizations Prevent Disease?

The microorganisms that cause disease or their toxins are weakened or killed and made into vaccines. These vaccines are then injected into the body or swallowed, as with the oral polio vaccine. The body reacts to these vaccines the same way that it responds to the disease itself, by producing antibodies. These antibodies last for a long time, often for life, to defend the body against disease.

What Childhood Diseases Can Be Prevented Through Immunization?

The reduction of childhood disease by immunization during the past 40 years has been dramatic. Eight childhood diseases can be prevented by routine immunization: measles, mumps, rubella (German measles), diphtheria, tetanus (lockjaw), pertussis (whooping cough), polio, *Haemophilus influenzae* type b (Hib) infections, and chickenpox (varicella). Except for tetanus,

all these diseases are contagious. They can be spread from child to child and from one community to another. And when children are not protected against them, serious outbreaks of disease can still occur.

Do Immunizations Have Side Effects?

Vaccines are among the safest and most reliable medications available. However, minor side effects may occur following administration of an immunization. They do not last long and may include a slight fever and irritability; redness, swelling, and soreness at the injection site; and a mild rash. On rare occasion, the effects can be more serious; therefore if any unusual symptoms occur following immunization, it is important to contact the physician immediately. Overall, the benefits of vaccines to prevent childhood diseases are greater than the possible risks for almost all children.

Are Immunizations Required by Law?

Every state has laws requiring vaccination against some or all of these diseases before children enter school. Children who get their vaccinations not only benefit from the protection these vaccinations provide, but they also contribute to the well-being of everyone by reducing the chance for disease to spread.

■ Encourage parents to have their children immunized.

■ Emphasize to parents the importance of maintaining an immunization record card documenting each of their children's immunizations.

■ Provide parents with educational materials on the importance of immunizations.

11

FIGURE 11–10. Immunization record card. (Courtesy of Mead, Johnson Nutritionals.)

Name _____ Sex ____ Date _____					
IMMUNIZATION AND SKIN TESTING RECORD					
	DATE	DATE	DATE	DATE	DATE
DTaP (Diphtheria, Tetanus, and Pertussis)					
IPV/OPV (Poliovirus Vaccine)					
MMR (Measles, Mumps, Rubella)					
HbPV (Haemophilius b Conjugate Vaccine)					
Varicella (Chicken pox)					
Tuberculin					
Tetanus Booster					
Other					

Provided courtesy of Mead, Johnson Nurtritionals, maker of Enfamil®, Prosobee®, and Nutramigen® full-year infant formulas; aspirin-free, alcohol-free Tempra®, Vi-Sol® vitamins; and Tri-Vi-Flor®/Poly-Vi-Flor® vitamin-fluoride supplements.

L-B980-11-90

11

Medical assistants should be completely familiar with each type of immunization that is given. They should have a knowledge of its use, precautions to be taken, common side effects and adverse reactions, the route of administration, the dosage, and the method of storage. The drug manufacturer includes a package insert with each vaccine or toxoid that contains valuable information about the drug. Drug references, such as the *Physician's Desk Reference*, also can be utilized to locate information on immunizations.

Once the immunization has been given, the medical assistant should make sure to record the information on the patient's chart. Included should be the date and time of administration, the product name, manufacturer, lot number, expiration date, the dosage given, the site and route of administration, and the signature and title of the individual administering the immunization.

It is helpful for parents to have an immunization record card (Fig. 11–10). They should be encouraged to bring this card on each visit so that their child's immunizations can be recorded. Parents should be informed of the possible normal side effects of each immunization and given instructions on how to respond to them if they occur.

NATIONAL CHILDHOOD VACCINE INJURY ACT

The National Childhood Vaccine Injury Act (NCVIA), which became effective in 1988, requires that parents be provided with information about the benefits and risks of childhood immunizations. To help medical offices comply with these regulations, the Centers for Disease Control developed Vaccine Information Statements (VISs) (Fig. 11–11). The VISs explain, in lay terminology, the benefits and risks of each specific vaccine.

DIPHTHERIA, TETANUS, AND PERTUSSIS VACCINES

W H A T   Y O U   N E E D   T O   K N O W

1 Why get vaccinated?

Diphtheria, pertussis, and tetanus are serious diseases.

Diphtheria
- Diphtheria causes a thick covering in the back of the throat.
- It can lead to breathing problems, paralysis, heart failure, and even death

Tetanus (Lockjaw)
- Tetanus causes painful tightening of the muscles, usually all over the body.
- It can lead to "locking" of the jaw so the person cannot open his mouth or swallow. Tetanus can lead to death.

Pertussis (Whooping cough)
- Pertussis causes coughing spells so bad that it is hard for infants to eat, drink, or breathe. These can last for weeks.
- It can lead to pneumonia, seizures (jerking and staring spells), brain damage, and death.

Diphtheria, tetanus, and pertussis vaccines prevent these diseases. Most children who get all their shots will be protected during childhood. Many more children would get these diseases if we stopped vaccinating.

2 Diphtheria, tetanus, and pertussis vaccines

DTP vaccine
- Protects against diphtheria, tetanus, and pertussis
- Used for many years

DTaP vaccine
- Protects against diphtheria, tetanus, and pertussis
- Newer than DTP

The Centers for Disease Control and Prevention (CDC) recommends DTaP over DTP. This is because DTaP is less likely to cause reactions than DTP.

Related vaccines
- Combinations: To reduce the number of shots a child must get, DTP or DTaP may be available in combination with other vaccines.
- DT protects against diphtheria and tetanus, *but not pertussis.* It only is recommended for children who should not get pertussis vaccine.

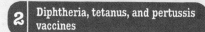

3 What are the risks from these vaccines?

- As with any medicine, vaccines carry a small risk of serious harm, such as a severe allergic reaction or even death.
- If there are reactions, they usually start within 3 days and don't last long.
- Most people have no serious reactions from these vaccines.

Possible reactions to these vaccines:

Mild Reactions (common)
- Sore arm or leg
- Fussy
- Tired
- Fever
- Less appetite
- Vomiting

Mild reactions are much less likely after DTaP than after DTP.

Moderate to Serious Reactions (uncommon)

Moderate to serious reactions have been uncommon with DTP vaccine:
- Non-stop crying (3 hours or more) . . . . 100 of every 10,000 doses
- Fever of 105 or higher . . . . 30 of every 10,000 doses
- Seizure (jerking or staring) . . . . 6 of every 10,000 doses
- Child becomes limp, pale, less alert . . . . 6 of every 10,000 doses

With DTaP vaccine, these reactions are much less likely to happen.

Severe Reactions (very rare)

There are two kinds of serious reactions:
- Severe allergic reaction (breathing difficulty, shock)
- Severe brain reaction (long seizure, coma or lowered consciousness)

Is there lasting damage?
- Experts disagree on whether pertussis vaccines cause lasting brain damage.
- If they do, it is very rare.

Most experts believe serious reactions will be *more rare* after DTaP than after DTP.

U.S. DEPARTMENT OF HEALTH & HUMAN SERVICES
Centers for Disease Control and Prevention
National Immunization Program

DTP/DTaP/DT (8/1 5/97)
Vaccine Information Statement
42 U.S.C. 300aa-26

11

(partially obscured left sheet)

4 When should my c[hild be] vaccinated?

Most children should get a dose at the[...]

2 Months   **4 Months**

12-18 Months

At 11-12 years of age and every 10 year[s...] booster to prevent diphtheria and tetan[us...]

5 What can be done [to] reduce possible fe[ver] after this vaccine[?]

Give your child an *aspirin-free* pain reli[...] for 24 hours after the shot.

This is important if your child has had a [...] seizure or has a parent, brother, or sister [...] who has had a seizure.

6 Some children sh[ould not get these] vaccines or shoul[d...]

Tell your doctor or nurse if your child:
- Ever had a moderate or serious reaction after getting vaccinated
- Ever had a seizure
- Has a parent, brother, or sister who has had a seizure
- Has a brain problem that is getting worse
- Now has a moderate or severe illness

Your doctor or nurse has information on what to do in this case (for example, give one of these vaccines, wait, give medicine to prevent fever).

■ **FIGURE 11–11.** Examples of vaccine information statements. (Courtesy of the Centers for Disease Control and Prevention, Atlanta, GA.)

Illustration continued on following page

MEASLES MUMPS & RUBELLA VACCINES

WHAT YOU NEED TO KNOW

1 Why get vaccinated?

Measles, mumps, and rubella are serious diseases.

Measles
* Measles virus causes rash, cough, runny nose, eye irritation, and fever.
* It can lead to ear infection, pneumonia, seizures (jerking and staring), brain damage, and death.

Mumps
* Mumps virus causes fever, headache, and swollen glands.
* It can lead to deafness, meningitis (infection of the brain and spinal cord covering), painful swelling of the testicles or ovaries, and, rarely, death.

Rubella (German Measles)
* Rubella virus causes rash, mild fever, and arthritis (mostly in women).
* If a woman gets rubella while she is pregnant, she could have a miscarriage or her baby could be born with serious birth defects.

You or your child could catch these diseases by being around someone who has them. They spread from person to person through the air.

Measles, mumps, and rubella (MMR) vaccine can prevent these diseases.

Most children who get their MMR shots will not get these diseases. Many more children would get them if we stopped vaccinating.

2 Who should get MMR vaccine and when?

Children should get 2 doses of MMR vaccine:

✔ The first at **12-15 months** of age
✔ and the second at **4-6 years** of age.

These are the recommended ages. But children can get the second dose at any age, as long as it is at least 28 days after the first dose.

Some **adults** should also get MMR vaccine: Generally, anyone 18 years of age or older, who was born after 1956, should get at least one dose of MMR vaccine, unless they can show that they have had either the vaccines or the diseases.

Ask your doctor or nurse for more information.

MMR vaccine may be given at the same time as other vaccines.

3 Some people should not get MMR vaccine or should wait

* People should not get MMR vaccine who have ever had a life-threatening allergic reaction to **gelatin**, the antibiotic **neomycin**, or a **previous dose of MMR vaccine.**

* People who are moderately or severely ill at the time the shot is scheduled should usually wait until they recover before getting MMR vaccine.

* Pregnant women should wait to get MMR vaccine until after they have given birth. Women should not get pregnant for 3 months after getting MMR vaccine.

* Some people should check with their doctor about whether they should get MMR vaccine, including anyone who:
  - Has HIV/AIDS, or another disease that affects the immune system
  - Is being treated with drugs that affect the immune system, such as steroids, for 2 weeks or longer.
  - Has any kind of cancer
  - Is taking cancer treatment with x-rays or drugs
  - Has ever had a low platelet count (a blood disorder)
  Over . . .

clude difficulty breathing, hives, paleness, weakness, a ss within a few minutes to ot. A high fever or seizure, n 1 or 2 weeks after the

person to a doctor right away. ppened, the date and time it vaccination was given. or health department to file a Reporting System (VAERS) urself at **1-800-822-7967.**

al Vaccine Injury ion Program

u or your child has a ccine, a federal program has pay for the care of those

ional Vaccine Injury all **1-800-338-2382** or visit

v/bhpr/vicp

learn more?

rse. They can give you the or suggest other sources of

e health department's

Disease Control and Prevention

(English)
(Español)

Visit the National Immunization Program's website at **http://www.cdc.gov/nip**

- Long-term seizures, coma, or lowered consciousness
- Permanent brain damage

5 What if there is a moderate or severe reaction?

What should I look for?

Any unusual conditions, such as a serious allergic reaction, high fever or behavior changes. Signs of a

U.S. DEPARTMENT OF HEALTH & HUMAN SERVICES
Centers for Disease Control and Prevention
National Immunization Program

Vaccine Information Statement	
MMR (12/16/98)	42 U.S.C. § 300aa-26

■ **FIGURE 11–11.** *Continued*

The NCVIA requires that the appropriate VIS be given to the parent or legal representative of a child receiving the following vaccines: DPT, MMR, polio, Hib, hepatitis B, and chickenpox. In addition, a notation must be made in the patient's medical record indicating that the VIS was provided at the time of the vaccination.

The NCVIA also requires that the following information be recorded in each patient's medical record: the date of administration of the vaccine, the manufacturer and lot number of the vaccine, and the name of the health care provider administering the vaccine. Refer to Fig. 11–12 for an example of a pediatric vaccine administrative record form used to record this information.

PEDIATRIC VACCINE ADMINISTRATION RECORD

Name _____
(first)   (MI)   (last)

D.O.B. _____ Today's date _____

Acct. # _____

Physician _____
(or attach label)

" I have read or had had explained to me information about the diseases and the vaccines listed below. I believe I understand the benefits and risks of the vaccines cited, and ask that vaccine(s) listed below be given to me or to the person named above for whom I am authorized to make this request. I grant permission for the record to be released to medical providers., health department, WIC agencies, schools, day care, facilities and others as is necessary."

Signature of Responsible Party _____

Vaccine	Date given	Vaccine Manufacturer	Vaccine Lot Number	Site Given	Signature of Vaccine Administrator
DTaP 1					
DTaP 2					
DTaP 3					
DTaP 4					
DTaP 5					
Hib 1					
Hib 2					
Hib 3					
Hib 4					
OPV/IPV 1					
OPV/IPV 2					
OPV/IPV 3					
OPV/IPV 4					
MMR 1					
MMR 2					
Hep B 1					
Hep B 2					
Hep B 3					
Mantoux					Reaction
Varivax #1					
Varivax #2					
Other					
Other					
Other					
Other					

■ FIGURE 11–12. Pediatric vaccine administration record.

THE PKU SCREENING TEST

☐ Phenylketonuria (PKU) is a congenital hereditary disease caused by a lack of the enzyme *phenylalanine hydroxylase.* This enzyme is needed to convert phenylalanine, an amino acid, into tyrosine, which is necessary for normal metabolic functioning. Without this enzyme, phenylalanine accumulates in the blood and, if the accumulation is left untreated, causes mental retardation and other abnormalities such as tremors and poor muscle coordination. In most cases, upon early detection, a special low-phenylalanine diet and close periodic monitoring can prevent adverse effects. Normal development usually occurs if treatment is started before the child reaches 3 to 4 weeks of age.

Phenylalanine can be detected in the blood of an afflicted child once the child has been on a breast or formula milk intake for several days. Most states require, by law, that infants undergo PKU screening. Although PKU is not a common condition (affecting 1 in every 10,000 births), early diagnosis and treatment lead to a better patient prognosis. Infants on formula can be tested earlier than breast-fed babies because formula contains phenylalanine whereas the "first breast-milk," or colostrum, does not. Therefore the test results of breast-fed babies are usually invalid until the mother begins producing milk.

PKU testing is performed within 2 to 7 days after birth. The testing procedure considered most accurate and used most often is the blood phenylalanine test performed on capillary blood obtained from the plantar surface of the infant's heel or from the big toe. The blood specimen is placed on a special filter paper attached to the PKU test card (Fig. 11–13) and mailed to an outside laboratory for analysis.

Along with PKU, additional tests are performed on the blood specimen to screen for other metabolic and endocrine diseases. These tests include congenital hypothyroidism, galactosemia, and homocystinuria.

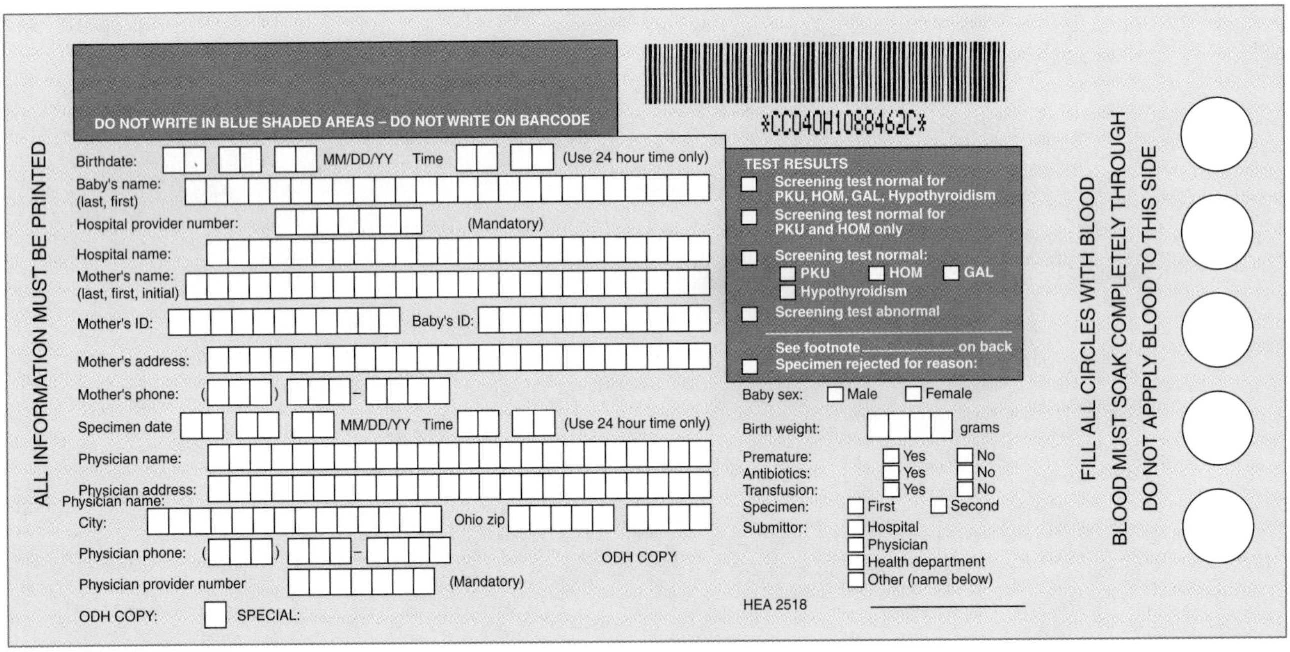
DO NOT WRITE IN BLUE SHADED AREAS – DO NOT WRITE ON BARCODE

CC040H1088462C

ALL INFORMATION MUST BE PRINTED

Birthdate: MM/DD/YY Time (Use 24 hour time only)
Baby's name: (last, first)
Hospital provider number: (Mandatory)
Hospital name:
Mother's name: (last, first, initial)
Mother's ID: Baby's ID:
Mother's address:
Mother's phone: ( ) -
Specimen date MM/DD/YY Time (Use 24 hour time only)
Physician name:
Physician address:
Physician name:
City: Ohio zip
Physician phone: ( ) -
Physician provider number (Mandatory)
ODH COPY: SPECIAL:
ODH COPY

TEST RESULTS
☐ Screening test normal for PKU, HOM, GAL, Hypothyroidism
☐ Screening test normal for PKU and HOM only
☐ Screening test normal: ☐ PKU ☐ HOM ☐ GAL ☐ Hypothyroidism
☐ Screening test abnormal
See footnote ________ on back
☐ Specimen rejected for reason:

Baby sex: ☐ Male ☐ Female
Birth weight: grams
Premature: ☐ Yes ☐ No
Antibiotics: ☐ Yes ☐ No
Transfusion: ☐ Yes ☐ No
Specimen: ☐ First ☐ Second
Submittor: ☐ Hospital ☐ Physician ☐ Health department ☐ Other (name below)
HEA 2518

FILL ALL CIRCLES WITH BLOOD
BLOOD MUST SOAK COMPLETELY THROUGH
DO NOT APPPLY BLOOD TO THIS SIDE

■ **FIGURE 11–13.** PKU test card.

PROCEDURE

11-5

PKU Screening Test

EQUIPMENT/SUPPLIES: Disposable gloves
Infant heel warmer or warm compress
Antiseptic wipe
Sterile 2×2 gauze pad

Sterile lancet
PKU test card and mailing envelope
Biohazard sharps container

1. **Procedural Step.** Wash the hands, and assemble the equipment.

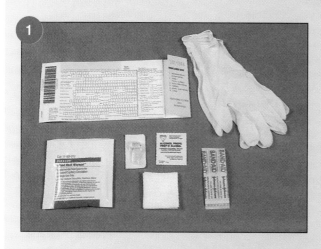

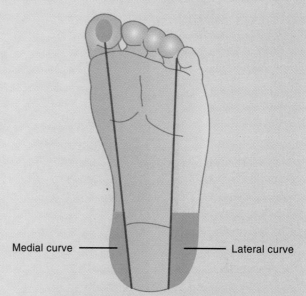

Medial curve ——————— Lateral curve

The shading indicates the appropriate area for marking the puncture.

2. **Procedural Step.** Greet the infant's parent, and identify the infant. Introduce yourself, and explain the procedure.

3. **Procedural Step.** Complete the information section of the PKU card.

4. **Procedural Step.** Apply gloves. Select an appropriate puncture site. The lateral and medial curves of the plantar surface of the heel and the big toe can be used.
Principle. The lateral and medial curves of the heel are used to avoid calcaneal complications.

5. **Procedural Step.** Warm the puncture site with a commercially available infant heel warmer or a warm compress for approximately 5 minutes.
Principle. Warming the puncture site increases capillary circulation and promotes bleeding.

6. **Procedural Step.** Cleanse the puncture site with an antiseptic wipe and allow it to dry.

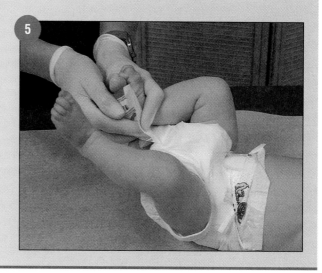

11

PROCEDURE 11–5

7. **Procedural Step.** Grasp the infant's foot around the puncture site and, without touching the cleansed site, make a puncture with the sterile lancet. The puncture should be made at a right angle to the lines of the skin. Dispose of the lancet in a biohazard sharps container.
Principle. Touching the site after cleansing will contaminate it and the cleansing process will have to be repeated.

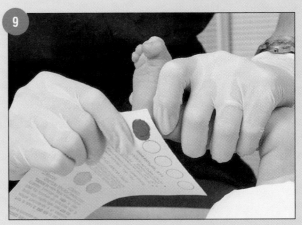

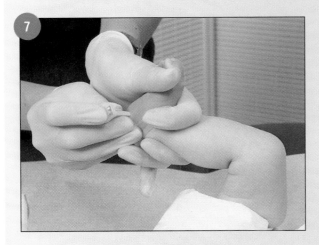

8. **Procedural Step.** Wipe away the first drop of blood with a gauze pad.
Principle. The first drop of blood is diluted with alcohol and tissue fluid and is not a suitable specimen.

9. **Procedural Step.** Use the second drop of blood for the test by placing the backside of the filter paper (side opposite the circles) against the baby's heel or toe and exerting gentle pressure without excessively squeezing the area.
Principle. Excessive squeezing will cause dilution of the blood sample with tissue fluid, leading to inaccurate test results.

10. **Procedural Step.** Completely fill each of the circles on the PKU test card with a large drop of blood. The proper amount of specimen is obtained when the blood can be observed soaking completely through the filter paper from one side to the other.
Principle. The circles must be completely filled to ensure enough of a blood sample to perform the test. Most repeat tests are required because of an inadequate blood specimen.

11. **Procedural Step.** Hold a piece of gauze or cotton over the puncture site and apply pressure to control the bleeding. Remain with the infant until the bleeding stops.

12. **Procedural Step.** Remove the gloves and wash hands.

13. **Procedural Step.** Allow the test card to dry for 2 hours at room temperature on a nonabsorbent surface. Cards should not be stacked together while drying.

14. **Procedural Step.** After the blood is completely dry, place the test card in its protective envelope and mail it to an outside laboratory for testing within 48 hours.
Principle. The test card should be mailed within 48 hours to ensure accurate test results.

15. **Procedural Step.** Chart the procedure. Include the date and time, the type of procedure, the puncture site location, and information regarding transfer to an outside laboratory.

CHARTING EXAMPLE	
Date	
8/15/2002	9:30 a.m. Blood specimen collected from Ⓡ lateral heel of foot. Sent to Newborn Screening Lab on 8/15/2002 for PKU test. —————————————— T. Powell, CMA

11

MEDICAL PRACTICE AND THE LAW

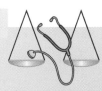

Pediatric patients are not small adults. They must be treated as individuals, according to their developmental level. Pediatric patients cannot give written or verbal consents, except for emancipated minors. Make sure a parent or legal guardian is available for consent. For example, a babysitter or grandparent cannot give consent for treatment without written permission from a par-

ent or legal guardian. Similarly, patient information can only be given to a parent or legal guardian.

If your office sees pediatric patients, you have a responsibility to be aware of developmental needs and milestones of children at various ages. This is necessary for accurate developmental assessment.

CERTIFICATION REVIEW

☐ Pediatrics is the branch of medicine dealing with the care and development of children and the diagnosis and treatment of diseases in children. A pediatrician is a medical doctor who specializes in pediatrics.

☐ There are two broad categories of pediatric patient office visits: the health maintenance visit and the sick child visit. The purpose of the health maintenance visit is to receive any necessary immunizations and to discover any abnormal conditions associated with the stage of development reached by the child. The sick child visit is to diagnose the condition of a child who is exhibiting the signs and symptoms of disease.

☐ To evaluate the progress of a child, the weight, height (or length), and head circumference are measured during each visit and plotted on a growth chart. The weight of a child is used to determine nutritional needs and the proper dosage of a medication to administer to the child. Growth charts provide a means for assessing the child's rate of growth; the physician investigates any significant change or rapid rise or drop in the child's growth pattern.

☐ A urine specimen may be required from a pediatric patient as part of a general physical examination, to assist in the diagnosis of a pathologic condition, or to evaluate the effectiveness of therapy. Collecting a urine specimen from an infant or young child who cannot urinate voluntarily involves the use of a pediatric urine collector.

☐ The same basic technique used to administer an IM injection to an adult is used for a child. The vastus lateralis site is recommended for infants and young children. It is large enough to accommodate the injected medication. The dorsogluteal site should not be used until the child has been walking for at least a year.

☐ Immunity is the resistance of the body to the effects of harmful agents such as pathogenic microorganisms or their toxins. Immunizations build up the body's defenses and protect an individual from attack by certain infectious diseases. Common immunizations administered to infants and children include: DPT vaccine, polio vaccine, MMR, *Haemophilus influenzae,* hepatitis B, and chickenpox.

☐ The National Childhood Vaccine Injury Act (NCVIA) requires that parents be provided with information about the benefits and risks of childhood immunizations through VISs (Vaccine Information Sheets) developed by the Centers for Disease Control and Prevention.

☐ Phenylketonuria (PKU) is a congenital hereditary disease. If left untreated, PKU can result in mental retardation and other abnormalities. Most states require that infants undergo PKU screening since early diagnosis and treatment can lead to a better patient prognosis. In addition to the PKU test, additional tests are performed on the blood specimen to screen for the presence of congenital hypothyroidism, galactosemia, and homocystinuria.

11

RESOURCE

ON THE WEB

For information on pediatrics:

American Academy of Pediatrics
www.aap.org

American SIDS Institute
sids-network.org

Children with Diabetes
www.childrenwithdiabetes.com

Dr. Greene's House Calls
www.drgreene.com

Kids Health
www.ama-assn.org/Kids-Health

Kids Health Organization
KidsHealth.org

The National Committee to Prevent Child Abuse
www.childabuse.org

Pediatrics Info
www.aub.edu/pedinfo

Tooth Fairy
www.asis.com/toothfairy

11

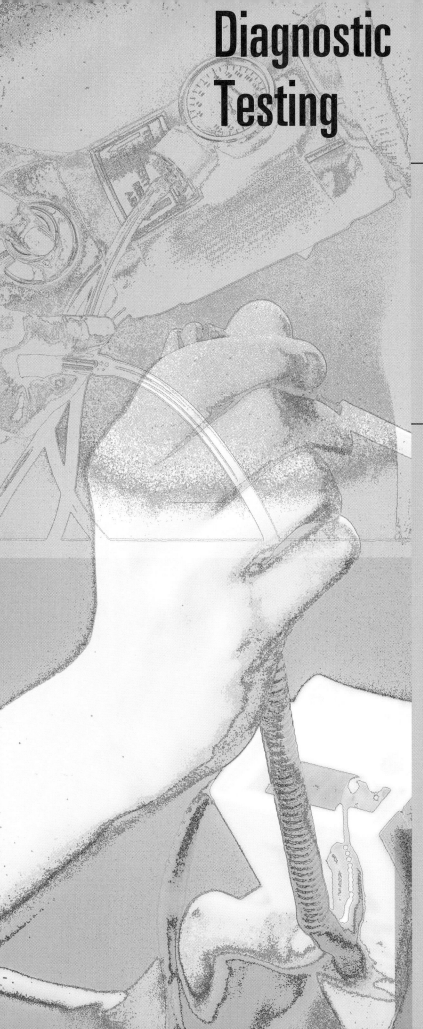

Diagnostic Testing

 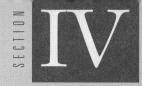
AAMA/CAAHEP COMPETENCIES INCLUDED IN THIS SECTION:

Clinical Competencies

Specimen Collection
- Instruct patients in the collection of fecal specimens.

Diagnostic Testing
- Perform electrocardiograms.
- Perform respiratory testing.

Patient Care
- Prepare and maintain examination and treatment areas.
- Prepare patient for and assist with routine and specialty examinations.

Transdisciplinary Competencies

Patient Instruction
- Instruct individuals according to their needs.
- Provide instruction for health maintenance and disease prevention.

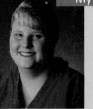

My name is

Janet Canterbury *and I am a Certified Medical Assistant. I graduated from an accredited medical assisting program with an associate's degree in Applied Science. I have worked as a medical assistant for 1 year. I run a medical laboratory, hook up and read Holter monitors, and perform pulmonary function tests and stress tests.*

The most interesting part of my job is the constant challenges that each patient presents. Every patient must be handled in a different way. I would like to go back to school one day to study physician assisting. When I first started school, I knew I wanted to continue my education, and medical assisting was the right first choice for me.

Cardiopulmonary Procedures

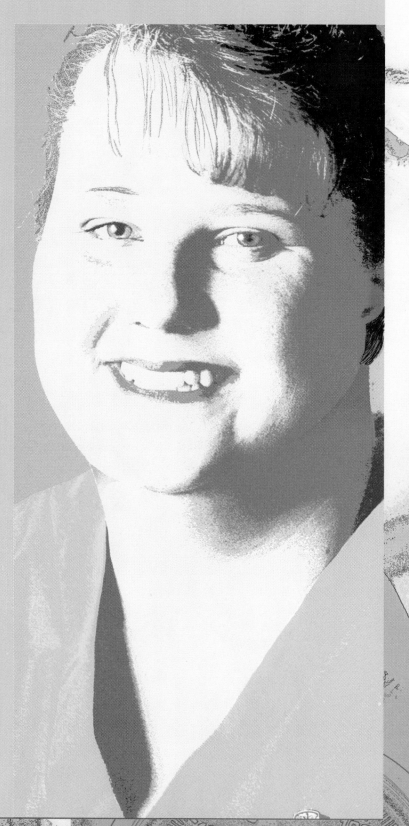

CHAPTER OUTLINE

Structure of the Heart
Conduction System of the
Heart
Cardiac Cycle
Waves
Baseline, Segments, and Intervals
Electrocardiograph Paper
Standardization of the Electrocardiograph
Electrocardiograph Leads
Bipolar Leads
Augmented Leads
Chest Leads
Maintenance of the Electrocardiograph
Electrocardiographic Capabilities
Three-Channel Recording
Capability
Telephone Transmission
Interpretive Electrocardiographs
Artifacts
Muscle
Wandering Baseline
Alternating Current
Interrupted Baseline
Holter Monitor Electrocardiography
Holter Monitor Electrode
Placement
Cardiac Arrhythmias
Atrial Premature Contraction
Paroxysmal Atrial Tachycardia
Atrial Flutter
Atrial Fibrillation
Premature Ventricular Contraction
Ventricular Tachycardia
Ventricular Fibrillation
Pulmonary Function Testing

OUTCOMES

After completing this chapter,
you should be able to demonstrate the proper procedures to
perform the following:

1. Record a 12-lead electrocardiogram.

2. Instruct a patient in the
   guidelines required for wearing a Holter monitor.
3. Apply a Holter monitor.

EDUCATIONAL OBJECTIVES

After completing this chapter,
you should be able to do the following:

1. Define the terms listed in
   the Key Terminology.
2. Trace the path the blood
   takes through the heart,
   starting with the right
   atrium.
3. Explain the conduction system of the heart.
4. State the purpose of electrocardiography.
5. Identify the following components on an electrocardiogram (ECG) and state what
   each represents: P wave,
   QRS complex, T wave, P–R
   interval, Q–T interval, P–R
   segment, S–T segment, and
   the baseline following the T
   (or U) wave.
6. State the purpose of the
   standardization mark.
7. State the function of the
   electrodes, amplifier, and
   galvanometer.
8. List the 12 ECG leads that
   are recorded and diagram
   the "picture" of the heart
   that each lead is taking.
9. Describe the function served
   by each of the following
   electrocardiographic capabilities: three-channel recorder,
   phone transmission, and interpretive electrocardiography.
10. Identify the following types
    of artifacts and state what
    may cause each to occur:
    muscle, wandering baseline,
    alternating current, and interrupted baseline.
11. Explain the purpose of Holter monitor electrocardiography.

12. List three reasons for applying a Holter monitor.
13. Explain the use of the patient diary in Holter monitor
    electrocardiography.
14. Identify the following cardiac arrhythmias and explain
    what causes each to occur:
    atrial premature contraction,
    paroxysmal atrial tachycardia,
    atrial flutter, atrial fibrillation, premature ventricular
    contraction, ventricular
    tachycardia, and ventricular
    fibrillation.
15. State the purpose of pulmonary function testing.

─────── **KEY TERMINOLOGY**

amplitude (AMP-li-TÛD): Refers to amount, extent, size, abundance, or fullness.

artifact: Additional electrical activity picked up by the electrocardiograph that interferes with the normal appearance of the ECG cycles.

baseline: The flat horizontal line that separates the various waves of the ECG cycle.

cardiac cycle: One complete heart beat.

ECG cycle: The graphic representation of a cardiac cycle.

electrocardiogram: The graphic representation of the electrical activity of the heart.

electrocardiograph (Ê-lek-trô-KAR-dê-ô-graf): The instrument used to record the electrical activity of the heart.

electrode (Ê-lek-TRÔD): A conductor of electricity, which is used to promote contact between the body and the electrocardiograph.

electrolyte (Ê-lek-TRÔ-lît): A chemical substance that promotes conduction of an electrical current.

interval: The length of a wave or the length of a wave with a segment.

ischemia (is-KÊM-ê-a): Deficiency of blood in a body part.

normal sinus rhythm: Refers to an electrocardiogram that is within normal limits.

segment: The portion of the ECG between two waves.

spirometer (SPÎ-rom-it-rê): An instrument for measuring air taken into and expelled from the lungs.

spirometry (SPÎ-rom-it-rê): Measurement of an individual's breathing capacity by means of a spirometer.

INTRODUCTION

12

☐ The **electrocardiograph** is an instrument used to record the electrical activity of the heart. The **electrocardiogram** (abbreviated ECG or EKG) is the graphic representation of this activity. The ECG exhibits the amount of electrical activity produced by the heart and the time required for the impulse to travel through the heart.

Electrocardiography is used for the following purposes: to detect an abnormal cardiac rhythm (arrhythmia); to help diagnose damage to the heart due to a myocardial infarction; to assess the effect on the heart of digitalis or other cardiac drugs; to determine the presence of an electrolyte imbalance; to assess the progress of rheumatic fever; and to determine the presence of hypertrophy of the heart chambers.

An ECG is not able to detect the presence of all cardiovascular disorders. In addition, it cannot always detect impending heart disease. The ECG is generally used in combination with other diagnostic and laboratory tests to assess cardiac functioning.

The medical assistant is frequently responsible for recording ECGs in the medical office. Because of this, knowledge and skill must be acquired in each of the following aspects of electrocardiography: preparation of the patient, operation of the electrocardiograph, identification and elimination of artifacts, labeling the completed ECG, and care and maintenance of the electrocardiograph.

Electrocardiographs are available in single-channel and three-channel recording formats. Because most medical offices use a three-channel ECG, the information presented in this chapter focuses on the three-channel electrocardiograph (Fig. 12–1).

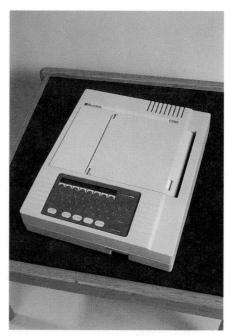

■ **FIGURE 12–1.** Example of a three-channel electrocardiograph.

STRUCTURE OF THE HEART

☐ The human heart consists of four chambers: the right and left atria are the upper chambers, and the right and left ventricles are the lower chambers (Fig. 12–2). Blood enters the right atrium from two large veins, the superior vena cava and the inferior vena cava, that bring it back from its circulation through the body. The blood entering the right atrium is deoxygenated, meaning it contains very little oxygen and is high in carbon dioxide.

From the right atrium, the blood enters the right ventricle. It is pumped from here to the lungs by way of the pulmonary artery. It picks up oxygen in the lungs in exchange for carbon dioxide and returns to the left atrium of the heart by way of the pulmonary veins. From the left atrium, the blood enters the left ventricle. This is the most powerful chamber of the heart and serves to pump blood to the entire body. Blood exits from the left ventricle by way of the aorta, which distributes it to all parts of the body to nourish the tissues with oxygen and nutrients.

CONDUCTION SYSTEM OF THE HEART

☐ The **sinoatrial node (SA node)** is located in the upper portion of the right atrium, just below the opening of the superior vena cava. It consists of a knot of modified myocardial cells that have the ability to send out an electrical impulse without an external nerve stimulus. In this way the SA node initiates and regulates the heart beat.

Each electrical impulse discharged by the SA node is distributed to the right and left atria and causes them to contract. This contraction forces blood through the open cuspid valves and into the ventricles. The impulse is then picked up by the **atrioventricular node (AV node),** another knot of modified myocardial cells located at the base of the right atrium. Its function is to transmit the electrical impulse to the **bundle of His.** The AV node delays the impulse momentarily to give the ventricles a chance to fill with blood from the atria.

The bundle of His divides into right and left branches known as the **bundle branches,** which then relay the impulse to the **Purkinje fibers.** The Purkinje fibers distribute the impulse evenly to the right and left ventricles, causing them to contract; this forces blood out of the ventricles and into the pulmonary artery and aorta. The entire heart relaxes momentarily. Then a new impulse is initiated by the SA node and the cycle repeats itself (Fig. 12–3).

CARDIAC CYCLE

☐ The **cardiac cycle** represents one complete heart beat. It consists of the contraction of the atria, the

12

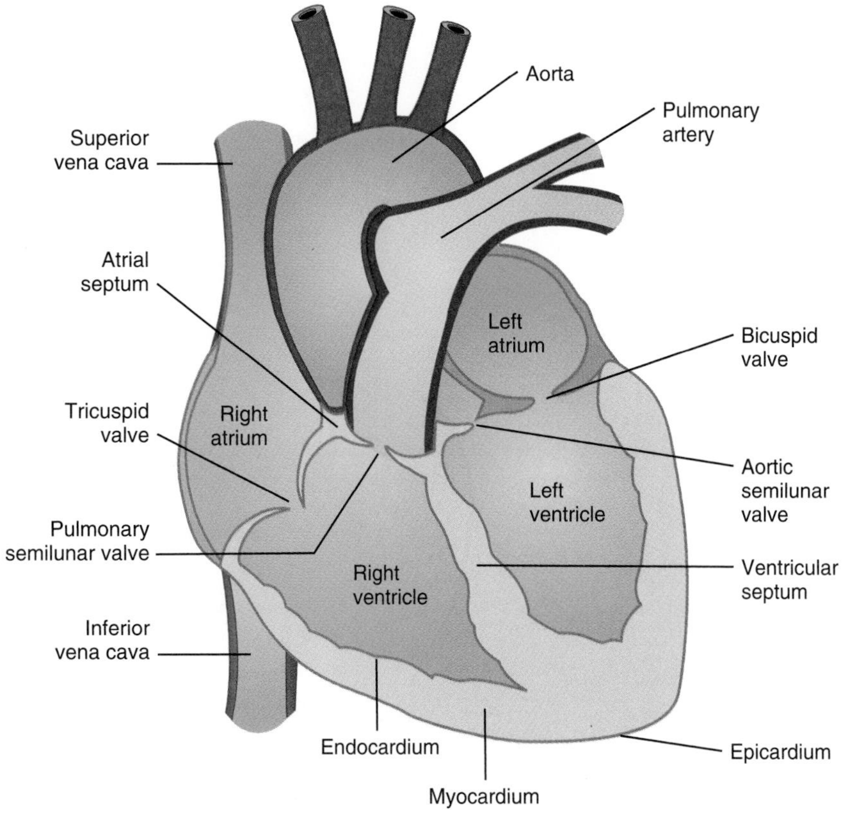

■ **FIGURE 12–2.** Diagram of the heart, identifying the structures.

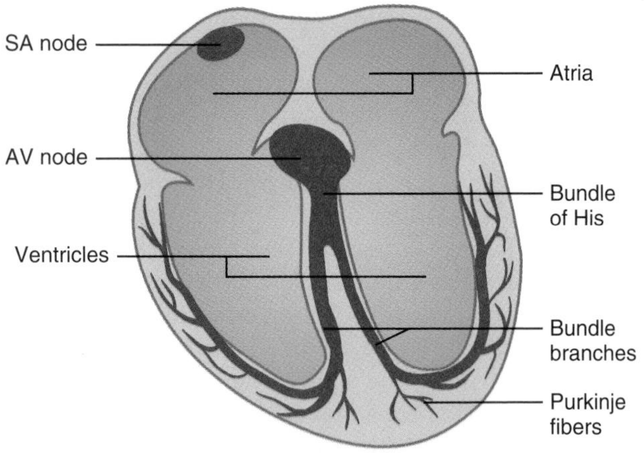

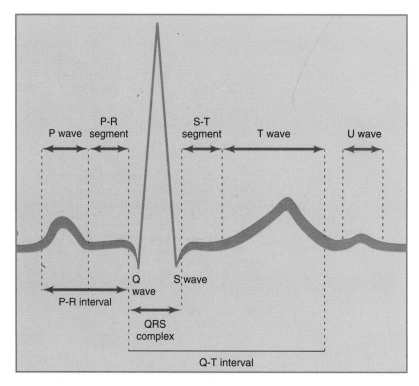

SA node

AV node

Ventricles

Atria

Bundle of His

Bundle branches

Purkinje fibers

■ **FIGURE 12–3.** Diagram of the heart, identifying the structures involved with the conduction of an electrical impulse through the heart.

WAVES

contraction of the ventricles, and the relaxation of the entire heart (as described previously). The electrocardiograph records the electrical activity that causes these events in the cardiac cycle to occur. The **ECG cycle** is the graphic representation of the cardiac cycle (Fig. 12–4).

WAVES

The normal ECG cycle consists of a P wave; the Q, R, and S waves (known as the QRS complex); and a T wave. The ECG cycle is recorded from left to right, beginning with the P wave.

P WAVE. The P wave represents the electrical activity associated with the contraction of the atria, or **atrial depolarization.**

QRS COMPLEX. The QRS complex represents the electrical activity associated with the contraction of the ventricles, or **ventricular depolarization.**

T WAVE. The T wave represents the electrical recovery of the ventricles, or **ventricular repolarization.** The muscle cells are recovering in preparation for another impulse.

U WAVE. Occasionally, a U wave is seen following the T wave. It is a small wave and is associated in some as yet undefined way with repolarization.

BASELINE, SEGMENTS, AND INTERVALS

The flat, horizontal line that separates the various waves is known as the **baseline.** The waves deflect either upward (positive deflection) or downward (negative deflection) from the baseline. The baseline is divided into segments and intervals for the purpose of interpretation and analysis of the ECG by the physician. A **segment** is the portion of the ECG between two waves, and an **interval** is the length of a wave or the length of a wave with a segment.

12

■ **FIGURE 12–4.** The ECG cycle.

P wave

P-R segment

S-T segment

T wave

U wave

Q wave

S wave

P-R interval

QRS complex

Q-T interval

P–R SEGMENT. The P–R segment represents the time interval from the end of the atrial depolarization to the beginning of the ventricular depolarization. It is the time needed for the impulse to travel from the AV node through the bundle of His and Purkinje fibers to the ventricles.

S–T SEGMENT. The S–T segment represents the time interval from the end of the ventricular depolarization to the beginning of repolarization of the ventricles.

P–R INTERVAL. The P–R interval represents the time lapse from the beginning of the atrial depolarization to the beginning of the ventricular depolarization.

Q–T INTERVAL. The Q–T interval is the time from the beginning of the ventricular depolarization to the end of repolarization of the ventricles. The baseline occurring after the T wave (or U wave, if present) represents the period when the entire heart returns to its resting, or **polarized,** state.

ELECTROCARDIOGRAPH PAPER

☐ Electrocardiograph paper is divided into two sets of squares for accurate and convenient measurement of the waves, intervals, and segments by the physician (Fig. 12–5). Each small square is 1 millimeter (mm) high and 1 mm wide. Each large square (made up of 25 small squares) is 5 mm high and 5 mm wide. By measuring the various waves, intervals, and segments of the graph cycle, the physician is able to determine whether the electrical activity of the heart falls within normal limits.

Electrocardiograph paper consists of a black or blue base with a white plastic coating. A black or red graph is printed on top of the plastic coating. A heated stylus moves over the heat-sensitive paper and melts away the plastic coating, resulting in the recording of the ECG cycles. In addition to being heat sensitive, the paper is pressure sensitive and should be handled carefully to avoid making impressions that would interfere with its proper reading.

STANDARDIZATION OF THE ELECTROCARDIOGRAPH

☐ The electrocardiograph machine must be standardized when recording an ECG. This ensures an accurate and reliable recording. It means that an ECG run on one electrocardiograph will compare with a tracing run on another machine.

By international agreement, 1 millivolt (mV) of electricity should cause the stylus to move 10 mm high in amplitude (10 small squares). A three-channel electrocardiograph automatically records standardization marks on the tracing. During the recording, the machine allows 1 mV to enter the electrocardiograph machine, which should result in an upward deflection of 10 mm. The marking on the ECG paper is known as the **standardization mark** (Fig. 12–6). The width of the mark made by the machine is approximately 2 mm (two small squares). If the standardization mark is more or less than 10 mm in amplitude, it can be adjusted. The instruction manual must be consulted for proper adjustment information. An electrocardiograph must never be adjusted for the first time without use of the instruction manual.

12

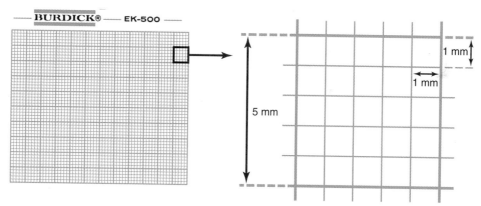

■ **FIGURE 12–5.** Diagram of ECG paper with a section enlarged to indicate the size of the large and small squares.

Highlight—Exercise Tolerance Testing (Stress Testing)

Exercise tolerance testing, also called stress testing, is a diagnostic procedure used to evaluate the cardiovascular system. It is usually performed in a hospital setting under the direction of a cardiologist and an exercise tolerance technician, so that emergency equipment and trained personnel are available to deal with unusual situations that may arise.

The purpose of exercise tolerance testing is as follows:

1. To diagnose ischemic heart disease that cannot be detected by a standard resting electrocardiogram. **Ischemic heart disease** is heart disease that occurs as a result of inadequate blood supply to the myocardium, as in a myocardial infarction and angina pectoris.
2. To assist in evaluating the cause of cardiac symptoms, such as chest discomfort and arrhythmias.
3. To assess the effectiveness of cardiac drug therapy.
4. To follow the course of rehabilitation after a myocardial infarction or a cardiac surgical procedure like a coronary bypass operation.
5. As a health screening measure to determine an individual's fitness for a strenuous exercise program, such as jogging.

Exercise tolerance testing involves the continuous electrocardiographic monitoring of an individual during physical exercise. The patient's blood pressure, heart rate, and physical symptoms are also monitored during the test. The exercising is accomplished by having the patient use a treadmill, stationary bicycle, or two-step staircase. The intensity of the physical exertion is gradually increased until the patient's target heart rate is reached unless the signs and symptoms of cardiac ischemia appear, in which case the test is stopped. These symptoms include claudication (severe leg pain), severe dyspnea, chest discomfort or pain, pallor, and dizziness.

The individual's response to the exercise tolerance testing is used to determine normal or abnormal results. For example, a normal response is a gradual increase in the patient's blood pressure as the level of physical exertion increases, whereas an abnormal response is a sudden increase or decrease of the patient's blood pressure. The electrocardiogram of a normal individual exhibits a shortened P–R interval and a compressed QRS complex. An abnormal tracing indicative of myocardial ischemia results in a depressed S–T segment and an inverted T-wave. An abnormal exercise tolerance test usually warrants further testing, such as cardiac arteriography.

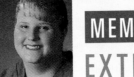

Normal Standard
Standardization mark is
10 mm high

■ **FIGURE 12–6.** Standardization mark.

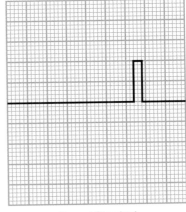

MEMORIES *from* EXTERNSHIP

JANET CANTERBURY: *On my last externship, I was at an urgent care facility in a fairly large city where anything could happen. One night as I was checking in patients, an elderly woman came in complaining of a severe headache. The woman was very disoriented and unable to give us any information. Her daughter told us that she was visiting from California and that she was a registered nurse. Aware that the woman had a history of strokes, the physician hooked her up to a heart monitor and examined her. While she was being examined she had a seizure. We called the ambulance to transport her to a local hospital. The whole time this was happening, I was trying to help the physician get an ECG, keep track of the heart monitor, and obtain health history information from the woman's daughter. That night I got a taste of what it would be like in an emergency room.*

12

ELECTROCARDIOGRAPH LEADS

☐ The standard electrocardiograph consists of 12 leads. Each lead records the heart's electrical activity from a different angle. The 12 leads provide an electrical "photograph" of the heart from different angles; this allows for a thorough three-dimensional interpretation of the heart's activity.

The electrical impulses given off by the heart are picked up by **electrodes** and conducted into the machine through lead wires. Electrodes are made of a substance that is a good conductor of electricity. The amount of electrical activity emitted by the body is very small. Therefore, to produce a readable ECG, it must be made larger, or amplified, by a device known as an **amplifier,** located within the electrocardiograph. The amplified voltages are changed into mechanical motion by the **galvanometer** and recorded on the electrocardiograph paper by a heated stylus (Fig. 12–7).

There are four limb electrodes, which include the right arm electrode (RA), the left arm electrode (LA), the right leg electrode (RL), and the left leg electrode (LL). The right leg electrode is known as the ground. It is not used for the actual recording but serves as an electrical reference point. The chest leads are abbreviated V or C and use six chest electrodes.

Disposable electrodes are typically used with a three-channel electrocardiograph. A disposable electrode consists of a self-adhesive tab containing an electrolyte. An **electrolyte** is a substance that facilitates the transmission of the electrical impulse given off by the heart. The electrode is applied to the skin and held in place with its adhesive backing and then thrown away after use.

BIPOLAR LEADS

The first three leads making up the 12-lead ECG are the bipolar leads; they are leads I, II, and III. The

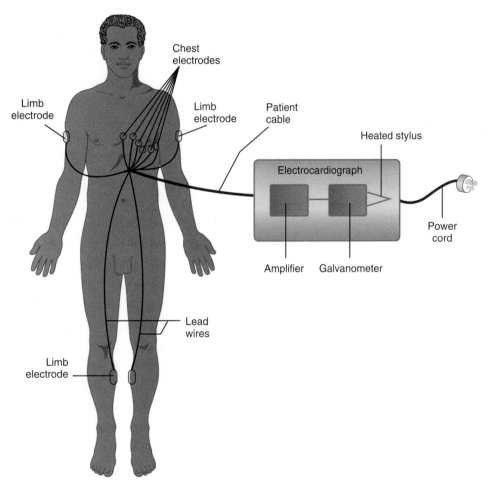

■ **FIGURE 12–7.** Diagram of the basic components of the electrocardiograph. The limb electrodes are attached to the fleshy parts of the limbs, and the lead wires are arranged to follow body contour. The patient cable is not dangling, and the power cord points away from the electrocardiograph.

bipolar leads use two of the limb electrodes to record the electrical activity given off by the heart. Lead I records the heart's voltage difference between the right arm and the left arm, lead II records the difference between the right arm and the left leg, and lead III records the difference between the left arm and the left leg (Fig. 12–8).

Lead II shows the heart's rhythm more clearly than the other leads. Because of this, the physician often requests a **rhythm strip,** which is a longer recording (approximately 12 inches) of lead II.

AUGMENTED LEADS

The next three leads are the augmented leads. They include aVR (augmented voltage—right arm), aVL (augmented voltage—left arm), and aVF (augmented voltage—left leg or foot). Lead aVR records the heart's voltage difference between the right arm electrode and a central point between the left arm and left leg. Lead aVL records the heart's voltage difference between the left arm electrode and a central point between the right arm and left leg. Lead aVF records the heart's voltage difference between the left leg electrode and a central point between the right arm and left arm. Leads I, II, III, aVR, aVL, and aVF record the voltage from side to side or from top to bottom of the heart (Fig. 12–8).

CHEST LEADS

The last six leads are the chest leads, or precordial leads. They are V_1, V_2, V_3, V_4, V_5, and V_6. These leads record the heart's voltage from the front to the back of the heart. The voltage is recorded from a central point from "within" the heart to a point on the chest wall at which the electrode is placed. These points are the location of each chest lead. Figure 12–9 shows the proper location of the six chest leads. The medical assistant should be able to locate each one accurately. When first learning to locate the chest leads, it helps to mark their location on the patient's chest with a felt-tipped pen.

Normally, the electrocardiogram is recorded with the paper moving at a speed of 25 mm/sec. Occasionally, the ECG cycles may be very close together, making the recording difficult to read. The medical assistant can change the paper speed to 50 mm/sec to help spread the cycles apart. To alert the physician to the change, he or she must make a notation of it by writing it on the recording.

MAINTENANCE OF THE ELECTROCARDIOGRAPH

☐ Electrocardiographs require very little preventive maintenance. The electrocardiograph should be

12

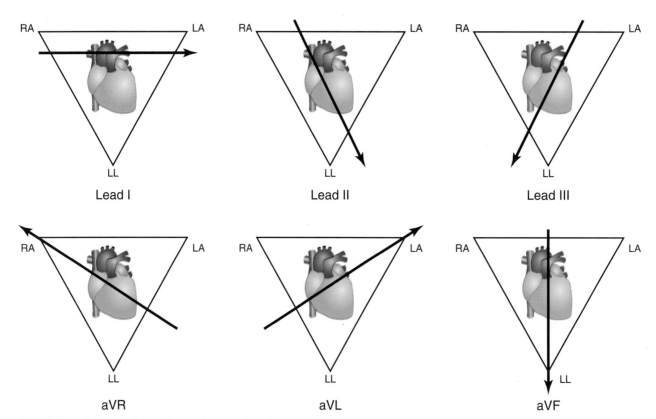

■ **FIGURE 12–8.** Diagram of the different pictures taken of the heart's voltage for leads I, II, III. aVR, aVL, and aVF.

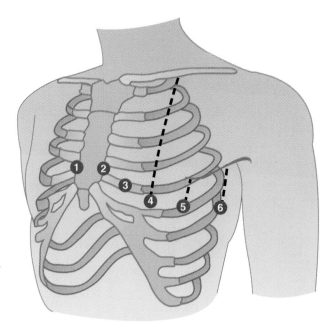

FIGURE 12–9. Recommended position for ECG chest leads:

V_1, Fourth intercostal space at right margin of sternum.
V_2, Fourth intercostal space at left margin of sternum.
V_3, Midway between position 2 and position 4.
V_4, Fifth intercostal space at junction of left midclavicular line.
V_5, At horizontal level of position 4 at left anterior axillary line.
V_6, At horizontal level of position 4 at left midaxillary line.

cleaned frequently with a mild detergent using a soft cloth to remove dust and dirt. Commercial solvents and abrasives should not be used as they can damage the finish.

The electrode cables should periodically be cleaned with a cloth saturated with a disinfectant cleaner. The cables should never be immersed in the cleaning solution as this could damage them.

ELECTROCARDIOGRAPHIC CAPABILITIES

☐ Electrocardiographs have a variety of capabilities that permit specific recording options. These capabilities are listed and described here.

THREE-CHANNEL RECORDING CAPABILITY

An electrocardiograph with a three-channel recording capability can simultaneously record three different leads. This is in contrast to a single-channel electrocardiograph, which records only one lead at a time. The advantage is that an ECG can be produced in a shorter period of time than would be required if each lead were being recorded separately.

The leads that are recorded simultaneously are Leads I, II, and III, followed by aVR, aVL, and aVF, followed by V_1, V_2, and V_3, followed by V_4, V_5, and

V_6. To record three leads at one time, a three-channel recording paper must be used, which is designed in a standard 8½ by 11 inch format. This type of printout fits easily into the patient's chart. Most three-channel electrocardiographs have a **copy capability** that quickly produces an accurate recording of the last ECG recorded. Refer to Figure 12–10 for an example of a three-channel ECG recording.

TELEPHONE TRANSMISSION

An electrocardiograph with telephone transmission capabilities can transmit a recording over the telephone line to an ECG data interpretation site. The electrocardiograph is equipped with a connector well interface for the attachment of the telephone headset. The recording is interpreted by a cardiologist or a computer at the data site, and a printout of the recording along with the interpretation is mailed back to the office the same day. Patient information and baseline data (e.g., age, sex, height, weight, medications) also need to be relayed to assist in the interpretation. This information is entered on the electrocardiograph and transmitted automatically.

INTERPRETIVE ELECTROCARDIOGRAPHS

An electrocardiograph with interpretive capabilities has a built-in computer program that analyzes the recording as it is being run. Interpretive electrocardiographs provide immediate information on the heart's activity, leading to earlier diagnosis and treatment. Patient data are used in the interpretation of the ECG and must therefore be entered into the computer before running the recording. The data generally required include the patient's age, sex, height, weight, and medications. The computer analysis of the ECG is printed out at the top of the recording along with the reason for each interpretation (Fig. 12–11). The results are then reviewed and further interpreted by the physician before diagnosis is made and treatment is initiated.

ARTIFACTS

☐ The medical assistant is responsible for producing a clear and concise ECG recording that can be easily read and interpreted by the physician. At times, structures appear in the recording that are not natural and that interfere with the normal appearance of the ECG cycles. They are known as **artifacts** and represent additional electrical activity that is picked up by the electrocardiograph. The medical assistant should be able to identify artifacts and correct them.

12

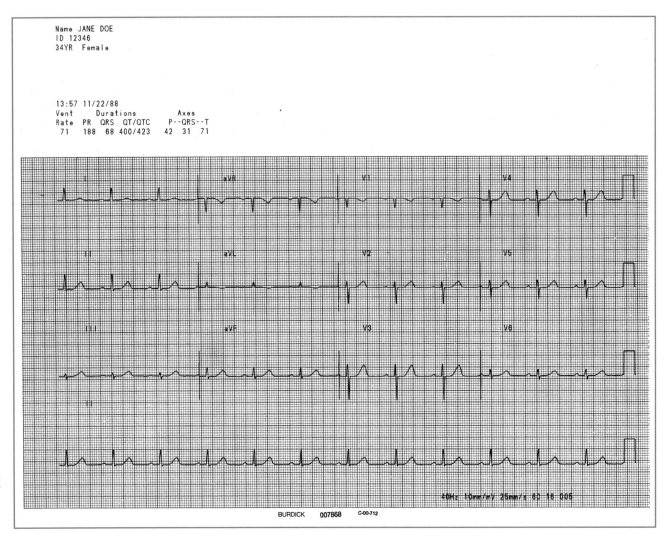

```
Name JANE DOE
ID 12346
34YR Female


13:57 11/22/88
Vent    Durations      Axes
Rate PR QRS QT/QTC   P--QRS--T
 71  188 68 400/423  42  31  71
```

BURDICK   007868   C-00-712

■ FIGURE 12–10. Example of a three-channel ECG. (Courtesy of the Burdick Corporation, Milton, Wisconsin.)

12

There are several types of artifacts; the most common ones are muscle, wandering baseline, and alternating current (AC) (Fig. 12–12).

In some circumstances, as when individuals have trouble holding still or in buildings with older electrical systems, normal methods to eliminate muscle and AC artifacts may not be successful. Electrocardiographs have an **artifact filter** that can be used to reduce artifacts when all else fails. However, because the artifact filter also affects the diagnostic accuracy of the ECG, it should be used as little as possible.

If the medical assistant is unable to correct an artifact, the physician should be consulted. It is possible that the machine itself is broken. If an electrocardiograph service technician has to be contacted, the medical assistant should have the following information available to aid the service technician in locating the problem:

1. What has already been done to locate and correct the problem.
2. Leads in which the artifacts occur.
3. A sample of the artifact as recorded by the machine.

MUSCLE

A muscle artifact (see Fig. 12–12A) can be identified by its fuzzy, irregular baseline. There are two types of muscle artifacts: those resulting from involuntary muscle movement (somatic tremor) and those resulting from voluntary muscle movement. Muscle artifacts may be caused by the following:

1. **An apprehensive patient.** Explaining the procedure and reassuring the patient that having an ECG recorded is a painless procedure can help reduce apprehension and relax muscles.

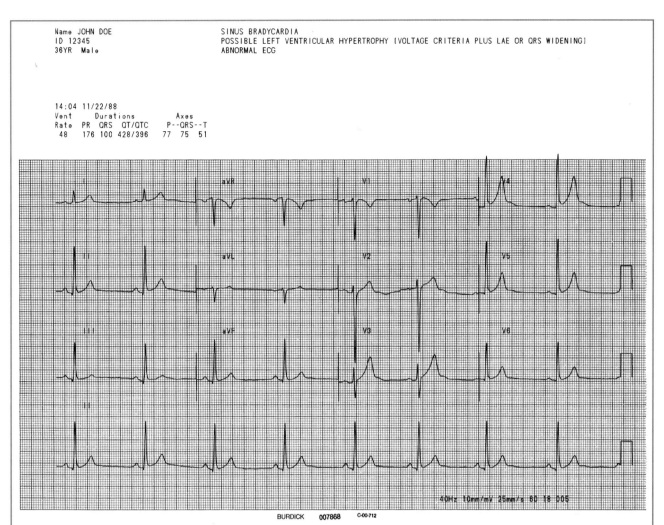

Name JOHN DOE
ID 12345
36YR Male

SINUS BRADYCARDIA
POSSIBLE LEFT VENTRICULAR HYPERTROPHY [VOLTAGE CRITERIA PLUS LAE OR QRS WIDENING]
ABNORMAL ECG

14:04 11/22/88

Vent	Durations		Axes
Rate	PR QRS QT/QTC		P--QRS--T
48	176 100 428/396		77 75 51

FIGURE 12–11. Example of an ECG recording that has been analyzed by an interpretive electrocariograph. The computer analysis is printed out at the top of the recording, along with the reason for each interpretation. (Courtesy of the Burdick Corporation, Milton, Wisconsin.)

2. **Patient discomfort.** Make sure the table is wide enough to support the patient's arms and legs adequately. The patient can be made more comfortable by placing a pillow under his or her head. Check to make sure that the room temperature is comfortable for the patient. A temperature that is warm enough for the medical assistant may be too cold for the patient who has removed clothing. This could result in shivering, which would also produce a muscle artifact on the ECG.

3. **Patient movement.** The patient must be instructed to lie still and not talk during the recording.

4. **A physical condition.** Several nervous system disorders, such as Parkinson's disease, prevent relaxation, and the patient trembles continually. The medical assistant must be understanding and try to record while the tremor is at a minimum.

WANDERING BASELINE

A wandering baseline (see Fig. 12–12B) may be caused by the following:

1. **Electrodes that are too loose.** The medical assistant should make sure the disposable adhesive electrodes are firmly attached to the patient's skin. If an electrode pulls loose, it can be reattached using nonallergenic tape. The alligator clips should be firmly attached to the electrodes; the patient cable should be firmly supported and should not be allowed to dangle (this prevents pulling or twisting of the cable).

2. **Body creams, oils, or lotions** present on the skin in the area where the electrode is applied. The medical assistant should remove these by rubbing with alcohol, using friction.

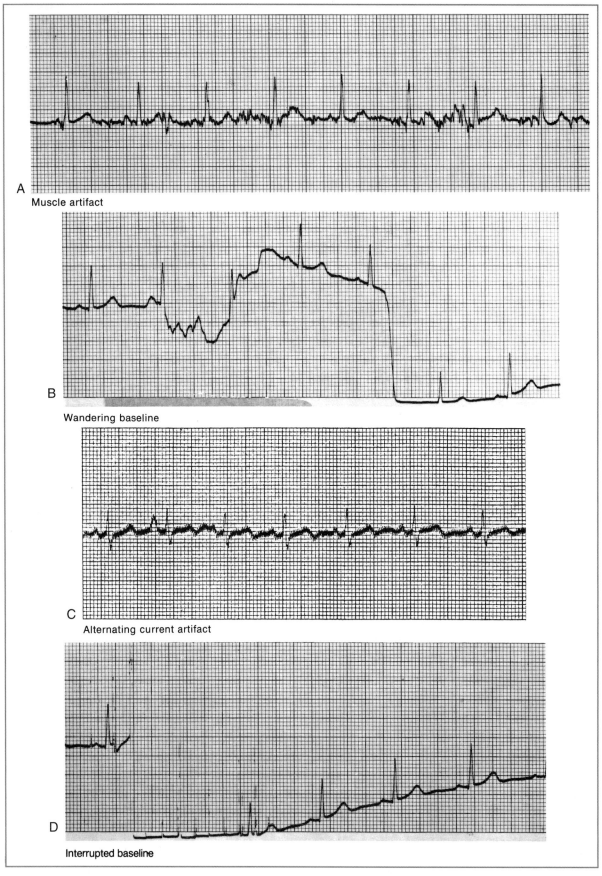

A
Muscle artifact

B
Wandering baseline

C
Alternating current artifact

D
Interrupted baseline

FIGURE 12–12. *A* to *D,* Examples of artifacts. (Courtesy of Burdick Corporation, Milton, Wisconsin.)

ALTERNATING CURRENT

Alternating current artifacts (see Fig. 12–12C) are caused by electrical interference. Alternating current can "leak" or spread out from the power used by other electrical appliances in the medical office. This current may be picked up by the patient and carried into the electrocardiograph, where it would show up on the ECG recording as an AC artifact. An AC artifact appears as small straight spiked lines that are consistent in nature. Alternating current artifacts may be caused by the following:

1. **Improper grounding of the electrocardiograph.** The machine is automatically grounded when it is plugged in. Make sure the plug is firmly secure to the wall outlet. The right leg electrode is not used for recording the leads but picks up alternating current present on the patient and carries it into the electrocardiograph. The alternating current is then carried away by the machine's grounding system.

2. **Electrical equipment present in the room.** Lamps, autoclaves, x-ray equipment, electrical examining tables, or other electrical equipment that is plugged in may be leaking alternating current. Unplug all nearby electrical equipment in the room.

3. **Wiring present in the walls, ceilings, or floors.** Try moving the patient table to a new location away from the walls.

4. **Lead wires not following body contour.** Dangling lead wires can pick up alternating current. Arrange the wires to follow body contour and to lie flat.

INTERRUPTED BASELINE

Occasionally, an interrupted baseline (see Fig. 12–12D) occurs that may be caused by the metal tip of a lead wire becoming detached or by a broken patient cable. If the latter is the case, the manufacturer should be contacted for directions on replacing the patient cable.

PROCEDURE

12–1

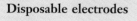

Running a 12-Lead Electrocardiogram—Three Channel

12

EQUIPMENT/SUPPLIES:	Three-channel electrocardiograph ECG paper	Disposable electrodes

1. **Procedural Step.** Work in a quiet, relaxing atmosphere away from nearby sources of electrical interference.

2. **Procedural Step.** Wash the hands. Greet and identify the patient. Introduce yourself, and explain the procedure.
   Principle. Explaining the procedure helps reassure apprehensive patients.

3. **Procedural Step.** Prepare the patient. Ask him or her to remove clothing from the waist up. The lower legs must also be uncovered. Properly drape the patient over the uncovered body parts to prevent exposure and to provide warmth. The patient should be placed in a supine position on the table. The table should support the arms and legs adequately, so that they do not dangle. A

pillow can be used to support the patient's head.
   Principle. The chest, upper arms, and lower legs must be uncovered to allow for proper placement of the electrodes. The patient should be kept warm, and the arms and legs should not be allowed to dangle; otherwise, muscle artifacts could result.

4. **Procedural Step.** Help the patient relax by explaining the procedure. Tell the individual that having an ECG recording is painless. Explain that he or she must lie still and not talk in order for an accurate recording to be obtained.
   Principle. The patient should be mentally and physically relaxed for an accurate ECG recording, because an apprehensive or moving patient produces muscle artifacts.

Continued

12

5. **Procedural Step.** Position the electrocardiograph so that the power cord points away from the patient and does not pass under the table. It is usually easier for the medical assistant to work on the left side of the patient.

Principle. Proper positioning of the electrocardiograph reduces AC artifacts.

6. **Procedural Step.** Prepare the patient's skin for application of the disposable electrodes. If the patient has oily skin or has used lotions, wipe the area to which the electrode will be applied with alcohol and allow it to dry.

Principle. The patient's skin must be dry and oil-free so that the adhesive backing of the electrodes will stick to the patient's skin and stay on during the procedure.

7. **Procedural Step.** Apply limb electrodes. Firmly apply the adhesive backing of the electrodes to the fleshy part of each of the four limbs (upper arms and lower legs). The tab of the arm electrodes should point downward, and the tab of the leg electrodes should point upward. The adhesive backing of the electrode allows it to adhere firmly to the patient's skin.

Principle. The tab of the electrodes should be positioned toward the cable to provide a more stable

connection when the lead wire is attached to the electrode and to prevent the lead wires from pulling and causing artifacts.

8. **Procedural Step.** Apply the chest electrodes. Properly locate each chest position and apply the electrode with the tab of the electrodes pointing downward.

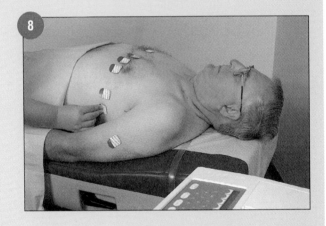

Principle. Positioning the tab of the electrodes downward prevents the lead wires from pulling and causing artifacts.

9. **Procedural Step.** Connect the lead wires to the electrodes. This is accomplished by inserting an alligator clip onto the metal tip of each electrode. The alligator clip is then attached to the tab of each electrode. The ends of the lead wires are usually color coded and identified with abbreviations to help the medical assistant connect the proper one to each electrode. Arrange the lead wires to follow body contour.

Principle. Arranging the lead wires to follow body contour reduces the possibility of AC artifacts.

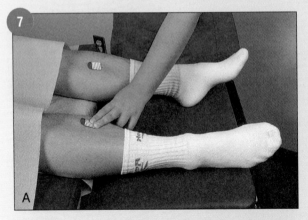

A

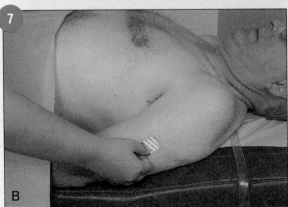

B

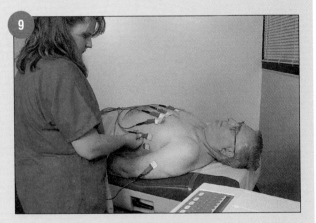

PROCEDURE 12–1

10. **Procedural Step.** Plug the patient cable into the machine. The cable should be supported on the table or on the patient's abdomen to prevent pulling or twisting.

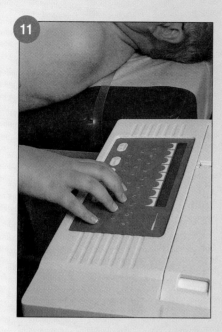

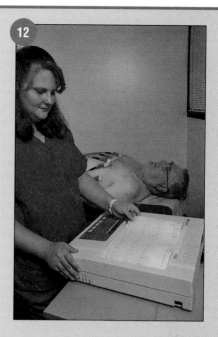

11. **Procedural Step.** Turn on the electrocardiograph. Enter patient data using the soft-touch keypad. Always use your fingertips to enter the data. Pencils or other sharp objects can damage the keyboard. As the data are entered, they will be displayed on the LCD screen. The patient data to be entered generally include the patient's name, a patient identification number, age, sex, height, weight, and medications.

Principle. The patient data are printed out at the top of the recording, along with the date and time of the recording. If the electrocardiograph is equipped with interpretive capabilities, this information is also used in the computer-assisted interpretation of the ECG.

12. **Procedural Step.** Press the AUTO (automatic) button and run the recording. The machine automatically inserts a standardization mark at the beginning of the recording, followed by the recording of

the 12-lead electrocardiogram in a three-channel format. Observe for artifacts appearing in the recording. If they occur, correct the problem and run another ECG.

13. **Procedural Step.** Turn the machine off. Disconnect the lead wires. Remove and discard the electrodes.

14. **Procedural Step.** Assist the patient in stepping down from the table.

15. **Procedural Step.** Wash the hands. Chart the procedure. Include the date and time and the name of the procedure (12-lead electrocardiogram). Place the recording in the appropriate place to be reviewed by the physician.

16. **Procedural Step.** Return all equipment to its proper place.

12

CHARTING EXAMPLE

Date	
6/12/2002	10:30 a.m. Completed a 12-lead ECG. ——————————— J. Canterbury, CMA

HOLTER MONITOR ELECTROCARDIOGRAPHY

☐ A Holter monitor is a portable ambulatory monitoring system for recording the cardiac activity of a patient over a 24-hour period. The system is designed so that the patient is able to maintain his or her usual daily activities with minimal inconvenience while being monitored. Holter monitor electrocardiography is an important noninvasive procedure used to diagnose cardiac rhythm and conduction abnormalities. It is most frequently used to evaluate patients with unexplained syncope, to discover cardiac arrhythmias that are intermittent in nature and not picked up on a routine 12-lead ECG, to assess the effectiveness of antiarrhythmic medications (e.g., digitalis and antianginal drugs), and to assess the effectiveness of the functioning of an artificial pacemaker.

The Holter monitor consists of electrodes that are placed on the patient's chest and a special portable magnetic tape recorder that continually monitors the heart's activity (Fig. 12–13). The lightweight, battery-powered recorder is held in a protective case, which is worn either on a belt around the patient's waist or hung over the patient's shoulder by a strap. Throughout the 24-hour period, the system continuously records the patient's heart beat on a magnetic tape. Depending on the brand of monitor, the magnetic tape may be either a cassette tape or a reel-to-reel tape.

An increasing number of physicians have Holter monitors in their offices. The medical assistant is responsible for preparing the patient, applying and removing the monitor, and instructing the patient in the guidelines for the procedure (Table 12–1).

The effectiveness of the monitor should be checked after hooking up the patient to make sure a clear signal is being relayed from the electrodes to the recorder. This is performed by attaching one end of an accessory device known as a **test cable** to the recorder and the other end to an electrocardiograph machine. A short baseline strip is then recorded and observed for correct waveforms and the absence of artifacts. If the waveforms are incorrect or if artifacts are present, the patient may not be hooked up properly, or a cable or lead malfunction may exist. The medical assistant

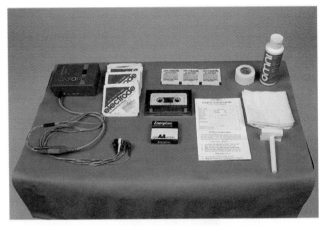

FIGURE 12–13. Holter monitor, including the supplies required for its application.

should reconnect the leads and reposition the electrodes. If a problem still exists, the monitor may be malfunctioning and in need of repair.

An important aspect of the Holter monitor procedure is the completion of an **activity diary** by the patient (Fig. 12–14). All activities and emotional states (e.g., stress, anger) must be recorded during the monitoring period, along with the time of their occurrence. In addition, any symptoms experienced by the patient, such as vertigo, syncope, palpitations, chest pain, and dyspnea, must be recorded, along with the time of their occurrence. As a result, any arrhythmia recorded on the magnetic tape can be compared with reports in the patient's diary to correlate patient symptoms with cardiac activity.

TABLE 12–1

Holter Monitor Patient Guidelines

The following guidelines must be relayed to the patient to ensure an accurate and reliable electrocardiographic recording

1. The electrodes and monitor must be kept dry to ensure an accurate recording and prevent damage to the recorder. The patient is not permitted to shower, bathe, or swim while wearing the monitor.
2. The electrodes should not be touched or moved during the monitoring period to prevent artifacts from appearing in the recording.
3. The monitor should not be handled or taken out of its carrying case.
4. The event marker should be depressed only momentarily when a significant symptom or event is recorded. Overuse of the marker may cause masking of the ECG signals that are being relayed from the electrodes.

5. An electric blanket should not be used during the monitoring period.
6. The patient must keep a diary of activities, emotional states, and symptoms (e.g., chest pain, nausea, dizziness) experienced during the monitoring period. The time of occurrence of each of the above must accompany each entry in the diary.
7. The patient should record the following activities in his or her diary: physical exercise, walking up or down stairs, emotional states, smoking, bowel movements, meals (including alcohol and caffeine beverages), sexual intercourse, medications consumed, and sleep periods.

PATIENT ACTIVITY DIARY		
TIME	ACTIVITY	SYMPTOM
AM PM	*Start recording*	
8:30 AM	Ate breakfast Smoked cigarette	
9:15 AM	Driving freeway	Chest pounding
10:35 AM	Argued with boss	Chest pounding
10:45 AM	Took medication	
12:30 PM	Ate lunch	Relaxed
1:15 PM	Walked up two flights of stairs	Stomach burning Pain in left arm

Page 1

PATIENT ACTIVITY DIARY		
TIME	ACTIVITY	SYMPTOM

Page 2

■ **FIGURE 12-14.** Holter monitor activity diary.

Some monitors have an **event marker** mounted on one end of the recorder; the event marker is used along with the patient diary for patient evaluation. The patient should be told to depress the event marker momentarily when experiencing a symptom. Depressing the marker places an electronic signal on the magnetic tape. This signal will later alert the technician to a significant event on the tape.

At the end of the 24-hour period, the Holter monitor system is removed from the patient, and the tape is evaluated either by displaying it on a special Holter scanning screen or by computer analysis. Printouts of any portion of the electrocardiographic recording can be obtained for further study. The tape must be analyzed where a trained technician and Holter scanner or computer are available. This may involve transferring the tape and diary to the cardiac department of a hospital for evaluation. The physician is provided with a written data report of the 24-hour period along with selected printouts of the patient's cardiac activity, including samples of any arrhythmias or abnormalities exhibited by the patient.

12

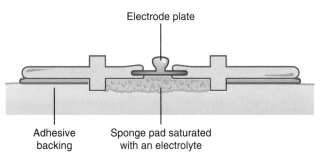

Electrode plate

Adhesive backing

Sponge pad saturated with an electrolyte

■ **FIGURE 12-15.** Electrode used with a Holter monitor.

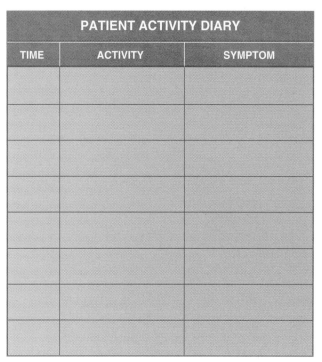

PUTTING IT ALL *into* PRACTICE

▶ **JANET CANTERBURY:** *One of the most unsettling experiences I had was while performing a stress test. The patient was an older woman. During the test, the patient is required to run on a treadmill. As the stress test started, the woman was unable to keep up. She fell off the machine and hit the floor. Everyone in the office was afraid that the woman was hurt. We helped the woman up, and she was able to stand. She was shaken but she was fine, although she had given us all the scare of our lives.*

■ **FIGURE 12–16.** Holter monitor electrode positions.

Right border of the sternum

Left border of the sternum

Right sternal border at the level of the fifth rib

Fifth rib space at the right anterior axillary line

Fifth rib space at the left anterior axillary line

HOLTER MONITOR ELECTRODE PLACEMENT

A special type of electrode is used with the Holter monitor. It consists of a round electrode plate with an adhesive backing and a central sponge pad containing an electrolyte gel (Fig. 12–15). This type of electrode is disposable and must be discarded after use.

Most Holter monitors are dual-channel systems, which means that two leads are recorded at the same time. A dual-channel monitor requires the use of five electrodes, one of which is the ground electrode. Some dual-channel monitors have the ground built into the monitor, in which case only four electrodes are required. The electrodes must be properly placed to ensure an accurate recording. Figure 12–16 shows the location of each of the electrode positions for the dual-channel Holter monitor. When one is learning to place these leads, it may help to mark their location on the patient's chest with a felt-tipped pen.

12

PROCEDURE

12–2

Applying a Holter Monitor

EQUIPMENT/SUPPLIES: Holter monitor   Alcohol swabs
                          Blank magnetic tape   Gauze
                          Battery   Razor
                          Carrying case   Nonallergenic tape
                          Belt or shoulder strap Patient diary
                          Disposable electrodes   Liquid skin abrasive

1. **Procedural Step.** Assemble the equipment.
2. **Procedural Step.** Prepare the equipment as follows; Remove the old battery from the recorder (if present), and install a new high-quality alkaline battery according to the markings on the battery holder. Insert a blank magnetic tape into the monitor according to the manufacturer's instructions.

Principle. A new battery must be installed each time the monitor is used to ensure sufficient power throughout the 24-hour monitoring period.

3. **Procedural Step.** Wash the hands. Greet and identify the patient.
4. **Procedural Step.** Introduce yourself, and explain the procedure. Tell the patient that the Holter monitor

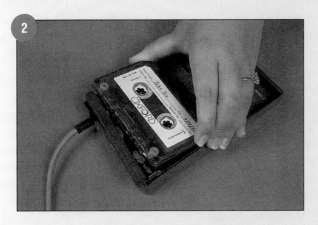

2

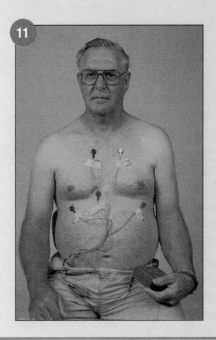

11

will record the heart beat without interfering with his or her daily activities. Tell the patient that, because of its small size, the monitor will be fairly inconspicuous. Instruct the patient in the guidelines for wearing a Holter monitor (see Table 12–1).
Principle. The patient guidelines must be followed carefully to ensure an accurate recording.

5. **Procedural Step.** Prepare the patient by asking him or her to remove clothing from the waist up.
Principle. Clothing must be removed for placement of the chest electrodes.

6. **Procedural Step.** Place the patient in a sitting position.

7. **Procedural Step.** Locate the electrode placement sites (see Fig. 12–16), and at each site prepare an area of skin slightly larger than an electrode as follows:
   a. If the patient's chest is hairy, dry shave it at each position site.
   b. Swab the skin with an alcohol wipe and allow the area to dry completely.
   c. Slightly abrade the skin with a 4 × 4-inch gauze square moistened with a liquid skin abrasive (e.g., Omni Prep) until the skin is visibly reddened. Rub the skin lightly with four or five small circular motions. On a patient with normal skin, use about the same pressure used to file the fingernails. Use less pressure on patients with sensitive skin or poor skin condition.

Principle. Shaving the chest improves the adherence of the electrodes and makes them easier to remove. The placement sites must be abraded with gauze to improve the adherence of the electrodes.

8. **Procedural Step.** Remove the electrodes from their package. Peel the electrode backing from one of the electrodes. Avoid touching the adhesive as much as possible to prevent loss of stickiness from the adhesive. Check to make sure the conducting gel is moist. If it is dry, a new electrode must be obtained.
Principle. The conducting gel should be moist to ensure good conduction of electrical impulses.

9. **Procedural Step.** Apply the electrode to the first electrode position site with the adhesive side facing downward. Apply firm pressure beginning at the center of the electrode and moving outward. Ensure a firm seal by running your finger around the outer edge of the electrode until it is firmly attached to the skin.
Principle. If pressure is applied by starting at one side and moving to the other, some of the conducting gel may be forced out from under the electrode, interfering with good conduction. The electrodes must be firmly attached to prevent distortion of the ECG recording.

10. **Procedural Step.** Repeat Procedural Step 8 until all five electrodes have been applied.
Principle. The electrodes pick up and conduct the electrical impulses given off by the heart.

11. **Procedural Step.** Attach the lead wires to the electrodes. Form a loop in each lead wire near the electrode, and attach the loop firmly to the patient with surgical tape.
Principle. The lead wires transmit the electrical impulses to the cardiac monitor. Forming a loop reduces artifacts caused by electrode movement.

12

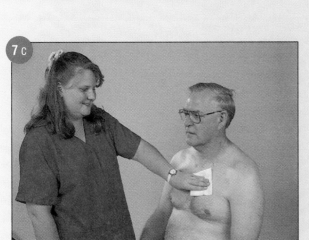

7 c

Continued

12. Procedural Step. Place a strip of nonallergenic tape over each electrode. Connect the lead wires to the patient cable.

Principle. Applying tape facilitates secure attachment of the electrodes by reducing strain and pulling on them.

13. Procedural Step. Check the recorder's effectiveness by connecting it to an electrocardiograph machine by way of the test cable and running a short baseline recording.

Principle. Checking the recorder verifies that the patient is properly hooked up and that no cable or lead malfunction exists.

14. Procedural Step. Tell the patient to redress while being careful not to pull on the lead wires. The electrode cable should extend from under the patient's garment or between buttons of the patient's garment.

15. Procedural Step. Insert the recorder into its carrying case and strap it over the patient's clothing, using either a waist belt or shoulder strap. Make sure the strap is properly adjusted so the weight of the recorder does not cause straining or pulling on the lead wires.

Principle. Straining or pulling on the lead wires may cause detachment of the electrodes.

16. Procedural Step. Plug the electrode cable into the recorder. Check the time and turn on the recorder according to the manufacturer's instructions. Record the starting time in the patient diary.

Principle. The beginning time must be recorded for later correlation of the patient diary with cardiac activity.

17. Procedural Step. Complete the patient information section of the diary notebook. Give the diary to the patient and provide him or her with instructions on completing it.

Principle. The patient diary is used to correlate patient symptoms with cardiac activity.

18. Procedural Step. Instruct the patient when to return for removal of the monitor. Be sure to remind the patient not to forget the diary.

19. Procedural Step. Wash the hands and chart the procedure in the patient's chart. Include the date and time, the name of the procedure (application of a Holter monitor), and the beginning time. Also chart instructions given to the patient.

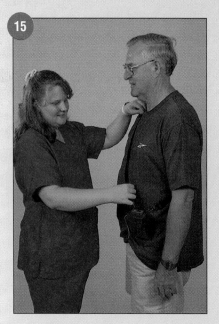

CHARTING EXAMPLE

Date	
6/15/2002	2:00 p.m. Applied Holter monitor.
	Starting time: 2:15 p.m. Instructed pt on
	recording data in diary. To return on
	6/16/2002 at 2:30 p.m. for removal of
	monitor. ———— J. Canterbury, CMA

CARDIAC ARRHYTHMIAS

☐ The normal ECG graph cycle consists of a P wave, a QRS complex, and a T wave, which repeats itself in a regular pattern (see Fig. 12–4). The term **normal sinus rhythm** refers to an ECG that is within normal limits. This means that the waves, intervals, segments, and cardiac rate fall within normal range. The normal heart rate ranges from 60 to 100 beats per minute. A rate falling below 60 beats per minute is termed **sinus bradycardia,** whereas a rate above 100 beats per minute is termed **sinus tachycardia.**

Each ECG graph cycle is separated from the next one by a flat length of baseline termed the T–P segment. Any change in the baseline distance between graph cycles indicates the presence of a cardiac abnormality falling into one of the following categories: (1) the presence of extra beats, (2) an abnormal rhythm, or (3) an abnormal heart rate. The medical assistant should be able to recognize basic cardiac arrhythmias

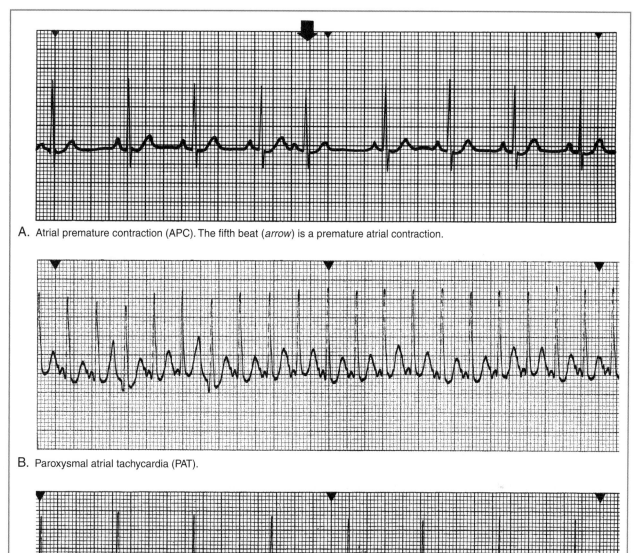

A. Atrial premature contraction (APC). The fifth beat (*arrow*) is a premature atrial contraction.

B. Paroxysmal atrial tachycardia (PAT).

C. Atrial flutter.

■ **FIGURE 12–17.** Cardiac arrhythmias. (*A, B, D* to *G* from Huang, S., et al.: *Coronary Care Nursing.* Philadelphia, W. B. Saunders, 1989. *C* and *H* from Johnson, R., Swartz, M. H.: *A Simplified Approach to Electrocardiography.* Philadelphia, W. B. Saunders, 1986.)

Illustration continued on following page

on an electrocardiographic recording for the purpose of alerting the physician to their presence. The arrhythmias the medical assistant should be able to identify are presented next, and a brief description of each and significant clinical aspects are included (see Fig. 12–17 for an illustration of each arrhythmia described).

ATRIAL PREMATURE CONTRACTION

DESCRIPTION. An atrial premature contraction (APC) is characterized by a beat that comes before the next normal beat is due. The most distinguishing feature is that the P wave of the premature beat has a different shape from the P wave of the normal beat. The APC

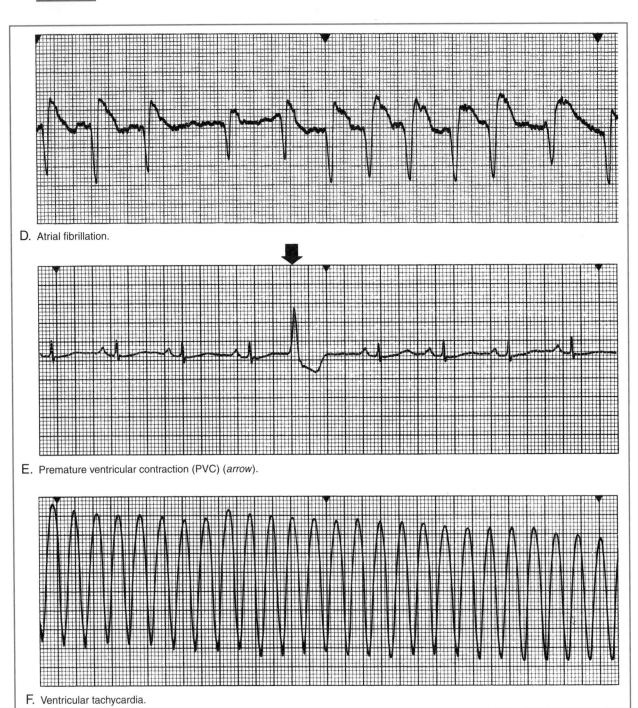

D. Atrial fibrillation.

E. Premature ventricular contraction (PVC) (*arrow*).

F. Ventricular tachycardia.

■ **FIGURE 12–17.** *Continued*

12

has a normal QRS complex and a normal T wave, similar to the other ECG graph cycles.

CLINICAL ASPECTS. Atrial premature contractions are common in healthy individuals and are often associated with the intake of stimulants such as caffeine or tobacco. They may also be associated with more serious atrial arrhythmias and structural heart disease.

PAROXYSMAL ATRIAL TACHYCARDIA

DESCRIPTION. Paroxysmal atrial tachycardia (PAT) is an abrupt episode of tachycardia with a constant heart rate that usually falls between 150 and 250 beats per minute. PAT is characterized by a rhythm that has a sudden onset and termination. The sudden increase in rate occurs in short bursts and lasts a few seconds only,

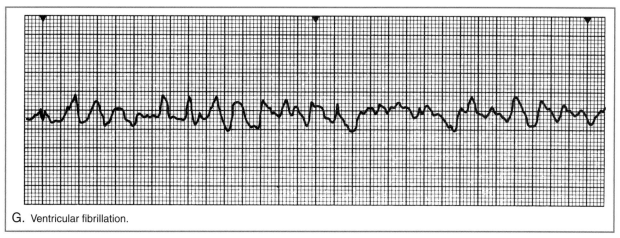

G. Ventricular fibrillation.

■ **FIGURE 12–17.** *Continued*

after which the rate returns to what it was before the PAT occurred. Because of the increase in heart rate, the ECG graph cycles are very close together. With PAT, the patient experiences a sudden pounding or fluttering of the chest associated with weakness or breathlessness and acute apprehension. Occasionally, the patient experiences syncope.

CLINICAL ASPECTS. PAT is one of the most common rhythm disorders, often occurring in healthy patients with no underlying heart disease and young adults with normal hearts. It may also occur in individuals with organic heart disease.

ATRIAL FLUTTER

DESCRIPTION. Atrial flutter is a rapid, regular fluttering of the atrium in which the heart rate falls between 250 and 350 beats per minute. More than one P wave precedes each QRS complex, and the P waves appear as saw-toothed spikes between the QRS complexes. The number of waves can range from just one extra P wave to as many as eight falling in rapid succession, but all have the same size and shape. The QRS complexes of an atrial flutter configuration are normal; however, the T wave is usually lost in the P waves.

CLINICAL ASPECTS. Atrial flutter is rarely seen in healthy individuals. It is found in patients with underlying heart disease. Atrial flutter is not specific for any particular type of heart disease and can occur in patients with mitral valve disease, coronary artery disease, acute myocardial infarction, chronic lung disease, hypertensive heart disease, and pulmonary emboli, and in those who have undergone cardiac surgery.

ATRIAL FIBRILLATION

DESCRIPTION. Atrial fibrillation is characterized by an ECG tracing in which the P waves have no definite pattern or shape. The P waves appear as irregular wavy undulations between the QRS complexes. The QRS complexes in atrial fibrillation are normal but do not have a definite pattern. It is difficult to measure accurately the atrial rate because the P waves are not discernible; however, the atria are contracting between 400 and 500 times per minute. The ventricular rate may be rapid (between 150 and 180 beats per minute) or relatively normal.

CLINICAL ASPECTS. Atrial fibrillation is a commonly seen arrhythmia and may occur both in healthy individuals and in patients with a variety of cardiac diseases. In healthy individuals, it can be initiated by emotional stress, excessive alcohol consumption, and vomiting. In individuals under 50 years of age, the common causes of atrial fibrillation are congenital heart disease and rheumatic heart disease with mitral valve involvement. In individuals over 50 years of age, atrial fibrillation is caused by diseases capable of producing ischemia or hypertrophy of the atria, such as coronary artery disease, mitral valve disease, and hypertensive heart disease.

PREMATURE VENTRICULAR CONTRACTION

DESCRIPTION. Premature ventricular contractions (PVCs) are among the most common rhythm disturbances seen on an ECG. The PVC is characterized by a beat that comes early in the cycle, is not preceded by a P wave, has a wide and distorted QRS complex, and has a T wave opposite in direction to the R wave of the QRS complex. Because of the unusual configura-

12

tion of the QRS complex, the PVC easily stands out from the normal ECG graph cycles. The baseline distance after the PVC is normally longer than the usual distance between the other cycles. In other words, the PVC is followed by a pause before the next normal beat occurs.

CLINICAL ASPECTS. PVCs are seen in normal individuals in all age groups and are caused by anxiety, smoking, caffeine, alcohol, and certain medications (epinephrine, isoproterenol, and aminophylline). PVCs may occur with virtually any type of heart disease but are seen most often in patients with hypertensive heart disease, ischemic heart disease, lung disease with hy-

poxia, and digitalis toxicity. PVCs are also common in individuals with mitral valve prolapse.

VENTRICULAR TACHYCARDIA

DESCRIPTION. Ventricular tachycardia consists of a series of three or more consecutive PVCs occurring at a rate of between 150 and 250 per minute. The tachycardia may occur paroxysmally and last only a short period of time, or it may persist for a long time. The QRS complexes are bizarre and widened, and no P waves are present. Sustained ventricular tachycardia is a life-threatening arrhythmia because the rapid ventricu-

PATIENT/TEACHING

ANGINA PECTORIS

■ Answer questions patients have about angina pectoris.

What Is Angina Pectoris?

Angina pectoris is actually a symptom rather than a disease. It comes from a Latin term meaning pain in the chest. Angina pectoris occurs when the muscle tissue of the heart does not receive enough oxygenated blood, resulting in discomfort or pain under the sternum.

What Causes Angina Pectoris?

In the majority of patients, the cause of angina is atherosclerosis. This is a condition in which fibrous plaques of fatty deposits and cholesterol build up on the inner walls of the coronary arteries, causing a narrowing and obstruction of the lumen of these arteries. This in turn results in a reduction of the blood flow carrying oxygen to the heart. In spite of the narrowing, enough oxygen may still reach the heart for normal needs. However, when situations occur that increase the work load of the heart, more oxygen is needed such as during physical activity, emotional stress, a heavy meal, or exposure to cold weather. If the coronary arteries cannot deliver enough oxygen during these times of increased need, angina pectoris results.

What Is Experienced During an Angina Episode?

Individuals experience angina in different ways, including the following: severe indigestion or burning, heaviness, ache, or squeezing or crushing pressure. The chest discomfort varies greatly. It can feel only mildly uncomfortable or it may be intense and accompanied by a feeling of suffocation and doom. The pain is usually felt beneath the sternum and may radiate to the neck, throat, jaw, left shoulder, and arm. In most cases, the pain lasts no longer than a few minutes and is

relieved by resting. Severe and prolonged anginal pain generally suggests a myocardial infarction (heart attack) and requires immediate medical attention.

What Type of Treatment May Be Prescribed by the Physician?

The goal of treating angina is to reduce the work load of the heart and to increase the oxygen supply to the heart. This is accomplished by resting when an angina attack occurs. In addition, the physician often prescribes medications, the most common one being nitroglycerin. Nitroglycerin is usually taken sublingually. It works by reducing the work load of the heart and increasing the oxygen supply to the heart by dilating the coronary arteries. Nitroglycerin can also be administered through patches worn on the skin or an ointment rubbed into the skin.

What Tests May Be Ordered by the Physician?

For patients exhibiting angina pectoris, the physician may order one or more of the following: a 12-lead electrocardiogram, chest x-ray, blood tests, and an exercise tolerance test. These tests assist in detecting the presence of coronary artery narrowing and blockage. To determine the exact location and extent of blockage, a more specific test may be performed known as cardiac arteriography. To help prevent more serious heart disease from developing, the physician generally recommends lifestyle changes such as a diet low in cholesterol and saturated fat, weight reduction, smoking cessation, and stress reduction. For patients with severe blockage of the coronary arteries, coronary artery bypass surgery or balloon angioplasty may be recommended.

■ Provide the patient with educational materials on angina pectoris and coronary artery disease.

12

lar rate prevents adequate filling time for the heart, leading to reduced cardiac output that often degenerates into ventricular fibrillation and cardiac arrest.

CLINICAL ASPECTS. Ventricular tachycardia is usually seen in patients with acute or chronic heart disease. Runs of ventricular tachycardia are indicative of coronary artery disease. Ventricular tachycardia also occurs as a complication of a myocardial infarction.

VENTRICULAR FIBRILLATION

DESCRIPTION. Ventricular fibrillation is the most serious arrhythmia. With this type of arrhythmia, the ventricles do not beat in any coordinated manner but instead they twitch or fibrillate. Because of this, virtually no blood is ejected into the systemic circulation. On an ECG recording, ventricular fibrillation is characterized by irregular, chaotic undulations of the baseline. There are no recognizable P waves, QRS complexes, or T waves in the irregular line of jagged spikes. Because the ventricles are twitching irregularly, there is no effective ventricular pumping action, resulting in no circulation. Ventricular fibrillation is a serious arrhythmia that must immediately be cared for because it can lead to sudden death.

CLINICAL ASPECTS. The most common cause of ventricular fibrillation is an acute myocardial infarction. It can also occur in patients with existing organic heart disease and cardiac arrhythmias. It may be preceded by an arrhythmia such as premature ventricular contractions or ventricular tachycardia, or it may occur spontaneously.

PULMONARY FUNCTION TESTING

☐ The purpose of a pulmonary function test (PFT) is to assess lung functioning, thus assisting in the detection and evaluation of pulmonary disease. The most frequently performed pulmonary function test is **spirometry.** Indications for performing spirometry include the following:

1. Patients exhibiting symptoms of lung dysfunction such as dyspnea
2. Individuals at high risk for lung disease because of smoking or exposure to environmental pollutants
3. Patients with existing lung disease, such as asthma, chronic bronchitis, emphysema, and bronchiectasis, to assess the progress of the disease
4. Patients undergoing surgery to assess lung performance during an operation

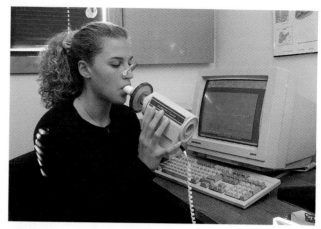

■ **FIGURE 12–18.** Spirometry.

5. As part of a routine physical examination to assess lung functioning for the early detection of problems

An instrument known as a **spirometer** is used to conduct the test. A spirometer measures how much air is pushed out of the lungs and how fast it is done. Spirometry should always be scheduled before meals or at least 1 hour after a meal. This is because the patient must exert his or her diaphragm muscles and food in the stomach may interfere with this action.

Spirometry is fairly simple to perform and is frequently performed in the medical office. To prepare for the test, the patient should loosen tight clothing such as neckties or tight collars. If the patient wears dentures, they should be removed. Nose clips are applied to the patient's nose to prevent air from escaping from the nostrils. A mouthpiece is placed in the patient's mouth with the lips sealed tightly around it so that all of the air leaving the mouth enters the mouthpiece (Fig. 12–18). Several different types of tests are performed during spirometry, as follows.

VC (VITAL CAPACITY). Vital capacity is measured by having the patient take a deep breath and exhale completely into the mouthpiece.

FVC (FORCED VITAL CAPACITY). Forced vital capacity is the maximum volume of air that can be expired when the patient exhales as forcefully and rapidly as possible. The patient is instructed to take a deep breath until the lungs are completely full. Following this, the patient is told to blow all the air out of the lungs and into the mouthpiece as hard and as fast as possible. A minimum of three acceptable efforts should be obtained.

12

MVV (MAXIMUM VOLUNTARY VENTILATION). To measure MVV, the patient must breathe as rapidly and forcefully as possible into the mouthpiece over a period of 10 to 15 seconds. The MVV is very strenuous and difficult to perform and therefore is not recommended for routine screening. Because of the rapid breathing involved with this test, the patient may experience symptoms such as lightheadedness, vertigo, arrhythmias, and fainting.

MEDICAL PRACTICE AND THE LAW

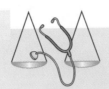

Cardiopulmonary procedures are frightening for many patients, because of the potential for unfavorable or life-threatening results. These results must never be given to the patient by the medical assistant. Only a physician can interpret results of an ECG or pulmonary function tests. If life-threatening results appear, your duty is to calmly notify the physician at once, without alarming the patient. All offices have emergency supplies; be aware of their location and use.

While you are attending to the machinery and technology, remember the humanity of the patient, and attend to all of his or her needs for privacy, comfort, respect, and caring.

CERTIFICATION REVIEW

12

☐ The electrocardiograph is used to record the electrical activity of the heart. An electrocardiogram (ECG) is the graphic representation of this activity.

☐ The heart consists of four chambers: the right and left atria and the right and left ventricles. The SA node consists of a knot of modified myocardial cells that have the ability to send out an electrical impulse, which initiates and regulates the heart beat. The AV node transmits the electrical impulse to the bundle of His and delays the impulse momentarily to give the ventricles a chance to fill with blood. The Purkinje fibers distribute the impulse evenly to the right and left ventricles, causing them to contract.

☐ The cardiac cycle represents one complete heart beat. It consists of the contraction of the atria, the contraction of the ventricles, and the relaxation of the entire heart. The electrocardiograph records the electrical activity that causes these events in the cardiac cycle to occur.

☐ The ECG cycle consists of a P wave, QRS complex, and T wave. The P wave represents the contraction of the atria; the QRS complex represents the contraction of the ventricles; and the T wave represents the electrical recovery of the ventricles.

☐ The electrocardiograph must be standardized when recording an ECG. This ensures an accurate and reliable recording. A normal standardization mark should be 10 mm high. If it is more or less than this, the electrocardiograph machine must be adjusted.

☐ The standard ECG consists of 12 leads. Each lead records the heart's activity from a different angle. The 12 leads are: I, II, III, aVR, aVL, aVF, V_1, V_2, V_3, V_4, V_5, and V_6.

☐ The electrical impulses given off by the heart are picked up by electrodes and conducted into the machine through lead wires. An electrolyte is also used to assist in transmitting the electrical impulse given off by the heart. An electrolyte consists of a chemical substance that promotes conduction of an electrical current.

☐ An electrocardiograph with a three-channel recording capability can simultaneously record three different leads. An electrocardiograph with telephone transmission capabilities can transmit a recording over the telephone line to an ECG data interpretation site. An electrocardiograph with interpretive capabilities has a built-in computer program that analyzes the recording as it is being run.

☐ Artifacts represent additional electrical activity that is picked up by the electrocardiograph. A muscle artifact has a fuzzy, irregular baseline and is caused by voluntary and involuntary muscle movement. A wandering baseline can be caused by electrodes that are too loose and by body creams, oils, or lotions present on the skin. Alternating current is caused by electrical interference and is characterized by small, straight spiked lines on the ECG. An interrupted baseline is caused by the metal tip of a lead wire becoming detached or by a broken patient cable.

☐ Holter monitor electrocardiography monitors the cardiac activity of a patient over a 24-hour period. It is used to evaluate patients with unexplained syncope, to discover cardiac arrhythmias that are intermittent in nature, and to assess the effectiveness of antiarrhythmic medications.

☐ Normal sinus rhythm refers to an ECG that is within normal limits. Cardiac abnormalities include the presence of extra beats, an abnormal rhythm, or an abnormal heart rate. Examples of cardiac arrhythmias include atrial premature contraction, paroxysmal atrial tachycardia, atrial flutter, atrial fibrillation, premature ventricular contraction, ventricular tachycardia, and ventricular fibrillation.

☐ The purpose of a pulmonary function test is to assess lung functioning, thus assisting in the detection and evaluation of pulmonary disease. The most frequently performed pulmonary function test is spirometry; an instrument known as a spirometer is used to conduct the test. A spirometer measures how much air is pushed out of the lungs and how fast that occurs.

RESOURCES

ON THE WEB

For information on cardiology:

American College of Cardiology
www.acc.org

American Heart Association
www.americanheart.org

The Chattanooga Heart Institute
www.heartinfo.com

Cut to the Heart
www.pbs.org/wgbh/nova/heart

For information on smoking cessation:

CDC's Office on Smoking and Health
www.cdc.gov/nccdphp/divoshoh.htm

Great American Smokeout
www.cancer.org/gasp

National Center for Tobacco-free Kids
www.tobaccofreekids.org

Oncolink
www.oncolink.upenn.edu//causeprevent/smoking

The Quit Net
www.quitnet.org

12

Colon Procedures

My name is

Megan Baer. *I am a medical assistant graduate from an accredited medical assisting program. I have an associate's degree in Applied Science. I work in a multiphysician office with specialities of family practice, proctology, allergy, and internal medicine.*

I have worked as a medical assistant for 3 years and plan to continue my education in the health care field. My primary job responsibility is Clinical Supervisor of the medical office. I oversee all clinical medical assistants including our "in-house" laboratory. I work closely with all physicians, especially the medical director, to meet the growing needs of the medical office. Other responsibilities include staff scheduling, product ordering, inventory, quality control, and patient care.

For me, one of the most interesting things about my job is the opportunity to take on new challenges. After my first year of being a medical assistant, I was given the opportunity to run a physician's office laboratory. I received weeks of training in different laboratory instruments and started our laboratory. Our office runs 85 percent of our own lab testing, including blood chemistry, hematology, and immunoassay. This has been a great experience for me.

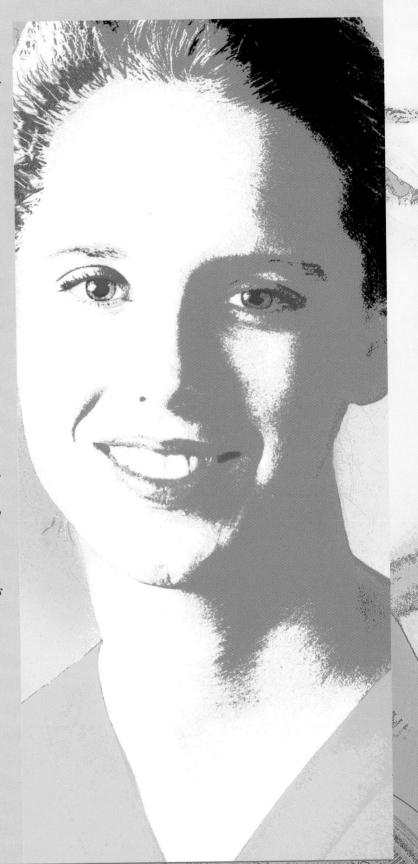

————— **OUTCOMES**

After completing this unit, you
should be able to demonstrate
the proper procedure to perform
the following:

1. Instruct an individual in the
   procedure for a fecal occult
   blood test.
2. Develop a fecal occult blood
   test.
3. Assist the physician with a
   proctoscopy.
4. Instruct a patient in the preparation required for a sigmoidoscopy.
5. Assist the physician with sigmoidoscopy.

————— **EDUCATIONAL OBJECTIVES**

After completing this unit, you
should be able to do the following:

1. Define the terms listed in the
   Key Terminology.
2. Explain the purpose of performing a fecal occult blood
   test.
3. Describe the patient preparation required for fecal occult
   blood testing and explain the
   purpose of each type of preparation.
4. Explain the purpose of performing the following: digital
   rectal examination, proctoscopy, and sigmoidoscopy.
5. Describe the patient preparation required for a sigmoidoscopy.

biopsy (BÎ-op-sê): The surgical removal and examination of tissue from the living body. Biopsies are generally performed to determine whether a tumor is benign or malignant.

endoscope (IN-dô-skôp): An instrument consisting of a tube and an optical system that is used for direct visual inspection of organs or cavities.

insufflate (IN-suf-flât): To blow a powder, vapor, or gas (such as air) into a body cavity.

melena (MA-lên-a): The darkening of the stool due to the presence of blood in an amount of 50 ml or greater.

occult blood (a-KULT blud): Blood occurring in such a small amount that it is not visually detectable to the unaided eye.

peroxidase (pur-OX-i-DÂs): (as it pertains to the guaiac slide test)—A substance that is able to transfer oxygen from hydrogen peroxide to oxidize guaiac, causing the guaiac to turn blue.

proctoscope (PROK-te-skôp): An endoscope that is specially designed for passage through the anus to permit visual inspection of the rectum.

proctoscopy (PROK-tos-KÔ-pê): The visual examination of the rectum using a protoscope.

sigmoidoscope (SIG-MÔID-ô-skôp): An endoscope that is specially designed for passage through the anus to permit visualization of the rectum and sigmoid colon.

sigmoidoscopy (SIG-môid-OS-kô-pê): The visual examination of the rectum and sigmoid colon using a sigmoidoscope.

INTRODUCTION

☐ Colon procedures are often performed in the medical office, the most common being proctoscopic and sigmoidoscopic examinations, and the fecal occult blood determination, all of which are presented in this chapter. The medical assistant helps the physician during each of these procedures in varying capacities. He or she should have a thorough knowledge of the responsibilities regarding each and perform them with skill and competence.

Obtaining the patient's cooperation helps make the examination proceed more smoothly and, as a result, makes the patient feel more comfortable. The medical assistant can help by explaining the purpose of the procedures to the patient. If the individual understands the beneficial results to be derived from the examination, he or she is more likely to participate as required.

FECAL OCCULT BLOOD TESTING

☐ Blood in the stool may be indicative of a number of pathologic conditions, including hemorrhoids, diverticulosis, polyps, upper gastrointestinal ulcers, and colorectal cancer. Some of these conditions produce visible red blood on the outside of the stool, making it easy to detect. Blood entering the stool from the upper gastrointestinal tract in an amount of 50 ml or greater causes the stool to exhibit **melena**, meaning it appears black and tarlike. The dark color is a result of the oxidation of the iron component of the blood (heme) by intestinal and bacterial enzymes. If blood is present in a minute quantity, however, it will not be detectable by the unaided eye. This hidden or nonvisible blood is termed **occult blood**, and its presence can be determined only through chemical or microscopic analysis.

Colorectal cancer is one of the most common forms of cancer in individuals over the age of 40 years. During the early asymptomatic stages, almost all neoplasms of the colon and rectum bleed a small amount on an intermittent basis, and this takes the form of occult blood. Assessing the presence of occult blood is of particular importance in the early diagnosis and treatment of colorectal cancer, which, in turn, increases the patient's survival rate. In most cases, when more pronounced symptoms of colorectal cancer start appearing (such as visible bleeding, a change in bowel habits, abdominal pain, and anemia) the condition has reached an advanced stage.

THE GUAIAC SLIDE TEST

Routine screening of stool specimens for occult blood is frequently performed in the medical office. The

13

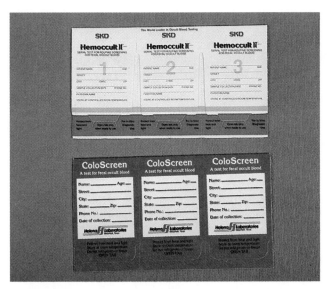

■ **FIGURE 13–1.** Examples of fecal occult blood testing kits. Hemoccult (*top*) and ColoScreen (*bottom*).

tinuing until all three slides have been prepared. The patient is placed on a high-fiber, meat-free diet. Meat contains animal blood that could lead to a false-positive test result. A high-fiber diet is used because it encourages bleeding from lesions that may bleed only occasionally. In addition, the fiber adds bulk, which promotes bowel elimination and ensures adequate specimen collection.

Certain medications cause irritation of the gastrointestinal tract, which may result in a small amount of bleeding; examples include aspirin, indomethacin, phenylbutazone, and corticosteroids. In addition, a vitamin C supplement (in excess of 250 mg/day) or an iron supplement may cause false-negative results and should also be discontinued before testing. Table 13–1 lists the specific patient preparation requirements and the purpose of each requirement.

Although the primary use of the guaiac slide test is to screen for colorectal cancer, other important uses

guaiac slide test is most often used and is commercially available with brand names of Hemoccult and Colo-Screen (Fig. 13–1). Fecal blood loss in excess of 5 ml/day results in a positive reaction. Patients may normally lose blood in amounts up to 3 ml/day in the feces, owing to minor insignificant abrasions of the nasopharynx and gastrointestinal tract. Thus, to allow for normal blood loss, the test does not show a positive reaction until it reaches 5 ml.

The guaiac slide test is a simple and inexpensive method to screen for the presence of occult blood; however, care must be taken to reduce the occurrence of false-positive or false-negative results. This test is designed to assess the presence of blood in stool specimens collected from three consecutive bowel movements or three bowel movements spaced closely in time. The purpose of using three specimens is to provide for the detection of blood from gastrointestinal lesions that exhibit intermittent bleeding, meaning they do not bleed every day. Because three stool specimens are required, most physicians prefer that the patient collect and process the specimens at home and return the prepared slides to the medical office for analysis. The medical assistant is responsible for providing the patient with instructions on patient preparation, collection, and processing of the specimens as well as proper care and storage of the slides until they are returned to the medical office.

Patient preparation plays an important role in ensuring accurate test results. The patient must follow a special diet, beginning 2 days before the test and con-

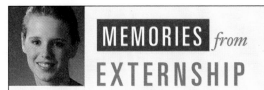

MEMORIES *from* EXTERNSHIP

MEGAN BAER: *One of the most terrifying things for me as a student was learning venipuncture. Even though I would practice during classroom lab hours and felt comfortable with it, it still scared me to know I would have to draw on a real person one day. When the day arrived to draw on my lab partner, I became sick to my stomach. In the end, we both got through it just fine and walked away without hurting each other. I spent days trying to prepare myself for that first experience, but after it was over, I felt more confident and relaxed that I could do this.*

At my externship site, I was able to perform several venipunctures a day, which raised my confidence level. Today, venipuncture is my favorite responsibility of all. I could sit and draw all day if I could. I know I could draw with my eyes closed but never would, of course!

13

TABLE 13 – 1

Patient Preparation for Fecal Occult Blood Testing

Beginning 2 days before obtaining the first stool specimen, the patient should follow the diet modifications listed below. The diet should be followed until all three slides have been prepared.

Meats. Eat no red or rare meat (beef and lamb) or processed meats and liver. Small amounts of well-cooked pork, poultry, and fish are permitted. Red meat contains animal blood that could cause a false-positive test result.

Vegetables. Eat moderate amounts of vegetables, both raw and cooked. Especially advised are lettuce, spinach, corn, and celery. Do not consume horseradish, turnips, broccoli, cauliflower, and radishes. These foods contain peroxidase, which could cause a false-positive test result.

Fruits. Eat moderate amounts of apples, bananas, oranges, peaches, pears, and plums. Do not consume melons because they contain peroxidase.

Miscellaneous High-Fiber Foods. Eat moderate amounts of whole wheat bread, bran cereal, and popcorn. Foods high in fiber provide roughage to promote bowel elimination and encourage bleeding from lesions that bleed only occasionally.

Medications. Do not take any medications that contain aspirin, iron, or vitamin C. In addition, based upon the patient's medication therapy, the physician may stipulate additional medication restrictions. Certain medications cause irritation of the gastrointestinal tract, which may result in a small amount of bleeding. (Aspirin and other nonsteroidal anti-inflammatory drugs should be avoided for at least 7 days before and continuing through the test period.)

Special Guidelines

Inform the physician and do not consume any of the food items listed above if they are known, from past experience, to cause severe gastrointestinal discomfort or serious diarrhea.

Make sure the diet modifications have been followed for 2 days (48 hours) before collecting the first stool specimen.

Do not initiate the test during a menstrual period or in the first three days after a menstrual period, or when bleeding from hemorrhoids is present. These conditions would result in false-positive test results.

Store the slides at room temperature and protect them from heat, sunlight, and fluorescent light to prevent deterioration of the active reagents on the slides.

13

include screening for occult blood for the detection of an upper gastrointestinal ulcer or for disorders causing gastric and intestinal irritation. A positive test result on the guaiac slide test indicates blood in the stool, although the cause of the bleeding must still be determined. Therefore, further diagnostic procedures must be performed before the physician can make a final diagnosis; these tests may include sigmoidoscopy, colonoscopy, and a double-contrast barium enema x-ray study.

QUALITY CONTROL

☐ Quality control methods must be employed with the guaiac slide test to ensure reliable and valid results. The quality control procedure should be performed after the patient's slide test has been developed, read, and interpreted. The Hemoccult slide test contains an on-slide performance monitor consisting of positive and negative monitor areas. This monitor is located on the developing side of the filter paper under the back flap of the cardboard slide. The positive monitor area contains a control chemical that has been impregnated into the filter paper during the manufacturing process.

The medical assistant should apply 1 drop of the developing solution between the positive and negative performance areas. The results must be read within 10 seconds after application of the developer. If the slide and developer are functional, the positive area will turn blue, whereas the negative area will show no color change. Failure of the expected control results to occur indicates an error and the test results are not considered valid; possible causes include the use of outdated cards or developing solution, an error in technique, or subjecting the slides to heat, sunlight, or strong fluorescent light.

ColoScreen uses a similar control method; the main difference is that the medical assistant must wait 30 seconds before reading the results.

13-1

PROCEDURE

Fecal Occult Blood Testing

> **EQUIPMENT/SUPPLIES:** Hemoccult slide testing kit

1. Procedural Step. Obtain a Hemoccult slide testing kit. Check the expiration date located on each cardboard slide.
Principle. Outdated slides may lead to inaccurate test results.

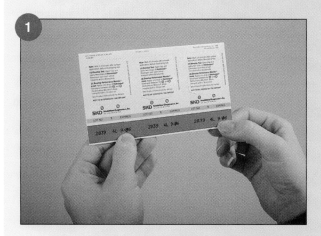

2. Procedural Step. Greet and identify the patient. Introduce yourself and explain the purpose of the test. Tell the patient that the test should not be conducted during a menstrual period or when hemorrhoidal bleeding is present.
Principle. Bleeding from other (identifiable) sources will invalidate the test results.

3. Procedural Step. Instruct the patient in the proper preparation for the test. Refer to Table 13–1 for the specific guidelines the patient should follow. Tell the patient to begin the diet modifications 2 days before collecting the first stool specimen. Encourage the patient to adhere to the diet modifications.
Principle. The diet modifications may discourage patient compliance. Therefore, the medical assistant should reinforce the importance of adhering to the diet requirements. Improper patient preparation may lead to inaccurate test results.

4. Procedural Step. Provide the patient with the envelope containing the Hemoccult slide test kit. The kit consists of three identical cardboard slides attached to one another; each slide contains two squares, labeled A and B. Three wooden applicator sticks and written instructions are also included in the testing kit.
Principle. Three slides are provided so that three stool specimens can be collected. The two squares in each slide (A and B) contain filter paper impregnated with guaiac, a chemical necessary for detection of blood in the stool.

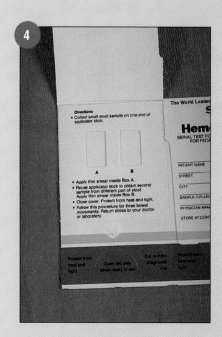

5. Procedural Step. Instruct the patient in the completion of the information required on the front flap of each card. This includes the patient's name, address, phone number, age, and the date of the specimen collection. A ball-point pen should be used to indicate this information.

Continued

13

13

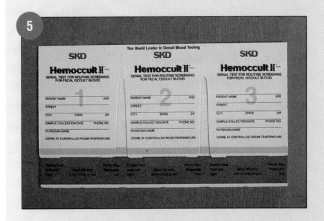

6. **Procedural Step.** Provide instructions on the proper care and storage of the slides. The patient should be told that the slides must be stored at room temperature and protected from heat, sunlight, and strong fluorescent light.

   Principle. Adverse storage conditions may result in deterioration of the active reagents impregnated on the filter paper, leading to inaccurate test results.

7. **Procedural Step.** Instruct the patient in the initiation of the test by telling him or her to begin the diet modifications and then to collect a stool specimen from the first bowel movement after the 2-day (48-hour) preparatory period.

8. **Procedural Step.** Instruct the patient in the proper collection and processing of the stool specimen:

   a. Using a wooden applicator, obtain a sample of the stool from the commode. The sample may be collected with the aid of a container or toilet tissue.

   c. Spread a very thin smear of the specimen over the filter paper in the square labeled A.

   d. Using the same wooden applicator, obtain another specimen from a different area of the stool.

   e. Spread a thin smear of the specimen over the filter paper in the square labeled B.

   f. Close the front flap of the cardboard slide and indicate the date in the space provided.

   g. Discard the wooden applicator in a waste container.

   Principle. Two squares are included in each slide to allow for specimen collection from different parts of the stool, because occult blood is not always equally distributed throughout the stool, as when bleeding occurs from the lower gastrointestinal tract. Thick specimens prevent adequate light penetration through the filter paper, making it difficult to interpret the test results.

9. **Procedural Step.** Instruct the patient to continue the testing period until all three specimens have been obtained and processed as outlined below.

   a. Repeat Procedural Step 8 after the bowel movement, using the cardboard slide located in the middle of the series of three.

   b. Repeat Procedural Step 8 after the third bowel movement, using the cardboard slide located to the right in the series of three.

   c. Allow the completed slides to air-dry overnight.

10. **Procedural Step.** Instruct the patient to place the cardboard slides in the envelope, seal carefully, and return them as soon as possible to the medical office.

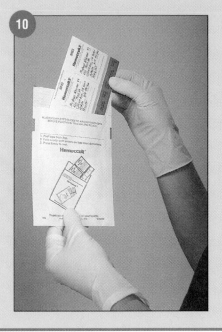

b. Open the front flap of the first cardboard slide (located on the left in the series of three).

PROCEDURE 13–1

11. Procedural Step. Provide the patient with an opportunity to ask questions; make sure the patient understands the instructions required for patient preparation, collection, and processing of the stool specimen and for storage of the slides.
Principle. Improper patient preparation and technique may lead to inaccurate test results.

12. Procedural Step. Record in the patient's chart. Include the date and documentation that the Hemoccult test and instructions were given to the patient.
Note: The ColoScreen guaiac slide test uses a procedure similar to that of Hemoccult.

PROCEDURE

13–2

Developing the Hemoccult Slide Test

EQUIPMENT/SUPPLIES: | Prepared cardboard slides | Reference card
Hemoccult developing solution | Biohazard waste container

1. Procedural Step. Assemble the equipment. The reference card provides an illustration of positive and negative test results, which can be used as a guide in interpreting results. *Note:* The slides may be prepared and developed immediately or prepared and stored for up to 14 days (at room temperature) before developing.

2. Procedural Step. Check the expiration date on the developing solution bottle. The developing solution contains hydrogen peroxide, should be stored away from heat and light, and should be tightly capped when not in use.
Principle. Outdated solution should not be used, because it may lead to inaccurate test results. The solution should be stored properly because it is flammable and evaporates easily.

3. Procedural Step. Apply gloves. Open the back flap of the cardboard slides. Apply 2 drops of the developing solution to the guaiac test paper underlying the back of each smear.
Principle. The developing solution will be absorbed through the filter paper and into the stool specimen. This solution could cause irritation to the skin and eyes; should contact occur, immediately rinse the area with water.

4. Procedural Step. Read the results within 60 seconds. Fecal blood loss in excess of 5 ml/day results in a positive reaction, which is indicated by any trace of blue appearing on or at the edge of the fecal smear. If no detectable color change occurs, the result is considered negative.

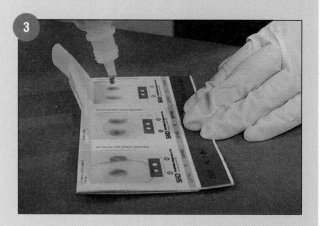

13

Continued

13

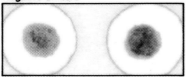

INTERPRETING THE HEMOCCULT® TEST

Negative Smears

Sample report: negative
No detectable blue on or at the edge of the smears indicates the test is negative for occult blood. (See **LIMITATIONS OF PROCEDURE.**)

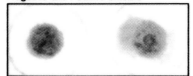

Negative and Positive Smears

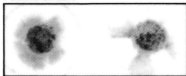

Positive Smears

Sample report: positive
Any trace of blue on or at the edge of one or more of the smears indicates the test is positive for occult blood.

SKD **SmithKline Diagnostics, Inc.**
A SMITHKLINE BECKMAN COMPANY
San Jose, CA 95134-1622

Principle. In the presence of hydrogen peroxide, the heme compound in hemoglobin oxidizes guaiac, causing it to turn blue within 60 seconds after adding the developer. The reading time is important because the color reaction may fade after 2 to 4 minutes.

5. **Procedural Step.** Perform the quality control procedure.
   Principle. Quality control procedures ensure the accuracy and reliability of the test results.

6. **Procedural Step.** Properly dispose of the Hemoccult slides in a biohazard waste container.
   Principle. The stool contains an abundant normal flora, and in some instances microorganisms making up the normal flora are capable of becoming pathogenic.

7. **Procedural Step.** Remove gloves and wash the hands. Chart the results. Include the date and time, the brand name of the test (Hemoccult), and the test results (recorded as positive or negative).

CHARTING EXAMPLE	
Date	
9/8/2002	9:00 a.m. Pt provided with a Hemoccult test and instructions for the procedure. ————————— M. Baer, CMA
9/14/2002	10:30 a.m. Hemoccult: Negative. ———— ————————— M. Baer, CMA

PROCTOSCOPY AND SIGMOIDOSCOPY

☐ Proctoscopy and sigmoidoscopy are procedures used to examine the lower intestines to diagnose and treat disorders of this part of the body. The physician may perform a proctoscopy or sigmoidoscopy as part of the physical examination or when the patient complains of a disorder of the bowel.

DIGITAL RECTAL EXAMINATION

A digital examination of the anal canal and rectum is performed before the proctoscopy or sigmoidoscopy, using a well-lubricated gloved index finger. The physician palpates the rectum for the presence of tenderness, hemorrhoids, polyps, or tumors. Any palpable abnormality will be viewed directly when the endoscope is inserted. The digital examination also helps relax the sphincter muscles of the anus and prepares the patient for the insertion of the endoscope.

Highlight on Colorectal Cancer

Colorectal cancer is the second leading cause of cancer-related deaths in the United States, with the most common being lung cancer. Each year approximately 150,000 individuals are diagnosed with colorectal cancer, and approximately 60,000 deaths a year are attributed to this disease. As the American population ages, these numbers will increase.

Approximately 5 percent of men and 6 percent of women will develop colorectal cancer at some time in the course of their life. Most colorectal cancer arises from polyps and small growths on the wall of the colon that gradually become malignant over a period of years.

The risk of colorectal cancer begins to increase after age 40 years and reaches a peak from age 60 to 75 years. Other factors that increase the risk of colorectal cancer include a family history of colorectal cancer, familial polyposis, and ulcerative colitis of more than 7 years' duration.

For the early detection of colorectal cancer, the American Cancer Society (ACS) recommends a yearly digital rectal examination for all individuals, starting at age 40 years, and a yearly fecal occult blood test for all individuals, beginning at age 50 years. The ACS also recommends that individuals undergo sigmoidoscopy for two consecutive years beginning at age 50 years; if both of these examinations are negative, sigmoidoscopy should then be performed every 3 to 5 years as long as the results continue to be negative and no other signs or symptoms of colorectal cancer develop. Individuals with risk factors are screened on a more frequent basis.

If colorectal cancer is detected and treated while the patient is still asymptomatic, the patient has an 80 percent chance of 5-year survival. By comparison, the 5-year survival rate for patients in whom colorectal cancer is diagnosed after the symptoms appear is only 40 percent. A digital rectal examination can detect approximately 10 percent of all colorectal cancers; and flexible fiberoptic sigmoidoscopy (using a 65-cm endoscope) can detect up to 65 percent of all colorectal cancers.

The exact cause of colorectal cancer is unknown, but studies have shown that there is a higher incidence of this disease in countries, such as the United States, whose populations have a diet that is high in meat and animal fat and low in fiber. This is further supported by the fact that in countries such as Japan, in which the diet is high in fiber and low in fat, the incidence of colorectal cancer is much lower.

PROCTOSCOPY

Proctoscopy is the visual examination of the rectum using a **proctoscope,** which is a rigid metal tubular instrument 15 cm in length containing a light and an obturator (Fig. 13–2). Proctoscopy may be performed to determine the presence of lesions, hemorrhoids, fissures, rectal bleeding, or other rectal disorders. The patient position for proctoscopy is the knee-chest position. The knee-chest position permits the abdominal contents to fall forward and away from the pelvis, making the procedure more comfortable for the patient and making it easier for the physician to insert the proctoscope.

Some physicians have specially designed proctologic tables that tilt the patient into the knee-chest position and provide support in this position (see Fig. 13–3). When using a proctologic table, the head and knee rests should be adjusted to fit each patient and then securely locked in place. The patient should be asked to kneel on the knee rest, bend at the hips, and place his or her body over the table in a manner that allows the patient's elbows and arms to lie against the head rest. The patient should be instructed to rest the head against the arms. The table is then slowly tilted into position.

During the procedure, a long cotton-tipped swab or suction equipment may be introduced through the lumen of the proctoscope to remove secretions such as mucus or particles of feces that interfere with proper visualization of the rectal mucosa. A biopsy may be taken from a suspicious area by inserting biopsy forceps (Fig. 13–2) through the lumen of the proctoscope.

Obtaining a biopsy is usually a painless procedure for the patient. Once the specimen is collected, it is placed in a sterile specimen container with a preservative and transported to the laboratory for histologic examination.

SIGMOIDOSCOPY

Sigmoidoscopy is the visual examination of the mucosa of the rectum and sigmoid colon using a flexible fiberoptic sigmoidoscope.

Sigmoidoscopy may be performed to detect the presence of lesions, polyps, hemorrhoids, fissures, infection and inflammation, or to determine the cause of rectal bleeding. It is especially valuable as a diagnostic procedure in the early detection of symptomatic and asymptomatic colorectal cancer. If a neoplasm is present, a biopsy is usually taken for histologic examination, using biopsy forceps. Early detection of colo-

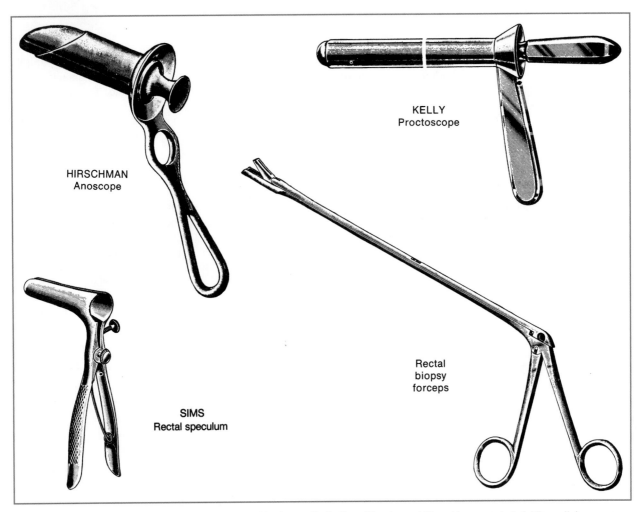

KELLY
Proctoscope

HIRSCHMAN
Anoscope

SIMS
Rectal speculum

Rectal
biopsy
forceps

13

■ **FIGURE 13–2.** Rectal instruments that may be used in the medical office. (Courtesy of Elmed Incorporated, Addison, IL.)

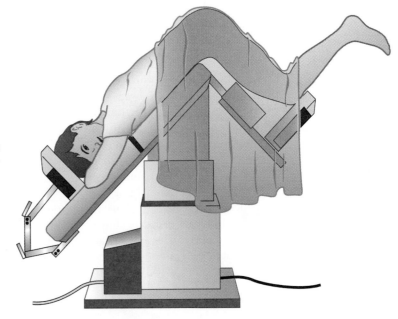

■ **FIGURE 13–3.** Proctologic table. A proctologic table tilts the patient into the knee-chest position and provides support in this position.

▶ **MEGAN BAER:** *Working with a proctologist has been very interesting and educational. When preparing a patient for an exam for flexible sigmoidoscopy, you must help the patient feel relaxed. This is an embarrassing situation for the patient, so you need to make him or her feel as comfortable as possible and maintain the patient's privacy and modesty. During the procedure, I talk to the patient about the weather, their pets, or interests to make them feel more relaxed and comfortable with me. This can help take their mind off of the procedure.*

One day I was assisting with a sigmoidoscopic exam, and a few minutes into the procedure, the look on the physician's face told me something was wrong. When the exam was finished, the physician and I left the room and went back to his office. He informed me that what he saw upon his exam was colorectal cancer, and at this stage, not much could

be done for the patient. The worst thing for a physician to have to do is give unpleasant news to a patient and to see the look on their face. This is something you don't forget, to go into a room of a patient who has just received life-threatening information. All you can do is be sympathetic, understanding, and be a good listener. You have to be strong and not show your emotions even though your heart is breaking for the patient and his or her family. Always let the patient know you are there for him or her.

Being with a patient who receives bad news about their health can make you think about your own life and how it not only affects you but also your family and friends. I often think of how I would feel about receiving such news. I try to put myself in the patient's place, and be sincere and understanding and willing to lend an ear, if needed.

13

rectal cancer leads to early diagnosis and treatment, which in turn increases the chance of survival for individuals with this disease.

Flexible Sigmoidoscope

The **flexible fiberoptic sigmoidoscope** is composed of extremely thin fibers of bendable glass that transmit light and images back to the physician. The image is magnified 10 times by the fiberoptic system and is viewed by the physician through the eye lens located in the handle of the sigmoidoscope. Videoscopes are also available for flexible sigmoidoscopy that permit viewing of the images on a display screen.

Flexible sigmoidoscopes consist of a control head and a long flexible insertion tube attached to a light source (Fig. 13–4). Flexible sigmoidoscopes are available in two lengths: 35 cm and 65 cm. The 65-cm length is generally preferred by most physicians because it offers the advantage of an increased range of visualization of the colon. To perform the procedure,

the distal end of the sigmoidoscope is lubricated and inserted into the anus and rectum, and then slowly advanced into the sigmoid colon.

A small amount of air is usually blown or **insufflated** into the colon through tubing attached to the air control valve located on the head of the sigmoidoscope. The function of the air is to distend the lumen of the colon for better visualization, similar to blowing air into a balloon.

In addition, suction equipment can be used to remove secretions such as mucus, blood, or liquid feces that interfere with proper visualization of the intestinal mucosa. The physician performs the visual examination of the intestinal mucosa as the sigmoidoscope is being inserted and also as it is being withdrawn.

Patient Preparation for Sigmoidoscopy

The physician may want the patient to prepare the bowel before the sigmoidoscopy. The preparation generally involves eating a light, low-residue meal the eve-

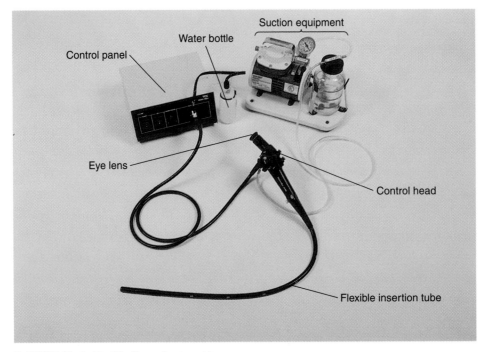

■ **FIGURE 13–4.** Flexible fiberoptic sigmoidoscope.

ning before the examination. Foods high in residue that should be avoided include raw fruits and vegetables and whole-grain breads and cereals. The patient may also be instructed to take a laxative and/or perform a sodium phosphate (Fleet's enema) or warm tap water cleansing enema the evening before the examination. On the morning of the examination, the patient should consume a light breakfast and perform another enema until the returns are clear. The fecal material

must be removed in order for the physician to visualize the mucosa of the bowel.

Some physicians prefer that the patient not take a laxative or perform an enema because it may change the appearance of the intestinal mucosa of the colon, making diagnosis difficult. In this case, the patient is examined after normal defecation. The medical assistant should consult with the physician to determine his or her preference.

13

PROCEDURE

13–3

Assisting with a Sigmoidoscopy

EQUIPMENT/SUPPLIES:
Disposable gloves
Flexible sigmoidoscope
Water soluble lubricant
Drape
Biopsy forceps

Sterile specimen container with a preservative
4 × 4 Gauze squares
Tissue wipes
Biohazard waste container

1. **Procedural Step.** Wash the hands.
2. **Procedural Step.** Assemble the equipment. Check to make sure the light source on the sigmoidoscope is working. Label the specimen container

with the patient's name, the date, and the source of the specimen.
3. **Procedural Step.** Greet and identify the patient. Introduce yourself and explain the procedure.

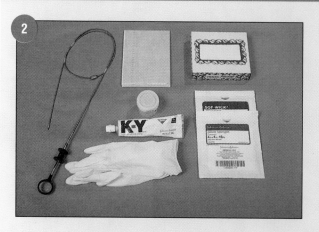

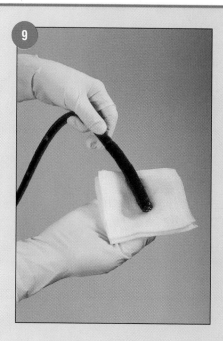

Principle. Explaining the procedure helps reduce patient apprehension.

4. **Procedural Step.** Ask the patient if he or she needs to empty the bladder before the examination. If a urine specimen is needed, the medical assistant requests that the patient void into a specimen container.
   Principle. An empty bladder makes the examination easier and is more comfortable for the patient.

5. **Procedural Step.** Instruct and prepare the patient for the examination. Ask him or her to remove all clothing from the waist down and to put on an examining gown with the opening positioned in back.

6. **Procedural Step.** Assist the patient onto the examining table using the footstool. The recommended position for flexible fiberoptic sigmoidoscopy is the Sims position or the left lateral position.

7. **Procedural Step.** Properly drape the patient so that only the anus is exposed. Some medical offices use fenestrated drapes with the circular opening placed over the anus.
   Principle. Draping the patient reduces exposure and provides warmth.

8. **Procedural Step.** Reassure the patient and help him or her relax the muscles of the anus and rectum by breathing slowly and deeply through the mouth. As the sigmoidoscope is inserted, the patient experiences a feeling of pressure and the urge to defecate. This pressure is caused by the insertion of the sigmoidoscope, and the patient should be reassured that although it is uncomfortable, it will last for only a short period of time.

9. **Procedural Step.** Assist the physician as required during the examination. The medical assistant may be responsible for the following:
   a. Lubricating the physician's gloved index finger for the digital examination.
   b. Placing lubricant on the distal end of the sigmoidoscope before insertion into the rectum. The sigmoidoscope should be well lubricated to facilitate insertion.
   c. Assisting with the suction equipment as required.

d. Assisting with the collection of a biopsy by handing the biopsy forceps to the physician and holding the specimen container to accept the biopsy. Do not touch the inside of the container, because it is sterile.

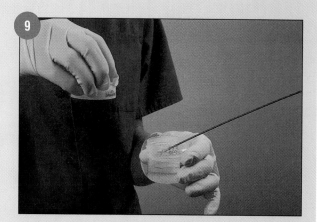

10. **Procedural Step.** Once the examination is completed, the medical assistant should apply gloves and clean the patient's anal region of any excess lubricant, using tissue wipes. Remove gloves and wash hands. Assist the patient off the examining table to prevent falls. Instruct him or her to get dressed.

11. **Procedural Step.** Transport any specimens that were taken (along with a laboratory request) to the laboratory to be examined by a pathologist.

12. **Procedural Step.** Clean the examining room in preparation for the next patient. The sigmoidoscope should be sanitized and disinfected according to the manufacturer's recommendations.

13

MEDICAL PRACTICE AND THE LAW

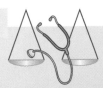

Colon procedures can be very embarrassing for the patient. Most colon procedures can be diagnostic for cancer. This combination makes for a very stressful event for the patient. Professionalism, compassion, and a caring attitude can alleviate many fears. Many invasive procedures require a written informed consent.

While assisting with a proctoscopy or sigmoidoscopy, assist the patient and maintain proper positioning as comfortably as possible. Be aware of the patient's condition, and inform the physician if he or she is not tolerating the procedure well.

Malpractice

Malpractice enforces a minimal level of care, and the value of doing good, or **beneficence.** Malpractice is a type of negligence, which is a tort, or wrong. Torts can be done intentionally or accidentally (negligently), and can be caused by something done, or something that was omitted.

CERTIFICATION REVIEW

13

☐ Blood in the stool may indicate a number of conditions, including hemorrhoids, diverticulosis, polyps, upper gastrointestinal ulcers, and colorectal cancer. Hidden or nonvisible blood in the stool is termed occult blood and its presence can be determined through fecal occult blood testing.

☐ Fecal occult blood testing is routinely performed in the medical office using the guaiac slide test (e.g., Hemoccult and ColoScreen). Patient preparation for the test is important in ensuring accurate test results. A positive test result warrants further diagnostic procedures such as sigmoidoscopy, colonoscopy, and a double-contrast barium enema x-ray study.

☐ Protoscopy and sigmoidoscopy are used to examine the lower intestines to diagnose and treat disorders of this part of the body. A digital examination of the anal canal and rectum is performed before the proctoscopy and sigmoidoscopy. The rectum is palpated for the presence of tenderness, hemorrhoids, polyps, or tumors.

☐ Proctoscopy is the visual examination of the rectum using a proctoscope. Proctoscopy may be performed to determine the presence of lesions, hemorrhoids, fissures, rectal bleeding, or other rectal disorders. A biopsy may be taken from a suspicious area by inserting biopsy forceps through the lumen of the proctoscope.

☐ Sigmoidoscopy is the visual examination of the mucosa of the rectum and sigmoid colon using a flexible fiberoptic sigmoidoscope. Sigmoidoscopy may be performed to detect the presence of lesions, polyps, hemorrhoids, fissures, infection and inflammation, or to determine the cause of rectal bleeding. It is especially valuable in the early detection of colorectal cancer.

RESOURCES

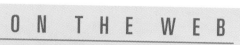

ON THE WEB

For information on colorectal cancer:

Medicine Online—Colon
    Cancer
www.meds.com

Cancernet
cancernet.nci.nih.gov

American Society of Clinical
    Oncology
www.asco.org

American Cancer Society
www.cancer.org

**For information on prostate
    cancer:**

The Prostate Cancer Infolink
www.comed.com/Prostate

The Prostatitis Foundation
www.prostatitis.org

13

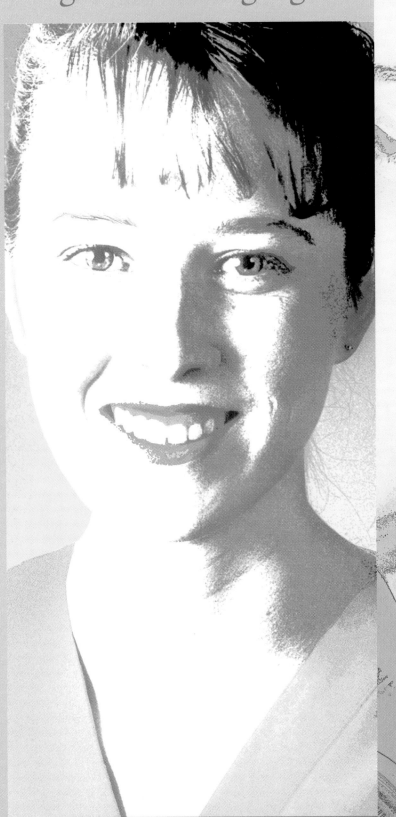

Michelle Shockey, *and I am a Certified Medical Assistant. I graduated from an accredited medical assisting program with an associate's degree in Applied Science. I graduated from the program in January of 1996 and started working at my last externship site, an orthopedic surgeon in a private practice.*

I assist the doctor in minor office surgery, dressing changes, joint injections, and cast applications. I work up patients by measuring vitals and taking patient histories. When the physician has surgery, I schedule the patients and do their preauthorizations. I have the opportunity to see a variety of problems from sprains and strains to surgical conditions.

Radiology and Diagnostic Imaging

OUTCOMES

After completing this chapter, you should be able to demonstrate the proper procedure to perform the following:

1. Instruct a patient in the proper preparation required for each of the following types of x-ray examinations: mammography, upper GI, lower GI, cholecystography, and intravenous pyelography.

2. Instruct a patient in the purpose and advance preparation for each of the following: ultrasonography, computed tomography, magnetic resonance imaging.

EDUCATIONAL OBJECTIVES

After completing this chapter, you should be able to do the following:

1. Define the words listed in the Key Terminology.

2. State the function of x-rays in medicine.

3. Explain why it is important for a patient to prepare properly for an x-ray examination.

4. Describe the following positions used for x-ray examinations: anteroposterior, posteroanterior, right and left lateral, supine, and prone.

5. Explain the function of a contrast medium.

6. Describe the purpose of a fluoroscope.

7. Explain the purpose of each of the following types of x-ray examinations: mammography, upper GI, lower GI, cholecystography, and intravenous pyelography.

8. Explain the purpose of each of the following diagnostic imaging procedures: ultrasonography, computed tomography, and magnetic resonance imaging.

contrast medium: A substance that is used to make a particular structure visible on a radiograph.

echocardiogram (Ek-Ô-kar-dê-ô-gram): An ultrasound examination of the heart.

enema: An injection of fluid into the rectum to aid in the elimination of feces from the colon.

fluoroscope (FLOOR-ô-skôp): An instrument used to view internal organs and structures directly.

fluoroscopy (FLOOR-os-KÔ-pê): Examination of a patient using the fluoroscope.

radiograph (RÂ-dê-Ô-graph): A permanent record of a picture of an internal body organ or structure produced on radiographic film.

radiography (RÂ-dê-OG-ra-fê): The taking of permanent records (radiographs) of internal body organs and structures by passing x-rays through the body to act upon a specially sensitized film.

radiologist (RÂ-dê-all-Ô-jist): A medical doctor who specializes in the diagnosis and treatment of disease using radiant energy such as x-rays, radium, and radioactive material.

radiology (RÂ-dê-all-Ô-gê): The branch of medicine that deals with the use of radiant energy in the diagnosis and treatment of disease.

radiolucent (RÂ-dê-Ô-lûs-nt): Describing a structure that permits the passage of x-rays.

radiopaque (RÂ-dê-Ô-pâk): Describing a structure that obstructs the passage of x-rays.

sonogram (SON-ô-gram): The record obtained by the use of ultrasonography.

ultrasonography (UL-TRA-sun-og-ra-fê): The use of high-frequency sound waves (ultrasound) to produce an image of an organ or tissue.

INTRODUCTION

☐ Wilhelm Konrad Roentgen, a German physicist, discovered x-rays on November 8, 1895, while working with a cathode ray tube. He noticed that these rays could pass through solid materials such as paper, wood, and human skin. He did not know what they were, so he named them x-rays. They have since been renamed **roentgen rays** after their discoverer; however, they are better known as **x-rays.**

X-rays are used to visualize internal organs and structures and serve as a diagnostic aid to determine the presence of disease. They are also used therapeutically to treat disease conditions such as malignant neoplasms.

The medical office may have its own x-ray machine, but more often the radiographs are taken in a hospital under the direction of radiology personnel. Some radiographs, such as a bone study, require no advance preparation, whereas others such as the barium enema require a great deal of special preparation. The medical assistant is usually responsible for instructing the patient in the type of preparation required for a particular x-ray examination and for making sure he or she understands the importance of the preparation. If the patient fails to prepare properly, a radiograph of poor quality may result. This may even necessitate rescheduling the procedure. This section provides an introduction to the study of x-rays, focusing on the patient preparation required for common radiographs.

X-RAYS

☐ X-rays are high-energy electromagnetic waves that are invisible and have a very short wavelength that enables them to penetrate solid materials. A special radiographic film is placed behind the part being examined, and a shadow or image of the internal body structure being photographed is produced on the film. **Radiograph** is the term given to the permanent record of the picture produced on the radiographic film.

Radiology is the branch of medicine that deals with the use of radiant energy in the diagnosis and treatment of disease. A **radiologist** is a medical doctor who specializes in the diagnosis and treatment of disease using any of various forms of radiant energy, such as x-rays, radium, and radioactive material.

CONTRAST MEDIA

☐ Radiography relies on differences in density between various body structures to produce shadows of varying intensities on the radiographic film. For example, there is a difference in density between bone and flesh (bone is denser than flesh). The bone absorbs more x-rays and does not allow them to reach the radiographic film. This leaves that part of the film unexposed and causes white areas to appear on the processed film. If the x-rays penetrate an organ or structure, it will appear black on the film. For example,

14

the lungs contain air and therefore x-rays are able to penetrate them easily; as a result, the lungs appear black on the processed film. The ribs, on the other hand, absorb many of the x-rays and appear as white shadows on the film (Fig. 14–1). A structure that permits the passage of x-rays, such as lung tissue, is **radiolucent.** A structure, such as bone, that obstructs the passage of x-rays and causes an image to be cast on the film is **radiopaque.**

In many cases, the natural densities of two adjacent organs or structures are similar. In this instance, in order to make a particular structure become visible on the radiograph, a **contrast medium** must be used. Substances used as contrast media are usually radiopaque chemical compounds that cause the body tissue or organ to absorb more radiation. This provides a contrast in density between the tissue or organ being filmed and the surrounding area. The tissue or organ becomes visible and appears white on the processed radiograph. Substances used as contrast media must be able to be ingested or injected into the body tissues or organs without causing harm to the patient.

Barium sulfate and inorganic iodine compounds are commonly used radiopaque contrast media. Barium sulfate is a chalky compound that is water insoluble and does not allow x-rays to penetrate it. It is frequently used for examination of the gastrointestinal tract, because barium is not absorbed into the body through the gastrointestinal (GI) tract and does not alter its normal function. Iodine salts are radiopaque and are combined with other compounds for x-ray examination of structures such as the gallbladder and kidneys. Iodine may sometimes produce an allergic reaction, and before it is administered, the patient should be asked whether he or she is allergic to iodine or foods containing iodine. Those patients who have known allergies may be given an iodine-sensitivity test as a precautionary measure.

Another type of contrast medium causes the structure to become less dense than the surrounding area. The x-rays are able to easily penetrate the structure, which appears as darker areas on the radiograph. This type of contrast medium includes such substances as air and carbon dioxide.

FLUOROSCOPY

☐ A **fluoroscope** is an instrument used in a darkened room to view internal organs and structures of the body directly. Examination of a patient using the fluoroscope is known as **fluoroscopy.** A radiopaque medium is often used with fluoroscopy to outline various parts of the body. The patient is positioned between the x-ray tube and a fluorescent screen composed of zinc cadmium sulfide crystals. When the x-rays pass

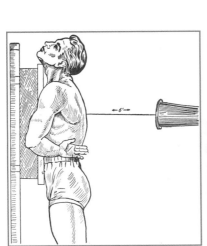

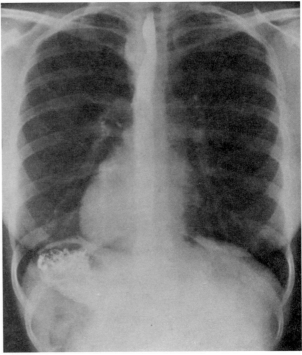

■ **FIGURE 14–1.** Posteroanterior view of the chest: position of patient and radiograph. (From Meschan, I.: *Synopsis of Radiologic Anatomy with Computed Tomography.* Philadelphia, W. B. Saunders Company, 1980.)

through the body and strike the crystals, they cause visible light to be given off so that the radiologist can view the action of body organs or structures such as the heart, stomach, and intestines on a television screen. During fluoroscopy, the radiologist can take radiographs that permit him or her to study the structure in detail and that also serve as a permanent record.

POSITIONING THE PATIENT

☐ The position of the patient is determined by the purpose of the examination and the part being examined. The patient is generally positioned so that several different views can be taken to provide a complete three-dimensional picture of the part being examined. Articles such as jewelry and hairpins must be removed so that they do not obscure the image on the radiograph. To prevent blurring of the image on the film, the patient must be instructed to maintain the position in which he or she is placed and not to move during the x-ray examination. Blurring prevents good visualization of the part and may warrant retaking of the film. The following types of x-ray views are used, and the methods used to position the patient for each are described.

Anteroposterior view (AP): The x-rays are directed from the front toward the back of the body. The patient is positioned with the anterior aspect of the body facing the x-ray tube and the posterior aspect facing the radiographic film.

Posteroanterior view (PA): The x-rays are directed from the back toward the front of the body. The patient is positioned with the posterior aspect of the body facing the x-ray tube and the anterior aspect facing the radiographic film (see Fig. 14–1).

Lateral view: The x-ray beam passes from one side of the body to the opposite side.

   Right lateral view (RL): The right side of the body is positioned next to the radiographic film, and the x-rays are directed through the body from the left to the right side.

   Left lateral view (LL): The left side of the body is positioned next to the radiographic film, and the x-rays are directed through the body from the right to the left side.

Oblique view: The body is positioned at an angle or in a semilateral position.

Supine position: The patient is positioned on his or her back with the face upward.

Prone position: The patient is positioned face down with the head turned to one side.

14

SPECIFIC RADIOGRAPHIC EXAMINATIONS

☐ The medical assistant should understand the purpose of commonly performed x-ray examinations and should be able to instruct a patient in the proper preparation for each (Fig. 14–2). Frequently performed radiographic examinations and the special advance preparation required for each are described here. The preparation may vary somewhat, depending on the medical office.

MAMMOGRAPHY

Mammography is an x-ray examination of the breasts, used to detect many forms of breast disease such as benign breast masses, breast calcification, fibrocystic breasts, and particularly breast cancer. It is also used to monitor the effects of surgery and radiation therapy on breast tumors.

Mammography uses low doses of x-rays, which pass

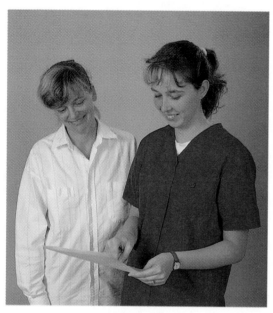

■ **FIGURE 14–2.** Michelle instructs a patient in the proper preparation for an x-ray.

through the breast and create an image on a film or plate. On the x-ray, an abnormal area appears noticeably different from normal breast tissue. Mammography can detect a breast tumor when the growth is less than 1 cm in diameter (about the size of a pea), which is before it is clinically palpable. If the lump is malignant, it can be removed at an early stage. This usually results in conservative treatment that is less deforming and has a high survival rate. In fact, if breast cancer is diag-

nosed and treated early, survival rates for women can be as high as 90 percent.

There is no specific preparation for mammography. The patient should be told not to wear any lotions, powders, or deodorants, since they may contain small amounts of metal that can be seen on the radiograph and may interfere with interpretation of the radiograph. To take the mammogram, the patient will be asked to remove clothing from the waist up; therefore, the patient should be told to wear a two-piece outfit to make the procedure easier and more comfortable.

The mammogram is generally taken by a radiology technician. The patient's breast is positioned on the mammography machine and pressure is applied with a plastic compression paddle that flattens the breast (Fig. 14–3). Compression of the breasts is necessary to obtain a clear radiograph and to lower the radiation dosage as much as possible. During the procedure, the patient must hold her breath and remain still momentarily while the x-ray is being taken. This is important because any type of motion, even breathing, can blur the image and make it necessary to repeat the radiograph.

Two radiographs are taken of each breast; one from above and one from the side. A radiologist then checks the mammogram (Fig. 14–4) and occasionally orders additional images to obtain a more complete view of the breast tissue. After the procedure, the radiologist will study the mammogram for any signs of breast cancer or other breast problems and send a written report of the findings to the patient's physician.

14

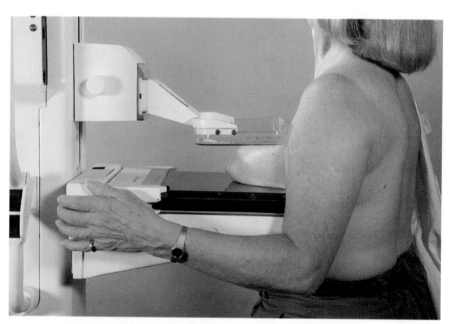

■ **FIGURE 14–3.** Patient positioning for mammography. (From Ballinger, P. W., Frank, E. D. [eds]: *Merrill's Atlas of Radiographic Positions and Radiologic Procedures,* Vol 2, 9th ed. St. Louis, Mosby, 1999.)

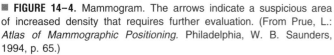

FIGURE 14–4. Mammogram. The arrows indicate a suspicious area of increased density that requires further evaluation. (From Prue, L.: *Atlas of Mammographic Positioning.* Philadelphia, W. B. Saunders, 1994, p. 65.)

PATIENT/TEACHING

14

MAMMOGRAPHY

■ Answer questions patients have about mammography:

What Is the Purpose of Mammography?

Mammography is a safe, low-dose x-ray examination used to screen for abnormal changes in the breasts. Mammography allows the physician to detect small lumps in the breast long before they can be felt. Although most breast lumps are not cancerous, when breast cancer is detected early, it can be removed at an early stage. This usually results in treatment that is less deforming and has a much higher survival rate.

Who Should Have a Mammogram?

The American Cancer Society recommends a baseline mammogram screening for women between 35 and 40 years of age. This baseline mammogram shows what is normal for that individual and gives the physician a means of comparison for future mammograms. Women between 40 and 49 years should have a mammogram every 2 years. Women age 50 years and over should have a mammogram annually, because the risk of breast cancer increases after this age. Women who have a family history of or other risk factors for breast cancer should follow the advice of the physician regarding mammography; the age guidelines do not apply since these women are examined on a more frequent basis.

What Occurs During the Mammography Procedure?

During mammography, the breast is positioned on a special machine and flattened with a compression paddle. Breast compression may be uncomfortable to some women. The discomfort can be reduced by avoiding caffeine several days before the procedure and by scheduling the mammography after a menstrual period when the breasts are less tender. Each breast is x-rayed from above and both sides. The resulting mammogram is then studied by a radiologist to detect any abnormalities. The results are reported to your physician who will then discuss the results with you.

Does Mammography Take the Place of Breast Self-Examination?

Mammography is not a substitute for breast self-examination. Women should continue to examine their breasts once a month and also have a periodic breast examination by a physician. Most breast lumps are detected by women themselves.

■ Encourage the patient to have a mammogram following the schedule recommended by the American Cancer Society.

■ Instruct the patient in the procedure for a breast self-examination.

■ Provide the patient with educational materials on breast self-examination and mammography.

GASTROINTESTINAL SERIES

Upper GI

This is an examination of the upper digestive tract using both fluoroscopy and radiography. It is helpful in diagnosing disorders of the esophagus, stomach, duodenum, and small intestine, such as peptic ulcers or benign and malignant tumors.

Proper patient preparation is very important for this procedure. The patient's stomach must be empty at the beginning of the study so that food does not obscure the radiographic image. To prepare for the examination, the patient must be instructed to eat a light evening meal only and then not to eat or drink anything, including water and medications, after midnight on the day before the examination. Food or fluid in the GI tract has a degree of density and could cause confusing shadows to appear on the radiograph.

The stomach varies little in density from the structures around it, and in order to make it show up on a radiograph, a contrast medium must be used. A suspension of barium mixed with water and a flavoring is given to the patient to drink. The mixture is known as the "barium swallow" and has a chalky taste. As the patient swallows the barium, the radiologist observes its passage down the esophagus and into the stomach and duodenum by fluoroscopy. Radiographs are taken periodically during the examination to allow a detailed study of the upper GI tract and to provide a permanent record. The patient's position is changed at various times so that the upper digestive tract can be visualized from different profiles. If the radiologist wants to observe the passage of the barium through the small and large intestines, the patient will have to return several times for additional radiographs.

The medical assistant should explain to the patient that the barium suspension will appear in his or her stool the following day, causing it to have a lighter color. The barium mixture may cause the patient to become constipated and require a laxative.

Lower GI

A lower GI involves filling the colon with a barium sulfate mixture by means of a tube inserted into the colon. The examination uses both fluoroscopy and radiography to observe and obtain permanent pictures of the colon (Fig. 14–5). A lower GI assists in diagnosing disorders of the lower intestines, such as polyps, tumors, lesions, and diverticulosis. The colon must be thoroughly cleansed in advance to remove gas and fecal

14

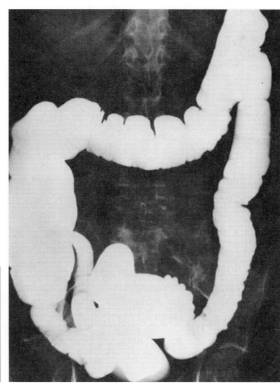

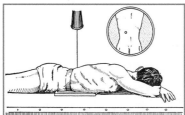

■ **FIGURE 14–5.** Lower GI. The colon is distended with barium: positioning of patient and radiograph. (From Meschan, I.: *Synopsis of Radiologic Anatomy with Computed Tomography.* Philadelphia, W. B. Saunders, 1980.)

material. Gas has a certain degree of density and shows up as confusing shadows on the radiograph. If fecal material appears on the film, it obscures the image of the colon.

The instructions a patient is given for cleansing the colon may vary somewhat from one medical office to another, but in general the patient is instructed to eat a light evening meal. A cathartic such as bisacodyl (Dulcolax) is taken on the day before the scheduled examination, and a cleansing enema may also be required. The patient must not eat anything after midnight on the day before the examination. Water may be taken when desired.

On the morning of the examination, the patient must perform a warm water cleansing enema. He or she should be instructed to use 500 to 1000 ml of tap water at a temperature of approximately 105°F (40.5°C). The enema solution container should be held approximately 12 to 18 inches above the anus. With the patient lying on the left side, one third of the enema solution is allowed to run slowly into the colon. The patient then turns on the right side for another third and finally turns on the back for the remainder of the solution. The patient retains the solution until the urge to defecate occurs, usually in 5 to 10 minutes. This procedure should be repeated until the returns are clear.

The patient reports at the scheduled time and is instructed to relax on one side while the rectal tube is inserted. As the barium enters the colon, the radiologist watches it on the fluoroscopic screen and periodically takes radiographs. The patient feels a sensation of fullness and the urge to defecate as the barium enters the colon. The patient is moved into various positions to allow the barium to fill the colon completely and to obtain better visualization of the colon. He or she is then allowed to evacuate, and another radiograph is taken to finish the x-ray study.

CHOLECYSTOGRAPHY

Cholecystography is an x-ray examination of the gallbladder to determine the presence of pathologic conditions such as gallstones.

The gallbladder is a pear-shaped sac located on the undersurface of the liver. It stores bile until it is needed by the body. Bile is produced by the liver and functions to break down fat. When fat enters the small intestine, the gallbladder contracts, releasing bile, which enters the small intestine by way of the common bile duct.

Because the gallbladder does not normally show up on a radiograph, a contrast medium must be used to

14

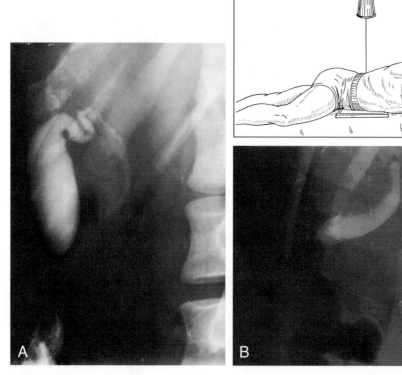

■ **FIGURE 14–6.** Cholecystography. Radiographic study of the gallbladder: positioning of patient and radiograph obtained before (A) and after (B) fatty stimulation. (From Meschan, I.: *Synopsis of Radiologic Anatomy with Computed Tomography.* Philadelphia, W. B. Saunders, 1980.)

make it radiopaque. The patient is instructed to eat an evening meal consisting of nonfatty food such as lean meat, fresh fruit and vegetables, toast or bread, jelly, and tea or coffee. The patient should not consume foods containing fat, such as milk, butter, cheese, cream, eggs, or chocolate, or fried or greasy foods. The reason for this is to prevent the gallbladder from functioning and contracting and thus emptying the contrast medium before the radiograph is taken.

The patient is given some tablets containing the contrast medium to take at regular intervals (generally 5 to 10 minutes) approximately 2 hours after the evening meal. Specific instructions are given with the tablets regarding how they should be taken. The contrast medium is absorbed by the gallbladder. Once the tablets have been taken, the patient should have nothing to eat or drink. The individual may also be instructed to cleanse the intestinal tract by means of a mild cathartic and cleansing enemas to prevent gas and fecal material from appearing on the radiograph and obstructing good visualization of the gallbladder.

The patient reports at the scheduled time, and a series of radiographs are taken. The individual is then given a meal containing fat to stimulate the gallbladder to empty, and another radiograph is taken to evaluate the functioning ability of the gallbladder (Fig. 14–6).

INTRAVENOUS PYELOGRAPHY

An intravenous pyelogram, more commonly known by its abbreviation IVP, is a radiograph of the kidneys and urinary tract (Fig. 14–7). It is used to assist in the diagnosis of kidney stones, blockage or narrowing of the urinary tract, and growths within or near the urinary system.

The patient should be instructed to eat a light evening meal and not to eat or drink anything after 9:00 P.M. He or she must remove gas and fecal material from the intestines with a cathartic (e.g., Dulcolax) and cleansing enemas. This permits proper visualization of the urinary tract. A contrast medium consisting of iodine must be used and is intravenously administered to the patient. Some patients are allergic to iodine; therefore, before the iodine is administered, the patient must be asked if he or she is allergic to iodine or foods containing iodine, such as seafood. As the iodine enters the bloodstream, the patient may feel warm and flushed and have a metallic or salty taste in the mouth. This is considered normal and lasts only for a few minutes.

OTHER TYPES OF RADIOGRAPHS

The following is a list of other types of radiographs that the medical assistant may encounter.

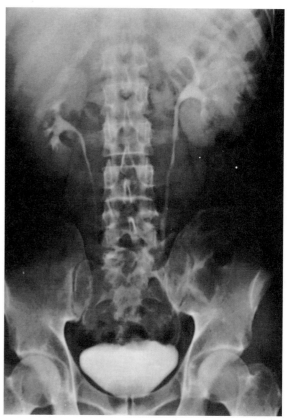

■ **FIGURE 14–7.** Intravenous pyelogram obtained 15 minutes after the intravenous injection of a suitable contrast agent. (From Meschan, I.: *Synopsis of Radiologic Anatomy with Computed Tomography.* Philadelphia, W. B. Saunders, 1980.)

14

Angiocardiogram	A radiograph of the heart in which valves and vessels are examined by x-ray and fluoroscopy after the introduction of a radiopaque contrast medium.
Bronchogram	A radiograph of the lungs taken after introduction of a radiopaque contrast medium.
Cardiac arteriogram	A radiograph of the coronary arteries after the injection of a radiopaque contrast medium.
Cerebral angiogram	A radiograph of the major arteries of the brain taken after injection of a radiopaque contrast medium.
Cholangiogram	A radiograph of the bile ducts taken after administration of a radiopaque contrast medium.
Cystogram	A radiograph of the urinary bladder taken after injection of a radiopaque contrast medium.
Hysterosalpingogram	A radiograph of the uterus and fallopian tubes taken af-

Retrograde pyelogram　ter injection of an oily radi-opaque contrast medium.
A radiograph of the kidneys and urinary tract taken after injection of radiopaque contrast medium directly into the ureter through a ureteral catheter. The dye flows to the kidneys through the ureters.

INTRODUCTION TO DIAGNOSTIC IMAGING

☐ Diagnostic imaging procedures are growing in use because they allow for the visualization of internal body structures in great detail. The most common procedures are ultrasonography, computed tomography, and magnetic resonance imaging. Diagnostic imaging procedures are almost always performed in a hospital setting; however, information may need to be relayed to a patient scheduled for such a procedure. Therefore, a medical assistant should have a basic knowledge of diagnostic imaging procedures and the preparation required for each.

ULTRASONOGRAPHY

Ultrasonography (US), also called ultrasound, is the oldest of the diagnostic imaging procedures. Ultrasonography uses high-frequency sound waves to study soft tissue structures. It is frequently used to diagnose conditions of the abdominal and pelvic organs, particularly the liver, gallbladder, spleen, pancreas, kidneys,

uterus, and ovaries. An ultrasound examination of the heart is called an **echocardiogram** and is used to determine the size, shape, and position of the heart and the movement of the heart valves and chambers.

Ultrasonography offers a number of advantages as a diagnostic imaging procedure. It shows movement, allows for continuous viewing of a structure, and uses sound waves rather than radiation. Ultrasonography does have some minor limitations. Because sound waves are unable to penetrate bone and gas-filled cavities such as the lungs, it cannot be used to evaluate these structures. In addition, ultrasonography may be difficult with obese patients because adipose tissue can interfere with sound wave transmission.

During ultrasonography, the examiner places a transducer firmly on the patient's skin surface and moves it over the body areas to be examined. The transducer generates sound waves that are directed into the patient's tissues. The sound waves are then reflected back to the transducer, similar to an echo. Deep structures of the body such as the kidneys are visualized by recording the reflections, or echoes, of the sound waves directed into the tissues (Fig. 14–8). The image is displayed on an oscilloscope, which is a special type of viewing screen. The image can also be permanently recorded on Polaroid film and video tape. The recording is called a **sonogram,** and the patient is often permitted to view the sonogram on the oscilloscope as the procedure is being performed.

Although ultrasonography is commonly used for a wide variety of noninvasive imaging procedures, individuals are most familiar with its use in obstetrics. **Obstetric ultrasonography** is most frequently used to determine gestational age of a fetus and confirm the due date; to detect congenital abnormalities, ectopic pregnancy, and multiple pregnancy; and to determine

14

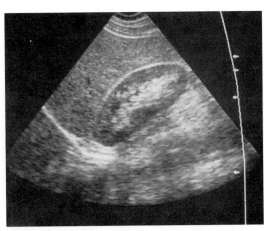

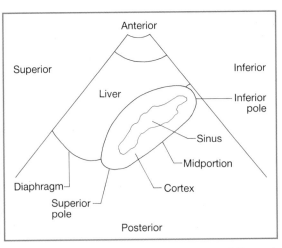

■ **FIGURE 14–8.** Sonogram of right kidney. (From Tempkin, B. B.: *Ultrasound Scanning: Principles and Protocols.* Philadelphia, W. B. Saunders, 1992, p. 103.)

PUTTING IT ALL *into* PRACTICE

▶ **MICHELLE SHOCKEY:** *When our patients come to our orthopedic office, they are usually in a lot of pain. Pain plays a big part in how our patients feel on that specific day. We see patients who have chronic problems that may never get better. There are also patients that come to our office in pain, but when their visits are over, they feel like they are on top of the world. Seeing a patient go from not being able to walk to being able to run a marathon is the best experience you can encounter.*

the baby's position and size late in pregnancy. Because the ultrasound machine is a compact unit, some obstetricians perform this procedure in their medical offices.

The medical assistant should tell the patient what to expect during ultrasonography and also instruct the patient in patient preparation:

1. Ultrasonography is a safe and painless procedure that takes approximately 15 to 45 minutes to complete, depending on the body part being examined.

2. The patient may be required to prepare for the procedure, depending on the part of the body to be examined. For example, ultrasonography of the gallbladder and liver require that the patient fast for 8 to 12 hours; obstetric ultrasound may require the patient to have a full bladder. This is accomplished by instructing the patient to consume approximately 32 ounces of fluid about an hour before the procedure.

3. The patient must remain still when requested during the procedure since movement can interfere with accurate results. In addition, the patient may be asked to change positions so the organs can be seen at different angles.

COMPUTED TOMOGRAPHY

Computed (axial) tomography, also known as a CT or CAT scan, is an advanced x-ray examination that uses only a minimal amount of radiation. It produces a series of cross-sectional images of a body part, permit-

ting the imaging of structures that cannot be visualized with conventional x-ray procedures. CT allows the radiologist to view the bones and organs of the head and body in fine detail and has been used most successfully in diagnostic studies of the brain. CT scans are used primarily to detect and evaluate tumors and other abnormalities and to monitor the effects of surgery, radiation therapy, or chemotherapy on tumors.

The scan is conducted by a skilled CT technician. The patient is positioned on a special motorized table (Fig. 14–9). From an adjoining room, the technician mechanically moves the table into a doughnut-shaped device known as the CT scanner until the part of the body to be examined is inside the tubular opening of the scanner.

During the scan, two examinations are often performed. The first is a plain scan, and the second is a repeat scan after a contrast dye has been injected through a vein in the arm. The dye makes it possible to obtain a sharper image of internal structures of the body. The CT scanner takes multiple x-ray pictures known as **tomograms** in a rapid sequence at different angles. The series of x-rays is processed by a computer to produce cross-sectional images, which are displayed on a video monitor and on film (Fig. 14–10).

The medical assistant should tell the patient what to expect during the CT scan and also instruct the patient in advance patient preparation:

1. If a contrast agent will be used, instruct the patient

14

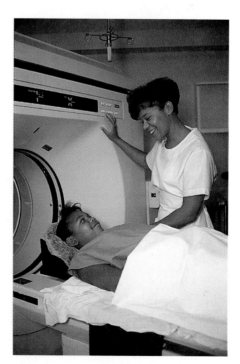

■ **FIGURE 14–9.** Positioning a patient for a CT scan. (From Kowalczyk N, Donnett K: *Integrated Patient Care for the Imaging Professional.* St. Louis, Mosby, 1996.)

to fast for 4 hours before the procedure. It is important to ask the patient if he or she is allergic to radiographic contrast media, iodine, or shellfish to avoid an adverse reaction to the contrast medium.

2. Before the procedure, the patient must remove all radiopaque objects such as metal and jewelry because they will interfere with a clear image of the part of the body being examined.

3. The patient must lie motionless and breathe normally during the procedure. The patient will hear mechanical clacking sounds coming from the scanner as it takes pictures.

MAGNETIC RESONANCE IMAGING

Magnetic resonance imaging (MRI) is the newest of the advanced diagnostic imaging procedures. It is used for imaging tissues of high fat and water content that cannot be seen with other radiologic techniques. Magnetic resonance imaging assists in the diagnosis of intracranial and spinal lesions and cardiovascular and soft tissue abnormalities such as herniated discs and joint diseases. MRI allows the examiner to see through bone and view fluid-filled soft tissue in great detail.

Magnetic resonance imaging is a safe and painless procedure that uses a strong magnetic field and ordi-

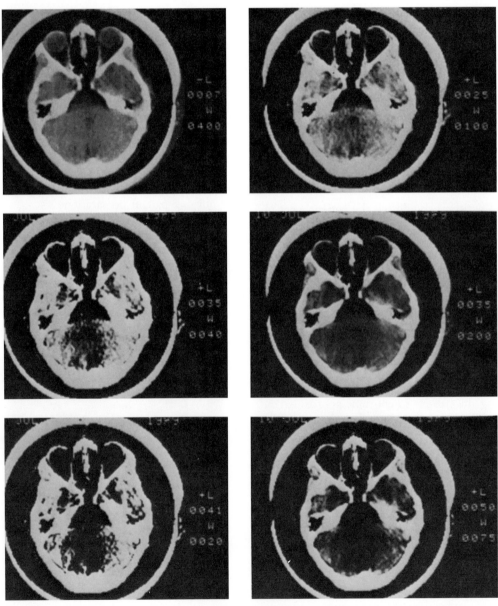

■ **FIGURE 14–10.** The CT scanner takes multiple cross-sectional x-ray pictures, known as tomograms. The tomograms shown here are cross-sectional pictures of the head used to evaluate orbits and sinuses. (From Snopek, A.: *Fundamentals of Special Radiographic Procedures,* 3rd ed. Philadelphia, W. B. Saunders, 1992, p. 116.)

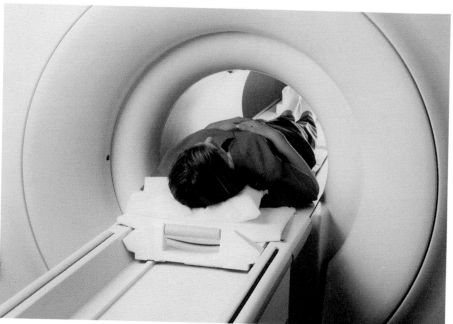

FIGURE 14–11. Magnetic resonance imaging. The patient lies on a table inside the bore of the cylindrical magnetic resonance machine while MRI technicians in an adjoining room monitor the procedure. (From Ballinger, P. W., Frank, E. D. [eds]: *Merrill's Atlas of Radiographic Positions and Radiologic Procedures,* Vol 2, 9th ed. St. Louis, Mosby, 1999.)

nary radio waves to produce computer-processed images of internal body structures. The patient lies on a table inside the bore of the cylindrical magnetic resonance machine while an MRI technician in an adjoining room monitors the procedure (Fig. 14–11). Because of the closed space, some patients may have difficulty with claustrophobia. For these patients, the physician may order a sedative.

High-resolution, three-dimensional images are obtained with magnetic resonance imaging; these are permanently recorded on film or magnetic tape. Because MRI does not involve the use of radiation, the FDA has classified the MRI machine as a low-risk device.

The medical assistant should tell the patient what to expect during MRI and also instruct the patient in advance patient preparation:

1. MRI is a safe and painless procedure that usually takes approximately 1 hour to complete.
2. No special preparation is required for the MRI examination. The patient may eat or drink before the examination and take any prescribed medication. The patient should wear loose, comfortable clothing for the procedure, such as a jogging suit.
3. Because the procedure involves the use of a strong magnet, the patient will be asked to remove any metal or magnetic-sensitive objects, such as watches, rings, or other metal jewelry and credit cards.
4. The patient must remain completely still for 15- to 20-minute intervals during the procedure. The patient will hear a metallic clacking sound that sounds like a muffled drumbeat during the procedure. Earplugs or headphones are available if the patient desires to use them.

MEDICAL PRACTICE AND THE LAW

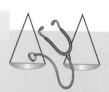

Radiology and diagnostic imaging involve high-technology equipment and procedures that can be frightening and uncomfortable to the patient. Be aware of the patient's reactions, and assist and comfort whenever possible. Be very specific in providing with instructions to ensure the best imaging results.

Procedures that involve injectable contrast media or that are invasive usually require written informed consent. Check with office policy for procedures requiring signed consent forms.

Whenever dealing with radiation, federal laws regulate usage and exposure testing and record keeping. The acronym ALARA, or As Low As Reasonably Able, reminds workers to minimize exposure to themselves and patients. Be sure to ask female patients if they may be pregnant before starting any radiologic procedure.

CERTIFICATION REVIEW

- ☐ X-rays are used to visualize internal organs and structures and serve as a diagnostic aid to determine the presence of disease. They are also used therapeutically to treat malignant neoplasms. Radiograph is the term for the permanent record of the picture produced on the radiographic film. Radiology is the branch of medicine that deals with the use of radiant energy in the diagnosis and treatment of disease.
- ☐ A structure that permits the passage of x-rays is radiolucent. A structure that obstructs the passage of x-rays is radiopaque. A contrast medium is used to make a particular structure become visible on the radiograph. A fluoroscope is an instrument used to view internal organs and structures of the body directly.
- ☐ The position of the patient is determined by the purpose of the examination and the part being examined. Different types of x-ray views include AP, PA, lateral, oblique, supine, and prone.
- ☐ Mammography is an x-ray examination of the breasts used to detect breast disease. Mammography can detect a breast tumor when the growth is less than 1 cm in diameter.
- ☐ An upper GI is an examination of the upper digestive tract using both fluoroscopy and radiography. It is used to diagnose disorders of the esophagus, stomach, duodenum, and small intestine.
- ☐ A lower GI involves filling the colon with a barium sulfate mixture by means of a tube inserted into the colon. The examination is used to diagnose disorders of the lower intestine, such as polyps, tumors, lesions, and diverticulosis.
- ☐ Cholecystography is an x-ray examination of the gallbladder to determine the presence of pathologic conditions such as gallstones.
- ☐ An IVP is a radiograph of the kidneys and urinary tract. It is used to assist in the diagnosis of kidney stones, blockage or narrowing of the urinary tract, and growths within or near the urinary system.
- ☐ Ultrasonography uses high-frequency sound waves to study soft tissue structures. It is frequently used to diagnose conditions of the abdominal and pelvic organs, particularly the liver, gallbladder, spleen, pancreas, kidneys, uterus, and ovaries. An ultrasound examination of the heart is called an echocardiogram. Ultrasonography shows movement and allows for continuous viewing of a structure. Obstetric ultrasonography is used to determine gestational age of a fetus and confirm date of delivery.
- ☐ CT, or CAT scan, is used to view the bones and organs of the head and body in fine detail. CT scans are used to detect and evaluate tumors and other abnormalities and to monitor the effects of surgery, radiation therapy, or chemotherapy on tumors.
- ☐ MRI is used to assist in the diagnosis of intracranial and spinal lesions, as well as cardiovascular and soft tissue abnormalities.

14

RESOURCE

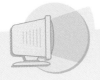

O N   T H E   W E B

For information on x-ray and diagnostic imaging:

Brigham RAD
www.brighamrad.
   harvard.edu

Journal of Digital Imaging
www.scar.rad.
   washington.edu

Whole Brain Atlas
www.med.harvard.edu/
   AANLIB/home.html

For information on breast cancer:

National Action Plan on
   Breast Cancer
www.napbc.org

American Cancer Society
www.cancer.org

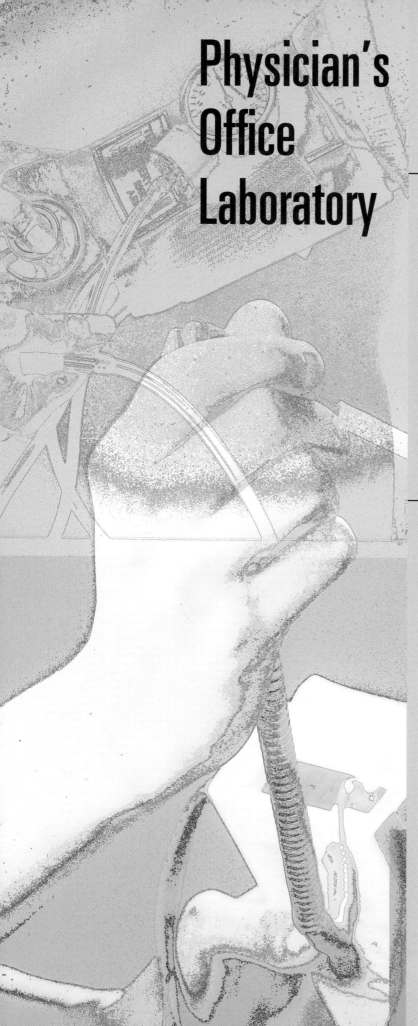

Physician's Office Laboratory

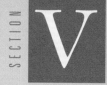

AAMA/CAAHEP COMPETENCIES INCLUDED IN THIS SECTION:

Clinical Competencies

Specimen Collection
- Perform venipuncture.
- Perform capillary puncture.
- Obtain throat specimen for microbiological testing.
- Perform wound collection procedure for microbiological testing.
- Instruct patients in the collection of a clean-catch mid-stream urine specimen.

Diagnostic Testing
- Use methods of quality control.
- Perform urinalysis.
- Perform hematology testing.
- Perform chemistry testing.
- Perform immunology testing.
- Perform microbiology testing.
- Screen and follow-up test results.

Transdisciplinary Competencies

Patient Instruction
- Instruct individuals according to their needs.
- Instruct and demonstrate the use and care of patient equipment.
- Provide instruction for health maintenance and disease prevention.
- Identify community resources.

Korey McGrew *and I am a Certified Medical Assistant. I received my associate's degree in medical assisting from an accredited medical assisting program. I have been working for the past year for a group of physicians in a family practice medical office. I work specifically with the group's nurse practitioner. Some of my duties include showing patients to examining rooms, taking the patient's vital signs, administering medications, dictation, filing, and many other miscellaneous duties that medical assistants perform. I have found that being a medical assistant has been a most challenging and rewarding occupation, and I wish you the best of luck in reaching your goals.*

Introduction to the Clinical Laboratory

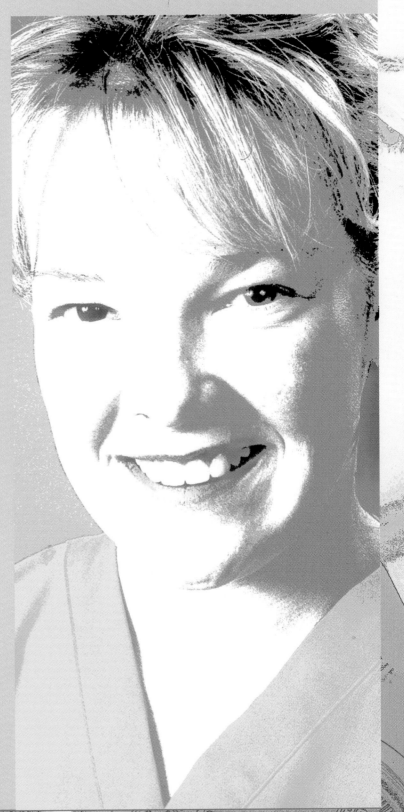

KEY TERMINOLOGY

automated method (*for testing laboratory specimens*): A method of laboratory testing in which the series of steps in the test method is performed by an automated analyzer.

fasting: Abstaining from food or fluids (except water) for a specified amount of time prior to the collection of a specimen.

homeostasis (HôM-ê-ô-STÂ-sis): The state in which body systems are functioning normally and the internal environment of the body is in equilibrium; the body is in a healthy state.

in vivo (IN-vêv-Ô): Occurring in the living body or organism.

laboratory test: The clinical analysis and study of materials, fluids, or tissues obtained from patients to assist in diagnosing and treating disease.

manual method: A method of laboratory testing in which the series of steps in the test method is performed by hand.

normal range (*for laboratory tests*): A certain established and acceptable parameter or reference range within which the laboratory test results of a healthy individual are expected to fall.

plasma (PLAZ-ma): The liquid part of the blood, consisting of a clear, yellowish fluid that makes up approximately 55 percent of the total blood volume.

profile: A number of laboratory tests providing related or complementary information used to determine the health status of a patient.

quality control: The application of methods to ensure that test results are reliable and valid and that errors are detected and eliminated.

routine test: Laboratory tests performed on a routine basis on apparently healthy patients to assist in the early detection of disease.

serum (SERE-um): Plasma from which the clotting factor fibrinogen has been removed.

specimen (SPES-i-men): A small sample of something taken to show the nature of the whole.

INTRODUCTION

☐ Clinical laboratory test results are often used along with a thorough health history and physical examination to provide essential data needed by the physician to diagnose accurately and to manage a patient's condition. Clinical laboratory tests provide objective and quantitative information regarding the status of body conditions and functions. When the body is in a healthy state, its systems will be functioning normally and a state of equilibrium of the internal environment is said to exist; this is termed **homeostasis.** When the body is in a state of homeostasis, the physical and chemical characteristics of the body substances (e.g., fluids, secretions, excretions) will be within a certain acceptable range known as the **normal** or **reference range.**

On the other hand, when a pathologic condition exists, biologic changes take place within the body, altering the normal physiology or functioning of the body and resulting in an imbalance. These changes cause the patient to experience the symptoms of that particular pathologic condition. For example, iron deficiency anemia will usually cause the patient to experience weakness, fatigue, pallor, irritability, and, in some cases, shortness of breath on exertion.

In addition, these changes in the body's biologic processes may cause an alteration in the characteristics of body substances, such as an alteration of the chemical content of the blood or urine; an alteration in the antibody level; an alteration in cell counts or cellular morphology; and so on.

The physical and chemical alterations of body substances are evidenced through abnormal values or results occurring in laboratory tests—in other words, values lying outside the accepted normal range or limit for that particular test. Just as certain pathologic conditions cause specific symptoms to occur, certain pathologic conditions cause abnormal values to occur for specific laboratory tests. For example, iron deficiency anemia causes an alteration in normal red blood cell morphology and a decreased hemoglobin level.

It is important to realize, however, that an abnormal value for a particular test may be seen with more than one pathologic condition. For example, a decrease in the hemoglobin level also is found with hyperthyroidism and cirrhosis of the liver. In this regard, the physician cannot rely solely on laboratory test results to make a final diagnosis but rather must rely upon the combination of the data obtained from the health history, the physical examination, and diagnostic and laboratory test results.

LABORATORY TESTS

☐ The number of laboratory tests ordered for a patient varies depending on the physician's clinical findings. A clinical diagnosis of a urinary tract infection, for example, usually requires only a urine culture to confirm it. Many diseases, however, exhibit more than one alteration in the physical and chemical characteristics of body substances; therefore, it is often necessary to order a series of laboratory tests to establish the pattern of abnormalities characteristic of a particular disease.

The medical assistant should realize that not all pathologic conditions require the use of laboratory test results to arrive at a final diagnosis; the information obtained from the patient's clinical signs and symptoms is sufficient to make a final diagnosis of some conditions. In these instances, the physician is so certain of the clinical diagnosis that therapy can be instituted without laboratory confirmation. For example, most physicians diagnose acute purulent otitis media using the information obtained from patient symptoms (earache, fever, feeling of fullness in the ear) and from an otoscopic examination of the tympanic membrane (the tympanic membrane is red and bulging). The information obtained through the clinical signs and symptoms is sufficiently specific to otitis media to allow the physician to make a final diagnosis and to prescribe treatment.

The medical assistant must acquire both knowledge and skill in basic clinical laboratory methods and techniques. It is important that the medical assistant have a knowledge of those laboratory tests that are performed most often, including the purpose of these tests, how to perform them, the normal value or range for each test, any advance patient preparation or special instructions, and any substances that might interfere with accurate test results, such as food or medication. The medical assistant frequently works with this information when collecting, handling, and storing specimens; performing laboratory tests; typing health histories; and receiving and filing laboratory reports. It is essential that the medical assistant appreciate the value of laboratory tests and alert the physician to any abnormal results as soon as the test is performed or the laboratory report is received.

This chapter is intended to serve as an introduction to the clinical laboratory by providing an overview of methods and general guidelines to follow and by focusing on the relationship between the medical office and an outside laboratory. Specific information for collection, handling, storing, and testing of biologic specimens is presented in the following chapters: Urinalysis, Phlebotomy, Hematology, Blood Chemistry and Serology, and Medical Microbiology.

PURPOSE OF LABORATORY TESTING

☐ The most frequent use of laboratory test results is to assist in the diagnosis of a patient's condition; however, they also have a number of other significant medical uses. A summary of the purpose and function of laboratory testing follows.

1. Laboratory tests are most frequently ordered by the physician to **assist in the diagnosis of pathologic conditions.** Along with the health history and the physical examination, laboratory test results provide the physician with essential data needed to arrive at the final diagnosis and to prescribe treatment. Following the health history and physical examination, the physician may order laboratory tests for these reasons:

   a. **To confirm a clinical diagnosis.** The patient's signs and symptoms may provide a strong clinical diagnosis of a particular condition, and the physician may order laboratory tests simply to confirm that diagnosis. For example, the patient may exhibit the typical signs and symptoms of diabetes mellitus, providing the physician with a fairly certain clinical diagnosis. In this instance, a glucose tolerance test is ordered to confirm the diagnosis and to institute therapy.

   b. **To assist in the differential diagnosis of a patient's condition.** Two or more diseases may have similar signs and symptoms; therefore, the physician will order laboratory tests to assist in the differential diagnosis of the patient's condition. For example, a final diagnosis of streptococcal sore throat must be made by a laboratory test to differentiate it from other pathologic conditions having similar signs and symptoms.

   c. **To obtain information regarding a patient's condition** when there is not enough concrete evidence to support a clinical diagnosis. At times, the patient may exhibit vague signs and symptoms, and laboratory tests are ordered to provide information on what may be causing the patient's problem. For example, the patient may complain of nonspecific abdominal pain, and the physical examination may not yield enough information to support a clinical diagnosis. In this case, the physician may order a series of tests that may include a number of laboratory tests (usually in the form of profiles) and special diagnostic procedures to assist in pinpointing the cause of the patient's problems.

2. Once the final diagnosis has been made, laboratory testing may be performed to **evaluate the patient's progress and to regulate treatment.** Based on the laboratory results, the therapy may need to be adjusted or further treatment prescribed. For example, a patient on iron therapy for iron deficiency anemia should have a complete blood count (CBC) performed every month to assess response to the treat-

ment and to make sure the condition is improving. Another example is a patient with thrombophlebitis who is taking warfarin sodium (Coumadin), an anticoagulant used to inhibit blood clotting. The patient must have a prothrombin time test at regular intervals to assess the clotting ability of the blood. Based on the test results, the medication may need to be adjusted to make sure the dosage is at a safe level. The diabetic patient who measures his or her blood glucose level each day to regulate insulin dosage is another example of using laboratory tests to regulate treatment.

3. Based on such factors as age, gender, race, and geographic location, individuals will have different normal levels within the established normal range for a particular test. In this respect, laboratory tests can also serve **to establish each patient's baseline or normal level** against which future results can be compared. For example, a patient who is going to be placed on warfarin sodium (Coumadin) therapy should have a blood specimen drawn for a prothrombin time test prior to administration of this anticoagulant. The results serve as a baseline recording for that particular patient against which future prothrombin time test results can be compared.

4. Laboratory tests can also help **prevent or reduce the severity of disease** by early detection of abnormal findings. Certain conditions, such as anemia and diabetes, are relatively common disorders and at times may exist undetected in a patient, especially early in the development of the disease. Laboratory tests known as **routine tests** are performed on a routine basis on apparently healthy patients (usually as part of a general physical examination) to assist in the early detection of disease. These tests are relatively easy to perform and present a minimal hazard to the patient. The most commonly used routine tests include urinalysis, CBC, and routine blood chemistries.

5. Another reason for performing a laboratory test is its **requirement by state law.** The statutes of most states require a gonorrhea culture and serology test for syphilis to be performed on pregnant women. The purpose of these tests is to protect the mother and fetus from harm by screening for the presence of these venereal diseases.

TYPES OF CLINICAL LABORATORIES

☐ The medical office may use an outside laboratory for testing, or the office may contain its own laboratory, known as a **physician's office laboratory (POL),** in which the medical assistant performs various tests; most medical offices use a combination of the two to fulfill the physician's needs for test results.

PHYSICIAN'S OFFICE LABORATORY

Generally speaking, laboratory tests that are convenient to execute and commonly required, such as the hematocrit determination and urinalysis, are performed in the POL. Most physicians consider it too time-consuming and expensive in terms of equipment, supplies, medical laboratory personnel, and quality control to perform in the medical office highly sophisticated and complex tests such as serologic studies and microbiologic studies. Therefore, these tests are usually performed at an outside laboratory. These laboratories use automated equipment to perform the tests, providing the medical offices with fast and reliable test results at a relatively low cost.

OUTSIDE LABORATORIES

Because the medical assistant usually works closely with an outside laboratory, it is important that she or he have a basic knowledge of the relationship between the medical office and the laboratory, as described in the following paragraphs.

Outside laboratories include **hospital** and **privately owned commercial laboratories,** which employ individuals specifically trained in clinical laboratory techniques and methods. The laboratory usually provides the medical office with the supplies and forms necessary to collect and transport specimens. The medical assistant is responsible for checking these supplies periodically and for reordering them from the laboratory as needed.

LABORATORY DIRECTORY

The outside laboratory provides the medical office with a **laboratory directory** that serves as a valuable reference source for the proper collection and handling of specimens. Directories vary in organization, depending on the laboratory; however, the following information is generally included: names of the tests performed by the laboratory, the normal range for each test, instructions on completion of forms, patient preparation required for each test, supplies required for the collection of each specimen, amount and type of specimen required by the laboratory, techniques to employ for the collection of the specimen, proper handling and storage of the specimen, and instructions for transporting specimens.

TABLE 15–1

Representative Tests from a Laboratory Directory

Test	Specimen Requirements	Normal Values
Albumin, serum	2 ml serum in a transfer tube or SST.	3.5–5.5 g/dl
ALT (alanine aminotransferase)	2 ml serum in a transfer tube or SST.	≤45 U/L
AST (aspartate aminotransferase)	2 ml serum in a transfer tube or SST.	≤40 U/L
Bilirubin, total	2 ml serum in a transfer tube or SST. Protect from light.	≤1.2 mg/dl
Blood group (ABO)	1–5 ml lavender-stopper tube	
BUN, serum	2 ml serum in a transfer tube or SST.	7–25 mg/dl
Calcium, serum	2 ml serum in a transfer tube or SST.	8.5–108 mg/dl
CBC with differential	1–5 ml lavender stoppered tube. Tube should be inverted 6–8 times immediately after drawing. 2 blood smears.	Values given with report
Chloride, serum	2 ml serum in a transfer tube or SST.	96–109 mmol/L
CPK (creatine phosphokinase)	3 ml serum in a transfer tube or SST.	Male: 54–186 IU/L Female: 41–117 IU/L
Creatinine, serum	2 ml serum in a transfer tube or SST.	Male: 0.2–0.7 mg/dl Female: 0.3–0.9 mg/dl
CRP (C-reactive protein)	1 ml serum in a transfer tube. Avoid hemolysis.	Negative
Glucose, plasma	1–5 ml gray stoppered tube. Tube should be inverted 6–8 times immediately after drawing.	65–115 mg/dl
LD (lactate dehydrogenase)	3 ml serum in a transfer tube or SST. Hemolysis invalidates results.	100–250 IU/L
Potassium, serum	2 ml serum in a transfer tube or SST. Hemolysis invalidates results.	3.5–5.3 mmol/L
Rapid plasma reagin (RPR)	2 ml serum in a white top transfer tube or SST.	Nonreactive
Sedimentation rate (ESR)	1–5 ml lavender stoppered tube. Tube should be inverted 6–8 times immediately after drawing.	Male: 0–15 mm/hour Female: 0–20 mm/hour
Sodium, serum	2 ml serum in a transfer tube or SST.	135–147 mmol/L
Tri-iodothyronine (T_3)	2 ml serum in a transfer tube or SST.	2.3–4.2 pg/ml
Thyroxine (T_4)	1 ml serum in a transfer tube or SST.	4.5–12 μg/dl
Total protein, serum	2 ml serum in a transfer tube or SST.	6.0–8.5 g/dl
Triglycerides	2 ml serum in a transfer tube. Patient should be fasting 12–14 hours.	<200 mg/dl
Uric acid, serum	2 ml serum in a transfer tube or SST.	Male: 2.2–8.7 mg/dl Female: 1.5–6.7 mg/dl
Urinalysis, routine	Random sample. First morning specimen preferred (10 ml).	

15

Table 15–1 is a sample of representative tests taken from a laboratory directory. If the medical assistant has a question regarding any aspect of the collection and handling of the specimen, she or he should call the laboratory before proceeding.

COLLECTION AND TESTING CATEGORIES

Collection and testing of a specimen can be categorized as follows: (1) the specimen is collected and tested at the medical office; (2) the specimen is collected at the medical office and transferred to an outside medical laboratory for testing; (3) the patient is given a laboratory request to have the specimen collected and tested at an outside laboratory. The responsibilities of the medical assistant depend on which of these modes is used in his or her medical office. For example, a specimen collected at the medical office and transferred to an outside laboratory for testing will involve a series of individual steps different from those followed when it is both collected and tested at the medical office.

The following clinical laboratory methods are presented in the remainder of this chapter to provide the student with the information needed to function competently in all three modes just described:

1. Completing laboratory request forms and reviewing laboratory reports.

15

2. Informing the patient of any necessary advance preparation or special instructions.
3. Collecting, handling, and transporting specimens.
4. Testing the specimens in the medical office.
5. Practicing quality control and laboratory safety.

LABORATORY REQUESTS

Purpose

Laboratory requests are printed forms containing a list of the most frequently ordered laboratory tests (Fig. 15–1). A laboratory request is required when the specimen is collected at the medical office and transferred to an outside laboratory for testing or when the specimen will be collected and tested at an outside laboratory, in which case the request is given to the patient at the medical office to take to the laboratory. The request provides the outside laboratory with essential information required for accurate testing, reporting of results, and billing. The organizational formats for the request forms vary, depending on the laboratory. In general, most outside laboratories find it more convenient and economical to provide the medical office with one form for designating all tests, with the possible exception of the Pap test, in which case a separate form, known as a cytology request, is provided.

PARTS OF A LABORATORY REQUEST FORM

Specific information that is required on the laboratory request form follows. This information should always be recorded in legible handwriting to avoid confusion or incomprehension by laboratory personnel.

1. **Physician's name and address.** The physician's name and address should be clearly indicated on the laboratory request form to facilitate the reporting of test results to the physician. Some laboratories provide request forms with the physician's name and address preprinted on the form. In addition, the forms may be prenumbered with the physician's account number, which assists in identification, reporting, and billing of laboratory tests.
2. **Patient's name.** The patient's name should be printed as requested by the laboratory; for example, the laboratory may want the patient's name written with the last name first, middle initial, first name. If the laboratory will be billing the patient directly or billing a third party, the patient's address is also required, including the city, state, and zip code.
3. **Patient's age and sex.** The normal ranges for some tests vary, depending on the patient's age and sex. For example, the normal range for hemoglobin concentration varies according to sex; it is 12 to 16 g/dl for a female, whereas for a male it is 14 to 18 g/dl.
4. **Date and time of collection of the specimen.** The date of the specimen collection indicates to the laboratory the number of days that have passed since the collection, thus providing the laboratory with information regarding the freshness of the specimen. Too long a time lapse between collection and testing of a specimen may affect the accuracy of some test results. The time of collection is significant with respect to selected laboratory tests. For example, the normal range for serum cortisol varies depending on whether the specimen is an A.M. specimen (collected in the morning) or a P.M. specimen (collected in the afternoon).
5. **Laboratory tests desired.** The tests desired by the physician are usually indicated by checking a box adjacent to those tests (see Fig. 15–1). The boxes should be clearly marked to avoid any confusion. A space designated as **additional tests** or **other tests** on the laboratory request form provides for writing in a test that is desired but that is not listed on the request form. As previously indicated, most laboratory request forms include only those tests most

Biomedical Laboratories, Inc.
100 Main Street
Athens, Georgia 45760

☐ Fax Send additional copy of report to:

☐ Call Client Number/Physician's Name ( ) Phone/Fax Number

☐ Mail Physician's Address City, State, Zip

Patient's Name (Last)	(First)	(M)	Sex	Date of Birth MO DAY YR	Collection Time : AM PM	Fasting ☐ YES ☐ NO	Collection Date MO DAY YR

NPI/UPIN	Physician's ID #	Patient's SS #	Patient's ID #	Urine hrs/vol hrs___ vol___

PATIENT / RESP. PARTY

Physician's Name (Last, First) x _____ Physician's Signature
Patient's Address Phone

Medicare # (Include prefix/suffix) ☐ Primary ☐ Secondary
City State ZIP

Medicaid # State Physician's Provider #
Name of Responsible Party (if different from patient)

Diagnosis/Signs/Symptoms in ICD-9 Format(Highest Specificity)
R E Q U I R E D
Address of Responsible Party APT #

City State ZIP

Patient's Relationship to Responsible Party ☐ 1 - Self ☐ 2 - Spouse ☐ 3 - Child ☐ 4 - Other

Performance Lab | Carrier | Group # | Employee # | Mem

INSURANCE

Insurance Company Name | Plan | Carrier Code
I hereby authorize the release of medical information related to the service described herein and authorize payment directed to LabCorp.
x _____
Patient's Signature Date

Subsciber/Member # | Location | Group #

Insurance Address | Physician's Provider #

MEDICARE ADVANCE BENEFICIARY NOTICE (ABN)

City | State | ZIP

I have read the ABN on the reverse. If Medicare denies payment, I agree to pay for the identified test(s).

Employer's Name or Number | Insured SS# (If Not Patient) | Worker's Comp ☐ Yes ☐ No
x _____
Patient's Signature Date

INDIVIDUAL COMPONENTS OF TEST COMBINATIONS/PROFILES LISTED IN THE SECTION ABOVE CAN BE ORDERED BELOW.

@ : Carrier-specific limited coverage test
# : Investigational test per Medicare

NOTE: WHEN ORDERING TESTS FOR WHICH MEDICARE OR MEDICAID REIMBURSEMENT WILL BE SOUGHT, PHYSICIANS SHOULD ONLY ORDER TESTS THAT ARE MEDICALLY NECESSARY FOR THE DIAGNOSIS OR TREATMENT OF THE PATIENT. COMPONENTS OF THE ORGAN OR DISEASE PANELS/COMBINATIONS PRINTED BELOW ARE SHOWN ON THE REVERSE SIDE AND MAY ALSO BE ORDERED INDIVIDUALLY BELOW. COMPONENTS MAY BE BILLED SEPARATELY PER CARRIER POLICY.

ORGAN OR DISEASE PANELS (See reverse for components)

303758	Basic Metabolic Panel	80049 (SST)
302085	Comp Metabolic Panel	80054 (SST)
303754	Electrolyte Panel	80051 (SST)
303755	Hepatic Function Panel	80058 (SST)
303744	Hepatitis Panel	80059 (SST)
303756	Lipid Panel	@ 80061 (SST)
235010	Lipid Panel w/LDL/HDL Ratio	@ 80061 (SST)
000455	Thyroid Panel	@ 80091 (SST)
000620	Thyroid Panel w/ TSH	@ 80092 (SST)

HEMATOLOGY

005009	CBC w Diff w Plt	85025 (LAV)
115907	CBC w Diff w/o Plt	@ 85022 (LAV)
028142	CBC w/o Diff w Plt	85027 (LAV)
005017	CBC w/o Diff w/o Plt	@ 85021 (LAV)
005058	Hematocrit	@ 85014 (LAV)
005041	Hemoglobin	@ 85018 (LAV)
005249	Platelet Count	85595 (LAV)
005033	RBC Count	85041 (LAV)
005025	WBC Count	85048 (LAV)
005090	WBC Differential	@ 85007 (LAV)

ALPHABETICAL/COMBINATION TESTS

006049	ABO and Rh (see reverse)	86900 86901 (LAV)
001081	Albumin	82040 (SST)
001107	Alkaline Phosphatase	84075 (SST)
001545	ALT (SGPT)	84460 (SST)
001396	Amylase	82150 (SST)
006254	Antinuclear Antibodies	86038 (SST)
001123	AST (SGOT)	84450 (SST)
000810	B12 and Folate (see reverse)	82607 82746 (SST)
001099	Bilirubin, Total	82250 (SST)

ALPHABETICAL TESTS CON'T

001040	BUN	84520 (SST)
001016	Calcium	82310 (SST)
007419	Carbamazepine (Tegretol®)	80156 (SER)
002139	CEA	82378 (SST)
001065	Cholesterol, Total	@ 82465 (SST)
001370	Creatinine	82565 (SST)
007385	Digoxin (Lanoxin)	@ 80162 (SER)
004515	Estradiol	82670 (SST)
004598	Ferritin	@ 82728 (SST)
100800	Fructosamine	@ 82985 (SST)
004309	FSH	83001 (SST)
028480	FSH and LH (see reverse)	83001 83002 (SST)
001958	GGT	82977 (SST)
001818	Glucose, Plasma	@ 82947 (GRY)
001032	Glucose, Serum	@ 82947 (SST)
002022	Glucose, 2-hr. PP	82950 (SST)
001693	Glycohemoglobin, Total	@ 83036 (LAV)
004556	hCG, Beta Subunit, Qual	84703 (SST)
004416	hCG, Beta Subunit, Quant	84702 (SST)
001925	HDL Cholesterol	@ 83718 (SST)
162289	Helicobacter pylori, IgG	86677 (SST)
006395	Hep B Surface Antibody	86706 (SST)
006510	Hep B Surface Antigen	87340 (SST)
140608	Hep C Antibody	86803 (SST)
001453	Hemoglobin A1c	@ 83036 (LAV)
083824	HIV Antibodies *	86701 (SST)
001339	Iron	@ 83540 (SST)
001321	Iron and IBC (see reverse)	83540 83550 (SST)
001115	LDH	83615 (SST)

ALPHABETICAL TESTS CON'T

004283	LH	83002 (SST)
001404	Lipase	83690 (SER)
007708	Lithium (Eskalith®)	80178 (SER)
001537	Magnesium	@ 83735 (SST)
007823	Phenobarbital (Luminal®)	80184 (SER)
0007401	Phenytoin (Dilantin®)	80185 (SER)
001180	Potassium	84132 (SST)
004465	Prolactin, Serum	84146 (SST)
010322	Prostate-Specific Antigen	@ 84153 (SST)
004747	Prostatic Acid Phos	84066 (SST)
001073	Protein, Total	84155 (SST)
005199	Prothrombin Time (PT)	85610 (BLU)
020321	PT and PTT Activated	85610 85730 (BLU)
005207	PTT Activated	85730 (BLU)
006502	Rheumatoid Arthritis Factor	86431 (SST)
006072	RPR	@ 86592 (SST)
006197	Rubella Antibodies, IgG	86762 (SST)
005215	Sed Rate, Westergren	85651 (LAV)
001198	Sodium	84295 (SST)
004226	Testosterone	84403 (SST)
007336	Theophylline	80198 (SER)
001149	Thyroxine (T4)	@ 84436 (SST)
001172	Triglycerides	@ 84478 (SST)
002188	Triiodothyronine (T3)	84480 (SST)
004259	TSH, High Sensitivity	@ 84443 (SST)
001057	Uric Acid	84550 (SST)
003038	Urinalysis Microscopic on Positives	81003 (URN)
003772	Urinalysis with Microscopic	81001 (URN)
007260	Valproic Acid (Depakene®)	80164 (SER)

MICROBIOLOGY - See Reverse Side

☐ ENDOCERVICAL ☐ THROAT ☐ URINE
☐ STOOL ☐ URETHRAL INDICATE SOURCE
OTHER _____

008649	Aerobic Bacterial Culture †	87070	Bact Trnspt
164160	Chlamydia/GC DNA Probe w/ Confirmation on Positives *	87490 87590	Probe Trnspt
096479	Chlamydia/GC DNA Probe without Confirmation	87490 87590	Probe Trnspt
164202	Chlamydia DNA Probe *	87490	Probe Trnspt
180745	Genital, Beta-Hemolytic Strep Cult, Group B	87081	Bact Trnspt
008334	Genital Culture, Routine †	87070	Bact Trnspt
180810	Lower Respiratory Culture †	87070	Steril Trnspt
164210	N. gonorrhoeae DNA Probe *	87590	Probe Trnspt
008623	Ova and Parasites	87015 87211	O & P Kit
008144	Stool Culture †	87081 X2 87045	Fecal Trnspt
008169	Throat, Beta-Hemolytic Strep Cult, Group A	87081	Bact Trnspt
008342	Upper Respiratory Culture, Routine †	87060	Bact Trnspt
008847	Urine Culture, Routine †	87086	Urn Cul Trnspt

† = ID/Susceptibility at Additional Charge
* = Confirmation at Additional Charge

Clinical Information/Comments

OTHER TESTS/INDIVIDUAL PROFILE COMPONENTS
TEST# TEST NAMES

15

LABCORP USE ONLY	STAT ☐ 998074	VENIPUNCTURE ☐ 998085	TRAVEL ☐ 998096	NON LABCORP ☐ 998239	VERBAL ORDER ☐ 998250	CHART ORDER ☐ 998261	HANDWRITTEN ☐ 998272	24 HR TUV ☐ 998283	PST/PSC #

CONTAINERS RECEIVED	SST SPUN	USST UNSPUN	SER SERUM TRNSPT	FRZ FRZ TRNS	RED RED	LAV LAVENDER	SLD SLIDE	BLU LT. BLUE	GRY GREY	GRN GREEN	RYB RYL BLU	YEL ACD	PLS PLASMA	URN URINE	24U 24 HR URINE	TA-U TART. ACID	FL FLUID	OT OTHER	BACT TRNSP	O & P KIT	PROBE TRNSP	URN CUL TRNSP	STERIL TRNSP	FECAL TRNSP	VIRAL TRNSP

300-0384

■ **FIGURE 15–1.** Laboratory Request Form.

TABLE 15-2

Laboratory Profiles

Profile	Tests Included	Use
Health screen profile	Glucose	General health screen
Diabetes assessment	Blood urea nitrogen (BUN)	Assessment of diseases of specific organs or disease states
Assessment of kidney function	Uric acid	
Assessment of infection and nutrition	Calcium Phosphorus	
Assessment of liver function	Total protein Albumin	
Assessment of tissue disease and cardiac function	Alkaline phosphatase Aspartate aminotransferase, AST Lactate dehydrogenase (LD) Bilirubin Cholesterol	
Liver function profile	Total bilirubin Total protein LD Albumin Globulin A/G ratio Alkaline phosphatase AST ALT	Detection of pathologic conditions affecting the liver
Thyroid function profile	T_4 RIA T_3 uptake T_7	Detection of pathologic conditions affecting the thyroid gland
Prenatal profile	Complete blood count ABO blood type Rh factor Serology (VDRL or RPR) Rubella titer Rh antibody titer Antibody screen if Rh−	Establishment of baseline recordings and screening of prenatal patients for disease or potential problems
Electrolyte profile	Sodium Potassium Chloride	
Rheumatoid profile	Antistreptolysin O (ASO) titer Rheumatoid factor (RA) test C-reactive protein (CRP) Uric acid	Detection of rheumatoid arthritis
Lipid profile	Total cholesterol Triglycerides HDL cholesterol LDL cholesterol Total cholesterol/HDL ratio	Detection of coronary heart disease
Hepatitis profile	HBsAg HBcAb—IgM HAvAb—IgM	Detection of viral hepatitis

frequently ordered. The laboratory directory contains a complete listing of all the tests performed.

Laboratory tests termed **profiles** contain a number of different tests; the profiles performed by the laboratory and the tests included in each are listed in the directory. A profile may be specific in nature; that is, all the tests included relate to a specific organ of the body or a particular disease state. A specific profile is usually ordered when the physician does not have a definite clinical diagnosis but has a good idea of what organ or organs are involved in the patient's condition. Most of these profiles are termed function tests, and the physician will order a function test of the organ in question. An example of this type of profile is the liver function profile, which is used to assess liver function and to assist in the diagnosis of a pathologic condition affecting the liver.

A profile may also be general in nature. A general profile contains a number of routine laboratory tests and is primarily used in a routine health screen of a patient. General health screen profiles are used to detect any changes in the body's biologic processes that may be present, even though the patient may not have experienced any symptoms to indicate that these changes have occurred. General profiles are also used when the patient's symptoms are so vague that the physician does not have enough concrete evidence to support a clinical diagnosis of a specific organ or disease state.

The medical assistant should have a knowledge of the names of common profiles and the tests generally contained in each, which are listed in Table 15–2. The specific tests contained in each profile may vary slightly from one laboratory to another, based on physicians' needs and the type of equipment utilized by the laboratory to perform the tests.

6. **Source of the specimen.** Certain tests require that the source of the specimen (e.g., throat, wound, ear, eye, urine, vagina) be recorded on the laboratory request form. The purpose of this is to identify the origin of the specimen for the laboratory because it is not possible to obtain this information by looking at the specimen. In many instances, the source dictates the test method used by the laboratory to evaluate the specimen for the presence of a possible pathogen. For example, the test method used to detect the presence of *Streptococcus* in a specimen obtained from the throat will be different from that used to detect *Candida albicans* in a vaginal specimen.

7. **Physician's clinical diagnosis.** The clinical diagnosis assists the laboratory in correlating the clinical laboratory data with the needs of the physician. In some instances, further testing is performed by the laboratory if one test method proves inconclusive with respect to providing the physician with the information necessary to confirm or reject the clinical diagnosis. Another function of the clinical diagnosis is to assure laboratory personnel that the test results are within the framework of the diagnosis. When the results of a test disagree with the physician's clinical diagnosis of the patient, the laboratory repeats the test on the same or another specimen. The clinical diagnosis also alerts laboratory personnel to the possibility of the presence of a potentially dangerous pathogen, such as the hepatitis virus. In addition, it is required for third-party billing by the laboratory. If the laboratory is billing an insurance company for the tests, the clinical diagnosis will be required on the insurance form. This facilitates the processing of insurance forms by having the information at hand and not having to contact the medical office to obtain it.

8. **Medications.** Certain medications the patient is taking may interfere with the accuracy and validity of the test results. Therefore, the laboratory should be notified of any medications being taken by the patient by listing them on the request form.

9. **STAT.** At times, the physician will want the laboratory test results reported as soon as possible. In this case, STAT should be clearly written in bold letters (or the appropriate STAT box checked) on the laboratory request form. Requests that are marked STAT are performed as soon as possible after being received by the laboratory, and the results are telephoned to the physician as soon as they are available.

Once the specimen has been collected, the completed request form must be placed with the specimen for transport to the outside laboratory. The medical assistant should realize the significance of this simple but important step. Numerous possible tests can be performed on one particular specimen, and without the request form, the laboratory does not have the information it needs to carry out the physician's orders, which causes delays in completing the tests and reporting results.

LABORATORY REPORTS

☐ The purpose of laboratory report forms is to relay the results of the laboratory tests to the physician (Fig. 15–2). The report may be in the form of a computer printout, or it may be a preprinted form with the test results written in by the laboratory technologist performing the tests. It will include certain types of information listed as follows:

NATIONAL HEALTH LABORATORIES, INC

DATE REPORTED	DATE RECEIVED	PATIENT NAME — I.D.		PHONE	AGE	SEX
4/12/2002	4/11/2002	Judith Johnson 08575		(614) 592-1100	26	F

DATE COLLECTED	TIME COLLECTED	HOSPITAL I.D.	REQUISITION NO.	ACCESSION NO.
4/11/2002	8:30 AM		91449	1235-G8

CLIENT NAME/ADDRESS	TEST REQUIRED
Woodside Medical Clinic 400 Main Street Athens, Ohio 45701	Health Screen Profile CBC

PHYSICIAN	VOLUME	FASTING	PATIENT SS #	COMMENTS
J. Camerson, M.D.		X	248-71-2669	

CHEMISTRY   RENAL   LIPIDS   ELECTROLYTES

GLUCOSE 65-115 mg/dL	B.U.N. 7-25 mg/dL	CREATININE 0.6-1.5 mg/dL	BUN/CREAT RATIO 6-20	CHOLESTEROL 130- • mg/dL (see back)	TRIGLYCERIDE 30-150 mg/dL	CALCIUM 8.5-10.8 mg/dL	PHOSPHORUS 2.5-4.5 mg/dL •	SODIUM 135-147 mmol/L	POTASSIUM 3.5-5.3 mmol/L	CHLORIDE 96-109 mmol/L	FERRITIN M 20-450 F 8-350 • ng/mL
91	24	1.3	18.5	185	69	9.8	3.3	140.6	4.45	105	

PROTEIN   LIVER

URIC ACID M 3.9-9.0 F 2.2-7.7 mg/dL	TOTAL PROTEIN 6.0-8.5 g/dL	ALBUMIN 3.5-5.5 g/dL	GLOBULIN 2.0-3.5 g/dL	ALB/GLB RATIO 1.0-2.4	TOTAL BILIRUBIN ≤ 1.2 mg/dL	ALK. PHOS. 25-140 U/L •	LD (LDN) ≤ 240 U/L	AST (SGOT) ≤ 40 U/L	ALT (SGPT) ≤ 45 U/L	GGT M 0-65 F 0-45 U/L	IONIZED CALCIUM 3.5-5.2 mg/dL
3.6	6.8	4.1		1.5	0.3	82	195	29	38		

THYROID

T3 UPTAKE 25-35%	T4 TOTAL 4.5-12 μg/dL	T7 (T3U × T4) 1.2-4.2	T3 by RIA 70-210 ng/dL	TSH 0.4-6.0 μg/mL	B₁₂ 200-1150 pg/mL	FOLATE 2.5-17.3 ng/mL	CORTISOL AM 7.0-25.0 PM 2.0-9.0 μg/dL	DIGOXIN 0.5-2.0 ng/mL	DILANTIN 10-20 μg/mL	PHENOBARB 10-35 μg/mL	THEOPHYLLINE 10-20 μg/mL

BLOOD CELL PROFILE   SEROLOGY

WBC 4.0-11.0 × 10³/μL	RBC M 4.4-6.2 F 3.8-5.4 × 10⁶/μL •	HGB M 13-18 F 11.5-16 g/dL •	HCT M 39-54 F 35-48 % •	MCV 80-100 fL	MCH 27-34 pg	MCHC 31-36 %	SYPHILIS SCREEN NON- REACTIVE	MONO TEST NEG	STREPTOZYME NEG	RHEUMATOID FACTOR < 1:10	C-RP NEG
12.3	4.27	13.4	39	91	31.3	34.5					

DIFFERENTIAL

NEUT 45-75	LYMPH 18-46	MONO ≤ 11	EOSIN ≤ 6	BASO ≤ 2	PLATELET COUNT 140-450 × 10³/μL	WINTROBE ESR M 0-10 F 0-20 mm/Hr	RUBELLA	BLOOD GROUP	Rhₒ(D)	Dᵁ	ANTIBODY SCREEN
83	12	3	2	0							

URINALYSIS

APPEARANCE CLEAR	COLOR YELLOW	SP. GRAVITY 1.005-1.035	pH 5.0-7.5	PROTEIN NEG	GLUCOSE NEG	KETONES NEG	BILIRUBIN NEG	BLOOD NEG	NITRATE NEG	UROBILINOGEN < 2	LEUKOCYTE TEST NEG

RESULT NAME	RESULT	UNITS	REFERENCE RANGE

■ **FIGURE 15–2.** Laboratory Report Form. (Courtesy of National Health Laboratories, Inc., San Diego, CA.)

1. Name, address, and telephone number of the laboratory
2. Physician's name and address
3. Patient's name, age, and gender
4. Patient accession number
5. Date the specimen was received by the laboratory
6. Date the results were reported by the laboratory
7. Names of the tests performed
8. Results of the tests
9. Normal range for each test performed

A patient **accession number** or laboratory number is assigned to each specimen received by the laboratory. Its purpose is to provide positive identification of each specimen within the laboratory and to allow easy access to the patient's laboratory records should a test result need to be located again. If the physician desires to have the laboratory test repeated, the accession number listed on the original report form must be included on the laboratory request form.

A **normal range,** rather than a single value, is necessary for laboratory test results because of individual differences among a general population due to factors such as age, gender, race, and geographic location. In addition, no test can be so accurate that a single value is possible. The normal range for each test varies slightly from one laboratory to another, depending on the test method, equipment, and reagents used to perform the test. In this regard, it is essential that the medical assistant compare the test results with the normal values supplied by the laboratory performing the test, rather than with a reference source such as a medical laboratory test.

Laboratory reports are either hand delivered or mailed to the medical office by the laboratory. Abnormal results posing a threat to the patient's health and laboratory reports marked STAT are telephoned to the medical office as soon as the tests are completed, and a written report follows immediately thereafter. The laboratory usually supplies the medical office with telephone reporting pads to transcribe the results from the telephone report to reduce errors.

The medical assistant may be responsible for reviewing the laboratory reports as they are received. He or she should compare the patient's test results with the normal ranges supplied by the laboratory and notify the physician of any abnormal test results. Many computer systems automatically identify abnormal results on the laboratory report; if not, the physician may want the medical assistant to identify them by circling them with a red pen. The reports are then reviewed by the physician, and the data obtained are correlated with the information obtained from the health history and physical examination of the patient. The physician indicates, usually by placing his or her initials on the report, when he or she is finished with it. The medical assistant is then responsible for filing the laboratory report in the patient's chart, according to the medical office policy.

PATIENT PREPARATION AND INSTRUCTIONS

☐ Factors such as food consumption, medication, activity, and time of day affect the laboratory results of certain tests. Therefore, for some laboratory tests advance patient preparation is necessary to obtain a quality specimen suitable for testing, which leads to accurate results and, in turn, assists the physician in accurate diagnosis and treatment. It is important to realize that the quality of the laboratory test results can be only as good as the quality of the specimen obtained from the patient. A specimen obtained from a patient who has not prepared properly may invalidate the test results and necessitate calling the patient back to collect the specimen again.

The medical assistant is usually responsible for instructing the patient in any advance preparation that might be required. A complete and thorough explanation of the instructions should be relayed clearly to the patient. The medical assistant should explain the reason for the advance preparation; in this way, the patient will be more likely to comply with the preparation required. It should be emphasized to the patient that the preparation is essential to obtain accurate test results and to avoid having to collect the specimen again.

Once the instructions have been explained, it is important to check to make sure the patient completely understands them and offer to answer any questions. It is also advisable to provide the patient with a written instruction sheet to serve as a reference, should he or she forget some of the information after leaving the medical office. Some specimen collections may require that the patient remain at the collection site for a specified period of time; an example of this is the glucose tolerance test, which requires several hours for the collection of multiple, timed specimens. The patient should be told in advance of the time requirement so that he or she can make any necessary arrangements with an employer, babysitter, and so on.

At times, the patient will be collecting the specimen himself or herself, either at home or at the medical office. The medical assistant is responsible for explaining detailed instructions to the patient on the proper techniques to use to collect the specimen. For example, if a first-voided morning urine specimen is required for the laboratory test, the medical assistant will need to provide the patient with the appropriate specimen container and to instruct the patient in the proper collection, handling, and storage of the specimen until it reaches the medical office.

The specific type of preparation required for a particular test depends on the test ordered and the method used to run it. If the medical office uses an outside laboratory, the patient preparation required for each test will be found in the laboratory directory. If the test is to be performed in the medical office, the medical assistant should consult the manufacturer's instructions that accompany the testing product to obtain specific information regarding patient preparation. Advance patient preparation is usually in the form of a diet modification (e.g., low-fat diet), fasting, or medication restrictions.

15

FASTING

Some venous blood specimens require the patient to fast before collection. The composition of blood is altered by consumption of food because the digested food is absorbed into the circulatory system, thus changing the results of certain laboratory tests. For example, food intake causes the blood glucose and triglyceride laboratory tests to yield falsely high results. Therefore, any individual test or profile including these tests, such as fasting blood sugar (FBS), a glucose tolerance test (GTT), or a health screen profile, requires the patient to fast before the specimen is collected.

Fasting involves abstaining from food and fluids (except water) for a specified amount of time before the collection of the specimen (usually 12 to 14 hours). Fasting specimens are usually collected in the morning, to allow the food from the previous evening meal to be completely digested and absorbed. In addition, collecting the specimen in the morning causes the least amount of inconvenience to the patient in terms of abstaining from food and fluid.

The medical assistant must be sure to give detailed instructions to the patient, making certain the patient understands that fasting includes abstaining from both food and fluid; however, the patient should be told that it is permissible—in fact advisable—to drink water, because dehydration caused by water abstinence can also alter certain test results.

The medical assistant should indicate a specific time to the patient for initiating the fast; if the specimen will be collected in the morning, the patient should be instructed to begin fasting at 6:00 P.M. on the previous evening. The patient must also be told the time to report for collection of the specimen.

MEDICATION RESTRICTIONS

Many medications affect the physical and chemical characteristics of body substances; therefore, medications the patient is taking may lead to inaccurate test results. For example, antibiotic therapy administered before collection of a throat specimen for culture may cause a falsely negative report. The physician generally asks the patient to avoid taking medication for a period of time before the collection of the specimen, if discontinuing the medication will not cause any health threat or serious discomfort to the patient.

Because medication is more likely to interfere with test results on urine than on blood, it is recommended that the patient discontinue medication 48 to 72 hours before the collection of a urine specimen and 4 to 24 hours prior to the collection of a blood specimen.

If the patient cannot be taken off medication, the information should be recorded on the laboratory request form for those specimens being transported to an outside laboratory for testing. This alerts the laboratory personnel to the presence of the medication. If the medication being taken by the patient interferes with the method normally used to perform the test, the laboratory may be able to use an alternate method to obtain valid results. If the test is being performed in the medical office, the medical assistant should consult the manufacturer's instructions that accompany the testing materials for the names of the medications that interfere with test results.

The physician determines the need for abstinence from the medication before specimen collection. The medical assistant is responsible for making sure the patient understands any instructions regarding restrictions on medication and for recording medications the patient is taking on the laboratory request form.

COLLECTING, HANDLING, AND TRANSPORTING SPECIMENS

☐ Clinical laboratory tests are performed on specimens obtained from the body. A **specimen** is a small sample or part taken from the body to represent the nature of the whole. The majority of laboratory tests are performed on specimens that are easily obtained from the body, such as blood, urine, feces, sputum, a cervical and vaginal scraping of cells, or a sample of a secretion or discharge from various parts of the body (e.g., nose, throat, wound, ear, eye, vagina, urethra) for microbiologic analysis. Other examples of specimens analyzed in the laboratory but more difficult to obtain from the body include gastric juices, cerebrospinal fluid, pleural fluid, peritoneal fluid, synovial fluid, and tissue biopsies. The source of the specimen may not necessarily be indicative of the pathologic condition in question; for example, T_3 and T_4 tests are performed on blood serum but are used to detect a condition affecting the thyroid gland.

The medical assistant is responsible for the collection of the majority of the specimens obtained from patients in the medical office; of these, blood and urine will constitute the largest percentage of specimens collected. Certain specimens, such as a sample of vaginal or urethral discharge, cerebrospinal fluid, or a tissue biopsy, must be collected by the physician; in this case, the medical assistant assists with the collection.

The most important aspect of specimen collection and handling is to provide the laboratory with a sample that is as biologically representative as possible of the body substance collected. If it is collected or handled improperly, the in vivo characteristics of the specimen may be adversely affected, which, in turn, may cause inaccurate and unreliable test results; this may interfere with accurate diagnosis and treatment of the patient's condition.

GUIDELINES

Specific guidelines that should be used regarding specimen collection and handling follow:

1. **Review and follow the OSHA Bloodborne Pathogens Standards** during specimen collection (see Chapter 1, OSHA Bloodborne Pathogens Standards).

2. **Review the requirements for collection and handling of the specimen,** which include the collection materials required, the type of specimen to be collected (e.g., serum, plasma, whole blood, clotted blood, urine), the amount required for laboratory analysis, the procedure to follow in collecting the specimen, and its proper handling and storage.

3. **Assemble the equipment and supplies.** Use only the appropriate specimen containers as specified by the medical office or laboratory. Substituting containers may not yield the proper type of specimen required or may affect the test results, as shown by the following examples: If serum is required and a tube containing an anticoagulant is used (instead of a plain tube not containing an anticoagulant), the blood separates into plasma and cells, rather than serum and cells, and the wrong type of blood specimen is obtained, which requires having to draw another specimen from the patient. Collecting a microbiologic specimen that may contain anaerobic pathogens with supplies meant for aerobic pathogens results in death of the anaerobic pathogen.

   The specimen container should be sterile, to prevent contamination of the specimen. Many specimens, especially microbiologic ones, are adversely affected by contaminants, such as extraneous microorganisms, which may affect the accuracy of the test results.

   The medical assistant should check each container before using it to make sure it is not broken, chipped, cracked, or otherwise damaged. Damaged containers are unsuitable for specimen collection and should be discarded. The medical assistant should be sure to label each tube and specimen container with the patient's name, the date, the medical assistant's initials, and any other information required by the laboratory, such as the source of the specimen. The information should be printed legibly and the medical assistant should be certain that the information is accurate, to avoid a mix-up of specimens.

4. **Identify the patient, and explain the procedure.** It is important for the medical assistant to identify the patient, to avoid collecting a specimen from the wrong patient by mistake. If the problem is not discovered, this could lead to invalid test results and could affect the patient's diagnosis and treatment. Explaining the procedure helps relax and reassure the patient, and gains the patient's confidence and cooperation, especially if it is the first time the patient has had a specimen collected.

   If the patient was required to prepare before having the specimen collected, determine whether this has been done properly. Improper preparation may lead to inaccurate test results. For example, if a test requiring fasting, such as an FBS, is performed on a nonfasting specimen, the results are altered; in this case, they are falsely high. If the patient has not prepared properly, inform the physician; the physician may want the patient to prepare properly and return, or the physician may tell the medical assistant to go ahead with the collection but to alert the laboratory to the situation by marking the information on the laboratory request. In the example just given, *nonfasting specimen* would be written on the request form.

5. **Collection of the specimen** involves a set of specific techniques for each type of specimen obtained. The information in this section is presented in general terms; the specific procedures for the collection of biologic specimens are included in this text in the following chapters: Urinalysis, Phlebotomy, Hematology, Blood Chemistry and Serology, and Medical Microbiology.

   Specimen collection involves a combination of medical and surgical aseptic techniques. Certain parts of collection materials, such as needles, swabs, and the inside of the specimen containers, must remain sterile. If a culture medium is being used to collect a microbiologic specimen, the medical assistant must make sure that the lid of the container is removed only when the specimen is being spread on the culture medium. Unnecessary removal of the lid results in contamination of the culture medium with extraneous microorganisms, which interferes with accurate test results. During the collection and handling of the specimen, the medical assistant also must be careful to use medical and surgical asepsis to prevent contamination of the specimen, the patient, or the self.

   The medical assistant must collect the specimen using proper technique. The procedure should be followed exactly to ensure a high-quality and reliable specimen. The proper type of specimen must be collected as designated either by the outside laboratory or by the instructions that accompany the testing materials. For example, the collection of a random urine specimen when a clean-catch midstream specimen is required will affect the accuracy of the test results.

The medical assistant must make sure to collect the amount required for the test, which varies, depending on the type of specimen being collected and the number of laboratory tests ordered. The medical assistant must refer to the appropriate reference material to determine the amount required for each test ordered by the physician. If the specimen is being transported to an outside laboratory, the amount required is listed next to each test in the laboratory directory (see Table 15–1). The amount required for those specimens being tested in the medical office is found in the manufacturer's instructions that accompany the testing materials. It is important that the medical assistant strictly observe

the stipulated amount requirements, especially for specimens being transported to an outside laboratory. If the medical assistant fails to collect the specified amount, the laboratory will be unable to perform the test and the laboratory request will be returned marked QNS (quantity not sufficient). This situation warrants calling the patient back for collection of another specimen.

Once the specimen has been collected, the medical assistant records the following information on the patient's chart: the date and time of the collection, the laboratory tests ordered by the physician, the type of specimen, and the source of the specimen. If the specimen is being transported to an outside laboratory, this information should be indicated in the patient's chart, including the date the specimen was transported to the laboratory, if it is different from the date of collection.

TABLE 15 – 3

Handling and Storage of Biologic Specimens

Specimen	Handling	Storage
Blood	***All Blood Specimens:*** Prevent hemolysis; Collect the specimen in a tube that is at room temperature ***Serum:*** Separate serum from blood within 30 to 45 minutes after collection ***Plasma:*** Mix anticoagulant gently but thoroughly with the blood specimen immediately after collection	For most blood specimens, refrigerate at 4°C (39°F) to retard alterations in the physical and chemical composition of the specimen; Plasma and serum may be frozen; however, whole blood should not be frozen because it will cause hemolysis
Urine	Avoid contamination of the inside of the specimen container; Do not leave the specimen standing out for more than 1 hour after collection	If the urine specimen cannot be tested within 1 hour after collection, refrigerate it or add an appropriate preservative
Microbiologic specimens	Avoid contamination of the swab used to collect the specimen; Avoid contamination of the inside of the microbiologic specimen container; Protect yourself from contamination from the microbiologic specimen; Protect anaerobic specimens from exposure to air	Transport the specimen as soon as possible. If not possible, place the specimen in a transport medium or inoculate it on the appropriate culture medium and (for most specimens) place it in the refrigerator at 4°C (39°F) to prevent drying and death of the specimen or overgrowth of the specimen with extraneous microorganisms
Stool	Collect the specimen in a clean container; For the detection of ova and parasites, keep the stool warm	For the most accurate test results, deliver the specimen to the laboratory immediately. If there will be a delay in transporting the specimen, mix the stool with an appropriate preservative or place it in a transport medium

For all specimens: Do not expose to extreme temperature changes.

6. **Properly handle and store the specimen** with care to preserve its in vivo qualities. Some specimens, such as microbiologic specimens, are more sensitive to environmental influences and must be handled with special care. Whenever possible, it is best to perform laboratory tests on fresh specimens (for most specimens, within 1 hour after collection), because they yield the most reliable test results. When this is not practical, as is usually the case, the specimen must be stored; it may require storage until pickup by an outside laboratory, mailing, or testing at the medical office. Storing a specimen involves properly preserving it so as to maintain its in vivo physical and chemical characteristics until it is analyzed. General guidelines for handling and storing biologic specimens most frequently collected in the medical office are presented in Table 15–3.

PROCEDURE

15–1

Collecting a Specimen for Transport to an Outside Laboratory

A summary of the series of individual steps required for collecting a specimen in the medical office and transporting it to an outside laboratory is presented in this procedure.

1. **Procedural Step.** Inform the patient of any advance preparation or special instructions, which may include
   a. Diet modification
   b. Fasting
   c. Medication restriction
   d. Collection of a specimen at home
   Explain the instructions thoroughly, and provide the patient with written instructions to take home as a reference. Notify the patient of the time of report to the medical office for the specimen collection.
   Principle. The patient must prepare properly in order to provide a quality specimen that will lead to accurate test results and avoid having to return to have another specimen collected.

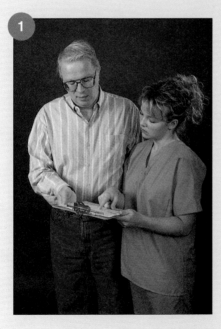

2. **Procedural Step.** Review the requirements in the laboratory directory for the collection and handling of the specimens ordered by the physician, which include
   a. Collection materials required
   b. Type of specimen to be collected
   c. Amount of the specimen required for laboratory analysis
   d. Procedure to follow to collect the specimen
   e. Proper handling and storage of the specimen
   Telephone the laboratory with any questions you have regarding any aspect of the collection or handling of the specimen.
   Principle. Reviewing the requirements beforehand prevents errors in collection and handling of the specimen.

3. **Procedural Step.** Complete the laboratory request form, which must include the following information printed in legible handwriting.
   a. Physician's name and address
   b. Patient's name (and address if required)
   c. Patient's age and sex
   d. Date and time of the collection
   e. Laboratory tests ordered by the physician
   f. Type of specimen
   g. Source of specimen
   h. Physician's clinical diagnosis
   i. Any medications the patient is taking
   j. When applicable, third-party billing information (e.g., Blue Cross, Blue Shield, Medicare, and so on)
   If the test results are needed by the physician as soon as possible mark STAT on the request in bold letters.
   Principle. The completed form provides the laboratory with the information necessary to perform the tests accurately.

15

Continued

15

4. **Procedural Step.** Wash the hands.
   Principle. Practicing medical asepsis helps protect the specimen from contamination.

5. **Procedural Step.** Assemble the equipment and supplies. Be sure to use the appropriate specimen container required by the outside laboratory. Make sure the container is sterile and check to make sure it is not broken, chipped, or cracked.
   Principle. The appropriate specimen container must be used to ensure the collection of the proper type of specimen required by the laboratory. Damaged specimen containers are unsuitable for collection and should be discarded.

6. **Procedural Step.** Clearly label the tubes and containers with the patient's name, the date, your initials, and any other information required by the laboratory, such as the source of the specimen.
   Principle. Properly labeled tubes and containers prevent mix-up of specimens.

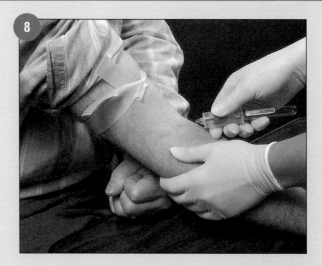

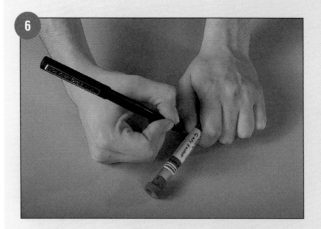

7. **Procedural Step.** Greet and identify the patient. Introduce yourself and explain the procedure. Make sure you have the correct patient. If the patient was required to prepare for the test, determine whether he or she has prepared properly.
   Principle. Identifying the patient prevents collecting a specimen from the wrong person by mistake. Specimen collection is often an anxiety-producing experience for the patient, and reassurance should be offered to help reduce apprehension.

8. **Procedural Step.** Collect the specimen, using the following guidelines:
   a. Follow the OSHA Standard.
   b. Collect the specimen using proper technique.
   c. Collect the proper type and amount of the specimen required for the test.
   d. Process the specimen further, if required by the outside laboratory (e.g., separating serum from whole blood).

e. Place the lid tightly on the specimen container.
f. Record information in the patient's chart, including the date and time of the collection, the type and source of the specimen, the laboratory tests ordered by the physician, and information indicating its transport to the outside laboratory, including the date the specimen was sent.
Principle. Proper collection of a specimen maintains its in vivo qualities and provides the laboratory with a biologically representative sample of the body substance collected.

9. **Procedural Step.** Properly handle and store (if necessary) the specimen, according to the laboratory specifications.

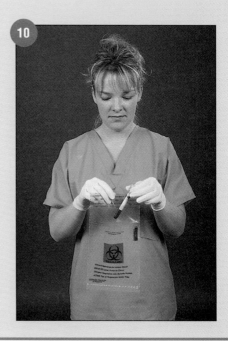

PROCEDURE 15-1

Principle. The specimen must be handled and stored properly to maintain the in vivo characteristics of the specimen.

10. **Procedural Step.** Prepare the specimen for transport to the outside laboratory. Be sure to include the completed laboratory request with the specimen.

Principle. The outside laboratory must have the completed request from to know which laboratory tests have been ordered by the physician.

11. **Procedural Step.** Review the laboratory report when it is returned to the medical office. Compare each test result with the normal range provided by the laboratory, and notify the physician of any abnormal results. File the laboratory report in the pa-

tient's chart after it has been reviewed by the physician.

CHARTING EXAMPLE	
Date	
3/10/2002	8:00 a.m. Venous blood specimen collected from (R) arm. Tests ordered: cholesterol, HDL, and triglycerides. Pt was in a fasting state. Courier pick-up by Medical Center Laboratory on 3/10/2002. ————— K. McGrew, CMA

CLINICAL LABORATORY IMPROVEMENT AMENDMENTS

PURPOSE OF CLIA 1988

In 1988, Congress passed the Clinical Laboratory Improvement Amendments (CLIA 1988) to improve the quality of laboratory testing in the United States. CLIA 1988 consists of federal regulations governing all facilities that perform laboratory tests for health assessment or for the diagnosis, prevention, or treatment of disease. CLIA 1988 includes facilities not previously covered under federal legislation, such as POLs and nursing homes. The regulations for implementing CLIA, developed by the Department of Health and Human Services (DHHS), consist of four separate sets of rules: laboratory standards, application and user fees, enforcement procedures, and approval of accreditation programs. The Health Care Financing Administration (HCFA) is a division of DHHS. HCFA is responsible for monitoring compliance with the CLIA regulations.

CATEGORIES OF LABORATORY TESTING

The CLIA regulations establish three categories of laboratory testing based on the complexity of the testing methods:

WAIVED TESTS. Waived tests are simple procedures, including those that patients can perform at home. Laboratories that perform only waived tests must apply

for a certificate of waiver from HCFA, which exempts them from many of the CLIA oversight requirements. Laboratories with certificates of waiver are still expected to adhere to good laboratory practices, which include following the manufacturer's recommended instructions for each product or testing kit. To assist individuals in keeping up with new waived test additions, and new methodologies for waived tests, the Centers for Disease Control and Prevention (CDC) maintain the following website: www.cdc.gov/phppo/dls/clia.htm. The following are examples of waived tests.

Dipstick or tablet reagent urinalysis (nonautomated) for bilirubin, glucose, hemoglobin, ketones, leukocytes, nitrite, pH, protein, specific gravity, and urobilinogen.
Fecal occult blood tests
Ovulation testing, using visual color comparisons
Urine pregnancy tests, using visual color comparisons
Erythrocyte sedimentation rate, nonautomated
Hemoglobin by copper sulfate method, nonautomated
Spun microhematocrit
Blood glucose determination with devices approved by the Food and Drug Administration (FDA) for home use
CLIA-approved strep A tests.

MODERATE-COMPLEXITY TESTS. Moderate-complexity tests account for 75 percent of the estimated 10,000 laboratory tests performed in the United States every day. Examples of moderate-complexity tests performed in the medical office include hematology and blood chemistry tests performed on an automated blood analyzer, Gram staining, pinworm preps, and microscopic analysis of urine sediment.

15

HIGH-COMPLEXITY TESTS. High-complexity tests include all procedures related to cytogenetics, histopathology, histocompatibility, and cytology (includes Pap testing). These tests are not usually performed in medical offices; most of these tests are done in laboratories already subject to federal regulation.

REQUIREMENTS FOR MODERATE- AND HIGH-COMPLEXITY TESTING

Laboratories performing moderate- or high-complexity tests or both must meet the CLIA regulations and are subject to unannounced inspections every 2 years by HCFA. The major components of the CLIA 1988 regulations relating to laboratory standards are listed here:

PATIENT TEST MANAGEMENT. A system must be established to maintain the optimal integrity and identification of patient specimens throughout the testing process and to ensure accurate reporting of results.

QUALITY CONTROL. To ensure accurate and reliable test results, each laboratory must establish and follow written quality control procedures that monitor and evaluate the quality of each testing process. These include developing a laboratory procedure manual, following the manufacturer's instructions for each product; performing and documenting calibration procedures at least every 6 months and two levels of controls daily; performing and documenting actions taken when problems or errors are identified; and documenting all quality control activities.

QUALITY ASSURANCE. Each laboratory must establish and follow written policies and procedures to monitor and evaluate the overall quality of the total testing process. This is done to ensure the accuracy and reliability of patient test results.

PROFICIENCY TESTING (PT). Proficiency testing is a form of external quality control in which laboratory specimens are prepared by an approved proficiency testing agency. Three times a year, the physician's laboratory must test a shipment of these unknown specimens using the same procedure as for testing a patient's specimen. The results are then forwarded to the proficiency testing agency for evaluation.

PERSONNEL REQUIREMENTS. The CLIA regulations specify qualifications and responsibilities for personnel for laboratory directors, technical consultants, clinical consultants, and testing personnel. The regulations list specific education and training qualifications for the various positions and also define the responsibilities for the persons who fill these positions. Personnel requirements are most stringent for high-complexity testing.

PUTTING IT ALL *into* PRACTICE

▶ **KOREY McGREW:** *As a practicing medical assistant, I had a very challenging venipuncture experience. The patient was a very kind and personable 64-year-old man who had hardening of the arteries. I tried two times to obtain the blood specimen from his arms but was not successful. The patient was very calm and not bothered at all by having two sticks. He said that it was hard to draw blood on him and to go ahead and try again. I decided to try taking blood from a vein on the back of his hand using a butterfly set-up. To my relief, I obtained the blood specimen. I think that I was more nervous about this experience than the patient. I think that it is important to try to remain calm on the outside around patients even if you are nervous on the inside.*

THE PHYSICIAN'S OFFICE LABORATORY

☐ As previously discussed, a POL consists of an in-house medical office laboratory. Testing a specimen in a POL involves following a series of steps to measure or identify the presence of a specific substance in the specimen, such as the measurement of a chemical or the identification of a microorganism. The medical assistant may be responsible for performing the laboratory tests and recording results, or the physician may employ a medical laboratory technician or a medical technologist to perform the tests. The decision is based on the number of tests performed in the medical office, the complexity of these tests, and the CLIA regulations. The medical assistant is qualified to perform basic laboratory tests; the more sophisticated tests require the knowledge and skill of the medical laboratory technician.

Laboratory tests can be classified by function into one of the following categories: hematology, clinical chemistry, serology and blood banking, urinalysis, microbiology, parasitology, cytology, and histology. Table 15–4 lists the definition of each of these categories and

TABLE 15 – 4

Categories of Laboratory Tests

Categories of laboratory tests are listed, including the definition of each and commonly performed tests or pathologic condition in each category. Those tests that are commonly known by their abbreviations are listed that way.

Hematology

Hematology is the science dealing with the study of blood and the blood-forming tissues. Laboratory analysis in hematology deals with the examination of blood for the detection of pathologic conditions and includes areas such as blood cell counts, cellular morphology, the clotting ability of the blood, and identification of cell types.

White blood cell count (WBC)
Red blood cell count (RBC)
Differential white blood cell count (Diff)
Hemoglobin (Hgb)
Hematocrit (Hct)
Prothrombin time (PT)
Erythrocyte sedimentation rate (ESR)
Platelet count

Clinical Chemistry

Laboratory analysis in clinical chemistry involves detecting the presence of chemical substances or determining the amount of substances present in body fluids, excreta, and tissues (e.g., blood, urine, cerebrospinal fluid). The largest area in clinical chemistry is blood chemistry.

Glucose
Blood urea nitrogen (BUN)
Creatinine
Total protein
Albumin
Globulin
Calcium
Inorganic phosphorus
Chloride
Sodium
Potassium
Bilirubin
Cholesterol
Triglycerides
Uric acid
Lactate dehydrogenase (LD)
Aspartate aminotransferase (AST)
Alanine aminotransferase (ALT)
Alkaline phosphatase
Phospholipids

Serology and Blood Banking

Laboratory analysis in serology and blood banking deals with studying antigen-antibody reactions to assess the presence of a substance and/or to determine the presence of disease.

Syphilis detection tests (VDRL, RPR)
C-reactive protein test (CRP)
ABO blood typing
Rh typing
Rh antibody titer test

Cross-match
Direct Coombs' test
Cold agglutinins
Rheumatoid factor (RA factor)
Mono test
Heterophil antibody titer test
Hepatitis tests
HIV tests: ELISA and Western blot
Antistreptolysin O (ASO) titer
Pregnancy tests

Urinalysis

Urinalysis involves the physical, chemical, and microscopic analysis of urine.

A. Tests included in the physical analysis of urine:
   Color
   Clarity
   Specific gravity
B. Tests included in the chemical analysis of urine:
   pH
   Glucose
   Protein
   Ketones
   Blood
   Bilirubin
   Urobilinogen
   Nitrite
   Leukocytes
C. Tests included in the microscopic analysis of urine
   Red blood cells
   White blood cells
   Epithelial cells
   Casts
   Crystals

Microbiology

Microbiology is the scientific study of microorganisms and their activities. Laboratory analysis in microbiology deals with the identification of pathogens present in specimens taken from the body (i.e., urine, blood, throat, sputum, wound, urethra, vagina, cerebrospinal fluid). Examples of infectious diseases diagnosed through identification of the pathogen present in the specimen include

Candidiasis
Chlamydia
Diphtheria
Gonorrhea
Meningitis
Pertussis
Pharyngitis
Pneumonia
Streptococcal sore throat
Tetanus

15

Continued

TABLE 15-4

Categories of Laboratory Tests *Continued*

Tonsillitis
Tuberculosis
Urinary tract infection

Parasitology

Laboratory analysis in parasitology deals with the detection of the presence of disease-producing human parasites or eggs present in specimens taken from the body (e.g., stool, vagina, blood). Examples of human diseases caused by parasites include

    Amebiasis
    Ascariasis
    Hookworm disease
    Malaria
    Pinworm disease (enterobiasis)
    Scabies
    Tapeworm disease (cestodiasis)

Toxoplasmosis
Trichinosis
Trichomoniasis

Cytology

Laboratory analysis in cytology deals with the detection of the presence of abnormal cells.
    Chromosome studies
    Pap test

Histology

Histology is the microscopic study of the form and structure of the various tissues making up living organisms. Laboratory analysis in histology deals with the detection of diseased tissues.
    Tissue analysis
    Biopsy studies

---

provides examples of commonly performed tests in each. Using these classifications makes it easier to refer to laboratory tests.

Specimens can be analyzed by either the **manual** or **automated** method. The method the physician uses to test biologic specimens in the medical office is based on the number and type of laboratory tests performed in the office.

Regardless of the method used, a series of basic steps must be followed in testing each specimen:

1. The specific amount of the specimen required for the test method is measured out of the specimen sample.
2. The necessary chemical reagents required for the test are combined with the specimen.
3. The specimen/reagents may require further processing, such as centrifugation, incubation, air drying, or heat fixing.
4. The substance undergoing assessment is manually or automatically measured or identified.
5. The results of the laboratory testing are obtained from a direct readout or by a mathematic calculation.
6. The results are recorded on a laboratory report form or in the patient's chart; the entry includes the patient's name, the date, the time, the name of each laboratory test, the results of the tests, and the name of the individual performing the tests.

These steps are stated in general terms, but they provide a basis for understanding the process of laboratory testing. Textbooks such as this one and the manufacturer's instructions included with testing equipment should be consulted as a reference source to obtain the procedure for performing specific tests. The medical assistant must be sure to follow the procedure exactly to ensure accurate and reliable test results.

MANUAL METHOD

The manual method of laboratory testing involves performing the series of steps included in the test method by hand, rather than using a self-operating system that performs them automatically. Testing kits, especially in urinalyses, are available to speed up the process, making it more convenient to perform the procedure using the manual method. Because each step in the procedure requires a physical manipulation and the application of clinical laboratory theory, the manual method requires a more thorough knowledge and skill in testing procedures than does the automated method. The medical assistant must be especially careful to avoid errors in technique, which may lead to inaccurate test results.

AUTOMATED ANALYZERS

There has been tremendous growth in the development of automated analyzer systems for performing laboratory tests, especially in the area of blood chemistry; automated systems are also available for certain tests in the areas of hematology, blood banking, serology, urinalysis, and microbiology. Highly sophisticated automated analyzers are almost always confined to an outside laboratory setting, because the smaller laboratory workload of the medical office does not justify the expense of such systems. However, automated systems have been developed that are more practical and economical for the medical office.

Automated systems designed for use in the medical office permit the processing of a specimen in a short period of time with accurate test results. Automated instruments take less time and provide greater precision than the manual method, because the steps in the testing procedure are automated. Such procedures include the measurement of the amount of the specimen required, the use of premeasured chemical reagents, measurement of the reaction, and calculation of results. The test results are obtained by a direct (digital display or printed) readout.

The ease in operating automated systems, however, should not lead to a false sense of security, because these systems have limitations that must be recognized—the most critical one being the mechanical failure of the equipment. Therefore, one of the most important aspects of utilizing an automated system is to be able to recognize signs that indicate the system is malfunctioning, because this may lead to inaccurate test results.

Numerous automated systems are available; they are continually growing in number and are being modified as new technology becomes available. The manufacturer of each automated system provides a detailed operating manual with the instrument that includes the information needed to collect, handle, perform quality control procedures, and test the specimen. In addition, the manufacturer has personnel available for on-site training and service. It is important that the medical assistant become completely familiar with all aspects of any automated system used to perform laboratory tests in his or her medical office.

Some examples of automated analyzer systems include the QBC hematology analyzer (Becton-Dickinson), the Reflotron blood chemistry analyzer (Boehringer Mannheim), and the Clinitek urine analyzer (Bayer Corporation).

QUALITY CONTROL

☐ The ultimate goal in the clinical laboratory is to make sure the laboratory test is accurately measuring what it is supposed to measure; this involves practicing and maintaining a quality control program. **Quality control** may be defined as the application of methods and means to ensure that test results are reliable and valid and that errors that may interfere with obtaining accurate test results are detected and eliminated. Quality control is an ongoing process that encompasses every aspect of patient preparation and specimen col-

lection, handling, transport, and testing. The quality control methods that should be employed to obtain precision and accuracy in these areas have already been presented in this chapter under their respective headings, with the exception of testing, which is discussed here.

Quality control methods employed in testing the specimen include

1. Using standards and controls to check the precision and accuracy of laboratory equipment and to detect any errors in technique of the individual performing the test.
2. Discarding outdated reagents.
3. Following the procedure exactly to test the specimen.
4. Performing tests in duplicate.
5. Periodically checking the accuracy of the test results with a reference laboratory (proficiency testing).
6. Maintaining equipment by having it checked periodically for proper working order.

Practicing quality control methods ensures that the test results represent the true status of the patient's condition and body functions and provides the physician with reliable information with which to make a diagnosis and prescribe treatment.

LABORATORY SAFETY

☐ Laboratory safety is an important aspect of clinical laboratory testing in the medical office. Many of the laboratory tests performed in the medical office involve the use of strong chemical reagents, the handling of specimens that may contain pathogens, and the use of laboratory equipment. Practicing good techniques in testing laboratory specimens and recognizing potential hazards help reduce accidents in the laboratory. Some areas specifically related to laboratory safety in the medical office are described here.

Carefully handle and store glassware to prevent breakage as follows:

1. Carefully arrange glassware in storage cabinets, to prevent breakage.
2. Carefully remove glassware from storage cabinets.
3. If glassware does break, dispose of it in a puncture-resistant container, to protect trash handlers from the sharps.

The medical assistant should handle all chemical reagents carefully by adhering to the following:

1. Make sure all reagent bottles are clearly and properly labeled.
2. If a label becomes loose, reattach it immediately.
3. Recap reagent bottles immediately after using, to prevent spills.

Laboratory specimens should be handled carefully as follows:

1. Follow the OSHA Standard when collecting and handling laboratory specimens.
2. The hands should be washed immediately if the medical assistant accidentally touches some of the material contained in the specimen.
3. Avoid hand-to-mouth contact while working with specimens.
4. Do not pipet any specimen by mouth (e.g., serum, plasma, blood).
5. Immediately clean up any specimen spilled on the work table and cleanse the table with a disinfectant.
6. Properly dispose of all contaminated needles, syringes, specimen containers, and infectious waste.
7. Cover any break in the skin, such as a cut or scratch, with a bandage.
8. Make sure all specimen containers are tightly capped, to prevent leakage.
9. Handle all laboratory equipment and supplies properly and with care, as indicated by the manufacturer. For example, when using a centrifuge, wait until it comes to a complete stop before opening it.

MEDICAL PRACTICE AND THE LAW

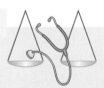

Laboratory procedures must be done precisely to obtain accurate results. Pay particular attention to each step in each procedure. Inaccurate laboratory results may cause the physician to misdiagnose and mistreat, opening both of you up for a lawsuit.

Many federal regulations govern laboratory testing, including those from the CLIA, OSHA, and CDC. These regulations help ensure standardization of laboratory tests and safe handling of reagents, blood and body fluids to prevent contamination of specimens and infection of health care workers. Know and follow all regulations. Failure to do so could result in a legal liability.

15

CERTIFICATION REVIEW

☐ The purpose of laboratory testing is to assist in the diagnosis of pathologic conditions, to evaluate a patient's progress, to regulate treatment, to establish a patient's baseline, to prevent or reduce the severity of disease, and because the test may be required by state law. A routine test is a laboratory test performed on a routine basis on apparently healthy people to assist in the early detection of disease.

☐ A POL consists of an in-house medical office laboratory. Laboratory tests that are convenient to execute and commonly required are often performed in the POL. Outside laboratories include hospital and privately owned commercial laboratories.

☐ A laboratory request is a printed form containing a list of the most frequently ordered laboratory tests. The laboratory request includes the physician's name and address, the patient's name, age and sex, the date and time of collection of the specimen, the laboratory tests desired, the source of the specimen, the clinical diagnosis, and medications being taken by the patient. A profile consists of a number of laboratory tests providing related information used to determine the health status of a patient.

☐ The purpose of the laboratory report is to relay the results of the laboratory tests to the physician. Information included on a laboratory report is as follows: the name, address, and telephone number of the laboratory, the physician's name and address, the patient's name, age, and sex, the patient accession number, the date the specimen was received by the laboratory, the date the results were reported by the laboratory, the names of the tests performed, the results of the tests, and the normal range for each test performed. The normal range is a certain established and acceptable parameter or reference range within which the laboratory test results of a healthy individual are expected to fall.

CERTIFICATION REVIEW *Continued*

☐ Laboratory safety is an important aspect of clinical laboratory testing in the medical office. Practicing good techniques in testing laboratory specimens and recognizing potential hazards helps reduce accidents in the laboratory.

☐ Some laboratory tests require advance patient preparation to obtain a quality specimen suitable for testing. A specimen obtained from a patient who has not prepared properly may invalidate the test results and necessitate calling the patient back to collect a specimen again. The specific type of preparation required for a particular test depends on the test ordered and the method used to run it. A common patient preparation requirement for laboratory testing is fasting. Fasting means that the patient must abstain from food or fluids (except water) for a specified amount of time (usually 12 to 14 hours) before the collection of a specimen.

☐ A specimen is a small sample taken from the body to represent the nature of the whole. Examples of specimens include the following: blood, urine, feces, sputum, a cervical and vaginal scraping of cells, and a sample of a secretion or discharge taken from various parts of the body such as the nose, throat, wound, ear, eye, vagina, or urethra.

☐ The purpose of the CLIA is to improve the quality of laboratory testing in the United States. The CLIA consists of federal regulations governing all facilities that perform laboratory tests for health assessment or for the diagnosis, prevention, or treatment of disease.

☐ The CLIA regulations establish three categories of laboratory testing, which include waived tests, moderate-complexity tests, and high-complexity tests. Laboratories performing moderate- or high-complexity tests must meet the CLIA regulations. Laboratories that perform only waived tests must apply for a certificate of waiver from HCFA, which exempts them from many of the CLIA requirements.

☐ Quality control is the application of methods to ensure that test results are reliable and valid and that errors are detected and eliminated. Quality control is an ongoing process that encompasses every aspect of patient preparation and specimen collection, handling, transport, and testing.

15

RESOURCES

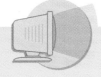

ON THE WEB

For information on aging:

National Institute on Aging
www.nih.gov/nia

Administration on Aging
www.aoa.dhhs.gov

American Association of Retired Persons
www.aarp.org

Social Security Administration
www.ssa.gov

Health Care Financing Administration (HCFA)
www.hcfa.gov

Medicare
www.medicare.gov

Growth House
www.growthhouse.org

Before I Die
www.pbs.org/wnet/bid

Urinalysis

MY NAME IS

Linda Proffitt, *and I am a Certified Medical Assistant. I graduated from a medical assisting program and have an associate's degree in Applied Science. I work for a urologist and his wife, who is a pediatrician. I have been working in this office for the past 11 years.*

I work primarily in the urology practice and only occasionally in pediatrics. I am responsible for having the charts ready when the patients are seen and for doing their urinalysis. Another one of my responsibilities is to assist with special procedures, such as catheter insertions, male and female dilations, ultrasound examinations of the bladder, and prostate examinations.

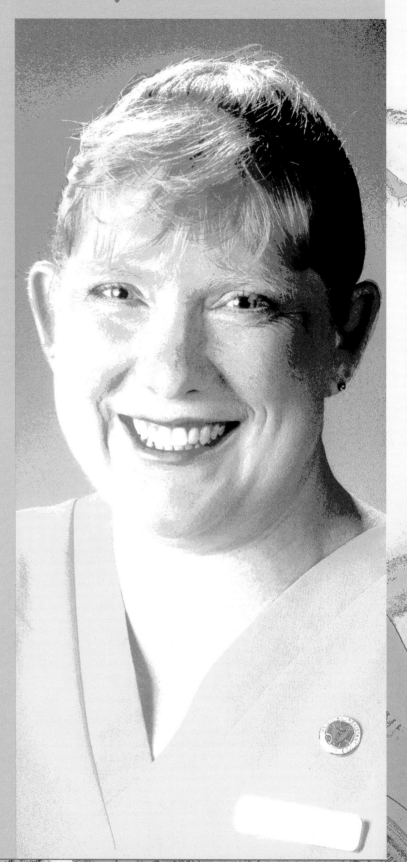

OUTCOMES

After completing this chapter, you should be able to demonstrate the proper procedure to perform the following:

1. Instruct an individual in the procedure for obtaining a clean-catch midstream urine specimen.
2. Instruct an individual in the procedure for obtaining a 24-hour urine specimen.
3. Assess the color and clarity of a urine specimen.
4. Measure the specific gravity of a urine specimen.
5. Perform a chemical assessment of a urine specimen.
6. Prepare the specimen, and identify the structures present in a microscopic examination of urine sediment.
7. Perform a rapid urine culture test.
8. Perform a urine pregnancy test.

EDUCATIONAL OBJECTIVES

After completing this chapter, you should be able to do the following:

1. Define the terms listed in the Key Terminology.
2. Describe the structures forming the urinary system and state the function of each.
3. List three conditions that may cause polyuria and three conditions that may cause oliguria.
4. Define the terms used to describe symptoms of the urinary system.
5. Explain why a first-voided morning specimen is often preferred for urinalysis.
6. Explain the purpose of collecting a clean-catch midstream specimen.
7. Explain the purpose of a 24-hour urine collection.
8. List changes that may occur if urine is allowed to remain standing for more than 1 hour.
9. List three factors that may cause urine to have an unusual color or to become cloudy.
10. Identify the various tests that are included in the physical and chemical examination of urine.
11. Explain the purpose of a rapid urine culture test.
12. Explain the basis for urine pregnancy tests.
13. List the guidelines that must be followed in performing a urine pregnancy test to ensure accurate test results.
14. Explain the principle underlying each step in the urinalysis procedures.

agglutination (a-GLÛT-in-Â-shun): The aggregation or uniting of separate particles into clumps or masses.

bilirubinuria (BILA-rû-bin-û-rêa): The presence of bilirubin in the urine.

glycosuria (GLÎ-kq-sur-ê-a): The presence of sugar in the urine.

ketonuria (KÊ-Tô-nur-ê-a): The presence of ketone bodies in the urine.

ketosis (KÊ-tô-sis): An accumulation of large amounts of ketone bodies in the tissues and body fluids.

meniscus (MEN-is-kus): The curved upper surface of a liquid in a container. The surface is convex if the liquid does not wet the container and concave if it does.

micturition (MIK-chur-ish-un): The act of voiding urine.

nephron (NEF-ron): The functional unit of the kidney.

oliguria (au-LIG-ur-ê-a): Decreased or scanty output of urine.

pH: The unit that describes the acidity or alkalinity of a solution.

polyuria (PAUL-ê-ur-ê-a): Increased output of urine.

proteinuria (PRÔ-têen-ur-ê-a): The presence of protein in the urine.

refractive index: The ratio of the velocity of light in air to the velocity of light in a solution.

refractometer (rê-FRAK-TOM-it-er) (clinical): An instrument used to measure the refractive index of urine, which is an indirect measurement of the specific gravity of urine.

renal threshold (RÊ-nul THRESH-hold): The concentration at which a substance in the blood that is not normally excreted by the kidneys begins to appear in the urine.

specific gravity: The weight of a substance as compared with the weight of an equal volume of a substance known as the standard. In urinalysis, the specific gravity refers to the measurement of the amount of dissolved substances present in the urine, as compared with the same amount of distilled water.

supernatant (SÛ-per-NÂ-tent): The clear liquid that remains at the top after a precipitate settles.

urinalysis (YUR-in-al-is-sis): The physical, chemical, and microscopic analysis of urine.

void: To empty the bladder.

16

STRUCTURE AND FUNCTION OF THE URINARY SYSTEM

☐ The function of the urinary system is to regulate the fluid and electrolyte balance of the body and to remove waste products. The structures making up the urinary system are the kidneys, the ureters, the urinary bladder, and the urethra (Fig. 16–1). The **kidneys** are bean-shaped organs approximately 4.5 inches (11.5 cm) long and 2 to 3 inches (5 to 8 cm) wide; they are located in the lumbar region of the body. Urine drains from the kidneys into the urinary bladder through two tubes known as **ureters.** Each ureter is approximately 10 to 12 inches in length and ½ inch in diameter. The urine produced by the kidneys is propelled into the urinary bladder by the force of gravity and the peristaltic waves of the ureters. The **urinary bladder** is a hollow, muscular sac that can hold approximately 500 milliliters (ml) of urine. Its function is to store and expel urine. The **urethra** is a tube that extends from the urinary bladder to the outside of the body. The **urinary meatus** is the external opening of the urethra. In males, the urethra functions in transporting urine

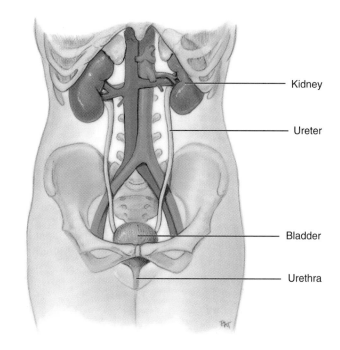

■ **FIGURE 16–1.** Structures making up the urinary system. (From Applegate, E. J.: *The Anatomy and Physiology Learning System.* Philadelphia, W. B. Saunders, 1995.)

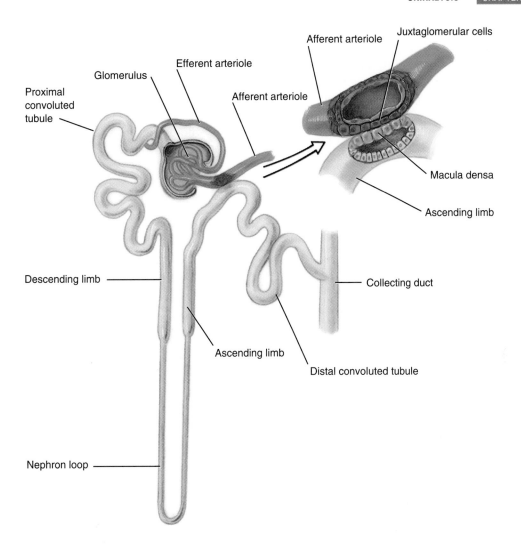

Proximal convoluted tubule

Glomerulus

Efferent arteriole

Afferent arteriole

Afferent arteriole

Juxtaglomerular cells

Macula densa

Ascending limb

Descending limb

Ascending limb

Distal convoluted tubule

Collecting duct

Nephron loop

■ FIGURE 16–2. Nephron. (From Applegate, E. J.: *The Anatomy and Physiology Learning System.* Philadelphia, W. B. Saunders, 1995.)

and reproductive secretions. In females, the urethra functions in urination only.

Each kidney is composed of approximately 1 million smaller units known as nephrons (Fig. 16–2). The **nephron** is the functional unit of the kidney. It filters waste substances from the blood and dilutes them with water to produce urine. Another function of the nephron is reabsorption. Some substances filtered by the nephron, such as water, glucose, and electrolytes, are needed by the body and are reabsorbed or returned to the body for future use.

COMPOSITION OF URINE

☐ A physiologic change in the body, such as that caused by disease, can cause a disturbance in one or more of the functions of the kidney. Detection of such

a disturbance can be made through the examination of urine as well as other body fluids such as blood.

Urine is composed of 95 percent water and 5 percent organic and inorganic waste products. Organic waste products consist of urea, uric acid, ammonia, and creatinine. Urea is present in the greatest amounts and is derived from the breakdown of proteins. Inorganic waste products include chloride, sodium, potassium, calcium, magnesium, phosphate, and sulfate.

The normal adult excretes approximately 750 to 2000 ml of urine per day. This amount varies according to the amount of fluid consumed and the amount of fluid lost through other means, such as perspiration and feces and water vapor from the lungs. An excessive increase in urine output is known as **polyuria,** with the urine volume exceeding 2000 ml in 24 hours. Polyuria may be caused by the excessive intake of fluids or the intake of fluids that contain

16

caffeine (e.g., coffee, tea, cola), which is a mild diuretic. Certain drugs, such as diuretics, and the pathologic conditions of diabetes mellitus, diabetes insipidus, and renal disease in which the kidney is unable to concentrate the urine may also result in polyuria. A decreased or scanty urine output is known as **oliguria.** In the case of oliguria, the urine volume will be less than 400 ml in 24 hours. Oliguria may occur with decreased fluid intake, dehydration, profuse perspiration, vomiting, diarrhea, or kidney disease. The normal act of voiding urine is known as **micturition.**

TERMS RELATING TO THE URINARY SYSTEM

The medical assistant should have a thorough knowledge of the following terms used to describe symptoms associated with the urinary system:

Anuria	Failure of the kidneys to produce urine
Diuresis	Secretion and passage of large amounts of urine
Dysuria	Difficult or painful urination
Frequency	The condition of having to urinate often
Hematuria	Blood present in the urine
Nocturia	Excessive (voluntary) urination during the night
Nocturnal enuresis	The inability of the patient to control urination at night during sleep (bedwetting)
Oliguria	Decreased output of urine
Polyuria	Increased output of urine
Pyuria	Pus present in the urine
Retention	The inability to empty the bladder. The urine is being produced normally but is not being voided
Urgency	The immediate need to urinate
Urinary incontinence	The inability to retain urine

COLLECTION OF URINE

☐ The advantage of testing urine is that it is readily available and does not require an invasive procedure or the use of special equipment to obtain. To obtain accurate test results, however, the medical assistant must adhere to proper urine collection procedures as well as obtain the proper specimen as ordered by the physician.

GUIDELINES FOR URINE COLLECTION

The guidelines listed next should be followed when collecting a urine specimen:

1. The medical assistant must make sure to obtain an adequate volume of urine as required for the type of test being run, which usually falls between 30 and 50 ml of urine.
2. Each specimen must be properly labeled with the patient's name, the date and time of collection, and the type of specimen (i.e., urine), to avoid any mixups in specimens.
3. Any medication the patient is taking should be recorded on the laboratory requisition and in the patient's chart, because some medications may interfere with the accuracy of the test results.
4. If possible, the collection of a urine specimen should be avoided in women during menstruation and for several days thereafter, because the specimen may become contaminated with blood.
5. The medical assistant should take into consideration that it is difficult for some patients to void under stress and anxiety. In these instances, understanding and patience should be relayed to the patient.
6. It may be difficult to obtain a urine specimen from a child, even with the assistance of the parents. In this case, the physician should be informed, because another collection method may be used, such as a urine collection bag, suprapubic aspiration, or catheterization of the patient.

URINE COLLECTION METHODS

The type of test to be performed often dictates the method used to collect the urine specimen. For example, a first-voided morning specimen is recommended for pregnancy testing, while a clean-catch midstream specimen is required to identify the presence of a urinary tract infection (UTI).

Most offices use disposable urine specimen containers made of plastic. These containers are available in different sizes and come with lids to reduce bacterial and other types of contamination.

Random Specimen

Urine testing in the medical office is often done on freshly voided, random specimens. The medical assistant instructs the patient to void into a clean, dry, wide-mouthed container, and the urine is tested immediately at the medical office.

First-Voided Morning Specimen

In many cases, a first-voided morning specimen may be desired for testing because it contains the greatest concentration of dissolved substances. Therefore, a small amount of an abnormal substance that is present would be more easily detected. The patient should be instructed to collect the first specimen of the morning after rising and to preserve the specimen by refrigerating it until it is brought to the medical office. It is helpful to provide the patient with a specimen container to prevent him or her from using a container that might harbor contaminants.

Clean-Catch Midstream Specimen

The urinary bladder and most of the urethra are normally free of microorganisms, whereas the distal urethra and urinary meatus normally harbor microorganisms. If the urine is being cultured and examined for bacteria, a **clean-catch midstream specimen** is required to prevent contamination of the specimen with these normally present microorganisms. Only those microorganisms that may be causing the patient's condition are desired in the urine specimen. A clean-catch midstream collection may be ordered for both the detection of a urinary tract infection (UTI) and the evaluation of the effectiveness of drug therapy in a patient being treated for such an infection.

The purpose of the clean-catch midstream collection is to remove microorganisms from the urinary meatus by thoroughly cleansing the area surrounding it and to flush out microorganisms in the distal urethra. The urine specimen is collected in a sterile container under medically aseptic conditions. A properly collected specimen reduces the possibility of having to perform a bladder catheterization or a suprapubic aspiration of the bladder. Bladder catheterization involves passing a sterile tube (the catheter) through the urethra and into the bladder to remove urine. Suprapubic aspiration involves passing a needle through the abdominal wall into the bladder to remove urine. Both of these procedures must be performed using sterile technique.

Guidelines

The following list contains guidelines that should be followed when collecting a clean-catch midstream specimen.

1. A clean-catch midstream specimen is collected by the patient at the medical office. The medical assistant must provide complete instructions for the collection of this specimen. Failure to instruct the patient adequately may necessitate his or her having to return to the medical office for the collection of another specimen, owing to bacterial contamination.

2. For reliable test results, the specimen should immediately be tested and not be allowed to stand. If this is not possible, the specimen should be refrigerated or a preservative should be added.

3. To assist the patient in obtaining a clean-catch midstream specimen, the medical assistant must first assemble the supplies needed by the patient for the specimen collection. The supplies include a sterile specimen container, a soap solution, and cotton balls. Midstream urine specimen kits are commercially available and include a sterile specimen container and label, antiseptic wipes, and absorbent tissues.

4. The medical assistant should prepare the supplies for the patient by setting them out on a flat surface near the toilet. The lid should be removed from the specimen container and placed with the open end facing up just prior to the collection of the specimen. Early removal of the lid could result in contamination of the sterile container with extraneous microorganisms present in the air, which interferes with accurate test results.

5. Once the specimen has been collected, the medical assistant should immediately cap and label the container with the patient's name, the date, the time of the collection, and the type of specimen (clean-catch midstream specimen).

6. If the specimen will be tested at an outside laboratory, it is necessary to complete a laboratory requisition to accompany it. Refer to Figure 16-3 for an example of a urinalysis laboratory request form.

7. The procedure is then completed by washing the hands and recording the procedure in the patient's chart. The information to be charted includes the date and time, type of specimen, and the laboratory tests ordered. Patient instructions for obtaining a clean-catch midstream specimen are presented in Procedure 16-1.

16

UR- 183900		
ICDA		
REQUESTING PHYSICIAN		
PHYSICIAN HAS SEEN-INITIAL		

N A M E   D A T E

	ROUTINE URINALYSIS - 001				MICROSCOPIC - 022			QUANTITATIVE	
	APPEARANCE COLOR				WBC'S	/HPF	024	SULKOWITCH	
023	SPECIFIC GRAVITY				RBC'S	/HPF	026	BILE	
004	PH				CASTS (Hyaline)	/LPF		PHENYLPYRUVIC ACID	
	PROTEIN				CASTS (Granular)	/LPF	027	PHENESTIX	
	GLUCOSE				CASTS (Cellular)	/LPF	028	UROBILINOGEN	
007	KETONES (ACETONE)				CASTS (Waxy)	/LPF	029	PORPHOBILINOGEN	
3	OCCULT BLOOD				EPITHELIAL CELLS	/LPF	030	PORPHYRIN	
	BILE				BACTERIA		031	BENCE-JONES	
	UROBILINOGEN				MUCUS		025	TOTAL PROTEIN 24HR. SPECIMEN	
	LEUKOCYTE				CRYSTALS			TOTAL VOLUME REQUIRED:	
COMMENTS					AMORPHOUS				
URINALYSIS					OTHER:			SIGNATURE:	
DMH-0067 (Rev. 3/83)			33	**F P N**				DATE:	

DMH-MedR-1065-A

■ **FIGURE 16–3.** Urinalysis laboratory request form.

16

PROCEDURE

16–1

Clean-Catch Midstream Specimen Collection Instructions

EQUIPMENT/SUPPLIES: Sterile specimen container and label   **Cotton balls**
Antiseptic solution

Instruct the female patient in the collection of the specimen as follows:

1. **Procedural Step.** Wash hands and assemble equipment.
2. **Procedural Step.** Greet and identify the patient. Introduce yourself and explain the procedure.
3. **Procedural Step.** Wash the hands, and remove undergarments.
4. **Procedural Step.** Expose the urinary meatus by spreading apart the labia with one hand.

5. **Procedural Step.** Cleanse each side of the urinary meatus with a front-to-back motion (from pubis to anus), using a fresh cotton ball on each side of the meatus. With the midstream specimen kit, an antiseptic wipe is used to cleanse each side of the meatus.
Principle. Cleansing removes microorganisms from the urinary meatus. A front-to-back motion must

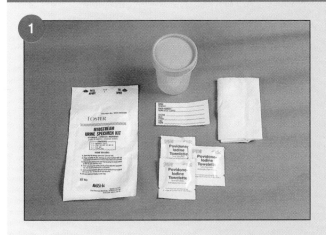

be used for cleansing to avoid drawing microorganisms from the anal region into the area that is being cleansed.

6. **Procedural Step.** Cleanse directly across the meatus (front to back), using a third cotton ball (or antiseptic wipe).

7. **Procedural Step.** Rinse with water to remove all traces of the soap.
   Principle. The soap solution must be completely removed to prevent its entrance into the urine specimen, which could affect the accuracy of the test results.

8. **Procedural Step.** Dry the area with a cotton ball, using a single front-to-back motion. (*Note:* With the midstream specimen kit, Steps 5 and 6 are not required.)

9. **Procedural Step.** Continue to hold the labia apart, and void a small amount of urine into the toilet.
   Principle. Voiding a small amount flushes microorganisms out of the distal urethra.

10. **Procedural Step.** Collect the next amount of urine by voiding into the sterile container. Be careful not to touch the inside of the container.
    Principle. Touching the inside of the container will contaminate it with microorganisms that normally reside on the skin.

11. **Procedural Step.** Void the last amount of urine into the toilet. This means that the first and last portion of the urine flow is not included in the specimen.

12. **Procedural Step.** Wipe the area dry with a tissue and wash the hands with soap and water.

13. **Procedural Step.** Provide the patient with instructions about what to do with the specimen once it has been collected (e.g., placing it on a designated shelf or directly handing it to the medical assistant).

Instruct the male patient as follows:

1. **Procedural Step.** Wash the hands and remove undergarments.

2. **Procedural Step.** Retract the foreskin of the penis (if uncircumcised).

3. **Procedural Step.** Cleanse the area around the meatus (glans penis) and the urethral opening (meatal orifice) by washing each side of the meatus with a separate cotton ball. With the midstream specimen kit, an antiseptic wipe is used to cleanse each side of the meatus.

4. **Procedural Step.** Cleanse directly across the meatus, using a third cotton ball (or antiseptic wipe).

5. **Procedural Step.** Rinse with water to remove all traces of the soap.

6. **Procedural Step.** Dry the area with a cotton ball, using a single front-to-back motion. (*Note:* If the midstream specimen kit it used, Steps 5 and 6 are not required.)

7. **Procedural Step.** Void a small amount of urine into the toilet.

8. **Procedural Step.** Collect the next amount of urine by voiding into the sterile container without touching the inside of the container with the hands or penis.

9. **Procedural Step.** Void the last amount of urine into the toilet.

10. **Procedural Step.** Wipe the area dry with a tissue and wash the hands with soap and water.

11. **Procedural Step.** Provide the patient with instructions about what to do with the specimen once it has been collected.

16

TWENTY-FOUR HOUR URINE SPECIMEN

A 24-hour urine specimen is used to measure specific urinary components quantitatively. By collecting urine over a 24-hour period, there is greater accuracy of measurement than there is with a random specimen. This is because body metabolism, exercise, and hydration can affect the excretion rate of substances in the urine. In addition, at certain times during a 24-hour period, there is an increased excretion of substances, such as electrolytes, hormones, proteins, and urobilinogen, and at other times, there is decreased excretion.

Examples of substances measured in a 24-hour specimen include calcium, creatinine, lead, potassium, protein, and urea nitrogen. A 24-hour specimen is often used to diagnose the cause of kidney stone formation as well as to assist in the control and prevention of new stone formation.

A large container (3000 ml) is used to collect the specimen. In order to prevent changes in the quality of the urine specimen, the specimen must be kept refrigerated or placed in an ice chest. Some containers also contain a preservative to assist in maintaining the quality of the specimen.

The medical assistant should provide the patient with both verbal and written instructions for the collection of the urine specimen. The patient should be advised to moderately limit the fluid intake during the collection period and to avoid alcohol intake for 24 hours before and during the collection period.

Certain medications such as thiazides, phosphorus-binding antacids, allopurinol, or vitamin C could alter results of the testing performed on the specimen. Because of this problem, the physician may want the patient to discontinue these medications for a week before the test.

16–2

Collection of a 24-Hour Urine Specimen

EQUIPMENT/SUPPLIES: **Large urine collection container** **Laboratory requisition**
Written instructions

1. **Procedural Step.** Wash hands, and assemble the equipment.
2. **Procedural Step.** Greet and identify the patient. Introduce yourself to the patient, and explain the procedure.

Instruct the patient in the collection of the specimen as follows:

3. **Procedural Step.** When you get up in the morning, empty your bladder into the commode just as you normally do. In other words, this urine is not to be saved. Make a note of what time it is, and write this information on a slip of paper.
4. **Procedural Step.** The next time you need to urinate, void the urine directly into the plastic container.
5. **Procedural Step.** Tightly screw the lid onto the container, and put the container into your refrigerator or into an ice chest.

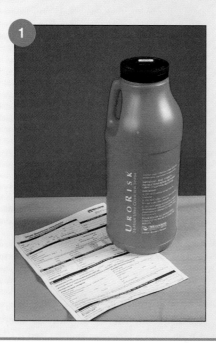

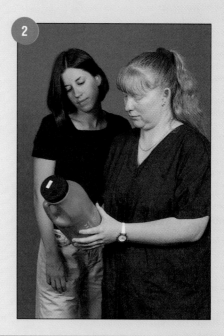

6. **Procedural Step.** Repeat Steps 4 and 5 each time you urinate.

7. **Procedural Step.** Emphasize the importance of the following to the patient:

   a. The urine must only be collected in the designated container.

   b. Make sure to collect all your urine during the 24-hour period. The information this test provides will be inaccurate if any urine from the 24-hour period doesn't go into the container.

   c. You must start the collection again from the beginning if any of the following occur:

   - You forget to urinate into the container at any time.
   - You spill some urine from the container.
   - The child wets the bed (if the specimen is being obtained from a child).

8. **Procedural Step.** On the following morning, get up at the same time (exactly 24 hours after beginning the test). Void into the container for the last time.

9. **Procedural Step.** Put the lid on the container tightly. Return the urine collection container to the office the same morning you complete the urine collection.

10. **Procedural Step.** Provide the patient with the collection container and written instructions. Chart this information in the patient's medical record.

Processing the Specimen

11. **Procedural Step.** When the patient returns the collection container, ask the patient whether he or she encountered any difficulty in following the instructions for the 24-hour collection. If any problems occurred that resulted in undercollection or overcollection of urine, the entire collection process must be repeated.

12. **Procedural Step.** Prepare the specimen for transport to the laboratory. Complete a laboratory request form.

13. **Procedural Step.** Chart the results. Include the date and time, the type of specimen, and information on sending the specimen to the laboratory.

CHARTING EXAMPLE	
Date	
3/26/2002	3:30 p.m. Container and verbal/written instructions provided on 24-hour specimen collection. ——————— L. Proffitt, CMA
3/28/2002	10:00 a.m. 24-hour urine specimen sent to Medical Center Laboratory for kidney stone risk analysis.———————L. Proffitt, CMA

ANALYSIS OF URINE

☐ **Urinalysis** is the analysis of urine and is usually the laboratory test most commonly performed in the medical office, because a urine specimen is readily obtainable and can be tested easily. Urinalysis consists of a **physical**, **chemical**, and **microscopic** examination. A deviation from normal in any of the three areas assists the physician in the diagnosis and treatment of pathologic conditions, not only of the urinary system but of other body systems as well. Urinalysis may be performed as a screening measure as part of a general physical examination or to assist in the diagnosis of a pathologic condition when the patient presents with symptoms. It may also assist in the evaluation of effectiveness of therapy once treatment has been initiated for a pathologic condition.

The urinalysis should be performed on a fresh or preserved specimen. If a specimen cannot be examined within 1 hour of voiding, it should be preserved at once in the refrigerator in a closed container and later returned to room temperature and mixed before testing. Chemical additives, such as toluene and thymol, are also used to preserve urine specimens, but they are generally used only with specimens that require prolonged storage, such as those that must be shipped a long distance. This is because the chemical preservative sometimes interferes with the chemicals used to perform the urine test.

If the urine is allowed to stand at room temperature for more than 1 hour, some of the following changes may take place:

1. Bacteria work on the urea present in the urine, converting it to ammonia. Because ammonia is alkaline, this causes an acid urine to become alkaline, raising the pH measurement. In addition, an alkaline pH may result in a false-positive result on the protein test.

2. Bacteria multiply rapidly in the urine, resulting in a cloudy specimen and a rise in the nitrite.

3. If glucose is present in the specimen, it will decrease in amount since microorganisms utilize the glucose as a source of food.

4. If any red or white blood cells are present, they may break down.

5. Casts decompose after several hours.

16

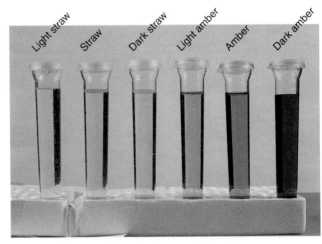

■ **FIGURE 16–4.** Color of urine.

PHYSICAL EXAMINATION OF THE URINE

The physical examination of the urine involves determination of the color, appearance, and specific gravity. The color and appearance of the urine specimen may be evaluated while it is being prepared for another testing procedure, such as the chemical testing of the urine, or before centrifuging the specimen in preparation for microscopic analysis. To make an accurate evaluation of the color and appearance, the urine specimen must be in a clear glass or plastic container.

Color

The normal color of urine ranges from almost colorless to dark yellow. Dilute urine tends to be a lighter yellow in color, whereas concentrated urine is a darker yellow. The first-voided morning specimen is usually the most concentrated because consumption of fluids is decreased during the night. The urine becomes more dilute as the day progresses and more fluids are consumed.

The color of the urine is due to the presence of a yellow pigment known as **urochrome**, produced by the breakdown of hemoglobin. It is not uncommon for the color of urine to vary among different shades of yellow within the course of a day. Classifications that can be used to describe the normal color of urine include light straw, straw, dark straw, light amber, amber, and dark amber (Fig. 16–4).

Abnormal colors may be due to the presence of hemoglobin or blood (resulting in a red or reddish color), bile pigments (resulting in a yellow-brown or greenish color), and fat droplets or pus (resulting in a milky color). Some drugs and foods may also cause the urine to change to an abnormal color. The color of the specimen assists in determining additional tests that may be required.

Appearance

The evaluation of the appearance of urine is usually performed at the same time as the color evaluation. Fresh urine is usually clear, or transparent, but becomes cloudy on standing. Cloudiness in a freshly voided specimen may be due to the presence of bacteria, pus, blood, fat, yeast, sperm, mucous threads, or fecal contaminants. A microscopic examination of the urine sediment should be performed on all cloudy specimens to determine what is causing the cloudiness. Cloudiness due to bacteria may be caused by a urinary tract infection.

Terms that may be used to describe the appearance of urine include clear, slightly cloudy, cloudy, and very cloudy (Fig. 16–5). The medical assistant should develop skill in recognizing the varying degrees of urine clarity.

Odor

Freshly voided urine normally should have a slightly aromatic odor. Urine that has been standing for a long period of time develops an ammonia odor owing to the breakdown of urea by bacteria in the specimen. The urine of patients with diabetes mellitus may have a fruity odor owing to the presence of ketones. The urine of patients with urinary tract infections is usually foul-smelling and becomes worse on standing. Certain

16

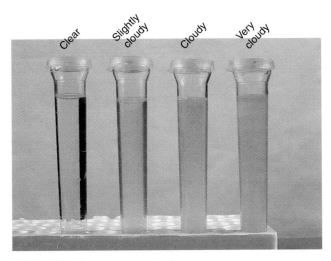

Clear　Slightly cloudy　Cloudy　Very cloudy

■ **FIGURE 16–5.** Appearance of urine.

foods, such as asparagus, can cause the urine to have a musty smell. Although the urine may have many characteristic odors, as a rule the odor of the urine is not generally used in the diagnosis of a patient's condition.

Specific Gravity

The specific gravity of urine measures the weight of the urine as compared with the weight of an equal volume of distilled water. Specific gravity indicates the amount of dissolved substances present in the urine, thus providing information on the ability of the kidneys to dilute or concentrate the urine. Specific gravity is decreased in conditions in which the kidneys cannot concentrate the urine, such as chronic renal insufficiency, diabetes insipidus, and malignant hypertension. The specific gravity is increased in patients with adrenal insufficiency, congestive heart failure, hepatic disease, diabetes mellitus with glycosuria, and conditions

causing dehydration such as fever, vomiting, and diarrhea.

Normal specific gravity may range from 1.003 to 1.030 but is usually between 1.010 and 1.025 (the specific gravity of distilled water is 1.000). Specific gravity varies greatly with fluid intake and the state of hydration of an individual. Dilute urine contains fewer dissolved substances and thus has a lower specific gravity. Concentrated urine, on the other hand, will have a higher specific gravity owing to the increased amount of dissolved substances. A urine specimen is generally more concentrated in the morning and becomes more dilute after fluid consumption.

Measurement of Specific Gravity

In the medical office, specific gravity is measured by one of the following methods.

REAGENT STRIP METHOD. One method involves a color comparison determination using a reagent strip that contains a reagent area for specific gravity. The reagent strip is dipped into the urine specimen, and the results are compared with a color chart (refer to Procedure 16–5, Chemical Testing of Urine Using the Multistix 10 SG Reagent Strip).

REFRACTOMETER METHOD. The amount of dissolved substances in urine can also be measured using a clinical refractometer, which is a hand-held optical instrument consisting of a lens and prism system. The refractometer measures the refractive index of urine, which is directly correlated with the specific gravity of urine; the results are read directly from a calibrated scale. The advantage of using a refractometer is that only 1 to 2 drops of urine are required to perform the test. The procedure for measuring the specific gravity of urine using a refractometer is presented on the following pages.

16

PROCEDURE

16–3

Measuring Specific Gravity of Urine—Refractometer Method

EQUIPMENT/SUPPLIES:

Disposable gloves
Refractometer
Urine specimen
Disposable pipet

Antiseptic wipe
Lint-free tissues
Biohazard waste container

16

1. **Procedural Step.** Wash the hands, and assemble the equipment. Make sure the surface of the prism is clean.
2. **Procedural Step.** Calibrate the refractometer according to the manufacturer's instructions. (Refer to the next procedure for information on calibration.)
3. **Procedural Step.** Apply gloves. Prepare the urine specimen. The urine specimen must be at room temperature. Mix the urine specimen using the disposable pipet.
   Principle. The specimen must be well mixed for accurate test results.

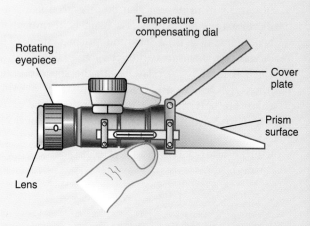

Rotating eyepiece

Temperature compensating dial

Cover plate

Prism surface

Lens

4. **Procedural Step.** Withdraw a small amount of urine into the disposable pipet. Holding the pipet in a vertical position, place a drop of urine on the surface of the prism. Depending on the brand of refractometer, this is accomplished in one of two ways as follows:
   a. Open the cover plate and place a drop of urine directly on the prism. Tightly close the cover plate.
   b. Close the cover plate and place a drop of urine at its notched part. The urine will be drawn across the prism surface (between the over plate and prism) by capillary action.

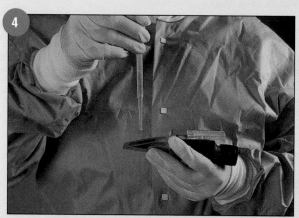

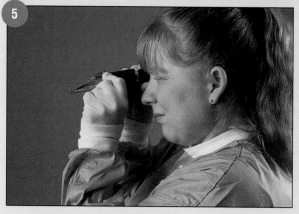

5. **Procedural Step.** Point the instrument toward a light source and rotate the eyepiece to bring the calibrated scale clearly into view. A light area (bottom) and a dark area (top) will be observed through the eyepiece.
6. **Procedural Step.** Read the value on the scale at the boundary line that shows the distinct division of the light and dark areas. (The specific gravity reading on this scale is 1.020.)

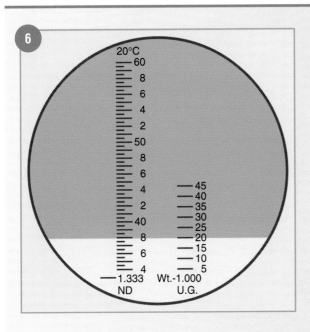

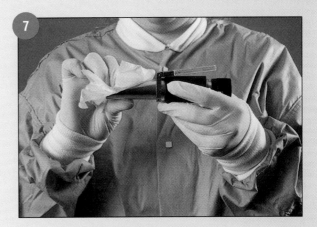

7. Procedural Step. Clean the prism surface with a soft lint-free tissue, being careful not to scratch the prism. Disinfect the prism surface with an antiseptic wipe.

8. Procedural Step. Remove the gloves and wash the hands.

9. Procedural Step. Chart the results. Include the date and time and the specific gravity reading.

CHARTING EXAMPLE

Date	
3/20/2002	10:15 a.m. SG: 1.020. ———— L. Proffitt, CMA

16–4

Quality Control: Calibration of the Refractometer

If the refractometer does not have a temperature compensating dial, it should be calibrated each day. Calibrating the refractometer compensates for day-to-day temperature variations to ensure accurate test results. The refractometer is calibrated as follows:

1. Procedural Step. Place a drop of distilled water on the surface of the prism using a disposable pipet.

2. Procedural Step. Point the instrument toward a light source and rotate the eyepiece to bring the calibrated scale clearly into view. A light area (bottom) and a dark area (top) will be observed through the eyepiece.

3. Procedural Step. Read the value on the scale at the boundary line that shows the distinct division of the light and dark areas. If the calibration of the refractometer is correct, the distilled water will have a specific gravity reading of 1.000 and the boundary line will fall exactly on the weight (wt) line.

4. Procedural Step. If the calibration of the refractometer is incorrect, the boundary line must be corrected to coincide with the weight line by turning an adjusting screw with a small screwdriver that is supplied by the manufacturer.

5. Procedural Step. Clean the prism surface with a soft lint-free tissue, being careful not to scratch the prism.

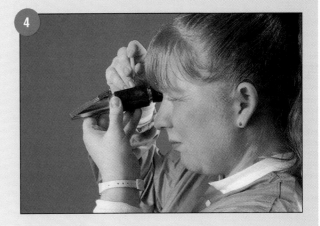

16

CHEMICAL EXAMINATION OF THE URINE

Substances present in excess (abnormal) amounts in the blood are usually removed by the urine. Therefore, the chemical testing of urine is an indirect means of detecting abnormal amounts of chemicals in the body, indicating a pathologic condition. The chemical examination of urine also can be used to detect the presence of substances that, in the absence of disease, do not normally appear in the urine, such as blood and nitrite.

Chemical tests that are routinely performed during a urinalysis include testing for pH, glucose, protein, and ketones. Other chemical tests that may be performed include testing for blood, bilirubin, urobilinogen, nitrite, and leukocytes.

QUALITATIVE TESTS. The chemical analysis of urine involves the use of both qualitative and quantitative tests. Qualitative tests provide an approximate indication of whether or not a substance is present in abnormal quantities. The interpretation of qualitative tests usually involves the use of a color chart, with results being recorded in terms of trace, 1+, 2+, or 3+; trace, small, moderate, or large; or negative or positive. Qualitative tests are useful for screening purposes in the medical office because they are easy to perform and can be used to screen large numbers of individuals, a procedure that otherwise might be too expensive and time consuming.

QUANTITATIVE TESTS. Quantitative tests indicate the exact amount of a chemical substance that is present; the results are reported in measurable units (e.g., milligrams per deciliter). Quantitative urine tests usually involve the use of more complex equipment and testing procedures than are found in the medical office; they are also more time consuming to run.

Commercial Testing Kits

Commercially prepared diagnostic testing kits are most frequently used in the medical office for the chemical testing of urine. These kits are usually preferred because they contain premeasured reagents, the procedure is easy to follow, and they provide an immediate answer. Most of these tests are qualitative, and a positive reading may indicate the need for further testing. The majority of the tests are manufactured in the form of reagent strips, and they rely on a color change for interpretation of results. A color chart is provided with the kit for making a visual comparison.

To ensure accurate and reliable test results, the medical assistant should carefully read and follow the instructions that accompany each kit. For example, test strips containing more than one reagent may require different time intervals for reading. Certain medications that the patient is taking may also interfere with the test results; these medications will be listed in the instructions.

Before a test is used, its expiration date must be checked. Test material must not be used if a color change has occurred or if the *tested* strip gives off a color that does not match the shades on the color chart. Light, heat, and moisture can alter the effectiveness of the strips; therefore, care must be taken to store the test materials in a cool, dry area. Most test materials are packaged in light-resistant containers to protect them from light. The test materials must never be transferred from their original container to another, because the other container may harbor traces of moisture, dirt, or chemicals that could affect the test results.

When results are recorded, the type of test that was used should be specified. A list of commercially available diagnostic kits for performing chemical tests on urine is presented in Table 16–1.

pH

The pH is the unit that indicates the acidity or alkalinity of a solution. The pH scale ranges from 0.0 to 14.0. The lower the number, the greater the acidity; the higher the number, the greater the alkalinity. A pH reading of 7.0 is neutral; a reading below 7.0 indicates acidity, and a reading above 7.0 indicates alkalinity.

The kidneys help regulate the acid-base balance of the body. To obtain an accurate pH reading of the urine, the measurement should be done on freshly voided urine. If the urine is allowed to remain standing, it becomes more alkaline as urea is converted to ammonia by bacterial action.

Although the pH of the urine can range from 4.5 to 8.0, the pH of a freshly voided specimen of a patient on a normal diet is usually acidic and has a pH reading of about 6.0. An abnormally high pH reading on a fresh specimen (that is, an alkaline urine) may indicate a bacterial infection of the urinary tract.

Glucose

Normally, no glucose should be detectable in the urine. Glucose in the blood is filtered through the nephrons and is reabsorbed into the body. If the glucose concentration in the blood becomes too high, the kidney is unable to reabsorb all of it back into the blood, the renal threshold is exceeded, and glucose is spilled into the urine—a condition known as **glycosuria.** (The **renal threshold** is the concentration at which a substance in the blood that is not normally excreted by the kidney begins to appear in the urine.)

TABLE 16-1

Diagnostic Kits Used for Chemical Testing of Urine

Brand Name	Function
Products of Bayer Corporation	
Acetest	Reagent tablet to detect ketones
Albustix	Reagent strip to detect protein
Bili-Labstix	Reagent strip to detect pH, protein, glucose, ketones, bilirubin, and blood
Clinistix	Reagent strip to detect glucose
Clinitest	Reagent tablet to detect glucose
Combistix	Reagent strip to detect pH, protein, and glucose
Diastix	Reagent strip to detect glucose
Hema-Combistix	Reagent strip to detect pH, protein, glucose, and blood
Hemastix	Reagent strip to detect blood
Ictotest	Reagent tablet to detect bilirubin
Keto-Diastix	Reagent strip to detect glucose and ketones
Ketostix	Reagent strip to detect ketones
Labstix	Reagent strip to detect pH, protein, ketones, and blood
Multisix	Reagent strip to detect pH, protein, glucose, ketones, urobilinogen, bilirubin, and blood
Multistix SG	Reagent strip to detect pH, protein, glucose, ketones, urobilinogen, bilirubin, blood, and specific gravity
Multistix 2	Reagent strip to detect leukocytes and nitrite
Multistix 7	Reagent strip to detect pH, protein, glucose, ketones, blood, leukocytes, and nitrite
Multistix 8 SG	Reagent strip to detect pH, protein, glucose, ketones, blood, leukocytes, nitrite, and specific gravity
Multistix 9	Reagent strip to detect pH, protein, glucose, ketones, urobilinogen, bilirubin, blood, leukocytes, and nitrite
Multistix 9 SG	Reagent strip to detect pH, protein, glucose, ketones, bilirubin, blood, leukocytes, nitrite, and specific gravity
Multistix 10 SG	Reagent strip to detect pH, protein, glucose, ketones, urobilinogen, bilirubin, blood, leukocytes, nitrite, and specific gravity
N-Multistix	Reagent strip to detect pH, protein, glucose, ketones, urobilinogen, bilirubin, blood, and nitrite
N-Multistix SG	Reagent strip to detect pH, protein, glucose, ketones, urobilinogen, bilirubin, blood, nitrite, and specific gravity
Uristix	Reagent strip to detect protein and glucose
Uristix 4	Reagent strip to detect protein, glucose, leukocytes, and nitrite
Products of Boehringer Mannheim Diagnostics	
Chemstrip 6	Reagent strip to detect pH, protein, glucose, ketones, blood, and leukocytes
Chemstrip 7	Reagent strip to detect pH, protein, glucose, ketones, bilirubin, blood, and leukocytes
Chemstrip 8	Reagent strip to detect pH, protein, glucose, ketones, urobilinogen, bilirubin, blood, and nitrite
Chemstrip 9	Reagent strip to detect pH, protein, glucose, ketones, urobilinogen, bilirubin, blood, leukocytes, and nitrite
Chemstrip 10 with SG	Reagent strip to detect pH, protein, glucose, ketones, urobilinogen, bilirubin, blood, leukocytes, nitrite, and specific gravity
Chemstrip UG	Reagent strip to detect glucose
Chemstrip 4 the OB	Reagent strip to detect glucose, protein, blood, and leukocytes
Chemstrip 2 GP	Reagent strip to detect protein and glucose
Chemstrip 2 LN	Reagent strip to detect leukocytes and nitrite
Chemstrip UGK	Reagent strip to detect glucose and ketones
Chemstrip K	Reagent strip to detect ketones

16

Highlight on Drug Testing in the Workplace

Statistics suggest that the problem of drug abuse is growing in the workplace. It is estimated that on any 1 day, 8.9 to 16 million employees will be working under the influence of drugs. The effects of on-the-job drug use extend into every segment of the population and touch every business and industry. OSHA (Occupational Safety and Health Administration) estimates that 65 percent of all work-related accidents can be traced to substance abuse. The Metropolitan Insurance Company states that drug abuse costs industry $85 billion annually due to absenteeism, lowered productivity, and higher health-care costs.

Because of these economic and safety factors, businesses across the country are adopting a less permissive attitude toward drug use and are beginning compulsory drug testing in the workplace. Approximately one third of American employers have implemented drug-testing programs in the workplace, including utility companies, transportation operations, sports associations, and governmental agencies. Currently many companies are testing both blue and white collar employees for drug use. Companies with drug-testing programs report a significant reduction in employee accidents, fewer sick days, and healthier employees.

A comprehensive drug-testing program includes the detection of drug use in the workplace, policies developed to discourage further abuse, and the referral of employees for treatment and rehabilitation. Drug testing may be performed for one or more of the following purposes: (1) pre-employment drug screening; (2) testing for probable cause following unexplained behavior or events; (3) random sample testing of the work force to detect use of controlled substances by employees on the job.

Blood testing is the best means for determining precise information concerning the amount of the drug used and when the drug was taken. However, blood tests are costly and time consuming to perform. Urine drug testing offers the next best alternative; it is noninvasive and technically easier and cheaper to perform. The current urine screening tests target the most common drugs of abuse: amphetamines, barbiturates, benzodiazepines, cocaine, marijuana, opiates, PCP, methaqualone, and methadone.

The usual procedure for urine drug testing involves screening the specimen and then confirming positive results with more specific urine tests. The specimen may be collected at the workplace, at the medical office, or at an outside laboratory. To help ensure reliable and valid drug-testing results, a security system or "chain of custody" must be followed in the collection and handling of the specimen. This typically includes ensuring the identification of the individual undergoing drug testing, taking precautions to avoid faked or tampered-with specimens, witnessing the collection of the specimen, properly labeling the urine specimen, sealing the sample in the specimen container after collection, and immediately sending the specimen to the laboratory for analysis or refrigerating it at once if there is any delay in transporting.

The main disadvantage of urine drug testing is that a positive test result indicates only the presence of a drug in the urine; it does not provide any information when the drug was taken. Drugs that are detected in the urine may or *may not* still be present in the blood where they can affect an individual's behavior and impair performance. Hence, a positive urine test result does not reveal whether an individual is impaired by drugs. In addition, the initial urine-screening tests are sometimes unreliable: unless positive results are confirmed with a more specific test, an individual may be unjustly accused of drug use. These factors, along with the violation of an individual's right to privacy, are the main areas of dispute for individuals who oppose drug testing in the workplace.

Companies with drug-testing programs have various options when results are positive, such as recommendations for drug treatment programs or disciplinary action. Many companies have established in-house employee assistance programs that include counseling and drug withdrawal therapy for employees desiring help. Most companies prefer to help current employees rehabilitate themselves instead of discharging them and hiring and training new employees. Studies show a 35 to 60 percent recovery rate for employees enrolled in drug treatment programs.

The renal threshold for glucose is generally between 160 and 180 mg/dl (100 ml of blood), but this figure may vary among individuals. Diabetes mellitus is the most common cause of glycosuria. Some individuals have a low renal threshold, and glucose may appear in their urine after the consumption of a large quantity of foods containing sugar. This condition is known as **alimentary glycosuria.** If glucose appears in a patient's urine, the physician may request that the medical assistant check several specimens at different times of the day to rule out alimentary glycosuria.

Common tests used to check for glycosuria include Clinitest, Clinistix, and Diastix.

Protein

An abnormally high amount of protein in the urine is known as **proteinuria.** Protein in the urine usually indicates a pathologic condition if it is found in several samples over time. A temporary increase in urine protein may be caused by stress or strenuous exercise. Some of the conditions that may cause proteinuria to occur include glomerular filtration problems, renal diseases, and bacterial infections of the urinary tract. If proteinuria occurs, the physician usually requests an examination of the sediment to aid in the determination of the patient's condition.

Commercially prepared diagnostic kits that test for protein in the urine include Albustix, Combistix (includes tests for protein, glucose, and pH), and Uristix (includes tests for protein and glucose).

Ketones

There are three types of ketone bodies: beta-hydroxybutyric acid, acetoacetic acid, and acetone. Ketones are the normal products of fat metabolism and can be used by muscle tissue as a source of energy. When more than normal amounts of fat are used, the muscles cannot handle all of the ketones that result. Large amounts of ketones, therefore, accumulate in the tissues and body fluids; this condition is known as **ketosis.** When excessive amounts of ketones also begin appearing in the urine, this is known as **ketonuria.** Conditions that may lead to ketonuria include uncontrolled diabetes mellitus, starvation, and a diet composed almost entirely of fat. Commercially prepared diagnostic kits that test for the presence of ketones in the urine include Acetest and Ketostix.

Bilirubin

The average life span of a red blood cell is 120 days. When a red blood cell breaks down, one of the substances released from the breakdown of hemoglobin is a vivid yellow pigment known as bilirubin. Normally, bilirubin is transported to the liver and excreted into the bile, leaving the body through the intestines. Certain liver conditions such as gallstones, hepatitis, and cirrhosis may result in the presence of bilirubin in the urine, or **bilirubinuria.** The urine becomes yellow-brown or greenish, and a yellow foam appears when the urine is shaken. A commercially prepared diagnostic kit for detecting bilirubinuria is Ictotest.

Urobilinogen

Normally, bilirubin is excreted by the liver into the intestinal tract. Bacteria present in the intestines convert it to urobilinogen. Approximately 50 percent of the urobilinogen is then reabsorbed into the body to be re-excreted by the liver. Small amounts may appear in the urine, but most of the urobilinogen is excreted in the feces. An increase in the production of bilirubin in turn increases the amount of urobilinogen excreted in the urine. Conditions such as excessive hemolysis of red blood cells, infectious hepatitis, cirrhosis, congestive heart failure, and infectious mononucleosis may increase the level of urobilinogen in the urine.

Blood

Blood is considered an abnormal constituent of urine, unless it is present as a vulval contaminant during menstruation. The condition in which blood is found in the urine is termed **hematuria.** It may be due to injury or to disorders such as cystitis, tumors of the bladder, urethritis, kidney stones, and certain kidney disorders. A commercially prepared diagnostic kit for detecting hematuria is Hemastix.

Nitrite

Nitrite in the urine indicates the presence of a pathogen in the (normally sterile) urinary tract, which results in a UTI. The pathogen possesses the ability to convert nitrate, which normally occurs in the urine, to nitrite, which is normally absent. The nitrite test must be performed using urine that has been in the bladder for at least 4 to 6 hours to ensure that bacteria have converted nitrate to nitrite. Therefore, it is recommended that a first-voided morning specimen be used. The test should *not* be performed on specimens that have been left standing out, because a false-positive result may occur owing to bacterial contamination from the atmosphere. Nitrite tests are to be considered only screening tests and must be followed by a quantitative culture and identification of the invading organism.

Leukocytes

The presence of leukocytes in the urine is known as **leukocyturia** and accompanies inflammation of the kidneys and the lower urinary tract. Examples of specific conditions include acute and chronic pyelonephritis, cystitis, and urethritis. Reagent strips are available containing a reagent area that permits the chemical detection of both intact and lysed leukocytes in the urine. The advantage of detecting lysed leukocytes is that these cells cannot be observed during a microscopic examination of urine sediment and would otherwise remain undetected. The recommended urine

16

TABLE 16–2

Urine Test Strip Parameters and the Diagnoses They Assist*

System/Source	Leukocytes	Nitrite	Urine pH		Protein
Genitourinary	Renal infection/inflammation • Acute/chronic pyelonephritis • Glomerulonephritis • Urolithiasis • Tumors • Lower urinary tract infection (cystitis, urethritis, prostatitis)	Bacteriuria • Urinary tract infection (cystitis, urethritis, prostatitis, pyelonephritis)	Up (>pH 6) in • Renal failure • Bacterial infection (e.g., *Proteus* bacteriuria) • Renal tubular acidosis		Renal/glomerular/tubular disease • Glomerulonephritis • Glomerulosclerosis (e.g., in diabetes) • Nephrotic syndrome • Pyelonephritis • Renal tuberculosis
Hepatobiliary					
Gastrointestinal			Up in • Pyloric obstruction • Vomiting	Down in • Diarrhea • Malabsorption	
Cardiovascular					Congestive heart failure
Hormonal, Metabolic, and Other Systems			Up in • Alkalosis (metabolic, respiratory)	Down in • Acidosis (metabolic, respiratory, diabetic) • Pulmonary emphysema • Dehydration	Gout Hypokalemia Pre-eclampsia Severe febrile infection
Environmental (diet, drugs, stress)	Phenacetin-induced nephritis		Up in • Diet high in vegetables, citrus fruits • Alkalizing drug use (sodium bicarbonate, acetazolamide)	Down in • Diet high in meats or other protein, cranberries • Starvation • Acidifying drug use (ammonium chloride, methenamine mandelate therapy)	Nephrotoxic drugs

*Reagent strip detection of an abnormal urine constituent or concentration characteristic of disease (e.g., glycosuria in diabetes mellitus) may provide a useful screen or monitor but requires confirmation by other laboratory and clinical evidence.

Modified from (1) Conn, H.F., Conn, R.B. (eds.): *Current Diagnosis 5*. Philadelphia, W. B. Saunders, 1977. (2) Davidson, I., Henry, J.B. (eds.): *Todd-Stanford Clinical Diagnosis by Laboratory Methods*, ed. 15. Philadelphia, W. B. Saunders, 1974. (3) Raphael, S.S. et al.: *Lynch's Medical Laboratory Technology*, ed. 3. Philadelphia, W. B. Saunders, 1976. (4) Wallach, J.: *Interpretation of Diagnostic Tests*, ed. 2. Boston, Little, Brown, 1974. (5) Widmann, F.K.: *Goodale's Clinical Interpretation of Laboratory Tests*, ed. 7. Philadelphia, F.A. Davis, 1973. Courtesy of Boehringer Mannheim Diagnostics, Indianapolis, Indiana.

Urine Test Strip Parameters and the Diagnoses They Assist* *Continued*

Glucose	Ketones	Urobilinogen	Bilirubin	Blood, Erythrocytes (Hematuria)	Hemoglobin
Renal glycosuria (e.g., during pregnancy) Renal tubular disease (e.g., in Fanconi's syndrome) Decreased renal glucose threshold (e.g., in old age)				Renal infection/ inflammation/ injury • Renal tuberculosis • Renal infarction • Calculi (urethral, renal) • Polycystic kidneys • Tumors (bladder, renal pelvis, prostate) • Salpingitis • Cystitis	Renal intravascular Hemolysis Acute glomerulonephritis
		Liver cell damage Chronic liver stasis Cirrhosis Dubin-Johnson syndrome Note: May be 0 or down in biliary obstruction	Biliary dysfunction • Gallstones Obstructive jaundice Hepatitis (viral toxic) Dubin-Johnson syndrome	Cirrhosis	
	Vomiting Diarrhea	Note: May be negative with inhibition of intestinal flora by antimicrobial agents		Colon tumor Diverticulitis	
Myocardial infarction Diabetes mellitus Hemochromatosis Hyperthyroidism Cushing's syndrome Pheochromocytomas	Diabetic ketosis Glycogen-storage disease Pre-eclampsia Acute fever	Sickle cell anemia Hemolytic disease • Pernicious anemia Leptospirosis	Hemolytic disease Leptospirosis	Bacterial endocarditis Blood dyscrasias • Hemophilia • Thrombocytopenia • Sickle cell anemia Disseminated lupus erythematosus Malignant hypertension	Hemolytic disease Plasmodium (malaria) Clostridia (tetanus) infection
Sudden shock or pain Steroid therapy	Weight-reducing diet Ketogenic diet (e.g., in anticonvulsant therapy) Starvation			Hemorrhagenic drugs (e.g., anticoagulant, salicylates) Nephrotoxic agents Internal injury or foreign body Vitamin C or K deficiency	Overexertion Exposure to cold Incompatible blood transfusion Drug-induced hemolysis

16

specimen, particularly for women, is a clean-catch midstream collection, to prevent contamination of the specimen with leukocytes from vaginal secretions leading to false-positive test results.

REAGENT STRIPS

In the medical office, reagent strips are the most commonly used diagnostic urine testing kit. Reagent strips consist of disposable plastic strips on which are affixed separated reagent areas for testing specific chemical constituents that may be present in the urine during pathologic conditions. The results provide the physician with information relating to the status of the patient's carbohydrate metabolism, kidney and liver function, acid-base balance, and bacteriuria. Reagent strips are considered qualitative tests, and a positive result requires further testing. (Refer to Table 16–2 for an outline of reagent strip parameters and the diagnoses in which they assist.)

The number and type of reagent areas included on the reagent strip depend on the particular brand of reagent strips. Multistix 10 SG (Bayer Corporation; formerly Ames), for example, contains ten reagent areas for testing pH, protein, glucose, ketones, bilirubin, blood, urobilinogen, nitrite, specific gravity, and leukocytes. Other brands and the tests included for each are listed in Table 16–1.

The reagent strip procedure in this chapter is specifically for Multistix 10 SG; however, it can be followed for the chemical testing of urine with most reagent strips. In all instances, the medical assistant should read the manufacturer's instructions before performing the test.

Guidelines for Reagent Strip Urine Testing

Testing urine with reagent strips is a relatively easy procedure to perform; however, specific guidelines must be employed to obtain accurate test results.

1. **Type of Specimen:** The best results are obtained by using a freshly voided urine specimen. Most reagent strips are designed to be used with a random specimen collection; however, clean-catch midstream and first-voided morning specimens are suggested for specific tests. For example, the nitrite test results are optimized by using a first-voided morning specimen, whereas a clean-catch midstream collection is recommended for the leukocyte test.
2. **Specimen Container:** The specimen container used must be thoroughly clean and free from any detergent or disinfectant residue, because cleansing agents contain oxidants that react with the chemicals on the reagent strip, leading to inaccurate test results.
3. **Storage of Reagent Strips:** The reagent strips are sensitive to light, heat, and moisture, and the bottle containing the strips must therefore be stored in a cool, dry area with the cap tightly closed to maintain reactivity of the reagent. The bottle may contain a desiccant, which should not be removed because its purpose is to promote dryness by absorbing moisture. The bottle of reagent strips must be stored at a temperature under 30°C (86°F) but should not be stored in the refrigerator or freezer. A tan-to-brown discoloration or darkening on the reagent areas indicates deterioration of the chemical reagent strips, which should not be used because the test results would be inaccurate.
4. **Interpretation of Results:** Of particular importance is the comparison of the reagent strip with the color chart. The reagent strip must be compared with the color chart in good lighting to obtain a good visual match of the color reactions with the color chart provided with the test kit.

Quality Control

Quality control should be employed when performing a chemical examination of urine using a reagent strip. Quality control ensures the reliability of test results by (1) determining if the reagent strips are reacting properly and (2) confirming that the test is being properly performed and accurately interpreted.

To check the reliability of Multistix reagent strips, Chek-Stix (Bayer Corporation) should be used. Each Chek-Stix consists of a firm plastic strip to which are affixed seven synthetic ingredients (Fig 16–6). The strip is reconstituted by immersing it in distilled water for 30 minutes, which allows the ingredients on the strip to dissolve in the water.

After reconstitution, the resulting solution is tested in the same manner as a urine specimen. The values to be expected are outlined on a sheet that accompanies the control strips.

Urine Analyzer

Urine analyzers are used to perform a chemical examination of urine automatically using reagent strips. They offer the advantage of being able to perform the chemical analysis quickly and to interpret results automatically. These analyzers are used most often in medical offices that perform moderate to large volume urine testing.

The Clinitek Analyzer (Bayer Corporation) is an example of a urine analyzer that automatically reads Mul-

16

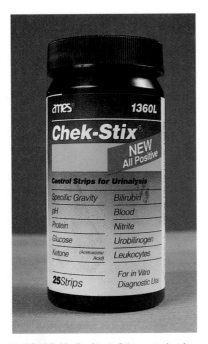

■ **FIGURE 16–6.** Chek-Stix control strips.

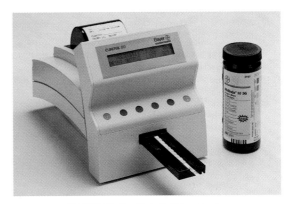

■ **FIGURE 16–7.** Clinitek Urine Analyzer.

tistix SG and other (Bayer) urinalysis reagent strips (Fig. 16–7). The results are printed out and abnormal results are highlighted to assist in reviewing results. There are different models available; some are able to perform a color and appearance analysis and a microscopic examination of the urine.

16–5

Chemical Testing of Urine Using the Multistix 10 SG Reagent Strip

| EQUIPMENT/SUPPLIES: | Disposable gloves
Multistix 10 SG reagent strips
Urine container | Biohazard waste container
Laboratory report form |

1. **Procedural Step.** Obtain a freshly voided urine specimen from the patient, using a clean container. The specimen should be well mixed, uncentrifuged, and at room temperature.
   Principle. The best results are obtained by using a freshly voided specimen. The container should be clean, because contaminants could affect the results. Well-mixed, uncentrifuged specimens assure a homogeneous sample.
2. **Procedural Step.** Wash the hands.
3. **Procedural Step.** Assemble the equipment. Check the expiration date of the reagent strips.
   Principle. Outdated reagent strips may lead to inaccurate test results.

4. **Procedural Step.** Apply gloves. Remove a reagent strip from the bottle and recap the bottle immediately. Do not touch the test areas with your fingers or lay the strip on the table. However, it is permissible to lay the reagent strip on a clean, dry paper towel.
   Principle. Recapping the bottle is necessary to prevent exposing the strips to environmental moisture, light, and heat, which cause altered reagent reactivity. Contamination of the test areas by the hands or table surface may affect the accuracy of the test results.
5. **Procedural Step.** Completely immerse the reagent strip in the urine specimen, and remove it immedi-

Continued

16

ately. While removing, run the edge of the strip against the rim of the urine container to remove excess urine.

Principle. The strip should be completely immersed to ensure that all test areas are moistened for accurate test results. Prolonged immersion of the reagent strip and failure to remove excess urine may cause the reagents to dissolve and leach onto adjacent test areas, affecting the accuracy of the test results.

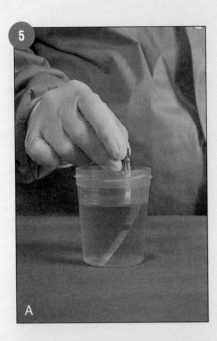

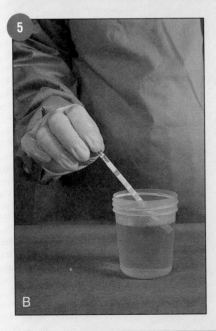

6. **Procedural Step.** Hold the reagent strip in a horizontal position and place it adjacent to the corresponding color blocks on the color chart. Do not lay the strip directly on the color chart because this will result in the urine's soiling the chart. Read the results carefully and at the exact reading times specified on the color chart and as indicated below.

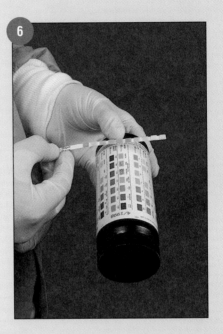

Glucose	30 seconds
Bilirubin	30 seconds
Ketones	40 seconds
Specific gravity	45 seconds
Blood	60 seconds
pH	60 seconds
Protein	60 seconds
Urobilinogen	60 seconds
Nitrite	60 seconds
Leukocytes	2 minutes

Principle. Holding the strip in a horizontal position avoids soiling the hands with urine and prevents reagents from running over into the adjacent testing areas, causing inaccurate test results. The strip must be read at the proper time to avoid dissolving out reagents, leading to inaccurate test results.

7. **Procedural Step.** Dispose of the strip in a biohazard waste container.

8. **Procedural Step.** Remove gloves, and wash the hands.

9. **Procedural Step.** Chart the results. The results should be charted following the interpretation guide provided above each color block on the color chart.

Be sure to include the date and time, the brand name of the test used (Multistix 10 SG), and the results.

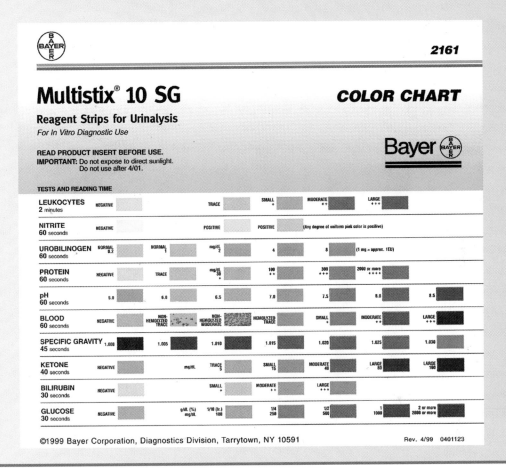

16

CELLS FOUND IN URINE

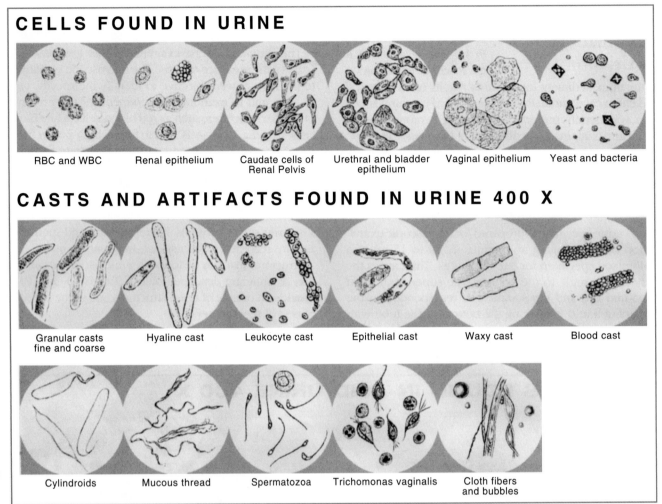

| RBC and WBC | Renal epithelium | Caudate cells of Renal Pelvis | Urethral and bladder epithelium | Vaginal epithelium | Yeast and bacteria |

CASTS AND ARTIFACTS FOUND IN URINE 400 X

| Granular casts fine and coarse | Hyaline cast | Leukocyte cast | Epithelial cast | Waxy cast | Blood cast |

| Cylindroids | Mucous thread | Spermatozoa | Trichomonas vaginalis | Cloth fibers and bubbles |

■ **FIGURE 16–8.** Urine sediment. (Courtesy of Bayer Corporation, Elkhart, Indiana.)

MICROSCOPIC EXAMINATION OF URINE

Urine sediment is the solid materials contained in the urine (Fig. 16–8). A microscopic examination of the urine sediment helps clarify results of the physical and chemical examination. A first-voided morning specimen is generally preferred, because it is more concentrated and contains more dissolved substances; therefore, small amounts of abnormal substances are more likely to be detected. It is important to use a fresh specimen, because changes will take place in a specimen left standing out, as previously discussed. These changes affect the reliability of the test results. The procedure for preparing a urine specimen for microscopic examination and examining the sediment under a microscope is presented at the end of this section.

Structures that may be found in a microscopic examination of urine are described below; Tables 16–3 to 16–6 provide an outline of these structures and of the possible causes of their presence.

Red Blood Cells

Red blood cells appear as round, colorless, biconcave discs that are highly refractile. The presence of 0 to 5 per high-power field is considered normal. More than this amount may indicate bleeding somewhere along the urinary tract. Refer to Table 16–3 for a list of possible causes of an abnormal number of red blood cells in the urine. Concentrated urine causes the red blood cells to become shrunken or **crenated,** whereas dilute urine causes them to swell and become rounded, which may cause them to hemolyze. If the red blood cells have hemolyzed, they will not be seen under the microscope. The presence of blood in the urine can still be identified, however, by the use of a reagent strip, such as Multistix, designed to detect free hemoglobin.

White Blood Cells

White blood cells are round and granular and have a nucleus. They are approximately 1.5 times as large as a red blood cell. The presence of 0 to 8 per high-power field is considered normal. More than this amount may indicate inflammation of the genitourinary tract. Refer to Table 16–3 for a list of possible causes of an abnormal number of white blood cells in the urine.

Epithelial Cells

Most structures making up the urinary system are composed of several layers of epithelial cells. The outer layer is constantly being sloughed off and replaced by the cells underneath it. **Squamous epithelial cells** are large, clear, flat cells with an irregular shape. They contain a small nucleus and come from the urethra, bladder, and vagina. Squamous epithelial cells are normally present in small amounts in the urine. **Renal epithelial cells** are round and contain a large nucleus. They come from the deeper layers of the urinary tract, and their presence in the urine is considered abnormal. Refer to Table 16–3 for a list of the types of epithelial cells and possible causes of the presence of abnormal amounts in the urine.

Casts

Casts are cylindric structures formed in the lumen of the tubules that make up the nephron. Materials in the tubules harden, are flushed out, and appear in the urine in the form of casts. Various types of casts may be present in the urine. Their presence generally indicates a diseased condition.

Casts are named according to what they contain. **Hyaline casts** are pale, colorless cylinders with rounded edges; they vary in size. **Granular casts** are hyaline casts that contain granules. They are described as "coarsely granular" or "finely granular," depending on the size of the granules. **Fatty casts** are hyaline casts that contain fat droplets. **Waxy casts** are light yellowish and have serrated edges. Their name is derived from the fact that they appear to be made of wax.

Cellular casts contain organized structures and are named according to what they contain. Examples include red blood cell casts, which are hyaline casts containing red blood cells; white blood cell casts, which are hyaline casts containing white blood cells; epithelial casts, which are hyaline casts containing epithelial cells; and bacterial casts, which are hyaline casts containing bacteria. Refer to Table 16–4 for a list of the types of casts and possible causes of their presence in urine.

Crystals

A variety of crystals may be found in the urine. The type and number vary with the pH of the urine. Abnormal crystals found include leucine, tyrosine, cystine, and cholesterol. Crystals that commonly appear in acid urine include amorphous urates, uric acid, and calcium oxalate. Those that commonly appear in alkaline urine include amorphous phosphate, triple phosphate, calcium phosphate, and ammonium urate crystals. Refer to Table 16–5 for a list of the types of urine crystals and their significance when found in urine.

Miscellaneous Structures

Mucous threads are normally present in small amounts in the urine. They appear as long, wavy, threadlike structures with pointed ends.

Bacteria should not normally exist in the urinary

Text continued on page 558

TABLE 16-3

Cells in Urine Sediment

Type	Presence in Normal Urine	Possible Causes of Abnormal Amounts of Cells in Urine	Microscopic Appearance
Red blood cells	0 to 5 cells per high-power field (depending on preparation of urine sediment)	Inflammatory diseases Acute glomerulonephritis Pyelonephritis Hypertension Renal infarction Trauma Stones Tumor Bleeding diseases Use of anticoagulants	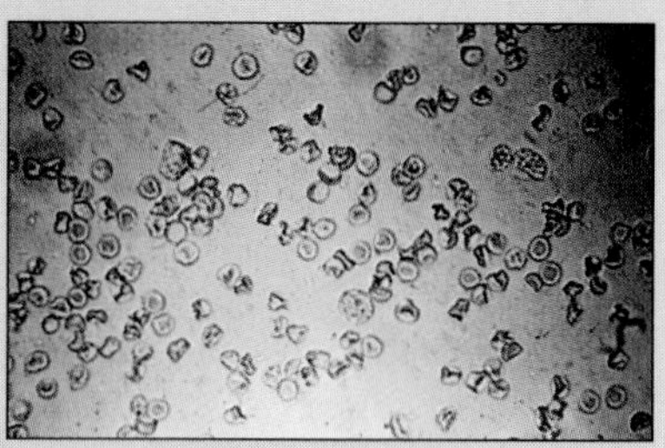
White blood cells	0 to 8 cells per high-power field (depending on preparation of urine sediment)	Pyelonephritis Cystitis Urethritis Prostatitis Transplant rejection (manifested by lymphocytes in urine) Tissue injury accompanied by severe inflammation (manifested by monocytes in urine) Inflammation, immune mechanisms, and other host defense mechanisms (manifested by histiocytes in urine)	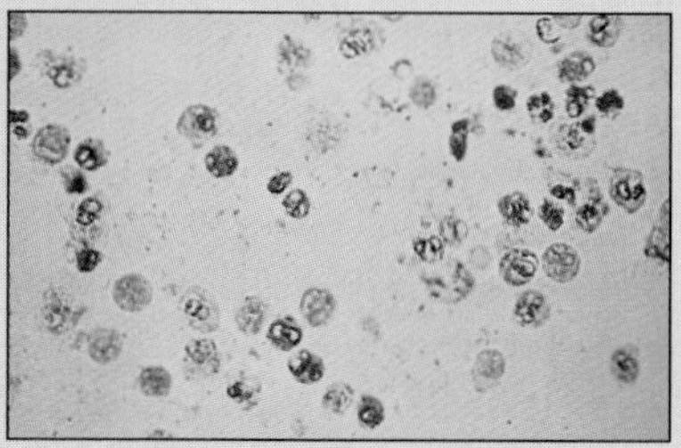
Squamous epithelial cells	Often present, depending upon collection technique	Vaginal contamination	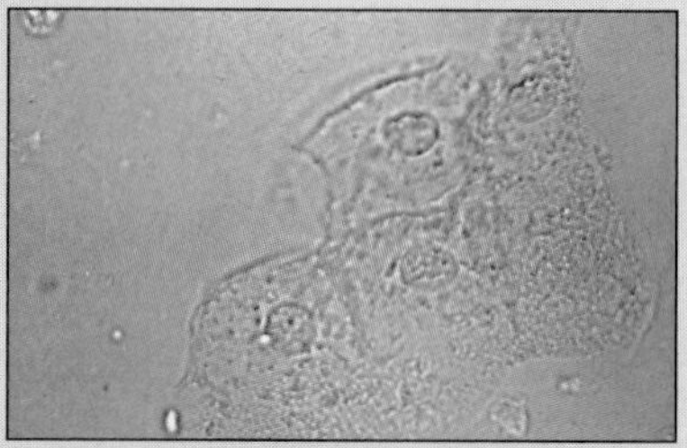
Transitional epithelial cells	Moderate number of cells present	Disease of bladder or renal pelvis Catheterization	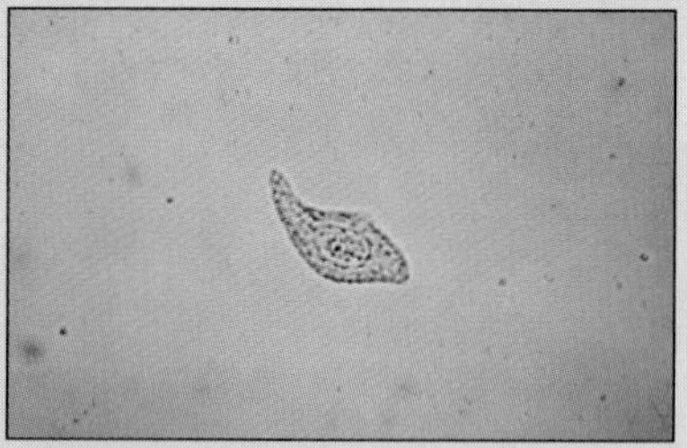
Renal tubular epithelial cells	Present in small numbers; higher numbers in infants	Acute tubular necrosis Glomerulonephritis Acute infection Renal toxicity Viral infection	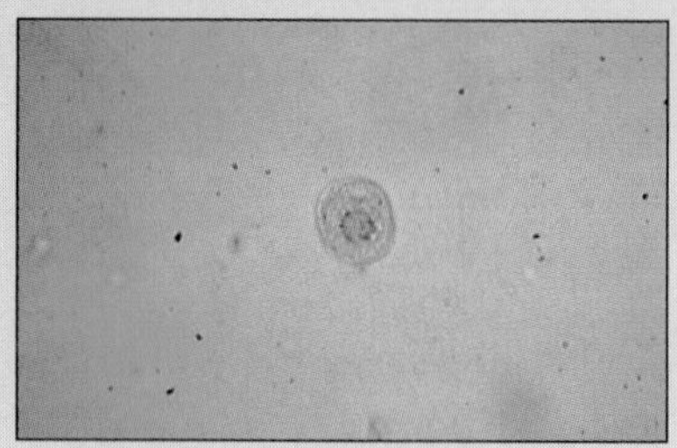

16

TABLE 16 – 3

Cells in Urine Sediment *Continued*

Type	Presence in Normal Urine	Possible Causes of Abnormal Amounts of Cells in Urine
Cytomegalic inclusion bodies	Not normally present in urine	Cytomegalic inclusion disease
Tumor cells	Not normally present in urine	Tumors of • Renal pelvis • Renal parenchyma • Ureters • Bladder

Text courtesy of Boehringer Mannheim Diagnostics, Indianapolis, Indiana.
Photomicrographs courtesy of Bayer Corporation, Elkhart, Indiana.

TABLE 16 – 4

Casts in Urine Sediment

Type	Description	Possible Causes	Microscopic Appearance
Hyaline casts	Colorless, transparent Low refractive index	Normal urine Strenuous exercise Acute glomerulonephritis Acute pyelonephritis Malignant hypertension Chronic renal disease	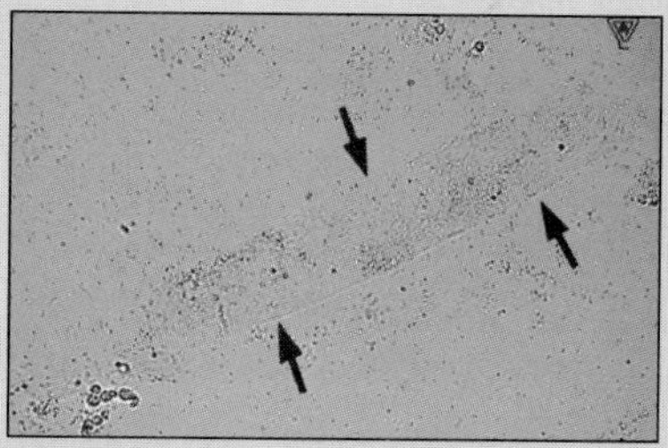 ‡
Red blood cell casts	Red cells in hyaline matrix Yellow-orange color High refractive index	Acute glomerulonephritis Lupus nephritis Severe nephritis Collagen diseases Renal infarction Malignant hypertension	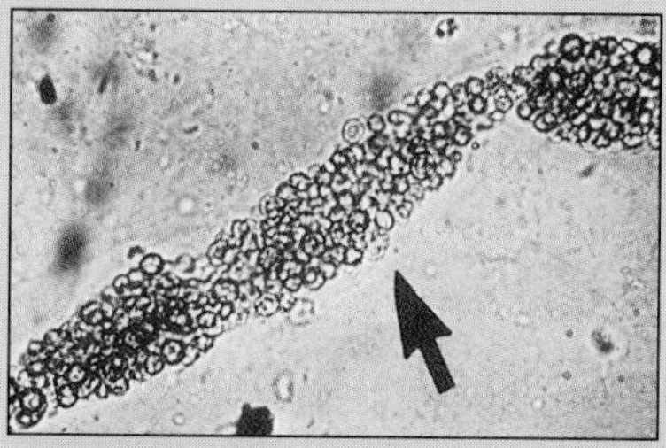 ‡
White blood cell casts	Neutrophils in hyaline matrix High refractive index	Acute pyelonephritis Acute glomerulonephritis Chronic renal disease	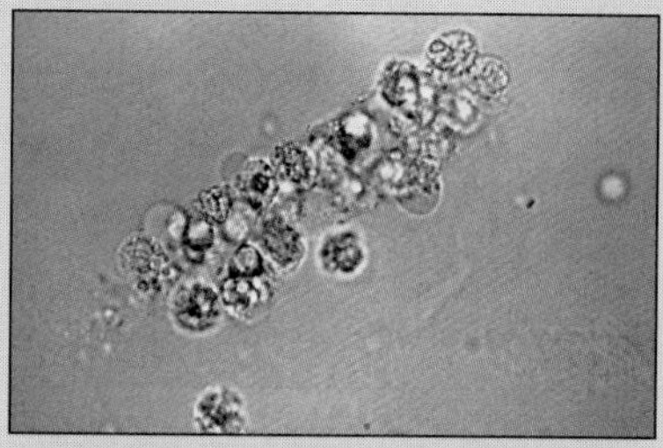 *
Epithelial cell casts	Renal tubular epithelial cells in hyaline matrix High refractive index	Glomerulonephritis Vascular disease Toxin Virus	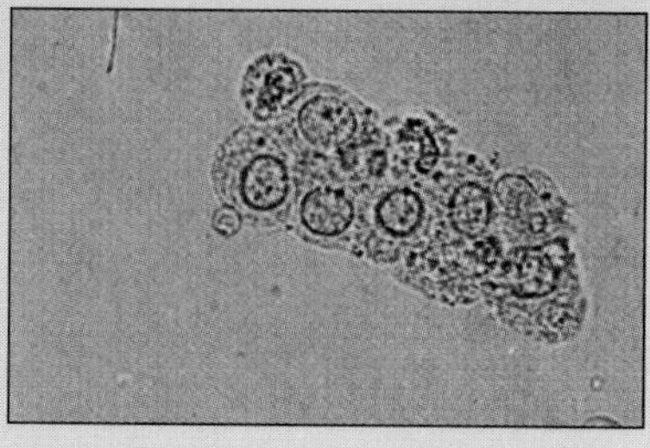 †

16

TABLE 16-4

Casts in Urine Sediment *Continued*

Type	Description	Possible Causes	Microscopic Appearance
Granular casts	Opaque granules in matrix	Heavy proteinuria (nephrotic syndrome) Orthostatic proteinuria Congestive heart failure with proteinuria Acute or chronic renal disease	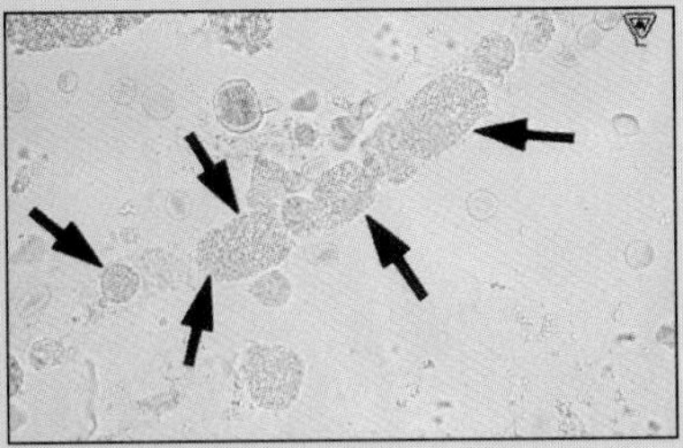 ‡
Waxy casts	Sharp, refractile outlines Irregular "broken off" ends Absence of differentiated structures	Severe chronic renal disease Malignant hypertension Kidney disease resulting from diabetes mellitus Acute renal disease	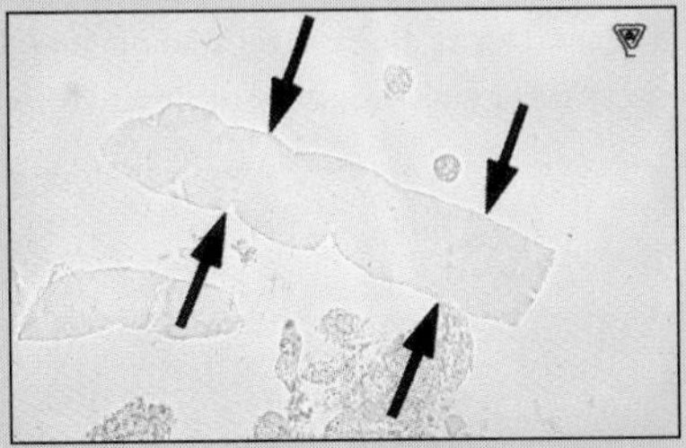 ‡
Fatty casts	Fat globules in transparent matrix	Nephrotic syndrome Diabetes mellitus Mercury poisoning Ethylene glycol poisoning	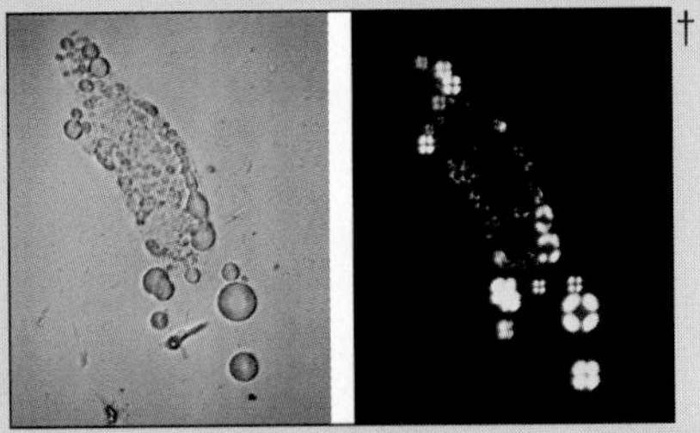 †
Broad casts	Larger diameter than other casts	Acute tubular necrosis Severe chronic renal disease Urinary tract obstruction	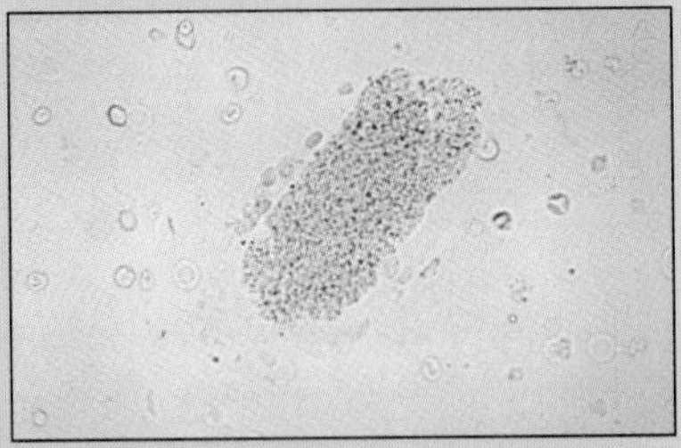 *
Mixed casts	Combination of any of the above	Any of the above, depending on cellular constituents	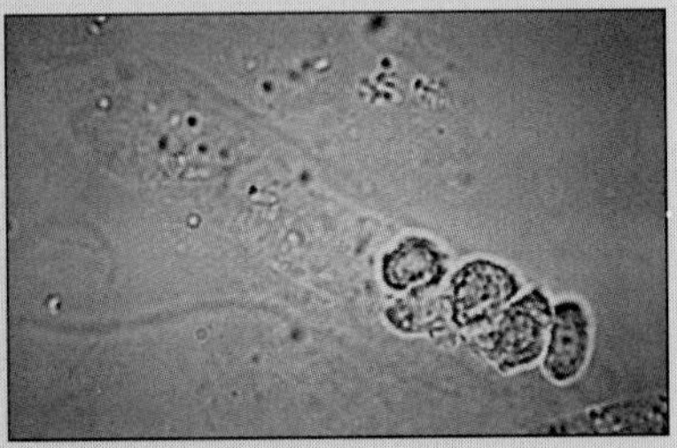 *

Text courtesy of Boehringer Mannheim Diagnostics, Indianapolis, Indiana.

*Photomicrographs courtesy of Bayer Corporation, Diagnostics Division, Elkhart, Indiana

†Photomicrographs from Henry J. B.: *Clinical Diagnosis and Management by Laboratory Methods.* ed. 19. Philadelphia, W. B. Saunders, 1996.

‡Photomicrographs from Stepp C. A., Woods M.: *Laboratory Procedures for Medical Office Personnel.* Philadelphia, W. B. Saunders, 1998.

16

TABLE 16-5

Urinary Crystals

Type of Urine	Type of Crystals	Description of Crystals	Significance When Found In Urine	Microscopic Appearance
Normal acid urine	Amorphous urate	Colorless or yellow-brown granules (pink macroscopically)	Nonpathologic	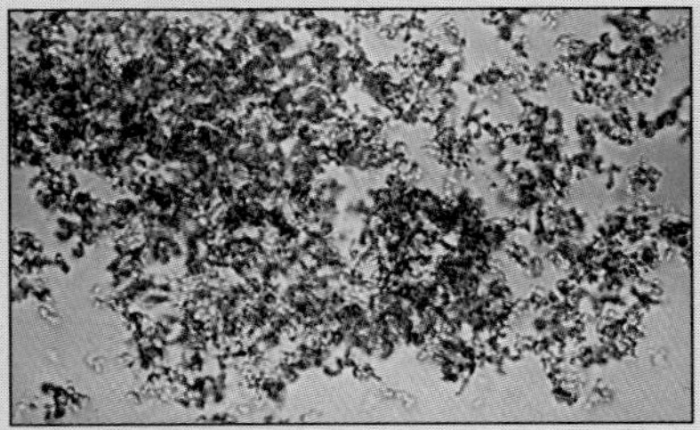 *
	Uric acid	Occur in many shapes; may be colorless, yellow-brown, or red-brown; and square, diamond-shaped, wedge-shaped, or grouped in rosettes	Usually nonpathologic; in large numbers, may indicate gout	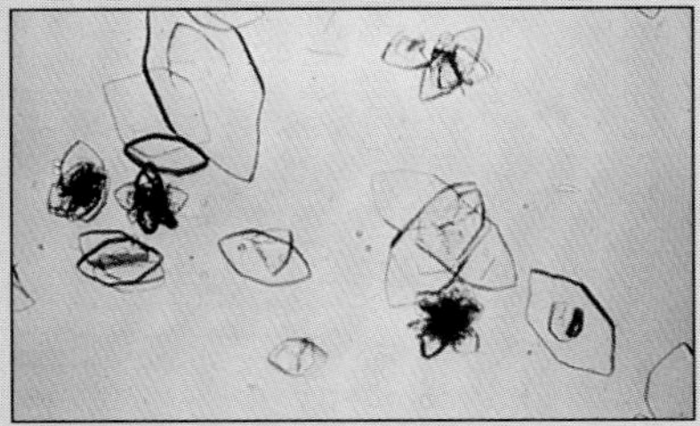 *
	Calcium oxalate	Octahedral or dumbbell-shaped; possess double refractive index	Usually nonpathologic; may be associated with stone formation	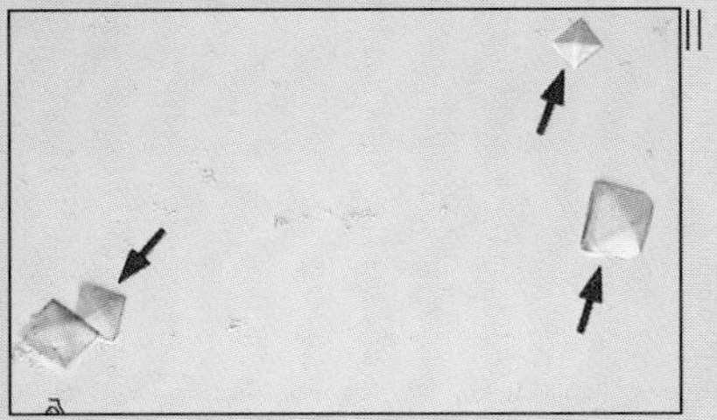 ‖
Normal alkaline urine	Amorphous phosphates	Small, colorless granules	Nonpathologic	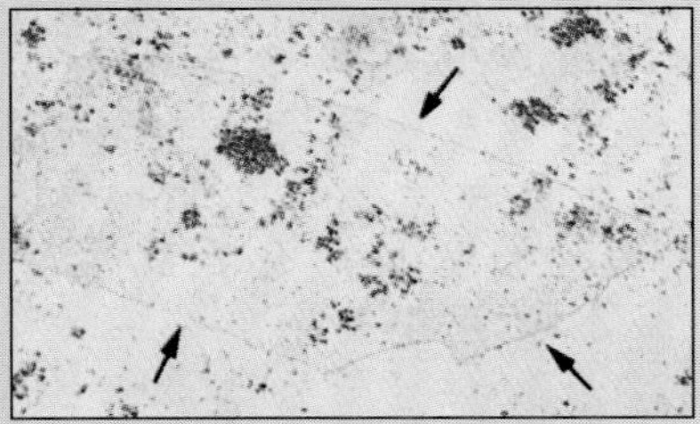 §

16

Continued

Urinary Crystals *Continued*

Type of Urine	Type of Crystals	Description of Crystals	Significance When Found In Urine	Microscopic Appearance
	Triple phosphates	Colorless prisms with three to six sides ("coffin lids") or feathery, shaped like fern leaves	Usually nonpathologic; may be associated with urine stasis or chronic urinary tract infection	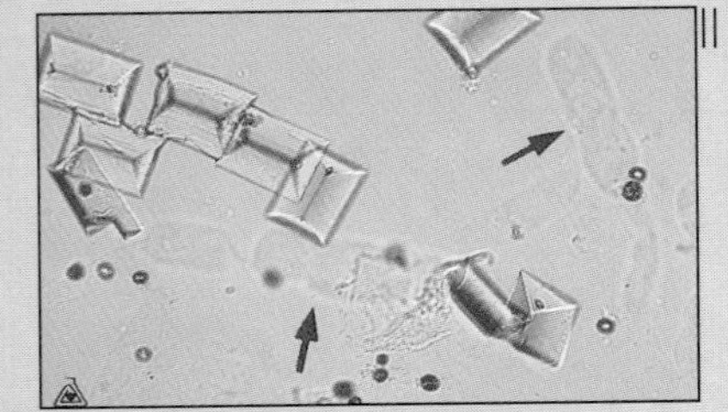
	Ammonium biurate	Yellow-brown "thorny apple" appearance or yellow-brown spheres	Nonpathologic	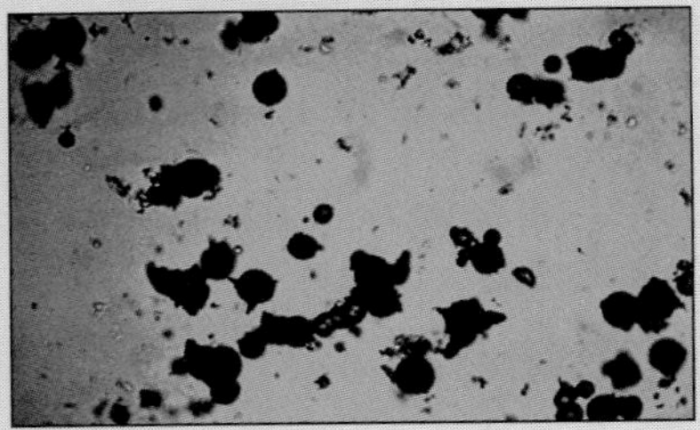
	Calcium phosphate	Colorless prisms or rosettes	Usually nonpathologic; may be associated with urine stasis or chronic urinary tract infection	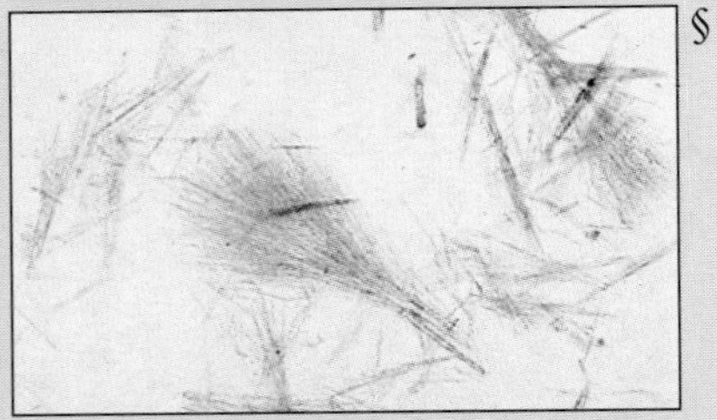
	Calcium carbonate	Usually appear colorless and amorphous; may be shaped like dumbbells, rhombi, or needles	Usually nonpathologic; may be associated with inorganic calculi formation	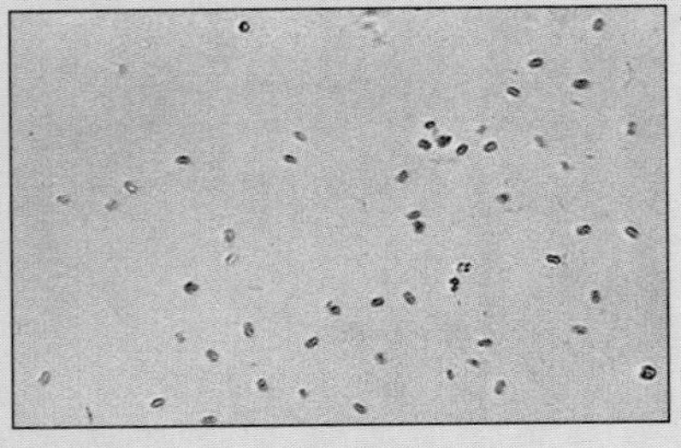

TABLE 16-5

554

Abnormal urine			
Tyrosine	Thin, dark needles, arranged in sheaves or clumps; usually colorless but may be pale yellow-brown	Liver disease or inherited metabolic disorder	*
Leucine	Yellow-brown spheres with radial striations	Liver disease or inherited metabolic disorder	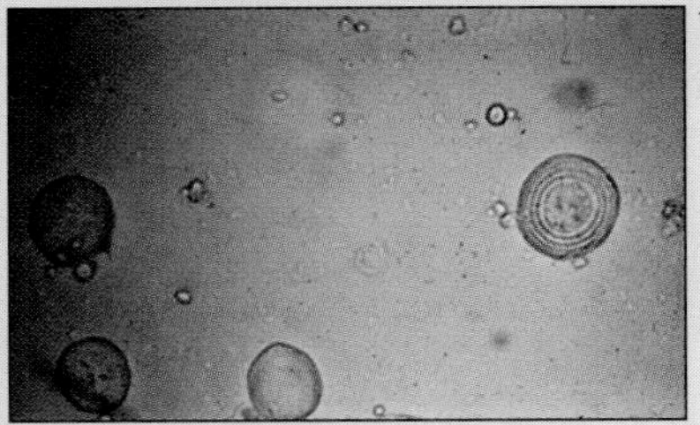 *
Cystine	Clear, hexagonal plates	Cystinuria	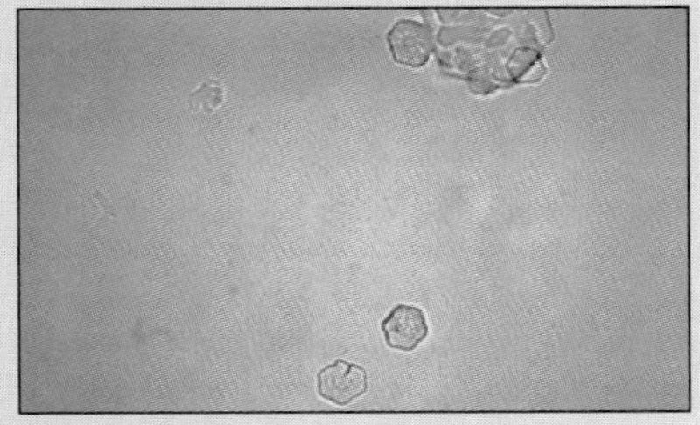 *
Hippuric acid	Star-shaped clusters of needles, rhombic plates, or elongated prisms; may be colorless or yellow-brown	Usually nonpathologic	‡

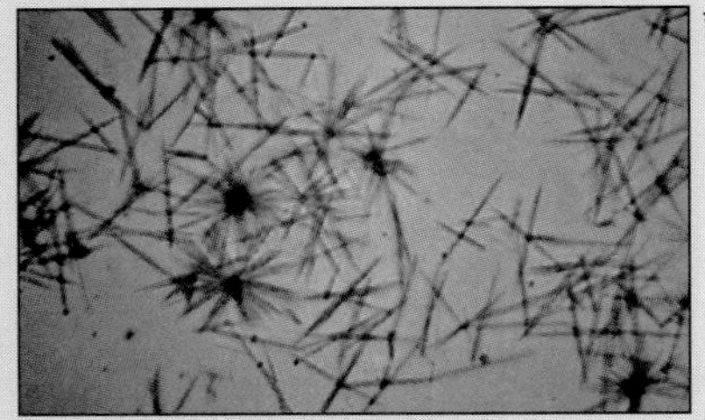

16

TABLE 16-5 Urinary Crystals *Continued*

Type of Urine	Type of Crystals	Description of Crystals	Significance When Found In Urine	Microscopic Appearance
	Bilirubin	Delicate needles or rhombic plates; red-brown in color; birefringent	Bilirubinuria	
	Cholesterol	Colorless, transparent plates with regular or irregular corner notches	Chyluria, urinary tract infections, nephrotic syndrome	
	Creatine	Pseudohexagonal plates with positive birefringence	Destruction of muscle tissue due to muscular dystrophies, atrophies, and myositis	
	Aspirin	Distinctive prismatic or starlike forms; usually colorless; show positive birefringence	Ingestion of aspirin or other salicylates	
	Sulfonamide	Yellow-brown dumbbells, asymmetric sheaves, rosettes, or hexagonal plates	Ingestion of sulfonamide drugs	

| Ampicillin | Long, thin, clear crystals | Parenteral administration of ampicillin § 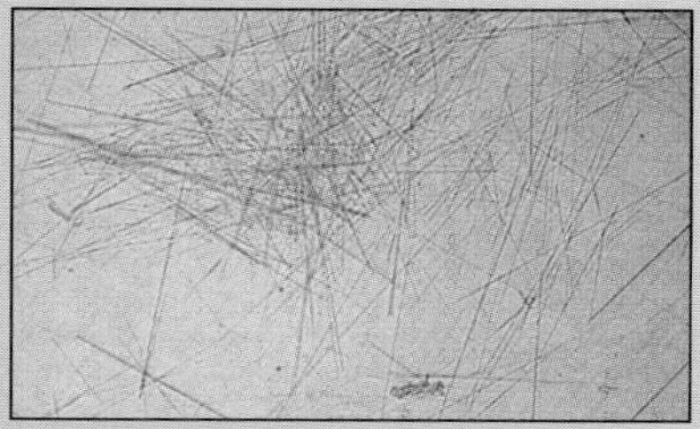|

| X-ray media | Long, thin rectangles or flat, four-sided, notched plates | X-ray procedure with contrast media * 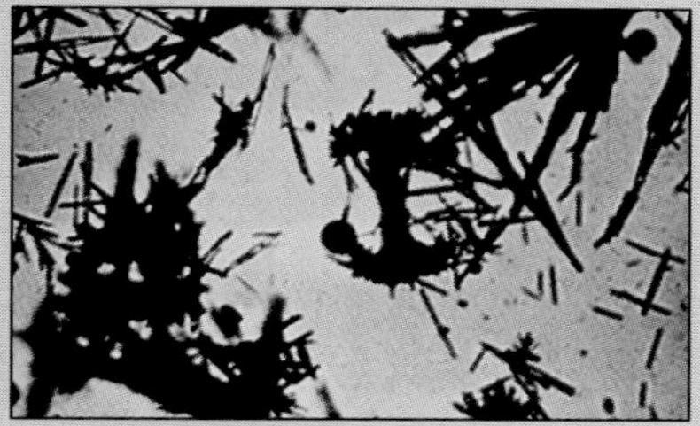|

Text courtesy of Boehringer Mannheim Diagnostics, Indianapolis, Indiana.

*Photomicrographs courtesy of Bayer Corporation, Diagnostics Division, Elkhart, Indiana.

†Photomicrograph from Brunzel, N. A.: *Fundamentals of Urine and Body Fluid Analysis*. Philadelphia, W.B. Saunders, 1994.

‡Photomicrograph from Lehmann, C. A.: Saunders *Manual of Clinical Laboratory Science*. Philadelphia, W.B. Saunders, 1998.

§Photomicrographs from Henry, J. B.: *Clinical Diagnosis and Management by Laboratory Methods*, ed. 19. Philadelphia, W.B. Saunders, 1996.

|| Photomicrographs from Stepp, C. A. Wood, M.: *Laboratory Procedures for Medical Office Personnel*. Philadelphia, W.B. Saunders, 1998.

TABLE 16–6

Microorganisms and Artifacts in the Urine

Microorganisms/Artifacts	Significance When Found in the Urine	Microscopic Appearance
Bacteria	More than 100,000 bacteria per ml indicates urinary tract infection 10,000 to 100,000 bacteria per ml indicates that tests should be repeated Less than 10,000 bacteria per ml may signify urine in which any bacteria are due to urethral organisms or contamination Bacteria accompanied by white blood cells and/or white cell or mixed casts may indicate acute pyelonephritis	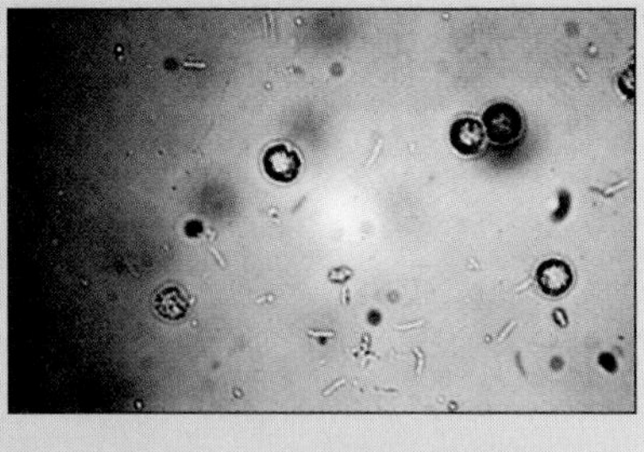
Yeast	May indicate contamination by yeasts from skin and hair May indicate diabetes mellitus or urinary tract infection *Candida albicans* may occur in patients with diabetes mellitus or in the contaminated urine of female patients with candidal vaginitis	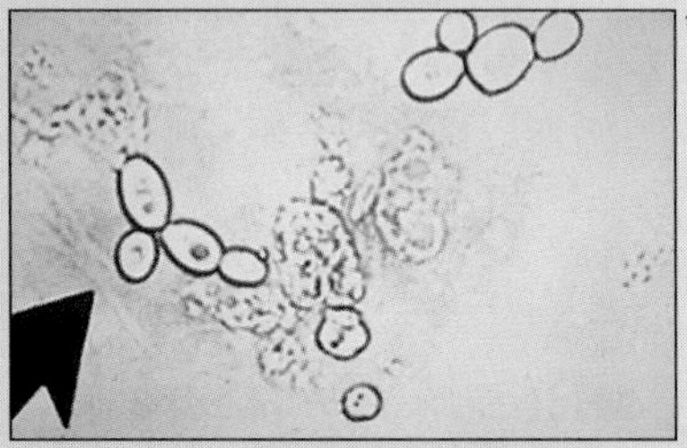
Parasites and parasitic ova	Usually indicate fecal or vaginal contamination and should be reported *Trichomonas* may be found in patients with urethritis and in the contaminated urine of women with *Trichomonas* vaginitis Pinworm is a common contaminant and should be reported	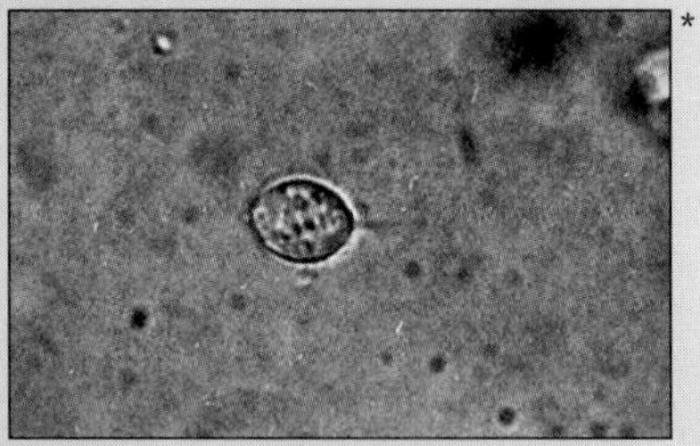
Spermatozoa	Nonpathologic	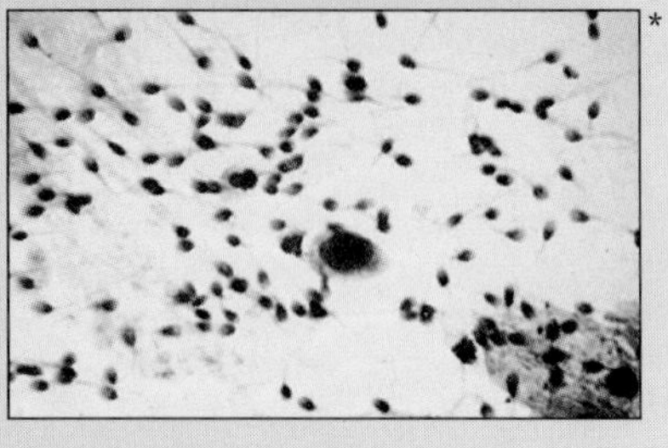

tract. The presence of more than a few bacteria may indicate either contamination of the specimen during collection or a UTI. Bacteria are small structures and may be rod shaped or round.

Yeast cells are smooth, refractile bodies that have an oval shape. A distinguishing feature of yeast cells is small buds projecting from the cells that are involved with reproduction. Yeast cells in the urine of female patients are usually a vaginal contaminant caused by the yeast *Candida albicans* and produce the vaginal in-

TABLE 16-6

Microorganisms and Artifacts in the Urine   *Continued*

Microorganisms/Artifacts	Significance When Found in the Urine	Microscopic Appearance

Urinary artifacts
  Hair (a)
  Starch from surgi-
  cal gloves
  Pollen grains
  Bubbles
  Oil droplets
  Fibers (b)
  Talc (c)
  Dust
  Threads (d)
  Mucus
  Glass particles
	Nonpathologic
	May result from improper urine collection, improper slide preparation, or outside contamination
		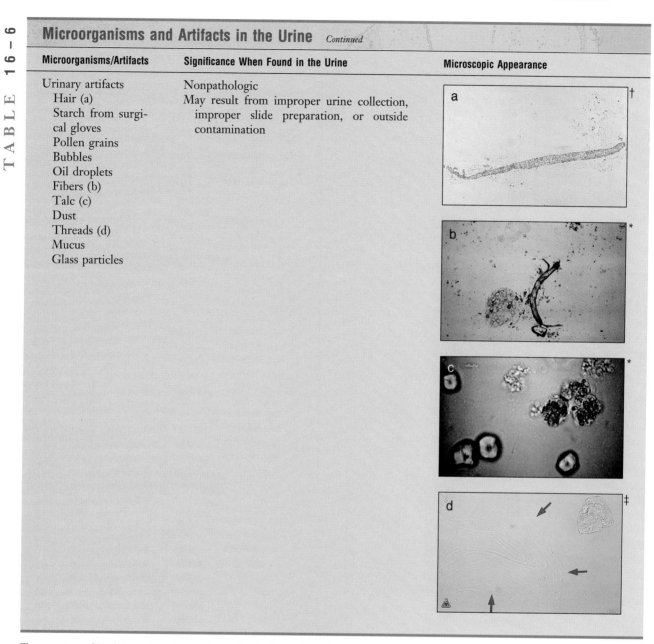

Text courtesy of Boehringer Mannheim Diagnostics, Indianapolis, Indiana.

*Photomicrographs courtesy of Bayer Corporation, Diagnostics Division, Elkhart, Indiana.

†Photomicrograph from Lehman C. A.: *Saunders Manual of Clinical Laboratory Science*, Philadelphia, W. B. Saunders, 1998.

‡Photomicrograph from Stepp C. A., Woods M.: *Laboratory Procedures for Medical Office Personnel*. Philadelphia, W. B. Saunders, 1998.

fection known as candidiasis. They may also be present in the urine of patients with diabetes mellitus.

Parasites may be present in the urine sediment as a contaminant from fecal or vaginal material. *Trichomonas vaginalis* is a parasite that causes Trichomonas vaginitis.

Spermatozoa may be present in the urine of a man or woman after coitus. The spermatozoa have round heads and long, slender, hairlike tails. Refer to Table 16-6 for a list of miscellanous structures that may be present in the urine and the significance when found.

Text continued on page 564

PUTTING IT ALL
into PRACTICE

 LINDA PROFFITT: *When I first started working in my urology office, I had to learn to assist with transrectal ultrasounds of the prostate in case the nurse was sick. When she retired, I inherited the position whether I wanted it or not.*

At first I dreaded doing them and would be so nervous that I would get the shakes and forget the order in which things were supposed to be done. My physician was very understanding and would

help me by talking me through it. I think the main reason I was so nervous was that sometimes the patients have trouble and we have to administer oxygen and run IVs. One time, the patient had a reaction to the pain medication we gave him before the procedure.

Time, practice, and confidence in myself have improved the nerves even with the occasional emergency situation.

PATIENT/TEACHING

URINARY TRACT INFECTIONS

Answer questions patients have about urinary tract infections.

What Is a UTI?

UTI is a general term for the presence of bacteria in any portion of the urinary tract. UTIs, particularly those involving the bladder (cystitis) and urethra (urethritis), are common and treatable. A UTI is usually treated with an antibiotic. It is important to take all the antibiotic for the full number of days prescribed by the physician, even if your symptoms disappear. If you stop taking the medication too soon, the infection may recur and be more difficult to treat than the original infection.

What Are the Symptoms of a UTI?

The symptoms of a simple UTI (cystitis) commonly include the frequent need to urinate, urgency (meaning the immediate need to urinate), a burning sensation during urination, and sometimes blood in the urine. The symptoms of a more complicated UTI involving the kidneys (pyelonephritis) include the preceding symptoms as well as lower abdominal discomfort, low back pain, fever, cloudy or foul-smelling urine, and blood in the urine.

Why Do Women Have UTIs More Frequently than Men?

Women are more prone to the type of UTI called cystitis than men. This is because the urethra of a woman is much shorter than that of a man, making it easier for bacteria to travel up the urethra and into the bladder. The most common source of infection is bacteria (*Escherichia coli*). This organism is normally found in the large intestine but can travel from the anal area to the urinary bladder, often as the result of poor hygienic practices. Cystitis occurs if *E. coli* are able to

overcome the body's natural defenses once the bacteria reach the urinary bladder and set up an infection.

What Can Women Do to Prevent a UTI?

The prevention measures that a woman prone to developing UTIs should practice are

Practice good hygienic measures by always cleaning the genital area from front to back after a bowel movement.

Avoid possible irritants such as bubble baths, perfumed soaps, feminine hygiene sprays, or the use of strong powders and bleaches for washing underclothes.

Avoid clothing that traps moisture and thereby encourages the growth of microorganisms, such as tight, constricting clothing, nylon panties, and panty hose.

Avoid activities that can contribute to irritation of the urinary meatus, such as prolonged bicycling, motorcycling, horseback riding, and traveling involving prolonged sitting.

Urinate as soon as possible when you feel the urge. Holding urine in the bladder gives the bacteria more time to grow, which can cause more infection. The more often you urinate, the quicker the bacteria will be removed from the bladder.

Seek prompt treatment if you experience any of the symptoms of a UTI.

- Encourage the patient with a UTI to drink plenty of water to help flush the bacteria out of the urinary tract.
- Emphasize to the patient the importance of taking all the antibiotic for the duration of time prescribed by the physician.
- Emphasize the importance of practicing preventive measures to prevent the occurrence of urinary tract infections.
- Provide the patient with educational materials on urinary tract infections.

16

PROCEDURE

16–6

Microscopic Examination of Urine—Kova Method

EQUIPMENT/SUPPLIES:

Disposable gloves
Urine specimen (first-voided morning specimen)
Kova urine centrifuge tube
Kova cap
Kova pipet
Kova slide

Kova stain
Test tube rack
Urine centrifuge
Mechanical stage microscope
Biohazard waste container

Preparing the Specimen

1. **Procedural Step.** Wash the hands, and assemble the equipment.

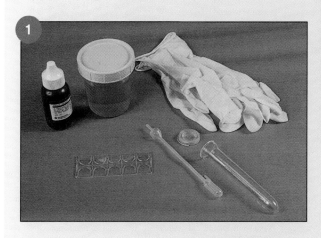

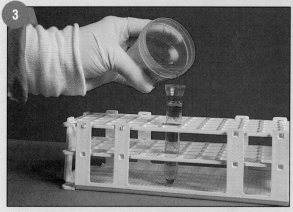

2. **Procedural Step.** Apply gloves. Mix the urine specimen using the Kova pipet.
   Principle. The specimen must be well mixed to ensure accurate test results.
3. **Procedural Step.** Pour the urine specimen into the urine centrifuge tube. Fill it to the 12-ml graduation mark, and cap the tube.
4. **Procedural Step.** Centrifuge the tube for 5 minutes at approximately 1500 revolutions per minute (rpm).
   Principle. Centrifuging the specimen causes the solid elements in the urine to settle to the bottom of the tube.
5. **Procedural Step.** Remove the urine tube from the centrifuge, being careful not to disturb or dislodge the sediment.
6. **Procedural Step.** Remove the cap. Insert the Kova pipet into the urine tube and push it to the bottom of the tube until it seats firmly. Make sure the clip

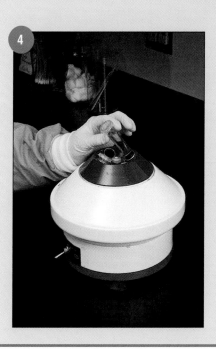

16

Continued

on the bulb is hooked over the outside edge of the tube.

Principle. Kova stain improves the detail of the sediment for better visualization of structures under the microscope.

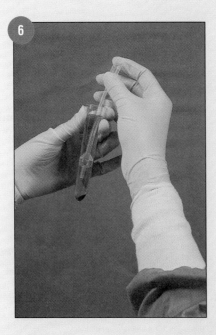

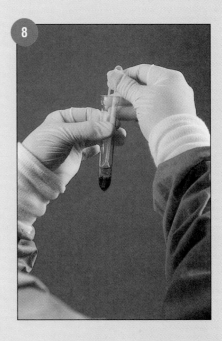

7. **Procedural Step.** Decant the specimen by inverting the tube and pouring off the supernatant fluid. Approximately 1.0 ml of sediment will be retained in the bottom of the tube.

8. **Procedural Step.** Remove the pipet from the tube. Add 1 drop of Kova stain to the tube. Place the pipet back in the tube, and mix the sediment and stain together vigorously using the pipet. Make sure the sediment and stain are well mixed. Place the urine tube in a test tube rack.

9. **Procedural Step.** Transfer a sample of the sediment to the Kova slide as follows:
   a. Place the Kova slide on a flat surface with the open "envelope" areas facing upward.
   b. Squeeze the bulb of the pipet to draw a sample of the sediment into the tip of the pipet.
   c. Place the tip of the pipet so that it just touches the notched corner edge of the slide.
   d. Gently squeeze the bulb to allow the specimen to fill the well. Do not overfill or underfill the well.
   e. Place the pipet in the urine tube.

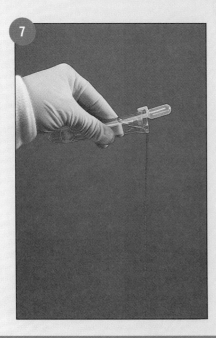

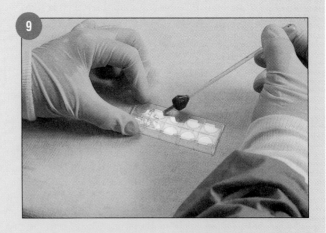

PROCEDURE 16–6

10. **Procedural Step.** Allow the specimen to sit for 1 full minute to permit the sediment to settle in the well. **Principle.** Allowing the sediment to settle prevents structures from moving when viewing the slide under the microscope.

Examining the Sediment

11. **Procedural Step.** Focus the specimen under low power as follows: (*Note:* Also refer to Chapter 20: Medical Microbiology [Procedure 20–1] for use of a microscope).
    a. Turn on the light source. Rotate the nosepiece of the microscope to the low-power objective (10×) making sure to click it into place.
    b. Place the slide on the microscope stage, and make sure it is secure.
    c. Look through the ocular. Use the coarse adjustment knob to bring the specimen into coarse focus.
    d. Use the fine adjustment knob to bring the specimen into a sharp clear focus.
    e. Decrease the light intensity using the iris diaphragm as needed to provide maximum focus and contrast.

12. **Procedural Step.** Examine the sediment under low power to scan for the presence of casts.

13. **Procedural Step.** Focus the specimen under high-power as follows:
    a. Rotate the nosepiece to the high-power objective (40×) making sure it clicks into place.
    b. Use the fine adjustment knob to bring the specimen into a precise focus. Do not use the coarse adjustment to focus the high-power objective, in order to prevent the objective from striking the slide.
    c. Adjust the light intensity using the iris diaphragm as needed to provide maximum focus and contrast.

14. **Procedural Step.** Examine the specimen under high power as follows:
    a. Identify the specific type of casts (if present).
    b. Examine the sediment for the presence of smaller structures, such as red blood cells, white blood cells, bacteria, or crystals. Ten to fifteen high-power fields should be examined and an average recorded.

15. **Procedural Step.** Turn off the light source, and remove the slide from the stage.

16. **Procedural Step.** Dispose of the slide and pipet in a biohazard waste container. Cap the urine centrifuge tube and dispose of it in a biohazard waste container.

17. **Procedural Step.** Remove the gloves and wash the hands.

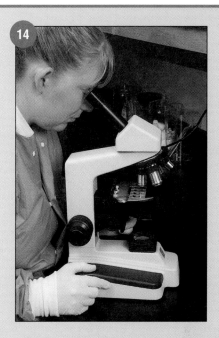

18. **Procedural Step.** Chart the results as follows:
    a. Record casts as the average number and type seen per low-power field.
    b. Record red blood cells, white blood cells, and epithelial cells as the average number viewed per high-power field.
    Record other structures such as crystals, bacteria, yeast, and spermatozoa as occasional, frequent, or many.

16

LAB REPORT

Date	Time	Name	
3/18/2002	10:00 a.m.	Tanya Howe	
	MICROSCOPIC		
	WBC'S		20 /HPF
	RBC'S		3 /HPF
	CASTS (Hyaline)		0 /LPF
	CASTS (Granular)		0 /LPF
	CASTS (Cellular)		0 /LPF
	CASTS (Waxy)		0 /LPF
	EPITHELIAL CELLS		0 /LPF
	BACTERIA		Freq
	MUCUS		Occ
	CRYSTALS		0
			L. Proffitt, CMA

RAPID URINE CULTURES

☐ A urine culture is used to assist in diagnosing a UTI and to assess the effectiveness of antibiotic therapy for a patient with a UTI.

Rapid urine culture tests are sometimes used in the medical office to culture a urine specimen; brand names include Uricult and Urichek. They provide more immediate results, compared with sending the specimen to an outside laboratory for culture. Rapid urine cultures consist of a slide attached to a screw cap. Each side of the slide is coated with an agar medium suitable for the growth of urinary bacteria. If the surface of the agar medium is dehydrated or if there is evidence of mold or bacterial growth, the culture test should not be used but discarded in an appropriate receptacle. The slide is suspended in a clean plastic vial, which protects it from contamination during inoculation, storage, or handling.

The type of voided urine specimen that provides the most accurate results is a clean-catch midstream specimen collected after the urine has been in the bladder at least 4 to 6 hours.

The procedure for performing a rapid urine culture test is presented on the following pages.

PROCEDURE

16–7

Performing a Rapid Urine Culture Test

EQUIPMENT/SUPPLIES: Disposable gloves
Rapid urine culture kit
Urine specimen (clean-catch midstream specimen)

Incubator
Biohazard waste container

16

Preparing the Specimen

1. **Procedural Step.** Wash the hands, and assemble the equipment. Check the expiration date on the rapid culture test. It should not be used if the expiration date has passed. Label the vial with the patient's name and the date and time of inoculation.

   Principle. An expired urine culture test may produce inaccurate test results.

2. **Procedural Step.** Apply gloves. Remove the slide from its protective vial by unscrewing the cap of the vial, being careful not to touch the culture media.

3. **Procedural Step.** Dip the agar-coated slide into the urine specimen; it must be completely immersed. If the urine volume is not sufficient to fully immerse the agar slide, the urine may be poured over the agar surfaces.

4. **Procedural Step.** Allow excess urine to drain from the slide.

5. **Procedural Step.** Immediately replace the inoculated slide in its protective vial. Screw the cap on loosely.

6. **Procedural Step.** Place the vial upright in an incubator for 18 to 24 hours at 93° to 100°F (35° to 38°C).

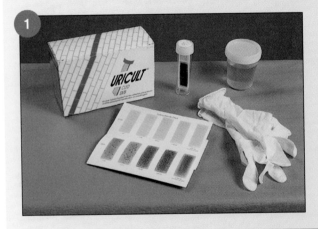

Continued

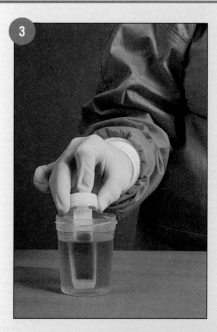

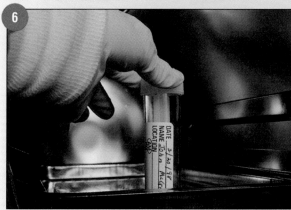

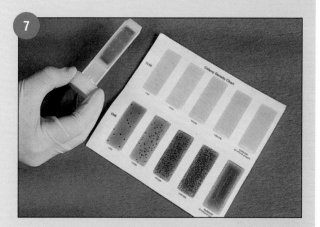

Principle. Incubation for more than 24 hours may cause erroneous test results.

Reading Test Results:

7. **Procedural Step.** Apply gloves. Remove the vial from the incubator following the incubation period. Remove the slide from its protective vial and compare the bacterial colony count density on the agar surface with the colony density reference chart provided by the manufacturer. The bacterial colony density on the agar surface should be matched with the printed example it most closely resembles on the colony density chart. (No actual bacterial colony counting is necessary.)

8. **Procedural Step.** Interpret results. The results of rapid urine tests are interpreted as follows:

Normal: Less than 10,000 bacteria/ml of urine. *Significance:* A normal result indicates the absence of infection

Borderline: 10,000 to 100,000 bacteria/ml of urine. *Significance:* A borderline result may be caused by chronic and relapsing infections, and it is recommended that the test be repeated.

Positive:

a. More than 100,000 bacteria/ml of urine.

b. Confluent growth, or complete coverage of the agar surface with bacterial colonies, which may occasionally occur when a colony count is more than 100,000 bacteria/ml. *Significance:* A positive result indicates that a bacterial infection is present.

9. **Procedural Step.** Return the slide to the vial and screw on the cap. (*Note:* To aid in the safe disposal of inoculated slides, it is recommended that the slide be immersed in a disinfectant solution, such as 3 percent phenol solution or Cidex, before placing the slide in the vial.)

10. **Procedural Step.** Dispose of the rapid culture test in a biohazard waste container. Remove the gloves, and wash the hands.

11. **Procedural Step.** Chart the results. Include the date and time, the name of the test (e.g., Uricult, Urichek), and the results.

16

CHARTING EXAMPLE

Date	
3/21/2002	10:00 a.m. Uricult: Normal. —— L. Proffitt, CMA

URINE PREGNANCY TESTING

☐ Determining whether or not a woman is pregnant can be accomplished in a number of ways. By the eighth week after fertilization, pregnancy can be confirmed through the medical history and physical examination. However, the physician may desire an earlier diagnosis through the use of a pregnancy test to initiate early prenatal care. A pregnancy test may also be required before certain medications are ordered or procedures are performed that may cause injury to a fetus.

In the medical office, immunologic tests are often used for pregnancy testing. These tests are performed on a concentrated urine specimen and rely upon the presence of a hormone known as human chorionic gonadotropin (HCG) for a positive reaction.

HCG

Human chorionic gonadotropin (HCG) is produced by the developing fertilized egg, and small amounts of it are secreted into the urine and blood. Immediately after conception and implantation of the fertilized egg, the plasma level of HCG rises rapidly and can be used to detect pregnancy approximately 1 to 5 days after the first missed menstrual period. The highest plasma levels of HCG occur at about the eighth week after conception. After this time, the production of HCG declines and remains at a lower level for the duration of the pregnancy. Within 72 hours of delivery, HCG disappears entirely from the plasma. As a result, pregnancy tests are more sensitive during the first trimester and may even show a negative reaction once the level of HCG begins to decline during the second and third trimester.

TESTING METHODS

The two main types of urine pregnancy tests are immunoassay enzyme tests and agglutination tests. These tests are used in the medical office because they are convenient to perform and provide immediate test results. Positive and negative reactions are evidenced by a specific visible reaction that is observed and interpreted by the individual performing the test.

Urine pregnancy tests are commercially available in kits that contain all the required reagents and supplies to perform the test. Each kit can be used to perform a specific number of tests, ranging between 10 and 100. The manufacturer's instructions may be carefully followed to prevent inaccurate test results. When used properly, urine pregnancy tests are 95 percent accurate.

Agglutination Tests

The **slide agglutination test** is sometimes used to perform pregnancy testing in the medical office. Positive test results are based on the inhibition of latex particle agglutination. The test takes place in two steps and can be performed in only 2 minutes. In the first step, a drop of the urine specimen is placed on a specially provided glass slide that comes with the kit. An HCG antiserum reagent (antibody) is then added to the urine specimen. If the patient's urine contains HCG, the antiserum combines with the HCG (antigen) in the urine specimen, resulting in an antigen-antibody reaction.

The next step involves the addition of an antigen reagent containing latex particles coated with HCG. If the antigen-antibody reaction has previously occurred in the first step of the procedure, no available HCG antiserum is left in the specimen to react with the latex particles. Therefore, the absence of agglutination on the slide test, known as agglutination inhibition, indicates a positive reaction for pregnancy. On the other hand, if agglutination occurs on the slide, the results are interpreted as negative (Fig. 16–9). Coating the HCG with latex permits visible agglutination that can be observed and interpreted as a negative reaction by the individual performing the test. Without the latex, agglutination would not be visible when the HCG antigen and antibody combine.

Immunoassay Tests

Immunoassay tests provide for the rapid, qualitative detection of HCG in a urine specimen; brand names include QuickVue, Clearview, Contrast, and AccuStat. Some brands of tests are able to detect pregnancy as early as 1 week after implantation, or 4 to 5 days before a first missed menstrual period. It is recommended however, that tests performed this early be repeated later to confirm the results.

Immunoassay tests take approximately 5 minutes to perform and are easier to read than agglutination tests, because the results are easily observed as a color change. Specific instructions for performing the test are included with each commercially available testing kit. The procedure for performing an immunoassay test using QuickVue (Quidel) is outlined in Procedure 16–8.

Slide agglutination method

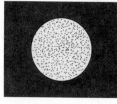

Negative   Positive

■ **FIGURE 16–9.** Urine pregnancy test results: slide agglutination method.

GUIDELINES FOR URINE PREGNANCY TESTING

Specific guidelines must be followed in performing a urine pregnancy test to ensure accurate test results. These guidelines are outlined here.

1. Use clean, preferably disposable, urine containers to collect the specimen. Traces of detergent in the specimen container may cause inaccurate test results.
2. Use a first-voided morning specimen, because it contains the highest concentration of HCG. If the urine specimen cannot be tested immediately after voiding, it should be preserved in the refrigerator. The patient who collects the specimen at home should be given instructions on preserving the specimen.
3. The specific gravity of the urine specimen should be determined before the test is performed. A specific gravity of less than 1.010 is considered too dilute for pregnancy testing, as it may lead to a false-negative test result.
4. The urine specimen should be at room temperature before the procedure is performed.
5. The urine pregnancy testing kit should be stored according to the manufacturer's instructions. Most testing kits can be stored either at room temperature or in the refrigerator. If a kit is stored in the refrigerator however, the reagents must be brought to room temperature before use to ensure accurate test results.
6. Testing kits past their expiration dates should not be used.

PROCEDURE

16–8

Performing a Urine Pregnancy Test

EQUIPMENT/SUPPLIES:
Disposable gloves
Urine pregnancy testing kit
(QuickVue by Quidel)

Urine specimen (first-voided morning specimen)
Biohazard waste container

16

1. **Procedural Step.** Wash the hands, and assemble the equipment. Check the expiration date on the urine pregnancy test. It should not be used if the expiration date has passed.
   Principle. An expired pregnancy test may produce inaccurate test results.

2. **Procedural Step.** Apply gloves. Remove the test cassette from its foil pouch, and place it on a clean, dry, level surface.
3. **Procedural Step.** Add 3 drops of urine to the round sample well on the test cassette using a disposable pipet supplied with the kit. The test cassette should not be handled again until the test is ready for interpretation. Dispose of the pipet in a biohazard waste container.
4. **Procedural Step.** Wait 3 minutes, and read the results by observing the result window.
5. **Procedural Step.** Interpret the test results as follows:
   Negative: The appearance of the blue procedural control line next to the letter "C" only and no pink-to-purple test line next the letter "T."
   Positive: The appearance of any pink-to-purple line next to the letter "T" along with a blue procedural control line next to the letter "C."
   No Result: If no blue procedural control line appears, the test result is invalid and the specimen must be retested.

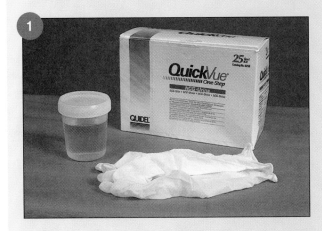

Continued

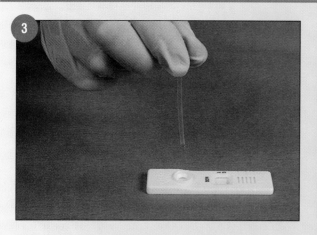

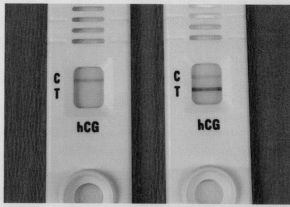

Negative   Positive

6. **Procedural Step.** Dispose of the test cassette in a biohazard waste container. Remove the gloves and wash the hands.
7. **Procedural Step.** Chart the results. Include the date and time of the patient's last menstrual period (LMP), the name of the test, and the results recorded as either positive or negative.

CHARTING EXAMPLE

Date	
3/25/2002	10:30 a.m. LMP: 2/20/2002.
	QuickVue preg test: Positive. ————
	———————————— L. Proffitt, CMA

(From Brunzel, N. A.: *Fundamentals of Urine and Body Fluid Analysis.* Philadelphia, W. B. Saunders; Lehmann, C. A.: *Saunders Manual of Clinical Laboratory Science.* Philadelphia, W. B. Saunders.)

SERUM PREGNANCY TEST

☐ The radioimmunoassay (RIA) for HCG is used to detect HCG in the serum of the blood. This test is more sensitive than a urine test and can detect pregnancy at approximately the eighth day after fertilization; therefore, the pregnancy can be detected even before the time of the missed menstrual period. This test uses a radioisotope technique and is capable of detecting minute amounts of HCG in the blood. This test is generally used to diagnose abnormalities such as ectopic pregnancy, to follow the course of early pregnancy when abnormalities of embryonic development are suspected, and to provide an early diagnosis of pregnancy in high-risk individuals such as diabetic patients.

MEDICAL PRACTICE AND THE LAW

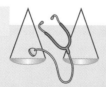

When collecting and analyzing patient urine, meticulous attention should be paid to patient instructions as to cleansing and to collecting first morning, midstream, or 24-hour specimens.

Patients are often embarrassed to have someone else see their urine, so handle urine specimens in a professional, matter-of-fact manner, using universal precautions to protect yourself.

As with all diagnostic procedures, care must be taken to perform the test correctly and treat results confidentially.

Civil Versus Criminal Law

Civil law involves a conflict with another person, and if found guilty by a preponderance of evidence (>50%), the loser may lose money or property. Malpractice is a type of civil law. Civil law is divided into **torts,** or wrongs, and **contracts,** or promises. Malpractice is a tort, and nonpayment for services is a contract.

Criminal law involves a conflict with society as a whole (local, state, or federal law). If found guilty beyond a reasonable doubt, the loser may lose money, property, freedom (jail), or life (execution). Violation of licensure laws and failure to report child abuse are criminal suits.

16

- The function of the urinary system is to regulate the fluid and electrolyte balance of the body and to remove waste products. The structures making up the urinary system are the kidneys, the ureters, the urinary bladder, and the urethra.

- The nephron is considered the functional unit of the kidney. Each kidney is composed of approximately 1 million nephrons. The nephron filters waste substances from the blood and dilutes them with water to produce urine. Another function of the nephron is reabsorption.

- Urine is composed of 95 percent water and 5 percent organic and inorganic waste products. The normal adult excretes approximately 750 to 2000 ml of urine per day.

- An excessive increase in urine output is known as polyuria and may be caused by the excessive intake of fluids, certain drugs, diabetes mellitus, and renal disease. A decreased output of urine is known as oliguria and may be caused by decreased fluid intake, dehydration, profuse perspiration, vomiting, diarrhea, or kidney disease.

- The type of test to be performed often dictates the method used to collect the urine specimen. A first-voided morning specimen contains the greatest concentration of dissolved substances and is recommended for the microscopic examination of urine. A clean-catch midstream specimen is recommended for the detection of a urinary tract infection. A 24-hour specimen is used to quantitatively measure specific substances in the urine.

- A complete urinalysis consists of a physical, chemical, and microscopic examination of urine. A deviation from normal in any of the three areas assists the physician in the diagnosis and treatment of pathologic conditions. A urine specimen should not be left standing out for more than 1 hour because changes take place that affect the test results.

- A physical examination of urine involves a determination of the color, appearance, and specific gravity of the urine. Dilute urine tends to be a lighter yellow in color, whereas concentrated urine is a darker yellow. Fresh urine is usually clear and transparent.

- The specific gravity of urine ranges from 1.003 to 1.030 but is usually between 1.010 and 1.025. Dilute urine contains fewer dissolved substances and has a lower specific gravity; concentrated urine has a higher specific gravity due to the increased amount of dissolved substances.

- The chemical testing of urine is a means of detecting abnormal amounts of chemicals in the body, which may indicate a pathologic condition. Chemical tests include pH, glucose, protein, ketones, blood, bilirubin, urobilinogen, nitrite, and leukocytes.

- A microscopic examination of the urine sediment helps clarify results of the physical and chemical examination. Structures that may be found in microscopic examination of urine include red and white blood cells, epithelial cells, casts, crystals, and miscellaneous structures such as mucous threads, bacteria, yeast cells, parasites, and spermatozoa.

- A urine culture is used to assist in diagnosing a urinary tract infection and to assess the effectiveness of antibiotic therapy for a patient with a UTI.

- HCG is produced by the developing fertilized egg, and small amounts of it are secreted into the urine and blood. Urine pregnancy tests are used to detect the presence of HCG and can be used to detect pregnancy approximately 1 to 5 days after the first missed menstrual period.

16

RESOURCES

ON THE WEB

For information on kidney disease:

National Kidney Foundation
www.kidney.org

National Institute of Diabetes and Digestive and Kidney Diseases
www.niddk.nih.gov

Renal Net

ns.gamewood.net/renal-net.html

For information on drug abuse:

National Institute on Drug Abuse
www.nida.nih.gov

American Council for Drug Education
www.acde.org

Research Institute on Addictions
www.ria.org

The U.S. Information Agency Gateway to Information on Substance Abuse
www.usia.gov/topical/global/drugs/subab.html

Phlebotomy

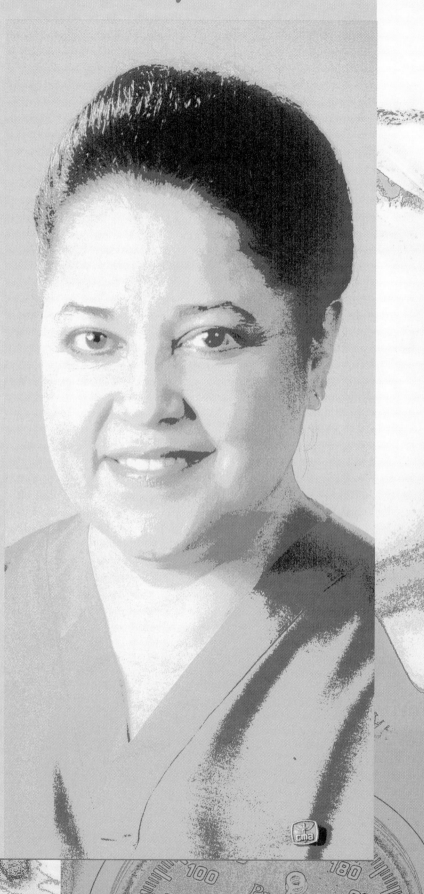

Dori Glover, *and I am a Certified Medical Assistant. I attended an accredited medical assisting program and received an associate's degree in Applied Science. After successfully passing the CMA examination, I received a certificate and my coveted pin!*

I work in a very busy, fast-paced family practice office for two wonderful physicians. My three co-workers are very well trained, efficient CMAs who also went through the same medical assisting program that I did. The atmosphere is professional but informal, with everyone able to do all jobs in the front and back office.

I take vital signs on all patients, assist with minor surgeries and Pap tests, run electrocardiograms, and perform allergy testing on site. In our laboratory, we perform urinalysis, prepare slides and culture plates, and do finger punctures for blood glucose levels and hematocrits. We administer a lot of injections ranging from immunizations for children to flu shots for the elderly, as well as allergy injections. In the front office, I schedule appointments and tests, take payments, make referrals, send faxes, call in prescriptions, and answer the ever-ringing phone! And of course there is always filing to be done.

I love my job. The physicians are great, with very different styles, the pace is fast, and the time flies by. I am constantly challenged, learning new things, meeting and helping people, and being a part of a team that works well together.

OUTCOMES

After completing this chapter, you should be able to demonstrate the proper procedures to perform the following:

1. Collect a venous blood specimen using the vacuum tube venipuncture method.
2. Collect a venous blood specimen using the butterfly venipuncture method.
3. Collect a venous blood specimen using the syringe venipuncture method.
4. Separate serum from a whole blood specimen.
5. Obtain a capillary blood specimen using a disposable lancet.
6. Obtain a capillary blood specimen using a disposable semi-automatic lancet.
7. Obtain a capillary blood specimen using a reusable semi-automatic lancet.

EDUCATIONAL OBJECTIVES

After completing this chapter, you should be able to do the following:

1. Define the terms listed in the Key Terminology.
2. List and describe the patient preparation required for venipuncture.
3. Explain how each of the following blood specimens is obtained: clotted blood, serum, whole blood, and plasma.
4. List the layers the blood separates into when an anticoagulant is added to the specimen.
5. List the layers the blood separates into when an anticoagulant is *not* added to the specimen.
6. List the OSHA safety precautions that must be followed during venipuncture and separating serum or plasma from whole blood.
7. State the additive content of the following vacuum tubes and list the type of blood specimens that can be obtained from each: red, lavender, gray, light blue, green, dark blue.
8. Identify and explain the order of draw for the vacuum tube method and butterfly method of venipuncture.
9. List and describe the guidelines to follow when using evacuated tubes.
10. Identify problems that may be encountered when performing a venipuncture.
11. List four ways to prevent a blood specimen from becoming hemolyzed.
12. Explain how the serum separator tube functions in the collection of a serum specimen.
13. Explain when a skin puncture would be preferred over a venipuncture.
14. Describe the following skin puncture devices: disposable lancet, disposable semi-automatic lancet, reusable semi-automatic lancet.
15. List and describe the guidelines to follow when performing a finger puncture.
16. Explain the principle underlying each step in the venipuncture procedures, the procedure for separating serum from whole blood, and the skin puncture procedures.

KEY TERMINOLOGY

antecubital space (AN-Ta-KŬB-it-al SPÂs): The surface of the arm in front of the elbow.

anticoagulant (an-tī-KÔ-ag-û-lant): A substance that inhibits blood clotting.

buffy coat: A thin, light-colored layer of white blood cells and platelets that lies between a top layer of plasma and a bottom layer of red blood cells when an anticoagulant has been added to a blood specimen.

evacuated tube: A closed glass or plastic tube containing a premeasured vacuum.

hematoma (HÊM-a-TOME-a): A swelling or mass of coagulated blood caused by a break in a blood vessel.

hemoconcentration (HÊM-o-kon-sen-trâ-shun): An increase in the concentration of the nonfilterable blood components such as red blood cells, enzymes, iron, and calcium as a result of a decrease in the fluid content of the blood.

hemolysis (he-maul-is-sis): The breakdown of blood cells.

osteochondritis (os-tê-ô-kun-drî-tis): Inflammation of bone and cartilage.

osteomyelitis (os-tê-Ô-Mî-lî-tis): Inflammation of the bone due to bacterial infection.

phlebotomist (FLA-bot-ta-mist): A health professional trained in the collection of blood specimens.

phlebotomy (FLA-bot-ta-mê): Incision of a vein for the removal or withdrawal of blood; the collection of blood.

plasma (PLAZ-ma): The liquid part of the blood consisting of a clear straw-colored fluid that makes up approximately 55 percent of the total blood volume.

serum (SERE-um): Plasma from which the clotting factor fibrinogen has been removed.

venipuncture (VÊ-na-punk-shur): Puncturing of a vein.

venous reflux (VÊ-nus RÊ-flux): The blackflow of blood (from an evacuated tube) into the patient's vein.

venous stasis (VÊ-nus STÂ-sis): The temporary cessation or slowing of the venous blood flow.

INTRODUCTION

☐ The purpose of phlebotomy is to collect a blood specimen for laboratory analysis. The word phlebotomy is derived from the Greek words for vein (*phlebos*) and incision (*tome*), and literally means making an incision into a vein. However, as used in the clinical laboratory sciences, **phlebotomy** is defined generally as the collection of blood. The individual collecting the blood sample is known as a **phlebotomist.**

Some blood specimens may be tested in the medical office, whereas others will be picked up and taken to a laboratory for testing. The latter specimens need to be accompanied by a laboratory request so that the laboratory personnel know what type of test the physician desires. The medical assistant may be responsible for filling out the laboratory request form. Included should be the physician's name and address; the patient's name, address, age, and sex; the date and time of collection of the specimen; the physician's clinical diagnosis; and a check mark next to the types of test to be performed.

Phlebotomy encompasses three major areas of blood collection: arterial puncture, venipuncture, and skin puncture. An arterial puncture is typically performed in a hospital setting to assess the oxygen levels, carbon dioxide levels, and acid-base balance of arterial blood; hence medical assistants do not perform arterial punctures. In the medical office, medical assistants perform venipunctures and skin punctures; therefore, this chapter focuses on these two areas of blood collection.

Venipuncture

The term **venipuncture** means the puncturing of a vein for the removal of a venous blood sample. In the medical office, a venipuncture is performed when a large blood specimen is needed for testing. Because it is not legal in every state for medical assistants to perform venipuncture, each assistant is responsible for checking the laws in his or her state before performing this procedure.

Venipuncture can be performed by the following three methods:

- Vacuum tube method
- Butterfly method
- Syringe method

The vacuum tube method is the fastest and most convenient of the three methods and is used most often. This method relies on the use of an **evacuated tube,** which is a closed glass or plastic tube containing a vacuum. The butterfly and syringe methods are used for difficult draws such as when a vein is small or sclerosed. The theory and procedure for each of these methods is presented in detail in this chapter.

GENERAL GUIDELINES FOR VENIPUNCTURE

☐ General guidelines that are common to all three methods of venipuncture include: preparing the patient for the venipuncture, positioning the patient, applying the tourniquet, selecting a site to perform the venipuncture, obtaining the type of blood specimen required, and following the OSHA safety precautions. These areas are discussed in the following sections.

PATIENT PREPARATION FOR VENIPUNCTURE

Depending on what the blood specimen is to be tested for, the patient should be given appropriate instructions on any advance preparation that may be required. Although most tests require no preparation at all, some tests require special preparation such as fasting or the avoidance of certain medications. If the medical assistant is unsure whether or not a laboratory test requires preparation, he or she should consult with an appropriate reference source. Reference sources consist of laboratory directories, instructions included with testing kits, or the laboratory testing the blood specimen.

When a laboratory test requires advance preparation, be sure to verify that the patient prepared properly before performing the venipuncture. If the patient has not prepared properly, the medical assistant should not collect the specimen unless directed otherwise by the physician. If the venipuncture is to be rescheduled, the medical assistant should carefully review the preparation requirements with the patient.

Venipuncture is often a frightening experience for the patient. For many patients the anticipation of the procedure is worse than the actual draw. The medical assistant should take time to explain the procedure to the patient in an unhurried and confident manner. This should help allay the patient's fears, which should help to relax the patient's veins. Relaxed veins make venipuncture easier to perform and result in less pain for the patient.

Instruct the patient to remain still and not move during the procedure. Explain to the patient that a small amount of pain is associated with a venipuncture but it will be of short duration. Never tell the patient that the venipuncture will *not* hurt. Just before insert-

ing the needle, tell the patient that he or she will "feel a small stick." This helps to avoid startling the patient, which could cause the patient to move. Movement causes pain for the patient and it may also damage the venipuncture site.

PATIENT POSITION FOR VENIPUNCTURE

The patient position for venipuncture is especially important to the successful collection of a blood specimen. Proper positioning allows easy access to the veins and is more comfortable for the patient. The patient position depends upon the vein to be used. The most common site for venipuncture is the antecubital space, and the information presented below refers to this site.

The patient should be seated comfortably in a chair. The arm should be extended in a downward position to form a straight line from the shoulder to the wrist with the palm facing up; the arm should not bend at the elbow. The arm should be well supported on the armrest by a rolled towel or by having the patient place the fist of the other hand under the elbow (Fig. 17–1).

A venipuncture should never be performed with the patient sitting on a stool or in a standing position. The possibility exists that the patient will faint and injure himself or herself. If the patient appears nervous or has fainted in the past from a venipuncture, it is best to place the patient in a semi-reclining position on the examining table. A pillow or a cushion should be placed under the patient's arm to support the arm in a straight line from the shoulder to the wrist.

Though unusual, it is possible for blood to flow from the evacuated tube back into the patient's vein during the procedure. This condition is known as

17

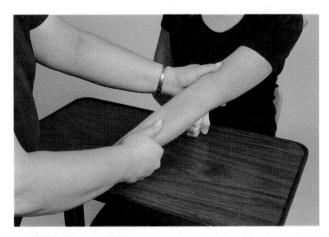

■ **FIGURE 17–1.** Patient position for obtaining blood specimen from the antecubital veins.

venous reflux. Venous reflux could cause the patient to have an adverse reaction to a tube additive, particularly if the additive in the tube is EDTA (ethylenediamine tetra-acetic acid). Venous reflux can only occur if the contents of the evacuated tube are in contact with the tube stopper while the specimen is being drawn. Venous reflux is prevented by keeping the patient's arm in a downward position (as described previously) so that the evacuated tube remains below the venipuncture site and fills from the bottom up.

APPLICATION OF THE TOURNIQUET

An important step in the venipuncture procedure is the application of the tourniquet. The purpose of the tourniquet is to make the patient's veins stand out so they are easier to palpate. The tourniquet acts as a "dam," which causes the venous blood to slow down and pool in the veins in front of the tourniquet. This pooling of blood causes the veins to become more prominent so that they are more visible and can be palpated.

When applying a tourniquet, it is very important to obtain the correct tourniquet tension. The tourniquet should be applied with enough tension to slow the venous flow without affecting the arterial flow. A tourniquet that is applied too tightly obstructs the arterial blood flow and the venous flow, which may result in a specimen that produces inaccurate test results. On the other hand, a tourniquet that is too loose fails to cause the veins to stand out enough to be palpated. A correctly applied tourniquet should fit snugly and not pinch the patient's skin.

Guidelines for Applying the Tourniquet

The following guidelines help to ensure the successful application of the tourniquet:

1. The tourniquet should not be applied over sores or burned skin.
2. The tourniquet should be placed 3 to 4 inches above the bend in the elbow. This allows adequate room for cleansing the site and performing the venipuncture without the tourniquet's getting in the way.
3. A tourniquet should be applied so that it is snug, but not so tight that it pinches the patient's skin or is otherwise painful to the patient.
4. When applying the tourniquet, ask the patient to clench his or her fist. This pushes blood from the lower arm into the veins and makes them easier to palpate. The patient can be asked to clench and unclench the fist a few times; however, vigorous pumping should be avoided as this could lead to

hemoconcentration, which may produce inaccurate test results.

5. The tourniquet should never be left on for more than 1 minute because it will be uncomfortable for the patient. In addition, prolonged application of the tourniquet causes the venous blood to stagnate, or stay in one place too long, a condition known as **venous stasis.** When venous stasis occurs, the plasma portion of the blood filters into the tissues, causing **hemoconcentration** or an increase in the concentration of nonfilterable blood components such as red blood cells, enzymes, iron, and calcium, which can alter test results.
6. Ideally the tourniquet should be removed as soon as a good blood flow is established; however, this may not be practical when first learning the venipuncture procedure. Removing the tourniquet may cause the needle to move so no more blood can be obtained and the blood has to be redrawn. Therefore, when first learning the venipuncture procedure, it is better to wait until just before the needle is removed before removing the tourniquet.
7. The tourniquet should always be removed before removing the needle from the patient's arm. If the needle is removed first, the pressure of the tourniquet causes blood to be forced out of the puncture site and into the surrounding skin, resulting in a hematoma.
8. After use, a tourniquet should be wiped thoroughly with a disinfectant such as alcohol. Disposable tourniquets are available that are thrown away after one use.

Types of Tourniquets

The most commonly used tourniquets are the **rubber tourniquet** and the **Velcro-closure tourniquet.** Rubber Penrose tubing is sometimes used; however, it has a tendency to cut into the patient's arm, causing patient discomfort. The type of tourniquet used is a matter of individual preference.

RUBBER TOURNIQUET. The rubber tourniquet consists of a flat, soft band of rubber approximately 1 inch (2.5 cm) wide and 15 to 18 inches (38 to 45 cm) long. It offers the advantage of being easily removable with one hand. The technique for applying a rubber tourniquet is described next and illustrated in Figure 17–2.

Procedure: Rubber Tourniquet

1. Hold each end of the tourniquet with one hand. Position the tourniquet 3 to 4 inches (7.5 to 10 cm)

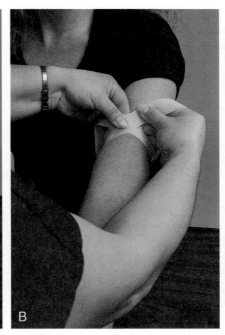

■ **FIGURE 17–2.** Application of a rubber tourniquet.

above the bend in the elbow, making sure that the tourniquet lies flat against the patient's skin. Pull the ends away from each other to create tension (Fig. 17–2*A*).

2. Bring the ends of the tourniquet toward each other and cross one over the other at the point of your grasp with enough tension so that the tourniquet is snug but not pinching the patient's skin (Fig. 17–2*B*).

3. Tuck a portion of the top length into the bottom length, forming a loop. This allows for a one-handed release of the tourniquet when pulled on one end. Make sure the flaps are directed upward so that they do not dangle into the working area (Fig. 17–2*C*).

VELCRO-CLOSURE TOURNIQUET. The Velcro-closure tourniquet consists of a band of rubber or elastic material with Velcro attached at the ends. This type of tourniquet is easier to apply and tends to be more comfortable for the patient. The disadvantage to the Velcro-closure tourniquet is that it is more difficult to remove with one hand than the rubber tourniquet. In addition, this type of tourniquet may not fit around the arms of extremely obese patients. The technique for applying a Velcro-closure tourniquet is described next and illustrated in Figure 17–3.

Procedure: Velcro-Closure Tourniquet

1. Hold each end of the tourniquet with one hand. Position the tourniquet 3 to 4 inches (7.5 to 10 cm) above the bend in the elbow.

17

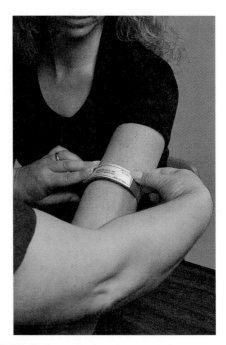

■ **FIGURE 17–3.** Application of a Velcro-closure tourniquet.

2. Wrap the tourniquet around the arm and secure it with the Velcro fastener. The tourniquet should be applied with enough tension so that it is snug but not pinching the patient's skin.

SITE SELECTION FOR VENIPUNCTURE

For most patients, the best site to use is the veins of the arm located in the antecubital space. (Fig. 17–4). If the patient has large, accessible antecubital veins, drawing blood is easy. On the other hand, if the patient has small veins or veins that cannot be palpated, obtaining a blood specimen can be quite a challenge, even for the most experienced medical assistant.

The **antecubital space** refers to the surface of the arm in front of the elbow. The antecubital veins generally have a wide lumen, are easily accessible, and are close to the surface of the skin. In addition, these veins typically have thick walls, making them less likely to collapse. Using the antecubital space spares the patient unnecessary pain because the skin is less sensitive there than in other sites (such as the back of the hand). The medical assistant should not be misled by the presence, in some patients, of many small very blue "spidery" veins that lie very close to the surface of the skin.

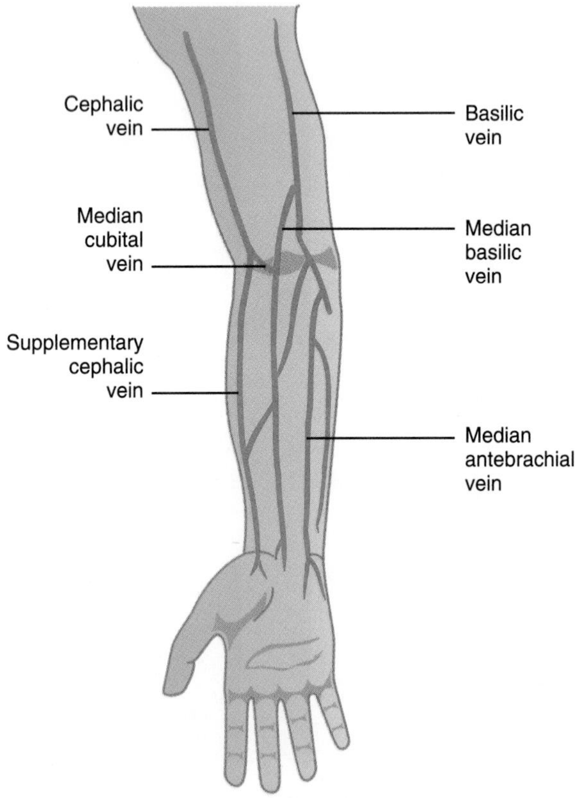

■ **FIGURE 17–4.** Antecubital veins.

These veins are not suitable for performing a venipuncture. The antecubital veins lie beneath these veins.

The best vein to use in the antecubital space is the **median cubital.** The median cubital is a prominent vein located in the middle of the antecubital space (see Fig. 17–4). At times, however, the median cubital vein cannot be used; for example, when it lies deep in the tissues and cannot be palpated or is scarred from repeated venipunctures.

The **basilic** and **cephalic** veins are located on either side of the antecubital space and are considered a second alternative when the median cubital vein is not available. The disadvantage of these "side" veins is that they tend to roll or move away from the needle, thereby escaping puncture. To prevent rolling, firm pressure should be applied below the vein to stabilize it as the needle is inserted.

The brachial artery is also located in the antecubital space. Before performing a venipuncture, palpate for the presence of this artery. Unlike a vein, an artery pulsates, is more elastic, and has a thicker wall than a vein. If the brachial artery is inadvertently punctured, the patient feels more than the usual amount of pain and the blood is bright red and comes out in pulsing movements. If this situation occurs, the tourniquet should be removed and then the needle. Pressure with a gauze pad should then be applied for 4 to 5 minutes.

Guidelines for Site Selection

There are specific guidelines that should be followed to facilitate the selection of a good vein. These guidelines are as follows:

1. Ensure that the lighting is adequate. Good lighting facilitates inspection of the veins.
2. Examine the antecubital veins of both arms. The best site to perform a venipuncture varies with each individual. Some patients have larger veins in one arm compared to the other. It is advisable to ask the patient if he or she has had a venipuncture before. Most adult patients have had previous venipunctures and know which of their veins are best to use and which should be avoided. Listen to and evaluate information offered by the patient.
3. Ensure that the veins "stand out" as much as possible. Before locating a venipuncture site, always apply the tourniquet and have the patient make a fist. This combination makes the veins more prominent.
4. Always feel for the median cubital vein first. It is usually bigger and anchored better and bruises less than the other veins. If the median cubital is good in both arms, select the one that appears the fullest. The cephalic vein is the second choice (over

the basilic vein) because it does not roll and bruise as easily as the basilic vein.

5. Inspection and *particularly* palpation should be used in the selection of a vein. A vein does not have to be seen in order to be a good selection. If you cannot see a vein, palpation alone can be used to locate it. A vein feels like an elastic tube that "gives" under the pressure of the fingertips.

6. Thoroughly assess the patient's veins. To assess a vein as a possible site for the venipuncture, place one or two fingertips (index and ring fingers) over it and press lightly then release pressure. Do not use your thumb to palpate the vein because it is not as sensitive as the index finger. To be considered a suitable site for a venipuncture, the vein should feel round, firm, elastic, and engorged. When you depress and release an engorged vein, it should spring back in a rounded, filled state.

7. Determine the size, depth, and direction of the vein. Once a suitable vein has been located, it should be thoroughly and carefully palpated to determine the direction of the vein and to estimate the size and depth of the vein. Palpate and trace the path of the vein several times by rolling your index finger back and forth over the vein to determine its size. Inspect and palpate the vein for problems. Some veins that appear suitable at first sight, feel small, hard, bumpy, or flat when palpated.

8. Map the location of the vein. After locating an acceptable vein, mentally "map" the location of the puncture site on the patient's arm. This technique is particularly helpful if the vein cannot be seen, but only palpated. For example, the puncture site may be located next to a freckle on the patient's arm, a small wrinkle, a pigmented area, and so on.

9. Do not leave the tourniquet on for more than 1 minute. When first learning the venipuncture procedure, you may need to perform a number of assessments of the patient's arms to locate the best vein. After each assessment, the tourniquet should be removed to prevent patient discomfort and hemoconcentration.

10. If a good vein cannot be found, the following techniques can be employed to make the veins more prominent:
    - Remove the tourniquet and have the patient dangle the arm over the side of the chair for 1 to 2 minutes.
    - Tap at the vein site sharply a few times with your index finger and second finger.
    - Gently massage the arm from the wrist to the elbow.
    - Apply a warm, moist washcloth to the area for 5 minutes.

ALTERNATIVE VENIPUNCTURE SITES

If it is not possible to locate a suitable vein in the antecubital space, alternative sites are available. These include the inner forearm, the wrist area above the thumb, and the back of the hand (Fig. 17–5). These alternative veins are smaller and have thinner walls than the antecubital veins and should only be used as a site when all other possibilities for obtaining the blood specimen have been considered. For example, if the medical assistant is able to palpate a small vein in the antecubital space, it may be possible to obtain blood there using the butterfly method of venipuncture.

The hand veins, in particular, should only be used as a last resort. The veins of the hand have a tendency to roll, because they are not supported by much tissue and are close to the surface of the skin. This makes them more difficult to stick. In addition, there is an abundant supply of nerves in the hands, which makes this procedure more uncomfortable for the patient. Hand veins tend to have thin walls, which makes them more susceptible to collapsing as well as bruising and phlebitis. However, in some patients, especially the obese and the elderly, the hand veins may be the only accessible site.

TYPES OF BLOOD SPECIMEN

The type of blood specimen required depends on the type of test to be performed. For example, serum is required for most blood chemistry studies, whereas whole blood is required for a complete blood count.

The various types of blood specimen that the medical assistant will be required to obtain through the venipuncture procedure are:

1. **Clotted blood.** Clotted blood is obtained from a tube to which an anticoagulant has not been added.
2. **Serum.** Serum is obtained from clotted blood by allowing the specimen to stand and then centrifuging it. This causes the specimen to separate into a top layer of serum and a bottom layer of clotted blood cells (Fig. 17–6A).
3. **Whole blood.** Whole blood is obtained by using a tube containing an anticoagulant to prevent clotting. It is important to mix the anticoagulant with the blood by gently inverting the tube eight to ten times.
4. **Plasma.** Plasma is obtained from whole blood that has been centrifuged. This causes the specimen to separate into a top layer of plasma, a middle layer (termed the buffy coat) that contains white blood

17

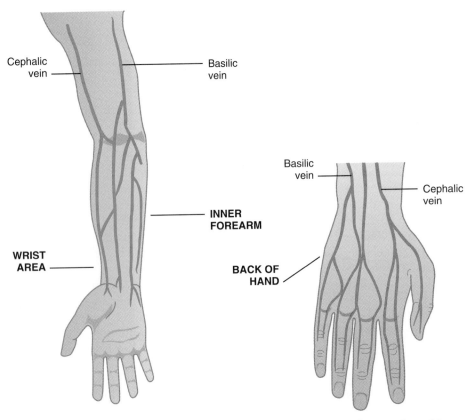

■ **FIGURE 17–5.** Alternative venipuncture sites. These include the inner forearm, the wrist area above the thumb, and the back of the hand.

17

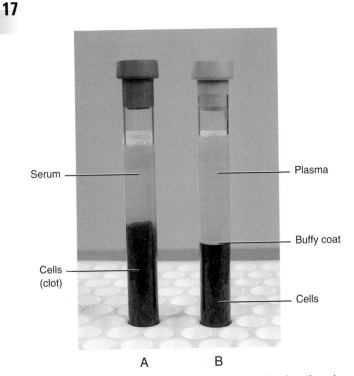

■ **FIGURE 17–6.** Layers the blood separates into A, when there is no anticoagulant and, B, when an anticoagulant is present.

cells and platelets, and a bottom layer of red blood cells (Fig. 17–6B).

OSHA SAFETY PRECAUTIONS

The OSHA Bloodborne Pathogens Standard presented in Chapter 1 must be carefully followed during a venipuncture procedure to avoid exposure to bloodborne pathogens. The following OSHA requirements apply specifically to the venipuncture procedure, as well as to separation of serum or plasma from whole blood (presented later in this chapter).

1. Wear gloves when it is reasonably anticipated that you will have hand contact with blood.
2. Face shields or masks in combination with eye protection devices must be worn whenever splashes, spray, spatter, or droplets of blood may be generated.
3. Perform all procedures involving blood in a manner so as to minimize splashing, spraying, spattering, and generating droplets of blood.
4. Bandage cuts and other lesions on the hands before gloving.

5. Wash hands as soon as possible after removing gloves.

6. If your hands or other skin surfaces come in contact with blood, wash the area as soon as possible with soap and water.

7. If your mucous membranes (e.g., eyes, nose, mouth) come in contact with blood, flush them with water as soon as possible.

8. Do not bend, break, or shear contaminated venipuncture needles.

9. A contaminated venipuncture needle may not be recapped. The venipuncture needle may be removed from its plastic holder using a mechanical device.

10. Immediately after use, place the contaminated venipuncture needle in a biohazard sharps container. Locate the sharps container as close as possible to the area of use.

11. Place blood specimens in containers that prevent leakage during collection, handling, processing, storage, transport, or shipping.

12. If you are exposed to blood, report the incident immediately to your physician-employer.

VACUUM TUBE METHOD OF VENIPUNCTURE

☐ The vacuum tube method is frequently used to collect venous blood specimens. This method is considered ideal for collecting blood from normal healthy antecubital veins that are adequate in size to withstand the pressure of the vacuum in the evacuated tube.

The vacuum tube system consists of a collection needle, a plastic needle holder, and an evacuated tube (Fig. 17–7). One such commercially available vacuum tube system is the Vacutainer, manufactured by Becton Dickinson. Each of the components of the vacuum tube system are described next.

NEEDLE

The needle used with the vacuum tube method consists of a double-pointed stainless steel needle with a threaded hub near its center (see Fig. 17–8). The needle is coated with silicon, enabling it to penetrate the skin smoothly. The threaded hub of the needle screws

---

Highlight on Vasovagal Syncope (Fainting)

Most individuals undergoing venipuncture do not experience any change in their sense of well-being. A very small percentage of individuals, however, experience a type of fainting known as vasovagal syncope.

Vasovagal syncope is caused by unpleasant physical or emotional stimuli such as pain, fright, or the sight of blood. A sudden pooling of blood occurs, which results in a sudden decrease in the blood pressure. This, in turn, momentarily deprives the brain of blood, causing a temporary loss of consciousness, usually lasting only 1 to 2 minutes. Vasovagal syncope usually occurs when an individual is in an upright position, as in standing or sitting. Before fainting, the patient usually experiences some warning signals, which include sudden light-headedness, nausea, weakness, yawning, paleness, blurred vision, a feeling of warmth, and sweating followed by drooping eyelids, weak, rapid pulse, and finally unconsciousness.

A person who is about to faint should be placed in a position that facilitates blood flow to the brain and told to breathe deeply. The preferred position is a lying-down (supine) position with the legs somewhat elevated and the collar and clothing loosened. This position may not always be possible, such as when a patient is seated and the venipuncture needle has already been inserted. In this case, the tourniquet and then the needle should be removed and the patient's head should be lowered between the legs. An individual who has fainted should be protected from injury from a fall and then be placed in a position that facilitates blood flow to the brain, as just described.

Fainting during or after venipuncture is more likely to occur in the following individuals: patients having a venipuncture for the first time; young patients; thin patients; patients with a low diastolic or high systolic blood pressure; patients with a history of fainting; patients exhibiting obvious nervousness or apprehension; and those who are very quiet or very talkative.

Fainting often can be prevented by identifying and closely observing those individuals who are more likely to faint (as described). Talking to the patient often helps relax the patient and divert attention from the venipuncture procedure. If a patient has a history of fainting, he or she should be placed in a lying-down position for the venipuncture procedure since people rarely faint in this position. Other factors contributing to fainting that should be avoided (if possible) include fatigue, lack of sleep, hunger, and environmental factors such as a noisy, crowded, or overheated room.

17

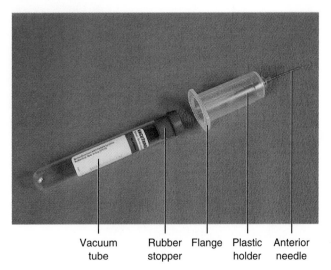

■ **FIGURE 17–7.** Vacuum tube system.

into the plastic holder. Vacuum tube needles are packaged in sealed twist-apart containers that are color-coded according to gauge for easy identification. The lot number and needle size are printed on the paper label covering the container (see Fig. 17–8). A needle should not be used if the seal has been broken prior to assembling the equipment.

The double-pointed needle consists of an anterior needle and a posterior needle. The **anterior needle** is longer and has a beveled point specially designed to facilitate entry into the skin and the vein. The **posterior needle** is shorter, and its purpose is to pierce the rubber stopper of the evacuated tube. The posterior

17

needle has a rubber sleeve that functions as a valve. Pushing an evacuated tube into the holder compresses the rubber sleeve and exposes the opening of the needle, allowing blood to enter the tube. When a tube is removed, the sleeve slides back over the needle opening and stops the flow of blood.

Vacuum tube needles are available in sizes 20 to 22 gauge, with 21-gauge needles most commonly used for a routine venipuncture. Vacuum tube needles come in two lengths: 1 inch and 1½ inch. The length used is based on individual preference; however, medical assistants often prefer the 1-inch needle for routine venipunctures. A 1-inch needle is less intimidating to the patient and tends to offer more control because it allows the medical assistant to rest the fourth and fifth fingers on the patient's arm for stability. On the other hand, a 1½-inch needle allows more room for stabilizing the vein.

PLASTIC HOLDER

The plastic holder consists of a plastic cylinder with two openings. The small opening is used to secure the double-pointed needle, while the large opening is used to hold the evacuated tube. The large opening has a plastic extension known as the flange. The flange assists in the insertion and removal of evacuated tubes and prevents the plastic holder from rolling when it is placed on a flat surface.

The plastic holder has an indentation about ½ inch from the hub of the needle. This marks the point at which the posterior needle starts to enter the rubber stopper of the tube. If a tube is inserted past this point before the vein is entered, the tube will fill with air, which will not allow blood to enter.

Plastic holders are available in two sizes: adult and pediatric (Fig. 17–9). Adult holders hold the regular

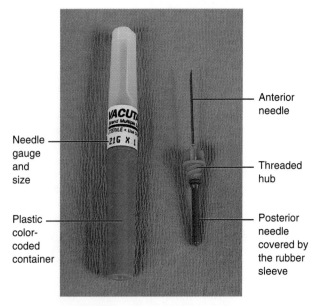

■ **FIGURE 17–8.** Vacuum tube needle in its container showing the size and gauge of the needle.

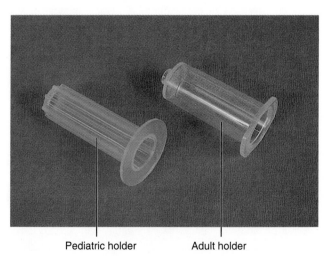

■ **FIGURE 17–9.** Adult and pediatric plastic needle holders.

Additive Content of Evacuated Tubes

The vacuum tube method utilizes a color-coded system for ease in identifying the additive content of each type of tube. The most frequently used vacuum tubes are classified here according to the color of the stopper and additive content.

1. **Red.** Red-stoppered tubes do not contain an anticoagulant and are used to obtain clotted blood or serum. Serum is required for serologic tests and most blood chemistries.
2. **Lavender.** Lavender-stoppered tubes contain the anticoagulant ethylenediaminetetraacetic acid (EDTA) and are used to obtain whole blood or plasma. The most common use is to collect a blood specimen for a complete blood count (CBC).
3. **Light Blue.** Light blue–stoppered tubes contain the anticoagulant sodium citrate and are used to obtain whole blood or plasma; the most common use is

for coagulation tests such as the prothrombin time (PT).
4. **Green.** Green-stoppered tubes contain the anticoagulant heparin and are commonly used to collect blood specimens to perform blood gas determinations and pH assays.
5. **Gray.** Gray-stoppered tubes contain the anticoagulant potassium oxalate and are used to obtain whole blood or plasma; the most common use is to collect blood specimens to perform a glucose tolerance test.
6. **Dark Blue.** Dark blue–stoppered tubes contain either heparin or no additive at all. These tubes are made of a specially refined glass and rubber stopper and are used for the detection of trace elements that are contracted through occupational or environmental exposure such as lead, zinc, arsenic, or copper.

---

diameter tubes and are used for routine venipunctures. The pediatric holders are smaller and hold small diameter tubes. They are used for pediatric patients or difficult draws.

Special holders designed to reduce the risk of accidental needlesticks are also available. They consist of a single-use holder with an outer sleeve that slides over the needle and locks in place after the needle is withdrawn from the vein. The entire holder assembly is then discarded in the sharps container.

EVACUATED TUBES

Evacuated tubes consist of a glass tube with a rubber stopper. The tube contains a premeasured vacuum that creates suction to pull the blood specimen into the tube. Evacuated tubes use a color-coded system for ease in identifying the additive content of each type of tube, which is described in the accompanying box and illustrated in Figure 17–10. The additive must not alter the blood components or affect the laboratory test

17

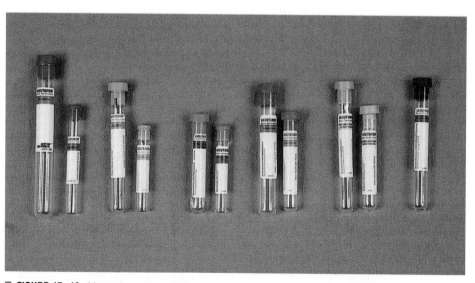

■ **FIGURE 17–10.** Vacutainer-evacuated tubes. The stoppers of the evacuated tubes are color coded for ease in identifying the additive content of each type of tube. The red-stoppered tubes contain no additive and are used to obtain clotted blood or serum. The lavender, light blue, green, gray, and dark blue tubes contain an anticoagulant and are used to obtain whole blood or plasma.

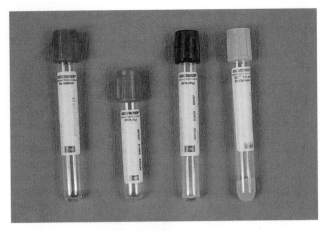

■ FIGURE 17–11. Hemogard tubes.

to be performed. Additive choice depends on the type of test to be performed. The medical assistant must be sure to use the additive specified by the test ordered. Additives must not be substituted for one another, because inaccurate test results will occur.

Evacuated tubes are available in varying capacities, the most common being the 2-, 3-, 5-, 7-, 10-, and 15-ml sizes (Fig. 17–10). The capacity of the tube used depends on the amount of the specimen required for the test. Information regarding additive content, expiration date, and tube capacity is found on the label of each box of vacuum tubes. In addition, most tubes have a label affixed to them indicating the additive content and expiration date of the tube.

Hemogard closure tubes, manufactured by Becton Dickinson, are a newer type of evacuated tube. After collecting a blood specimen, the medical assistant may need to gain access to the blood in the tube for testing it or for further processing such as in separating serum from whole blood. A regular evacuated tube "pops" as the top is removed to access the specimen, creating an aerosol mist that could be inhaled by the medical assistant. The Hemogard tube is made of plastic and has a plastic shield that fits over the rubber stopper to contain any aerosols that might be dispersed when the cap is removed (Fig. 17–11). It should be noted that the color coding of Hemogard stoppers varies slightly from that of rubber stoppers.

ORDER OF DRAW FOR MULTIPLE TUBES

When using the vacuum tube system and when multiple tubes are to be drawn, the following order of draw is recommended

1. **Blood culture tubes** (and other tests requiring sterile specimens)

Rationale: To prevent contamination of the specimen by other tubes, which may lead to inaccurate test results.
2. **Red-stoppered or red/gray-stoppered tube:** non-additive and gel separator, respectively
Rationale: To prevent contamination of nonadditive tubes by additive tubes.
3. **Coagulation tubes** (light blue stopper)
Rationale: To prevent erroneous test results. When the needle penetrates the patient's skin, thromboplastin, a clotting factor, may be released. Thromboplastin can enter the blood specimen, affecting the test results. (Note: If a light blue–stoppered tube is the first or only tube to be drawn, a 5-ml red-stoppered tube should be drawn first and discarded to eliminate contamination from tissue thromboplastin picked up during needle penetration.)
4. **Additive tubes** in this order: green, lavender, gray
Rationale: To prevent cross-contamination between different types of additive tubes, which may lead to inaccurate test results.

EVACUATED TUBE GUIDELINES

Certain guidelines should be followed when using evacuated tubes. These include the following:

1. Select the proper evacuated tubes according to the tests to be performed and amount of specimen required.
2. Check to make sure the tube is not cracked. A cracked tube will no longer have a vacuum.
3. Check the expiration date of each tube. Outdated tubes may no longer contain a vacuum, and, as a result, they may not be able to draw blood into the tube.
4. Label each tube with the patient's name, the date, and your initials. Proper labeling avoids mix-up of specimens. Recent advances in specimen identification include the use of computer bar codes to identify specimens (Fig. 17–12). The laboratory instruments that do the testing are able to read the bar codes and automatically record results onto the laboratory report.
5. Before using tubes that contain powdered additives, gently tap the tube just below the stopper so that all the additive is dislodged from the stopper. If an additive remains trapped in the stopper, erroneous test results may occur.
6. Take precautions to avoid premature loss of the tube's vacuum. Premature loss of vacuum can occur from dropping the tube or partially pulling the needle out of the arm after penetrating the patient's skin.

PUTTING IT ALL *into* PRACTICE

▶ **DORI GLOVER:** *While performing a routine finger stick for a blood glucose determination (a procedure I have performed many, many times), I accidentally stuck myself while removing the lancet from an automatic lancet device. I could see the blood inside my glove and I could see the patient's blood clinging to the point—my heart sank. I placed the lancet in the sharps container and tried to keep my cool and not alarm the patient. I mentally assessed the patient. He was an older man from a rural community, but I know you cannot always judge a book by its cover.*

I excused myself and immediately proceeded to wash my hands thoroughly with soap and water and rinse, rinse, rinse! I then notified the physician. The physician questioned the patient regarding recent operations he had in the previous year. He had undergone bypass surgery, and had received two units of blood. Although blood is effectively screened, I thought about that one-in-a-zillion chance that it could have been contami-

nated. Thankfully, I had received the hepatitis B immunization series, but there was still concern regarding hepatitis C and, of course, HIV.

The patient was gracious and complied with our request to be tested for hepatitis and HIV. The physician and I discussed the situation and we determined the risk to be low, but he nonetheless offered me the option of getting the post-exposural prophylactic treatment. The window of time for this to be effective is only 1 to 2 hours after the stick. It is very toxic and therefore, not something you want to receive needlessly. I declined and proceeded to wait 5 agonizing days for the patient's test results. The word relief *hardly describes how I felt when the laboratory results came back negative!*

This incident confirmed the importance of getting the hepatitis B immunization as well as paying attention to good technique when performing procedures involving blood.

17

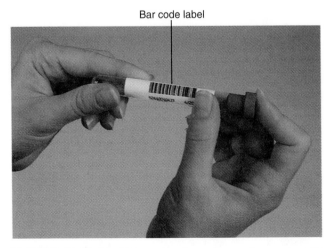

Bar code label

■ **FIGURE 17–12.** Identifying a blood specimen using a computer bar code.

7. When multiple tubes are to be drawn, follow the proper **order of draw.** This prevents contamination of nonadditive tubes by additive tubes as well as cross-contamination between different types of additive tubes, which could lead to inaccurate test results.
8. Fill evacuated tubes until the vacuum is exhausted, as evidenced by the cessation of the blood flow into the tube. The tube will be almost, but not quite, full when the vacuum is exhausted. If the evacuated tube is removed before the vacuum is exhausted, a rush of air enters the tube, damaging the red blood cells. A tube containing an additive must be filled completely to ensure the proper ratio of additive to blood.
9. Remove the last tube from the plastic holder be-

fore removing the needle. This prevents blood from dripping out of the tip of the needle after it is withdrawn from the patient's skin.

10. Mix tubes containing an anticoagulant immediately after drawing by gently inverting the tube eight to ten times. This provides adequate mixing without causing hemolysis. Inadequate mixing may result in clotting, leading to inaccurate test results.

11. After performing the venipuncture, the top of the stopper may contain residual blood. Be sure to take precautions following the OSHA Standard when handling these tubes.

17–1

Venipuncture Using the Vacuum Tube Method (Collection of Multiple Tubes)

EQUIPMENT/SUPPLIES:

Disposable gloves
Tourniquet
Antiseptic wipe
Double-pointed needle
Plastic holder

Evacuated tubes with labels
Sterile 2 × 2 gauze pad
Adhesive bandage
Biohazard sharps container

1. **Procedural Step.** Wash the hands.
2. **Procedural Step.** Greet and identify the patient, and introduce yourself. If the patient was required to prepare for the test (e.g., fasting, medication restriction), determine whether he or she has prepared properly. If the patient has not followed the patient preparation requirements, notify the physician for instructions on handling this situation. **Principle.** It is important to make sure you have the correct patient. The patient must prepare properly in order to obtain a quality specimen that will lead to accurate test results.

3. **Procedural Step.** Assemble the equipment. Be sure to select the proper evacuated tubes according to the tests to be performed. Check the expiration date of the tubes. Label each tube with the patient's name, the date, and your initials. If the specimen will be tested at an outside laboratory, complete a laboratory request form. **Principle.** Outdated tubes may no longer contain a vacuum, and, as a result, they may not be able to draw blood into the tube. Proper labeling of blood specimens avoids a mix-up of specimens.

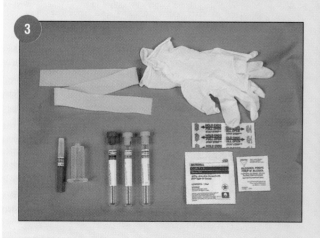

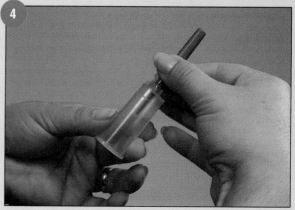

PROCEDURE 17–1

4. Procedural Step. Prepare the vacuum tube system. Insert the posterior needle into the plastic holder. Screw the needle into the plastic holder and tighten it securely.
Principle. An unsecured needle can fall out of its plastic holder.

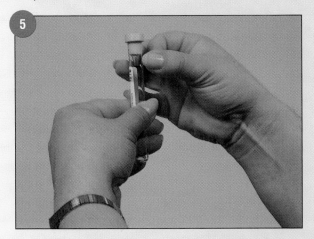

5. Procedural Step. Open the sterile gauze packet, and place the gauze pad on the inside of its wrapper. Position the evacuated tubes in the correct order of draw. If the evacuated tube contains a powdered additive, tap the tube just below the stopper to release any additive adhering to the stopper.
Principle. If an additive remains trapped in the stopper, erroneous test results may occur.

6. Procedural Step. Place the first tube loosely in the plastic holder. Place the remaining supplies within comfortable reach of your nondominant hand.
Principle. Items used during the procedure should be positioned so that you do not have to reach over the patient and possibly move the needle.

7. Procedural Step. Explain the procedure to the patient, and reassure the patient. Perform a preliminary assessment of both arms to determine the best vein to use. It is also helpful to ask the patient which arm has been used in the past to obtain blood.
Principle. Venipuncture is often a frightening experience for the patient, and reassurance should be offered to help reduce apprehension.

8. Procedural Step. Apply the tourniquet. Position the tourniquet 3 to 4 inches above the bend in the elbow. The tourniquet should be snug but not tight. Ask the patient to clench the fist of the arm to which the tourniquet has been applied.
Principle. The combined effect of the pressure of the tourniquet and the clenched fist should cause the antecubital veins to stand out so that accurate selection of a puncture site can be made.

9. Procedural Step. With a tourniquet in place, thoroughly assess the veins of first one arm and then the other to determine the best vein to use. Never leave the tourniquet on an arm for more than 1 minute at a time. (Note: If you need to perform several assessments to locate the best vein, the tourniquet can be applied and reapplied as required.)
Principle. Leaving the tourniquet on for more than 1 minute is uncomfortable for the patient and may alter the test results.

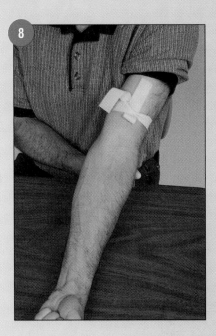

10. Procedural Step. Position the patient's arm. The arm with the vein selected for the venipuncture should be extended and placed in a straight line from the shoulder to the wrist with the antecubital veins facing anteriorly. The arm should be supported on the armrest by a rolled towel or by having the patient place the fist of the other hand under the elbow.
Principle. This position allows for easy access to the antecubital veins.

11. Procedural Step. Thoroughly palpate the selected vein. Gently palpate the vein with the fingertips to determine the direction of the vein and to estimate the size and depth of the vein.

12. Procedural Step. Cleanse the site with an antiseptic. Cleansing should be done in a circular motion, starting from the inside and moving away from the puncture site. Allow the site to air dry and do not touch the area after cleansing or fan the area with your hand.

17

Continued

17

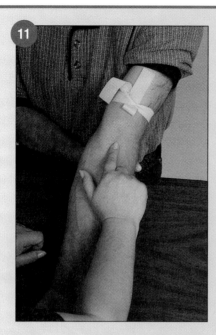

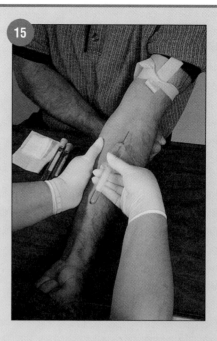

Principle. Using a circular motion helps carry foreign particles away from the puncture site. The site must be allowed to dry because alcohol entering the blood specimen contaminates it, leading to inaccurate test results. In addition, the alcohol causes the patient to experience a stinging sensation. Touching or fanning the area causes contamination, and the cleansing process has to be repeated.

13. **Procedural Step.** Apply gloves. Remove the cap from the needle. Hold the vacuum tube system by placing the thumb and index finger of the dominant hand on the plastic holder while supporting the rest of the holder and evacuated tube with the remaining three fingers. The needle should be positioned with the bevel facing up. Position the evacuated tube so that the label is facing downward.
    Principle. Gloves are a precaution that provides a barrier against bloodborne pathogens. Positioning the needle with the bevel up allows for easier entry into the skin and the vein. With the label facing downward, you will be able to observe the blood as it fills the tube, which allows you to know when the tube is full.

14. **Procedural Step.** Anchor the vein. Grasp the patient's arm with the nondominant hand. Your thumb should be placed 1 to 2 inches below and to the side of the puncture site. Using your thumb, draw the skin taut over the vein in the direction of the patient's hand.
    Principle. The thumb helps hold the skin taut for easier entry and helps stabilize the vein to be punctured.

15. **Procedural Step.** Position the needle at a 15-degree angle to the arm. Make sure the needle points in the same direction as the vein to be entered.
    Principle. An angle of less than 15 degrees may cause the needle to enter above the vein, preventing puncture. An angle of more than 15 degrees may cause the needle to go through the vein by puncturing the posterior wall. This could result in a hematoma.

16. **Procedural Step.** The needle should be positioned so that it enters the vein approximately ¼ inch below the place where the vein is to be entered. Tell the patient that he or she will "feel a small stick," and with one continuous motion, enter the skin and then the vein.
    Principle. Using one continuous motion helps to prevent tissue damage.

17. **Procedural Step.** Firmly grasp the holder between the thumb and the underlying fingers to prevent the needle from moving. With the nondominant hand place two fingers on the flange of the plastic holder and with the thumb slowly push the tube forward to the end of the holder. This allows the posterior needle to puncture the rubber stopper. Blood will begin flowing into the tube if the (anterior) needle is in a vein.
    Principle. Firmly grasping the holder prevents the needle from moving deeper into the vein when inserting an evacuated tube. Moving the needle is painful for the patient.

18. **Procedural Step.** Allow the evacuated tube to fill to the exhaustion of the vacuum as indicated by the cessation of the blood flow into the tube. The

PROCEDURE 17–1

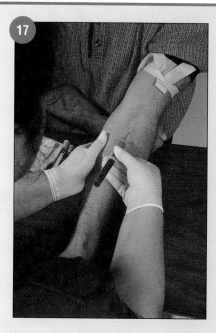

suction action of the evacuated tube automatically draws the blood into the tube.

Principle. If the evacuated tube is removed before the vacuum is exhausted, a rush of air enters the tube, damaging the red blood cells. Also, a tube containing an additive such as an anticoagulant must be filled completely to ensure accurate test results.

19. **Procedural Step.** Using the flange, remove the tube

from the plastic holder, being careful not to change the position of the needle in the vein. If the tube contains an additive, gently rotate the tube approximately eight to ten times before laying it down.

Principle. The rubber sheath covers the point of the needle, stopping the flow of blood until the next tube is inserted. The tube containing an additive must be inverted immediately to prevent the blood from clotting. Careful mixing of the blood with the additive prevents hemolysis.

20. **Procedural Step.** Carefully insert the next tube into the holder using the flange. Continue in this manner until the last tube has been filled.

21. **Procedural Step.** Remove the tension from the tourniquet and ask the patient to unclench the fist.

Principle. The tourniquet tension must be removed before the needle. Otherwise, the pressure on the vein from the tourniquet could cause internal and external bleeding around the puncture site.

22. **Procedural Step.** Remove the last tube from the holder.

Principle. This prevents blood from dripping out of the tip of the needle.

23. **Procedural Step.** Place a sterile gauze pad over the site and slowly withdraw the needle at the same angle as that for penetration. Do not apply any pressure to the puncture site until the needle is completely removed.

Principle. Placing the gauze pad over the puncture site helps prevent tissue movement as the needle

17

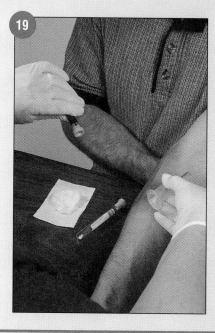

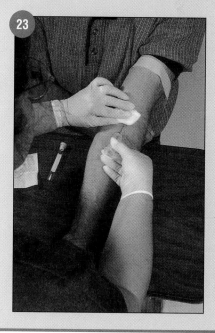

Continued

is withdrawn and reduces patient discomfort. Careful withdrawal prevents further tissue damage.

24. **Procedural Step.** Apply pressure with the gauze pad. Ask the patient to apply pressure with the gauze pad for 1 to 2 minutes. The arm can be elevated to facilitate clot formation. Do not allow the patient to bend the arm at the elbow as this increases blood loss from the puncture site.
Principle. Applying pressure reduces the leakage of blood from the puncture site either externally or internally. Internal leakage of blood into the tissues could result in a hematoma.

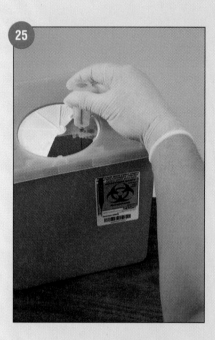

25. **Procedural Step.** Properly dispose of the needle in a biohazard sharps container. The needle may be removed from the plastic holder using a biohazard sharps container with a special serrated adapter that mechanically unscrews the needle from the plastic holder, allowing it to drop into the container. If the plastic holder is contaminated with blood, it should be disposed of or decontaminated with bleach.
Principle. Proper disposal is required by the OSHA Standard to prevent accidental needlestick injuries.

26. **Procedural Step.** The medical assistant should stay with the patient until the bleeding has stopped. Apply an adhesive bandage to the puncture site. As an alternative, the gauze pad can be folded into quarters and taped on the puncture site to be used as a pressure bandage. Instruct the patient not to pick up anything for about an hour. (Note: If any swelling or discoloration occurs, apply an ice pack to the site after bandaging it.)
Principle. Lifting a heavy object causes pressure on the puncture site, which could result in bleeding.

27. **Procedural Step.** Remove the gloves, and wash the hands.

28. **Procedural Step.** Chart the procedure. Include the date and time, which arm and vein were used, and any unusual patient reaction.

29. **Procedural Step.** Test, transfer, or store the blood specimen according to the medical office policy. If the specimen is to be transported to an outside laboratory for testing, record this information in the patient's chart, including the date the specimen was transported to the laboratory.

CHARTING EXAMPLE	
Date	
4/5/2002	9:00 a.m. Venous blood specimen collected from Ⓛ arm. Picked up by Medical Center Laboratory on 4/5/2002. —— D. Glover, CMA

BUTTERFLY METHOD OF VENIPUNCTURE

☐ The butterfly method of venipuncture is also called the **winged infusion method.** This is because a winged infusion set is used to perform the procedure. The term "butterfly" is derived from the plastic "wings" located between the needle and the tubing of the winged infusion set (Fig. 17–13).

The butterfly method is used to collect blood from patients who are difficult to stick by conventional methods. This includes adult patients with small antecubital veins and children, who typically have small antecubital veins. The butterfly method is also used when the antecubital veins are not available and the veins in the forearm, wrist area, or back of the hand are used, as may occur with elderly and obese patients

The gauge of the winged infusion needle ranges from 21 to 23, and the length of the needle ranges from ½ to ¾ inches. The needle is short and very sharp, making it easier to stick difficult veins. For

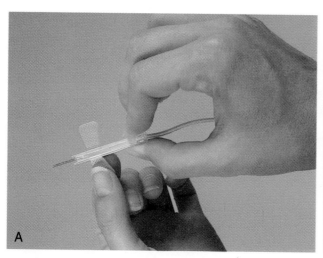

Hub adapter

Luer adapter

■ **FIGURE 17–13.** Winged infusion set. *A,* Luer adapter with evacuated tube. *B,* Hub adapter with syringe.

extremely small veins, a 23-gauge needle should be used to prevent rupture of the vein by a larger needle. In this case, it is preferable to use smaller volume tubes (e.g., 2-ml evacuated tubes) because large evacuated tubes may put too much vacuum pressure on the vein, causing it to collapse.

The winged infusion needle is attached to a 6- or 12-inch length of tubing and a **Luer adapter,** attached to a (posterior) needle with a rubber sleeve. A plastic evacuated tube holder is screwed onto the Luer adapter (Fig. 17–13). Winged infusion sets are also available with a **hub adapter** that allows them to be used with a syringe (Fig. 17–13). The evacuated tube adapter is generally preferred because of the safety haz-

ard involved with transferring blood from a syringe to an evacuated tube. Safety needles are also available that have a shield that covers the contaminated needle after it is withdrawn from the patient's vein (Fig. 17–14).

GUIDELINES FOR THE BUTTERFLY METHOD

Certain guidelines should be followed when performing the butterfly method of venipuncture. These include the following:

1. The patient should be positioned according to the site selected for the venipuncture as follows:

   Antecubital, Wrist and Forearm Veins. Position the arm in a straight line from the shoulder to the wrist as described in the vacuum tube method of venipuncture.

   Hand Veins. Position the patient's hand on the arm rest and ask the patient to make a loose fist or to grasp a rolled towel. This combination causes the hand veins to stand out so that accurate selection of a puncture site can be made. Locate a suitable vein between the knuckles and the wrist bones. Hand veins are usually visible and easy to locate.

2. The tourniquet should be positioned according to the venipuncture site as follows: If the veins of the forearm or wrist are used, the tourniquet should be applied to the forearm, approximately 3 inches above the puncture site. For hand veins, the tourniquet should be positioned on the arm just above the wrist bone (Fig. 17–15).

3. The needle should be grasped by compressing the plastic wings together. The needle should be in-

17

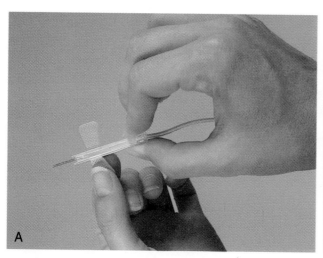

A

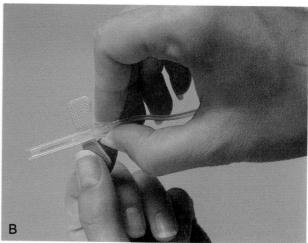

B

■ **FIGURE 17–14.** Butterfly safety needle. The safety needle has a shield that covers the contaminated needle after it is withdrawn from the patient's vein. *A,* The medical assistant has covered half of the needle with the shield. *B,* The needle is completely covered with the shield.

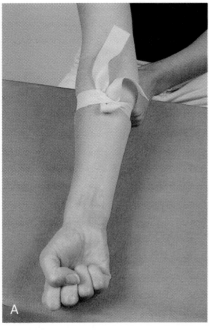 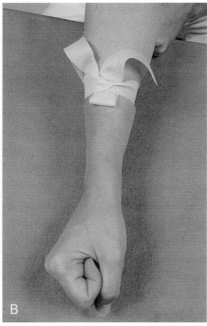 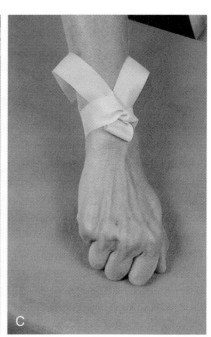

Forearm   Wrist   Hand

FIGURE 17–15. Application of the tourniquet for alternative venipuncture sites: *A*, forearm; *B*, wrist; *C*, hand.

serted with the bevel facing up at a 15-degree angle to the skin. Once the vein has been entered, the angle should be decreased to 5 degrees.

4. After inserting the needle, it should be slowly threaded inside the vein an additional ¼ inch. This anchors the needle in the center of the vein.

5. To prevent venous reflux, keep the evacuated tube and holder in a downward position as in the vacuum tube venipuncture procedure. This technique en-

sures that the blood fills from the bottom up and not near the rubber stopper.

6. When multiple tubes are to be drawn, follow the proper order of draw. The order of draw for the butterfly method is identical to that of the vacuum tube method (refer to page 582). Following this order of draw prevents contamination of nonadditive tubes as well as cross-contamination between different types of additive tubes.

Text continued on page 595

17–2

Venipuncture Using the Butterfly Method (Collection of Multiple Tubes)

EQUIPMENT/SUPPLIES:

Disposable gloves
Tourniquet
Antiseptic wipe
Winged-infusion set with a Luer adapter and a multiple draw needle

Plastic holder
Evacuated tubes with labels
Sterile 2 × 2 gauze pad
Adhesive bandage
Biohazard sharps container

1. **Procedural Step.** Wash the hands.
2. **Procedural Step.** Greet and identify the patient, and

introduce yourself. If the patient was required to prepare for the test (e.g., fasting, medication re-

striction), determine whether he or she has prepared properly. If the patient has not followed the patient preparation requirements, notify the physician for instructions on handling this situation.
Principle. It is important to make sure you have the correct patient. The patient must prepare properly in order to obtain a quality specimen that will lead to accurate test results.

3. **Procedural Step.** Assemble the equipment. Be sure to select the proper evacuated tubes according to the tests to be performed. Check the expiration date of the tubes. Label each tube with the patient's name, the date, and your initials. If the specimen will be tested at an outside laboratory, complete a laboratory request form.

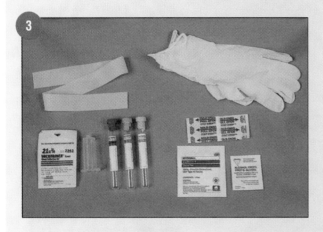

Principle. Outdated tubes may no longer contain a vacuum, and, as a result, they may not be able to draw blood into the tube. Proper labeling of blood specimens avoids mix-up of specimens.

4. **Procedural Step.** Prepare the winged infusion set. Remove the winged infusion set from its package. Extend the tubing to its full length and stretch it slightly to prevent it from coiling back up. Insert the Luer adapter and attached needle into the plastic holder. Screw the plastic holder onto the adapter and tighten it securely.
Principle. Extending the tubing straightens it to permit a free flow of blood in the tubing. An unsecured needle can fall out of its plastic holder.

5. **Procedural Step.** Open the sterile gauze packet, and place the gauze pad on the inside of its wrapper. Position the evacuated tubes in the correct order of draw. If the evacuated tube contains a powdered additive, tap the tube just below the stopper to release any additive adhering to the stopper.
Principle. If an additive remains trapped in the stopper, erroneous test results may occur.

6. **Procedural Step.** Place the first tube loosely in the plastic holder with the label facing downward. Place the remaining supplies within comfortable reach.
Principle. With the label facing downward, you will be able to observe the blood as it fills the tube, which allows you to know when the tube is full. Items used during the procedure should be positioned so that you do not have to reach over the patient and possibly move the needle.

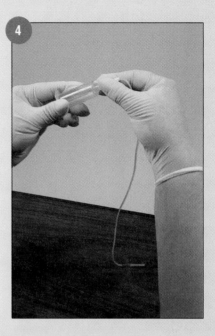

7. **Procedural Step.** Explain the procedure to the patient, and reassure the patient. Perform a preliminary assessment of both arms to determine the best vein to use. It is also helpful to ask the patient which arm has been used in the past to obtain blood.
Principle. Venipuncture is often a frightening experience for the patient, and reassurance should be offered to help reduce apprehension.

8. **Procedural Step.** Apply the tourniquet. Position the tourniquet 3 to 4 inches above the bend in the elbow. The tourniquet should be snug but not tight. Ask the patient to clench the fist of the arm to which the tourniquet has been applied.
Principle. The combined effect of the pressure of the tourniquet and the clenched fist should cause the antecubital veins to stand out so that accurate selection of a puncture site can be made.

9. **Procedural Step.** With a tourniquet in place, thoroughly assess the veins of first one arm and then the other to determine the best vein to use. Never leave the tourniquet on an arm for more than 1 minute at a time. (Note: You may need to perform several assessments to locate the best vein by applying and removing the tourniquet several times.)

17

17

10. **Procedural Step.** Position the patient's arm. The arm with the vein selected for the venipuncture should be extended and placed in a straight line from the shoulder to the wrist with the antecubital veins facing anteriorly. The arm should be supported on the armrest by a rolled towel or by having the patient place the fist of the other hand under the elbow.
Principle. This position allows for easy access to the antecubital veins.

11. **Procedural Step.** Thoroughly palpate the selected vein. Gently palpate the vein with the fingertips to determine the direction of the vein and to estimate the size and depth of the vein.

12. **Procedural Step.** Cleanse the site with an antiseptic. Cleansing should be done in a circular motion, starting from the inside and moving away from the puncture site. Allow the site to air dry and do not touch the area after cleansing or fan the area with your hand.
Principle. Using a circular motion helps carry foreign particles away from the puncture site. The site must be allowed to dry, because alcohol entering the blood specimen contaminates it, leading to inaccurate test results. In addition, the alcohol causes the patient to experience a stinging sensation. Touching or fanning the area causes contamination, and the cleansing process has to be repeated.

gether. Remove the protective shield from the needle of the infusion set. The needle should be positioned with the bevel facing up.
Principle. Gloves are a precaution that provide a barrier against bloodborne pathogens. Positioning the needle with the bevel up allows for easier entry into the skin and the vein.

14. **Procedural Step.** Anchor the vein. Grasp the patient's arm with the nondominant hand. The thumb should be placed 1 to 2 inches below and to the side of the puncture site. Using the thumb, draw the skin taut over the vein in the direction of the patient's hand.
Principle. The thumb helps hold the skin taut for easier entry and helps stabilize the vein to be punctured.

15. **Procedural Step.** Position the needle at a 15-degree angle to the arm. Make sure the needle points in the same direction as the vein to be entered.
Principle. An angle of less than 15 degrees may cause the needle to enter above the vein, preventing puncture. An angle of more than 15 degrees may cause the needle to go through the vein by puncturing the posterior wall. This could result in a hematoma.

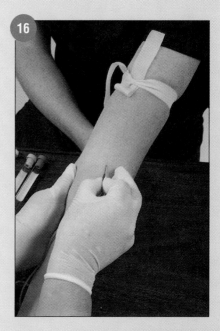

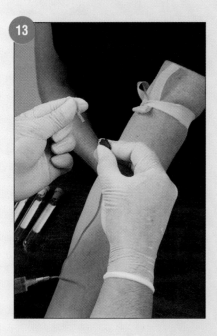

13. **Procedural Step.** Apply gloves. Grasp the winged infusion set by compressing the butterfly tips to-

16. **Procedural Step.** The needle should be positioned so that it enters the vein approximately ¼ inch below the place where the vein is to be entered. Tell the patient that he or she will "feel a small stick," and with one continuous motion, enter the skin and then the vein. After penetrating the vein,

decrease the angle of the needle to 5 degrees. If the needle is in the vein, a flash of blood will appear in the tubing.

Principle. Using one continuous motion helps to reduce tissue damage.

17. **Procedural Step.** Seat the needle by threading it up the lumen (central area) of the vein slightly so that it will not twist out of the vein, even if you let go of it. Securely rest the needle flat against the skin. Be sure that the needle does not move.

Principle. Seating the needle anchors the needle in the center of the vein. Moving the needle is painful for the patient.

18. **Procedural Step.** Keep the tube and holder in a downward position so that the tube fills from the bottom up and not near the rubber stopper. Using the flange, slowly push the tube forward to the end of the holder. This allows the needle to puncture the rubber stopper. Blood will begin flowing into the tube. Allow the evacuated tube to fill to the exhaustion of the vacuum as indicated by the cessation of the blood flow into the tube. The suction action of the evacuated tube automatically draws the blood into the tube.

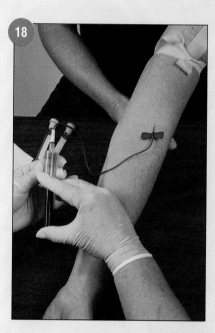

Principle. The tube must fill from the bottom up to prevent venous reflux. If the evacuated tube is removed before the vacuum is exhausted, a rush of air enters the tube, damaging the red blood cells. Also, a tube containing an additive such as an anticoagulant must be filled completely to ensure accurate test results.

19. **Procedural Step.** Using the flange, remove the tube from the plastic holder, being careful not to change the position of the needle in the vein. If the tube contains an additive, gently rotate the tube approximately eight to ten times before laying it down.

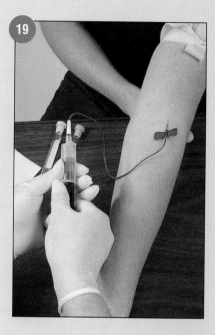

Principle. The rubber sheath covers the point of the needle, stopping the flow of blood until the next tube is inserted. The tube containing an additive must be inverted before laying it down to prevent the blood from clotting. Careful mixing of the blood with the additive prevents hemolysis.

20. **Procedural Step.** Carefully insert the next tube into the holder using the flange. Continue in this manner until the last tube has been filled.

21. **Procedural Step.** Remove the tension from the tourniquet and ask the patient to unclench the fist.

Principle. The tourniquet tension must be removed before the needle. Otherwise, the pressure on the vein from the tourniquet could cause internal and external bleeding around the puncture site.

22. **Procedural Step.** Remove the last tube from the holder.

Principle. This prevents blood from dripping out of the tip of the needle.

23. **Procedural Step.** Place a sterile gauze pad over the site. Grasp the wings and slowly withdraw the needle at the same angle as that for penetration. Do not apply any pressure to the puncture site until the needle is completely removed.

17

Continued

Principle. Placing the gauze pad over the puncture site helps prevent tissue movement as the needle is withdrawn and reduces patient discomfort. Careful withdrawal prevents further tissue damage.

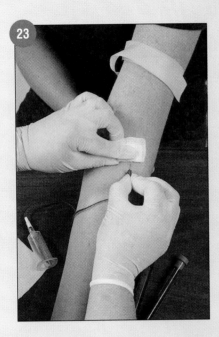

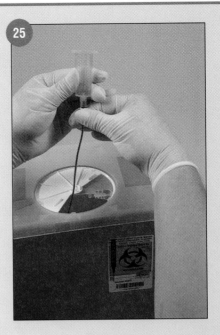

17

24. **Procedural Step.** Apply pressure with the gauze pad. Ask the patient to apply pressure with the gauze pad for 1 to 2 minutes. The arm can be elevated to facilitate clot formation. Do not allow the patient to bend the arm at the elbow because this increases blood loss from the puncture site.
    Principle. Applying pressure reduces the leakage of blood from the puncture site either externally or internally. Internal leakage into the tissues could result in a hematoma.

25. **Procedural Step.** Properly dispose of the winged infusion set. Drop the needle and tubing in a biohazard sharps container while holding onto the plastic holder. Twist and disconnect the plastic holder at the Luer adapter so that everything but the plastic holder is discarded. If the plastic holder is contaminated with blood, it should be disposed of or decontaminated with bleach.
    Principle. Proper disposal of the needle is required by the OSHA Standard to prevent accidental needlestick injuries.

26. **Procedural Step.** The medical assistant should stay with the patient until the bleeding has stopped.

Apply an adhesive bandage to the puncture site. As an alternative, the gauze pad can be folded into quarters and taped on the puncture site to be used as a pressure bandage. Instruct the patient not to pick up anything for about an hour. (Note: If any swelling or discoloration occurs, apply an ice pack to the site after bandaging it.)
Principle. Lifting a heavy object causes pressure on the puncture site, which could result in bleeding.

27. **Procedural Step.** Remove the gloves, and wash the hands.

28. **Procedural Step.** Chart the procedure. Include the date and time, which arm and vein were used, and any unusual patient reaction.

29. **Procedural Step.** Test, transfer, or store the blood specimen according to the medical office policy. If the specimen is to be transported to an outside laboratory for testing, record this information in the patient's chart, including the date the specimen was transported to the laboratory.

CHARTING EXAMPLE

Date	
4/10/2002	10:30 a.m. Venous blood specimen collected from Ⓛ arm. Picked up by Medical Center Laboratory on 4/10/2002. —— D. Glover, CMA

SYRINGE METHOD OF VENIPUNCTURE

☐ The syringe method is the least used method of venipuncture. This is because once the blood specimen is obtained, it must be transferred from the syringe to an evacuated tube, which presents the risk of an accidental needlestick.

The syringe method is primarily used to obtain blood from small veins that are likely to collapse. Because the rate of flow of blood into the syringe is not dictated by the premeasured vacuum of an evacuated tube, the syringe method offers more control than other methods of venipuncture. Once the vein has been punctured, the specimen is obtained by pulling back on the plunger of the syringe. Pulling the plunger back slowly minimizes pressure against the vein wall and the vein is less likely to collapse.

The set-up for the syringe method includes a disposable needle and syringe. The gauge of the needle ranges from 21 to 23, and the length of the needle ranges from 1 to 1½ inches. For extremely small veins, a 23-gauge needle should be used to prevent rupture of the vein by a larger needle. The capacity of the syringe depends upon the amount of specimen required and ranges from 5 ml (cc) to 20 ml (cc). If more than 20 ml is required, a second venipuncture must be performed; this is another disadvantage of this method.

After collecting the blood specimen, it must be transferred to an evacuated tube. For safety reasons, the tube should always be placed in a test tube rack. The tube should *never* be held in the hand during the transfer because of the danger of a needlestick injury.

If more than one evacuated tube is being filled, a specific "order of fill" is required as follows: blue, lavender, green, gray, and red. It should be noted that this order is reversed as compared to the vacuum tube and butterfly methods (i.e., the tubes with additives are filled first followed by the tubes without additives). The reason for this is to combine the blood with the additive as soon as possible after collection to prevent clotting. Tubes with additives should be inverted eight to ten times immediately after filling them.

PROCEDURE

17–3

Venipuncture Using the Syringe Method

EQUIPMENT/SUPPLIES: Disposable gloves
Tourniquet
Antiseptic wipe
Syringe and needle
Evacuated tubes with labels

Test tube rack
Sterile 2 × 2 gauze pad
Adhesive bandage
Biohazard sharps container

1. **Procedural Step.** **Follow Steps 1 through 3 of the Butterfly Method of Venipuncture (Procedure 17–2).**
2. **Procedural Step.** Prepare the needle and syringe, making sure to keep the needle and inside of the syringe sterile. Break the seal on the syringe by moving the plunger back and forth several times. Loosen the cap on the needle and check to make sure that the hub is screwed tightly into the syringe.
3. **Procedural Step.** Place the evacuated tubes to be filled in a test tube rack on a work surface. If an evacuated tube contains a powdered additive, tap the tube just below the stopper to release any additive adhering to the stopper. Make sure the

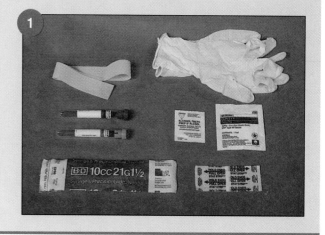

17

Continued

tubes are placed in the correct order to be filled. Open the sterile gauze packet and place the gauze pad on the inside of its wrapper.

Principle. If an additive remains trapped in the stopper, erroneous test results may occur.

4. **Procedural Step. Follow Steps 7 through 12 of the Butterfly Method of Venipuncture.**

5. **Procedural Step.** Apply gloves. Remove the cap from the needle. Hold the syringe by placing the thumb and index finger of the dominant hand near the needle hub while supporting the barrel of the syringe with the three remaining fingers. The needle should be positioned with the bevel facing up.

Principle. Gloves are a precaution that provides a barrier against bloodborne pathogens. Positioning the needle with the bevel up allows for easier entry into the skin and the vein.

6. **Procedural Step.** Anchor the vein. Grasp the patient's arm with the nondominant hand. The thumb should be placed 1 to 2 inches below and to the side of the puncture site. Using the thumb, draw the skin taut over the vein in the direction of the patient's hand.

Principle. The thumb helps hold the skin taut for easier entry and helps stabilize the vein to be punctured.

7. **Procedural Step.** Position the needle at a 15-degree angle to the arm. Make sure the needle points in the same direction as the vein to be entered.

Principle. An angle of less than 15 degrees may cause the needle to enter above the vein, preventing puncture. An angle of more than 15 degrees may cause the needle to go through the vein by puncturing the posterior wall. This could result in a hematoma.

8. **Procedural Step.** The needle should be positioned so that it enters the vein approximately ¼ inch below the place where the vein is to be entered. Tell the patient that he or she will "feel a small stick," and with one continuous motion, enter the skin and then the vein.

Principle. Using one continuous motion helps to prevent tissue damage.

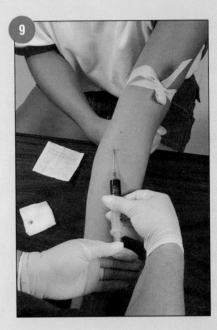

9. **Procedural Step.** Securely grasp the syringe firmly between the thumb and the underlying fingers. Blood may spontaneously enter the top of the syringe. If not, pull back gently on the plunger until blood begins to enter the syringe. Do not move the needle once the venipuncture has been made.

Principle. Moving the needle is painful for the patient.

10. **Procedural Step.** Remove the desired amount of blood by pulling back slowly and gently on the plunger. Care should be taken while pulling back on the plunger to avoid the accidental withdrawal of the needle from the patient's arm.

Principle. Pulling back on the plunger causes a suction effect, which draws the blood into the syringe. The blood should be withdrawn slowly from the vein to prevent hemolysis and to prevent the vein from collapsing.

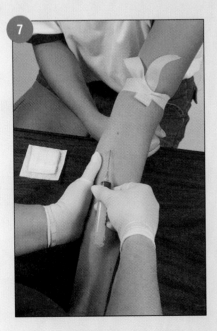

17

11. **Procedural Step.** Remove the tension from the tourniquet and ask the patient to unclench the fist.
    Principle. The tourniquet tension must be removed before the needle. Otherwise, the pressure on the vein from the tourniquet could cause internal and external bleeding around the puncture site.

12. **Procedural Step.** Place a sterile gauze pad over the site and slowly withdraw the needle at the same angle as that for penetration. Do not apply any pressure to the puncture site until the needle is completely removed.
    Principle. Placing the gauze pad over the puncture site helps prevent tissue movement as the needle is withdrawn and reduces patient discomfort. Careful withdrawal prevents further tissue damage.

13. **Procedural Step.** Apply pressure with the gauze pad. Ask the patient to apply pressure with the gauze pad for 1 to 2 minutes. The arm can be elevated to facilitate clot formation. Do not allow the patient to bend the arm at the elbow because this increases blood loss from the puncture site.
    Principle. Applying pressure reduces the leakage of blood from the puncture site either externally or internally. Internal leakage into the tissues could result in a hematoma.

14. **Procedural Step.** Transfer the blood to the labeled evacuated tubes as soon as possible as follows:

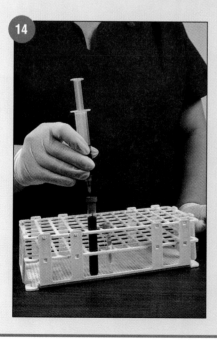

Double-check to make sure the tubes are in the correct order of fill in the rack.
Insert the needle through the center of the rubber stopper and allow the vacuum to fill the tube. Do not apply pressure to the plunger of the syringe.
If the blood is added to a tube containing an additive, it must be mixed immediately by gently inverting the tube eight to ten times.
Principle. A delay in transferring the blood to the evacuated tubes causes clotting of the blood in the syringe. To avoid an accidental needlestick, the tubes should not be held in the hand when the needle is inserted through the stopper. The suction action of the vacuum tube will automatically draw the blood into the tube. The tube containing an anticoagulant must be inverted immediately to prevent the blood from clotting. Careful mixing of the blood with the anticoagulant prevents hemolysis.

15. **Procedural Step.** Properly dispose of the needle and syringe in a biohazard sharps container.
    Principle. Proper disposal is required by the OSHA Standard to prevent accidental needlestick injuries.

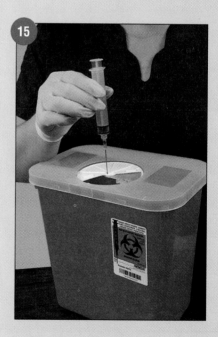

16. **Procedural Step. Follow Steps 26 through 29 of the Butterfly Method of Venipuncture.**

17

PROBLEMS ENCOUNTERED WITH VENIPUNCTURE

☐ At times, the medical assistant will encounter problems when attempting to draw blood from a patient. The appropriate response depends on the type of problem encountered.

FAILURE TO OBTAIN BLOOD

Periodically, even those highly skilled at performing venipuncture have difficulty in obtaining blood. Although large and prominent veins make it easier to collect the blood specimen, conditions often exist that make the procedure more difficult.

Problems in obtaining blood are often encountered with obese patients who have small, superficial veins and whose veins suitable for venipuncture are buried deeper in adipose tissue. Elderly patients with arteriosclerosis may have veins that are thick and hard, making them difficult to puncture. Other patients have veins that are small or have a thin wall, making the veins likely to collapse. After two unsuccessful attempts at venipuncture, the medical assistant should notify the physician to get advice or assistance regarding alternative puncture sites.

Factors that result in a failure to obtain blood once the needle has been inserted include not inserting the needle far enough, preventing it from entering the vein (Fig. 17–16B); insertion of the needle too far, causing it to go through the vein (Fig. 17–16C); and the bevel opening's becoming lodged against the wall of the vein. In these instances, most authorities recommend removal of the needle rather than trying to probe the vein. Probing is often uncomfortable for the patient and also can affect the integrity of the blood specimen. Occasionally, an evacuated tube loses its vacuum due to a manufacturing defect or through improper handling of the tube. If suspected, this problem can be corrected by removing the defective tube and inserting another vacuum tube.

INAPPROPRIATE PUNCTURE SITES

If a patient complains of pain or soreness in a potential venipuncture site, this area should be avoided. In addition, any skin areas that are scarred, bruised, burned, or adjacent to areas of infection should not be used. An arm in a cast or affected by a radical mastectomy should be avoided.

SCARRED AND SCLEROSED VEINS

One who has had many venipunctures over a period of years often develops scar tissue in the wall of the vein. Elderly patients may have veins that have become thickened from arteriosclerosis. In both cases, the veins feel stiff and hard when palpated. A scarred or sclerosed vein is difficult to stick and the blood return may be poor due to a narrowed lumen; therefore, it is recommended that another vein be used for the venipuncture. If this is not possible, the needle should be inserted with careful pressure to avoid going completely through the vein.

ROLLING VEINS

The median cubital vein, located in the center of the antecubital space, is considered the best vein to use for a venipuncture. At times, however, it is not possible to use this vein; for example, when it lies deep in the tissues and cannot be palpated or is scarred from repeated venipunctures. The veins on either side of the median cubital can be used; however, they have a tendency to "roll," or move away from the needle, thereby escaping puncture. To prevent rolling, firm pressure should be applied below the vein to stabilize it as the needle is inserted.

COLLAPSING VEINS

Veins are most likely to collapse in people who have small veins or veins with thin walls. This is particularly true when the vacuum tube method is being used. The "sucking action" exerted on the vein when the pressure in the vacuum is released causes the vein to collapse, thereby blocking the flow of blood into the tube (see Figure 17–16D). Because better control is possible, it is recommended that the butterfly or syringe method of venipuncture be used to obtain the specimen in patients with small veins.

PREMATURE NEEDLE WITHDRAWAL

Patient movement or improper venipuncture technique may cause the needle to come out of the vein prematurely. Because of the pressure exerted by the tourniquet, blood may be forced out of the puncture site, and immediate action is required to prevent a hematoma. The tourniquet should be removed at once, a gauze pad placed on the puncture site, and pressure applied until the bleeding has stopped.

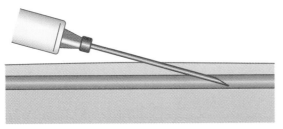

A   Correct insertion of the needle into the vein.

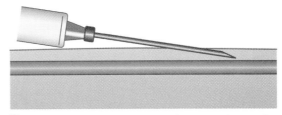

B   Improper angle of insertion (<15°), causing the needle to enter above the vein.

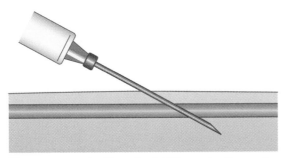

C   Improper angle of insertion (>15°), causing the needle to go through the vein.

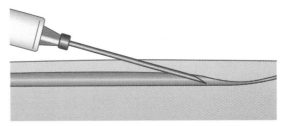

D   Collapsed vein (most likely to occur in persons with small veins).

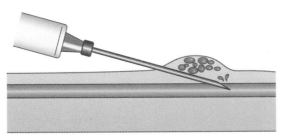

E   The beveled opening is partially within and partially outside of the vein, causing a hematoma.

■ **FIGURE 17–16.** Problems encountered with venipuncture.

HEMATOMA

A hematoma is caused by blood leaking from the vein and into the surrounding tissues, resulting in a bruise. A hematoma is caused by a needle that is inserted too far and that goes through the vein; a bevel opening that is partially within the vein and partially out of the vein (Fig. 17–16E); and applying insufficient pressure to the puncture site after removing the needle. When a hematoma is developing, the first sign is a sudden swelling in the area around the puncture site. If this occurs, the tourniquet and needle should be removed immediately, and pressure should be applied to the puncture site until the bleeding stops.

HEMOLYSIS

The blood specimen should be handled carefully at all times. Blood cells are fragile, and rough handling may cause **hemolysis,** or breakdown of the blood cells. Hemolyzed blood specimens produce inaccurate test results. To prevent hemolysis, these guidelines should be followed:

1. Store the vacuum tubes at room temperature, because chilled tubes can result in hemolysis.
2. Do not use a small-gauge needle to collect the specimen; a needle with a gauge between 20 and 22 should be used.
3. Practice good technique in collecting the specimen;

MEMORIES *from* EXTERNSHIP

DORI GLOVER: *While on externship in an office specializing in internal medicine, I had an experience that made me feel that all my schooling and hard work were worthwhile. A patient who had a colostomy had an embarrassing "accident." I took her into a room and cleaned her up, rinsed her colostomy bag, and helped her put it back on. She apologized profusely and asked me if I minded or felt repulsed. I replied that I was learning and getting experience in helping people. She told me that at the nursing home where she lived, some of the aides told her that it was disgusting and that it made them sick. She said she could not help it and that she felt very ashamed. I reassured her that it was nothing to be ashamed about. She then told me that she wished I could be the one to take care of her all the time. When I reached out to shake her hand and say good-bye, she pulled me down and whispered in my ear that she loved me. I was very moved and knew at that moment that I had chosen the right profession.*

17

excessive trauma to the blood vessel can result in hemolysis.

4. Always handle the blood specimen carefully; do not shake it or handle it roughly.

FAINTING

Occasionally a patient experiences dizziness or fainting during or after a venipuncture. Should this occur, the most immediate concern is to protect the patient from injury due to falling. The patient should then be placed in a position that promotes blood flow to the brain, and the physician should be notified for further treatment. (Refer to the earlier Highlight on Vasovagal Syncope.)

OBTAINING A SERUM SPECIMEN

SERUM

Serum is plasma from which the clotting factor fibrinogen has been removed. A brief discussion of serum is presented here, and a thorough discussion of plasma is presented under Obtaining a Plasma Specimen later in this chapter.

Serum contains numerous dissolved substances such as glucose, cholesterol, lipids, sodium, potassium, chloride, antibodies, hormones, and enzymes. As a result, many laboratory tests require a serum specimen to determine whether these substances are within normal limits and also to detect the presence of any substances that should not normally be present in the serum and that, if present, indicate a pathologic condition. To perform laboratory tests on serum, it must be separated from the blood specimen, which is usually the responsibility of the medical assistant.

TUBE SELECTION

A tube containing no additives (red-stoppered) must be used to collect the blood specimen, to allow the specimen to separate into serum and blood cells in a fibrin clot, known as the "clot." Since the amount of serum recovered is only a portion of the total specimen collected, a blood specimen must be drawn that is 2½ times the amount required for the test. For example, if 2 ml of serum is required, a 5-ml blood specimen must be collected; if 4 ml of serum is required, a 10-ml tube is collected, and if 6 ml of serum is required, a 15-ml tube is needed.

PREPARATION OF THE SPECIMEN

Once the blood specimen has been collected, the tube must be allowed to stand at room temperature in an upright position for 30 to 45 minutes before being centrifuged. The purpose of this is to allow clot formation, which will yield more serum from the specimen. If the specimen is centrifuged immediately after collection, the clotting factors do not have an opportunity to settle down into the cell layer to form a whole blood clot. The result of this is the formation of a **fibrin clot** in the serum layer consisting of the clotting factors. A fibrin clot is a spongy substance that occupies space, interfering with adequate serum collection. However, the blood specimen should not be allowed to stand for longer than 1 hour, because changes will take place in the specimen that will lead to inaccurate test results.

REMOVAL OF SERUM

Once clot formation has occurred, the specimen is centrifuged and the serum is then removed from the clot and placed in a separate transfer tube. It is important that proper technique be employed in removing the serum, to avoid disturbing the cell layer of the clot and drawing red blood cells into the serum. If cells do enter the pipet, the entire specimen must be recentrifuged.

When the serum has been removed from the blood specimen, the medical assistant should hold the specimen up to good light to inspect it for the presence of intact red blood cells or hemolyzed blood; in both cases, the specimen has a reddish appearance. Any specimen having a reddish appearance must be recentrifuged. If the specimen contains intact red blood cells, they settle to the bottom of the tube and the serum can be removed. If the blood is hemolyzed, recentrifugation will not make the red color disappear, because the red blood cells have ruptured and released hemoglobin into the serum. Hemolyzed serum is unsuitable for laboratory tests because the results will be inaccurate; therefore, another blood specimen must be collected.

Procedure 17–4 presents the method for separating serum from whole blood using a conventional vacuum tube.

PROCEDURE

17–4

Separating Serum from Whole Blood

EQUIPMENT/SUPPLIES: Red-stoppered vacuum tube venipuncture set-up
Test tube rack
Disposable pipet with a rubber bulb
Transfer tube and label
Disposable gloves
Face shield or mask and an eye protection device
Centrifuge
Biohazard sharps container

1. **Procedural Step.** Collect the blood specimen following the venipuncture procedure. A tube containing no additives (red-stoppered) should be used to collect the specimen. The tube selected should have a capacity of 2½ times the amount of serum required. Be sure to label *both* the red-stoppered tube and the transfer tube with the patient's name, the date, and your initials. In addition, the transfer tube should bear the word *serum*. Allow the tube to fill until the vacuum is exhausted.
Principle. To obtain serum, a tube containing no additives must be used. The tube must be allowed to fill completely in order to obtain the proper amount of serum. Several different types of specimen such as serum, plasma, and urine are straw colored; therefore, the transfer tube containing serum must be labeled as such to avoid confusion and mix-up among these specimens.

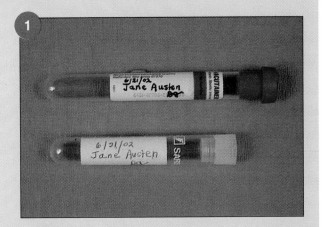

2. **Procedural Step.** Place the blood specimen tube in an upright position for 30 to 45 minutes at room

Continued

17

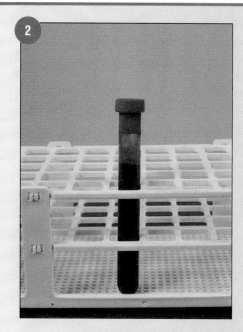

trifugation. Centrifuge the specimen for 10 to 15 minutes.

Principle. Centrifuging packs the cells and causes them to settle to the bottom of the tube, thereby yielding more serum. If the centrifuge is not balanced, it may vibrate and move across the table top. An unbalanced centrifuge may also cause specimen tubes to break.

4. **Procedural Step.** Put on a face shield or a mask and an eye protection device such as goggles or glasses with solid side-shields. Apply gloves. Carefully remove the tube from the centrifuge without disturbing the contents.

Principle. The OSHA Standard requires the use of personal protective equipment whenever spraying or splashing of blood may be generated. Disturbing the contents may cause the cells to enter the serum, and the specimen will need to be recentrifuged.

5. **Procedural Step.** Carefully remove the stopper from the tube, pointing the stopper away from you. Squeeze the bulb of the pipet to push the air out; then insert it into the serum. Place the tip of the pipet against the side of the tube approximately ¼ inch above the cell layer. Release the bulb to suction serum into the pipet. Do not allow the tip of the pipet to touch the cell layer.

Principle. The air should be removed from the bulb before inserting the pipet into the serum to prevent disturbance of the cell layer. If the cell layer is disturbed, red blood cells will enter the serum and the specimen will need to be recentrifuged.

temperature. Do not remove the stopper from the tube, to prevent evaporation of the serum sample.

Principle. Specimens must be placed in an upright position and allowed to stand to permit clot formation, which will yield more serum from the specimen. Evaporation of the sample will lead to falsely elevated test results.

3. **Procedural Step.** Place the specimen in the centrifuge, stopper end up. Balance the specimen with the same type and weight of tube or another specimen tube. Make sure the tube is stoppered to prevent evaporation of the sample during cen-

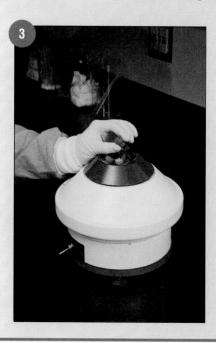

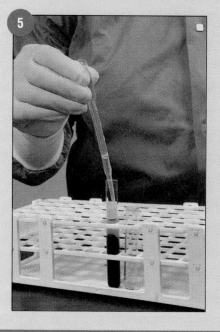

Pointing the stopper away prevents accidental spraying or splashing of the specimen onto the medical assistant.

6. **Procedural Step.** Transfer the serum in the pipet to the transfer tube. Continue pipetting until as much serum as possible is removed without disturbing the cell layer. Tightly cap the transfer tube to prevent sample evaporation.

7. **Procedural Step.** Hold the specimen up to the light and examine it for the presence of hemolysis. Make sure the proper amount of serum has been obtained.

   Principle. Hemolyzed serum is unsuitable for laboratory testing.

8. **Procedural Step.** Properly dispose of equipment. Following the OSHA Standard, the vacuum tube (containing the blood specimen) and the disposable pipet must be discarded in a biohazard sharps container.

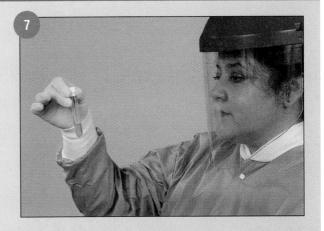

9. **Procedural Step.** Remove the gloves, and wash the hands.

10. **Procedural Step.** Test, transfer, or store the specimen according to the medical office policy.

SERUM SEPARATOR EVACUATED TUBES

A serum separator tube (SST) is a specially designed evacuated tube used to facilitate the collection of a serum specimen. The SST glass tube is identified by a red and slate-gray stopper and is used for both the collection and separation of blood. The serum separator tube contains a thixotropic gel, which is in a solid state in the bottom of the unused tube (Fig. 17–17A).

The blood specimen is collected and processed following the appropriate venipuncture method. The specimen must then be allowed to stand in an upright position for proper clot formation and then centrifuged as previously described. During centrifugation, the gel temporarily becomes fluid and moves to the dividing point between the serum and cells, where it re-forms into a solid gel, thus serving as a physical and chemical barrier between the serum and clot (Fig. 17–17B).

The serum can be transported or stored in the separator tube; however, the medical assistant must inspect the tube carefully to ensure that the gel barrier is firmly attached to the glass wall. If a complete barrier has not formed, the serum specimen must be placed in a transfer tube to prevent leaching of substances from the cell layer into the serum, thereby affecting the accuracy of the test results.

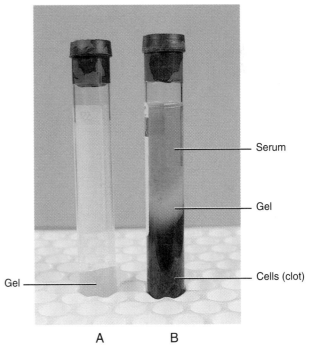

Serum

Gel

Cells (clot)

Gel

A   B

■ **FIGURE 17–17.** Serum separator tubes. *A,* A tube containing the thixotropic gel in the bottom of the unused tube. *B,* A tube that has been used to collect a blood specimen. During centrifugation, the gel temporarily becomes fluid and moves to the dividing point between the serum and blood cells in a fibrin clot.

17

OBTAINING A PLASMA SPECIMEN

PLASMA

Plasma is the straw-colored liquid portion of the blood. It serves as a transportation medium in which various substances are dissolved and blood cells are suspended for circulation through the body. Approximately 92 percent of plasma consists of water; the remaining 8 percent is dissolved solid substances (solutes) that are carried by the blood to and from the tissues.

The solutes present in greatest amounts are the **plasma proteins,** which include serum albumin, globulins, fibrinogen, and prothrombin. Serum albumin is synthesized in the liver and functions in regulating the volume of plasma within the blood vessels. Globulins play an important role in the immunity mechanism of the body, and fibrinogen and prothrombin are essential for proper blood clotting.

Various **electrolytes** are carried by the plasma and are needed for normal cell functioning and the maintenance of the normal fluid and acid-base balance of the body. Some of these electrolytes are sodium, chloride, potassium, calcium, phosphate, bicarbonate, and magnesium. **Nutrients** derived from the breakdown of food substances are carried by the plasma to nourish the tissues of the body and include glucose, amino acids, and lipids. **Waste products** formed as the byproducts of metabolism and carried by the plasma to be excreted include urea, uric acid, lactic acid, and creatinine. **Respiratory gases** dissolved in and carried by the plasma include carbon dioxide and a small amount of oxygen. Substances present in the plasma that help regulate and control the functions of the body include hormones, antibodies, enzymes, and vitamins.

TUBE SELECTION

At times a plasma specimen may be required for the performance of a laboratory test. The procedure for separating plasma from whole blood is essentially the same as that for separating serum from whole blood with minor variances, which are described here.

A tube containing an anticoagulant must be used to obtain plasma. The medical assistant should check the laboratory directory or the medical office laboratory procedures manual to determine the type of anticoagulant to be used; it is usually specified by the color of the tube stopper. The tube used to collect the specimen *and* the transfer tube should be properly labeled with the patient's name, the date, and the medical assistant's initials. In addition, the transfer tube should bear the word *plasma.*

PREPARATION AND REMOVAL OF THE SPECIMEN

As with serum, a blood specimen must be collected that is 2½ times the amount required for the test. Before collecting the specimen, the vacuum tube should be tapped just below the stopper to release any of the anticoagulant that may have adhered to the stopper. It is important to allow the specimen to fill to the exhaustion of the vacuum to ensure the proper ratio of anticoagulant to blood, which, in turn, will ensure accurate test results.

Immediately after drawing the specimen, invert the tube eight to ten times to mix the anticoagulant with the blood specimen. The specimen is then placed in a centrifuge with the stopper on for 10 to 15 minutes. (The specimen does not need to stand before it is centrifuged.) Centrifuging the specimen packs the blood cells and causes it to separate into three layers: a top layer of plasma, a middle layer termed the buffy coat, and a bottom layer of red blood cells. The plasma is then separated from the blood specimen using the same procedure as that outlined for the separation of serum from whole blood.

On the laboratory request form, the medical assistant should indicate the color of the tube stopper (e.g., lavender, gray, green, or light blue) into which the specimen was originally drawn.

Skin Puncture

A skin puncture is used to obtain a capillary blood specimen and, therefore, is also called a **capillary puncture.** Laboratory testing of a capillary blood specimen is usually done at the medical office. Examples of such tests include: hemoglobin, hematocrit, and glucose using a glucose meter.

The reason for performing a skin puncture rather than a venipuncture is as follows. A skin puncture is performed when a test requires only a small blood specimen. Skin puncture is the method preferred for obtaining blood from infants and very young children. Collecting blood in this age group by venipuncture is difficult and may damage veins and surrounding tissues. In addition, infants and young children have such a small blood volume that removing large quantities of blood may cause anemia. A skin puncture might also be performed as a last resort on an adult when a blood specimen is needed and there are no accessible veins.

Before collecting a capillary blood specimen, the medical assistant must (1) select a puncture site, (2) select the skin puncture device, and, finally, (3) obtain the proper microcollection device to collect the specimen. Each of these topics is described next.

PUNCTURE SITE

☐ The puncture site varies depending on the age of the patient. The fingertip is the preferred site for a skin puncture on an adult. In the past, the earlobe was also recommended as a skin puncture site for an adult. This is no longer true. Blood obtained by puncturing the earlobe has been found to contain a higher concentration of hemoglobin than fingertip blood. In addition the earlobe produces a slower flow of blood, making it more difficult to obtain a blood specimen.

In an infant (birth to one year), the skin puncture should be performed on the plantar surface of the heel or plantar surface of the big toe. A finger puncture should *never* be performed on this age group. The amount of tissue between skin surface and bone is so small that an injury to the bone is very likely. Once a child is walking, the skin puncture should be performed on the finger.

SKIN PUNCTURE DEVICES

☐ A skin puncture can be performed using the following devices: a disposable lancet, a disposable semi-automatic lancet, or a reusable semi-automatic lancet. The device used to perform the skin puncture is a matter of personal preference, while the technique for performing the puncture depends upon the choice of equipment. A description of skin puncture devices is presented next and the procedure for using each of the previously mentioned devices is presented at the end of this section.

Regardless of the skin puncture device used, the depth of the puncture must not penetrate deeper than 3.1 mm on an adults and 2.4 mm on infants and children. If the puncture is deeper than this, the bone may be penetrated, which could result in the painful and serious conditions of osteochondritis or osteomyelitis. **Osteochondritis** is the inflammation of bone and cartilage, and **osteomyelitis** is an inflammation of the bone due to bacterial infection. To avoid these complications, a number of companies manufacture special skin puncture devices that control the depth of puncture as will be described later in this chapter.

DISPOSABLE LANCET

A disposable lancet is a sterile, sharp-pointed device used to pierce the skin (Fig 17–18*A*). The skin puncture is made by pushing the point of the lancet into the skin. A disadvantage to the lancet is that patients may become apprehensive and flinch when they see the point of the lancet coming. Children may even pull their hand out of the medical assistant's grasp. In either case, this could cause the medical assistant to accidentally stick herself or himself.

DISPOSABLE SEMI-AUTOMATIC LANCET

A disposable semi-automatic lancet consists of a spring-loaded plastic holder with a metal blade. Different sized blades are available to control the depth of the puncture. The blade is approximately 1.0 mm wide and produces a small cut that results in a good blood flow. The plastic holder conceals the blade so the patient cannot see the blade during the puncture. An example of one such lancet device is the Microtainer Brand Safety Flow Lancet, manufactured by Becton Dickinson (Fig. 17–18*B*). Another example is the Tenderlette, manufactured by International Technidyne Corporation.

To perform the skin puncture, the lancet device is placed on the patient's skin and a plunger is depressed. The spring forces the blade into the skin followed by retraction of the blade. The concealed blade and automatic puncture tend to result in less patient apprehen-

17

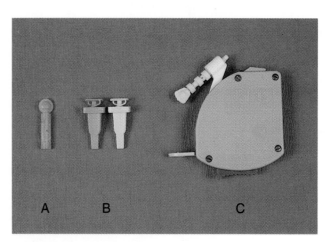

■ **FIGURE 17–18.** Lancet devices. *A*, Disposable lancet. *B*, Microtainer brand safety flow lancet. *C*, Autolet II.

sion. After performing the puncture, the entire lancet device is discarded in a biohazard sharps container. For safety reasons, disposable lancet devices are preferred over other skin puncture devices because not only is the device disposable, but the retractable blade eliminates the possibility of an accidental needlestick.

REUSABLE SEMI-AUTOMATIC LANCET

A wide variety of semi-automatic lancets are commercially available; however, not all are appropriate for use in the medical office. Some of these devices are suitable only for use by an individual patient performing home blood glucose monitoring, and when used on more than one patient in the medical office they have been associated with the transmission of hepatitis B. The safest reusable device is one that can be autoclaved. An example of this is the Autolet II by Ulster Scientific, Inc.

The Autolet II consists of a plastic spring-loaded device containing a lancet and platform (Fig. 17–18C). The plastic device is reusable and the lancet and platform are disposable and meant for only one use. It has a lancet held in place by a spring-loaded arm. When released, the blade penetrates the skin to a depth of 2 to 3 mm, depending on the choice of platform used.

The platform regulates the depth of the puncture. There are two types of platform available: standard and extra puncture. The **standard type** is used for infants, children, and most adults; it produces a puncture to a maximum penetration of 2.4 mm. The **extra puncture** type is used for patients with thick or callused skin; it produces a puncture to a maximum penetration of 3.0 mm. Following the procedure, both the lancet and the platform can be ejected from the reusable holder, which prevents a needlestick injury and possible infection from a contaminated lancet and platform.

MICROCOLLECTION DEVICES

☐ Once the skin has been punctured, a capillary blood specimen must be collected. The blood specimen may simply be collected directly onto a reagent strip such as occurs with blood glucose meters. It may also be collected in a small container known as a **microcollection device.** The device used depends on the laboratory equipment running the test. Common examples of microcollection devices are capillary tubes and microcollection tubes, which are discussed here.

MICROCOLLECTION TUBES. A microcollection tube consists of a small plastic tube with a removable blood

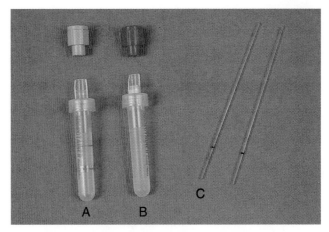

■ **FIGURE 17–19.** Microcollection devices. *A* and *B,* Microcollection tubes. *C,* Capillary tubes.

collector tip. The tip is specially designed to collect capillary blood from a skin puncture and results in a relatively large blood specimen. After collecting the specimen, the collector tip is removed and discarded and replaced by a plastic plug. Microcollection tubes are available with or without additives. The plugs are color-coded and correspond to the colored-coded evacuated tube system used in venipuncture. An example of one such device is the Microtainer by Becton-Dickinson (Fig. 17–19A and B). Other examples include Capiject tubes by Termumo TMG and Samplette capillary blood collectors by Sherwood Medical.

CAPILLARY TUBES. A capillary tube consists of a disposable glass or plastic tube (Fig. 17–19C). Depending on the size of the tube, it can hold between 5 and 75 microliters of blood. In the medical office, a capillary tube is used to collect a blood specimen for performing a hematocrit determination. This procedure is presented in the next chapter.

GUIDELINES FOR PERFORMING A FINGER PUNCTURE

☐ The following guidelines should be followed when performing a finger puncture.

1. If a laboratory test requires advance preparation, be sure to verify that the patient prepared properly before performing the finger puncture. If the patient has not prepared properly, the medical assistant should not collect the specimen unless directed otherwise by the physician. If the finger puncture

is to be rescheduled, the medical assistant should carefully review the preparation requirements with the patient.

2. The patient should be seated comfortably in a chair. The arm should be firmly supported and extended with the palmar surface of the hand facing up. A skin puncture should never be performed with the patient sitting on a stool or in a standing position. The possibility exists that the patient will faint and injure himself or herself.

3. Instruct the patient to remain still and not move during the procedure. Explain to the patient that the procedure should be relatively quick and only slightly uncomfortable. Just before making the puncture, tell the patient that he or she will "feel a small stick." This will help to avoid startling the patient, which could cause the patient to move.

4. Use the lateral part of the tip of the third or fourth fingers (middle and ring fingers) of the non-dominant hand for the puncture site. The capillary bed in these fingers is large and the skin is easy to penetrate. The puncture site should be free of lesions, scars, bruises, or edema. The index finger and the little finger are not recommended as puncture sites. The index finger is more callused and, therefore, harder to penetrate than the other fingers. Also, the patient uses that finger more and will notice the pain longer. The tissue of the little finger is much thinner than that of the others and using this finger as a puncture site could result in an injury to the bone.

5. After the puncture site has been selected, the site may be warmed, to increase the blood flow to the capillary bed. Warming the site can be accomplished by gently massaging the finger five or six times from base to tip or by placing the hand in warm water for a few minutes (108°F or 42°C). Warming the site promotes bleeding after an effective puncture.

6. Cleanse the site with an antiseptic wipe and allow it to dry thoroughly. The site must be dry to allow a round drop of blood to form. Otherwise the drop will leach out on the patient's skin and be difficult to collect. In addition, alcohol entering the capillary specimen contaminates it, leading to inaccurate test results. Alcohol causes the patient to experience a stinging sensation when the puncture is made.

7. Firmly grasp the finger in front of the most distal knuckle joint. The puncturing area should be hard and red so that adequate penetration and depth of puncture can occur.

8. The puncture should be made in the central, fleshy portion of the finger, slightly to the side of center.

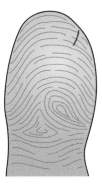

■ **FIGURE 17–20.** Recommended site for a finger puncture.

To avoid an injury to the bone, do not puncture the side or very tip of the finger. The puncture should be performed perpendicular to the lines of the fingerprint rather than parallel to the fingerprint (Fig. 17–20). This facilitates the formation of a well-formed drop of blood that is easy to collect. Punctures that are not perpendicular will be difficult to collect because the blood flow will follow the lines of the fingerprint and run down the finger, making collection difficult.

9. Perform the puncture. If a good puncture has been made, the blood will flow freely. When first learning this procedure, many individuals tend not to press hard enough. If this occurs, a poor blood flow results and the patient has to be punctured again. A deep puncture hurts no more than a superficial one and provides a much better blood flow.

10. Wipe away the first drop of blood with a gauze pad. The first drop of blood is diluted with alcohol and tissue fluid and is not a suitable specimen.

11. Allow a large drop of blood to form by applying continual gentle pressure near the puncture site. Collect the blood specimen using the appropriate microcollection device. If the required amount of blood is not obtained, the tissue surrounding the puncture site can be massaged gently. The area should not be squeezed or massaged excessively because doing so causes dilution of the blood specimen with tissue fluids.

12. Check the puncture site to make sure the bleeding has stopped. An adhesive bandage can be applied, if needed. A bandage is not recommended for children under 2 years of age. The bandage may irritate the skin of a young child, and the child might put the bandage in his or her mouth, aspirate it, and choke.

17

PROCEDURE

17–5

Skin Puncture Using a Disposable Lancet

EQUIPMENT/SUPPLIES:　Disposable gloves　Sterile 2 × 2 gauze pad
Antiseptic wipe　Biohazard sharps container
Disposable lancet

1. **Procedural Step.** Wash the hands.
2. **Procedural Step.** Greet and identify the patient, and introduce yourself. If the patient was required to prepare for the test (e.g., fasting, medication restriction), determine whether he or she has prepared properly. If the patient has not followed the patient preparation requirements, notify the physician for instructions on handling this situation.

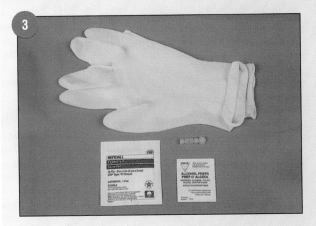

3. **Procedural Step.** Assemble the equipment. Open the sterile gauze packet and place the gauze pad on the inside of its wrapper.
4. **Procedural Step.** Explain the procedure to the patient and reassure the patient.
   Principle. Reassurance should be offered to help reduce apprehension.
5. **Procedural Step.** Seat the patient comfortably in a chair. The patient's arm should be firmly supported and extended with the palmar surface of the hand facing up.

6. **Procedural Step.** Select an appropriate puncture site using the lateral part of the tip of the third or fourth finger of the nondominant hand. If the patient's finger is cold, it can be warmed by gently massaging the finger five or six times from base to tip or by placing the hand in warm water for a few minutes.
   Principle. Warming the site increases the blood flow to the area and promotes bleeding from the puncture site.
7. **Procedural Step.** Cleanse the site with an antiseptic wipe. Allow the site to air dry and do not touch the area after cleansing it or fan the area with your hand.
   Principle. The site must be dry to prevent a stinging sensation when the puncture is made and to allow a round drop of blood to form. Alcohol entering the capillary specimen contaminates it, leading to inaccurate test results. Touching or fanning the site after cleansing contaminates it, and the cleansing process has to be repeated.
8. **Procedural Step.** Apply gloves. Remove the plastic cover from the end of the lancet using a twisting motion; this exposes its sterile point. If the tip becomes contaminated, a new lancet must be obtained.
   Principle. Gloves provide a barrier precaution against bloodborne pathogens.
9. **Procedural Step.** Without touching the puncture site, firmly grasp the patient's finger and make a puncture with the sterile lancet, using a quick jabbing motion. The puncture should be made perpendicular to the lines of the fingerprint and should be approximately 2 to 3 mm deep for an adult. A well-made puncture results in a free-flowing wound that needs only slight pressure to make it bleed.

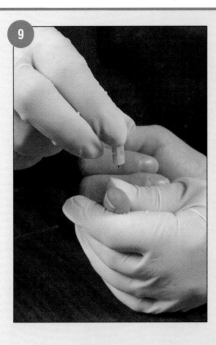

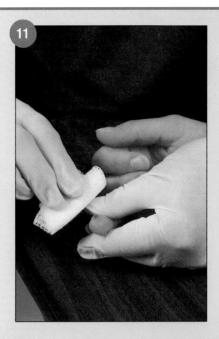

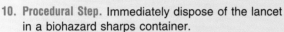

10. **Procedural Step.** Immediately dispose of the lancet in a biohazard sharps container.
   Principle. Proper disposal of contaminated sharps is required by the OSHA Standard to prevent exposure to bloodborne pathogens.

11. **Procedural Step.** Wait a few seconds to allow blood flow to begin. Wipe away the first drop of blood with a gauze pad.
   Principle. The first drop of blood is diluted with alcohol and tissue fluid and is not a suitable specimen.

12. **Procedural Step.** Use the second drop of blood for the test. Allow a large well-rounded drop of blood to form by applying gentle continuous pressure without squeezing the finger. The tissue surround-

ing the puncture site can be massaged firmly but gently to encourage blood flow.
   Principle. Squeezing or massaging the site excessively causes dilution of the blood sample with tissue fluid; inaccurate test readings result.

13. **Procedural Step.** Collect the blood specimen in the appropriate microcollection device.

14. **Procedural Step.** Have the patient hold a gauze pad over the puncture site and apply pressure until the bleeding stops. Remain with the patient until the bleeding stops as a safety precaution. If needed, apply an adhesive bandage.

15. **Procedural Step.** Test the blood specimen as required by the test being performed.

16. **Procedural Step.** Remove the gloves, and wash the hands.

17

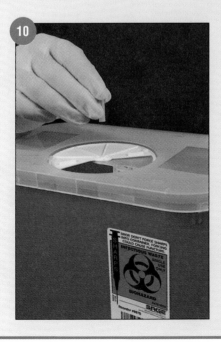

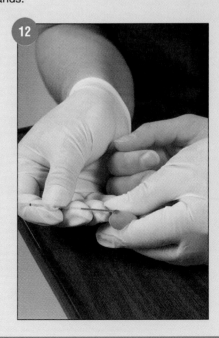

Skin Puncture Using a Disposable Semi-Automatic Lancet Device

EQUIPMENT/SUPPLIES: Disposable gloves
Antiseptic wipe
Microtainer brand safety flow lancet

Sterile 2 × 2 gauze pad
Biohazard sharps container

17

1. **Procedural Step. Follow Steps 1 through 7 of the Disposable Lancet Method of Skin Puncture (Procedure 17–5).**

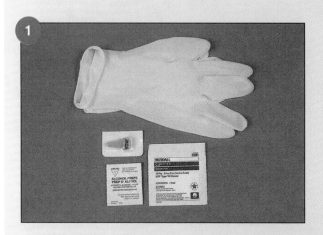

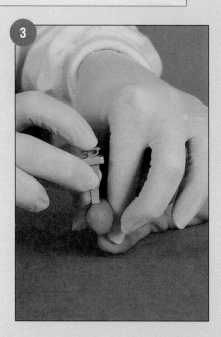

2. **Procedural Step.** Remove the semi-automatic lancet from its plastic packet. The blue (1.9-mm puncture depth) Microtainer lancet should be used for a finger puncture. Apply gloves.
Principle. Gloves provide a barrier precaution against bloodborne pathogens.

3. **Procedural Step.** Without touching the puncture site, firmly grasp the patient's finger. Place the plastic holder on the patient's finger with moderate pressure. The puncture should be made perpendicular to the lines of the fingerprint. Depress the plunger with the index finger. While still holding the lancet on the puncture site, immediately release the plunger. A well-made puncture results in a free-flowing wound that needs only slight pressure to make it bleed.

4. **Procedural Step.** Immediately dispose of the semi-automatic lancet in a biohazard sharps container.
Principle. Proper disposal of contaminated sharps is required by the OSHA Standard to prevent exposure to bloodborne pathogens.

5. **Procedural Step. Follow Steps 11 through 16 of the Disposable Lancet Method of Skin Puncture.**

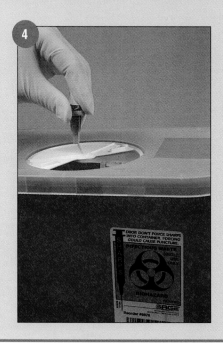

Skin Puncture Using a Reusable Semi-Automatic Lancet Device

EQUIPMENT/SUPPLIES:

Disposable gloves
Antiseptic wipe
Autolet II semi-automatic lancet device
Disposable platform

Sterile lancet
Sterile 2 × 2 gauze pad
Biohazard sharps container

1. **Procedural Step.** Wash the hands.
2. **Procedural Step.** Greet and identify the patient, and introduce yourself. If the patient was required to prepare for the test (e.g., fasting, medication restriction), determine whether he or she has prepared properly. If the patient has not followed the patient preparation requirements, notify the physician for instructions on handling this situation.
3. **Procedural Step.** Assemble the equipment. Pull the spring-loaded arm of the Autolet back toward the activating button until it clicks into position. Once the arm clicks into place, it will be held stationary until the activating button is pressed.

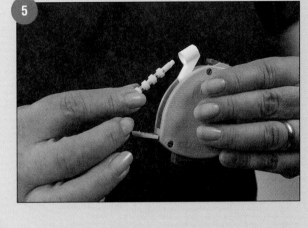

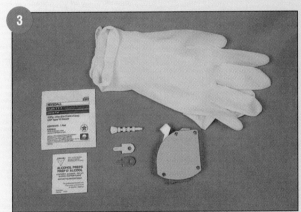

4. **Procedural Step.** Insert the appropriate single-use platform into the proper slot of the Autolet with the flat side up. The standard (yellow) platform is used for children and most adults, and the extra puncture (orange) platform is used for patients with thick or callused skin.
5. **Procedural Step.** Insert the lancet into the lancet socket located at the end of the arm. Push it firmly into place. Open the sterile gauze packet and place the gauze pad on the inside of its wrapper.

6. **Procedural Step.** Explain the procedure to the patient, and reassure the patient.
   Principle. Reassurance should be offered to help reduce apprehension.
7. **Procedural Step.** Seat the patient comfortably in a chair. The patient's arm should be firmly supported and extended with the palmar surface of the hand facing up.
8. **Procedural Step.** Select an appropriate puncture site using the lateral part of the tip of the third or fourth finger of the nondominant hand. If the patient's finger is cold, it can be warmed by gently massaging the finger five or six times from base to tip or by placing the hand in warm water for a few minutes.
   Principle. Warming the site increases the blood flow to the area and promotes bleeding from the puncture site.
9. **Procedural Step.** Cleanse the site with an antiseptic wipe. Allow the site to air dry and do not touch the area after cleansing it or fan the area with your hand.
   Principle. The site must be dry to prevent a stinging sensation when the puncture is made and to allow a round drop of blood to form. Alcohol entering the capillary specimen contaminates it, leading

17

Continued

to inaccurate test results. Touching or fanning the site after cleansing contaminates it, and the cleansing process has to be repeated.

10. **Procedural Step.** Apply gloves. Remove the plastic cover from the end of the lancet using a twisting motion; this exposes its sterile point. If the tip becomes contaminated, a new lancet must be obtained.

    Principle. Gloves provide a barrier precaution against bloodborne pathogens.

11. **Procedural Step.** Without touching the puncture site, firmly grasp the patient's finger. Place the platform firmly against the puncture site so that the tissue protrudes into the hole in the center of the platform. The puncture should be made perpendicular to the lines of the fingerprint.

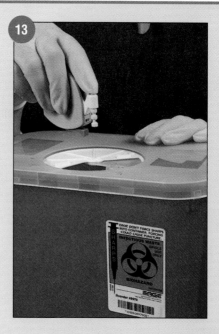

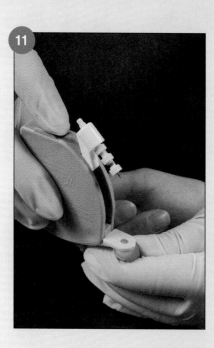

17

12. **Procedural Step.** Press the release button with a slight pressure, which permits the lancet to puncture the skin. A well-made puncture results in a free-flowing wound that needs only slight pressure to make it bleed.

13. **Procedural Step.** Immediately dispose of the platform and lancet into a biohazard sharps container. Eject the platform by pushing the slider forward and letting the platform drop into the biohazard container. Eject the lancet by pushing it out of the socket directly into the biohazard container.

    Principle. Proper disposal of contaminated items is required by the OSHA Standard to prevent exposure to bloodborne pathogens.

14. **Procedural Step.** Wait a few seconds to allow blood

flow to begin. Wipe away the first drop of blood with a gauze pad.

Principle. The first drop of blood is diluted with alcohol and tissue fluid and is not a suitable specimen.

15. **Procedural Step.** Use the second drop of blood for the test. Allow a large well-rounded drop of blood to form by applying gentle continuous pressure without squeezing the finger. The tissue surrounding the puncture site can be massaged firmly but gently to encourage blood flow.

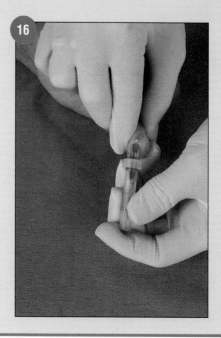

Principle. Squeezing or massaging the site excessively causes dilution of the blood sample with tissue fluid; inaccurate test readings result.

16. **Procedural Step.** Collect the blood specimen in the appropriate microcollection device.

17. **Procedural Step.** Have the patient hold a gauze pad over the puncture site and apply pressure until the bleeding stops. Remain with the patient until the bleeding stops as a safety precaution. If needed, apply an adhesive bandage.

18. **Procedural Step.** Test the blood specimen as required by the test being performed.

19. **Procedural Step.** Remove the gloves, and wash the hands.

20. **Procedural Step.** Sanitize and sterilize the Autolet II according to the medical office policy. The Autolet II should be stored with the arm in its resting position to prolong its lifespan.

MEDICAL PRACTICE AND THE LAW

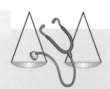

Phlebotomy is an invasive procedure that can result in harm to the patient if performed incorrectly. Sharps and medical waste contaminated with blood must be disposed of according to federal regulations. Laboratory tests involving blood must be performed correctly for accurate results. Incorrect results can lead to an inaccurate diagnosis and treatment. Currently, performing HIV testing requires the patient's written consent. If the patient has questions regarding HIV, refer him or her to the physician for discussion. Never give out laboratory results without checking with the physician. HIV results should be given only by the physician. Never speculate to the patient or coworkers your opinion on the results of any test. All test results must remain confidential.

Use appropriate personal protective equipment to prevent the transmission of bloodborne pathogens to protect yourself, your coworkers, and your patients.

17

CERTIFICATION REVIEW

☐ Phlebotomy is defined as the collection of blood, and the individual collecting the blood sample is known as a phlebotomist. The term venipuncture means the puncturing of a vein for the removal of a venous blood sample. Venipuncture can be performed by the following methods: vacuum tube, butterfly, and syringe.

☐ The antecubital space is generally used as the site for drawing blood. The antecubital veins typically have a wide lumen, are easily accessible, and are close to the surface of the skin. The best vein to use in the antecubital space is the median cubital. The basilic and cephalic veins are located on either side of the antecubital space and are considered a second alternative when the median cubital vein is not available.

☐ The various types of blood specimen that the medical assistant will be required to obtain through the venipuncture procedure include clotted blood, serum, whole blood, and plasma. The blood specimen should be handled carefully at all times. Blood cells are fragile and rough handling may cause hemolysis. Hemolyzed blood specimens produce inaccurate test results.

☐ The vacuum tube method is frequently used to collect venous blood specimens. Vacuum tube needles are available in sizes 20 to 22 gauge and come in two lengths: 1 inch and 1½ inch. Evacuated tubes consist of a glass tube with a rubber stopper and contain a vacuum to pull the blood specimen into the tube. Evacuated tubes use a color-coded system to identify their additive content.

☐ The butterfly method of venipuncture is also called the winged infusion method. It is used to collect blood from patients who are difficult to stick by conventional methods, such as adult patients with small antecubital veins and children.

☐ The syringe method is the least used method of venipuncture. This is because once the blood specimen is obtained, it must be transferred from the syringe to an evacuated tube, which presents the risk of an accidental needlestick. The syringe method is primarily used to obtain blood from small veins.

☐ Plasma is the straw-colored liquid portion of the blood. It serves as a transportation medium in which various substances are dissolved in blood and in which blood cells are suspended for circulation through the body. Approximately 92 percent of plasma consists of water; the remaining 8 percent is dissolved solid substances that are carried by the blood to and from the tissues.

☐ A skin puncture is used to obtain a capillary blood specimen. A skin puncture is performed when a test requires only a small blood specimen. Also, skin puncture is the method preferred for obtaining blood from infants and very young children. The fingertip is the preferred site for a skin puncture on an adult.

☐ Once the skin has been punctured, a capillary blood specimen must be collected. The blood specimen may be collected directly onto a reagent strip or it may be collected in a microcollection device. Examples of microcollection devices are capillary tubes and microcollection tubes.

17

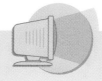

ON THE WEB

RESOURCES

For information on phlebotomy:

American Society for Clinical
Laboratory Science
(ASCLS)
www.ascls.org

American Society of Clinical
Pathologists (ASCP)
www.ascp.org

American Society of Phlebotomy Technicians (ASPT)
www.aspt.org

Becton Dickinson
www.bd.com

National Phlebotomy Association (NPA)
www.scpt.com/npa.htm

17

Hematology

Latisha Sharpe, *and I am a Certified Medical Assistant. I graduated from an accredited medical assisting program and have an associate's degree in Applied Science. I work in a multi-physician office as a laboratory technician. I have worked in the office for 2 years. My job duties include venipuncture, preparing blood for transport to an outside laboratory, operating laboratory equipment, and performing laboratory tests.*

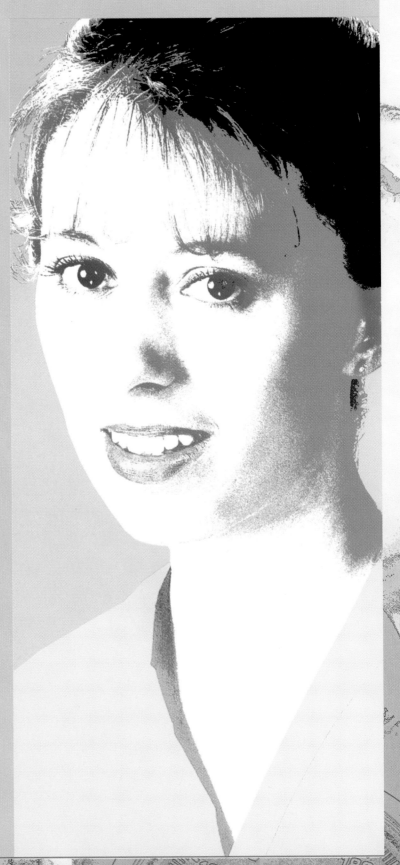

OUTCOMES

After completing this unit, you should be able to demonstrate the proper procedures to perform the following:

1. Perform a hemoglobin determination using an automated analyzer and instruction manual.
2. Perform a hematocrit determination.
3. Perform a white blood cell count using an automated blood cell counter and an instruction manual.
4. Prepare a blood smear.

EDUCATIONAL OBJECTIVES

After completing the unit, you should be able to do the following:

1. Define the terms listed in the Key Terminology.
2. List the tests included in a complete blood count (CBC).
3. Describe the shape of an erythrocyte and explain how it acquires this shape.
4. Describe the composition of hemoglobin and explain its function.
5. Describe the normal appearance of leukocytes and explain how they work to fight infection in the body.
6. State the normal value or range for each of the following hematologic tests: hemoglobin, hematocrit, red and white blood cell counts, and the differential cell count.
7. State the purpose of the hematocrit, and list the layers the blood separates into after it has been centrifuged to obtain a hematocrit reading.
8. Explain the purpose of the differential cell count, and list and describe the appearance of each of the five types of white blood cells.

INTRODUCTION

18

☐ Hematology involves the study of blood, including the morphologic appearance, function, and diseases of the blood and blood-forming tissues. Laboratory analysis in hematology is concerned with the examination of blood for the purpose of detecting pathologic conditions. It includes performing blood cell counts, evaluating the clotting ability of the blood, and identifying cell types. These tests are valuable tools that allow the physician to determine whether each of the blood components falls within its normal value or range.

Examples of hematologic tests include the white blood cell count, red blood cell count, differential white blood cell count, hemoglobin, hematocrit, prothrombin time, erythrocyte sedimentation rate, and platelet count. Table 18–1 summarizes common hematologic tests, including specimen requirements, normal values, and conditions leading to abnormal test results.

Hematologic laboratory tests are often performed in the medical office. Advances in automated blood analyzers specially designed for use in the medical office have made this possible. Automated blood analyzers perform laboratory tests in a very short period of time with accurate test results. Each automated analyzer is accompanied by a detailed instruction manual explaining its operation, test parameters, care, and maintenance.

The most frequently performed hematologic laboratory test is the **complete blood count (CBC)**. A CBC is routinely performed on new patients and on patients with a pathologic condition. The test results provide valuable information to assist the physician in making a diagnosis, evaluating the patient's progress, and regulating treatment. The tests included in a CBC are as follows:

- White blood cell count (WBC count)
- Red blood cell count (RBC count)
- Platelet count
- Hemoglobin (Hgb)
- Hematocrit (Hct)
- Differential white blood cell count (Diff)
- Red blood cell indices

COMPONENTS AND FUNCTION OF BLOOD

☐ Blood consists of two parts: liquid and solid. The liquid portion of the blood, consisting of a clear yellowish fluid, is known as the **plasma** and makes up approximately 55 percent of the total blood volume. The function of the plasma is to transport nutrients to the tissues of the body to nourish and sustain them. The plasma picks up wastes from the tissues, and the wastes are eliminated through the kidneys. The plasma also transports antibodies, enzymes, and hormones to help regulate normal body functioning.

Common Hematologic Tests

TABLE 18-1

Name of Test and Specimen Requirement	Abbreviation	Purpose	Normal Range	Increased With	Decreased With
White blood cell count (whole blood)	WBC	Used to assist in the diagnosis and prognosis of disease	4,500–11,000/mm³ (SI Units: 4.5–11.0 cells × 10⁹/L)	**Leukocytosis** Acute infections (appendicitis, chickenpox, diphtheria, infectious mononucleosis, meningitis, pneumonia, rheumatic fever, smallpox, tonsillitis) Hemorrhaging Trauma Malignant disease Leukemia Polycythemia vera	**Leukopenia** Viral infections Hypersplenism Bone marrow depression Infectious hepatitis Cirrhosis Chemotherapy Radiation therapy
Red blood cell count (whole blood)	RBC	Used to assist in the diagnosis of anemia and polycythemia	Male: 4.5–6.2 million/mm³, or 10¹² cells/L Female: 4–5.5 million/mm³, or 10¹² cells/L MCV 81–99 μm³ MCH 27.0–31.0 pg MCHC 32.0–36.0%	Polycythemia vera Secondary polycythemia Severe diarrhea Dehydration Acute poisoning Pulmonary fibrosis Severe burns	Iron-deficiency anemia Hodgkin's disease Multiple myeloma Leukemia Hemolytic anemia Pernicious anemia Lupus erythematosus Addison's disease
Differential white blood cell count (fresh whole blood)	Diff	Used to assist in the diagnosis and prognosis of disease	Neutrophils 50–70% Eosinophils 1–4% Basophils 0–1% Lymphocytes 20–35% Monocytes 3–8%	**Neutrophilia** Acute bacterial infections Parasitic infections Liver disease **Eosinophilia** Allergic conditions Parasitic infections Addison's disease Lung and bone cancer	**Neutropenia** Acute viral infections Blood diseases Hormone diseases Chemotherapy **Eosinopenia** Infectious mononucleosis Hypersplenism Congestive heart failure Aplastic and pernicious anemia

Continued

619

TABLE 18-1

Common Hematologic Tests *Continued*

Name of Test and Specimen Requirement	Abbreviation	Purpose	Normal Range	Increased With	Decreased With
Differential white blood cell count (fresh whole blood) *(Continued)*				***Basophilia*** Leukemia Chronic inflammation Polycythemia vera Hemolytic anemia Hodgkin's disease ***Lymphocytosis*** Acute and chronic infections Hematopoietic disorders Addison's disease Carcinoma Hyperthyroidism ***Monocytosis*** Viral infections Bacterial and parasitic infections Collagen diseases Cirrhosis Polycythemia vera	***Basopenia*** Acute allergic reactions Hyperthyroidism Steroid therapy ***Lymphopenia*** HIV infection Cardiac failure Cushing's disease Hodgkin's disease Leukemia ***Monocytopenia*** Prednisone treatment Hairy cell leukemia
Hemoglobin (whole blood)	Hgb	Used to screen for the presence and severity of anemia and to monitor the response to treatment	Male: 14–18 g/dl (SI Units: 2.17–2.79 mmol/L) Female: 12–16 g/dl (SI Units: 1.86–2.48 mmol/L)	Polycythemia Severe burns Chronic obstructive pulmonary disease Congestive heart failure	Anemia Hyperthyroidism Cirrhosis Severe hemorrhage Hemolytic reactions Hodgkin's disease Leukemia
Hematocrit (whole blood)	Hct, HCT	Assists in the diagnosis and evaluation of anemia	Male: 40–54% Female: 37–47%	Polycythemia vera Severe dehydration Shock Severe burns	Anemia Leukemia Hyperthyroidism Cirrhosis Acute blood loss Hemolytic reactions

Test	Reference Values	Description		
Prothrombin time (whole blood) — PT	11–16 sec	Used to screen for the presence of coagulation disorders and to regulate treatment of patients on oral anticoagulant therapy with warfarin sodium (Coumadin)	***Thrombocytosis*** Prothrombin deficiency, Vitamin K deficiency, Hemorrhagic disease of the newborn, Liver disease, Anticoagulant therapy, Biliary obstruction, Acute leukemia, Polycythemia vera	***Thrombocytopenia*** Acute thrombophlebitis, Diuretics, Multiple myeloma, Pulmonary embolism, Vitamin K therapy
Erythrocyte sedimentation rate (whole blood) — ESR	Westergren's method Male: <50 yr, 0–15 mm/hr; ≥50 yr, 0–20 mm/hr Female: <50 yr, 0–20 mm/hr; ≥50 yr, 0–30 mm/hr	Used as a nonspecific test for connective tissue diseases, malignancy, and infectious diseases. Also used to evaluate the progress of inflammatory diseases. (Elevated test results warrant further testing)	Collagen diseases, Infections, Inflammatory diseases, Carcinoma, Cell or tissue destruction, Rheumatoid arthritis	Polycythemia vera, Sickle cell anemia, Congestive heart failure
Platelet count (whole blood)	150,000–400,000/mm^3 (SI Units: 150–400 $\times 10^9$/L)	Assists in the evaluation of bleeding disorders that occur with liver disease, thrombocytopenia, uremia, and anticoagulant therapy	***Thrombocytosis*** Cancer, Leukemia, Polycythemia vera, Splenectomy, Acute blood loss, Rheumatoid arthritis, Trauma (fractures, surgery)	***Thrombocytopenia*** Pernicious anemia, Aplastic anemia, Hemolytic anemia, Pneumonia, Allergic conditions, Infection, Bone marrow–depressant drugs

18

The solid portion of the blood consists of three different types of cells: erythrocytes, leukocytes, and thrombocytes, which are described next in detail. The solid portion of the blood accounts for 45 percent of the total blood volume. The average adult body contains 10 to 12 pints (5 to 6 liters) of blood.

ERYTHROCYTES

In the adult, erythrocytes, or red blood cells, are formed in the red bone marrow of the ribs, sternum, skull, and pelvic bone and in the ends of the long bones of the limbs. The immature form of an erythrocyte contains a nucleus. As the cell develops and matures, however, it loses its nucleus and therefore acquires the shape of a biconcave disc, thicker at the rim than at the center. This shape provides the erythrocyte with a greater surface area for the exchange of substances. An erythrocyte is approximately 7 to 8 micrometers in diameter. The average number of erythrocytes in the adult female ranges from 4 to 5.5 million per cubic millimeter of blood and in the adult male from 4.5 to 6.2 million per cubic millimeter of blood.

A major portion of the erythrocyte consists of a complex compound called **hemoglobin,** which functions to transport oxygen and is also responsible for the red color of the erythrocyte. The amount of hemoglobin in the blood averages 12 to 16 g per 100 ml (or g/dl) for the adult female and 14 to 18 g per 100 ml for the adult male. A hemoglobin molecule consists of a globin or protein part and an iron-containing pigment called heme. One hemoglobin molecule loosely combines with four oxygen molecules in the lungs to form a substance called **oxyhemoglobin.** Oxyhemoglobin is transported and distributed to the tissues, where the oxygen is easily released from the hemoglobin. The blood then picks up carbon dioxide, a waste product, and transports it back to the lungs to be expelled. When oxygen combines with hemoglobin, a bright red color results that is characteristic of arterial blood. Venous blood has a darker red color, owing to its lower oxygen content.

The average life span of a red blood cell is 120 days. Toward the end of this time, it becomes more and more fragile and eventually ruptures and breaks down; this process is known as **hemolysis.** Hemoglobin, liberated from the red blood cell, also breaks down. The iron is stored and later reused to form new hemoglobin, and the protein is metabolized by the body. **Bilirubin** is formed from metabolism of the

heme units and transported to the liver, where it is eventually excreted as a waste product in the bile.

LEUKOCYTES

Leukocytes, or white blood cells, are clear, colorless cells that contain a nucleus. The average number of leukocytes in the adult ranges from 4,500 to 11,000 per cubic millimeter of blood. **Leukocytosis** is the name given to the condition of an abnormal increase in the number of leukocytes (more than 11,000 per cubic millimeter), and the term **leukopenia** is used to describe an abnormal decrease in the number of leukocytes (below 4,500 per cubic millimeter).

The function of leukocytes is to defend the body against infection. Pathogens may gain entrance to the body in a variety of ways (review the Infection Process Cycle in Chapter 1). Leukocytes attempt to destroy the invading pathogens and remove them from the body. Unlike erythrocytes, leukocytes do their work in the tissues; they are transported to the site of infection by the circulatory system. During inflammation, the blood vessels in the infected area dilate, resulting in an increased blood supply. More oxygen, nutrients, and white blood cells can then be delivered to the infected area to aid in the healing process. The cells making up the wall of the capillaries spread apart, enlarging the pores between the cells. White blood cells squeeze through the pores by ameboid movement and move out into the tissues to fight the infection. This movement of the leukocytes through the pores of the capillaries and out into the tissues is known as **diapedesis.**

Leukocytes (especially the granular forms) are phagocytic, and once they arrive at the site of infection they begin engulfing and destroying the pathogens and damaged cells through a process known as **phagocytosis.** In some conditions pus may form in the infected area (suppuration); pus contains dead leukocytes, dead bacteria, and dead tissue cells.

THROMBOCYTES

Platelets, also known as thrombocytes, are small and clear and shaped like discs. They lack a nucleus and are formed in the red bone marrow from giant cells known as megakaryocytes. Platelets function by participating in the blood-clotting mechanism. The average number of platelets in the adult is 150,000 to 400,000 per cubic millimeter of blood.

18

HEMOGLOBIN DETERMINATION

☐ Hemoglobin (abbreviated Hgb or Hb) is a major component of red blood cells. Hemoglobin functions to transport oxygen to the tissue cells of the body and is also responsible for the red color of the red blood cell.

The hemoglobin determination is used to measure indirectly the oxygen-carrying capacity of the blood. The normal range for the adult woman is 12 to 16 g per 100 ml, and the normal range for the adult man is 14 to 18 g per 100 ml (or g/dl). A hemoglobin determination may be performed as an individual test or as part of the CBC. A hemoglobin determination is often performed as a routine test on individuals at risk for developing anemia, such as children under 2 years of age and pregnant women.

A decreased hemoglobin level occurs with anemia (especially iron-deficiency anemia), hyperthyroidism, cirrhosis of the liver, severe hemorrhaging, hemolytic reactions, and certain systemic diseases such as leukemia and Hodgkin's disease. Increased levels of hemoglobin are present with polycythemia, chronic obstructive pulmonary disease (COPD), and congestive heart failure.

The hemoglobin determination may be performed on either capillary blood or venous blood. The most accurate and reliable method for measuring hemoglobin concentration involves the use of a blood analyzer. A blood analyzer permits the processing of the specimen in a short period of time, allowing the physician to evaluate the patient's condition while still at the medical office.

HEMATOCRIT

☐ The hematocrit (abbreviated Hct) is a simple, reliable, and informative test that is frequently performed in the medical office. The word hematocrit means "to separate blood." The solid or cellular elements are separated from the plasma by centrifuging an anticoagulated blood specimen. The heavier red blood cells become packed and settle to the bottom of a tube. The top layer contains the clear, straw-colored plasma. Between the plasma and the packed red blood cells is a small, thin, yellowish-gray layer known as the **buffy coat,** which contains the platelets and white blood cells (Fig. 18–1).

The purpose of the hematocrit is to measure the percentage volume of packed red blood cells in whole

18

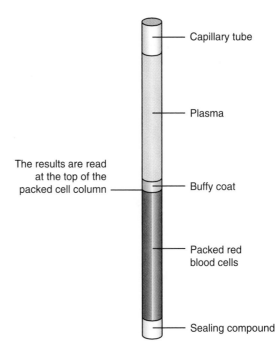

The results are read at the top of the packed cell column — Buffy coat

Capillary tube
Plasma
Packed red blood cells
Sealing compound

■ **FIGURE 18–1.** Hematocrit test results. The cellular elements are separated from the plasma by centrifuging an anticoagulated blood specimen, and the results are read at the top of the packed cell column.

blood. The normal hematocrit range for the adult woman is 37 to 47 percent and for the adult man is 40 to 54 percent. A low hematocrit reading may indicate **anemia,** whereas a high reading may indicate **polycythemia.** The hematocrit, used in conjunction with other hematologic tests, is useful as an aid to the physician in the diagnosis of a patient's condition. The hematocrit is also used as a screening measure for the early detection of anemia and therefore is often included as part of a general physical examination.

The microhematocrit method is most often utilized in the medical office to perform a hematocrit determination. Through capillary action, blood is drawn directly from a free-flowing skin puncture into a disposable capillary tube lined with an anticoagulant. An anticoagulated blood specimen collected by other means such as venipuncture can also be used. The microhematocrit centrifuge spins the blood at an extremely high speed and requires only 3 to 5 minutes (as designated by the manufacturer) to pack the red blood cells. The results are then read at the top of the packed cell column.

PROCEDURE

18–1

Hematocrit

EQUIPMENT/SUPPLIES: **Personal protective equipment, including disposable gloves**
Lancet
Antiseptic wipe
Gauze pads
Capillary tubes
Sealing compound
Microhematocrit centrifuge
Biohazard sharps container

1. **Procedural Step.** Assemble the equipment. Wash the hands, and put on personal protective equipment, including gloves.
2. **Procedural Step.** Greet and identify the patient. Introduce yourself, and explain the procedure. Perform a finger puncture and dispose of the lancet in a biohazard sharps container.
   Principle. Personal protective equipment and proper disposal of the lancet are required by the OSHA Standard to prevent exposure to blood-borne pathogens.
3. **Procedural Step.** Wipe away the first drop of blood with a gauze pad. Fill the capillary tube by holding one end of it horizontally, but slightly downward, next to the free-flowing puncture. Keep the tip of the capillary tube in the blood, but do not allow it to press against the skin of the patient's finger.
   Calibrated tubes are filled to the calibration line, whereas uncalibrated tubes are filled approximately three quarters (within 10 to 20 mm of the end of the tube). The blood will be drawn into the

tube through capillary action. Fill a second tube using the method just described.

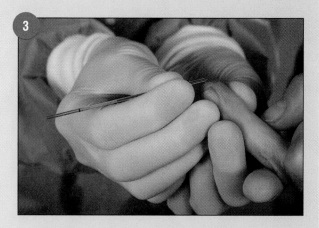

Principle. Not keeping the tip of the capillary tube in the blood may result in air bubbles in the stem of the tube, which lead to inaccurate test results. Allowing the capillary tube to press against the skin will close off the opening of the capillary tubes and not allow blood to enter the capillary tubes.

The type of tube used (calibrated or uncalibrated) is based on the method used to read the test results. The hematocrit should be performed in duplicate to ensure accurate and reliable test results.

4. **Procedural Step.** Seal one end of each tube with a small amount of putty or a commercially prepared sealing compound (e.g., Critoseal, Hemato-Seal).

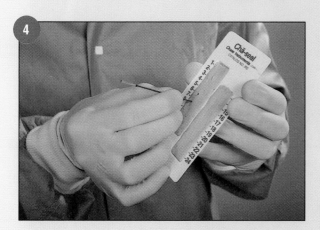

Principle. The capillary tubes must be properly sealed to prevent leakage of the blood specimen during centrifugation.

5. **Procedural Step.** Place the capillary tubes in the microhematocrit centrifuge with the sealed end facing the outside. Balance one tube with the other capillary tube placed on the opposite side of the centrifuge.

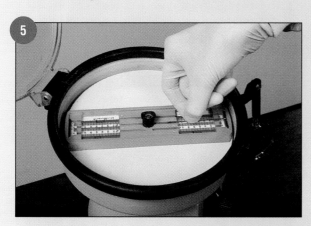

Principle. Placing the sealed end toward the outside prevents the blood specimen from spinning out of the capillary tube when the centrifuge is in operation.

6. **Procedural Step.** Place the cover on the centrifuge and lock it securely. Centrifuge the blood specimen for 3 to 5 minutes at a speed of 10,000 rpm. **Principle.** Centrifuging the blood specimen causes the red blood cells to become packed and to settle on the bottom of the tube.

7. **Procedural Step.** Allow the centrifuge to come to a complete stop. Read the results, as follows:

Calibrated Tube. If a capillary tube with a calibration line was used, the results are read using the special graphic reading device that is con-

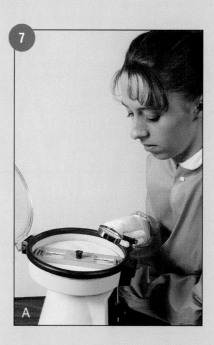

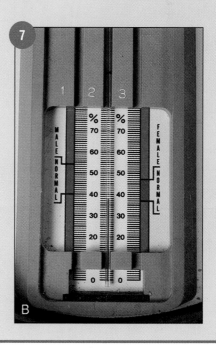

18

PROCEDURE 18–1

tained as part of the centrifuge. Adjust the capillary tube so that the bottom of the red blood cell column (just above the sealing compound) is placed on the 0 line. The results are read at the top of the packed red blood cell column, using a magnifying glass, and are read directly as a percentage on the reading device.

Uncalibrated Tube. If an uncalibrated tube was used, a microhematocrit reader card must be used to determine the results; the top of the plasma column is placed on the 100 percent mark and the bottom of the cell column is placed on the 0 line. The results are read on the scale, which corresponds to the top of the packed cell column.

In both cases, the buffy coat should not be included in the reading. The answer represents the percentage of the total volume of blood occupied by the red blood cells. (The hematocrit determination on this reading device is 38.)

Principle. Stopping the centrifuge by using the hands may injure the medical assistant and may also damage the machine.

8. Procedural Step. Read the second tube in the manner just described; the results of the tubes should agree within 4 percentage points. If not, the hematocrit procedure must be repeated. If they are within 4 percentage points, the two values are averaged together to derive the test results.

9. Procedural Step. Properly dispose of the capillary tubes in a biohazard sharps container. Remove personal protective equipment, including gloves, and wash the hands. Chart the results. Include the date and time and the hematocrit results.

10. Procedural Step. Return the equipment.

CHARTING EXAMPLE

Date	
5/5/2002	11:15 a.m. Hct: 38%. ———L. Sharpe, CMA

18

PATIENT/TEACHING

IRON-DEFICIENCY ANEMIA

■ Answer questions patients have about iron-deficiency anemia:

What Is Anemia?

Anemia is a shortage of red blood cells or hemoglobin. Hemoglobin is the part of the blood that gives red blood cells their color and carries oxygen to all the cells in the body. There are many different types of anemia; of these, iron-deficiency anemia by far is the most common. Other types of anemia include pernicious anemia, sickle cell anemia, hemolytic anemia, and aplastic anemia.

What Causes Iron-Deficiency Anemia?

In general, iron-deficiency anemia is caused by conditions that deplete the iron that is stored in the body such as from an increased need for iron by the body or an increased loss of iron from the body. Iron-deficiency anemia may occur in children under 2 years of age if there is not enough iron in their diet to meet their demands of rapid growth. This is especially true in children whose main source of nutrition during these years is breast milk or bottle milk, because milk does not naturally contain iron. Adolescent girls are prone to iron-deficiency anemia because of their growth spurts during puberty, along with the added loss from menstruation. In adults, the most common cause of anemia is chronic blood loss such as a bleeding ulcer or hemorrhoids or from heavy menstrual bleeding. Pregnant women are also at increased risk because of the demands of the growing baby.

What Can Be Done for Individuals Who Are at Risk for Developing Iron-Deficiency Anemia?

Individuals prone to developing iron-deficiency anemia are encouraged to increase foods in their diet that contain iron, such as beef, liver, spinach, eggs, and iron-fortified breads and cereals. As a preventive measure, the physician usually prescribes vitamin supplements for individuals who are at increased risk for developing iron-deficiency anemia, such as pregnant women, infants, and young children. Also, infant formulas and cereals are available that have been supplemented with iron.

What Are the Symptoms of Anemia?

All types of anemia have the same general symptoms. Often these symptoms do not develop right away and when they do develop, feeling tired and run down may be the only sign that anemia is present. Other symp-

What Are the Symptoms of Anemia?

toms that may occur, particularly as the anemia becomes worse, are paleness of the skin, fingernail beds, and mucous membranes; shortness of breath, especially during physical activity; dizziness; headache; irritability; and inability to concentrate. These symptoms result from the diminished ability of the blood to carry oxygen to the cells of the body. Blood tests are necessary to diagnose anemia and to determine the specific type of anemia present.

How Is Iron-Deficiency Anemia Treated?

The most important part of treating anemia is to determine what is causing it and to correct that condition—such as not enough iron being consumed in the diet or chronic blood loss. An iron supplement is usually prescribed by the physician to replace the iron that has been depleted from the body. It is generally prescribed in oral form, but it also may be given through an injection in special situations. An oral iron supplement causes the stool to turn black or green. This is

normal and should not be a cause for concern. Also, an effort should be made to consume foods high in iron content.

- For patients who have had a vitamin supplement prescribed to *prevent* iron-deficiency anemia, such as children under 2 years of age and pregnant women: Emphasize the importance to the patient of taking the vitamin supplement each day to prevent the development of iron-deficiency anemia.
- For patients who have had an iron supplement prescribed to *treat* iron-deficiency anemia: Emphasize to the patient the importance of taking the iron supplement for the period of time prescribed by the physician, since replacement of iron takes time.
- Instruct the patient to keep iron supplements out of the reach of children to prevent iron poisoning.
- Provide the patient with written educational materials on anemia.

WHITE BLOOD CELL COUNT

☐ The white blood cell count (WBC) is used by the physician to assist in the diagnosis and prognosis of disease. The white blood cell count is an approximate measurement of the total number of white blood cells in the circulating blood. The normal range for a white blood count is 4,500 to 11,000 white blood cells per cubic millimeter of blood, which is expressed as 4.5 to 11.0 ($\times 10^3/mm^3$) on laboratory reports. An increase in the white blood count, or **leukocytosis,** is most commonly seen in acute infection such as appendicitis, chickenpox, diphtheria, infectious mononucleosis, meningitis, and rheumatic fever. A normal elevation in the white blood cell count can occur with pregnancy, strenuous exercise, stress, and treatment with corticosteroids. Conditions resulting in **leukopenia,** or a decrease in the white blood cell count, include viral infections and chemotherapy and radiation therapy treatments.

If the white blood cell count is performed in the medical office, a blood cell counter is used. Blood cell counters are also able to perform a red blood count, platelet count, hemoglobin, hematocrit, differential white blood cell count, and calculation of red blood cell indices. Examples of blood cell counters include the Coulter (Coulter Company) (Fig. 18–2), the B-D-Q-BC (Becton-Dickenson), and the Cell-Dyn (Abbott).

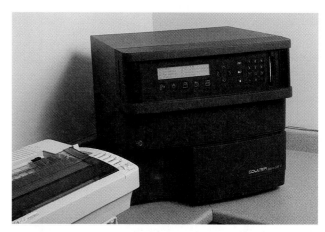

■ **FIGURE 18–2.** Coulter blood cell counter.

18

RED BLOOD CELL COUNT

☐ The red blood cell (RBC) count is a measurement of the total number of red blood cells in whole blood. The normal range for the red blood count in the adult woman is 4 to 5.5 million red blood cells per cubic millimeter of blood, expressed as 4.0–5.5 ($\times 10^6/mm^3$) on laboratory reports. The normal range for the adult man is 4.5 to 6.2 million red blood cells per cubic millimeter of blood, expressed as 4.5–6.2 ($\times 10^6/mm^3$)

PUTTING IT ALL *into* PRACTICE

▶ **LATISHA SHARPE:** *When I first started working in a physician's office, the patients were a bit apprehensive about someone new drawing their blood. It made me a little nervous since they were questioning my ability to perform the procedure. I explained to the patients that I had the proper training and showed that I was confident I could perform the procedure with success. By doing this, I gained their trust. Before long, they were requesting that I draw their blood.*

on a laboratory report. In the medical office, the red blood count is performed using a blood cell counter.

Conditions that cause a decrease in the red blood cell count include anemia, Hodgkin's disease, and leukemia; conditions that cause an increase include polycythemia, dehydration, and pulmonary fibrosis.

WHITE BLOOD CELL DIFFERENTIAL COUNT

☐ There are five types of white blood cells, or leukocytes, each having a certain size, shape, appearance, and function (Fig. 18–3). The purpose of the differential cell count is to identify the five types of white blood cells present in a representative blood sample. An increase or decrease in one or more types may occur in pathologic conditions, which assists the physician in making a diagnosis.

The differential cell count can be performed automatically or manually. The automatic method is faster and more convenient and, because of this, is growing in popularity. Both of these methods are described next.

AUTOMATIC METHOD. The automatic method involves the use of a blood cell counter such as the Coulter cell counter (see Fig. 18–2). The specimen requirement is an EDTA-anticoagulated blood specimen, which is obtained through venipuncture using a lavender tube. The blood cell counter automatically performs the dif-

ferential cell count, and the results are printed out on a laboratory report.

MANUAL METHOD. The manual method requires that the medical assistant make two peripheral blood smears. The procedure for preparing a blood smear is outlined in Procedure 18–2. Fresh whole blood is preferred for making the blood smears; however, a satisfactory smear may be made from an EDTA-anticoagulated blood specimen, provided the smear is made within 2 hours after collection. Other anticoagulants should not be used, since they may alter the morphology and staining reaction of the white blood cells. After preparing the blood smear, the medical assistant places the slides in a protective container for transportation to an outside laboratory. The blood smear is evaluated at the laboratory by medical laboratory personnel. Because white blood cells are clear and colorless, they must be stained first with an appropriate dye (usually Wright's stain) before performing a differential count. The nucleus, cytoplasm, and any granules present in the cytoplasm take on the characteristic color of their cell type, which aids in proper identification. A minimum of 100 white blood cells is identified on the blood smear, and each is assigned to its appropriate category (neutrophil, eosinophil, basophil, lymphocyte, and monocyte). The number of each type of leukocyte is recorded as a percentage and reflects the overall distribution of the white blood cells present in the patient's bloodstream.

TYPES OF WHITE BLOOD CELLS

Leukocytes are classified into two major categories—granular and nongranular. **Granular leukocytes** contain distinct granules in the cytoplasm and include neutrophils, eosinophils, and basophils. **Nongranular leukocytes** contain few or no granules in the cytoplasm and include lymphocytes and monocytes. Each of the five types of white blood cells is described here, along with their staining reaction to Wright's stain.

The **neutrophils** are the most numerous of the white blood cells. They have a purple, multilobed nucleus that may contain from three to five lobes or segments; therefore, they are also known as "segs." The cytoplasm of a neutrophil stains a faint pink and contains many fine granules that stain a violet-pink. Neutrophils exhibit a high degree of ameboid movement and are actively phagocytic. Immature forms of leukocytes are known as **bands** or **stabs** and can be identified by their curved, nonsegmented nucleus. Normally, from zero to five of the neutrophils present will be in the immature band form. When the percentage

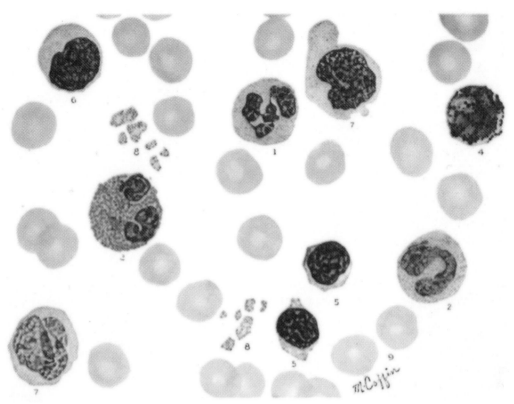

FIGURE 18-3. Types of human blood cells. 1 to 7, White cells (or leukocytes) stained as they are in the laboratory to show the many different types. They play the active role in immune response, or in defense against disease. (1, neutrophil; 2, neutrophilic band; 3, eosinophil; 4, basophil; 5, lymphocyte; 6 Lange lymphocyte; 7, monocyte). 8, Platelets (thrombocytes), which are responsible for clotting. 9, Red blood cells (erythrocytes), which carry oxygen. (From Custer. R.P.: *An Atlas of the Blood and Bone Marrow,* 2nd ed. Philadelphia, W.B. Saunders, 1974.)

18

of band forms increases, this condition is often referred to as a "shift to the left." An increase in the number of neutrophils, including band forms, is generally seen during an acute infection.

Eosinophils contain a segmented nucleus, generally of no more than two lobes. Large granules are found in the cytoplasm; these stain a bright reddish-orange. An increase in eosinophils is often seen in allergic conditions and parasitic infestations.

Basophils are the least numerous of the white blood cells and contain an S-shaped nucleus. The cytoplasm contains large, coarse, dark bluish-black granules that almost completely obscure the details of the nucleus.

Lymphocytes are the smallest of the white blood cells. They have a round or slightly indented nucleus that almost completely fills the cell and stains a deep purplish blue. There is a small rim of sky-blue cytoplasm around the nucleus that contains few or no granules. Lymphocytes are involved with the immune system and the production of antibodies. An increase

in lymphocytes generally occurs with certain viral diseases, including infectious mononucleosis, mumps, chickenpox, rubella, and viral hepatitis.

Monocytes are the largest of the white blood cells and have a large nucleus that is usually kidney- or horseshoe-shaped but may be round or oval. They contain abundant cytoplasm that stains grayish blue.

Normal Range

The normal adult range for each type of white blood cell making up the total number of leukocytes is listed here:

Neutrophils	50 to 70 percent
Eosinophils	1 to 4 percent
Basophils	0 to 1 percent
Lymphocytes	20 to 35 percent
Monocytes	3 to 8 percent

PROCEDURE

18–2

Preparation of a Blood Smear for a Differential Cell Count

EQUIPMENT/SUPPLIES: Personal protective equipment, including disposable gloves
Supplies to perform a finger puncture or venipuncture
Slides with a frosted edge
Slide container
Biohazard sharps container

1. **Procedural Step.** Assemble the equipment. Using a pencil, label the slides on the frosted edge with the patient's name and the date.
   Principle. Most laboratories request the preparation of two blood smears.
2. **Procedural Step.** Wash the hands, and put on personal protective equipment, including gloves.
3. **Procedural Step.** Greet and identify the patient. Introduce yourself, and explain the procedure. Place a drop of fresh whole blood on each slide as follows:
   From a venipuncture. The blood specimen can be obtained from the fresh whole blood left in the needle immediately after performing a venipuncture as follows: After withdrawing the needle from the patient's arm, deposit the drop of blood remaining in the needle onto the middle of each slide, approximately ¼ inch from the frosted edge of the slide.
   From a skin puncture. Perform a finger puncture and wipe away the first drop of blood. Place a drop of blood from the patient's finger in the middle of each slide, approximately ¼ inch from the frosted edge of the slide, by touching the slide to the drop of blood. Do not allow the patient's finger to touch the slide.
   Principle. If the patient's finger touches the slide, it will cause the blood specimen to spread out, producing an uneven smear. In addition, the patient's finger may contain moisture or oil that would interfere with the smear.
4. **Procedural Step.** Hold a second "spreader" slide in front of the drop of blood and at a 30-degree angle to the first slide. Move the spreader slide until it touches the drop of blood. The blood distributes itself along the edge of the spreader by capillary action. Using a smooth, continuous motion, spread the blood thinly and evenly across the surface of the first slide, ending the motion by lifting the spreader slide off the specimen in a smooth, low arc. The length of the smear should be approximately 1½ inches. The blood smear is thickest at the beginning and gradually thins out to a very fine

"feathered" edge. If the blood smear has been prepared correctly, it exhibits the following characteristics: (1) it is smooth and even with no ridges, holes, lines, streaks, or clumps; (2) it is not too thick or too thin; (3) there is a feathered edge at the thin end of the smear; and (4) there is a margin on all sides of the smear. Repeat this step with the other slide.

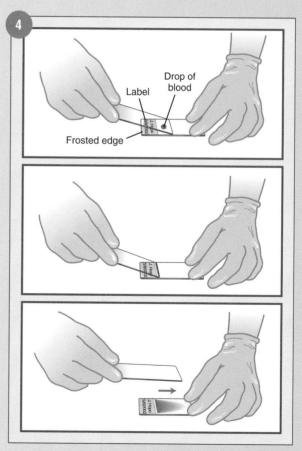

(From Rodak, B. F.: *Diagnostic Hematology.* Philadelphia, W. B. Saunders, 1995.)

18

PROCEDURE 18-2

Unacceptable blood smears:

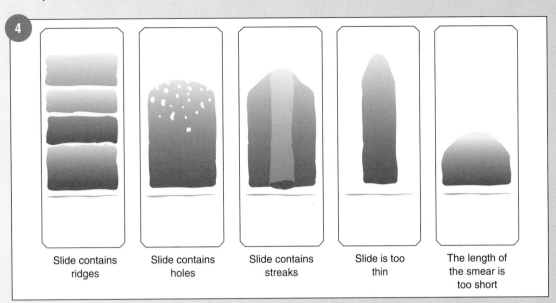

| Slide contains ridges | Slide contains holes | Slide contains streaks | Slide is too thin | The length of the smear is too short |

Principle. An angle of more than 30 degrees causes the smear to be too thick; the cells overlap, do not stain well, and are smaller than normal, making them difficult to count. If the angle is less than 30 degrees, the smear will be too thin and the cells will be spread out, increasing the time needed to count them.

5. **Procedural Step.** Dispose of the spreader slide in a biohazard sharps container.

6. **Procedural Step.** Quickly dry the blood smears by waving them gently back and forth. Never blow on the slides.

Principle. The blood smears must be dried immediately to prevent shrinkage of the blood cells, which makes them difficult to identify. Blowing on the slide may cause exhaled water droplets to make holes on the slide.

7. **Procedural Step.** Prepare the slides for transportation to the laboratory by placing them in a protective slide container.

8. **Procedural Step.** Remove the gloves, and wash the hands.

18

MEDICAL PRACTICE AND THE LAW

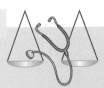

Whenever dealing with blood, be aware that any specimens can contain bloodborne pathogens such as hepatitis B and HIV. Use personal protective equipment including gloves, mask, and goggles if spraying or splashing of blood is a possibility.

Laboratory test results are confidential. Giving out results without the patient's permission can result in an invasion of privacy lawsuit. Usually, only the physician gives these results, so he or she can explain their meaning to the patient.

18

CERTIFICATION REVIEW

☐ Hematology involves the study of blood, including the morphologic appearance, function, and diseases of the blood and blood-forming tissues. The most frequently performed hematologic laboratory test is the complete blood count (CBC). The tests included in a CBC include hemoglobin, hematocrit, white blood cell count, red blood cell count, differential white blood cell count, and red blood cell indices.

☐ Blood consists of plasma and cells. The function of the plasma is to transport nutrients to the tissues of the body and to pick up wastes from the tissues.

☐ The three different types of cells in the blood are erythrocytes, leukocytes, and thrombocytes. Erythrocytes are formed in the red bone marrow. The average number of erythrocytes in the adult female ranges from 4 to 5.5 million per cubic millimeter of blood and in the adult male from 4.5 to 6.2 million per cubic millimeter of blood.

☐ Hemoglobin functions to transport oxygen and is also responsible for the red color of the erythrocyte. The amount of hemoglobin in the blood averages 12 to 16 g/dl for the adult female and 14 to 18 g/dl for the adult male. The average life span of a red blood cell is 120 days.

☐ Leukocytes are clear, colorless cells that contain a nucleus. The average number of leukocytes in the adult ranges from 4,500 to 11,000 per cubic millimeter. Leukocytosis is an abnormal increase in the number of leukocytes, and leukopenia is an abnormal decrease in the number of leukocytes. The function of leukocytes is to defend the body against infection.

☐ Thrombocytes, or platelets, function by participating in the blood-clotting mechanism. The average number of platelets in the adult is 150,000 to 400,000 per cubic millimeter.

☐ The hemoglobin determination is used to measure indirectly the oxygen-carrying capacity of the blood. A hemoglobin determination is often performed as a routine test on individuals at risk for developing anemia, such as children under 2 years of age and pregnant women.

☐ The purpose of the hematocrit is to measure the percentage volume of packed red blood cells in whole blood. The normal hematocrit range for the adult woman is 37 to 47 percent, and for the adult man, it is 40 to 54 percent. A low hematocrit reading may indicate anemia, whereas a high reading may indicate polycythemia.

☐ The white blood cell count is used to assist in the diagnosis and prognosis of disease. Leukocytosis is most commonly seen in acute infection. Conditions resulting in leukopenia include viral infections and chemotherapy and radiation therapy treatments.

☐ The red blood cell count is a measurement of the total number of red blood cells in whole blood. Conditions that cause a decrease in the red blood cell count include anemia, Hodgkin's disease, and leukemia. Conditions that cause an increase include polycythemia, dehydration, and pulmonary fibrosis.

☐ The purpose of the differential cell count is to identify the five types of white blood cells present in a representative blood sample. An increase or decrease in one or more types may occur in pathologic conditions, which assists the physician in making a diagnosis.

☐ The five types of white blood cells include neutrophils, eosinophils, basophils, lymphocytes, and monocytes. Neutrophils are the most numerous of the white blood cells. An increase in the number of neutrophils is generally seen during an acute infection. Basophils are the least numerous of the white blood cells. Lymphocytes are the smallest of the white blood cells and are involved with the immune system and the production of antibodies. An increase in lymphocytes generally occurs with certain viral diseases. Monocytes are the largest of the white blood cells.

RESOURCE

ON THE WEB

For information on stress and stress management:

The American Institute of
   Stress
www.stress.org

The Medical Basis of Stress,
   Depression, Anxiety, Sleep
   Problems, and Drug Use
www.teachhealth.com

Panic Attacks
**www.algy.com/anxiety/
   index.html**

International Stress Management Association
**www.stress-management-
   isma.org**

Stress: Basic Concepts
**www.aomc.org/
   stressBC.html**

Michelle Villers, *and I am a Certified Medical Assistant. I graduated from a medical assisting program and have an associate's degree in Applied Science. I am currently working for a physician in an internal medicine medical office. I have been working in the field of medical assisting for 10 months after recently graduating. My primary job responsibility includes running the laboratory at the office. I mainly draw blood and perform blood chemistry tests. I also work up patients, run electrocardiograms, apply Holter monitors, and perform pulmonary function tests, along with many other medical assisting procedures. In addition to working as a medical assistant, I recently returned to school to further my education.*

Blood Chemistry and Serology

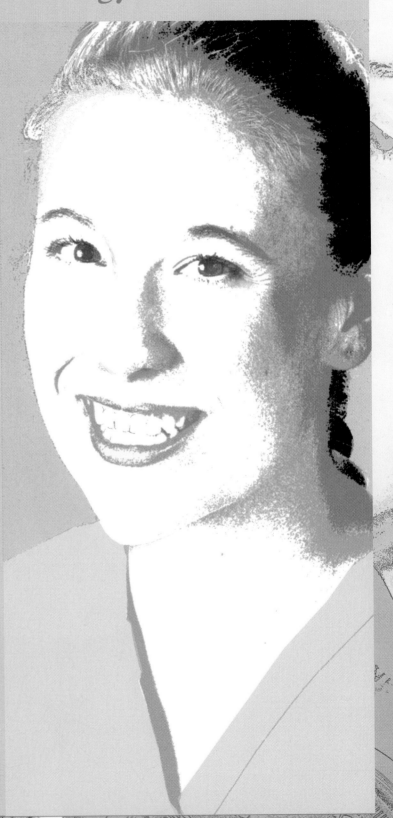

OUTCOMES

After completing this chapter, you should be able to demonstrate the proper procedures to do the following:

1. Perform blood chemistry testing, using an automated blood chemistry analyzer and operating manual.
2. Perform a FBS (fasting blood sugar) using a glucose monitor.
3. Instruct a patient in the procedure for determining blood glucose using a glucose monitor.
4. Demonstrate the proper care and maintenance of a glucose monitor.
5. Perform a rapid mononucleosis test.

EDUCATIONAL OBJECTIVES

After completing this chapter, you should be able to do the following:

1. Define the terms listed in the Key Terminology.
2. Explain the purpose of performing a blood chemistry test.
3. Describe the function of LDL cholesterol and HDL cholesterol in the body.
4. State the desirable ranges for each of the following tests: total cholesterol, LDL cholesterol, and HDL cholesterol.
5. State the patient preparation required for a triglyceride test.
6. Explain the function of glucose and insulin in the body.
7. State the patient preparation required for a fasting blood sugar.
8. Identify the normal range for a fasting blood sugar.
9. State the purpose of the following tests: fasting blood sugar, 2-hour postprandial glucose test, glucose tolerance test.
10. Describe the procedure for performing a 2-hour postprandial glucose test.
11. Identify the patient preparation required for a glucose tolerance test.
12. State the restrictions that must be followed by the patient during the glucose tolerance test.
13. Explain the storage requirements for blood glucose reagent strips.
14. List three advantages of self-monitoring of blood glucose by diabetic patients at home.
15. Explain the principle underlying each step in the procedure for the measurement of blood glucose.
16. Explain the purpose of each of the following serologic tests: hepatitis tests, syphilis tests, mono test, rheumatoid factor, antistreptolysin test, C-reactive protein, cold agglutinins, ABO and Rh blood typing, and Rh antibody titer.
17. List the symptoms of infectious mononucleosis.
18. Identify the location of the blood antigens and antibodies.
19. Tell how the blood antigen-antibody reaction is used as the basis for blood typing in vitro.
20. List the antigens and antibodies that are present in each of the following blood types: A, B, AB, and O.
21. Explain the difference between Rh+ and Rh− blood.

KEY TERMINOLOGY

agglutination (AG-lû-tin-â-shun): (as it pertains to blood) Clumping of blood cells.

antibody: A substance that is capable of combining with an antigen, resulting in an antigen-antibody reaction.

antigen: A substance capable of stimulating the formation of antibodies.

antiserum (pl. antisera): A serum that contains antibodies.

blood antibody: A protein present in the blood plasma that is capable of combining with its corresponding blood antigen to produce an antigen-antibody reaction.

blood antigen: A protein present on the surface of red blood cells that determines the blood type of an individual.

donor: One who furnishes something such as blood, tissue, or organs to be used in another person.

gene: A unit of heredity.

glycogen (GLÎ-kô-jen): The form in which carbohydrate is stored in the body.

HDL cholesterol: A lipoprotein consisting of protein and cholesterol, which removes excess cholesterol from the cells.

hyperglycemia (HÎ-PER-glî-sê-mê-a): An abnormal increase in the glucose level in the blood.

hypoglycemia (HÎ-Pô-glî-sê-mê-a): An abnormally low level of glucose in the blood.

in vitro (IN-VÊ-trô): Occurring in glass. Refers to tests performed under artificial conditions, as in the laboratory.

in vivo (IN-vêv-ô): Occurring in the living body or organism.

LDL cholesterol: A lipoprotein consisting of protein and cholesterol, which picks up cholesterol and delivers it to the cells.

lipoprotein (LÎ-Pô-prô-têên): A complex molecule consisting of protein and a lipid fraction such as cholesterol. Lipoproteins function in transporting lipids in the blood.

recipient: One who receives something, such as a blood transfusion, from a donor.

19 INTRODUCTION

Blood chemistry and serologic laboratory tests are often performed in the medical office. Over the past decade, advances in automated blood analyzers specially designed for use in the medical office have made this possible. Automated blood analyzers perform laboratory tests in a very short period of time with accurate test results. Each automated analyzer is accompanied by a detailed instruction manual explaining its operation, test parameters, care, and maintenance.

This chapter is divided into two units: The first presents blood chemistry laboratory tests, and the second presents serologic tests.

The material presented in this chapter on blood testing is intended only to serve as a basic guide for the medical assistant and should be supplemented by much well-supervised practice in a classroom laboratory or the medical office or both.

Blood Chemistry

Blood chemistry testing involves the quantitative measurement of chemical substances present in the blood.

These chemicals are dissolved in the liquid portion of the blood; therefore, most blood chemistry tests require a serum specimen for analysis. There are numerous types of blood chemistry tests; the type of test (or tests) ordered depends upon the physician's clinical diagnosis. Table 19–1 provides a listing of common blood chemistry tests, including specimen requirements, normal values, and conditions resulting in abnormal test results. The blood chemistry tests that are most frequently performed are described in more detail in this chapter.

AUTOMATED BLOOD CHEMISTRY ANALYZERS

In the medical office, automated blood chemistry analyzers are often used to perform blood chemistry testing. A blood chemistry analyzer consists of a reflectance photometer that quantitatively measures the amount of chemical substances or **analytes** in the blood. Specifically, a reflectance photometer measures light intensity to determine the exact amount of an analyte present in a specimen.

Examples of blood chemistry analyzers used in the medical office include the ATAC Lab System (Bio-

Text continued on page 641

TABLE 19–1

Common Blood Chemistry Tests

Name of Test and Specimen Requirement	Abbreviation	Purpose	Normal Range		Increased With	Decreased With
Alanine aminotransferase	ALT	To detect liver disease	≤45 U/L		Hepatocellular disease Active cirrhosis Metastatic liver tumor Obstructive jaundice Pancreatitis	
Alkaline phosphatase (serum)	ALP	Assists in the diagnosis of liver and bone diseases	20–70 U/L		Liver disease Bone disease Hyperparathyroidism Infectious mononucleosis	Hypophosphatasia Malnutrition Hypothyroidism Chronic nephritis
Aspartate aminotransferase	AST	To detect tissue damage	≤40 U/L		Myocardial infarction Liver disease Acute pancreatitis Acute hemolytic anemia	Beriberi Uncontrolled diabetes mellitus with acidosis
Blood urea nitrogen (serum)	BUN	A screening test to detect renal disease, especially glomerular functioning	7–18 mg/dl (SI Units: 2.5–6.4 mmol/L)		Kidney disease Urinary obstruction Dehydration Gastrointestinal bleeding	Liver failure Malnutrition Impaired absorption
Calcium (serum)	Ca	To assess parathyroid functioning and calcium metabolism, and to evaluate malignancies	8.4–10.2 mg/dl (SI Units: 2.1–2.55 mmol/L)		*Hypercalcemia* Hyperparathyroidism Bone metastases Multiple myeloma Hodgkin's disease Addison's disease Hyperthyroidism	*Hypocalcemia* Hypoparathyroidism Acute pancreatitis Renal failure
Chloride (serum)	Cl	Assists in diagnosing disorders of acid-base and water balance	98–106 mmol/L		Dehydration Cushing's syndrome Hyperventilation Pre-eclampsia Anemia	Severe vomiting Severe diarrhea Ulcerative colitis Pyloric obstruction Severe burns Heat exhaustion

19

Continued

TABLE 19–1

Common Blood Chemistry Tests *Continued*

Name of Test and Specimen Requirement	Abbreviation	Purpose	Normal Range		Increased With	Decreased With
Cholesterol (serum)	CH Chol	To screen for the presence of atherosclerosis related to coronary heart disease (CHD). Also used as a secondary aid in the study of thyroid and liver functioning	**Total Cholesterol** Below 200 mg/dl 200–239 mg/dl 240 mg/dl or higher (SI Units): Below 5.18 mmol/L 5.18–6.19 mmol/L 6.22 mmol/L or higher **LDL Cholesterol** Below 130 mg/dl 130–159 mg/dl 160 mg/dl or higher (SI Units): Below 3.37 mmol/L 3.37–4.12 mmol/L 4.14 mmol/L or higher **HDL Cholesterol** 35 mg/dl or above Below 35 mg/dl (SI Units): 0.91 mmol/L or above Below 0.91 mmol/L	Desirable Borderline high High Desirable Borderline high High Desirable Borderline high High Desirable Borderline high High Acceptable Increased risk for CHD Acceptable Increased risk for CHD	Atherosclerosis Cardiovascular disease Obstructive jaundice Hypothyroidism Nephrosis	Malabsorption Liver disease Hyperthyroidism Anemia
Creatinine (serum)	creat	A screening test of renal functioning	0.2–0.8 mg/dl (SI Units: 15–61 μmol/L)		Impaired renal function Chronic nephritis Obstruction of the urinary tract Muscle disease	Muscular dystrophy
Globulin (serum)	glob	To identify abnormalities in the rate of protein synthesis and removal	1.0–3.5 g/dl (SI Units: 10–35 g/L)		Brucellosis Chronic infections Rheumatoid arthritis Dehydration Hepatic carcinoma Hodgkin's disease	Agammaglobulinemia Severe burns

19

TABLE 19–1

Common Blood Chemistry Tests *Continued*

Name of Test and Specimen Requirement	Abbreviation	Purpose	Normal Range		Increased With	Decreased With
Glucose Fasting blood sugar Two-hour post-prandial blood sugar Glucose tolerance test (serum)	FBS 2-hr PPBS GTT	To detect disorders of glucose metabolism	**FBS:** 70–110 mg/dl (SI Units: 3.9–6.1 mmol/L) **2-hr PPBS** <140 mg/dl (SI Units: <7.8 mmol/L) *Glucose Tolerance Test (mg/dl)*		*Hyperglycemia* Diabetes mellitus Hepatic disease Brain damage Cushing's syndrome	*Hypoglycemia* Excess insulin Addison's disease Bacterial sepsis Carcinoma of the pancreas Hepatic necrosis Hypothyroidism

Glucose Tolerance Test (mg/dl)

	Normal	Diabetic
FBS	70–110	>120
30 min	150–160	>200
1 hr	160–170	>200
2 hr	≤120	>140
3 hr	70–110	>140

(SI Units: mmol/L)

		Diabetic
FBS	3.9–6.1	>6.7
30 min	8.4–8.9	>11.1
1 hr	8.9–9.5	>11.1
2 hr	≤6.7	>7.8
3 hr	3.9–6.1	>7.8

Name of Test and Specimen Requirement	Abbreviation	Purpose	Normal Range	Increased With	Decreased With
Lactate dehydrogenase, 30°C (serum)	LD	To assist in confirming a myocardial or pulmonary infarction. Also used in the differential diagnosis of muscular dystrophy and pernicious anemia	≤240 U/L	Acute myocardial infarction Acute leukemia Muscular dystrophy Pernicious anemia Hemolytic anemia Hepatic disease Extensive cancer	
Phosphorus (serum)	P	Assists in the proper evaluation and interpretation of calcium levels. Used to detect disorders of the endocrine system, bone diseases, and kidney dysfunction	3.0–4.5 mg/dl (SI Units: 0.97–1.45 mmol/L)	*Hyperphosphatemia* Renal insufficiency Severe nephritis Hypoparathyroidism Hypocalcemia Addison's disease	*Hypophosphatemia* Hyperparathyroidism Rickets and osteomalacia Diabetic coma Hyperinsulinism

19

Continued

TABLE 19-1

Common Blood Chemistry Tests *Continued*

Name of Test and Specimen Requirement	Abbreviation	Purpose	Normal Range	Increased With	Decreased With
Potassium (serum)	K	To diagnose disorders of acid-base and water balance in the body	3.5–5.1 mmol/L	*Hyperkalemia* Renal failure Cell damage Acidosis Addison's disease Internal bleeding	*Hypokalemia* Diarrhea Pyloric obstruction Starvation Malabsorption Severe vomiting Severe burns Diuretic administration Chronic stress Liver disease with ascites
Sodium (serum)	Na	To detect changes in water and salt balance in the body	136–146 mmol/L	*Hypernatremia* Dehydration Conn's syndrome Primary aldosteronism Coma Cushing's disease Diabetes insipidus	*Hyponatremia* Severe burns Severe diarrhea Vomiting Addison's disease Severe nephritis Pyloric obstruction
Total bilirubin (serum)	TB	To evaluate liver functioning and hemolytic anemia	0.2–1.0 mg/dl (SI Units: 3.4–17.1 μmol/L)	Liver disease Obstruction of the common bile or hepatic duct Hemolytic anemia	
Total protein (serum)	TP	A screening test for diseases that alter the protein balance and to assess the state of body hydration	6.0–8.0 g/dl (SI Units: 60–80 g/L)	Dehydration (vomiting, diarrhea) Chronic infections Acute liver disease Multiple myeloma Lupus erythematosus	Severe hemorrhaging Hodgkin's disease Severe liver disease Malabsorption
Total thyroxine T_4 (serum)	Total T_4	To assess thyroid functioning and to evaluate thyroid replacement therapy	5–12 μg/dl (SI Units: 64–155 nmol/L)	Hyperthyroidism Graves' disease Thyrotoxicosis Thyroiditis	Hypothyroidism Cretinism Goiter Myxedema Hypoproteinemia

19

TABLE 19-1

Common Blood Chemistry Tests *Continued*

Name of Test and Specimen Requirement	Abbreviation	Purpose	Normal Range	Increased With	Decreased With
Triglycerides (serum)	Trig	To evaluate patients with suspected atherosclerosis (Elevated triglycerides along with elevated cholesterol are risk factors for atherosclerosis)	Desirable level: 40–150 mg/dl (SI Units: 0.4–1.5 g/L)	Liver disease Nephrotic syndrome Hypothyroidism Poorly controlled diabetes Pancreatitis	Malnutrition Congenital lipoproteinemia
Uric acid (serum)	UA	To evaluate renal failure, gout, and leukemia	Male: 3.4–7.0 mg/dl (SI Units: 202–416 μmol/L) Female: 2.4–6.0 mg/dl (SI Units: 143–357 μmol/L)	Renal failure Gout Leukemia Severe eclampsia Lymphomas	Patients undergoing treatment with uricosuric drugs

Chem) (Fig. 19–1), DuPont Analyst (DuPont Diagnostics), and the Reflotron Analyzer (Boehringer Mannheim).

The manufacturer of each automated analyzer provides a detailed operating manual with the instrument that includes the information needed to collect, handle, and to perform quality control procedures, and test the specimen. In addition, the manufacturer has personnel available for on-site training and service.

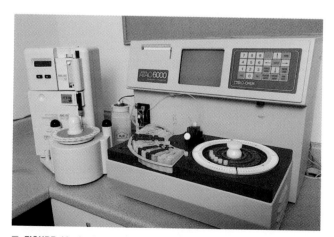

■ **FIGURE 19–1.** An example of a blood chemistry analyzer (ATAC Lab System by Bio-Chem).

QUALITY CONTROL

☐ Quality control consists of methods and means to ensure that the test results are reliable and valid. Two very important quality control measures must be performed routinely when using a blood chemistry analyzer: calibration of the instrument and running controls.

Calibration involves the use of a standard to check the precision of the blood chemistry analyzer. If an analyzer is not properly calibrated, it will be unable to produce accurate test results. If this occurs, the operating manual should be consulted to determine the action that should be taken to correct the problem. Calibration of a blood chemistry analyzer can be compared with placing a scale at zero before weighing a patient. In other words, if the scale is not at zero, the results will not be accurate.

A **control** consists of a sample of a known value. The control is processed in the same manner as a patient specimen, and the results should fall within a specified range as indicated on a reference sheet that accompanies each control. Both normal and abnormal controls are commercially available. Normal controls fall within normal range whereas abnormal controls fall outside normal range. Low abnormal controls fall below the normal range, and high abnormal controls fall

19

above the normal range. If the control does not fall within its specified range, problems or errors exist, either with the analyzer itself or with the technique used to perform the procedure. The operating manual should be consulted to determine the action to take to correct the situation. A control can be compared with placing an object with a known weight of 5 pounds on a scale. The scale should weigh the object at 5 pounds, otherwise the results are not considered valid.

The Clinical Laboratory Improvement Amendments of 1988 (CLIA 1988) require that the calibration procedure be performed and documented at least every 6 months and that two levels of control be performed daily (e.g., running a normal control and a high control). In addition, when problems or errors are identified, the action taken to correct them must be documented.

CHOLESTEROL

☐ Cholesterol is a white, waxy, fatlike substance (lipid) that is essential for normal functioning of the body. It is an important component of cell membranes and is used in the production of hormones and bile. Most of the cholesterol circulating in the blood is manufactured by the liver; however, a portion of it comes from an

individual's diet and is known as **dietary cholesterol.** Dietary cholesterol is found only in animal products, such as organ meats, egg yolk, and dairy products.

High blood cholesterol means there is an excessive amount of cholesterol in the blood. An individual's cholesterol level is determined by his or her genetic makeup and also by the amount of dietary cholesterol and saturated fat consumed. High blood cholesterol may cause fatty deposits, or plaque, to build up on the walls of the arteries, a condition known as **atherosclerosis.** As the atherosclerosis progresses, the arteries become more occluded, which eventually could lead to a heart attack or stroke. Because of this, high blood cholesterol is considered a major risk for coronary heart disease and efforts should be made to lower the cholesterol level (see Highlight on Lowering Cholesterol).

HDL AND LDL CHOLESTEROL

Cholesterol is transported in the blood as a complex molecule known as a **lipoprotein.** Two types of lipoproteins containing cholesterol are termed low-density lipoprotein cholesterol (LDL cholesterol) and high-density lipoprotein cholesterol (HDL cholesterol).

LDL cholesterol picks up cholesterol from ingested fats and from the liver and delivers it to blood vessels

19

Highlight on Coronary Heart Disease (CHD)

Coronary heart disease affects 6.6 million Americans, or one fourth of the U.S. population. The chief forms of CHD are atherosclerosis, high blood pressure, heart attacks, strokes, congestive heart failure, congenital heart disease, and rheumatic heart disease. These various forms of heart disease are interrelated and have elements in common; for example, atherosclerosis can lead to a stroke or heart attack.

Heart disease is the number one killer of adults in the United States today. Because of the recent national focus on heart disease and cholesterol reduction, the last 15 years have seen a decline in heart attacks by 25 percent and strokes by nearly 40 percent; however, the death rate from heart disease is likely to remain the number one cause of death until more Americans adopt a more heart-healthy lifestyle.

Not everyone is equal when it comes to coronary heart disease. Some individuals have a much higher risk of developing it than others. The following are risk factors for CHD:

• High total blood cholesterol (above 200 mg/dl confirmed by repeated measurement)
• High blood pressure
• Cigarette smoking (more than 10 cigarettes per day)

• Family history of premature coronary heart disease (definite heart attack or sudden death in a parent or sibling before age 55 years)
• Diabetes mellitus
• History of blood vessel disease
• Obesity (30 or more percent overweight)
• Low HDL cholesterol (below 35 mg/dl confirmed by repeated measurement)
• Being a man over 45 years of age
• Being a woman over 55 years of age or post-menopausal

Some of these risk factors can be modified, while others cannot, such as age, gender, and a family history of CHD. The three major risk factors for CHD are high total blood cholesterol, high blood pressure, and cigarette smoking, which fortunately are all modifiable.

Each person's overall risk of coronary heart disease must be assessed individually by the physician, based on the type and number of risk factors present. For example, a 47-year-old man with a cholesterol level of 220 mg/dl who smokes a pack of cigarettes a day and is overweight is at greater risk than a 28-year-old man who is within normal weight, does not smoke, and exercises regularly but has a cholesterol level of 250 mg/dl.

and muscles, where it is deposited in the cells. LDL cholesterol is often referred to as "bad" cholesterol because an excess amount of it in the blood (over 130 mg/dl) can cause plaque to build up on the arterial walls, resulting in atherosclerosis.

HDL cholesterol removes excess cholesterol from the cells and carries it to the liver to be excreted. Because HDL removes excess cholesterol from the walls of the blood vessels, it is protective and beneficial to the body and is often called "good" cholesterol. A high HDL cholesterol level has been shown to reduce the risk of heart disease, whereas a low level of HDL cholesterol (less than 35 mg/dl) is considered a definite risk factor for coronary heart disease.

CHOLESTEROL TESTING

All adults over 20 years of age should have a cholesterol test at least once every 5 years. Initial testing includes a **total cholesterol** determination, which is a combined measurement of the amount of LDL cholesterol and HDL cholesterol in the blood. To obtain a more complete picture of a patient's cholesterol status, most physicians also order an HDL cholesterol determination, which measures only the amount of HDL cholesterol in the blood. Both these tests are considered screening tests, and elevated results *always* require confirmation through repeated testing and further testing before a diagnosis of high blood cholesterol can be made.

INTERPRETATION OF RESULTS

Cholesterol test results are interpreted as follows: Total cholesterol levels under 200 mg/dl are considered desirable. Levels between 200 and 239 are considered borderline high, and 240 and above are considered high. Based on confirmed testing, individuals in the high category are clearly at increased risk for coronary heart disease, and individuals in the borderline high category are at increased risk if they have other risk factors such as being overweight or smoking. An HDL cholesterol level above 35 mg/dl is considered acceptable, while a level below 35 mg/dl has been determined to be a risk factor for coronary heart disease.

PATIENT PREPARATION

Since the total cholesterol and the HDL cholesterol determinations are not affected significantly by food consumption, the patient is usually not required to fast before the collection of the blood specimen. However, some physicians prefer the patient to be in a fasting state.

If the total cholesterol level is 200 mg/dl or higher, the physician usually orders a **lipid profile,** which includes total cholesterol, triglycerides, HDL cholesterol, and LDL cholesterol. (The LDL cholesterol level is usually determined as a calculation from the results of the triglyceride and HDL cholesterol levels.) Because triglyceride levels are affected by the consumption of food, the patient must be instructed to fast for at least 12 hours before collection of this blood specimen. An elevated triglyceride level (over 250 mg/dl) places an individual at an increased risk for coronary heart disease, particularly when the LDL cholesterol is high (over 130 mg/dl) and the HDL cholesterol is low (less than 35 mg/dl).

Although the primary use of cholesterol testing is to screen for the presence of high blood cholesterol related to coronary heart disease, this test is also used as a secondary aid in the study of thyroid and liver function. Refer to Table 19–1 for a list of specific conditions causing abnormal cholesterol test results.

BLOOD UREA NITROGEN

☐ The blood urea nitrogen (BUN) is a kidney function test. Urea is the end product of protein metabolism and is normally present in the blood. However, certain kidney diseases may interfere with the ability of the body to excrete the urea properly, causing an increased level of urea in the blood. Refer to Table 19–1 for a list of specific conditions causing abnormal BUN test results.

BLOOD GLUCOSE

☐ Glucose is the end product of carbohydrate metabolism; its function is to serve as the chief source of energy for the body. Body energy is needed to carry out normal body functions and to assist in maintaining body temperature. The body maintains a constant blood glucose level to ensure a continuous source of energy for the body. Glucose taken in that is not needed for energy can be stored in the form of **glycogen** in muscle and liver tissue for later use. When no more tissue storage is possible, excess glucose is converted to fat and stored as adipose tissue.

Insulin is a hormone secreted by the beta cells of the pancreas and is required for normal utilization of glucose in the body. Insulin enables glucose to enter the body's cells and be converted to energy. Insulin is also needed for the proper storage of glycogen in liver and muscle cells.

Highlight on Lowering Cholesterol

Research has shown, beyond doubt, that high total blood cholesterol is a major risk factor for coronary heart disease, and the higher the cholesterol, the greater the risk. The National Institutes of Health (NIH) has established guidelines on safe levels of blood cholesterol. The NIH recommends that adults not exceed 200 mg/dl of blood cholesterol.

The National Cholesterol Educational Program (NCEP) was established in 1985 by the federal government to reduce the prevalence of elevated blood cholesterol levels in the United States by educating the public about the health risks associated with high blood cholesterol, and to make recommendations for helping individuals lower their cholesterol levels. It has been shown that for every 1 percent that an individual lowers his or her total blood cholesterol, the risk of coronary heart disease is lowered by 2 percent. The following are measures that individuals can take to lower their level of "bad" LDL cholesterol and raise their level of "good" HDL cholesterol.

DIET

Dietary therapy is considered the first line of treatment of high blood cholesterol. The NCEP recommends that all individuals (over 2 years of age) reduce dietary cholesterol and saturated fats. Many foods high in fat tend to be high in cholesterol. Reading nutrition labels on packaged products helps provide information on the cholesterol and fat content of a food.

DIETARY CHOLESTEROL.
The body manufactures all the cholesterol it needs for normal functioning, and therefore dietary intake of foods containing cholesterol only serves to increase the blood cholesterol. According to the NCEP, dietary cholesterol should be limited to 300 mg daily, which is slightly more than the amount of cholesterol in one egg (270 mg). Cholesterol is found only in animal foods and shellfish. Egg yolks, dairy products, and organ meats such as liver and kidneys are especially high in cholesterol.

SATURATED FAT.
The intake of saturated fat is the single most important dietary factor leading to high blood cholesterol, even more so than consuming dietary cholesterol. In general, the more saturated a fat is, the harder and more solid it is at room temperature. The main source of saturated fat is animal products, including meat fat, poultry skin, and the fat in dairy products (butter, cream, ice cream, cheese, whole milk). Unsaturated fats have little or no effect on the blood choles-

terol level and include olive oil, canola oil, peanut oil, and sunflower, safflower, and corn oil. The NCEP recommends that no more than 30 percent of the total calories consumed each day should come from fat, with no more than 10 percent of calories coming from saturated fat, and the remaining 20 percent from unsaturated fat.

SOLUBLE FIBER.
Soluble fiber has been shown to lower the cholesterol level by keeping the cholesterol consumed from being absorbed by the body. Examples of foods high in soluble fiber are bran, oats, and beans.

WEIGHT REDUCTION

It is estimated that one in four Americans is overweight. For these individuals, it is recommended that a sensible eating plan along with an exercise program be followed to reach and maintain desirable weight. Losing weight helps lower both total cholesterol and triglyceride levels. People who are overweight or obese are at higher risk for CHD because their hearts have to work harder to pump blood through the body.

EXERCISE

An aerobic exercise program is especially beneficial for weight control, improving cardiovascular fitness and lowering blood cholesterol level. People who exercise regularly generally have higher HDL cholesterol levels in their blood. Health experts recommend exercising three times a week for 20 to 30 minutes at your target heart rate.

SMOKING CESSATION

Smoking is one of the three main risk factors for coronary heart disease. By quitting smoking, an individual may be able to strengthen the heart and lower the cholesterol level. Also, nonsmokers tend to have higher HDL levels in their blood. A variety of smoking cessation programs are usually offered in the community. Some people have succeeded by using nicotine patches, which help them adjust gradually to lower levels of nicotine.

Generally the cholesterol level begins to drop 2 to 3 weeks after beginning a cholesterol-lowering diet and other cholesterol-lowering measures. Over time, it is possible to reduce the total cholesterol level by 30 to 55 mg/dl or even more through these lifestyle changes. If the blood cholesterol level cannot be lowered to an acceptable level, cholesterol-lowering medications may be prescribed by the physician along with the continuation of the aforementioned measures.

Measuring the amount of glucose present in a blood specimen is one of the most commonly performed blood chemistry tests. It is used to detect abnormalities in carbohydrate metabolism such as occur in diabetes mellitus, hypoglycemia, and liver and adrenocortical dysfunction. Blood glucose measurement is performed using several different testing methods, which include the fasting blood sugar, the 2-hour postprandial glucose test, and the glucose tolerance test. Each of these methods serves a specific role in diagnosing and evaluating abnormalities in carbohydrate metabolism and is described in more detail here.

FASTING BLOOD SUGAR

Blood glucose is usually measured when the patient is in a fasting state. This type of test is termed a fasting blood sugar (FBS), which involves collecting a fasting blood sample and measuring the amount of glucose in it. The patient should not have anything to eat or drink, except water, for 12 hours preceding the test. Certain medications, such as oral contraceptives, salicylates, diuretics, and steroids, may affect the test results; therefore, the physician may also place the patient on medication restrictions for a specific period of time before the test—usually for 3 days. The patient should be scheduled for the test in the morning to minimize the inconvenience of abstaining from food and fluid.

The normal range for a fasting blood sugar varies among laboratories and with the specific type of test utilized, but it usually falls between 70 and 110 mg of glucose per 100 ml of blood (or mg/dl). An FBS is often performed on diagnosed diabetics to evaluate their progress and regulate treatment and as a routine screening procedure to detect diabetes mellitus. An FBS above 120 mg/dl is considered the dividing point between normal and hyperglycemic values and is indicative of diabetes mellitus. An elevated test result warrants further testing with the glucose tolerance test.

TWO-HOUR POSTPRANDIAL BLOOD SUGAR

The 2-hour postprandial blood sugar (2-hour PPBS) test is used to screen for the presence of diabetes mellitus and to monitor the effects of insulin dosage in diagnosed diabetics. The patient is required to fast, beginning at midnight preceding the test and continuing until breakfast. For breakfast, the patient must consume a prescribed meal containing 100 grams of carbohydrate, consisting of orange juice, cereal with sugar, toast, and milk. An alternative to this is the consumption of a 100-gram test-load glucose solution. A blood specimen is collected from the patient exactly 2 hours after consumption of the meal or glucose solution.

In the nondiabetic patient, the glucose level returns to the fasting level within 1½ to 2 hours from the time of glucose consumption, whereas the glucose level in the diabetic patient does not return to the fasting level. A postprandial glucose level of 140 g/dl or higher is suggestive of diabetes mellitus and warrants further testing, such as the glucose tolerance test.

GLUCOSE TOLERANCE TEST

The glucose tolerance test (GTT) provides more detailed information about the ability of the body to metabolize glucose by assessing the insulin response to a glucose load. The GTT is used to assist in the

MEMORIES *from* **EXTERNSHIP**

MICHELLE VILLERS: *During my externship experience, I was assigned to a four-physician pediatric practice. The office was constantly busy with screaming children. As if I was not nervous enough, I was asked to assist in the removal of sutures. When I walked into the room with the physicians, beads of sweat began to form on my forehead. A child was lying on the examining table—a little boy no more than 7 years of age. He was here to have sutures removed from a recent surgery. The sutures had been tied very well, and it was difficult for the physician to cut them. The little boy lay there with tears streaming down his cheeks. I reassured him and talked to him, and his tears began to subside. "A few more minutes and it will be all over," I told him. And within those next few minutes, the physician cut the last suture. The little boy eagerly hopped down off the examining table and gave me a big hug. I learned that day how a little reassurance can make everyone involved feel better.*

19

diagnosis of diabetes mellitus, hypoglycemia, and liver and adrenocortical dysfunction. It provides a more thorough analysis of glucose utilization than either the FBS or the 2-hour PPBS test.

Testing Requirements

The patient is usually required to consume a high-carbohydrate diet for 3 days before the glucose tolerance test, consisting of 150 grams of carbohydrate per day. The patient must be in a fasting state when the test begins. On the morning of the test, a blood specimen is drawn from the patient (FBS) and a urine specimen is taken to measure the amount of glucose in each of these samples. If the FBS indicates hyperglycemia, the physician should be notified, because this situation contradicts the administration of a large test load of glucose.

After the FBS has been performed, the patient is instructed to drink a measured amount of a glucose solution (1.75 grams of glucose per kilogram of body weight, or the standard adult dose of 100 grams). Thereafter, at regular intervals (generally 30, 60, 120, and 180 minutes), blood and urine samples are taken to determine the patient's ability to handle the increased amount of glucose. Each blood and urine specimen must be labeled carefully with the exact time of collection. The patient is permitted to eat and drink normally at the completion of the test.

It is important that the patient adhere to certain restrictions during the test to ensure accurate results. Since food and fluid affect blood glucose levels, the patient must not eat or drink anything during the test, except water. In fact, consumption of water should be encouraged to make it easier for the patient to produce a urine specimen. Smoking is not permitted during the test because it acts as a stimulant that increases the blood glucose level. The patient should remain at the testing site so that he or she is present when needed for the collection of the blood and urine specimens and to minimize activity. Activity affects the test results by utilizing glucose; therefore, the patient should remain relatively inactive during the test. Sitting and reading, for example, is an activity that would be recommended.

Side Effects

The patient may experience some normal side effects, particularly during the second and third hours of the test, including weakness, a feeling of faintness, and perspiration. These are considered normal reactions of the body to a fall in the glucose level as insulin is secreted in response to the glucose load. The patient should be reassured that this is a temporary condition that will go away. Serious symptoms indicative of severe hypoglycemia should immediately be reported to the physician and include headache; pale, cold, and clammy skin; irrational speech or behavior; profuse perspiration; and fainting.

Interpretation of Results

The test results are interpreted by evaluating the data obtained for each collection period. If the glucose level is abnormally increased compared with established norms for the various blood collection times, a disorder of glucose metabolism such as diabetes mellitus may be present. Individuals with diabetes are unable to remove glucose from the bloodstream at the same rate as a nondiabetic individual.

As glucose is absorbed into the bloodstream, the blood glucose level of a nondiabetic rises to a peak level between 160 and 180 mg/dl approximately 30 to 60 minutes after the glucose solution is consumed. The pancreas secretes insulin to compensate for this rise, and the blood glucose returns to the fasting level within 2 to 3 hours from the time of ingestion of the glucose solution. In addition, the urine specimens exhibit negative test results for glucose.

The individual with diabetes does not exhibit the normal utilization of glucose just described. Rather, the blood glucose peaks at a much higher level, and glucose is present in the urine. In addition, glucose levels are above normal throughout the test because of the lack of insulin. Refer to Table 19–1 for normal and diabetic glucose values.

The glucose tolerance test is generally not used for diagnostic purposes in patients with an FBS above 140 mg/dl or a 2-hour postprandial test result above 180 mg/dl, because results greater than these values would qualify for the diagnosis of diabetes mellitus and the GTT would not be required.

Hypoglycemia

Hypoglycemia is a condition in which the glucose in the blood is abnormally low. During the GTT, patients with this condition exhibit an abnormally low blood glucose level beginning at the 2-hour interval and continuing up to 4 or 5 hours. Hypoglycemia results from glucose removal from the blood at an excessive rate or from a decreased secretion of glucose into the blood, which may be caused by an overdose of insulin, Addison's disease, bacterial sepsis, carcinoma of the pancreas, hepatic necrosis, or hypothyroidism.

GLUCOSE MONITORS

In the medical office, a glucose monitor is often used to quantitatively measure the blood glucose level. The specific test most frequently performed using the glucose monitor is the FBS, although a significant number of offices also perform the GTT and the 2-hour postprandial test. Glucose monitors are commercially available with brand names that include the Accu-Chek Advantage (Boehringer Mannheim) and the Glucometer Elite (Bayer Corporation). By measuring the blood glucose concentration in the medical office, better patient care can be provided. On-site testing eliminates the time required for an outside laboratory to provide the results, thus allowing the physician to make decisions immediately regarding patient diagnosis, treatment, and follow-up care.

Reagent Strips

A reagent strip must be used with the glucose monitor; it consists of a plastic strip with a reaction pad. The pad contains chemicals that react with the glucose in whole blood to determine the blood glucose level in milligrams per deciliter. Through an electronic signal, the glucose results are displayed as a digital read-out. The manufacturer's instructions accompanying the glucose monitor must be followed exactly to ensure accurate and reliable test results.

It is important to store the container of reagent strips properly to prevent their deterioration, which affects the test results. The reagents on the strips are sensitive to heat, light, and moisture and must therefore be stored in a cool, dry area at room temperature (under 90°F or 32°C) with the cap tightly closed. Strips that are discolored or that have darkened should be discarded to prevent inaccurate test results. The container of test strips includes a desiccant. Its purpose is to promote dryness by absorbing moisture.

Care and Maintenance

The glucose monitor should be handled carefully. It is a delicate instrument, and a severe physical jar could result in a malfunction. The glucose monitor should not be placed in an area of high humidity, such as a bathroom. Exposing the instrument to severe variations in environmental temperature, such as leaving it in a closed vehicle on a hot or cold day, should be avoided.

Proper cleaning of the glucose monitor is essential for ensuring its accurate and reliable operation. On a regular basis, the exterior of the glucose monitor, including the display screen, should be cleaned with a soft, clean cloth slightly dampened with a mild cleaning agent, and it should be dried thoroughly. Do not allow water or detergent to run into the glucose monitor, which could damage the internal components.

Because glucose monitors are battery operated, periodic replacement of the battery is required. The glucose monitor alerts the user to low battery voltage by displaying a special notation on the screen. The type of battery required is specified in the operator's manual, along with directions for installation.

Calibration Procedure

The purpose of calibrating the glucose monitor is to ensure accurate and reliable test results by compensating for variables that exist in the manufacturing process of each container of reagent strips. Calibration programs the electronics of the glucose monitor to match the reactivity of the container of strips that are in current use.

The calibration procedure for the Accu-Chek Advantage is performed using a plastic code key that accompanies each container of Advantage reagent strips. Accu-Chek requires lot-specific calibration, meaning that the calibration procedure needs to be performed only once per container of test strips. This is possible because the Accu-Chek glucose monitor has a built-in memory system that enables it to retain a point of reference, once it has been calibrated. This reference point is retained until the glucose monitor is reprogrammed for a new container of test strips. The calibration procedure delineated next should be followed when a new container of test strips is opened.

1. Make sure the monitor is turned off.
2. Turn the monitor over so that the back of the monitor is facing you.
3. Remove the old code key if one is installed.
4. Insert a new code key until it snaps into place (Fig. 19–2A).
5. Turn the monitor on. A three-digit code number appears on the display screen. This number must match the code number of the vial of reagent strips (Fig. 19–2B). If it does not, repeat Steps 1 through 3.

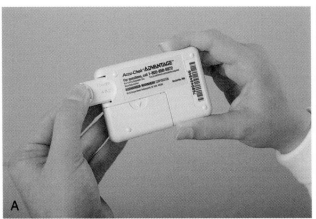
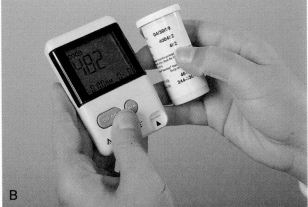

■ **FIGURE 19–2.** Accu-Chek Advantage Calibration Procedure: *A,* The code key is inserted into the monitor. *B,* The code number must match the code number of the vial of reagent strips.

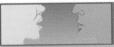

PATIENT/TEACHING

OBTAINING A CAPILLARY BLOOD SPECIMEN

The medical assistant may need to instruct the patient in the procedure for obtaining and testing a capillary blood specimen for blood glucose measurement. Properly educating the patient to perform the procedure is the most important factor in obtaining accurate test results.

1. **Obtaining the capillary blood specimen.** Inform the patient of the sites available for obtaining the blood specimen. These include the fingers and the side of the hand where there are no calluses. Most patients prefer to use an automatic lancet device to perform the skin puncture. Using such a device makes the puncture less painful, and the preset puncture depth generally assures a successful stick. For a finger puncture, instruct the patient to obtain the blood specimen from the lateral side of the tip of the finger, because this area contains fewer nerve endings and less pain results. If the patient's hands are cold, tell him or her to rub them together or place them in warm water, which improves the blood flow to the area. Instruct the patient in the proper procedure for obtaining a large drop of blood to ensure accurate test results.

2. **Performing the blood glucose test.** The patient performs the test with a reagent strip using a glucose monitor. Instruct the patient in the proper procedure for performing the test, making sure he or she understands that accurate test results assist in greater glucose control. Patients should also be given detailed instructions on the proper care and maintenance of the glucose monitor.

3. **Recording results.** Instruct the patient to record each test result in a log book to provide a permanent record between office visits. In addition, most glucose monitors are equipped with a memory system that stores test results for later retrieval. The following information should be included with each recording:
   a. Date and time.
   b. Number of hours since the patient last ate.
   c. Time of the last insulin injection or oral hypoglycemic medication.
   d. Any feeling of physical or emotional stress.
   e. How much exercise the patient has undergone.

   Keeping track of these factors helps explain a shift in the blood glucose level and provides the basis for sound self-management decisions.

Quality Control Check

A quality control should be performed to ensure that the test results are reliable and valid and that errors that may interfere with obtaining accurate test results are detected and eliminated. A quality control check is

PUTTING IT ALL *into* PRACTICE

▶ **MICHELLE VILLERS:** *When performing a venipuncture, you need to make sure all the necessary equipment is on hand and ready. Sometimes you may have a vacuum tube that has no vacuum in it. In cases like these, it is always better to have a couple of spare tubes on hand. I recently had an experience in which one of my tubes had no vacuum. Luckily I had a few extra tubes within arm's reach so I did not have to interrupt the procedure to get a new one. Basically I have learned that you can never be too prepared.*

performed on the Accu-Chek Advantage using commercially available glucose control solutions. Two levels of controls should be used (high, normal, or low).

A quality control check should be performed under the following circumstances:

1. Daily, before using the monitor for the first time
2. When a new container of reagent strips is opened
3. If the monitor is dropped
4. If a test has been repeated and the blood glucose result is still lower or higher than expected

SELF-MONITORING OF BLOOD GLUCOSE

☐ Diabetic patients taking insulin must monitor blood glucose levels at home to provide for effective management of their condition. Based upon the results, decisions can be made regarding insulin and dietary adjustments that may be necessary to maintain normal glucose levels and to avoid the extremes of hypoglycemia or hyperglycemia. Satisfactory control of the blood glucose level reduces symptoms of the disease and helps decrease or delay long-term complications that can occur with diabetes mellitus, such as retinopathy and peripheral vascular disease.

Research shows that frequent blood glucose monitoring is the most effective means of maintaining normal blood glucose levels and preventing long-term complications associated with diabetes mellitus. Because of the necessity of performing a finger puncture, however, and the fact that the patient must assume more responsibility in self-management decisions, the medical assistant may need to reinforce the advantages of home blood glucose monitoring:

1. **Convenience of testing.** The patient is able to test his or her blood at any time of the day without a physician's order. Before the development of glucose monitors, patients could obtain a blood glucose test only through a laboratory order from the physician. Because of the cost and inconvenience involved in this process, most patients did not comply with the testing requirements needed to achieve and maintain satisfactory control. In addition, the patient was unable to obtain the test when the office or laboratory was closed. With some patients, the lowest blood glucose level occurs from 3:00 to 5:00 a.m. when most laboratory facilities are closed. Testing at home also lets the patient check his or her blood glucose when a side effect common to diabetes mellitus occurs, such as hypoglycemia.

2. **More involvement in self-management decisions.** The patient is able to become more involved in self-management decisions regarding insulin dosage, meal planning, and physical activity. Initially, some patients may lack confidence in making insulin and dietary adjustments based upon the blood glucose test results. The medical assistant should provide encouragement and stress the benefits to be derived in terms of improved regulation of the blood glucose level.

3. **Reliable decisions regarding insulin dosage.** More reliable decisions regarding insulin needs can be made during situations that affect the blood glucose level, such as illness, emotional stress, increased physical activity, or suspected hypoglycemia.

4. **Decrease or delay in long-term complications.** Diabetic patients maintaining good blood glucose control generally experience fewer symptoms and decrease or delay long-term complications of the disease; these results can lead to a longer life expectancy. Having a record of the patient's daily blood glucose values also assists the physician in making decisions regarding treatment and follow-up care.

The frequency of the blood glucose testing depends upon a number of factors, including the severity of the diabetes, the presence of special conditions such as pregnancy, and variations in activity level. Ideally, the blood glucose level should be monitored four times a day: in the morning (after an 8-hour fast), before lunch and dinner, and at bedtime. The FBS test result (obtained in the morning) is the best overall indicator of control, and the other determinations provide guidance for adjusting insulin dosage, diet, and exercise. Some physicians may periodically recommend a 2-hour postprandial specimen to further assist in maintaining good control by detecting hyperglycemia that might otherwise be missed.

Overall, self-monitoring of the blood glucose level at home provides an important feedback mechanism to maintain normal blood glucose levels and to assist the diabetic patient in anticipating and treating fluctuations in glucose levels brought on by food, exercise, stress, and infection.

19

PROCEDURE

19–1

Blood Glucose Measurement Using the Accu-Chek Advantage Glucose Monitor

EQUIPMENT/SUPPLIES: Personal protective equipment, including disposable gloves
Accu-Chek Advantage glucose monitor
Accu-Chek Advantage reagent strips
Lancet
Antiseptic wipe
Gauze pad
Biohazard sharps container

1. **Procedural Step.** Wash hands. Assemble the equipment. Check the expiration date on the container of reagent strips.

Principle. Outdated reagent strips can cause inaccurate test results.

2. **Procedural Step.** Greet and identify the patient. In-

Continued

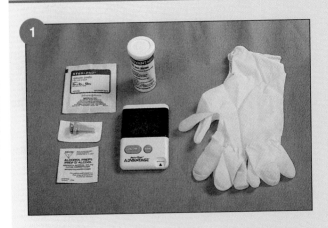

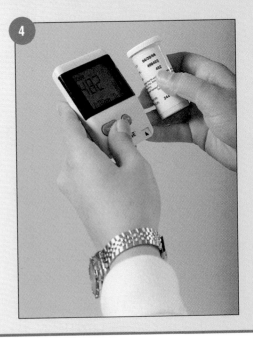

5. Procedural Step. Remove a test strip from the container. Promptly replace the lid of the container to prevent the strips from being exposed to moisture. **Principle.** The reagent pads are moisture sensitive and could be affected by environmental moisture, leading to inaccurate test results.

6. Procedural Step. Within 30 seconds, gently insert the test strip with the yellow target area facing up into the test strip guide. Once the strip is correctly inserted, a blood drop symbol flashes on the display.

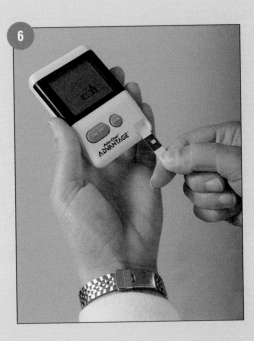

troduce yourself, and explain the procedure. If a fasting specimen is required, ask the patient if he or she has had anything to eat or drink (besides water) for the past 12 hours.
Principle. Consumption of food or fluid increases the blood glucose level, leading to inaccurate interpretation of FBS test results.

3. Procedural Step. Ask the patient to wash his or her hands in warm water and thoroughly dry them.
Principle. Washing the hands cleans the fingers and stimulates the flow of blood. The hands must be completely dry to encourage the formation of a hanging drop of blood which assists in the transfer of the blood to the reagent pad.

4. Procedural Step. Turn the monitor on. Check that the code number displayed matches the code number on the vial of test strips that you are using. When the test strip symbol flashes on the display, the monitor is ready to accept a test strip.

7. Procedural Step. Cleanse the puncture site with an antiseptic wipe and allow it to air dry. Put on personal protective equipment, including gloves, and perform a finger puncture. Dispose of the lancet in a biohazard sharps container.
Principle. The antiseptic must be allowed to dry to prevent it from reacting with the chemicals on the reagent pad, leading to inaccurate test results. Gloves are a precaution that provide a barrier against bloodborne pathogens.

8. Procedural Step. Once the puncture has been made, wipe away the first drop of blood with a gauze pad. Place the hand in a dependent position (palm facing down), and gently squeeze the finger around the puncture site until a large drop of blood forms.
Principle. The first drop of blood contains a large amount of serum, which dilutes the specimen and leads to inaccurate test results. A large drop of blood is needed to completely cover the target area of the reagent strip.

9. Procedural Step. Touch the drop of blood to the center of the yellow target area. Do not smear the

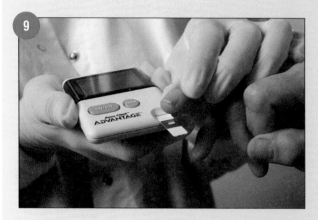

blood with your finger on the target area. If any yellow mesh is still visible after you have applied the initial drop of blood, a second drop of blood

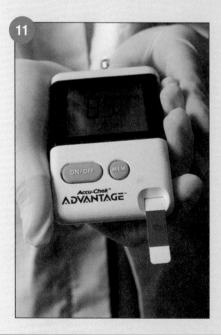

may be applied to the target area within 15 seconds of the first drop. If more than 15 seconds has passed, the test result may be erroneous and you should discard the test strip and repeat the test. When the blood is correctly applied to the strip, a box rotates on the display until the measurement is completed.

Principle. The entire yellow target area must be completely covered with blood to ensure accurate and reliable test results.

10. Procedural Step. Have the patient hold a gauze pad over the puncture site and apply pressure until the bleeding stops.

11. Procedural Step. After a short period of time, the glucose value is displayed in milligrams per deciliter. If the glucose value is higher or lower than expected or if the screen displays something other than the glucose value, refer to the Trouble-Shooting Guide section of the operator's manual to obtain instructions for correcting the problem. (The glucose result indicated on this glucose meter is 89 mg/dl.)

12. Procedural Step. Remove the reagent strip from the monitor and discard it in a biohazard waste container. Turn the monitor off.

13. Procedural Step. Remove the personal protective equipment, including gloves, and wash the hands. Chart the results. Include the date and time, when the patient last ate, the type of test (e.g., FBS, random), and the glucose test result. If the patient has diabetes mellitus, also record the time of his or her last insulin injection or last consumption of oral hypoglycemic medication.

14. Procedural Step. Properly store the glucose meter according the manufacturer's instructions.

19

CHARTING EXAMPLE

Date	
5/18/2002	8:30 a.m. FBS: 89 mg/dl. Pt last ate on
	5/17 @ 7:00 p.m. —— M. Villers, CMA

Serology

In the simplest terms, **serology** is defined as the scientific study of the serum of the blood. More specifically, however, serology deals with the study of antigen and antibody reactions.

An **antigen** is a substance that is capable of stimulating the formation of antibodies in an individual. An-tigens may consist of protein, glycoprotein, complex polysaccharides, or nucleic acid. Specific examples of antigens include bacteria and viruses, bacterial toxins, allergens, and blood antigens. An **antibody** is a substance that is capable of combining with an antigen, resulting in an antigen-antibody reaction.

Laboratory testing in serology deals with studying antigen-antibody reactions to assess the presence of a substance (e.g., ABO blood typing) or to assist in the diagnosis of disease (e.g., mononucleosis testing). Serologic tests are often used for the early diagnosis of disease and are also used to follow the course of the disease.

SEROLOGIC TESTS

☐ Some specific examples of serologic tests are listed and described here:

HEPATITIS TESTS. Hepatitis testing is performed to detect the presence of viral hepatitis. There are five types of viral hepatitis: A, B, C, D, and E, which are described in detail in Chapter 1: Medical Asepsis and Infection Control. Hepatitis testing not only detects the presence of viral hepatitis, but it also determines the specific type of hepatitis present.

SYPHILIS TESTS. Syphilis is a sexually transmitted disease (STD) caused by the microorganism *Treponema pallidum*. The tests most commonly used to detect the presence of syphilis are the Venereal Disease Research Laboratories (VDRL) test and the rapid plasma reagin (RPR) test. The test results are reported as nonreactive, weakly reactive, or reactive. Weakly reactive and reactive results are considered positive for the presence of syphilis antibodies. These tests are considered screening tests, and a positive result warrants more specific testing to arrive at a diagnosis for syphilis.

MONO TEST. This test is used to detect the presence of infectious mononucleosis. The theory and procedure for this test are given in detail in this chapter.

RHEUMATOID FACTOR. Rheumatoid arthritis is a chronic inflammatory disease that affects the joints of the body. The blood of individuals with rheumatoid arthritis contains a type of antibody called rheumatoid factor (RF). This test is used to detect the presence of the rheumatoid factor's antibodies and thereby assist in the diagnosis of rheumatoid arthritis.

ANTISTREPTOLYSIN O TEST. The antistreptolysin O (ASO) test is used to detect the presence of ASO antibodies in the serum. This is the most widely used serologic test for the detection of conditions resulting from streptococcal infections and diseases that occur secondary to a streptococcal infection. This test is useful in assisting in the diagnosis of rheumatic fever, glomerulonephritis, bacterial endocarditis, and scarlet fever.

C-REACTIVE PROTEIN. During inflammation and tissue destruction, an abnormal protein called C-reactive protein (CRP) appears in the blood. Patients with inflammatory conditions or disorders accompanied by tissue destruction will have a positive result to this test. Because of this, the CRP test is used to assist in diagnosing or charting the progress of such conditions as rheumatoid arthritis, acute rheumatic fever, widespread malignancy, and bacterial infections.

COLD AGGLUTININS. This test is used to detect the presence of antibodies called cold agglutinins. The cold agglutinins test is performed by incubating the patient's serum with erythrocytes at cold temperatures. If cold agglutinins are present, this causes agglutination of the erythrocytes. Cold agglutinins are found in patients with infectious mononucleosis, mycoplasmal pneumonia, chronic parasitic infections, and lymphoma.

ABO AND Rh BLOOD TYPING. Blood typing is performed to determine an individual's ABO and Rh blood type. The purpose of blood typing is to prevent transfusion and transplant reactions, to identify problems such as hemolytic disease of the newborn, and to determine parentage. The theory and procedure for ABO and Rh blood typing are presented in this chapter.

Rh ANTIBODY TITER. This test detects the amount of circulating Rh antibodies against red blood cells. These antibodies can occur in a pregnant woman who is Rh− and is carrying an Rh+ fetus. Therefore, this test is most frequently used to detect the presence of an Rh incompatibility problem with a mother and her unborn child.

RAPID MONONUCLEOSIS TESTING

☐ Infectious mononucleosis is an acute infectious disease caused by the Epstein-Barr virus (EBV). Infectious mononucleosis most frequently affects children and young adults. It is transmitted through saliva by direct oral contact, and because of this, it is often called the "kissing disease." Symptoms of infectious mononucleosis include mental and physical fatigue, fever, sore throat, severe weakness, headache, and swollen lymph nodes.

The rapid mono test is often performed in the medical office and is used to assist in the diagnosis of infectious mononucleosis. Rapid mono tests are easy to perform and provide reliable results in a short period of time.

Individuals with infectious mononucleosis produce an antibody called heterophile antibody, usually by the sixth to the tenth day of the illness. Rapid mono tests are able to detect the presence of this antibody. The presence of the heterophile antibody along with patient symptoms can provide the basis for the diagnosis of infectious mononucleosis. The procedure for performing a rapid monotest using the Cards O. S. Mono Test by Pacific Biotech, Inc. (a subsidiary of Quidel Corporation), is outlined in Figure 19–3.

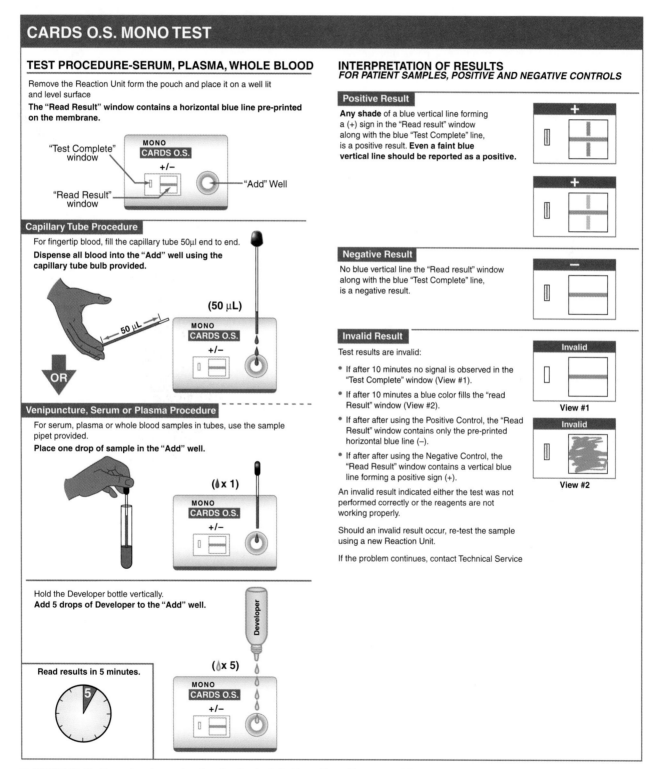

■ FIGURE 19–3. Procedure for performing the Cards O.S. Mono Test. (Courtesy of Quidel Corporation, San Diego, CA.)

19

BLOOD TYPING

BLOOD ANTIGENS

Each individual has a blood type. Blood type depends upon the presence of certain factors, or antigens, on the surface of the red blood cells. **Blood antigens** consist of protein and are inherited through genes, which program the body to produce a particular antigen. If a blood antigen is present, it will appear on the surface of all the red blood cells in the body.

Many different types of antigen can appear in the blood. These antigens can be grouped into categories known as blood group systems. The blood group systems that are most likely to cause problems in blood transfusions and in Rh disease of the newborn are the ABO and Rh blood group systems. Therefore, these are the blood group systems most commonly tested for in the medical laboratory.

Within the ABO blood group system, there are four main blood types: A, B, AB, and O. The blood type depends on which antigens are present on the surface of the red blood cells.

If the A antigen is present, the blood type is A.

If the B antigen is present, the blood type is B.

If both the A and B antigens are present, the blood type is AB.

If neither the A nor the B antigen is present, the blood type is O. Figure 19–4 helps illustrate this principle.

19

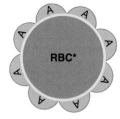

Type A blood:
A antigen is present

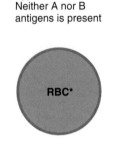

Type B blood:
B antigen is present

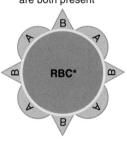

Type AB blood:
A and B antigens
are both present

Type O blood:
Neither A nor B
antigens is present

* Red blood cell

■ **FIGURE 19–4.** Blood type depends on which antigens are present on the surface of the red blood cells.

BLOOD ANTIBODIES

Blood antibodies are proteins that are naturally present in the plasma of the blood. An **antibody** is a substance that is capable of combining with an antigen. The body never produces an antibody to combine with its own blood antigen. For example, if the blood type is A, the plasma does not contain the A antibody. However, the B antibody naturally occurs in that plasma. The B antibody cannot combine with the A antigen. If a blood antigen and its corresponding antibody combine (in this case, the A antigen combining with the A antibody), a serious antigen-antibody reaction will take place that could pose a threat to life.

■ If the blood type is A, the plasma contains the B antibody.
■ If the blood type is B, the plasma contains the A antibody.
■ If the blood type is AB, neither the A nor the B antibodies appear in the plasma.
■ If the blood type is O, both the A and B antibodies appear in the plasma. Remember, type O blood has neither the A nor the B antigen on the surface of its

red blood cells. The A and B antibodies appearing in the plasma would not have an A or B antigen to combine with them (Table 19–2).

THE Rh BLOOD GROUP SYSTEM

In 1940, Landsteiner and Wiener discovered the Rh blood group system while working with rhesus monkeys. Approximately 85 percent of the white population has the Rh antigen present on the red blood cells and therefore has Type Rh+ blood. The remaining 15 percent of the population does not have the Rh antigen present on the red blood cells and thus has Type Rh− blood. The Rh antibodies do not normally occur in the plasma as do the A and B antibodies.

TABLE 19–2

ABO Blood Group System		
Blood Type	**Antigen Present on the Red Blood Cell**	**Antibody Present in the Plasma**
A	A	B
B	B	A
AB	A, B	Neither A nor B
O	Neither A or B	A, B

Highlight on Blood Donor Criteria

Each year, approximately 5 million Americans require blood transfusions, resulting in 13.5 million units of blood being transfused. A safe, readily available blood supply is essential for lifesaving medical procedures, such as replacing blood loss from hemorrhages or surgical procedures, replacing plasma in burn and shock victims, and providing platelets to control bleeding. In an average population, 75 percent of the people are physically and medically eligible to donate blood; however, only 5 percent of those eligible decide to donate.

Basic blood donor criteria have been established on a national basis to ensure donor safety and a quality blood donation. All blood collection facilities, such as the American Red Cross, must follow these regulations. In general, blood donors must be in good health and be of a certain age and weight.

HEALTH HISTORY. To protect both the donor and recipient, each donor is asked to give a brief health history. The prospective donor is asked to provide information relating to diseases that may be transmitted through the blood (such as hepatitis and AIDS) and medications being taken that could affect the quality of the blood donation. Information is also obtained relating to medical conditions that might jeopardize the health of the donor if he or she were to donate.

Based on this information, a prospective donor could be **temporarily deferred** from donating blood because of the following: recent immunizations, pregnancy, certain medical conditions such as cancer or a recent heart attack, certain prescription medications being taken, recent tattooing, and travel to a malaria-prone area. Individuals who are temporarily deferred will be told how long they must wait and are encouraged to donate blood once the waiting period is over. The waiting period varies based on the specific condition or situation; for example, for pregnancy, there is a 6-week waiting period following delivery, whereas there is only a 48-hour wait following the last dose of an antibiotic medication.

A prospective donor is **permanently deferred** from giving blood because of any of the following: a history of hepatitis, infection with the AIDS virus (HIV infection), and behavior that is associated with the spread of the AIDS virus.

AGE. An individual must be at least 18 years of age or older to donate blood. With written parental consent, however, 17-year-old individuals may donate blood.

Also, some states require that people over the age of 65 years have their physician's written consent to donate blood.

DATE OF LAST DONATION. At least 56 days (8 weeks) must elapse between donations.

WEIGHT. The donor must weigh at least 110 pounds. (In some states, the minimum weight is 105 pounds.) For the average individual, the total volume of blood is approximately 8 percent of the body weight. Underweight donors are not accepted because a full donation would result in a proportionately greater reduction in blood volume and could possibly precipitate a reaction.

TEMPERATURE. Body temperature of donors may not exceed 99.5°F (37.5°C). The primary purpose of temperature measurement is to eliminate donors who are ill.

PULSE. The acceptable range for the pulse rate is 50 to 110 beats per minute. If the pulse rate appears to be elevated because of physical exertion, the donor may be asked to remain seated for 5 to 10 minutes, with a recheck taken after the resting period.

BLOOD PRESSURE. The acceptable limit for blood pressure is a reading no higher than 180 mm Hg for the systolic pressure and a reading no higher than 100 mm Hg for the diastolic pressure.

HEMOGLOBIN. The hemoglobin must be 12.5 g/dl or higher for women and 13.5 g/dl or higher for men.

BLOOD-DONATING PROCESS

It takes approximately 1 hour to complete the blood donation process, which begins with the health history, followed by a mini-physical check of temperature, pulse, blood pressure, and hemoglobin level. Next, a unit (1 pint) of blood is collected using a sterile needle and a sterile plastic bag containing an additive. A donor should feel no pain during the blood collection procedure, which takes approximately 8 to 10 minutes. It is not possible to contract AIDS or any other infectious disease by donating blood. Following the collection of the unit of blood, the donor is encouraged to have refreshments to begin replenishing the fluids and nutrients temporarily lost during the donation.

PROCESSING THE BLOOD

Each blood donation is tested for AIDS, hepatitis, and syphilis. Any unit of blood that tests positive is rejected for transfusion. The unit of blood is typed and then labeled with its ABO and Rh blood type. It is then available for distribution to hospitals for transfusing.

19

BLOOD ANTIGEN AND ANTIBODY REACTIONS

☐ When a blood antigen and its corresponding antibody unite, the result is the clumping, or **agglutination,** of red blood cells. Agglutination of red blood cells can be serious and even fatal if it occurs in vivo (in the living body). The clumped red blood cells cannot pass through the small tubules of the kidneys, and this may lead to kidney failure. Also, the clumping of the red blood cells eventually leads to **hemolysis,** or breakdown of the red blood cells.

Blood antigen-antibody reactions can occur if the wrong blood type is administered to an individual during a blood transfusion. If an individual with type A blood is given a transfusion of type B blood, the B antibody of the recipient (person receiving the blood) would combine with the B antigen of the donor (person donating the blood), and an antigen-antibody reaction would occur, resulting in agglutination of red blood cells. Therefore, we say that type A blood is incompatible with type B blood.

AGGLUTINATION AND BLOOD TYPING

☐ Agglutination of red blood cells is the basis for the ABO and Rh blood typing procedure. The antigen-antibody reaction occurs in vitro, or "in glass" in the laboratory, so there is no threat to life.

To test for the ABO blood group system, a commercially prepared antiserum is used. An **antiserum** is a serum containing antibodies. An antiserum containing the A antibody is added to an unknown blood specimen. If the A antigen is present, it combines with the A antibody, resulting in agglutination. An antise-

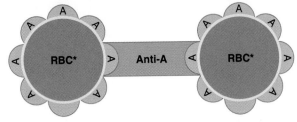

The bridge forming between the antigen and antibody represents the antigen-antibody reaction. This reaction leads to agglutination of red blood cells, which is visible to the naked eye.

■ **FIGURE 19–5.** The antigen-antibody reaction that occurs in vitro when the unknown blood sample is Type A.

rum containing the B antibody is added to another sample of the unknown blood. If the B antigen is present, it will combine with the B antibody, resulting in agglutination. If agglutination occurs in both instances, the sample is type AB. If no agglutination occurs, this indicates the absence of blood antigens, or type O blood. Agglutination that occurs in vitro is visible to the naked eye.

The antigen-antibody reaction that occurs when the unknown blood sample is type A is diagrammed in Figure 19–5.

19

MEDICAL PRACTICE AND THE LAW

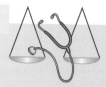

When running laboratory tests, you must make sure all equipment is functioning properly. This is done by the periodic calibration or running of controls on each piece of equipment. Know how and how often to calibrate or run controls and document appropriately. Without these quality controls, results cannot be trusted to be accurate. Inaccurate results can lead to an inaccurate diagnosis and treatment.

Use personal protective equipment appropriate to each test to avoid transmission of disease and cross-contamination of specimens.

Who Can Sue?

Anyone can sue for anything. The important thing to know is, can they win? The person filing the lawsuit is called the plaintiff, and the one being sued is called the defendant. In order to win a malpractice lawsuit, four things are necessary:

1. The defendant must have had a duty to the plaintiff, that is, a doctor-patient relationship must exist.

2. Care must have been provided that was not consistent with that of a "reasonably prudent" physician or medical assistant. In other words, a mistake was made and the individual making it should have known better. If you work in a specialty area, you are expected to know more about that specialty than if you worked in a general practice office. Therefore, be very familiar with your office's policy and procedure manual.
3. The plaintiff must prove proximate cause. This means the patient's problem is a direct cause of the physician's or medical assistant's actions.
4. The plaintiff must have been injured by the mistake. Damages may include pain and suffering, loss of income, and medical bills.

To avoid personal lawsuits, practice good care, document everything you do, and maintain good relationships with patients. Few patients who are hurt will sue, but most patients who are hurt and are angry *will* sue.

19

CERTIFICATION REVIEW

☐ Blood chemistry testing involves the quantitative measurement of chemical substances present in the blood. These chemicals are dissolved in the liquid portion of the blood; therefore, most blood chemistry tests require a serum specimen for analysis. In the medical office, automated blood chemistry analyzers are often used to perform blood chemistry testing.

☐ Quality control consists of methods and means to ensure that the test results are reliable and valid.

☐ Calibration involves the use of a standard to check the precision of the blood chemistry analyzer. If an analyzer is not properly calibrated, it will be unable to produce accurate test results. A control consists of a sample of a known value. Normal controls fall within normal range whereas abnormal controls fall outside normal range.

☐ Cholesterol is a white, waxy, fatlike substance that is essential for normal functioning of the body. Most of the cholesterol circulating in the blood is

Continued

CERTIFICATION REVIEW *Continued*

manufactured by the liver; however, a portion of it is dietary cholesterol. Dietary cholesterol is found only in animal products.

☐ High blood cholesterol may cause fatty deposits, or plaque, to build up on the walls of the arteries, a condition known as atherosclerosis. LDL cholesterol is often referred to as "bad" cholesterol because an excess amount of it in the blood can cause plaque to build up on the arterial walls, resulting in atherosclerosis. HDL cholesterol removes excess cholesterol from the walls of the blood vessels and is protective and beneficial to the body.

☐ Cholesterol test results are interpreted as follows: Total cholesterol levels under 200 mg/dl are considered desirable. Levels between 200 and 239 mg/dl are considered borderline high, and levels of 240 mg/dl and above are considered high. An HDL cholesterol level above 35 mg/dl is considered acceptable, while a level below 35 mg/dl has been determined to be a risk factor for coronary heart disease.

☐ Glucose is the end product of carbohydrate metabolism; its function is to serve as the chief source of energy for the body. Glucose taken in that is not needed for energy can be stored in the form of glycogen in muscle and liver tissue for later use. Insulin is a hormone secreted by the pancreas and is required for normal utilization of glucose in the body.

☐ Measuring the amount of glucose present in a blood specimen is one of the most commonly performed blood chemistry tests. It is used to detect abnormalities in carbohydrate metabolism such as occur in diabetes mellitus, hypoglycemia, and liver and adrenocortical dysfunction.

☐ Blood glucose is usually measured when the patient is in a fasting state. This type of test is termed a fasting blood sugar (FBS). The patient should not have anything to eat or drink, except water, for 12 hours preceding the test. The normal range for a fasting blood sugar is 70 to 110 mg/dl. An FBS is often performed on patients with diabetes to evaluate their progress and regulate treatment, and as a routine screening procedure to detect diabetes mellitus.

☐ The 2-hour postprandial blood sugar (2-hour PPBS) test is used to screen for the presence of diabetes mellitus and to monitor the effects of insulin dosage in diagnosed diabetics. The glucose tolerance test (GTT) provides more detailed information about the ability of the body to metabolize glucose by assessing the insulin response to a glucose load. The GTT is used to assist in the diagnosis of diabetes mellitus, hypoglycemia, and liver and adrenocortical dysfunction.

☐ Serology is defined as the scientific study of the serum of the blood. Examples of serologic tests include hepatitis tests, syphilis tests, mono test, rheumatoid factor, antistreptolysin O test, C-reactive protein, cold agglutinins, ABO and Rh blood typing, and Rh antibody titer.

☐ Infectious mononucleosis is an acute infectious disease caused by the Epstein-Barr virus (EBV). Symptoms include mental and physical fatigue, fever, sore throat, severe weakness, headache, and swollen lymph nodes.

☐ Blood antigens consist of protein and are inherited through genes. Within the ABO blood group system, there are four main blood types: A, B, AB, and O. Blood antibodies are proteins that are naturally present in the plasma of the blood. An antibody is a substance that is capable of combining with an antigen. When a blood antigen and its corresponding antibody unite, the result is the clumping, or agglutination, of red blood cells. Agglutination of red blood cells can be serious and even fatal if it occurs in the living body.

19

RESOURCE

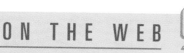

ON THE WEB

For information on diabetes:

American Diabetes Association
www.diabetes.org

Diabetes Well
www.diabeteswell.com

Joslin Diabetes Center
www.joslin.org

National Diabetes Education
Initiative
www.ndei.org

The National Institute of Diabetes
www.niddk.nih.gov

19

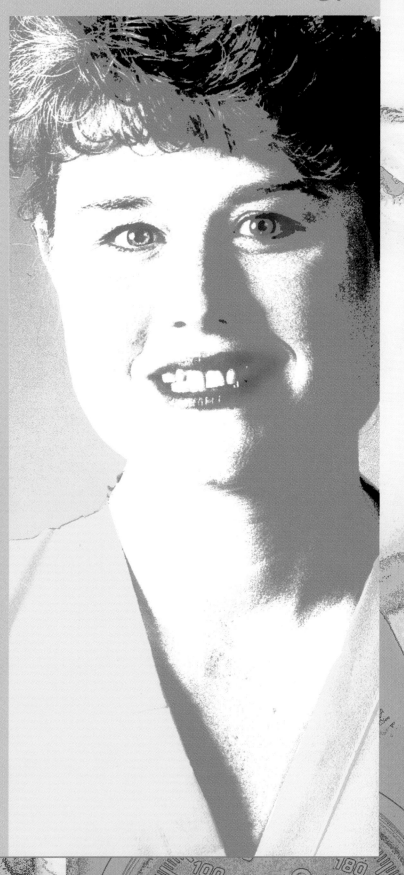

Natalie Moorehead, *and I am a Certified Medical Assistant. I graduated from an accredited medical assisting program and have an associate's degree in Applied Science. I am employed by a physician who specializes in family practice, and I have been on staff at this facility for 4 years.*

For the past year, my primary responsibilities have been working in both the front and back office. I handle all of our workers' compensation patients with active claims. I schedule patient appointments, make referrals, process the mail, and perform countless other tasks involved with running the front office properly. It is not uncommon for me to talk on the phone to an insurance company one minute and then the next minute to be taking vital signs or performing a venipuncture on a patient. I have had to learn to separate the two and to concentrate on one thing at a time. It gets kind of crazy at times, but I work for a physician who tells me that I am a valuable asset because I can work anywhere in the office. To me this means one thing—job security.

I enjoy my job. There is something new and different every day, but I would have to say what keeps my job interesting is the patients. They come from all walks of life. I have established many friendships, and through these people, my education continues.

OUTCOMES

After completing this chapter, you should be able to demonstrate the proper procedures to perform the following:

1. Use a compound microscope.
2. Properly handle and care for a microscope.
3. Obtain a specimen for a throat culture.
4. Perform a streptococcus test, using a rapid strep test.
5. Perform a streptococcus test, using the bacitracin susceptibility test.
6. Prepare a wet mount.
7. Prepare a hanging drop slide.
8. Prepare a microbiologic smear.

EDUCATIONAL OBJECTIVES

After completing this chapter, you should be able to do the following:

1. Define the words listed in the Key Terminology.
2. List and explain the stages in the course of an infectious disease.
3. List and describe the three classifications of bacteria based on shape.
4. Give examples of infectious diseases caused by the following types of cocci: staphylococci, streptococci, and diplococci.
5. State examples of infectious diseases caused by bacilli, spirilla, and viruses.
6. Explain the function of the following parts of a compound microscope: base, arm, stage, light source, substage condenser, iris diaphragm, body tube, coarse adjustment, and fine adjustment.
7. Identify the function of each of the following microscope lenses: low power, high power, and oil immersion.
8. List five guidelines that should be followed for proper care of the microscope.
9. Explain the purpose of obtaining a specimen, and identify five body areas from which a specimen may be taken for microbiologic examination.
10. List two ways to prevent contamination of a specimen by extraneous microorganisms.
11. Explain what types of precautions a medical assistant should take to prevent infection from a pathogenic specimen.
12. Explain the purpose and describe the procedure for culturing a microbiologic specimen.
13. Explain the importance of the early diagnosis of streptococcal pharyngitis.
14. Explain the purpose and describe the procedure for performing a sensitivity test.
15. Explain the purpose of making a microbiologic smear.
16. Explain the purpose of Gram staining.
17. Identify four infectious diseases caused by gram-positive bacteria and four caused by gram-negative bacteria.
18. Give examples of methods to prevent and control infectious diseases in the community.
19. Explain the principle underlying each step in the microbiologic procedures.

bacilli (ba-SILL-î) **(singular, bacillus):** Bacteria that have a rod shape

cocci (COCK-sî) **(singular, coccus):** Bacteria that have a round shape

colony: A mass of bacteria growing on a solid culture medium that have arisen from the multiplication of a single bacterium.

contagious: Capable of being transmitted directly or indirectly from one person to another.

culture: The propagation of a mass of microorganisms in a laboratory culture medium.

culture medium: A mixture of nutrients on which microorganisms are grown in the laboratory.

false negative: A test result denoting that a condition is absent when, in actuality, it is present.

false positive: A test result denoting that a condition is present when, in actuality, it is absent.

fastidious (FAS-stid-ê-us): Extremely delicate, difficult to culture, therefore involving specialized growth requirements.

immunization (IM-Û-nis-â-shun): The process of becoming protected from a disease through vaccination.

incubate (INK-û-bâte): In microbiology, the act of placing a culture in a chamber (incubator), which provides optimal growth requirements for the multiplication of the organisms, such as the proper temperature, humidity, and darkness.

incubation period: The interval of time between the invasion by a pathogenic microorganism and the appearance of first symptoms of the disease.

infectious disease: A disease caused by a pathogen that produces harmful effects on its host.

inoculate (IN-ok-û-lâte): To introduce microorganisms into a culture medium for growth and multiplication.

inoculum (IN-ok-û-lum) The specimen used to inoculate a medium.

microbiology: The scientific study of microorganisms and their activities.

mucous membrane: A membrane lining body passages or cavities that open to the outside.

normal flora: Harmless, nonpathogenic microorganisms that normally reside in many parts of the body but do not cause disease.

prodrome (PRÔ-drôm): A symptom indicating an approaching disease.

resistance: The natural ability of an organism to remain unaffected by harmful substances in its environment.

sequela (SA-kwêl-ya): A morbid (secondary) condition occurring as a result of a less serious primary infection.

smear Material spread on a slide for microscope examination.

specimen (spess-a-men): A small sample or part taken from the body to show the nature of the whole.

spirilla **(singular, spirillum):** Bacteria that have a spiral shape.

streaking: In microbiology, the process of inoculating a culture to provide for the growth of colonies on the surface of a solid medium. Streaking is accomplished by skimming a wire inoculating loop containing the specimen across the surface of the medium, using a back and forth motion.

streptolysin (STREP-tô-lî-sin): An exotoxin produced by beta-hemolytic streptococci, which completely hemolyzes red blood cells.

susceptible Easily affected, lacking resistance.

INTRODUCTION

☐ **Microbiology** is the scientific study of microorganisms and their activities. As described in Chapter 1 microorganisms are tiny living plants and animals that cannot be seen by the naked eye but must be viewed under the microscope. Anton van Leeuwenhoek (1632–1723) designed a magnifying glass strong enough for viewing microorganisms. He was the first individual to observe and describe protozoa and bacteria (Fig. 20–1). Leeuwenhoek's magnifying glass was the precursor of the modern microscopes used today for studying microorganisms. A microscope allows the observer to see individual microbial cells and thereby to differentiate and identify microorganisms.

For the most part, microbiology deals with unicellular, or one-celled, microscopic organisms. All of the life processes needed to sustain the microbe are performed by one cell. Among them are the ingestion of

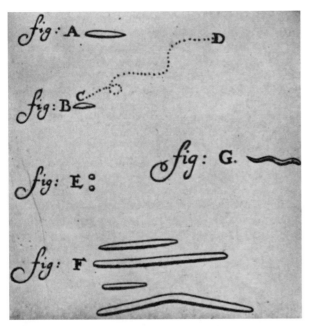

■ FIGURE 20–1. Drawings of bacteria made by van Leeuwenhoek in 1684. (From Fuerst, R.: *Frobisher and Fuerst's Microbiology in Health and Disease,* ed. 15. Philadelphia, W. B. Saunders, 1983.)

food substances and their utilization for energy, growth, reproduction, and excretion.

Microorganisms are **ubiquitous;** they are found almost everywhere—in the air, in food and water, in the soil, and in association with plant, animal, and human life. Although there are vast numbers of microorganisms, only a relatively small minority are pathogenic and able to cause disease.

When a pathogen infects a host, it often produces a specific set of symptoms peculiar to that disease. For example, scarlet fever is frequently characterized by a sore throat, swelling of the lymph nodes of the neck, a red and swollen tongue, and a bright red rash covering the body. These symptoms aid the physician in diagnosing the disease. The medical assistant must be alert to any symptoms described in the patient and relay this information to the physician. Microbiologic laboratory tests are also used to help the physician identify the pathogen causing the disease. Identification of the pathogen leads to the proper treatment of the disease.

Although most microbiologic tests are performed in the hospital or the medical laboratory, the medical assistant is frequently responsible for the collection of specimens. This chapter provides an introduction to the field of microbiology, including a description of those techniques that may be performed in the medical office. Before undertaking this study, the medical assistant should review Chapter 1, which discusses introductory concepts that are basic to this chapter.

THE NORMAL FLORA

☐ Each individual has a **normal flora,** which consists of the harmless, nonpathogenic microorganisms that normally reside in many parts of the body but do not cause disease. The surface of the skin, the mucous membrane of the gastrointestinal tract, and parts of the respiratory and genitourinary tracts all have an abundant normal flora. The microorganisms making up the normal flora may sometimes be beneficial to the body, such as those contained in the intestinal tract that feed on other potentially harmful microscopic organisms. Other examples are those microorganisms found in the intestinal tract that synthesize vitamin K, an essential vitamin needed by the body for proper blood clotting. In rare instances, if the opportunity arises, such as in a condition of lowered body resistance, certain microorganisms making up the normal flora are capable of becoming pathogenic and causing disease.

INFECTION

☐ The invasion of the body by pathogenic microorganisms is known as **infection.** Under conditions favorable to the pathogens, they grow and multiply, resulting in an **infectious disease** that produces harmful effects on the host. However, not all pathogens that enter a host are able to cause disease. When a pathogen enters the body, it attempts to invade the tissues so it can grow and multiply. The body, in turn, tries to stop the invasion with its second line of natural defense mechanisms,* which includes inflammation, phagocytosis by white blood cells, the production of antibodies, and others. These defense mechanisms work to destroy the pathogen and remove it from the body. If the body is successful, the pathogens are destroyed and the individual suffers no adverse effects. If the pathogen is able to overcome the body's natural defense mechanisms, an infectious disease results.

Many infectious diseases are **contagious,** meaning that the pathogen causing the disease can be spread from one person to another either directly or indirectly. Frequently, **droplet infection** is the mode of transmission of pathogens. This is the inhalation of pathogens from a fine spray emitted by a person already infected with the disease. When the infected individual exhales, as during breathing, talking, coughing, or sneezing, the pathogens are dispersed into the air on minute liquid particles. Therefore, infected individuals should cover their mouths or noses while cough-

20

---

*The first line of natural defense mechanisms that works to *prevent* the entrance of pathogens into the body (e.g., coughing and sneezing) has already been described in Chapter 1.

ing or sneezing. Refer to Figure 1–1, the Infection Process Cycle, for examples of other means of pathogen transmission.

STAGES OF AN INFECTIOUS DISEASE

Once a pathogen becomes established in the host, a series of events generally ensues. The stages of an infectious disease are

1. The **infection** is the invasion and multiplication of pathogenic microorganisms in the body.
2. The **incubation period** is the interval of time between the invasion by a pathogenic microorganism and the appearance of the first symptoms of the disease. Depending on the type of disease, the incubation period may range in duration from only a few days to several months.
3. The **prodromal period** is a short period in which the first symptoms that indicate an approaching disease occur. Headache and a feeling of illness are common prodromal symptoms.
4. The **acute period** is when the disease is at its peak and symptoms are fully developed. Fever is a common symptom of many infectious diseases.
5. The **decline period** is when the symptoms of the disease begin to subside.
6. The **convalescent period** is the stage in which the patient regains strength and returns to a state of health.

20

MICROORGANISMS AND DISEASE

☐ The groups of microorganisms known to contain species capable of causing human disease include bacteria, viruses, protozoa, fungi (including yeasts), and animal parasites. Bacteria and viruses are most frequently responsible for causing disease in humans and are discussed next.

BACTERIA

Bacteria are microscopic organisms. Of the 1700 species known to dwell in humans, only approximately 100 produce human disease. The discovery of antibiotics has helped immensely in combating and controlling infections caused by bacteria. It must be remembered, however, that antibiotics are not effective against viral infections.

Bacteria can be classified into three basic groups, according to their shape (Fig. 20–2). Bacteria having a

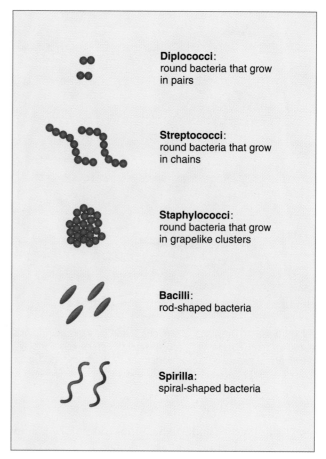

Diplococci: round bacteria that grow in pairs

Streptococci: round bacteria that grow in chains

Staphylococci: round bacteria that grow in grapelike clusters

Bacilli: rod-shaped bacteria

Spirilla: spiral-shaped bacteria

■ **FIGURE 20–2.** Classification of bacteria based on shape.

round shape are known as **cocci.** The cocci can be further divided into diplococci, streptococci, and staphylococci, depending on their pattern of growth. Bacteria having a rod shape are termed **bacilli.** Those having a spiral shape are known as **spirilla,** and they include spirochetes and vibrios.

The Cocci

Staphylococci are round bacteria that grow in grapelike clusters (Fig. 20–3*A*). The species *Staphylococcus epidermidis* is widely distributed and is normally present on the surface of the skin and the mucous membranes of the mouth, nose, throat, and intestines. *S. epidermidis* is usually nonpathogenic; however, a cut, abrasion, or other break in the skin may result in the invasion of the tissues by the organism, resulting in a mild infection.

Staphylococcus aureus is the species commonly associated with pathologic conditions such as boils, carbuncles, pimples, impetigo, abscesses, *Staphylococcus* food poisoning, and wound infections. Infections caused by

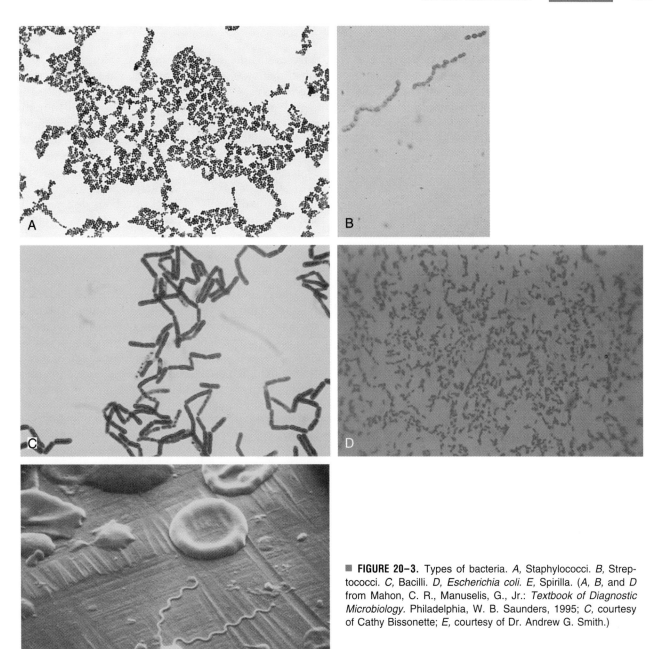

20

■ **FIGURE 20–3.** Types of bacteria. *A,* Staphylococci. *B,* Streptococci. *C,* Bacilli. *D, Escherichia coli. E,* Spirilla. (*A, B,* and *D* from Mahon, C. R., Manuselis, G., Jr.: *Textbook of Diagnostic Microbiology.* Philadelphia, W. B. Saunders, 1995; *C,* courtesy of Cathy Bissonette; *E,* courtesy of Dr. Andrew G. Smith.)

staphylococci usually cause much pus formation (suppuration) and are termed pyogenic infections.

Streptococci are round bacteria that grow in chains (Fig. 20–3*B*). Before the advent of antibiotics, streptococcal infections were one of the major causes of death in humans. Some of the diseases caused by different types of streptococci include streptococcal sore throat ("strep throat"), scarlet fever, rheumatic fever, pneumonia, puerperal sepsis, erysipelas, and skin conditions such as carbuncles and impetigo.

Diplococci are round bacteria that grow in pairs. Pneumonia, gonorrhea, and meningitis are examples of infectious diseases caused by different types of diplococci.

The Bacilli

Bacilli are rod-shaped bacteria that are frequently found in the soil and air (Fig. 20–3C). Some bacilli are able to form spores, a characteristic that enables them to resist adverse conditions such as heat and disinfectants. Some of the diseases caused by different types of bacilli include botulism, tetanus, gas gangrene, gastroenteritis produced by *Salmonella* food poisoning, typhoid fever, pertussis (whooping cough), bacillary dysentery, diphtheria, tuberculosis, leprosy, and the plague.

Escherichia coli is the name of one type of bacillus that is found among the normal flora of the intestinal tract in enormous numbers (Fig. 20–3D). It is normally a harmless bacterium; however, if it enters the urinary tract as a result of lowered resistance or poor hygienic practices, or both, it may cause a urinary tract infection.

THE SPIRILLA

Spirilla are spiral bacteria. *Treponema pallidum*, a spirochete, is the causative agent of syphilis (Fig. 20–3E). This microorganism cannot be grown in commonly available culture media; therefore, the diagnosis of syphilis is generally made using serologic tests. A serologic test is performed on the serum of the blood. Cholera is caused by another type of spirillum, *Vibrio cholerae*. Immunization and proper methods of sanitation and water purification have all but eliminated cholera epidemics in the United States.

VIRUSES

Viruses are the smallest living organisms. They are so small that an electron microscope must be used to view them. Viruses infect plants and animals as well as humans and use nutrients inside the host's cells for their metabolic and reproductive needs. Some of the human infectious diseases caused by different types of viruses include influenza, chickenpox, rubeola (measles), rubella (German measles), mumps, poliomyelitis, smallpox, rabies, herpes simplex, herpes zoster, yellow fever, hepatitis, and the majority of infectious diseases of the upper respiratory tract, including the common cold.

THE MICROSCOPE

☐ Many kinds of microscopes are available, but the type used most often for office laboratory work is the **compound microscope.** The compound microscope consists of a two-lens system, and the magnification of one system is increased by the other. A source of bright light is required for proper illumination of the object to be viewed. This combination of lenses and light permits visualization of structures that cannot be seen with the unaided eye, such as microorganisms and cellular forms. The compound microscope consists of two main components: the support system and the optical system, each of which includes a number of parts discussed next. The medical assistant should be able to identify the parts of a microscope (Fig. 20–4) and be able to properly use and care for it.

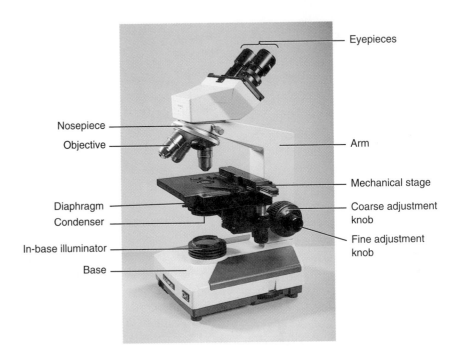

■ **FIGURE 20–4.** Parts of the microscope.

20

SUPPORT SYSTEM

Frame

The working parts of the microscope are supported by a sturdy frame consisting of a **base** for support and an **arm** for carrying it without damaging the delicate parts. The arm is also needed to support the magnifying and adjusting systems.

Stage

The stage of a microscope is the flat, horizontal platform on which the microscope slide is placed. It is located directly over the condenser and beneath the objective lenses. The stage has a small round opening in the center that permits light from below to pass through the object being viewed and up into the lenses above. The slide should be placed on the stage; the object to be viewed is positioned over this opening so that it is satisfactorily illuminated by the light source below. Standard microscope stages have metal clips attached to the stage to hold the glass slide securely in place. With this type of stage, the slide must be moved by hand to examine various areas on it.

Other types of microscope have a **mechanical stage** that allows movement of the slide in a vertical or horizontal position by using adjustment knobs. The mechanical stage provides precise positioning of the slide, which is essential for performing certain procedures such as differential white blood counts and inspection of gram-stained smears.

Light Source

The light source is located at the base of the microscope and consists of a built-in illuminator (or bulb), along with a switch for turning it on. The light is directed to the condenser above it and then through the object to be viewed.

Condenser

Compound microscopes have a lens system between the light source and object, known as the **substage condenser.** A commonly used condenser is the **Abbé condenser,** which consists of two lenses used to illuminate objects with transmitted light. The condenser collects and concentrates the light rays and directs them up, bringing them to a focus on the object so that it is well illuminated.

Diaphragm

The amount of light focused on the object can also be controlled by the **iris diaphragm,** located beneath or within the condenser. The diaphragm consists of a series of horizontally arranged interlocking plates with a central opening, or aperture. The iris diaphragm has a lever that is used to increase or decrease the amount of light admitted by increasing or decreasing the size of the aperture. The diaphragm aperture opening is combined with the movement of the substage condenser to control the light intensity.

Appropriate adjustment of the light intensity is essential for properly viewing the specimens, especially at a higher magnification. A general rule is that, as the desired magnification increases, the more intense the light must be. For example, increased light intensity is required for good visualization of a specimen with the oil-immersion objective. On the other hand, when using the low-power objective, the light must be somewhat diminished in order to produce the appropriate contrast for specimen detail and to reduce glare. The degree of illumination is also influenced by the density of the object; therefore, stained structures (e.g., a gram-stained smear of bacteria) usually require more light than do unstained ones.

Adjustment Knobs

There are two adjustment knobs that are used to bring the specimen into focus: the coarse adjustment knob and the fine adjustment knob. The **coarse adjustment** is used to obtain an approximate focus quickly. The **fine adjustment** is then used to obtain the precise focusing necessary to produce a sharp, clear image. On some microscope models, the adjustment knobs are mounted as two separate knobs; on others, they may be placed together with the smaller fine adjustment knob extending from a larger coarse adjustment wheel.

OPTICAL SYSTEM

Compound microscopes have a two-lens magnification system. **Magnification** is defined as the ratio of apparent size of an object when viewed through the microscope to the actual size of the object.

The Eyepiece

The first lens system is the eyepiece or ocular lens located at the top of the body tube and marked with 10×, meaning that it magnifies 10 times. Microscopes that have one eyepiece only are called **monocular** microscopes, and those with two eyepieces are called **binocular.** A binocular microscope is recommended for medical office laboratory work because it causes less eye fatigue than the monocular type. The binocular eyepieces can be adjusted to each individual by moving the eyepieces apart or together as needed.

Objective Lenses

The second lens system consists of three objective lenses located on the revolving **nosepiece,** each with a different degree of magnification. The metal shaft of each objective lens differs in length and is identified with its power of magnification. The short objective is known as the **low-power objective** and has a magnification of 10×. The **high-power objective** is also known as the high-dry objective because it does not require the use of immersion oil; it has a magnification of 40×. The **oil-immersion objective** has the highest power of magnification, which is 100×.

Some microscope manufacturers identify the objective lenses by variously colored rings. For example, green is used for low power, yellow for high power, and red or black for oil immersion. If the objective is not color coded, it can be identified by the length of the metal shaft; the low-power objective is the shortest, whereas the oil-immersion objective is the longest.

The objective lens magnifies the specimen, and the ocular lens magnifies the image produced by the objective lens. The **total magnification** of each objective is determined by multiplying the ocular magnification by the objective magnification. The total magnification of the low-power objective is 100 times the actual size of the object being viewed (10 × 10). The total magnification of the high-power objective is 400× (10 × 40), and the oil-immersion magnification is 1000 (10 × 100).

Focus

Depending on the type of microscope, there are two ways to focus a specimen. Some microscopes are equipped with a **barrel focus.** With this type of microscope, the body tube (or barrel) moves and the stage is stationary during focusing. Other microscopes focus the specimen using **stage focus.** With this type of microscope, the stage moves and the body tube is stationary during focusing.

Low and High Power

The low-power objective is used for the initial focusing and light adjustment of the microscope. The **low-power objective** is also used for the initial observation and scanning requirements needed for most microscopic work. For example, urine sediment is first examined using the low-power objective to scan the specimen for the presence of casts. The **high-power objective** is used for a more thorough study, such as observing cells and urinary sediment in more detail. The **working distance,** defined as the distance between the tip of the lens and the slide, is short when using this objective. Because of this, care must be taken in focusing the high-power objective to prevent it from striking and breaking the slide or damaging the lens.

Most compound microscopes are **parfocal.** This means that once the specimen is focused with the low-power objective, the nosepiece can be rotated to the high-power objective and focused simply through the use of the fine adjustment knob.

Oil Immersion

The oil-immersion objective provides the highest magnification and is used to view very small structures, such as microorganisms and blood cells. The oil-immersion objective has a very short working distance, and when it is in use, the lens nearly rests on the microscope slide itself. A special grade of oil known as **immersion oil** must be used with this lens. Oil has the advantage of not drying out when exposed to air for a long period of time. A drop of the oil is placed on the slide and resides between the oil-immersion objective and the slide. The oil provides a path for the light to travel on between the slide and the lens, and prevents the scattering of light rays, which, in turn, permits clear viewing of very small structures. The oil also improves the resolution of the objective lens, that is, its ability to provide sharp detail, which is particularly necessary at high magnifications. Examples of procedures requiring oil immersion include differential white blood cell counts and examination of Gram-stained smears.

CARE OF THE MICROSCOPE

The microscope is a delicate instrument and must be handled carefully. These guidelines should be followed to care for the microscope properly:

1. The microscope should always be carried with two hands. One hand should be placed firmly on the arm, and the other hand should be placed under the base for support. Place the microscope down gently to prevent jarring it, which could cause damage to its delicate parts.

2. The microscope should always be handled in such a way that the fingers do not touch the lenses, to avoid leaving fingerprints on them. Wearing mas-

MEMORIES *from* EXTERNSHIP

NATALIE MOOREHEAD: *During my externship, I remember having to observe my first minor office surgery. It was a lesion removal. The lesion was located on the calf of the patient's left leg. I helped in setting up the surgical tray and prepared and draped the site. I tried to explain to the patient what was going on to prepare her for the procedure. I think the patient was calmer than I was about the whole thing. The doctor entered the room with a medical assistant on hand. I helped him with his surgical gloves and in numbing the site. However, I was in the room primarily to observe. I watched the doctor make the incision and cut out and remove a rather large cyst.*

Everything was going smoothly until the doctor started to suture the wound. I felt like someone had turned the heat up really high and the room seemed to get really hot. I started to feel dizzy. I smiled at the doctor and excused myself. He just smiled back at me and I left the room. I went outside the room and caught my breath. I regained my composure and re-entered the room. The doctor was still suturing the wound. As I watched him run the needle through the skin and pull the suture tight, it really got to me. I smiled and told the doctor that I would wait outside until they were done. After the doctor left the room, I went back to help clean up. I felt so stupid. Later that day, the doctor looked at me and said: "Got a little warm in there, didn't it?" He just laughed and said that what I did was normal and not to worry about it. He made me feel better about myself. After that incident, I went in alone and helped him with lesion removals and it didn't bother me at all.

20

cara should be avoided when one is using a microscope, because this substance is difficult to remove from the ocular lens.

3. When it is not in use, the microscope should be covered with its plastic dust cover and stored in a case or cupboard. The microscope should be stored with the nosepiece rotated to the low-power objective and as close as possible to the stage.

4. The microscope should be cleaned periodically by washing the enameled surfaces with mild soap and water and drying them thoroughly with a soft cloth. Alcohol should never be used on the enameled surfaces because it may remove the finish.

5. The metal stage should be wiped clean after each use with gauze or tissue. If immersion oil comes in contact with the stage, it should be removed with a piece of gauze that is slightly moistened with xylene.

6. The ocular, objectives, and condenser consist of hand-ground optical lenses, which must be kept spotlessly clean by using clean, dry lens paper. Optical glass is softer than ordinary glass; therefore, tissues or gauze should not be used, in order to prevent scratching of the lens. If the lenses are especially dirty, a commercial lens cleaner or xylene should be used in the cleaning process. A small amount of cleaner is applied to the lens paper, followed by thorough drying and polishing with a clean piece of lens paper.

7. The light source should be kept free of dust, lint, and dirt by periodic polishing with lens paper.

8. A malfunctioning microscope should be repaired only by a qualified service person. Attempting to fix the microscope yourself may result in further damage.

PROCEDURE

20–1

Using the Microscope

EQUIPMENT/SUPPLIES: Microscope
Lens paper
Specimen slide
Tissue or gauze

Immersion oil
Xylene
Soft cloth

These steps should be followed for proper use of the microscope:

1. **Procedural Step.** Clean the ocular and objective lenses with lens paper.

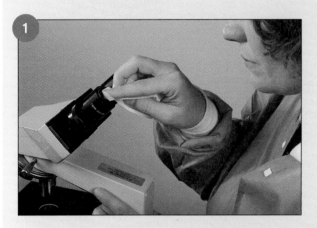

2. **Procedural Step.** Turn on the light source.
3. **Procedural Step.** Rotate the nosepiece to the low-power objective (10×), making sure to click it into place. Use the coarse adjustment knob to provide sufficient working space for placing the slide on the stage and to avoid damaging the objective lens as follows:
   a. **Barrel focus:** Raise the objective all the way up using the coarse adjustment knob.
   b. **Stage focus:** Lower the stage all the way down using the coarse adjustment knob.
4. **Procedural Step.** Place the slide on the stage specimen side up and make sure it is secure.
5. **Procedural Step.** Position the low-power objective until it almost touches the slide using the coarse adjustment knob. Be sure to observe this step to prevent the objective from striking the slide.
6. **Procedural Step.** Look through the ocular. If a monocular microscope is being used, both eyes should be kept open to prevent eyestrain. With a binocular microscope adjust the two oculars to the width between your eyes until a single circular field of vision is obtained.
7. **Procedural Step.** Bring the specimen into coarse focus as follows:

20

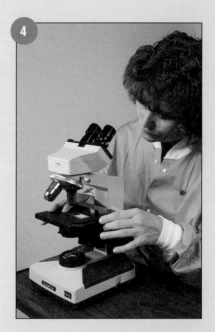

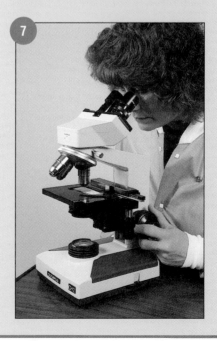

a. **Barrel focus:** Slowly raise the objective using the coarse adjustment knob.

b. **Stage focus:** Slowly lower the stage using the coarse adjustment knob.

Observe the specimen through the ocular until comes into focus.

8. **Procedural Step.** Use the fine adjustment knob to bring the specimen into a sharp, clear focus.

9. **Procedural Step.** Adjust the light as needed, using the iris diaphragm to provide maximum focus and contrast.

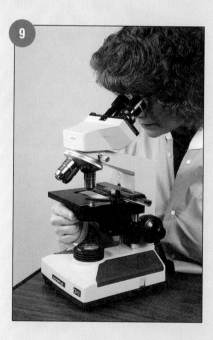

10. **Procedural Step.** Rotate the nosepiece to the high-power objective, making sure it clicks into place. Proper focusing with the low-power objective ensures that the objective does not hit the slide during this operation. Use the fine adjustment knob to bring the specimen into a precise focus. Do not use the coarse adjustment to focus the high-power objective in order to prevent the objective from moving too far and striking the slide.

11. **Procedural Step.** Examine the specimen as required by the test or procedure being performed.

12. **Procedural Step.** Turn off the light after use, and remove the slide from the stage.

13. **Procedural Step.** Clean the stage with a tissue or gauze.

14. **Procedural Step.** Properly care for and store the microscope.

Using the Oil Immersion Objective

The following steps should be followed for proper use of the oil-immersion objective.

1. **Procedural Step.** Rotate the nosepiece to the oil-immersion objective. Do not click it into place but move it to one side.

2. **Procedural Step.** Place a drop of immersion oil on the slide directly over the center opening in the stage.

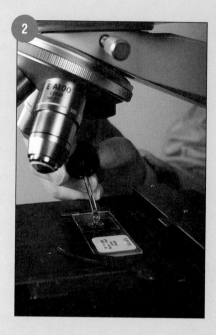

3. **Procedural Step.** Move the oil-immersion objective into place until a click is heard. Make sure that the objective does not touch the stage or slide.

4. **Procedural Step.** Using the coarse adjustment, slowly position the oil-immersion objective until the tip of the lens touches the oil but does not come in contact with the slide. A pop of light will be observed. Be sure to observe carefully this step of the procedure.

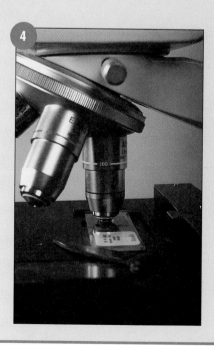

20

PROCEDURE 20-1

5. **Procedural Step.** Look through the eyepiece, and focus slowly using the coarse adjustment until the object is visible.

6. **Procedural Step.** Use the fine adjustment to bring the object into sharp focus to view fine details.

7. **Procedural Step.** Adjust the light as needed, using the iris diaphragm to provide maximum focus and contrast. Increased light intensity is required for good visualization of the specimen with the oil-immersion objective.

8. **Procedural Step.** Examine the specimen as required by the test or procedure being performed.

9. **Procedural Step.** Turn off the light after use. Remove the slide from the stage, being careful not to get oil on the high-power objective or the stage.

10. **Procedural Step.** Using a piece of clean, dry lens paper gently clean the oil-immersion objective. The lens must be immediately cleaned after use to prevent oil from drying on the lens surface. In addition, the oil may seep into the lens and perhaps loosen it.

11. **Procedural Step.** Clean the oil from the slide by immersing it in xylene and wiping it off with a soft cloth.

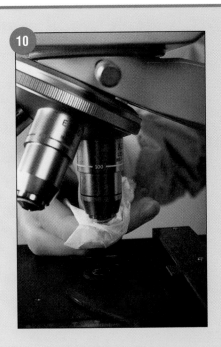

MICROBIOLOGIC SPECIMEN COLLECTION

20

☐ If the physician suspects that a particular disease is caused by a pathogen, he or she may want to obtain a specimen for microbiologic examination. This will identify the specific pathogen causing the disease and aid in the diagnosis. For example, if a urinary tract infection is suspected, a urine specimen is obtained for bacterial examination. In this instance, a clean-catch midstream collection is required to obtain a specimen that excludes those microorganisms making up the normal flora of the urethra and urinary meatus.

A **specimen** is a small sample or part taken from the body to represent the nature of the whole. The medical assistant is often responsible for collecting specimens from certain areas of the body, such as the throat, nose, or wound areas. He or she may also be responsible for assisting the physician in the collection of specimens from other areas, such as the eye, ear, cervix, vagina, urethra, or rectum. In most instances, a swab is used to collect the specimen. A **swab** is a small piece of cotton wrapped around the end of a slender wooden or plastic stick. It is passed across a suspected area to obtain a specimen from a body surface or opening for microbiologic analysis.

Good techniques of medical and surgical asepsis must be practiced when a specimen is obtained, to prevent inaccurate test results. The medical assistant must be careful not to contaminate the specimen with **extraneous microorganisms.** These are undesirable microorganisms that may enter the specimen in various ways; they grow and multiply, and possibly obscure and prevent identification of any pathogens that may be present. To prevent extraneous organisms from contaminating the specimen, all supplies used to obtain the specimen, such as swabs and specimen containers, must be sterile. In addition, the specimen should not contain any microorganisms from areas surrounding the collection site. For example, when obtaining a throat specimen, the swab should not be allowed to touch the inside of the mouth.

The OSHA Bloodborne Pathogens Standards presented in Chapter 1 should be carefully followed when performing microbiologic procedures. Specifically, the medical assistant must wear gloves when it is reasonably anticipated that hand contact may occur with blood or other potentially infectious materials. Eating, drinking, and smoking are strictly forbidden when one is working with microorganisms, because pathogens can be transmitted to the medical assistant through this type of hand-to-mouth contact. In addition, labels for specimen containers should not be licked, and any break in the skin, such as a cut or scratch, must be covered with a bandage. If the medical assistant accidentally touches some of the material contained in the specimen, the area of contact should be washed immediately and thoroughly with soap and water. If the specimen comes in contact with the worktable, the table should be cleansed immediately with a suitable disinfectant such as phenol. The worktable should also be cleaned with a disinfectant at the end of each day.

After collection, the specimen must be placed in its proper container with the lid securely fastened. The container must be clearly labeled with the patient's name, the date, the source of the specimen, the medical assistant's initials, and any other information that may be required.

HANDLING AND TRANSPORTING MICROBIOLOGIC SPECIMENS

Once the specimen has been collected, care should be taken in handling and transporting it. Delay in processing the specimen may cause the death of any pathogens that may be present or the overgrowth of the specimen by microorganisms that are part of the normal flora usually collected along with the pathogen from the specimen site. If the specimen is to be analyzed in the medical office, it should be examined under the microscope or cultured immediately. Otherwise, it should be preserved (if possible) with the method used by the medical office. Some microorganisms, such as gonococci, are extremely fastidious outside the host and need to be cultured immediately.

The specimens that are to be transported to an outside medical laboratory through a courier pick-up service are usually placed in a transport medium. The transport medium prevents drying of the specimen and preserves it in its original state until it reaches its destination. An example of a commercially available transport medium is the Culturette.

Outside laboratories provide the medical office with specific instructions on the care and handling of specimens being transported to them. A laboratory request designating the physician's name and address; the patient's name, age, and sex; the date and time of collection; the type of microbiologic examination requested; the source of the specimen (e.g., throat, wound, and urine); and the physician's clinical diagnosis must accompany all specimens being transported to an outside laboratory. There is usually a space on the form to indicate whether the patient is receiving antibiotic therapy. Antibiotics may suppress the growth of bacteria, a factor that could produce falsely-negative results.

PROCEDURE

20–2

Taking a Specimen for a Throat Culture

A specimen for a throat culture is obtained by using a sterile swab. It is commonly used to aid in the diagnosis of infections such as streptococcal sore throat, pharyngitis, and tonsillitis. Less frequently, it is used to diagnose whooping cough and diphtheria. These latter diseases are not prevalent today because of the availability of immunizations against them.

The following procedure outlines the steps necessary to obtain a throat specimen that will be used to perform a rapid streptococcus test, which is discussed later in the chapter.

EQUIPMENT/SUPPLIES: **Disposable gloves**   **Sterile dacron swab**
  Tongue depressor   **Biohazard waste container**

1. **Procedural Step.** Wash hands and assemble the equipment.
2. **Procedural Step.** Greet and identify the patient. Introduce yourself, and explain the procedure.
3. **Procedural Step.** Position the patient, and adjust the light to provide clear visualization of the throat.

Principle. The throat must be clearly visible so the medical assistant is able to determine the proper area for obtaining the specimen.

4. **Procedural Step.** Apply gloves. Remove the sterile swab from its peel-apart package, being careful not to contaminate it.

Continued

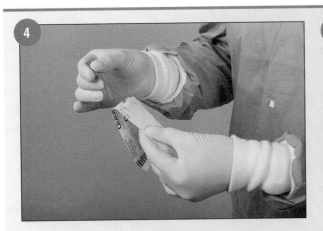

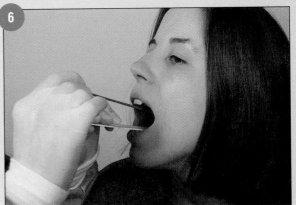

Principle. Contamination of the swab may lead to inaccurate test results.

5. **Procedural Step.** Depress the tongue with the tongue depressor.

   Principle. The tongue depressor holds the tongue down and facilitates access to the throat.

6. **Procedural Step.** Place the swab at the back of the throat (posterior pharynx) and firmly rub it over any lesions or white or inflamed areas of the mucous membrane of the tonsillar area and posterior pharyngeal wall. The swab should be rotated constantly as the specimen is obtained, making sure there is good contact with the tonsillar area. Do not allow the swab to touch any areas other than the throat such as the inside of the mouth.

   Principle. The swab should be rubbed over suspicious-looking areas where pathogens are likely to be found. A rotating motion is used to deposit the maximum amount of material possible on the swab. Touching it to any areas other than the throat contaminates the specimen with extraneous microorganisms.

7. **Procedural Step.** Keeping the patient's tongue depressed, withdraw the swab and remove the tongue depressor from the patient's mouth.

8. **Procedural Step.** Properly dispose of the tongue depressor in a biohazard waste container to prevent transmission of microorganisms.

9. **Procedural Step.** Process the swab according to the directions accompanying the rapid strep test.

10. **Procedural Step.** Remove gloves, and wash the hands. Chart the test results.

CHARTING EXAMPLE

Date	
7/12/2002	10:30 a.m. Throat specimen collected from tonsillar area. QuickVue Strep Test: Positive. ———————— N. Moorehead, CMA

Wound Specimens

Wound specimens are collected using many of the techniques described previously. In many cases, two swabs are used to collect the specimen. The specimen is obtained by inserting the swab into the area of the wound that contains the most drainage and gently rotating the swab from side to side to allow it completely to absorb any microorganisms present. The swab is placed in the specimen container, and the process is then repeated using a second swab. It is important to collect a specimen from within the wound, rather than from the surface, to obtain accurate and reliable test results.

COLLECTION AND TRANSPORT SYSTEMS

Microbiologic collection and transport systems are commercially available to facilitate the collection of a specimen that is to be transported to an outside laboratory for analysis; examples include Culturette (Marion Scientific Corporation) (Fig. 20–5) and Precision Culture CATS (Precision Dynamics Corporation). These systems consist of a plastic tube containing a sterile swab and transport medium. The medium is effective for 72 hours once the swab has been immersed in it; therefore, it is important that the specimen reach the laboratory within this time. The tube comes packaged in a peel-apart envelope and should be stored at room

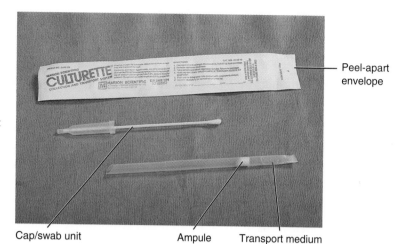

Peel-apart
envelope

Cap/swab unit   Ampule   Transport medium

■ **FIGURE 20–5.** Culturette Collection and Transport System.

temperature. The procedure for the utilization of a microbiologic collection and transport system is outlined next.

1. Complete a laboratory request form.
2. Wash the hands, and apply gloves.
3. Check the expiration date on the peel-apart envelope.
4. Peel open approximately one third of the length of the envelope.
5. Remove the plastic collection tube from the envelope, and label it with the patient's name, the date, the source of the specimen (e.g., throat, wound), and your initials.

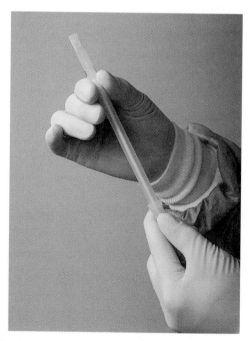

■ **FIGURE 20–6.** Natalie is crushing the ampule of the Culturette to immerse the swab in the transport medium.

6. Using a twisting motion, remove the cap/swab unit from the tube. The cap is permanently attached to the sterile swab.
7. Collect the specimen using aseptic technique. Do not allow the swab to touch any area other than the collection site.
8. Return the cap/swab unit to the plastic tube.
9. Completely immerse the swab in the transport medium. Using the Culturette system, this is accomplished by squeezing the plastic tube to crush an ampule that separates the transport medium from the rest of the tube (Fig. 20–6). The cap/swab unit is then pushed forward to bring the swab in contact with the moistened pledget). With the Precision system, the swab must be pushed in as far as it will go; this automatically opens a seal separating the transport medium from the rest of the tube.
10. Remove the gloves, and wash the hands.
11. Chart the procedure.
12. Transport the specimen to the laboratory within 72 hours.

CULTURES

☐ Once a microbiologic specimen is taken, it must be examined to determine the type of microorganisms present. Because most specimens generally contain only a small number of pathogens, it is often desirable to induce any pathogens that may be present to grow and multiply.

Most microorganisms, especially bacteria, may be grown on a culture medium. A **culture medium** is a mixture of nutrients on which microorganisms are grown in the laboratory. The culture medium and the environment in which it is placed must contain the necessary requirements to support and encourage the growth of the suspected pathogen. These growth re-

20

quirements include either the presence or the absence of oxygen (depending on the microorganism); proper nutrition, temperature, and pH; and the presence of moisture.

The culture medium may be in a solid or a liquid form. Blood agar is one of the most frequently used solid culture media. It is prepared by adding sheep's blood to a substance known as **agar,** which is transparent and colorless. Blood added to the agar provides nutrients that support the growth of a variety of bacteria. When heated, it melts and becomes a liquid. On cooling, agar solidifies, forming a firm surface on which microorganisms can be grown. A liquid culture medium is often referred to as a broth and is usually contained in a tube; an example is nutrient broth. Culture media must be stored in the refrigerator and then warmed to room temperature before using. A cold culture medium must not be used, because the cold temperature results in the death of microorganisms placed on it.

A **Petri plate** is frequently used to hold solid culture medium. The plate consists of a shallow circular dish made of glass or clear plastic with a cover, the diameter of which is greater than that of the base. Microorganisms can be cultured on the surface of the medium contained in the plate (Fig. 20–7). Petri plates allow for the examination of a culture and at the same time prevent microorganisms from entering or escaping. A **culture** is defined as a mass of microorganisms growing in a laboratory culture medium.

Most medical offices use commercially prepared culture media contained in disposable plastic Petri plates. The plates come packaged in a plastic bag and must be stored in the refrigerator with the medium side facing upward. The plastic bag prevents the medium from drying out; storing the plates medium side upward prevents condensation on the medium surface. The plate will have an expiration date that must be checked before using; Plates that are past the expiration date or are dried out or contaminated should not be used.

The solid culture medium contained in a Petri plate is inoculated by lightly rolling the swab containing the specimen over the surface of the medium; this process is known as **streaking.** The cover of the Petri plate should be removed only when the specimen is being spread on the culture medium. Unnecessary removal of the cover results in contamination of the medium with extraneous microorganisms. The culture is then incubated for 24 to 48 hours, using the proper conditions to encourage the growth of the suspected pathogen.

PUTTING IT ALL *into* PRACTICE

▶ **NATALIE MOOREHEAD:** *Working as a medical assistant, one can encounter many challenges. One experience that I had involved a 4-year-old boy. The patient came into the office with a very sore throat and a high fever. The little fellow did not think that his office visit had gone too badly until he found out that the doctor had ordered a rapid strep test to check for strep throat. That's when he decided he did not care for me, my tongue depressor, or my swab. He decided to protest by keeping his mouth tightly shut. Rather than forcing the procedure on the child, I took my time and kept my patience. I managed to convince the child that even though the procedure was uncomfortable and tasted bad, it was the only way we would know if he was really sick or not. I also explained that the test was the only way the doctor would know what kind of medicine to prescribe so he could get well and feel like playing again. It took a while, but we got our specimen and the patient received the right antibiotic that he needed to get better.*

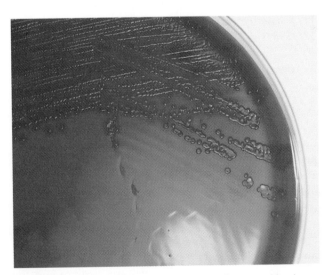

■ **FIGURE 20–7.** Streptococcal colonies growing on a blood agar culture medium contained in a Petri plate. (From Mahon, C. R., Manuselis, G., Jr.: *Textbook of Diagnostic Microbiology.* Philadelphia, W. B. Saunders, 1995.)

Most specimens taken for analysis contain a mixture of different organisms because of the presence of normal flora in most parts of the body. When this is the case, the resulting culture is known as a **mixed culture,** or one that contains two or more different types of microorganisms. To analyze most microbiologic specimens, the suspected pathogen must be separated from the mixed culture and permitted to grow alone. This establishes a **pure culture,** or a culture that contains only one type of microorganism. After the culture has grown sufficiently, the appropriate tests are performed to identify the pathogen.

It is not possible to grow viruses by this method; rather, they must be cultured on living tissue or identified using serologic tests.

STREPTOCOCCUS TESTING

☐ The most commonly occurring streptococcal condition is streptococcal sore throat (streptococcal pharyngitis), which primarily affects children and young adults. The causative agent of streptococcal pharyngitis is a Group A beta-hemolytic streptococcus known as *Streptococcus pyogenes.* Streptococcal pharyngitis is a potentially serious condition because some patients develop a poststreptococcal sequela. A **sequela** is a morbid secondary condition that occurs as a result of a less serious primary infection. A small percentage of patients with streptococcal pharyngitis (primary infection) develop rheumatic fever; the rheumatic fever is considered a poststreptococcal sequela. Owing to the risk of sequela, early diagnosis and treatment of streptococcal pharyngitis is important. In the medical office, commercially available tests are often used for identification of Group A beta-hemolytic streptococci. The most frequently used testing methods are presented next.

RAPID STREPTOCOCCUS TESTS

Rapid streptococcus tests directly detect Group A streptococcus from a throat swab in a very short period of time. Most tests require only 4 to 10 minutes to process; therefore, diagnosis can often be made and antibiotics prescribed, if necessary, before the patient leaves the office.

The most frequently used rapid streptococcus test is the direct antigen identification test, which confirms the presence of Group A streptococcus through an antigen-antibody reaction. The test works by combining particles sensitized to the streptococcus antibody with the throat specimen. If Group A streptococcal antigen is in the specimen, it combines with the antibody-sensitized particles to produce either agglutina-

tion or a color change that can be observed with the unaided eye.

The advantage of the direct antigen identification test is that it provides the physician with immediate test results rather than requiring an overnight culture. Specific instructions are included with each commercially available antigen identification test; examples of these tests include Strep A Cards OS (Quidel), Clearview Strep A (Wampole Laboratories), and QuickVue In Line Strep A (Quidel) (Fig. 20–8).

HEMOLYTIC REACTION AND BACITRACIN SUSCEPTIBILITY TEST

Streptococci are classified into three types, according to their hemolytic properties exhibited on a blood agar medium: **alpha, beta,** and **gamma.** They are further divided according to their antigenic properties into 15 subgroups designated by the letters "A" through "O." The hemolytic reaction and bacitracin susceptibility test is a biochemical culture test that relies on these hemolytic and antigenic properties of streptococci for the interpretation of the test results.

The testing procedure involves placing a filter paper disc impregnated with 0.04 U of bacitracin on the surface of a sheep-blood agar medium previously inoculated with the throat specimen. The medium is then incubated for 18 to 24 hours to allow for the growth of the bacteria and also to permit diffusion of the bacitracin into the culture medium surrounding the disc.

After the 18- to 24-hour incubation period, the plate is examined for its **hemolytic reaction.** As stated, the causative agent of streptococcal pharyngitis is a (Group A) beta-hemolytic streptococcus. Beta-hemolytic streptococci produce and secrete streptolysin, an exotoxin that completely hemolyzes red blood cells; therefore, a clear, wide, colorless zone of hemolysis (with no intact red blood cells) around the bacterial colonies indicates their presence. On the other hand, a greenish halo around the colonies indicates the less pathogenic alpha-hemolytic streptococci. The generally nonpathogenic gamma-type streptococci will not cause a reaction on the blood agar medium.

If the hemolytic property exhibited is of the beta type, the area around the bacitracin disc is next inspected for **bacitracin susceptibility.** Group A streptococci are susceptible or sensitive to bacitracin, whereas Groups B, C, and G (which are also beta-hemolytic) are resistant to the bacitracin. If Group A is present, a clear zone of inhibition appears around the disc (Fig. 20–9*A*). Because Groups B, C, and G are resistant to the bacitracin, the bacteria grow right up to the edge of the disc; that is, a zone of inhibition is not present (Fig. 20–9*B*).

20

20

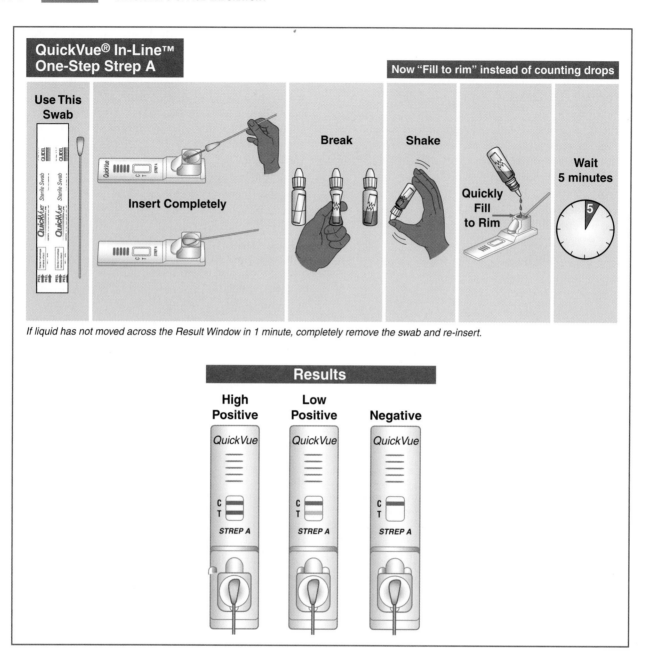

FIGURE 20-8. Procedure for performing the QuickVue In-Line One-Step Strep A test. (Courtesy of Quidel Corporation, San Diego, California.)

Therefore, hemolysis of the blood agar surrounding the bacterial colonies combined with any zone of inhibition around the bacitracin disc is considered presumptive positive for Group A beta-hemolytic streptococci. The test is considered presumptive because a small percentage of bacterial strains included in Groups B, C, and G are sensitive to bacitracin; therefore, a fraction (less than 5 percent) of the test results obtained will be false positive. A **false positive** is a test result denoting that a condition is present when, in fact, it is not.

The bacitracin disc test is a convenient, reliable, and cost-effective method used in the medical office to de-

termine the presence of streptococcal pharyngitis. However, it is not used as frequently as it once was, owing to the development of the rapid streptococcus tests.

SENSITIVITY TESTING

☐ The physician may request not only that the laboratory identify the infecting pathogen but also that a sensitivity test be performed on it to determine the best antibiotic to treat the condition. These tests must always be performed on pure cultures rather than on mixed cultures. A sensitivity test determines the sus-

A   B

Zone of   Bacitracin   Sheep blood
inhibition   disk   agar medium

■ **FIGURE 20–9.** Hemolytic reaction and bacitracin susceptibility test. *A*, A positive reaction for Group A beta-hemolytic streptococcus, as evidenced by a clear zone of inhibition present around the bacitracin disc. *B*, A negative reaction as evidenced by the bacteria growing right up to the edge of the disc. (From Mahon, C. R., Manuselis, G., Jr.: *Textbook of Diagnostic Microbiology.* Philadelphia, W. B. Saunders, 1995.)

ceptibility of pathogenic bacteria to various antibiotics; therefore, only the growth of the infectious pathogen is desired on the culture.

The most commonly used method for sensitivity testing is the **disc-plate method** (Fig. 20–10). Commercially prepared discs impregnated with known concentrations of various antibiotics are dropped on the surface of a solid culture medium in a Petri plate inoculated with the pathogen. The culture is then incubated, allowing the antibiotics to diffuse out into the culture medium. If the pathogen is susceptible or sensitive to an antibiotic, there is a clear zone without bacterial growth around the disc. This indicates that the antibiotic was effective in destroying the pathogen. If the pathogen is unaffected by or resistant to the antibiotic, there is not a clear zone around the disc, indicating that the antibiotic was unable to kill the pathogen.

Sensitivity testing enables the physician to decide which antibiotics will most likely be effective against the infectious disease in question.

PATIENT/TEACHING

20

STREP THROAT
■ Answer questions patients have about strep throat:

What Is Strep Throat?
Strep throat is a contagious and acute infection that is medically known as streptococcal pharyngitis. It is caused by a bacterium known as Group A streptococcus. Strep throat is transmitted directly from one person to another through droplets of saliva or nasal secretions. It most frequently occurs in children between the ages of 5 and 10 years and during the months of October through April. Strep infections are different from most other infectious diseases because one strep infection does not prevent the development of another at a future date.

What Are the Symptoms of Strep Throat?
The symptoms of strep throat include a sore throat with severe pain on swallowing, a bright red pharynx (called beefy red pharynx), fever, white patches on the tonsils, swollen glands in the neck, muscular aches and pains, and a feeling of tiredness.

How Is Strep Throat Diagnosed and Treated?
Strep throat is diagnosed by taking a throat specimen and running a laboratory test on it to determine whether Group A streptococcus is present. Strep throat is usually treated by antibiotics taken orally for 10 days. It is important to take all the antibiotic prescribed by the physician to prevent complications that can occur from strep throat. The patient with strep throat should also rest in bed and avoid contact with others to prevent spreading it.

What Are the Complications of Strep Throat?
Severe complications can result from strep throat if it is not adequately treated. These include rheumatic fever and glomerulonephritis, which is a kidney disorder. Fortunately, these complications do not occur very often since most patients seek early treatment for strep infections.
■ Encourage the patient to complete the entire prescribed course of antibiotics.
■ Instruct the patient to notify the physician if any new symptoms develop.
■ Provide the patient with educational materials on strep throat.

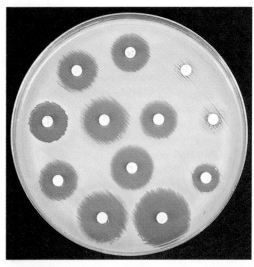

■ FIGURE 20–10. Sensitivity testing. *Enterobacter aerogenes* tested by the disk diffusion method. Zone measurements confirm that the isolate is susceptible to all agents tested except ampicillin (positioned at 1 o'clock) and cefazolin (positioned at 2 o'clock). No zones are present for either of these agents. (From Mahon, C. R., Manuselis, G., Jr.: *Textbook of Diagnostic Microbiology.* Philadelphia, W. B. Saunders, 1995.)

MICROSCOPIC EXAMINATION OF MICROORGANISMS

20

☐ Microorganisms may be examined under a microscope in the fixed state or in the living state. Examination in the fixed state involves the preparation of a smear through heat fixation, followed by a staining process such as Gram's stain, which is discussed later in this chapter. Most microorganisms are examined in the fixed state because it is easier to examine them when they are stained.

Some microorganisms require examination in the living state, however, owing to special circumstances such as their inability to be readily stained or difficulty in culturing them. The living state also allows visualization of the movement of motile microorganisms. This is especially helpful in the identification of certain motile microorganisms such as *Trichomonas vaginalis*. To observe the motility of a microorganism, it must first be suspended in a liquid medium so that it is free to move about.

The two most common methods of examining microorganisms in the living state are the wet mount method and the hanging drop preparation, which are described next.

WET MOUNT METHOD

In the wet mount method, a drop of fluid containing the organism is placed on a glass slide, which is cov-

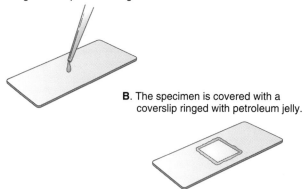

A. A drop of fluid containing the organism is placed on a glass slide.

B. The specimen is covered with a coverslip ringed with petroleum jelly.

■ FIGURE 20–11. Wet mount method of slide preparation for examining microorganisms in the living state.

ered with a coverslip (Fig. 20–11). The coverslip may be ringed with petroleum jelly to provide a seal between the slide and coverslip. The purpose is to reduce the rate of evaporation through air currents that lead to drying and possible death of the specimen.

The slide is then placed under the microscope for examination, using the high-power objective. For satisfactory visualization, the intensity of the light must be diminished by partially closing the diaphragm of the microscope. The slide and coverslip should then be properly disposed of in a biohazard container.

SMEARS

A smear consists of material spread on a slide for microscopic examination. It may be prepared directly from the specimen collected on the swab, or the specimen may first be grown on a culture medium and a smear then prepared. Most smears must be stained before they can be viewed under the microscope, using one of a number of available staining techniques. Smears are often helpful when time is a factor, because a smear can be prepared immediately from the specimen. This procedure gives the physician a preliminary clue to the causative agent while other, more time-consuming tests are being performed.

THE GRAM STAIN

Bacteria contained in a smear are colorless and usually are difficult to identify under the microscope unless some type of staining technique is used. Staining them allows the observer to view directly the size, shape, and growth patterns of the bacteria.

20–3

Preparing a Hanging Drop Slide

This method is performed using a hanging drop slide, which consists of a thick glass slide with a depression in its center (see illustrations below). The hanging drop preparation is made as outlined.

EQUIPMENT/SUPPLIES: Disposable gloves   Hanging drop slide
Coverslip   Petroleum jelly
Microscope   Biohazard waste container

1. **Procedural Step.** Spread a small amount of petroleum jelly around the edge of the coverslip.

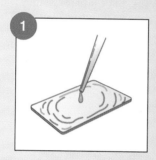

2. **Procedural Step.** Place the coverslip on a clean, dry surface with the petroleum jelly facing up.

3. **Procedural Step.** Apply gloves and transfer a drop of the specimen to the center of the coverslip.
4. **Procedural Step.** Place the hanging drop slide over the coverslip so that the center of the depression lies directly over the drop.
5. **Procedural Step.** Apply slight pressure to the slide to ensure satisfactory contact between the coverslip and slide. The petroleum jelly seals the coverslip to the slide to hold it in place and prevent evaporation through air currents.
6. **Procedural Step.** Invert the slide quickly so that the drop to be examined hangs from the bottom of the coverslip.
7. **Procedural Step.** Place the slide under the microscope.

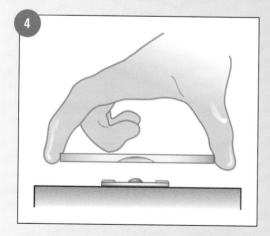

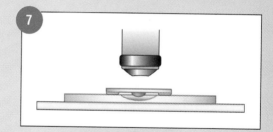

8. **Procedural Step.** Examine the specimen with the high-power objective. The amount of light must be reduced by partially closing the diaphragm.
9. **Procedural Step.** Properly dispose of the slide and coverslip in a biohazard waste container.

A very commonly employed staining method is the Gram stain. In 1883, Christian Gram, a Danish physician, discovered a way to differentiate bacteria on the basis of their color reactions to various stains.

Gram staining is based on the fact that when treated with crystal violet dye, certain bacteria permanently retain this dye after undergoing a decolorization process. These bacteria exhibit a purple color when

PROCEDURE

20–4

Preparing a Smear

EQUIPMENT/SUPPLIES:

Clean gloves
Bunsen burner
Clean glass slide
Microbiologic specimen

Slide forceps
Sterile swab or inoculating needle
Biohazard waste container

1. **Procedural Step.** Wash the hands.
2. **Procedural Step.** Assemble the equipment. Label the slide with the patient's name and the date.
   Principle. Scratches and dirt on the slide may be mistaken for microorganisms. Greasy slides result in an unsatisfactory smear, because the bacteria are harder to spread out.
3. **Procedural Step.** Apply gloves. Hold the edges of the slide between your thumb and index finger. Starting at the right side and using a rolling motion, gently and evenly spread the material from the specimen over the slide. The material should cover approximately one-half to two-thirds of the slide. Do not rub the material vigorously over the slide. Properly dispose of the contaminated swab in a biohazard waste container.

position for at least one-half hour. Heat should not be applied at this time.
   Principle. Air drying allows the bacterial cells to dry slowly. Applying heat at this stage would burst the bacterial cells resulting in an inappropriate smear.
5. **Procedural Step.** Holding the slide with the slide forceps heat fix the smear by quickly passing the slide back and forth (approximately three times) through the flame of a Bunsen burner. The slide has been fixed properly if the back of the slide feels uncomfortable (but not too hot) when touched to the back of your hand. Excessive heat should be avoided. Allow the slide to cool completely. An alternative to heat fixing the slide is to apply ethyl alcohol to the slide and allow it to air dry.

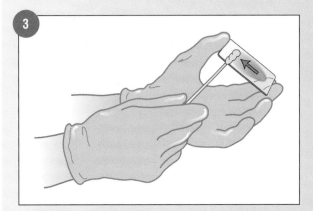

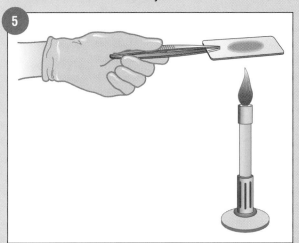

Principle. The specimen may contain pathogens that are capable of infecting the medical assistant; therefore, it is important to don gloves. A rolling motion is used to deposit the maximum amount of material possible on the slide. Rubbing may disintegrate the cellular structures making up the microorganisms in the specimen.

4. **Procedural Step.** Allow the smear to air dry in a flat

Principle. Heat fixing the slide kills the microorganisms and attaches them firmly to the slide so they do not wash off during the staining process. An excessive amount of heat could result in distortion of the bacterial cells.

6. **Procedural Step.** Examine the smear under the microscope or stain it according to your medical office policy.

viewed under the microscope and are known as **gram-positive** bacteria (Fig. 20–12*A*). Other bacteria are unable to retain this dye after being decolorized and become colorless. They must be counterstained with a

contrasting hue to become visible under the microscope. These bacteria exhibit a pink or red color and are known as **gram-negative** bacteria (Fig. 20–12*B*). These staining characteristics are due to differences

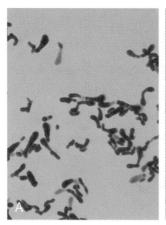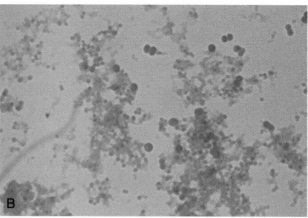

■ **FIGURE 20–12.** Gram-positive and gram-negative bacteria. *A,* Diphtheria is caused by a gram-positive bacillus; *B,* gonorrhea is caused by a gram-negative diplococcus. (*A,* courtesy of Cathy Bissonette; *B,* from Mahon, C. R., Manuselis, G., Jr.: *Textbook of Diagnostic Microbiology.* Philadelphia, W. B. Saunders, 1995.)

in the chemical composition of the bacterial cell walls.

Gram staining allows for the division of most bacteria into two large groups; gram positive and gram negative. Some of the infectious diseases caused by gram-positive bacteria are streptococcal sore throat, scarlet fever, rheumatic fever, diphtheria, lobar pneumonia, tetanus, and botulism. Infectious diseases caused by gram-negative bacteria include whooping cough, gonorrhea, meningitis, bacillary dysentery, cholera, typhoid fever, and the plague.

Bacteria undergoing Gram staining are also observed for their characteristic shape and fall into one of the following categories: gram-positive rods, gram-negative rods, gram-positive cocci, or gram-negative cocci. For example, the causative agent of gonorrhea is a gram-negative diplococcus.

Gram staining is often used in combination with culture tests to help in the diagnosis and treatment of infectious diseases. The medical assistant may be responsible for preparing a Gram-stained smear for ex-amination by the physician. Proper timing of the various reactions is a critical factor in the preparation of a well-stained smear.

PREVENTION AND CONTROL OF INFECTIOUS DISEASES

☐ Individuals in the community can help prevent and control infectious diseases by practicing good techniques of medical asepsis, by obtaining proper nutrition and rest, and by using good hygienic measures. In addition, infected individuals should contact their physicians in an effort to ensure early diagnosis and treatment of the disease. Immunizations are available for a wide range of infectious diseases and function to prevent the disease. The medical assistant has a responsibility to help educate community members in the use of practices that reduce the transmission of pathogens and help control and prevent infectious diseases.

20

MEDICAL PRACTICE AND THE LAW

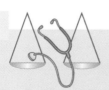

This chapter deals with the collection and identification of microorganisms that cause infections. You must maintain standard precautions whenever handling potentially infectious material to protect yourself, your co-workers, and your patients. Microbiology is an exact science—one stray microorganism can contaminate the entire specimen. Wash hands thoroughly, and apply new gloves between handling specimens to avoid cross-contamination. If specimen contamination occurs, immediately discard it and collect a new one. Be precise in your labeling—a mislabeled specimen can cause unnecessary concern for and or treatment for the patient.

Maintain confidentiality of information—certain infectious diseases must be reported to the Centers for Disease Control and Prevention (CDC) or local board of health, but do not give information to anyone else but the patient or legal guardian.

CERTIFICATION REVIEW

- ☐ Microbiology is the scientific study of microorganisms and their activities. Each individual has a normal flora, which consists of the harmless, non-pathogenic microorganisms that normally reside in many parts of the body but do not cause disease.

- ☐ The invasion of the body by pathogenic microorganisms is known as infection. Many infectious diseases are contagious, meaning that the pathogen causing the disease can be spread from one person to another either directly or indirectly. Frequently, droplet infection is the mode of transmission of pathogens.

- ☐ The incubation period is the interval of time between the invasion by a pathogenic microorganism and the appearance of the first symptoms of the disease. The prodromal period is when the first symptoms that indicate an approaching disease occur. The acute period is when the disease is at its peak and the symptoms are fully developed. The decline period is when the symptoms of the disease begin to subside. The convalescent period is the stage in which the patient regains strength and returns to a state of health.

- ☐ Bacteria can be classified into three basic groups, according to their shape. Staphylococci are round bacteria that grow in grapelike clusters. Streptococci are round bacteria that grow in chains. Diplococci are round bacteria that grow in pairs. Bacilli are rod-shaped bacteria that are frequently found in the soil and air. Spirilla are spiral bacteria. Viruses are the smallest living organisms, and an electron microscope must be used to view them.

- ☐ A compound microscope is used for office laboratory work. It contains three objective lenses. The low-power objective has a magnification of 10× and is used for the initial observation and scanning requirements needed for most microscopic work. The high-power objective has a magnification of 40× and is used for a more thorough study. The oil-immersion objective has the highest power of magnification, which is 100×.

- ☐ A specimen is a small sample taken from the body to represent the nature of the whole. Throat specimens are frequently collected in the medical office to aid in the diagnosis of streptococcal sore throat. Specimens may also be collected from wounds, the eye, ear, cervix, vagina, urethra, and rectum.

- ☐ A culture medium is a mixture of nutrients on which microorganisms are grown in the laboratory. A culture is a mass of microorganisms growing in a laboratory culture medium. A mixed culture contains two or more different types of microorganisms. A pure culture contains only one type of microorganism.

- ☐ The most commonly occurring streptococcal condition is streptococcal sore throat. A sequela is a morbid secondary condition that occurs as a result of a less serious primary infection. A small percentage of patients with streptococcal pharyngitis develop rheumatic fever; rheumatic fever is considered a poststreptococcal sequela.

- ☐ A sensitivity test determines the best antibiotic to treat a condition caused by a pathogenic bacterium. A sensitivity test must be performed on a pure culture.

- ☐ Microorganisms may be examined under a microscope in the fixed state or in the living state. Examination in the fixed state involves the preparation of a smear followed by a staining process such as Gram's stain. A smear consists of material spread on a slide for microscopic examination. The wet mount method and the hanging drop preparation are used to examine microorganisms in the living state.

- ☐ Gram staining is used to differentiate bacteria on the basis of their color reactions to various stains. Bacteria exhibiting a purple color when they are viewed under the microscope are known as gram-positive bacteria. Bacteria exhibiting a pink or red color are known as gram-negative bacteria.

20

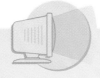

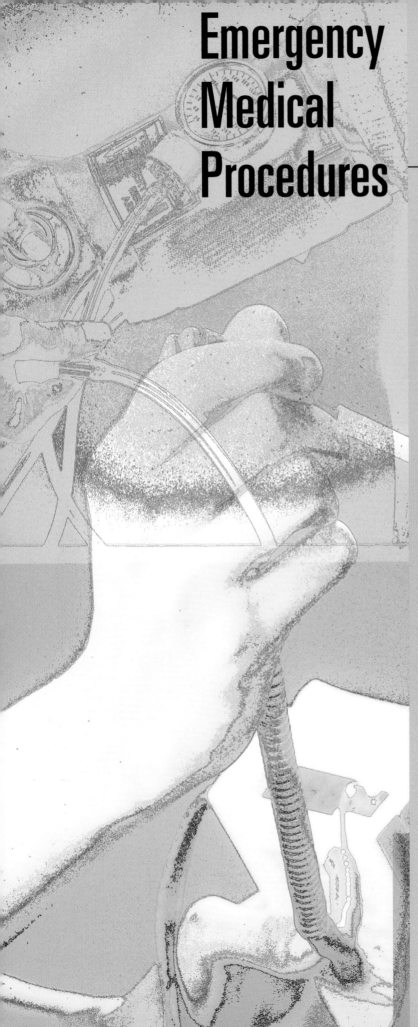

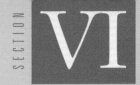
Emergency Medical Procedures

AAMA/CAAHEP COMPETENCIES INCLUDED IN
THIS SECTION:

Clinical Competencies

Patient Care
■ Obtain CPR certification and first aid training.

Emergency Medical Procedures

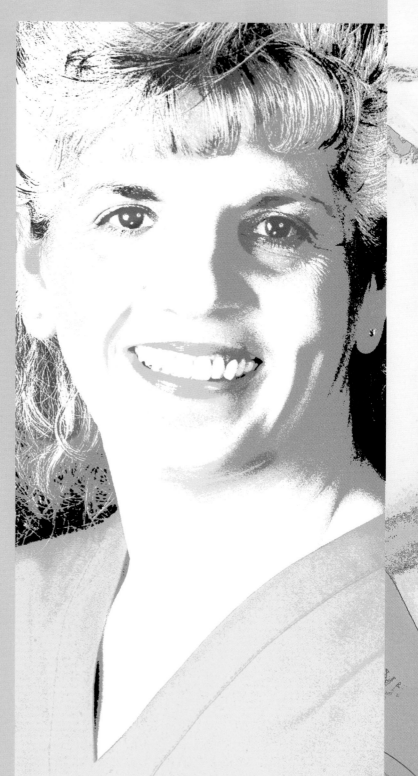

Judy Markins. *I am a Certified Medical Assistant with an associate's degree in Applied Science. I graduated from a medical assistant program when I was 35 years old. Although it was difficult managing classes and a home life with a husband and five children, we made it. With their support and encouragement, I accomplished my goal. After almost 11 years working as a certified medical assistant, I am still satisfied with my career choice.*

I work at a large clinic in the family medicine department with 12 physicians. We also have 6 to 10 physicians that do their internship and residency program with us. I've been with this department for 8 years. Before that I worked in obstetrics and gynecology for 2 ½ years. I have had the opportunity to work in other areas of the clinic, but I enjoy family medicine because of the wide variety of people and situations encountered. We treat newborns through prenatal and geriatric patients. With the popularity of health maintenance organizations (HMOs) and preferred provider organizations (PPOs), many patients are required to see their family physician first, so the symptoms, conditions, and diseases we encounter vary widely.

Most of my time I spend working on the floor triaging the patients, assisting the physician, drawing blood, performing electrocardiograms (ECGs), assisting with minor office surgery, giving injections, and educating patients.

OUTCOMES

After completing this chapter, you should be able to demonstrate the proper procedures to perform the following:

1. Open an airway.
2. Perform rescue breathing.
3. Perform the Heimlich maneuver.
4. Perform one-rescuer CPR.

EDUCATIONAL OBJECTIVES

After completing this chapter, you should be able to do the following:

1. Define the terms listed in the Key Terminology.
2. State the purpose of first aid.
3. Explain the purpose of the emergency medical services (EMS) system.
4. List the OSHA Standards that should be followed when administering first aid.
5. Explain the purpose and identify the components of the primary assessment.
6. List examples of conditions that cause respiratory arrest and respiratory distress.
7. Identify factors that increase the likelihood of a respiratory obstruction.
8. Explain how the Heimlich maneuver helps relieve a respiratory obstruction.
9. List examples of the conditions that cause cardiac arrest.
10. Explain the purpose of cardiopulmonary resuscitation (CPR).
11. Explain the cause of each of the following types of shock: cardiogenic, neurogenic, anaphylactic, and psychogenic.
12. Identify and describe the three classifications of external bleeding.
13. Explain the difference between an open wound and a closed wound.
14. Describe the characteristics of each of the following types of fracture: impacted, greenstick, transverse, oblique, comminuted, and spiral.
15. Identify the characteristics of each of the following types of burns: superficial, partial thickness, and full thickness.
16. Explain the difference between a partial seizure and a generalized seizure.
17. List examples of the following types of poisoning: ingested, inhaled, absorbed, and injected.
18. Identify factors that place an individual at higher risk for developing heat- and cold-related injuries.
19. Describe the difference between Type I and Type II diabetes mellitus.
20. Explain the cause of insulin shock and diabetic coma.
21. Identify the symptoms and describe the emergency care for each of the following conditions: breathing emergencies, cardiac arrest, heart attack, stroke, shock, bleeding, wounds, musculoskeletal injuries, burns, seizures, poisoning, heat and cold exposure, and diabetic emergencies.

KEY TERMINOLOGY

burn: An injury to the tissues caused by exposure to thermal, chemical, electrical, or radioactive agents.

cardiac arrest: A condition in which the heart has stopped beating or beats too irregularly to circulate blood effectively through the body.

crash cart: A specially equipped cart for holding and transporting medications, equipment, and supplies needed for performing life-saving procedures in an emergency.

crepitus (KREP-it-us): A grating sensation caused by fractured bone fragments rubbing against each other.

dislocation: An injury in which one end of a bone making up a joint is separated or displaced from its normal anatomic position.

emergency medical services (EMS) system: A network of community resources, equipment, and personnel that provides care to victims of injury or sudden illness.

first aid: The immediate care that is administered to an individual who is injured or suddenly becomes ill before complete medical care can be obtained.

fracture (FRAK-shur): Any break in a bone.

hypothermia (HÎ-po-ther-mê-a): A life-threatening condition in which the temperature of the entire body falls to a dangerously low level.

poison: Any substance that causes illness, injury, or death if it enters the body.

pressure point: A site on the body where an artery lies close to the surface of the skin and can be compressed against an underlying bone to control bleeding.

seizure (SÊ-zhur): A sudden episode of involuntary muscular contractions and relaxation, often accompanied by a change in sensation, behavior, and level of consciousness.

shock: The failure of the cardiovascular system to deliver enough blood to all the vital organs of the body.

splint: Any device that will immobilize a body part.

sprain: Trauma to a joint, which causes tearing of ligaments.

strain: A stretching or tearing of muscles or tendons caused by trauma.

wound: A break in the continuity of an external or internal surface, caused by physical means.

INTRODUCTION

☐ Medical emergencies often arise both in and outside of the workplace that can result in the sudden loss of life or permanent disability. If the emergency situation occurs in the medical office, the physician provides immediate medical care for the patient. Some medical offices maintain a crash cart for this purpose, which is discussed next. In these situations, the medical assistant may be required to assist the physician in providing the emergency medical care.

The medical assistant may need to administer first aid for medical emergencies occurring outside of the medical office environment. **First aid** is defined as the immediate care that is administered to an individual who is injured or suddenly becomes ill before complete medical care can be obtained. The medical assistant is most likely to administer first aid to a family member or friend. The purpose of first aid is to save a life, reduce pain and suffering, prevent further injury, reduce the incidence of permanent disability, and increase the opportunity for an early recovery.

To function effectively in providing first aid, the medical assistant should be able to recognize emergency situations, provide artificial ventilation and circulation (CPR), control bleeding, protect injuries from infection and other complications, and arrange for medical assistance and transportation.

This chapter focuses on common emergency situations that the medical assistant may encounter and the first aid required for each. It is not intended, however, as a substitute for thorough first aid instruction through the American Red Cross, National Safety Council, or the American Heart Association.

THE OFFICE CRASH CART

☐ A crash cart is a specially equipped cart for holding and transporting medications, equipment, and supplies needed for performing life-saving procedures in an emergency situation. A growing number of physicians are incorporating crash carts into their medical offices. Patients who are injured or suddenly become ill may be brought to the medical office for emergency medical care. In addition, a patient may develop a sudden illness while at the medical office that requires emergency medical care. Examples of these situations include life-threatening cardiac arrhythmias, shock, cardiac arrest, poisoning, and traumatic injury.

The items included on an office crash cart vary widely among medical offices depending on the extent of the emergency medical care that needs to be administered. This, in turn, is directly related to how long it takes for emergency medical personnel to arrive and the location of the nearest hospital. Table 21–1 provides a general list of the medications, equipment, and supplies that may be included on an office crash cart. The medical assistant may be responsible for checking the crash cart on a regular basis to replenish supplies and to check the expiration date on medications.

TABLE 21–1

The Office Crash Cart

Name	Drug Category	Emergency Use
Medications Used in Cardiovascular Emergencies		
Epinephrine (Adrenalin)	Sympathomimetic*	Helps restore cardiac rhythm in cardiac arrest
Sodium bicarbonate	Alkalinizing agent	To correct metabolic acidosis after a cardiac arrest
Lidocaine (Xylocaine)	Antiarrhythmic	For rapid control of acute ventricular arrhythmias following a myocardial infarction
Bretylium tosylate	Antiarrhythmic	For treatment of ventricular fibrillation or ventricular tachycardia that fails to respond to lidocaine
Procainamide (Pronestyl)	Antiarrhythmic	An alternative drug when lidocaine fails to suppress ventricular arrhythmias
Atropine	Parasympatholytic†	For treating bradycardia associated with hypotension
Isoproterenol (Isuprel)	Sympathomimetic	To increase the heart rate in bradycardia that fails to respond to atropine
Dopamine (Intropin)	Sympathomimetic	One of the most commonly used agents for the treatment of hypotension associated with cardiogenic shock.
Dobutamine (Dobutrex)	Sympathomimetic	To manage congestive heart failure when an increase in heart rate is not desired
Nitroprusside (Nitropress)	Antihypertensive-vasodilator	For immediate reduction of blood pressure in hypertensive crisis and cardiogenic shock
Norepinephrine (Levophed)	Sympathomimetic	To increase blood pressure in cardiogenic shock and other hypotensive emergencies
Adenosine (Adenocard)	Antiarrhythmic	To manage complex paroxysmal supraventricular tachycardia
Verapamil (Calan, Isoptin)	Antiarrhythmic	For treatment of supraventricular tachycardia that fails to respond to adenosine
Furosemide (Lasix)	Diuretic	For treatment of congestive heart failure and acute pulmonary edema
Nitroglycerin (Nitrostat)	Coronary vasodilator	For treatment of chest pain associated with both angina pectoris and acute myocardial infarction
IV Solutions		
Dextrose, 5% (D5W)	Glucose	A solution of 5% glucose in water used to replace fluid and nutrients
Isotonic saline	Electrolyte	A solution of sodium chloride in purified water used to replace lost fluid, sodium, and chloride

21

Continued

TABLE 21-1

The Office Crash Cart *Continued*

Name	Drug Category	Emergency Use
Lactated Ringer's solution	Electrolyte	A sterile solution of sodium chloride, potassium chloride, and calcium chloride in purified water, used for fluid and electrolyte replacement

Medications Used in Breathing Emergencies

Name	Drug Category	Emergency Use
Epinephrine (Adrenalin)	Sympathomimetic	For symptomatic relief in acute attacks of bronchial asthma or bronchospasm associated with chronic bronchitis and emphysema
Terbutaline (Brethine)	Sympathomimetic	For symptomatic relief of bronchial asthma and reversible bronchospasm associated with bronchitis, and emphysema
Aminophylline	Bronchodilator	For symptomatic relief in acute attacks of bronchial asthma or reversible bronchospasm associated with chronic bronchitis and emphysema
Albuterol (Proventil, Ventolin)	Sympathomimetic	For symptomatic relief of bronchial asthma and reversible bronchospasm associated with chronic bronchitis and emphysema

Medications Used in Anaphylactic Reactions

Name	Drug Category	Emergency Use
Epinephrine (Adrenalin)	Sympathomimetic	For treatment of hypersensitivity reactions caused by medications, allergens, or insect stings
Diphenhydramine (Benadryl)	Antihistamine	To counteract histamine in the treatment of hypersensitivity reactions
Methylprednisolone (Solu-Medrol)	Glucocorticoid	For severe anaphylactic reactions when epinephrine does not effect a satisfactory response

Medications Used for Poisoning

Name	Drug Category	Emergency Use
Ipecac syrup	Emetic	To induce vomiting of ingested poisons
Activated charcoal	Antidote, adsorbent	Used as a general purpose antidote to adsorb swallowed poisons. To decrease the absorption of the poison or drug by binding with any unabsorbed drug from the digestive tract
Naloxone (Narcan)	Narcotic antagonist	For the treatment of overdoses caused by narcotics or synthetic narcotic agents

Medications Used in Neurologic Emergencies

Name	Drug Category	Emergency Use
Diazepam (Valium)	Anticonvulsant, antianxiety	For the treatment of convulsions in major motor seizures, status epilepticus, and acute anxiety states
Phenytoin (Dilantin)	Anticonvulsant	For controlling status epilepticus. For management of generalized tonic-clonic seizures, complex partial seizures, and critical focal seizures
Phenobarbital	Anticonvulsant, sedative/ hypnotic	For management of generalized tonic-clonic seizures and partial seizures, and in the control of acute convulsive episodes (status epilepticus, febrile seizures)

Medications Used in Metabolic Emergencies

Name	Drug Category	Emergency Use
Glucose (e.g., orange juice)	Glucose	To provide glucose for conscious patients with hypoglycemia

TABLE 21-1

The Office Crash Cart *Continued*

Name	Drug Category	Emergency Use
Dextrose, 50%	Glucose	To provide glucose for unconscious patients with hypoglycemia

Equipment and Supplies

Cardiac Equipment
Defibrillator
Defibrillator pads

IV Equipment
Tourniquet
Surgical tape
IV catheters
IV cannulas
IV tubing and needles
Armboard
IV cut-down tray
   Scalpel
   Curved and straight hemostats
   Needle holder
   Tissue forceps
   Small scissors
   Local anesthetic
   Gauze squares

Airway Equipment
Suction equipment:
   Suction pumps
   Suction tubing
   Suction catheters
Oral and nasal airways
Oxygen equipment:
   Oxygen
   Oxygen face mask
   Nasal cannula
   Oxygen tubing
Laryngoscope handle and blades
Endotracheal tubes
Lubricant

Miscellaneous Supplies
Sterile gloves
Clean gloves
Biohazard containers
Syringes (assorted sizes)
Needles (assorted sizes)
Filter needles
Tubex syringe
Alcohol swabs
Betadine swabs
Sterile dressings
Roller gauze (various widths)
Adhesive tape
Band-Aids
Bandage scissors
Local anesthetic (Xylocaine)
Lidocaine ointment

21

Continued

TABLE 21-1

The Office Crash Cart *Continued*		
Name	**Drug Category**	**Emergency Use**
Lidocaine spray		
Lubricant		
Tongue blades		
Flashlight		
Cold packs		
Sphygmomanometer		
Stethoscope		

* A drug that stimulates the sympathetic nervous system (also called an adrenergic).

† A drug that inhibits the action of the parasympathetic nervous system (also called an anticholinergic).

EMERGENCY MEDICAL SERVICES SYSTEM

☐ The **emergency medical services (EMS) system** is a network of community resources, equipment, and medical personnel that provides emergency care to victims of injury or sudden illness. An **emergency medical technician-basic (EMT-B)** is a professional provider of prehospital emergency care, which includes care both at the scene and during transportation to the hospital. An EMT-B has received formal training and is certified to provide basic life support measures. An **EMT-Paramedic (EMT-P)** is qualified to provide advanced life support care, including advanced airway maintenance, starting intravenous drips, administration of medication, cardiac monitoring and interpretation, and cardiac defibrillation.

Activating the emergency medical services is often the most important step the medical assistant can take in an emergency. The rapid arrival of emergency medical technicians increases the patient's chances of surviving a life-threatening emergency. In the majority of urban and in some rural areas in the United States, the medical assistant can activate the local emergency medical services by dialing **911** on the telephone. Other areas will have a local seven-digit number, and it is important to keep the number at hand.

When calling local emergency medical services, the medical assistant will speak with an **emergency medical dispatcher (EMD).** An EMD has had formal training in handling emergency situations over the phone. The responsibility of the EMD is to answer the emergency call, listen to the caller, obtain needed information, determine what help is needed, and send the appropriate personnel and equipment. The EMD is also responsible for relaying instructions to the caller about providing emergency care until the emergency medical technicians arrive.

These guidelines should be followed when calling the emergency medical services:

- Speak clearly and calmly to the EMD. Identify the problem as accurately and concisely as possible so that proper equipment and personnel can be sent. The EMD will want to be informed of the number of victims involved, the condition of the victim or victims, and the emergency care that has already been administered.
- The EMD will ask you for your phone number and address. In responding, be sure to relay the exact location of the victim to the dispatcher, including the correct street name and house number, and (if applicable) the building name, the floor, and the room number. With the 911 emergency system, the address automatically appears on a monitor: however, there is a chance that the address may not show up on the monitor. In addition, the emergency may not be in the same location as the caller. If possible, have someone meet the ambulance personnel and direct them to the scene.
- Do not hang up until the EMD gives you permission to do so. The dispatcher may need to obtain additional information or may need to provide you with instructions on treating the patient until emergency medical technicians arrive.

FIRST AID KIT

☐ It is important that the medical assistant acquire and maintain a first aid kit. A first aid kit contains basic supplies needed to provide emergency care to individuals experiencing injury or sudden illness (Fig. 21–1). It is recommended that a first aid kit be kept both at home and in the car.

First aid kits are commercially available at most drug stores or from the local Red Cross chapter. It is

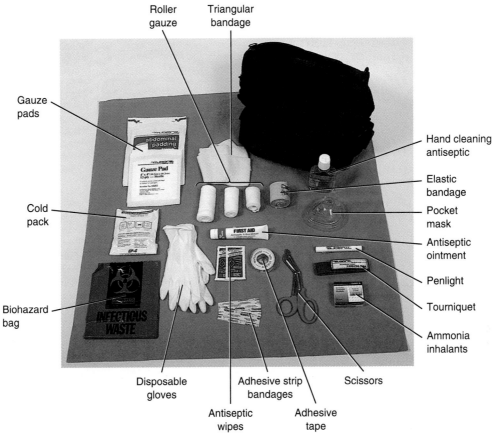

Roller gauze

Triangular bandage

Gauze pads

Cold pack

Biohazard bag

Hand cleaning antiseptic

Elastic bandage

Pocket mask

Antiseptic ointment

Penlight

Tourniquet

Ammonia inhalants

Disposable gloves

Antiseptic wipes

Adhesive strip bandages

Adhesive tape

Scissors

■ **FIGURE 21–1.** First-aid kit.

21

also possible to make your own. Along with the items shown in Figure 21–1, the first aid kit should include the phone numbers of the local emergency medical service, the regional poison control center, and the police and fire departments. It is important to check the first aid kit on a regular basis and replace needed supplies.

OSHA SAFETY PRECAUTIONS

☐ To avoid exposure to bloodborne pathogens and other potentially infectious materials, the OSHA Bloodborne Pathogens Standards presented in Chapter 1 should be followed when performing first aid. The following guidelines help reduce or eliminate the risk of infection:

1. Make sure that your first aid kit contains personal protective equipment such as gloves, a face shield and mask, and a pocket mask.
2. Wear gloves when it is reasonably anticipated that you will have hand contact with the following:

blood and other potentially infectious materials, mucous membranes, nonintact skin, and contaminated articles or surfaces.

3. Perform all first aid procedures involving blood or other potentially infectious materials in a manner so as to minimize splashing, spraying, spattering, and generation of droplets of these substances.
4. Wear protective clothing and gloves to cover cuts or other lesions of the skin.
5. Wash hands as soon as possible after removing gloves.
6. Avoid touching objects that may be contaminated with blood or other potentially infectious materials.
7. If your hands or other skin surfaces come in contact with blood or other potentially infectious materials, wash the area as soon as possible with soap and water.
8. If your mucous membranes (e.g., eyes, nose, mouth) come in contact with blood or other potentially infectious materials, flush them with water as soon as possible.
9. Avoid eating, drinking, and touching your mouth, eyes, or nose while providing emergency care or before you wash your hands.

10. If you are exposed to blood or other potentially infectious materials, report the incident as soon as possible to your physician so that postexposure procedures can be instituted.

THE PRIMARY ASSESSMENT

☐ When the medical assistant encounters an emergency, the situation must be assessed immediately to identify the presence of any serious conditions that may pose a threat to the patient's life. This initial assessment to detect life-threatening conditions is called a **primary assessment** and is described below in more detail. The following questions must be answered when performing the primary assessment:

- Is the patient responsive?
- Does the patient have an open airway?
- Is the patient breathing?
- Does the patient have a pulse?
- Is the patient bleeding severely?

ASSESSING RESPONSIVENESS

To determine whether the patient is responsive, the medical assistant should gently tap the patient and shout: "Are you okay?" The medical assistant should not jar or move the patient unnecessarily, to prevent further injury from occurring. A patient who can speak or cry is conscious, is breathing, and has a pulse.

If the patient is unable to respond, he or she may be unconscious. Unconsciousness should be a warning to the medical assistant that a life-threatening condition may exist. When a patient is unconscious, the lower jaw relaxes and may cause the tongue to fall on the back of the pharnyx, resulting in a blockage of the airway. This can cause breathing to stop and, if not corrected, will progress to cardiac arrest and death.

The current guidelines issued by the American Heart Association state that emergency medical services should be activated immediately for an adult patient who is unresponsive (Fig. 21–2). Studies have shown that ventricular fibrillation is the most common initial heart rhythm for adults in nontraumatic cardiac arrest. In these instances, rapid defibrillation is the key to their survival.

AIRWAY AND BREATHING ASSESSMENT

In the unresponsive patient, the medical assistant should continue the primary assessment by assessing the **ABCs: airway, breathing, and circulation.** Although airway and breathing are listed as two separate

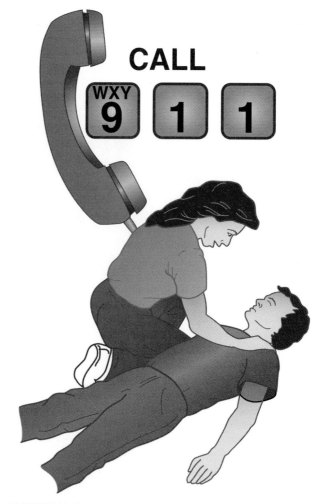

■ **FIGURE 21–2.** The emergency medical services should be activated immediately for an adult patient who is unresponsive. (Reproduced with permission. *Basic Life Support Heartsaver Guide, 1993.* Copyright American Heart Association.)

components of the ABCs, they are evaluated together. If possible, the patient should be assessed in the position found, particularly if the medical assistant suspects that the patient has suffered a head or neck injury. Improper movement of the patient with these conditions may cause further injury or even permanent paralysis.

To determine whether the patient is breathing and has an open airway, the medical assistant should **look, listen,** and **feel** as follows: Look for the rise and fall of the chest associated with breathing; listen for air entering and leaving the nose and mouth; and feel for air moving out of the nose or mouth. This evaluation should take about 5 seconds to perform. *Remember, if the patient can speak or cry, she or he has an open airway, is breathing, and has a pulse.*

A patient who is not breathing is said to be in

respiratory arrest. The first step in the care of such a patient is to ensure an open airway so that air can enter the lungs. This may be all that is necessary to allow the patient to resume breathing spontaneously. The airway must be opened with the patient in a supine position on a firm, flat surface. If the patient is not in a supine position, gently roll the patient over, making sure to keep the head and spine in as straight a line as possible.

The airway can be opened by one of the following methods: the **head tilt–chin lift maneuver** or the **jaw-thrust maneuver** (refer to Procedure 21–1). The head tilt–chin lift maneuver should not be used with a patient who has suffered a head, neck, or spinal injury because further injury or permanent paralysis could result from the rotating force involved with this maneuver. In this case, the jaw-thrust maneuver should be used to open the patient's airway.

PROCEDURE

21–1

Opening the Airway*

Head Tilt–Chin Lift Maneuver

1. **Procedural Step.** Place one hand on the forehead and the fingers of the hand closest to the feet along the patient's jawbone.

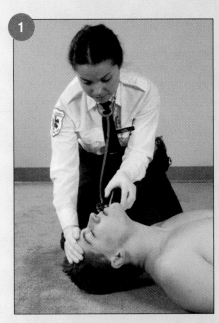

(From Henry, M., Stapleton, E.: *EMT Prehospital Care,* 2nd ed. Philadelphia, W. B. Saunders, 1997.)

2. **Procedural Step.** Apply a gentle, rotating force to the forehead while lifting the jaw upward until the teeth are touching but the mouth is not completely closed. The thumb may be used to distract the lower lip away from the upper lip, if necessary.

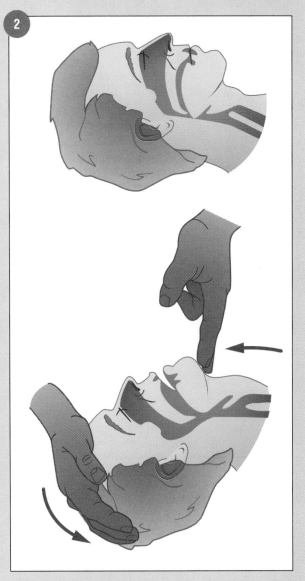

(From Henry, M., Stapleton, E.: *EMT Prehospital Care,* 2nd ed. Philadelphia, W. B. Saunders, 1997.)

*From Henry, M., Stapleton, E.: *EMT Prehospital Care.* Philadelphia, W. B. Saunders, 1997, page 155, Fig. 7-9A.

Jaw-Thrust Maneuver

1. Procedural Step. Place both thumbs on the patient's *maxillae* (cheekbones) and your index and middle fingers on both sides of the *mandible* (lower jaw) where it angles toward the ear.

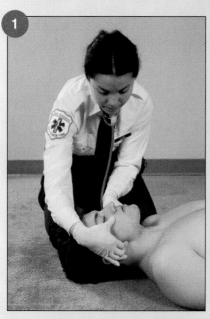

(From Henry, M., Stapleton, E.: *EMT Prehospital Care,* 2nd ed. Philadelphia, W. B. Saunders, 1997.)

2. Procedural Step. While using the cheekbones to stabilize the head, lift the jaw upward, *without tilting the head or flexing the cervical spine.*

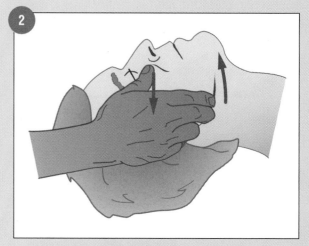

(From Henry, M., Stapleton, E.: *EMT Prehospital Care,* 2nd ed. Philadelphia, W. B. Saunders, 1997.)

21

If the patient is still not breathing after opening the airway, the medical assistant must breathe for him or her. The process of breathing for the patient is known as **rescue breathing,** also termed artificial ventilation, mouth-to-mouth breathing, and pulmonary resuscitation. Rescue breathing is illustrated and described in this chapter under Respiratory Arrest.

ASSESSMENT OF CIRCULATION

The next step in the primary assessment is to check the patient's circulation. If the heart is not beating, blood is unable to circulate through the body. Without an adequate blood supply, irreversible brain damage will occur in just 4 to 6 minutes and brain death will usually occur within 10 minutes.

To assess circulation, the medical assistant should check for the presence of a carotid pulse, which is located on the anterior side of the neck slightly to one side of the midline. If the medical assistant cannot feel a pulse, the patient is in cardiac arrest and requires **cardiopulmonary resuscitation (CPR).** CPR involves a combination of rescue breathing to transfer oxygen into the patient's lungs and chest compressions to circulate blood containing oxygen to the brain. CPR is illustrated and described in this chapter under Cardiopulmonary Resuscitation.

In cases of traumatic injury, the patient should also be assessed for the presence of severe bleeding. Bleeding is considered severe when blood spurts from a wound or when bleeding cannot be controlled. Check for severe bleeding by looking at the patient from head to toe for signs of external bleeding. Severe bleeding must be controlled; otherwise, it will quickly progress to hypovolemic shock and death (refer to Bleeding).

GUIDELINES FOR PROVIDING EMERGENCY CARE

☐ The remainder of this chapter presents specific emergency situations that maybe encountered by the medical assistant and the emergency care for each. The following guidelines should be followed when providing emergency care:

1. Remain calm, and speak in a normal tone of voice. These measures help calm and reassure the patient.

2. Make sure that the scene is safe before approaching the patient. It is important that you protect yourself from harm in an emergency situation.

3. Before administering emergency care to a conscious patient, you must first have permission or consent. To obtain consent, you must inform the patient who you are, your level of training, and what you are going to do to help. *Never* administer care to a conscious patient who refuses it. When a life-threatening condition exists and the patient is unconscious or otherwise unable to give consent, consent is assumed or implied. Under law, it is implied that if the patient could give consent to care, he or she would.

4. Perform a primary assessment to detect and care for life-threatening conditons before proceeding with emergency care of conditions that are not life-threatening.

5. Follow the OSHA Standards when providing emergency care to reduce or eliminate exposure to bloodborne pathogens or other potentially infectious materials.

6. Know how to activate your local emergency medical services (EMS) system. Activating the EMS is often the most important step you can take to help a patient who has experienced an injury or sudden illness.

7. Do not move the patient unnecessarily. Unnecessary movement can result in further injury or even be life-threatening to a patient with a serious condition.

8. Obtain information as to what happened from the patient, family members, coworkers, bystanders, and so on.

9. Look for a medical alert tag on the patient's wrist or neck. A medical alert tag provides information on a medical condition the patient may have.

10. Continue caring for the patient until more highly trained personnel arrive. On the arrival of emergency medical personnel or a physician, relay the condition in which you found the patient and the emergency care that has been administered.

BREATHING EMERGENCIES

☐ The body requires a constant supply of oxygen to survive. Oxygen is breathed in through the nose and mouth, and travels down the pharynx, through the trachea, and into the lungs. Once oxygen reaches the lungs, it is picked up by the circulatory system and

Highlight on Good Samaritan Laws

In most states, Good Samaritan laws have been enacted to provide immunity to individuals, such as the medical assistant, who administer first aid at the scene of an emergency. These laws were enacted to encourage individuals to help others in an emergency. They assume that an individual would do her or his best to save a life or prevent further injury.

The legal immunity provided by Good Samaritan laws protects an individual from being sued and found financially responsible for a patient's injury. The individual is immune from liability (except for "gross negligence") if he or she acts in good faith and uses a reasonable level of skill that does not exceed the scope of the individual's training.

Good Samaritan laws do not mean that an individual *cannot* be sued for administering first aid. An individual is *not* protected from liability if he or she is grossly careless or reckless in handling the situation. Because the components of Good Samaritan laws vary from state to state, the medical assistant must become familiar with the laws that govern his or her state.

transported to all the tissues of the body. A breathing emergency interferes with this normal process, and therefore, prompt action must be taken. The major types of breathing emergencies are described next, along with the emergency care for each.

RESPIRATORY ARREST

Respiratory arrest means that an individual has ceased breathing altogether and therefore is not receiving an oxgyen supply. Signs that indicate a patient is in respiratory arrest include the absence of chest movement or chest movements that are minimal or uneven in nature, the absence of air moving in or out of the nose or mouth, and cyanosis of the skin, lips, tongue, or ear lobes. Without treatment, irreparable damage to vital organs, such as the brain, will occur in a matter of minutes. A number of conditions can result in respiratory arrest:

Airway obstruction
Heart attack or heart disease
Stroke
Emphysema and asthma
Pneumonia
Poisoning
Drug overdose

21

Electrocution
Shock
Drowning
Traumatic injury
Anaphylactic shock
Suffocation

A patient in respiratory arrest is in need of **rescue breathing.** Rescue breathing provides the patient with oxygen and allows carbon dioxide to be removed to keep the patient alive until more advanced techniques can be applied. Procedure 21–2 presents the procedure for performing rescue breathing.

PROCEDURE

21–2

Rescue Breathing*

1. **Procedural Step.** Open the airway with the head tilt–chin lift or modified jaw thrust.

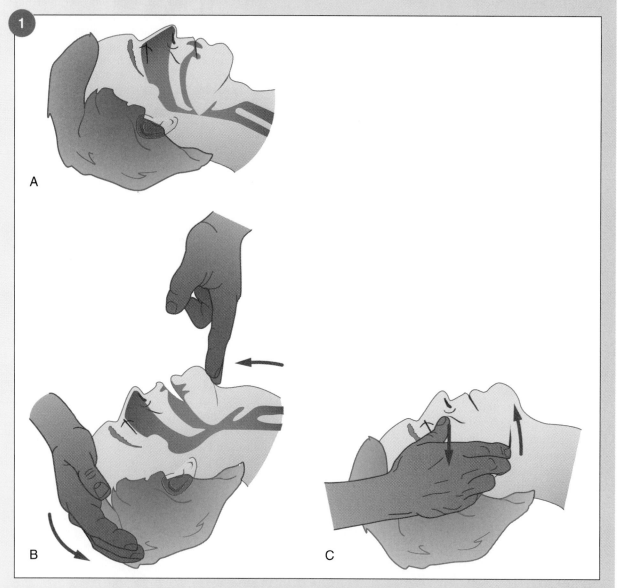

A

B

C

(From Henry, M., Stapleton, E.: *EMT Prehospital Care,* 2nd ed. Philadelphia, W. B. Saunders, 1997.)

21

*From Henry, M., Stapleton, E.: *EMT Prehospital Care.* Philadelphia, W. B. Saunders, 1992, pp. 111 and 112.

PROCEDURE 21-2

2. Procedural Step. Once the need for rescue breathing has been established, seal your mouth completely around the victim's mouth while pinching the nose and maintaining an airway.

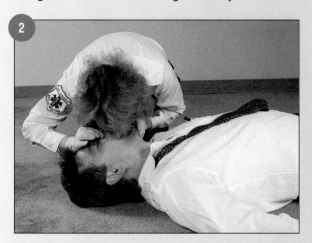

(From Henry, M., Stapleton, E.: *EMT Prehospital Care*, 2nd ed. Philadelphia, W. B. Saunders, 1997.)

3. Procedural Step. When using the modified jaw thrust, seal the nose with your cheek during ventilation.

4. Procedural Step. Give two smooth breaths while observing for chest rise out of the corner of your eye. Each breath should take 1.5 to 2 seconds to deliver. Take your mouth away from the patient's mouth after each breath so that you can take another breath. Avoid breathing the exhaled air from the patient.

5. Procedural Step. Assuming that the pulse is present, administer one breath every 5 seconds for the adult and 1 breath every 3 seconds for the infant or child until the patient begins to breathe adequately.

6. Procedural Step. If the patient is breathing at an adequate rate but inadequate depth, assist ventilations by providing a breath each time the patient attempts to breathe, thereby synchronizing your efforts with the patient's.

AIRWAY OBSTRUCTION (CHOKING)

An airway obstruction interferes with the movement of air through the upper or lower airway.

The patient's airway may be blocked by an anatomic obstruction such as the tongue or swollen tissues of the mouth and throat. Examples of conditions resulting in an anatomic obstruction include unconsciousness, an injury to the neck, and anaphylactic shock.

An airway obstruction also occurs when the airway is blocked by a foreign object such as a piece of food or a small object, or fluids such as vomit, blood, mucus, saliva, or water. Certain factors increase the likelihood of a foreign object's becoming lodged in the airway. These include trying to swallow large, poorly chewed pieces of food, drinking alcohol before or during a meal, eating too fast, talking excitedly or laughing while eating, and talking, playing, or running with food or objects in the mouth.

Foreign objects may cause either a partial or a complete airway obstruction. With a **complete airway obstruction,** the patient is unable to speak, breathe, or cough and requires immediate care in order to survive.

A **partial airway obstruction** allows for some air exchange. The patient's ability to breathe will depend on how much air can get past the obstruction. The narrowed airway often causes a high-pitched sound (stridor) as air moves in and out of the lungs. The air usually allows the patient to cough, which may help dislodge and expel the object. The patient may also be able to speak if she or he is able to move air past the vocal cords.

EMERGENCY CARE FOR AN AIRWAY OBSTRUCTION

If the patient is conscious, the first step in determining the presence of an airway obstruction is to ask the patient: "Are you choking?" An individual with an airway obstruction is usually able to nod in response and may also clutch the throat with one or both hands. Clutching the throat is recognized as the universal distress signal for choking, and the public is encouraged to use this signal if choking occurs (Fig. 21-3).

If the patient is coughing forcefully, do not interfere with these attempts to dislodge and expel the object. An individual who has enough air to cough forcefully or speak also has enough air entering the lungs to breathe. Remain calm, and encourage the patient to continue coughing to clear the obstruction. If this fails to expel the foreign object, EMS should be activated.

If a complete airway obstruction is present, there will be no movement of air and the individual is unable to speak, breathe, or cough. The Heimlich maneuver is recommended for relieving a complete airway obstruc-

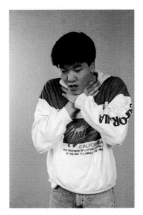

■ **FIGURE 21–3.** Clutching the throat is the universal distress signal for choking. (From Henry, M., Stapleton, E.: *EMT Prehospital Care.* Philadelphia, W. B. Saunders, 1997.)

tion or a partial airway obstruction in which there is very little air exchange.

HEIMLICH MANEUVER

The Heimlich maneuver consists of a series of manual thrusts to the abdomen to force residual air from the lungs. The residual air creates an "artificial cough" that may be enough to expel the foreign object. It may be necessary to repeat the abdominal thrust multiple times to clear the airway. Each individual thrust should be administered with the intent of relieving the obstruction. The method for performing the Heimlich maneuver is presented in Procedure 21–3.

MEMORIES *from* **EXTERNSHIP**

JUDY MARKINS: *As it turned out, one of my most terrible moments during my externship was a great learning experience.*

I was drawing blood (which was not my favorite procedure) and missed the vein—not once, but twice! You could see the sweat under my gloves. My stomach was in my throat, and I did not want to try again. Thank goodness my patient was understanding and I had an excellent externship supervisor. She insisted that I try again, encouraging me that I could and providing some suggestions that she had learned from her many years of experience. I got the blood specimen along with some newfound confidence.

In most situations, someone can help you if you have questions. Use your resources when you need to. Be honest, know your procedure, and have confidence in yourself.

21–3

PROCEDURE

Performing the Heimlich Maneuver*

When Victim is Conscious and Standing or Sitting

1. **Procedural Step.** Stand behind the victim and wrap your arms around the victim's waist. The rescuer should stand directly behind the victim and with an open stance. This provides a secure position for support should the victim become unconscious.
2. **Procedural Step.** Grasp one fist with your other hand, and place the thumb of that fist against the

victim's abdomen, slightly above the navel and below the xiphoid process.
3. **Procedural Step.** Press your fist into the victim's abdomen with a quick upward thrust.
4. **Procedural Step.** Repeat until the obstruction is relieved or until the victim becomes unconscious.

*From Henry, M., Stapleton, E.: *EMT Prehospital Care.* Philadelphia, W. B. Saunders, 1997.

PROCEDURE 21–3

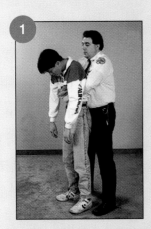

(From Henry, M., Stapleton, E.: *EMT Prehospital Care,* 2nd ed. Philadelphia, W. B. Saunders, 1997.)

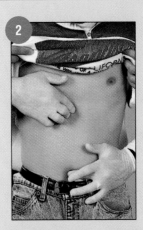

(From Henry, M., Stapleton, E.: *EMT Prehospital Care,* 2nd ed. Philadelphia, W. B. Saunders, 1997.)

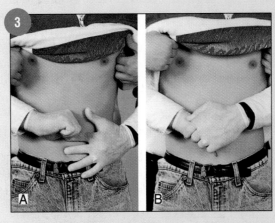

(From Henry, M., Stapleton, E.: *EMT Prehospital Care,* 2nd ed. Philadelphia, W. B. Saunders, 1997.)

21

RESPIRATORY DISTRESS

Respiratory distress indicates that the patient is breathing but is having great difficulty in doing so. Respiratory distress may sometimes lead to respiratory arrest. It is therefore important that the medical assistant be alert for the signs and symptoms of respiratory distress. These signs and symptoms may include noisy breathing, such as gasping for air, or rasping, gurgling, or whistling sounds; breathing that is unusually fast or slow; and breathing that is painful. The general care for respiratory distress is to place the patient in a comfortable position that facilitates breathing. Most patients prefer a sitting or semi-reclining position. Remain calm, and reassure the patient to help reduce anxiety. Calming the patient may help the patient

breathe easier. If the patient's condition worsens or does not resolve within a few minutes, activate the local emergency medical services.

Examples of conditions frequently causing respiratory distress are described next.

Asthma

Asthma is a condition characterized by wheezing, coughing, and dyspnea. During an asthmatic attack, the bronchioles constrict and become clogged with mucus, which accounts for many of the symptoms of asthma.

Asthma may occur at any age, but it is more common in children and young adults. If the condition is not treated, it can lead to serious complications such as permanent lung damage. It is frequently, but not always, associated with a family history of allergies. Any of the common allergens, such as house dust, pollens, molds, or animal danders, may trigger an asthmatic attack. Asthmatic attacks also may be caused by nonspecific factors such as air pollutants, tobacco smoke, chemical fumes, vigorous exercise, respiratory infections, exposure to cold, and emotional stress. Normally, an individual with asthma easily controls attacks with medications. These medications stop the muscle spasms and open the airway, making breathing easier.

Some patients may develop a severe prolonged asthma attack that is life-threatening, which is known as **status asthmaticus.** These patients can move only a small amount of air. Because so little air is being moved, the typical breathing sounds associated with asthma may not be audible. The patient may have a bluish discoloration of the skin and extremely labored breathing. Status asthmaticus is a true emergency and requires immediate transportation of the patient to an emergency care facility by the fastest way possible.

Emphysema

Emphysema is a progressive lung disorder in which the terminal bronchioles that lead into the alveoli become plugged with mucus. Because of this problem, the alveoli become damaged, resulting in less surface area to diffuse oxygen into the blood. Eventually, this condition results in a loss of elasticity of the alveoli, causing inhaled air to become trapped in the lungs. This makes breathing difficult, particularly during exhalation.

Emphysema usually develops over many years and is found most frequently in heavy smokers. It also occurs in patients with chronic bronchitis and in elderly patients whose lungs have lost their natural elasticity.

Chronic emphysema is one of the major causes of death in the United States. As the lungs progressively become less efficient, breathing becomes more and more difficult. Patients with advanced cases may go into respiratory or cardiac arrest.

Hyperventilation

Hyperventilation literally means "overbreathing." Hyperventilation is a manner of breathing in which the respirations become rapid and deep, causing an individual to exhale too much carbon dioxide. In fact, the low carbon dioxide levels in the body account for many of the symptoms of hyperventilation.

Hyperventilation is often the result of fear or anxiety and is more likely to occur in people who are tense and nervous. It is also caused by serious organic conditions such as diabetic coma, pneumonia, pulmonary edema, pulmonary embolism, head injuries, high fever, and aspirin poisoning.

In addition to rapid and deep respirations, the signs and symptoms of hyperventilation include dizziness, faintness, light-headedness, visual disturbances, chest pain, tachycardia, palpitations, fullness in the throat, and numbness and tingling of the fingers, toes, and the area around the mouth. Despite their rapid breathing efforts, patients complain that they cannot get enough air. They often think they are having a heart attack.

Treatment for hyperventilation caused by emotional factors is as follows: Calm and reassure the patient, and encourage him or her to slow the respirations, thereby allowing the carbon dioxide level to return to normal. In the past, breathing into a paper bag was advocated as a remedy for hyperventilation. Recent studies no longer recommend this practice because it could be harmful if an underlying medical condition exists or if the patient is not actually hyperventilating. If the medical assistant suspects that hyperventilation has been caused by an organic problem, the emergency medical services should be activated immediately.

CARDIAC ARREST

☐ Cardiac arrest means that the heart has stopped beating or beats too irregularly to circulate the blood effectively through the body. Conditions that can result in cardiac arrest include a heart attack, stroke, airway obstruction, near-drowning, drug overdose, trauma, and suffocation.

The primary assessment is used to determine whether a patient is in cardiac arrest. An individual in cardiac arrest is unresponsive, is not breathing, and does not have a pulse. Three important emergency care measures significantly increase the chance of survival for a patient in cardiac arrest: early activation of the emergency medical services, early initiation of cardiopulmonary resuscitation, and early defibrillation.

EMS should be activated immediately for an adult patient found to be unresponsive. If a bystander is present, the medical assistant should instruct that person to activate EMS, which permits the medical assistant to continue the primary assessment. If it is determined that the patient does not have a pulse, cardiopulmonary resuscitation should be started immediately and continued until emergency medical personnel arrive to defibrillate the patient. **Defibrillation** is the application of an electric current to the patient's heart, which can shock the heart out of ventricular fibrillation and allow it to resume beating normally. Traditionally, health-care providers trained in the interpretation of ECG rhythms delivered defibrillation.

However, new technology called **automated external defibrillators (AED)** permits defibrillation by minimally trained individuals including lay people. An *automated external defibrillator* is a computerized defibrillator that can recognize a shockable rhythm and direct the operator using voice prompts and lighted indicators whether the rhythm should be shocked. This highly reliable technology will allow for widespread early defibrillation in public buildings, stadiums, clinics and other facilities throughout the United States. Training in the use of AEDs is available in a 4- to 8-hour course offered by the American Heart Association, American Red Cross, or National Safety Council.

CARDIOPULMONARY RESUSCITATION

Cardiopulmonary resuscitation (CPR) is a combination of rescue breathing and chest compressions. The purpose of rescue breathing is to transfer oxygen to the lungs, while the purpose of chest compressions is to circulate blood containing oxygen to the patient's brain.

CPR must be performed with the patient in a supine position on a firm, flat surface. When possible, CPR should be performed using a pocket mask or other barrier device as protection against infectious diseases. The procedure for performing CPR is presented here.

Performing One-Rescuer CPR*

1. **Procedural Step.** Establish unresponsiveness, and position the patient.

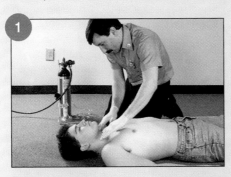

(From Henry, M., Stapleton, E.: *EMT Prehospital Care,* 2nd ed. Philadelphia, W. B. Saunders, 1997.)

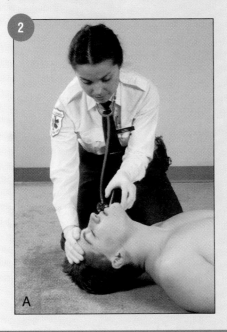

2. **Procedural Step.** Open the airway using head tilt–chin lift or jaw-thrust maneuver.

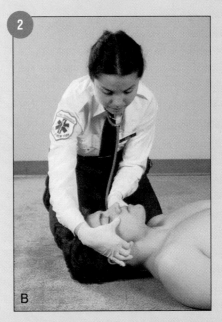

(From Henry, M., Stapleton, E.: *EMT Prehospital Care,* 2nd ed. Philadelphia, W. B. Saunders, 1997.)

3. **Procedural Step.** Look, listen, and feel for breathing.
4. **Procedural Step.** Provide positive-pressure ventilation (two breaths), and observe chest rise.
5. **Procedural Step.** Check for carotid pulse.

Continued

*From Henry, M., Stapleton, E.: *EMT Prehospital Care.* Philadelphia, W. B. Saunders, 1992, pp. 244–246.

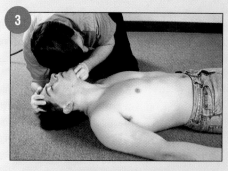

(From Henry, M., Stapleton, E.: *EMT Prehospital Care,* 2nd ed. Philadelphia, W. B. Saunders, 1997.)

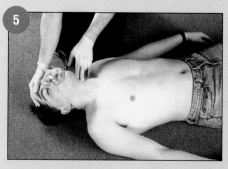

(From Henry, M., Stapleton, E.: *EMT Prehospital Care,* 2nd ed. Philadelphia, W. B. Saunders, 1997.)

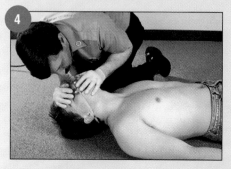

(From Henry, M., Stapleton, E.: *EMT Prehospital Care,* 2nd ed. Philadelphia, W. B. Saunders, 1997.)

6. **Procedural Step.** Locate the correct hand position by *(A)* placing your index and middle fingers of the hand closest to the patient's feet along the margin of the ribs and *(B)* sliding up to the bottom of the breast bone. *(C)* Place the heel of the hand closest to the patient's head next to your fingers, and *(D)* place the heel of the other hand directly over the hand on the sternum and interlock your fingers to avoid pressure in the area of the ribs.

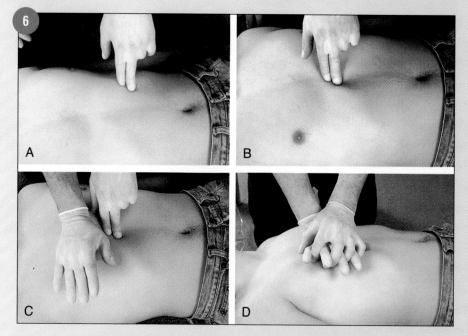

(From Henry, M., Stapleton, E.: *EMT Prehospital Care,* 2nd ed. Philadelphia, W. B. Saunders, 1997.)

21

7. **Procedural Step.** Maintain correct body position. While performing chest compressions, your shoulders, elbows, and the heels of your hands should be in alignment directly over the patient's sternum.
8. **Procedural Step.** Perform four cycles of 15 compressions/2 ventilations.
9. **Procedural Step.** Recheck the pulse after four cycles and every few minutes thereafter.

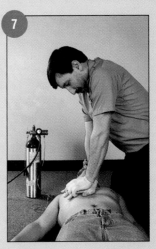

(From Henry, M., Stapleton, E.: *EMT Prehospital Care*, 2nd ed. Philadelphia, W. B. Saunders, 1997.)

HEART ATTACK

☐ A heart attack, also known as a myocardial infarction (MI), is caused by partial or complete obstruction of one or both of the coronary arteries or their branches. In most cases, the severity of the attack depends on the size of the artery that is obstructed and, in turn, the amount of myocardial tissue nourished by the artery. For example, if a small branch of a coronary artery is obstructed, the myocardial damage and symptoms may be mild, whereas the damage is usually extensive and the symptoms intense if a coronary artery is completely blocked.

The principal symptom of a heart attack is chest pain or discomfort. The chest pain is described by patients as squeezing or crushing pressure, severe indigestion or burning, heaviness, or aching. The chest discomfort can range in severity from feeling only mildly uncomfortable to being intense and accompanied by a feeling of suffocation and doom. The pain is usually felt behind the sternum and may radiate to the neck, throat, jaw, both shoulders, and arms. The pain associated with a heart attack is prolonged and is usually not relieved by resting or taking nitroglycerin. Other signs and symptoms of a heart attack include shortness of breath, profuse perspiration, nausea, and fainting.

If the medical assistant suspects that the patient is having a heart attack, EMS should be activated imme-

diately. Meanwhile, loosen tight clothing and have the patient rest in a comfortable position that facilitates breathing. If cardiac arrest occurs, the medical assistant should begin CPR immediately.

STROKE

☐ A stroke, also called a cerebrovascular accident (CVA), results when an artery to the brain is blocked or ruptures, causing an interruption of the blood flow to the brain.

The signs and symptoms of a stroke include sudden weakness or numbness of the face, arm, or leg on one side of the body; difficulty in speaking; dimmed vision or loss of vision in one eye; double vision; dizziness; confusion; severe headache; and loss of consciousness.

If the medical assistant suspects that the patient is having a stroke, EMS should be activated immediately. Meanwhile, loosen tight clothing and have the patient rest in a comfortable position. If respiratory arrest or cardiac arrest or both occur, begin rescue breathing or CPR, or both, as required.

SHOCK

☐ To function properly, adequate blood flow must be maintained to all the vital organs of the body. This is

21

accomplished by the three important cardiovascular functions:

- Adequate pumping action of the heart,
- Sufficient blood circulating in the blood vessels, and
- Blood vessels being able to respond to blood flow.

When an individual suffers a severe injury or illness, one or more of these cardiovascular functions may be affected, which can lead to shock.

Shock is defined as the failure of the cardiovascular system to deliver enough blood to all the vital organs of the body. Shock accompanies many types of emergency situations: hemorrhaging, a myocardial infarction, a severe allergic reaction.

The five major types of shock are categorized according to cause: hypovolemic, cardiogenic, neurogenic, anaphylactic, and psychogenic. Each type of shock is described in this section. If they are not treated, most types of shock become life threatening. This is because shock is progressive; once reaching a certain point, it becomes irreversible and the patient's life cannot be saved.

The signs and symptoms of shock are caused by the failure of the vital organs to receive enough oxygen and nutrients. The organs most affected are the heart, brain, and lungs, which can be irreparably damaged in just 4 to 6 minutes. The general signs and symptoms of shock include weakness, restlessness, anxiety, disorientation, pallor, cold, clammy skin, rapid breathing, and rapid pulse.

If they are not treated, these symptoms can rapidly progress to a significant drop in the blood pressure, cyanosis, loss of consciousness, and death. It is important to know that the signs and symptoms of shock may be subtle or pronounced. In addition, no single sign or symptom will determine accurately the presence or severity of the shock. Because of this, it is extremely important to consider the nature of the illness or injury in determining whether the patient is a potential victim of shock. For example, if a patient suffers a traumatic injury to the abdomen, shock should be considered as a possibility, even if the patient's signs and symptoms do not suggest shock.

Shock requires immediate medical care (with the exception of psychogenic shock). The medical assistant should activate the emergency medical services without delay, so that proper medical care can be obtained as soon as possible.

HYPOVOLEMIC SHOCK

Hypovolemic shock is caused by a loss of blood or other body fluids. Conditions that may result in this type of shock include external and internal hemorrhaging, plasma loss from severe burns, and severe dehydration from vomiting, diarrhea, or profuse perspiration. The first priority of hypovolemic shock is to control bleeding. The patient in hypovolemic shock must have the volume of fluid that was lost replaced and therefore must be transported to an emergency care facility immediately.

CARDIOGENIC SHOCK

Cardiogenic shock is caused by the failure of the heart to pump blood adequately to all the vital organs of the body. This type of shock occurs when the heart has been injured or damaged. Cardiogenic shock is most frequently seen with myocardial infarction. Other causes include arrhythmias, severe congestive heart failure, acute valvular damage, and pulmonary embolism. Once a patient develops cardiogenic shock, it is very difficult to reverse and, therefore, has a high fatality rate (80 to 90 percent).

NEUROGENIC SHOCK

Neurogenic shock occurs when the nervous system is unable to control the diameter of the blood vessels. In normal situations, the nervous system instructs the blood vessels to constrict or dilate, which controls blood pressure. In neurogenic shock, that control is lost and the blood vessels dilate, causing the blood to pool in peripheral areas of the body away from vital organs.

This type of shock is most often seen with brain and spinal injuries. The blood vessels become dilated, and there is not enough blood in the circulatory system to fill the dilated vessels, causing the blood pressure to drop significantly.

ANAPHYLACTIC SHOCK

Anaphylactic shock is a very serious and life-threatening reaction of the body to an allergen or substance to which an individual is highly allergic. Examples of allergens that are most apt to result in anaphylaxis include drugs (e.g., penicillin), insect venoms, foods, and allergen extracts used in hyposensitization injections.

An anaphylactic reaction causes the release of large amounts of histamine, resulting in dilation of the blood vessels throughout the entire body and a drop in the blood pressure. The symptoms of anaphylactic shock begin with sneezing, hives, itching, angioedema, erythema, and disorientation and progress to difficulty in breathing, dizziness, faintness, and loss of consciousness. Medical care should be obtained immediately, because most fatalities occur within the first 2 hours.

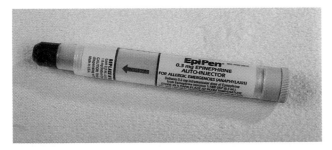

FIGURE 21–4. Anaphylactic emergency epinephrine injection.

The emergency care for anaphylactic shock is the administration of epinephrine. Because time is a factor, individuals known to have a severe allergy are provided with an anaphylactic emergency treatment kit containing injectable epinephrine (Fig. 21–4) and oral antihistamines. With the kit, treatment for a severe allergic reaction can be started immediately.

PSYCHOGENIC SHOCK

Psychogenic shock is the least serious type of shock. It is caused by unpleasant physical or emotional stimuli, such as pain, fright, or the sight of blood.

With psychogenic shock, a sudden dilation of the blood vessels causes the blood to pool in the abdomen and extremities. This, in turn, temporarily deprives the brain of blood, causing a temporary loss of consciousness (fainting). usually only lasting 1 to 2 minutes. Fainting generally occurs when an individual is in an upright position. Before fainting, the patient usually experiences some warning signals that include sudden light-headedness, pallor, nausea, weakness, yawning, blurred vision, a feeling of warmth, and sweating.

An individual who is about to faint should be placed in a position that facilitates blood flow to the brain and

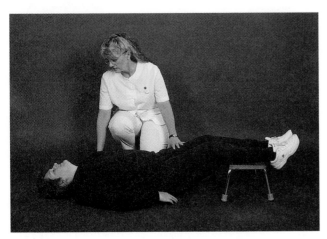

FIGURE 21–5. Prevention and treatment of fainting.

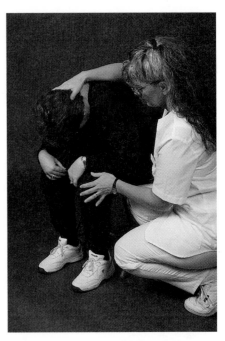

FIGURE 21–6. Prevention of fainting.

told to breathe deeply. The preferred position is to move the patient into a supine position with the legs elevated approximately 12 inches and the collar and clothing loosened (Fig. 21–5). This position may not always be possible, such as when a patient is seated; in this case, the patient's head should be lowered between the legs (Fig. 21–6). A patient who has fainted should be placed in the supine position with the legs elevated. It is recommended that a patient who has experienced fainting contact her or his physician for further evaluation.

BLEEDING

☐ Bleeding, or hemorrhaging, is the escape of blood from a severed blood vessel. Bleeding can range from being very minor to very serious, which could lead to shock and death. The amount of blood that can be lost before bleeding becomes life threatening varies according to each individual. In general, a loss of 25 to 40 percent of an individual's total blood volume can be fatal. This equates to approximately 2 to 4 pints of blood for the average adult.

EXTERNAL BLEEDING

External bleeding is bleeding that can be seen coming from a wound. Common examples of external bleeding include bleeding from open fractures, lacerations, and the nose.

21

Individuals with serious external bleeding will exhibit the following symptoms: obvious bleeding, restlessness, cold and clammy skin, thirst, increased and thready pulse, rapid and shallow respirations, a drop in the blood pressure (a late symptom), and decreasing levels of consciousness.

There are three types of external bleeding classified according to the type of blood vessel that has been injured: capillary, venous, and arterial.

CAPILLARY BLEEDING. Capillary bleeding is the most common type of external bleeding and consists of a slow oozing of blood that is bright red. This type of bleeding occurs with minor cuts, scratches, and abrasions.

VENOUS BLEEDING. Venous bleeding occurs when a vein has been punctured or severed. This type of bleeding is characterized by a slow and steady flow of blood that is dark red.

ARTERIAL BLEEDING. Arterial bleeding is the most serious type of external bleeding and occurs when an artery is punctured or severed. Fortunately, it is the least common type of bleeding, since arteries are situated deeper in the body and are protected by bone. Arterial bleeding is characterized by bleeding that comes in spurts and is bright red. The arteries most frequently involved in accidents are the carotid, brachial, radial, and femoral.

Emergency Care for External Bleeding

The most effective way to control bleeding is through the application of direct pressure to the bleeding site.

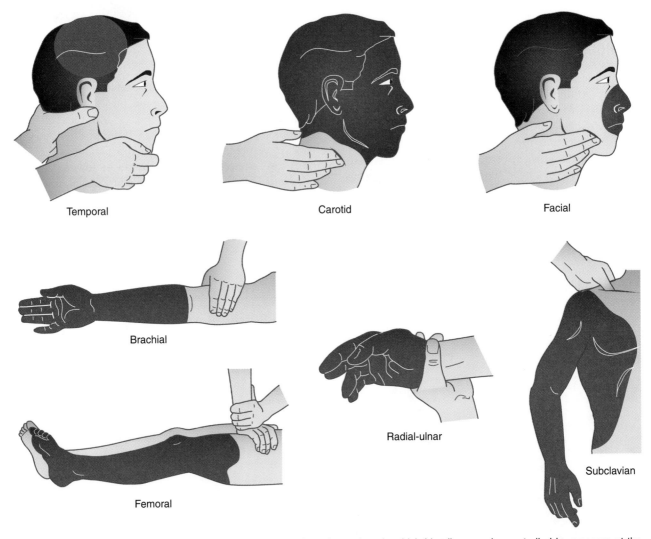

Temporal

Carotid

Facial

Brachial

Femoral

Radial-ulnar

Subclavian

■ **FIGURE 21–7.** Location of pressure points. Shaded areas show the regions in which bleeding may be controlled by pressure at the points indicated. (From Miller, B. F., Keane, C. B.: *Encyclopedia and Dictionary of Medicine, Nursing, and Allied Health*, 6th ed. Philadelphia, W. B. Saunders, 1997, p. 1275.)

21

The pressure functions by either slowing down or stopping the flow of blood altogether. The amount of pressure required depends on the type of bleeding involved. A small amount of pressure is usually sufficient to control capillary bleeding, whereas significant pressure is often required to control arterial bleeding.

If bleeding cannot be controlled with direct pressure, a pressure point can be used. A **pressure point** is a site on the body where an artery lies close to the surface of the skin and can be compressed against an underlying bone. Refer to Figure 21–7 for an illustration of pressure points. Using a pressure point helps slow or stop the flow of blood to the wound. The pressure points used most often are the brachial and femoral arteries. The brachial artery is located on the inside of the upper arm midway between the elbow and shoulder. Squeezing the brachial artery helps control severe bleeding in the arm. The femoral artery is located in the groin and helps control severe bleeding in the leg.

The specific steps for controlling bleeding are:

1. Apply direct pressure to the wound with a clean covering such as a large, thick gauze dressing (Fig. 21–8A). If gauze is not available, a clean material such as a sanitary napkin, washcloth, handkerchief, or sock can be used. If the wound is located on an extremity, elevate the limb while continuing to apply direct pressure.
2. Apply additional dressings if needed. If the dressing soaks through, apply another dressing over the first one and continue to apply pressure (Fig. 21–8B). (Never remove a dressing once it has been applied as this could result in more bleeding.) If the bleeding cannot be controlled with direct pressure, apply pressure to the appropriate pressure point while continuing to apply direct local pressure.
3. Apply a pressure bandage. When bleeding has been controlled, apply a bandage snugly over the dressing to maintain pressure on the wound (Fig. 21–8C).
4. Transport the patient to an emergency care facility, or, if the case is serious enough, activate the local emergency medical services.

NOSEBLEEDS

A nosebleed, or epistaxis, is a common form of external bleeding and is usually not serious but is more of a

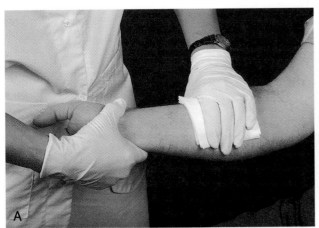
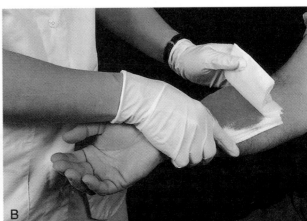
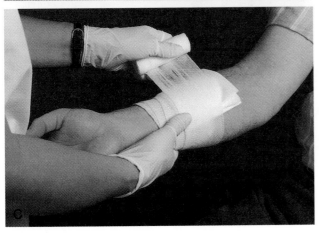

■ **FIGURE 21–8.** Control of bleeding. *A,* Apply direct pressure to the wound with a large, thick gauze dressing. *B,* If blood soaks through the dressing, apply another dressing over the first one and continue to apply pressure. *C,* When bleeding has been controlled, apply a pressure bandage.

nuisance. Nosebleeds are usually caused by an upper respiratory infection but can also result from a direct blow from a blunt object, hypertension, strenuous activity, and exposure to high altitudes.

Emergency Care for a Nosebleed

1. Position the patient in a sitting position with the head tilted forward. This prevents the blood from running down the back of the throat, which may result in nausea.
2. Apply direct pressure by pinching the nostrils together (Fig. 21–9A). Do not release the pressure too soon, because the bleeding may resume. It usually takes about 15 minutes for adequate clot formation to occur. An ice pack can also be applied to the bridge of the nose to help control the bleeding (Fig. 21–9B). If these measures do not control the bleeding, apply pressure on the upper lip, just below the nose.
3. After the bleeding has stopped, tell the patient not to blow the nose for several hours as this could loosen the clot, causing the bleeding to start again.
4. If bleeding cannot be controlled, transport the patient to an emergency care facility for further treatment.

INTERNAL BLEEDING

Internal bleeding is bleeding that flows into a body cavity, an organ, or between tissues. It may be minor, as in the case of a contusion, or it may be very serious, such as a severe, blunt blow to the abdomen.

Severe internal bleeding is a life-threatening emergency. Because there is no obvious blood flow, the nature of the injury and the signs and symptoms of bleeding must be used in recognizing internal bleeding. Signs and symptoms include bruises, pain, tenderness, or swelling at the site of the injury; rapid weak pulse; cold and clammy skin; nausea and vomiting; excessive thirst, a drop in the blood pressure; and decreased levels of consciousness.

If a patient is suspected of having internal bleeding, the local emergency medical services should be activated immediately. Until emergency medical personnel arrive, the patient should be kept quiet and treated for shock.

WOUNDS

☐ A **wound** is a break in the continuity of an external or internal surface, caused by physical means. Wounds are either open or closed.

OPEN WOUNDS

An open wound is a break in the skin surface or mucous membrane that exposes the underlying tissues. Because the skin is broken, hemorrhaging and wound contamination are a primary concern with open wounds. Examples of open wounds include incisions, lacerations, punctures, and abrasions (Fig. 21–10). An

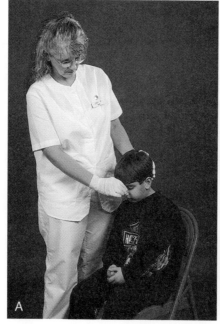
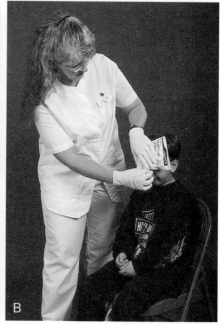

■ **FIGURE 21–9.** Care of a nosebleed. *A,* Apply direct pressure by pinching the nostrils together. *B,* An ice pack can be applied to the bridge of the nose to help control the bleeding.

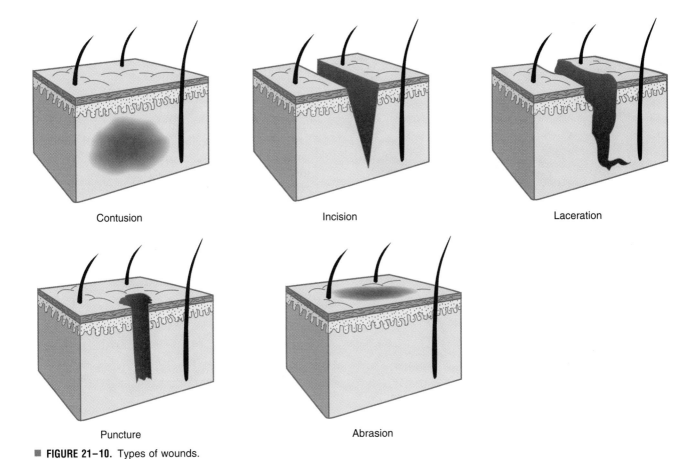

FIGURE 21–10. Types of wounds.

Contusion

Incision

Laceration

Puncture

Abrasion

individual with an open wound should receive prompt medical attention by a physician if any of the following occur: spurting blood, bleeding that cannot be controlled, a break in the skin that is deeper than just the outer skin layers, embedded debris or an embedded object in the wound, involvement of nerves, muscles, or tendons, and occurrence on the mouth, tongue, face, genitals, or other area where scarring would be apparent.

INCISIONS AND LACERATIONS

An incision is a clean, smooth cut caused by a sharp cutting instrument such as a knife, razor, or a piece of glass. Deep incisions are accompanied by profuse bleeding; in addition, damage to muscles, tendons, and nerves may occur. Because the edges of the wound are smooth and straight, incisions usually heal better than lacerations.

A laceration is a wound in which the tissues are torn apart, rather than cut, leaving ragged and irregular edges. Lacerations are caused by dull knives, large objects that have been driven into the skin, and heavy machinery. Deep lacerations result in profuse bleeding,

and a scar often results from the jagged tearing of the tissues.

Emergency Care for Incisions and Lacerations

Minor Incisions and Lacerations

1. Assess the length, depth, and location of the wound.
2. Control bleeding by covering the wound with a dressing and applying firm pressure.
3. Clean the wound with soap and water to remove dirt and other debris (Fig. 21–11).
4. Cover the wound with a dry, sterile dressing. Instruct the patient to check the wound for redness, swelling, discharge, or increase in pain and to contact a physician if any of these problems occur.

Serious Incisions and Lacerations

1. Control bleeding by covering the wound with a large, thick gauze dressing and applying firm pressure. Do not clean or probe the wound as this may result in more bleeding.
2. Transport the individual to a physician or, if the wound is serious enough, activate the local EMS.

21

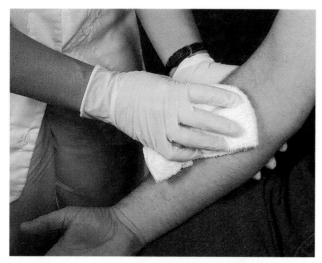

■ **FIGURE 21–11.** Minor incisions and lacerations should be cleaned with soap and water to remove dirt and other debris.

PUNCTURES

A puncture is a wound made by a sharp, pointed object piercing the skin layers and sometimes the underlying structures. Examples of objects causing a puncture wound include a nail, splinter, needle, wire, knife, bullet, or animal bite. A puncture wound has a very small external skin opening, and for this reason bleeding is usually minor. A tetanus booster may be administered, because the tetanus bacteria grow best in a warm, anaerobic environment, as would be found in a puncture wound.

Emergency Care for Puncture Wounds

1. Allow the wound to bleed freely for a few minutes to help wash out bacteria.
2. Clean the wound with soap and water.
3. Apply a dry, sterile dressing to prevent contamination.
4. Transport the individual to a physician so that medical care can be provided to prevent infection and to ensure that the patient's tetanus toxoid immunization is up to date.

ABRASIONS

An abrasion, or scrape, is a wound in which the outer layers of the skin are scraped or rubbed off. Blood and underlying structures may ooze from ruptured capillaries; however, the bleeding is not usually severe. Abrasions are caused by falls, resulting in floor burns and skinned knees and elbows. Dirt and other debris are frequently rubbed into the wound; therefore, it is important to clean scrapes thoroughly to prevent infection.

Emergency Care for Abrasions

1. Rinse the wound with cold running water.
2. Wash the wound gently with soap and water to remove dirt and other debris. Embedded debris should be removed by a physician.
3. Cover large abrasions with a dry, sterile dressing. Small minor abrasions do not require a dressing.
4. Instruct the patient to check the wound for signs of inflammation, including redness, swelling, discharge, or increase in pain and to contact a physician if they occur.

CLOSED WOUNDS

A closed wound involves an injury to the underlying tissues of the body without a break in the skin surface or mucous membrane; an example is a contusion or bruise.

A contusion results when the tissues under the skin are injured (Fig. 21–10) and is often caused by a sudden blow or force from a blunt object. Blood vessels rupture, allowing blood to seep into the tissues, resulting in a bluish discoloration of the skin and swelling. Most contusions heal without special treatment, but cold compresses may reduce bleeding and thus reduce swelling and discoloration and relieve pain. After several days, the color of the contusion turns greenish or yellow, owing to oxidation of blood pigments. Contusions commonly occur with injuries such as fractures, sprains, strains, and black eyes. These injuries, along with the corresponding emergency care, are discussed next.

MUSCULOSKELETAL INJURIES

☐ The musculoskeletal system is made up of all the bones, muscles, tendons, and ligaments of the body. Injuries that affect the musculoskeletal system include fractures, dislocations, sprains, and strains.

FRACTURE

A fracture is any break in a bone. The break may range in severity from a simple chip or a crack to a complete break or shattering of the bone. Fractures can occur anywhere on the surface of the bone, includ-

PUTTING IT ALL *into* PRACTICE

▶ **JUDY MARKINS:** *As a medical assistant you come in contact with a wide variety of people, cultures, personalities, and medical problems. You need to keep an open mind and not let your personal feelings and ideas interfere with the care that you give.*

One experience that has probably affected me more than any other was while I was working in obstetrics and gynecology. A full-term prenatal patient came in for a routine weekly appointment late one afternoon. By this stage of pregnancy, you have seen them often enough to develop a more personal relationship. I was obtaining her vital signs and asking the routine questions when she responded "I haven't felt the baby move for 2 days." This immediately sent up a red flag, but I was mindful to hide my concern until I was out of her room. The physician was unable to pick up any fetal heart tones, so she did an ultrasound right there. It showed that the fetus had died. The patient was alone and extremely upset. I stayed with her until her family came.

Although there was little medical treatment given during this time, I do believe that my medical assistant training and experience made a difference in knowing what to do and say to help comfort the patient through this crisis.

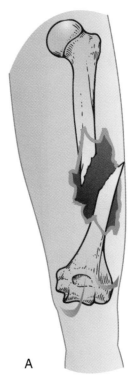 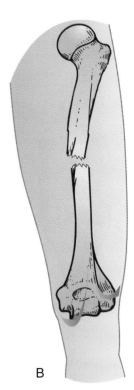

■ **FIGURE 21–12.** Fractures. *A,* Open fracture. *B,* Closed fracture. (From Connolly J. F.: *DePalma's The Management of Fractures and Dislocations: An Atlas.* Philadelphia, W. B. Saunders, 1981.)

21

break in a bone but no break in the skin's surface over the fracture site. An **open fracture** involves a break in the bone along with a penetration of the overlying skin surface. Open fractures are more serious due to the risk of blood loss and contamination leading to infection.

The signs and symptoms of a fracture include pain and tenderness, deformity, swelling and discoloration, loss of function of the body part, and numbness or tingling. The patient usually guards the injured part and may relay to you that he or she heard the bone break or snap or felt a grating sensation. This grating sensation, known as **crepitus,** is caused by the bone fragments rubbing against each other.

Fractures can also be classified according to the nature of the break: impacted, greenstick, transverse, oblique, comminuted, and spiral. Figure 21–13 illustrates and describes each of these types of fracture.

DISLOCATION

A dislocation is an injury in which one end of a bone making up a joint is separated or displaced from its normal position. A dislocation is caused by a violent pulling or pushing force that tears the ligaments. Dis-

ing across the surface of a joint such as the wrist or ankle. Fractures are caused by a direct blow, a fall, bone disease, or a twisting force as may occur in a sports injury. Although fractures often cause severe pain, they are seldom life-threatening.

The two basic types of fracture are closed fractures and open fractures (Fig. 21–12). A **closed fracture** is the most common type and occurs when there is a

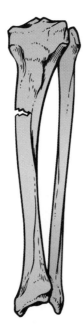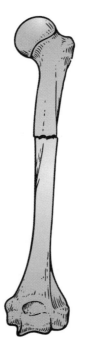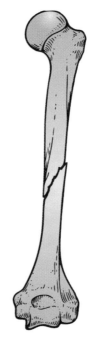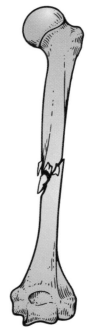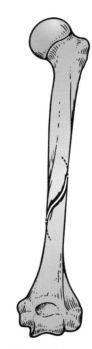

Impacted Fracture	**Greenstick Fracture**	**Transverse Fracture**	**Oblique Fracture**	**Comminuted Fracture**	**Spiral Fracture**
The broken ends of the bones are forcefully jammed together.	The bone remains intact on one side, but broken on the other, in much the same way a that a "green stick" bends; common in children, whose bones are more flexible than those of adults.	The break occurs perpendicular to the long axis of the bone.	The break occurs diagonally across the bone; generally the result of a twisting force.	The bone is splintered or shattered into three or more fragments; usually caused by an extremely traumatic direct force.	The bone is broken into a spiral or S-shape; caused by a twisting force.

■ **FIGURE 21–13.** Types of fractures. (Adapted from Copass, M., Soper, R., Eisenberg, M.: *EMT Manual,* 2nd ed. Philadelphia, W. B. Saunders, 1991.)

21

locations usually result from falls, sports injuries, and motor vehicle accidents. The signs and symptoms of a dislocation include significant deformity of the joint, pain and swelling, and loss of function.

SPRAIN

A sprain is a tearing of ligaments at a joint. Sprains may result from a fall, a sports injury, or a motor vehicle accident. The joints most commonly sprained are the ankle, knee, wrist, and fingers. The signs and symptoms of a sprain include pain, swelling, and discoloration. Sprains can vary in seriousness from mild to severe, depending on the amount of damage occurring to the ligaments.

STRAIN

A strain is a stretching and tearing of muscles or tendons. Strains are most likely to occur when an individ-

ual lifts a heavy object or overworks a muscle, as during exercise. The muscles most commonly strained are those of the neck, back, thigh, and calf. The signs and symptoms of a strain are pain and swelling. Strains do not usually cause the intense symptoms associated with fractures, dislocations, and sprains.

Emergency Care for a Fracture

It is often difficult to determine whether a patient has a fracture, dislocation, or sprain because the symptoms of these injuries are similar. Because of this, any serious musculoskeletal injury to an extremity should be treated as if it were a fracture.

The primary goal of emergency care for a fracture is to immobilize the body part to prevent motion. Immobilization reduces pain and prevents further damage. A **splint** is the term used for any item that will immobilize a body part. In an emergency situation, a length of wood, cardboard, or rolled newspapers or magazines are items that can be used for splinting. The splint should be padded with a soft material such as a rolled-up towel.

The body part should be splinted in the position in which you found it. However, severely angulated fractures may have to be straightened before splinting. If you attempt to straighten an angulated fracture, be careful not to force the affected part. A dislocated bone end can become "locked" and will have to be realigned at the hospital. If you straighten an angulated bone and encounter pain, stop and splint it in the position in which you found it. The splint should also immobilize the area above and below the injury. For example, when splinting an injury to the wrist, the hand and forearm also should be immobilized (Fig. 21–14A). When splinting an injury to the shaft of the bone, the joints both above and below the injury should be immobilized. For example, when splinting the forearm, both the elbow joint and the wrist joint should be immobilized.

The splint should be held in place with a roller gauze bandage or other suitable material such as neck-ties, scarves, or strips of cloth (Fig. 21–14A). The splint should be applied snugly but not so tightly that it interferes with proper circulation. After applying the splint, check the pulse below the splint to make sure the splint has not been applied too tightly. If you cannot detect a pulse, immediately loosen the splint until you can feel the pulse (Fig. 21–14B).

Whenever possible, elevate an injured extremity after it has been immobilized to reduce swelling (Fig. 21–14C). An ice pack may also be applied to the injured part. The cold limits the accumulation of fluid in the body tissues by constricting blood vessels and reducing leakage of fluid into the tissues. In addition, cold temporarily relieves pain because of its anesthetic or numbing effect, which reduces stimulation of nerve receptors.

Once you have properly immobilized the injury, transport the patient to an emergency care facility, or if the injury is serious enough, activate the local emergency medical services. In any situation in which an injury to the spine is suspected, activate the local EMS system.

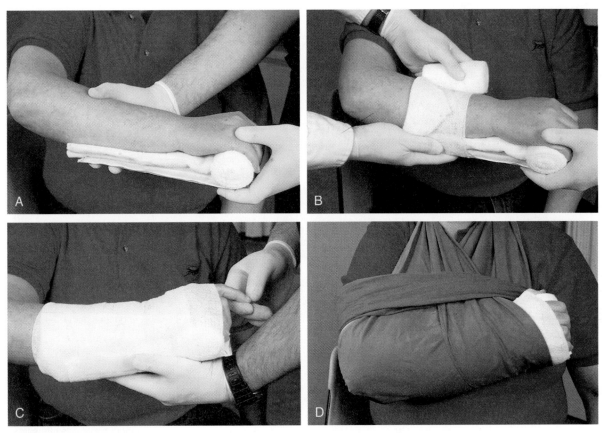

■ **FIGURE 21–14.** Emergency care of a fracture. *A,* The splint should immobilize the area above and below the injury. *B,* The splint is held in place with a gauze roller bandage. *C,* After the splint is applied, check the pulse below the splint to make sure the splint has not been applied too tightly. *D,* A sling can be used to elevate the extremity to reduce swelling. (From Henry, M., Stapleton, E.: *EMT Prehospital Care.* Philadelphia, W.B. Saunders, 1997.)

BURNS

□ A burn is an injury to the tissues caused by exposure to thermal, chemical, electrical, or radioactive agents. The severity of a burn depends on the depth of the burn, the percentage of the body involved, the type of agent causing the burn, the duration and intensity of the agent, and the part of the body.

Burns are classified according to the depth of tissue injury, as illustrated in Figure 21–15, and are described as follows:

SUPERFICIAL BURNS (FIRST-DEGREE BURN).
A superficial burn is the most common type of burn. It involves only the top layer of skin, the epidermis. With this type of burn, the skin appears red, is warm and dry to the touch, and is usually painful. Sunburn is a common example of a superficial burn. A superficial burn heals in 2 to 5 days of its own accord and does not cause scarring.

PARTIAL-THICKNESS BURNS (SECOND-DEGREE BURN).
A partial-thickness burn involves the epidermis and extends into the dermis but does not pass through the dermis to the underlying tissues. The burned area usually appears red, mottled, and blistered. In most cases, the blisters should not be broken as they provide a protective barrier against infection. Partial thickness burns are usually very painful, and the area often swells. This type of burn usually heals within 3 to 4 weeks and may result in some scarring.

FULL-THICKNESS BURNS (THIRD-DEGREE BURN).
A full-thickness burn completely destroys both the epidermis and the dermis and extends into the underlying tissues such as fat, muscle, bone, and nerves. The affected area appears charred black, brown, and cherry red, with the damaged tissues underneath often appearing pearly white. The patient may experience intense pain; however, if there has been substantial damage to the nerve endings, the patient may not feel any pain at all. Dur-

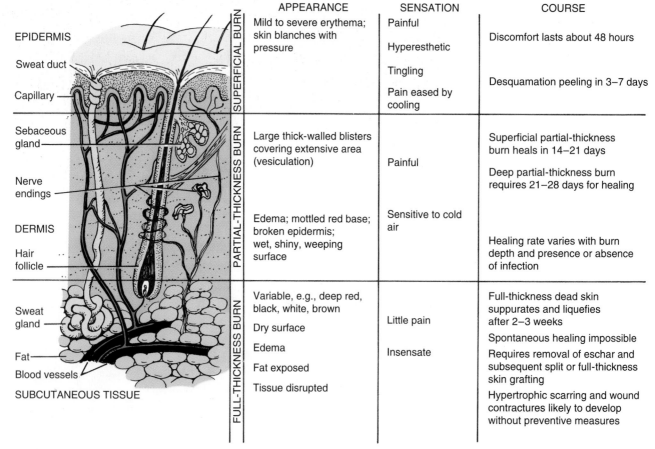

		APPEARANCE	SENSATION	COURSE
SUPERFICIAL BURN		Mild to severe erythema; skin blanches with pressure	Painful / Hyperesthetic / Tingling / Pain eased by cooling	Discomfort lasts about 48 hours / Desquamation peeling in 3–7 days
PARTIAL-THICKNESS BURN		Large thick-walled blisters covering extensive area (vesiculation)	Painful	Superficial partial-thickness burn heals in 14–21 days / Deep partial-thickness burn requires 21–28 days for healing
		Edema; mottled red base; broken epidermis; wet, shiny, weeping surface	Sensitive to cold air	Healing rate varies with burn depth and presence or absence of infection
FULL-THICKNESS BURN		Variable, e.g., deep red, black, white, brown / Dry surface / Edema / Fat exposed / Tissue disrupted	Little pain / Insensate	Full-thickness dead skin suppurates and liquefies after 2–3 weeks / Spontaneous healing impossible / Requires removal of eschar and subsequent split or full-thickness skin grafting / Hypertrophic scarring and wound contractures likely to develop without preventive measures

Skin labels (left side): EPIDERMIS, Sweat duct, Capillary, Sebaceous gland, Nerve endings, DERMIS, Hair follicle, Sweat gland, Fat, Blood vessels, SUBCUTANEOUS TISSUE

■ **FIGURE 21–15.** Types of burns. (From Polaski, A. L., Tatro, S. E.: *Luckmann's Core Principles and Practice of Medical-Surgical Nursing.* Philadelphia, W. B. Saunders, 1996.)

ing the healing process, dense scars typically result. Infection is a major concern, and the patient must be carefully monitored.

THERMAL BURNS

Thermal burns usually occur in the home, often as a result of fire, scalding water, or coming into contact with a hot object such as a stove or curling iron.

EMERGENCY CARE FOR MAJOR THERMAL BURNS

1. Stop the burning process to prevent further injury. If the individual is on fire, wrap him or her in a blanket, rug, or heavy coat and push him or her to the ground to help smother the flames. If a covering is not available, shout at the individual to drop to the ground and roll around to smother the flames.
2. Cool the burn, using large amounts of cool water from a faucet or garden hose. Do not use ice or ice water because this may result in further tissue damage; it also causes heat loss from the body. If the burn covers a large surface area (greater than 20 percent), do not use water. The loss of a large amount of skin surface places the patient at risk for hypothermia (generalized body cooling). With large surface area burns you may cool the most painful areas but not an area greater than 20 percent of the body (i.e., two arms, one leg, and so on).
3. Activate your local EMS.
4. Cover the patient with a clean, nonfuzzy material such as a tablecloth or sheet. The cover serves to maintain warmth, reduce pain, and reduce the risk of contamination. Do not apply any type of ointment, antiseptic, or other substance to the burned area.

EMERGENCY CARE FOR MINOR THERMAL BURNS

1. Immerse the affected area in cold water for 2 to 5 minutes. Be careful not to break any blisters because they provide a protective barrier against infection.
2. Cover the burn with a dry sterile dressing.

CHEMICAL BURNS

Chemical burns occur both in the workplace and at home. The severity of the burn depends on the type and strength of the chemical and the duration of exposure to the chemical. The main difference between a chemical burn and a thermal burn is that the chemical continues to burn the patient's tissues as long as it is on the skin. Because of this factor, it is important to remove the chemical from the skin as quickly as possible and then to activate the local emergency medical services.

Liquid chemical burns should be treated by flooding the area with large amounts of cool running water until emergency personnel arrive. If a solid substance such as lime has been spilled on the patient, it should be brushed off before flooding the area with water. This is because a dry chemical may be activated by contact with water.

SEIZURES

☐ A seizure is a sudden episode of involuntary muscular contractions and relaxation, often accompanied by a change in sensation, behavior, and level of consciousness. A seizure results when the normal electrical activity of the brain is disturbed, causing the brain cells to become irritated and overactive. Specific conditions that may trigger a seizure include epilepsy, encephalitis, a recent or old head injury, high fever in infants and young children, drug and alcohol abuse or withdrawal, eclampsia associated with toxemia of pregnancy, diabetic conditions, and heat stroke.

Seizures can be classified according to the location of the abnormal electrical activity in the brain as partial or generalized.

Partial seizures are the most common type of seizures, occurring in approximately 80 percent of individuals who have seizures. With a partial seizure, the abnormal electrical activity is localized into very specific areas of the brain; therefore, only the brain functions in those area are affected.

Partial seizures are further classified as simple or complex depending on whether the patient's level of conciousness is affected. The symptoms of a **simple partial seizure** include twitching or jerking in just one part of the body. This type of seizure lasts less than a minute, and the patient remains awake and alert during the seizure. With a **complex partial seizure,** the patient's level of consciousness is affected, and the patient has little or no memory of the seizure afterward.

The symptoms of this type of seizure include abnormal behavior such as confusion, a glassy stare, aimless wandering, lip smacking or chewing, or fidgeting with clothing, which lasts for a few seconds up to a minute or two. Both a simple and a complex partial seizure can progress to a generalized seizure.

With a **generalized seizure,** the abnormal electrical activity spreads throughout the entire brain. The best-known type of generalized seizure is a **tonic-clonic seizure** (formerly known as a grand mal seizure). With this type of seizure, the patient exhibits tonic-clonic activity followed by a postictal state. During the tonic phase, the patient suddenly loses consciousness and exhibits rigid muscular contractions, which result in odd posturing of the body. Respirations are inhibited, which may cause cyanosis around the mouth and lips. The patient may lose control of the bladder or bowels, resulting in involuntary urination and defecation. The tonic phase lasts for up to 30 seconds, followed by the clonic phase. During the clonic phase, the patient's body jerks about violently. The patient's jaw muscles contract, which may cause the patient to bite the tongue or lips. The final phase of the seizure is the postictal state, lasting between 10 and 30 minutes, in which the patient exhibits a depressed level of consciousness, is disoriented, and often has a headache. The patient generally has little or no memory of the seizure and feels confused and exhausted for several hours after the seizure is over.

In some instances of seizures, particularly in patients with epilepsy, an aura precedes the seizure. An **aura** is a sensation perceived by the patient that something is about to happen: examples include a strange taste, smell, or sound, a twitch, or a feeling of dizziness or anxiety. An aura provides the patient with a warning signal that a seizure is about to begin.

Although seizures are frightening to observe, they are usually not as bad as they look. Most patients fully recover within a few minutes after the seizure begins. An exception to this is **status epilepticus,** in which the seizures are prolonged or come in rapid succession without full recovery of consciousness between the seizures. Status epilepticus is a potentially life-threatening situation that requires immediate medical care.

Emergency Care for Seizures

The most important criterion in caring for a patient in a seizure is to protect the patient from harm. Remove hazards from the immediate area to prevent the patient from injury by striking a surrounding object. Do not restrain the patient. Loosen restrictive clothing that may interfere with breathing, such as collars, neckties, scarves, and jewelry. It is important to realize that the seizure will occur no matter what you do; therefore, restraining the patient could seriously injure the patient's muscles, bones, or joints. Do not insert anything into the patient's mouth during the seizure as this could damage the teeth or mouth or interfere with breathing. In addition, it could trigger the gag reflex, causing the patient to vomit and possibly aspirate the vomitus into the lungs. If the patient vomits, roll him or her onto one side so that the vomitus can drain from the mouth.

If you are uncertain as to the cause of the seizure or suspect that the patient is having status epilepticus, activate your local emergency medical services immediately. Otherwise, transport the patient to an emergency medical care facility for further evaluation and treatment once the seizure is over.

POISONING

☐ A **poison** is any substance that causes illness, injury, or death if it enters the body. Most poisoning episodes take place in the home, are accidental, and occur in children under the age of 5 years. Poisoning usually involves common substances such as cleaning agents, medications, and pesticides. For most poisonous substances, the reaction is more serious in children and the elderly than in adults.

Poison control centers are valuable resources that are easily accessible to medical personnel and the community. There are over 500 regional poison control centers across the United States: most are located in the emergency departments of large hospitals. These centers are staffed by personnel who have access to information about almost all poisonous substances. Most of the centers are staffed 24 hours a day, and calls are toll free.

A poison may enter the body in four ways: ingestion, inhalation, absorption, or injection. Each of these is described here along with the corresponding emergency care.

INGESTED POISONS

Poisons that are ingested enter the body by being swallowed. Ingestion is the most common route of entry for poisons. Examples of poisons that are often ingested include cleaning products, pesticides, contaminated food, petroleum products (e.g., gasoline, kerosene), and poisonous plants. The abuse of drugs or alcohol or both also can result in poisoning from an accidental or intentional overdose.

The signs and symptoms of poisoning by ingestion are based on the specific substance that has been consumed but often include strange odors, burns or stains around the mouth, nausea, vomiting, abdominal pain, diarrhea, difficulty in breathing, profuse perspiration, excessive salivation, dilated or constricted pupils, unconsciousness, and convulsions.

Emergency Care for Poisoning by Ingestion

1. Acquire as much information as possible about the type of poison, how much was taken, and when it was taken.
2. Call your regional poison control center or local emergency medical services. *Never* induce vomiting unless directed to do so by a medical authority. Vomiting is often contraindicated: for example, when an individual is unconscious, has swallowed a petroleum product, or has swallowed a corrosive poison such as a strong acid or base. Corrosive poi-

sons may cause more injury to the esophagus, throat, and mouth if they are vomited back up. If it is available, you may be directed by the poison control center to administer activated charcoal. Activated charcoal is used to absorb the poison that remains in the stomach and prevents absorption by the intestine.

3. If the individual vomits, collect some of the vomitus for transport with the patient to the hospital for analysis by a toxicologist, if necessary. In addition, bring along containers of any substances ingested, such as empty medication bottles and household cleaner containers because the label of the container often lists the ingredients in the product.

INHALED POISONS

A poison that is inhaled is breathed into the body by an individual in the form of gas, vapor, or spray. The most commonly inhaled poison is carbon monoxide, such as from car exhausts, malfunctioning furnaces, and fires. Other examples of inhaled poisons include carbon dioxide from wells and sewers and fumes from household products such as glues, paints, insect sprays, and cleaners (e.g., ammonia, chlorine).

The signs and symptoms of inhaled poisoning often include severe headache, nausea and vomiting, coughing or wheezing, shortness of breath, chest pain or tightness, facial burns, burning of the mouth, nose, eyes, throat or chest, cyanosis, confusion, dizziness, and unconsciousness.

Emergency Care for Inhaled Poisons

1. Determine whether it is safe to approach the patient. Toxic gases and fumes can also be dangerous to individuals helping the patient.
2. Remove the individual from the source of the poison and into fresh air as quickly as possible.
3. Call your regional poison control center or local emergency medical services.
4. If oxygen is available, you may be directed to administer it under the supervision of a physician. Oxygen is the primary antidote for carbon monoxide poisoning.

ABSORBED POISONS

A poison that is absorbed enters the body through the skin. Examples of absorbed poisons include fertilizers and pesticides used for lawn and garden care. The signs and symptoms of absorbed poisoning include irritation, burning and itching, burning of the skin or eyes, headache, and abnormal pulse or respiration or both.

Emergency Care for Absorbed Poisons

1. Remove the patient from the source of the poison. Be sure to avoid contact with the toxic substance.
2. Call your regional poison control center or local emergency medical services. In most cases, you will be instructed to flood the area that has been exposed to the poison with water. Dry chemicals should be brushed from the skin before flooding with water.

INJECTED POISONS

An injected poison enters the body through bites, through stings, or by a needle. Examples of injected poisons include the venom of insects, spiders, snakes, and marine creatures such as jellyfish; and the bite of rabid animals. The poison may also be a drug that is self-administered with a hypodermic needle, such as heroin.

The general signs and symptoms of injected poisoning include an altered state of awareness; evidence of stings, bites, or puncture marks on the skin; mottled skin; localized pain or itching; burning, swelling, or blistering at the site; difficulty in breathing; abnormal pulse rate; nausea and vomiting; and anaphylactic shock.

The emergency care for specific types of injected poisons is described in more detail in the following paragraphs.

INSECT STINGS

It is estimated that 1 of every 125 Americans is allergic to insect stings. Approximately 40 people in the United States die each year from a severe allergic reaction to insect stings. The incidence of deaths is low because most people know they need to obtain medical attention immediately if an allergic reaction begins to occur.

Almost all the insects whose venom can cause allergic reactions belong to a group call *Hymenoptera*, which includes honeybees and bumblebees, wasps, yellow jackets, and hornets. When a honeybee stings, its stinger remains imbedded in the skin of the victim, causing the bee to die as it tries to tear itself away. Wasps, yellow jackets, and hornets are more aggressive than bees and can sting repeatedly. Hornets are the most aggressive of the group and may sting even when not provoked. Yellow jackets are close behind in aggressiveness, while wasps usually sting only if someone interferes with them near their nest.

21

If an insect sting does not cause an allergic reaction within 30 minutes, chances are excellent that no problem will occur. A normal reaction to an insect sting includes localized pain, redness, swelling, and itching lasting 1 to 2 days. Any generalized reaction not arising directly from the area of the sting is almost certain to be an allergic reaction, which begins with such symptoms as sneezing, hives, itching, angioedema, erythema, and disorientation and progresses to difficulty in breathing, dizziness, faintness, and loss of consciousness.

Medical care should be sought immediately, because these are the symptoms of an anaphylactic reaction, and most fatalities occur within the first 2 hours after the sting. Because time is a factor, individuals known to have a severe allergy to insect stings are provided with an anaphylactic emergency treatment kit containing injectable epinephrine and oral antihistamines (see Fig. 21–4). With this kit, treatment for a severe allergic reaction can be started immediately.

Emergency Care for Insect Stings

1. Remove the stinger and attached venom sac. Scrape the stinger off the patient's skin with your fingernail or a plastic card such as a credit card (Fig. 21–16). Do not use tweezers or forceps as squeezing the venom sac may cause more venom to be injected into the patient's tissues.

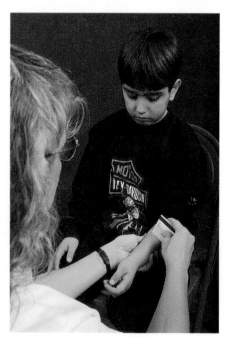

■ **FIGURE 21–16.** Removing a honeybee stinger and venom sac using the edge of a credit card.

2. Wash the site with soap and water.
3. Apply a cold pack on the affected area to reduce pain and swelling.
4. Observe the patient for the signs of an anaphylactic reaction.

SPIDER BITES

Although spiders are numerous throughout the United States, most do not cause injuries or serious complications. Only two spiders have bites that cause serious or even life-threatening reactions: the black widow spider and the brown recluse spider. Both these spiders prefer dark, out-of-the way places such as woodpiles, brush piles, under rocks, and in dark garages and attics. Because of this, bites usually occur on the hands and arms of individuals reaching into places where the spiders are hiding. Often the individual does not know that she or he has been bitten until she or he begins to feel ill or notices swelling and a bite mark on the skin.

The black widow spider is approximately 1 inch long and is black with a distinctive bright red hourglass shape on its abdomen. The venom injected when this spider bites an individual is toxic to the central nervous system. The signs and symptoms of a black widow bite include swelling and a dull pain at the injection site; nausea and vomiting; a rigid, boardlike abdomen; fever; rash; and difficulty in breathing or swallowing. Although the symptoms are severe, they are not usually fatal. An antivenin is available; however, because of its undesirable and frequent side effects, it is generally only administered to individuals with severe bites and to individuals who may have a heightened reaction, such as elderly people and children under the age of 5 years.

The brown recluse spider is light brown with a dark brown violin-shaped mark on its back. The bite of a brown recluse causes severe local effects including tenderness, redness, and swelling at the injection site. On the other hand, systemic effects, such as difficulty in breathing or swallowing, seldom occur.

Emergency Care for Spider Bites

1. Wash the wound.
2. Apply a cold pack to the affected area to reduce pain and swelling.
3. Obtain medical help immediately if you suspect the individual has been bitten by a black widow spider or a brown recluse spider or if a severe reaction begins to occur.

SNAKEBITES

Snakebites kill very few people in the United States. Each year, approximately 45,000 persons are bitten by a snake; however only 7,000 of these bites involve a poisonous snake, and fewer than 15 of the individuals die.

The species of snakes that are poisonous in the United States include rattlesnakes, copperheads, cottonmouths (water moccasins), and coral snakes. However, other poisonous species may be privately owned by individuals, zoos, or labs. Rattlesnakes account for most snakebites and nearly all fatalities from snakebites. Most snakebites occur near the home, as opposed to in the wild. Because it is often difficult to identify a snake, any unidentified snake should be considered to be poisonous.

The general signs and symptoms of a bite from a poisonous snake include puncture marks on the skin, pain and swelling at the puncture site, rapid pulse, nausea, vomiting, unconsciousness, and convulsions.

Emergency Care for Snakebites

1. Wash the bite area gently with soap and water.
2. Immobilize the injured part and position it below the level of the heart.
3. Call emergency personnel. Do not apply ice to a snakebite. Do not apply a tourniquet or cut or suction the wound.
4. If the snake is dead, inform emergency personnel of its location so that it can be transported to the hospital for identification.

ANIMAL BITES

Bites and other injuries from animals may range in severity from minor to serious and may even prove to be fatal. Most people who are bitten by animals do not report the bite to a physician. Because of this factor, the incidence of animal bites in the United States each year is not known but has been estimated at approximately 1 to 2 million for dog bites and 400,000 for cat bites.

The most serious type of bite is one from an animal with rabies. Rabies is a viral infection transmitted through the saliva of an infected animal. If the condition is not treated, rabies is generally fatal.

Certain animals tend to have a higher incidence of rabies than others. These include skunks, bats, raccoons, cats, dogs, cattle, and foxes. On the other hand, hamsters, gerbils, guinea pigs, chipmunks, rats, mice, gophers, and rabbits are rarely infected with the rabies virus.

An individual who has been bitten by an animal that has rabies or is suspected of having rabies must obtain medical care. To prevent rabies, a rabies vaccine is administered to the individual, which produces antibodies to fight the rabies virus.

Emergency Care for Animal Bites

FOR MINOR ANIMAL BITES. Wash the wound with soap and water. Apply an antibiotic ointment and a dry sterile dressing. Transport the individual to a physician so that medical care can be provided to prevent infection and to ensure that the patient's tetanus toxoid immunization is up to date.

FOR SERIOUS ANIMAL BITES. If the wound is bleeding heavily, first control the bleeding with direct pressure. Do not clean the wound because this may result in more bleeding. Transport the patient to a physician, or if the bite is serious enough, call the local emergency medical service.

FOR ALL ANIMAL BITES. If you suspect that the animal has rabies, relay this information to the appropriate authorities, such as medical personnel, the police, or animal control personnel. If possible, try to remember what the animal looked like and the area in which you last saw it.

HEAT AND COLD EXPOSURE

☐ Exposure to excessive environmental heat or cold can result in injury to the body ranging in severity from minor to life-threatening.

Heat-related injuries are most apt to occur on very hot days that are accompanied by high humidity with little or no air movement. The three conditions caused by overexposure to heat are heat cramps, heat exhaustion, and heat stroke.

The two major types of cold-related injuries are frostbite and hypothermia. Although cold-related injuries are most apt to occur in the winter months, they may also occur at other times of the year, such as when an individual is exposed to cold water in a near-drowning incident.

Certain individuals are at higher risk for developing heat- and cold-related injuries:

- Elderly people
- Young children, particularly infants
- Individuals who work or exercise outdoors
- Individuals with medical conditions that cause poor blood circulation, such as diabetes mellitus and cardiovascular disease

■ Individuals who have had heat- or cold-related injuries in the past
■ Individuals under the influence of drugs or alcohol

HEAT CRAMPS

Heat cramps are the least serious of the three types of heat-related injuries. Heat cramps are most apt to occur when an individual is exercising or working in a hot environment and fails to replace lost fluids and electrolytes. Lost electrolytes can be replaced with a commercial sports drink (e.g., Gatorade).

The signs and symptoms of heat cramps include painful muscle spasms, particularly of the legs, calves, and abdomen; hot, sweaty skin; weakness; and a rapid pulse. These symptoms serve as a warning signal that an individual is having a problem with the heat. If the problem is ignored, heat cramps may progress to a more serious condition, such as heat exhaustion or heat stroke.

Treatment of heat cramps consists of removal of the patient to a cool environment, rest, and replacement of fluids and electrolytes. If the patient's conditon does not improve, she or he should be transported to an emergency care facility for further treatment.

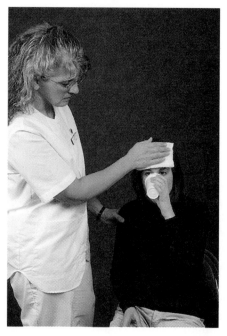

■ **FIGURE 21–17.** Treatment of heat exhaustion consists of removing the patient to a cool environment, giving fluid and electrolyte replacement, and applying a cold compress to the forehead; the patient should then rest.

HEAT EXHAUSTION

21

Heat exhaustion is the most common heat-related injury. It occurs most often in individuals involved in vigorous physical activity on a hot and humid day, such as athletes and construction workers. It may also occur in people who are wearing too much clothing on a hot and humid day.

The signs and symptoms of heat exhaustion are very similar to those of influenza: cold and clammy skin that is pale or gray, profuse sweating, headache, nausea, dizziness, weakness, and diarrhea.

Treatment of heat exhaustion consists of removal of the patient to a cool environment, fluid and electrolyte replacement, application of a cold compress to the forehead, and rest (Fig. 21–17). Tight clothing should be loosened and excessive layers or clothing should be removed. In most cases, these measures will improve the patient's condition in approximately 30 minutes. If the patient's condition does not improve, however, he or she should be transported to an emergency care facility.

to occur in elderly people during a heat wave and in athletes who overexert in a hot and humid environment. Heat stroke can occur in a very short period of time, as when a child has been left to wait in a closed car on a hot day.

During heat stroke, the body becomes so overheated that the heat-regulating mechanism breaks down and is unable to cool the body effectively. The body temperature rises to a dangerous level, causing the destruction of tissues. The signs and symptoms of heat stroke include a body temperature of 105°F (40°C) or higher; red, hot dry skin; a rapid weak pulse; dizziness and weakness; rapid, shallow breathing; decreased levels of consciousness; and seizures.

Heat stroke is a life-threatening emergency and requires immediate transport of the patient to an emergency care facility by the fastest way possible. If not treated, heat stroke is always fatal. During transport, every attempt possible should be made to lower the body temperature, such as setting the air conditioner to its maximum capacity, covering the victim with cool, wet sheets, or fanning the victim.

HEAT STROKE

Heat stroke is the least common, but most serious, of the three heat-related injuries. Heat stroke is most apt

FROSTBITE

Frostbite is the localized freezing of body tissue due to exposure to cold. The severity of the frostbite depends on the environmental temperature, the duration of exposure, and the wind-chill factor. Frostbite most commonly affects the hands, fingers, feet, toes, ears, nose, and cheeks. Although frostbite is not life-threatening, it can cause severe tissue damage that may require amputation of the affected body part. The signs and symptoms of frostbite include loss of feeling in the affected area, cold and waxy skin, and white, yellow, or blue discoloration of the skin.

Treatment of frostbite requires rewarming of the affected body part to prevent permanent damage. This is best accomplished in an emergency care facility since improper rewarming can result in further tissue damage. To transport the patient, loosely wrap warm clothing or blankets around the affected body part. The frozen area can also be placed in contact with another body part that is warm. It is very important to handle the affected area gently. Do not rub or massage the affected area, as this can result in further damage to the frozen tissue.

HYPOTHERMIA

Hypothermia is a serious life-threatening emergency in which the temperature of the entire body falls to a dangerously low level. Hypothermia may occur rapidly, such as when an individual falls through the ice on a frozen lake. It may also occur slowly when an individual is exposed to a cold environment for a prolonged period of time, such as a hiker lost in the woods.

When the core body temperature falls too low, the body loses its ability to regulate its temperature and to generate body heat. The signs and symptoms of hypothermia include shivering, numbness, drowsiness, apathy, a glassy stare, and decreased levels of consciousness.

Treatment of hypothermia should focus on preventing further heat loss. Remove the patient from the cold, or if this is not possible, wrap him or her in blankets. Do not attempt to rewarm the patient such as through immersion in warm water. Rapid rewarming can result in serious respiratory and cardiac problems. The patient should be transported immediately to an emergency care facility.

DIABETIC EMERGENCIES

☐ Glucose is the end-product of carbohydrate metabolism. Its function is to serve as the chief source of energy to carry out normal body functions and to assist in maintaining body temperature. The body maintains a constant blood glucose level to ensure a continuous source of energy for the body. Glucose taken in that is not needed for energy can be stored in the form of glycogen in muscle and liver tissue for later use. When no more tissue storage is possible, excess glucose is converted to fat and stored as adipose tissue.

Insulin is a hormone secreted by the beta cells of the pancreas and is required for normal utilization of glucose in the body. Insulin enables glucose to enter the body's cells and be converted to energy. Insulin is also needed for the proper storage of glycogen in liver and muscle cells.

Diabetes mellitus is a disease in which the body is unable to use glucose for energy due to a lack of insulin in the body. There are two types of diabetes: a severe form, usually appearing in childhood, known as Type I diabetes, and a mild form, appearing in adulthood, known as Type II diabetes. Most individuals with diabetes (90 percent) have Type II diabetes. There is no cure for diabetes mellitus, but significant advances have been made in controlling the disease through a combination of drug therapy, diet therapy, and activity. The goal for the diabetic patient is to balance food intake and level of activity with the body's insulin.

Two types of emergencies can be experienced by a diabetic patient: hypoglycemia, commonly referred to as insulin shock, and diabetic ketoacidosis, commonly known as diabetic coma.

Insulin shock (hypoglycemia) occurs when there is too much insulin in the body and not enough glucose. Insulin shock can be caused by administration of too much insulin, skipping meals, and unexpected or unusual exercise. The symptoms of insulin shock include normal or rapid respirations; pale, cold, and clammy skin; sweating; dizziness and headache; full rapid pulse; normal or high blood pressure; extreme hunger; aggressive or unusual behavior; fainting; and seizure or coma. The onset of insulin shock occurs rapidly, usually over a period of 5 to 20 minutes, after the blood glucose level begins to fall. Because the brain requires a constant supply of glucose for proper functioning, permanent brain damage or even death can result from severe hypoglycemia.

Diabetic coma (diabetic ketoacidosis) occurs when there is not enough insulin in the body. This causes the blood glucose level to rise in the body, resulting in hyperglycemia. When glucose cannot be used for energy, fat is broken down. This results in a build-up of acid waste products in the blood, known as **ketoacidosis.** The combined effect of the hyperglycemia and ketoacidosis causes the following symptoms: polyuria, excessive thirst and hunger, vomiting, abdominal pain, dry, warm skin, rapid and deep sighing respirations, a sweet or fruity (acetone) odor to the breath, and a rapid, weak pulse.

If the condition is not treated, diabetic coma can

21

progress to dehydration, hypotension, coma, and death. Unlike insulin shock, however, the onset of diabetic coma is gradual, usually developing over a period of 12 to 48 hours. Diabetic coma may be caused by illness and infection, overeating, forgetting to administer an insulin injection, or administering an insufficient amount of insulin.

Most individuals with diabetes have a thorough knowledge of their disease and manage it effectively. Because of this, diabetic emergencies are most apt to occur when there is an unusual upset in the insulin/glucose balance in the body, such as might be caused by illness or infection. An emergency situation may also arise in an individual who has diabetes but in whom the condition has not yet been diagnosed.

It may be difficult to tell the difference between insulin shock and diabetic coma because the symptoms are similar. Often a patient suffering from either of these conditions may appear to be intoxicated. If he or she is conscious, the diabetic patient usually knows what the trouble is; therefore, you should listen carefully to the patient to determine what may have caused the problem (e.g., not eating, forgetting to administer an insulin injection). If the patient is unconscious, and

therefore unable to communicate, you should observe the patient's respirations. A patient in insulin shock has normal or rapid respirations, whereas a patient in diabetic coma has deep, labored respirations.

Most diabetic patients carry an emergency medical identification to alert others to their condition when they cannot; examples include a medical alert bracelet or necklace, and a wallet card (Fig. 21–18).

EMERGENCY CARE IN DIABETES

Insulin Shock (Hypoglycemia)

A patient in insulin shock needs sugar immediately. For the conscious patient, glucose should be administered by mouth in the form of fruit juice (e.g., orange juice), nondiet soft drinks, candy, honey, or table sugar dissolved in water (Fig. 21–19). Improvement is usually fairly rapid after the glucose has been consumed. If the patient is unconscious, do not give anything by mouth because it may be aspirated into the lungs. Instead, provide the fastest possible transportation of the patient to an emergency care facility.

Diabetic Coma (Diabetic Ketoacidosis)

The patient in diabetic coma needs insulin and therefore must be transported as soon as possible to an emergency care facility.

21

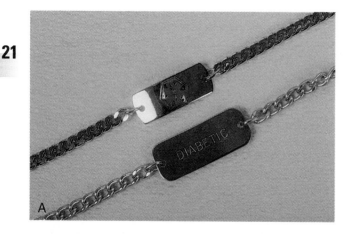

I HAVE TYPE I DIABETES

If I appear to be intoxicated or am unconscious, I may be having a reaction to diabetes or its treatment.

EMERGENCY TREATMENT

If I am able to swallow, please give me a beverage that contains sugar, such as orange juice, cola or even sugar in water. Then please send me to the nearest hospital **IMMEDIATELY.**

B

■ **FIGURE 21–18.** Diabetic medical identification. *A,* Diabetic medical alert bracelet. *B,* Diabetic wallet card.

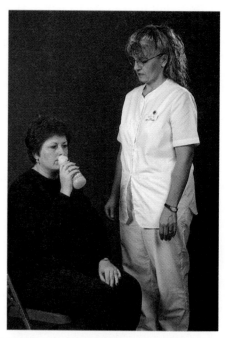

■ **FIGURE 21–19.** Orange juice is administered to a diabetic patient with the signs and symptoms of insulin shock.

Doubtful Situations

If you ever have doubt as to whether a patient is developing insulin shock or diabetic coma, give sugar, even though the final diagnosis actually may be diabetic coma. This is because insulin shock develops much more rapidly than diabetic coma and can quickly cause permanent brain damage or death. If you give sugar to a patient in diabetic coma, there is very little risk of making the condition worse because a patient can withstand a high blood glucose level longer than he or she can tolerate a low blood glucose level.

MEDICAL PRACTICE AND THE LAW

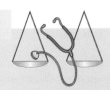

Emergency medicine is one of the most litigious (lawsuit-prone) areas of health care. Owing to the nature of emergencies, there is little time to plan your actions, and one misstep could cause damage. Keep in mind that your actions will be compared in court to those of a "reasonably prudent medical assistant with similar education and experience." Do not perform procedures you are not comfortable performing.

Whenever possible, obtain written consent for all procedures. In a life or death situation, this may not be possible. In this case, you are held accountable to try to save the life of the patient, even without consent.

Many times, patients or families become hysterical during emergencies. As a health care professional, you are expected to keep a cool head and calm the patient and family while attending to the emergency situation.

If you are out of the office and encounter an emergency situation, many states have a "Good Samaritan" law that protects you from legal action if you perform only procedures with which you are familiar, such as emergency first aid or CPR.

CERTIFICATION REVIEW

☐ First aid is the immediate care that is administered to an individual who is injured or suddenly becomes ill before complete medical care can be obtained. The emergency medical services (EMS) system is a network of community resources, equipment, and medical personnel that provides emergency care to victims of injury or sudden illness.

☐ A primary assessment is an initial assessment to detect life-threatening conditions of an individual in an emergency situation. A patient who is not breathing is said to be in respiratory arrest. The airway can be opened using the head tilt–chin lift maneuver or the jaw-thrust maneuver. The process of breathing for a patient is called rescue breathing.

☐ Cardiopulmonary resuscitation (CPR) involves a combination of rescue breathing to transfer oxygen into the patient's lungs and chest compressions to circulate blood containing oxygen to the brain.

☐ An airway obstruction interferes with the movement of air through the upper or lower airway. A complete airway obstruction means that the patient is unable to speak, breathe, or cough and requires immediate care in order to survive. A partial airway obstruction allows for some air exchange, and the patient's ability to breathe will depend on how much air can get past the obstruction. The Heimlich maneuver is recommended for relieving a complete airway obstruction or a partial airway obstruction in which there is very little air exchange.

☐ Respiratory distress indicates that the patient is breathing but is having great difficulty in doing so. Asthma is a condition characterized by wheezing, coughing, and dyspnea. Emphysema is a progressive lung disorder in which the terminal bronchioles that lead into the alveoli become plugged with mucus. Hyperventilation is a manner of breathing in which the respirations become rapid and deep, causing an individual to exhale too much carbon dioxide.

☐ Cardiac arrest means that the heart has stopped beating or beats too irregularly to circulate the blood effectively through the body. Conditions that can result in cardiac arrest include a heart attack, stroke, airway obstruction, near-drowning, drug overdose, trauma, and suffocation. Defibrillation is the application of an electric current to the pa-

Continued

□ tient's heart, which can shock the heart out of ventricular fibrillation and allow it to resume beating normally.

□ A heart attack, also known as a myocardial infarction (MI), is caused by partial or complete obstruction of one or both of the coronary arteries or their branches. The principal symptom of a heart attack is chest pain or discomfort. The pain is usually felt behind the sternum and may radiate to the neck, throat, jaw, both shoulders, and arms.

□ A stroke results when an artery to the brain is blocked or ruptures causing an interruption of the blood flow to the brain. The signs and symptoms of a stroke include sudden weakness or numbness of the face, arm, or leg on one side of the body; difficulty in speaking; dimmed vision or loss of vision in one eye; double vision; dizziness; confusion; severe headache; and loss of consciousness.

□ Shock is defined as the failure of the cardiovascular system to deliver enough blood to all the vital organs of the body. Shock accompanies many types of emergency situations: hemorrhaging, a myocardial infarction, a severe allergic reaction. There are five major types of shock: hypovolemic, cardiogenic, neurogenic, anaphylactic, and psychogenic. The general signs and symptoms of shock include weakness, restlessness, anxiety, disorientation, pallor, cold, clammy skin, rapid breathing, and rapid pulse.

□ Hypovolemic shock is caused by a loss of blood or other body fluids. Cardiogenic shock is caused by the failure of the heart to pump blood adequately to all the vital organs of the body. Neurogenic shock occurs when the nervous system is unable to control the diameter of the blood vessels. Anaphylactic shock is a very serious and life-threatening reaction of the body to an allergen. Psychogenic shock is caused by an unpleasant experience or emotional stimuli, such as pain, fright, or the sight of blood.

□ Bleeding or hemorrhaging is the escape of blood from a severed blood vessel. External bleeding is bleeding that can be seen coming from a wound. The most effective way to control bleeding is through the application of direct pressure to the bleeding site. If bleeding cannot be controlled with direct pressure, a pressure point can be used. A pressure point is a site on the body where an artery lies close to the surface of the skin and can be compressed against an underlying bone. Internal bleeding is bleeding that flows into a body cavity, an organ, or between tissues.

□ A wound is a break in the continuity of an external or internal surface caused by physical means. An open wound is a break in the skin surface or mucous membrane that exposes the underlying tissues; examples include incisions, lacerations, punctures, and abrasions.

□ An incision is a clean, smooth cut caused by a sharp cutting instrument such as a knife, a razor, or a piece of glass. A laceration is a wound in which the tissues are torn apart, rather than cut, leaving ragged and irregular edges. A puncture is a wound made by a sharp, pointed object piercing the skin layers and sometimes the underlying structures. An abrasion is a wound in which the outer layers of the skin are scraped or rubbed off.

□ A closed wound involves an injury to the underlying tissues of the body without a break in the skin surface or mucous membrane; an example is a contusion or bruise.

□ A fracture is any break in a bone. A closed fracture occurs when there is a break in a bone but no break in the skin's surface over the fracture site. An open fracture involves a break in the bone along with a penetration of the overlying skin surface. The signs and symptoms of a fracture include pain and tenderness, deformity, swelling and discoloration, loss of function of the body part, and numbness or tingling.

□ A dislocation is an injury in which one end of a bone making up a joint is separated or displaced from its normal position. A sprain is a tearing of ligaments at a joint. A strain is a stretching and tearing of muscles or tendons. A splint is any item that will immobilize a body part.

□ A burn is an injury to the tissues caused by exposure to thermal, chemical, electrical, or radioactive agents. A superficial burn (first-degree burn) involves only the epidermis; an example is sunburn. A partial-thickness burn (second-degree burn) involves the epidermis and extends into the dermis. A full-thickness burn (third-degree burn) completely destroys both the epidermis and the dermis and extends into the underlying tissues such as fat, muscle, bone, and nerves.

□ A seizure is a sudden episode of involuntary muscle contractions and relaxation often accompanied by a change in sensation, behavior, and level of consciousness. Seizures are classified as partial and generalized. In a partial seizure, the abnormal electrical activity is localized into very specific areas of the brain; therefore, only the brain functions in those areas are affected. With a generalized

21

CERTIFICATION REVIEW *Continued*

seizure, the abnormal electrical activity spreads throughout the entire brain.

☐ A poison is any substance that causes illness, injury, or death if it enters the body. Poisons that are ingested enter the body by being swallowed. A poison that is inhaled is breathed into the body by an individual in the form of gas, vapor, or spray. A poison that is absorbed enters the body through the skin. An injected poison enters the body through bites, through stings, or by a needle.

☐ Heat cramps are most apt to occur when an individual is exercising or working in a hot environment and fails to replace lost fluids and electrolytes. The symptoms include painful muscle spasms, particularly of the legs, calves, and abdomen; hot, sweaty skin; weakness; and a rapid pulse.

☐ Heat exhaustion occurs most often in individuals involved in vigorous physical activity on a hot and humid day. The symptoms of heat exhaustion include cold and clammy skin, profuse sweating, headache, nausea, dizziness, weakness, and diarrhea.

☐ Heat stroke is the most serious heat-related injury and is most apt to occur in elderly people during a heat wave and in athletes who overexert in a hot and humid environment. The symptoms of heat stroke include a body temperature of 105°F or higher; red, hot, dry skin; a rapid, weak pulse; dizziness and weakness; rapid, shallow breathing; decreased levels of consciousness; and seizures.

☐ Frostbite is the localized freezing of body tissue due to exposure to cold. Frostbite commonly affects the hands, fingers, feet, toes, ears, nose, and cheeks. Hypothermia is a serious life-threatening emergency in which the temperature of the entire body falls to a dangerously low level.

☐ Diabetes mellitus is a disease in which the body is unable to use glucose for energy due to a lack of insulin in the body. Insulin shock (hypoglycemia) occurs when there is too much insulin in the body and not enough glucose. Diabetic coma occurs when there is not enough insulin in the body. This causes the blood glucose level to rise in the body, resulting in hyperglycemia.

21

RESOURCES

ON THE WEB

For information on emergency medicine:

American Red Cross
www.crossnet.org

Federal Emergency Management Agency
www.fema.gov

Global Emergency Medical Services
www.globalmed.com

Medical Abbreviations

a̅a̅	of each
AAL	anterior axillary line
AAMA	American Association of Medical Assistants
Ab	abortion
abd	abdomen
ABE	acute bacterial endocarditis
ABG	arterial blood gases
ABO	blood groups
abs	absent
ac	acute
	before meals
ACTH	adrenocorticotropic hormone
AD	right ear
ADH	antidiuretic hormone
ADL	activities of daily living
ad lib	as desired
adm	admission
Adr	adrenalin
AF	atrial fibrillation
A/G	albumin-to-globulin ratio
AGA	appropriate for gestational age
agg	agglutination
AGN	acute glomerular nephritis
AHA	American Heart Association
AHD	arteriosclerotic heart disease
	atherosclerotic heart disease
AI	aortic insufficiency
AIDS	acquired immunodeficiency syndrome
AJ	ankle jerk
alb	albumin
ALP	alkaline phosphatase
AM	before noon (ante meridiem)
AMA	against medical advice
	American Medical Association
AMI	acute myocardial infarction
amp	ampule
amt	amount
anes	anesthesia
	anesthetist
ant	anterior
AODM	adult-onset diabetes mellitus
AOM	acute otitis media
AP	apical pulse
A & P	anterior and posterior
	auscultation and palpation
	auscultation and percussion
APB	atrial premature beat
approx	approximately
aq	water
AR	apical-radial (pulse)
	at risk
ARC	American Red Cross
ARD	acute respiratory disease

ARF	acute renal failure
	acute respiratory failure
	acute rheumatic fever
AS	left ear
ASA	acetylsalicylic acid
ASAP	as soon as possible
ASCAD	arteriosclerotic coronary artery disease
ASCVD	arteriosclerotic cardiovascular disease
	atherosclerotic cardiovascular disease
ASHD	arteriosclerotic heart disease
ATR	Achilles tendon reflex
AU	in each ear
AVH	acute viral hepatitis
AVR	aortic valve replacement
A & W	alive and well
ax	axillary
BA	backache
	bronchial asthma
Ba	barium
Bab	Babinski (reflex)
BAC	blood alcohol concentration
BBB	bundle branch block
BBT	basal body temperature
BC	birth control
BCP	birth control pills
bd	twice a day
BE	bacterial endocarditis
	barium enema
BG	blood glucose
BHS	beta-hemolytic streptococcus
bid	twice a day
BIL	bilirubin
bil	bilateral
BJ	biceps jerk
B & J	bone and joint
BJM	bones, joints, and muscles
BK	below knee (amputation)
BM	basal metabolism
	bowel movement
BMR	basal metabolic rate
BNO	bladder neck obstruction
	bowels not open
BOM	bilateral otitis media
BP	blood pressure
	British Pharmacopoeia
BS	blood sugar
	bowel sounds
	breath sounds
BSL	blood sugar level
BSN	bowel sounds normal
BSR	blood sedimentation rate
BTL	bilateral tubal ligation
BUN	blood urea nitrogen

A

BW	below waist		**CS**	cerebrospinal
	birth weight			cesarean section
	body weight		**C & S**	culture and sensitivity
Bx	biopsy		**CSF**	cerebrospinal fluid
C	Celsius		**CT**	computed tomography
	centigrade		**CTS**	carpal tunnel syndrome
c̄	with		**cu cm**	cubic centimeter
C1	first cervical vertebra		**cu mm**	cubic millimeter
C2	second cervical vertebra		**CV**	cardiovascular
CA	cancer			cerebrovascular
	carcinoma		**CVA**	cerebrovascular accident
Ca	calcium		**CVP**	central venous pressure
	cancer		**CW**	chest wall
CAD	coronary artery disease		**Cx**	cervix
CAHD	coronary atherosclerotic heart disease		**CXR**	chest x-ray
caps	capsules		**cysto**	cystoscopic examination
CAT	computed axial tomography			cystoscopy
cath	catheter		**DB**	date of birth
CB	chronic bronchitis		**DBM**	diabetic management
CBC	complete blood count		**DBP**	diastolic blood pressure
CBD	common bile duct		**dc**	discontinue
CBR	complete bed rest		**D & C**	dilation and curettage
CC	chief complaint		**DD**	differential diagnosis
cc	cubic centimeter		**DDD**	degenerative disc disease
CCF	congestive cardiac failure		**DEA**	Drug Enforcement Agency
CCMSU	clean catch midstream urine		**dec**	decrease
CCU	coronary care unit		**def**	deficiency
C & D	cystoscopy and dilation		**deg**	degeneration
CDC	Centers for Disease Control and Prevention		**del**	delivery
cerv	cervical, cervix		**DI**	diabetes insipidus
CH	cholesterol		**diab**	diabetic
CHD	childhood disease		**diag**	diagnosis
	congenital heart disease		**diff**	differential white blood cell count
	congestive heart disease		**dil**	dilute
	coronary heart disease		**dis**	disabled
CHF	congestive heart failure			disease
CHO	carbohydrate		**disp**	dispense
chol	cholesterol		**DKA**	diabetic ketoacidosis
chr	chronic		**dl**	deciliter
ck	check		**DM**	diabetes mellitus
Cl	chloride, chlorine		**DNR**	do not resuscitate
CLD	chronic liver disease		**DOA**	dead on arrival
	chronic lung disease		**DOB**	date of birth
cldy	cloudy		**DOD**	date of death
cm	centimeter		**DOE**	dyspnea on exertion
cm³	cubic centimeter		**DOI**	date of injury
CMA	Certified Medical Assistant		**dos**	dosage
CNS	central nervous system		**DP**	diastolic pressure
c/o	complains of		**DPT**	diphtheria, pertussis, and tetanus
CO₂	carbon dioxide		**DR**	delivery room
COD	cause of death		**dr**	dram
COPD	chronic obstructive pulmonary disease		**DRG**	diagnostic-related group
CP	cerebral palsy		**DSD**	dry sterile dressing
	cleft palate		**dsg**	dressing
CPN	chronic pyelonephritis		**DT**	diphtheria and tetanus toxoid
CPR	cardiopulmonary resuscitation			delirium tremens
CRD	chronic renal disease		**DTR**	deep tendon reflex
	chronic respiratory disease		**D & V**	diarrhea and vomiting
CRF	chronic renal failure		**DVA**	distance visual acuity
crit	hematocrit		**DW**	distilled water

D/W	dextrose in water		gen	general
Dx	diagnosis		ger	geriatrics
ea	each		GI	gastrointestinal
EAM	external auditory meatus		glu	glucose
EBL	estimated blood loss		g	gram
EBV	Epstein-Barr virus		GP	general practitioner
ECF	extracellular fluid		gr	grain
	extended care facility		GTT	glucose tolerance test
ECG	electrocardiogram		gtt(s)	drop (drops)
Echo	echocardiogram		GU	genitourinary
	echoencephalogram		GYN	gynecology
E. coli	Escherichia coli		H	height
ECT	electroconvulsive therapy		h	hour
ED	emergency department		HA	headache
EDD	expected date of delivery		HBP	high blood pressure
EEG	electroencephalogram		HC	head circumference
EENT	eyes, ears, nose and throat		HCG	human chorionic gonadotropin
EFA	essential fatty acid		HCl	hydrochloric acid
eg	for example		Hct	hematocrit
EH	enlarged heart		HCVD	hypertensive cardiovascular disease
	essential hypertension		HDL	high density lipoprotein
elix	elixir		HEENT	head, eyes, ears, nose, and throat
EMG	electromyography		H & H	hemoglobin and hematocrit
ENT	ear, nose, and throat		HHD	hypertensive heart disease
eos	eosinophil		HIV	human immunodeficiency virus
ER	emergency room		H & L	heart and lungs
ESR	erythrocyte sedimentation rate		HMO	health maintenance organization
Ez	eczema		H/O	history of
F	Fahrenheit		H$_2$O	water
FA	fatty acid		H & P	history and physical
FB	finger breadth		hpf	high-power field
	foreign body		hs	at bedtime
FBP	femoral blood pressure		HT	hypertension
FBS	fasting blood sugar		ht	height
FD	fatal dose		HVD	hypertensive vascular disease
	forceps delivery		Hx	history
FDA	Food and Drug Administration		IBP	iron-binding protein
FFA	free fatty acids		IBS	irritable bowel syndrome
FFI	free from infection		IBW	ideal body weight
FFP	fresh frozen plasma		IC	irritable colon
FH	family history		ICCU	intensive coronary care unit
FHR	fetal heart rate		ICD	International Classification of Diseases (of the World Health Organization)
FHT	fetal heart tones			
flex	flexion		ICDA	International Classification of Diseases, Adapted
FMP	first menstrual period			
FOB	fetal occult blood		ICU	intensive care unit
FP	family practice		ID	intradermal
freq	frequent		I & D	incision and drainage
FSH	follicle-stimulating hormone		IM	Internal Medicine
ft	foot			intramuscular
FTT	failure to thrive		imp	impression
FWB	full weight bearing		inf	infant
fx	fracture		I & O	intake and output
G	gravida		IPPB	intermittent positive-pressure breathing
g	gram		IU	international unit
GA	gastric analysis		IUD	intrauterine device
	general anesthesia		IUFD	intrauterine fetal death
	gestational age		IUGR	intrauterine growth rate
GB	gallbladder		IV	intravenous
GC	gonorrhea		IVP	intravenous pyelogram

A

IVSD	interventricular septal defect
JAMA	*Journal of the American Medical Association*
jaund	jaundice
JODM	juvenile onset diabetes mellitus
JRA	juvenile rheumatoid arthritis
JV	jugular vein
K	potassium
KA	ketoacidosis
KB	ketone bodies
KCl	potassium chloride
ket	ketones
kg	kilogram
kj	knee jerk
KLS	kidney, liver, and spleen
KOH	potassium hydroxide
KUB	kidneys, ureters, and bladder
L	liter
l	length
LA	left arm
	left atrium
lac	laceration
LAO	left anterior oblique
lap	laparotomy
lat	lateral
lax	laxative
lb	pound
LB	low back
LBBB	left bundle branch block
LBM	lean body mass
LBP	low back pain
LBW	low birth weight
L & D	labor and delivery
LDL	low-density lipoprotein
LE	lupus erythematosus
	lower extremity
LFT	liver function test
liq	liquid
LKS	liver, kidneys, and spleen
LL	left leg
LLE	left lower extremity
LLQ	left lower quadrant
LMP	last menstrual period
LOC	loss of consciousness
LOM	loss of motion
LP	lumbar puncture
lpf	low-power field
LRQ	lower right quadrant
LSD	low-salt diet
LSK	liver, spleen, and kidneys
lt or L	left
LUQ	left upper quadrant
LV	left ventricle
L & W	living and well
lymphs	lymphocytes
m	meter
	minim
MCH	mean corpuscular hemoglobin and red cell indices
MCHC	mean corpuscular hemoglobin concentration
MCL	midclavicular line

MCV	mean corpuscular volume
MD	muscular dystrophy
	doctor of medicine
MDR	minimum daily requirement
meds	medications
mEq/L	milliequivalents per liter
MG	myasthenia gravis
mg	milligram
MH	marital history
	medical history
	menstrual history
MHx	medical history
MI	myocardial infarction
	maturation index
ML	midline
ml	milliliter
MM	multiple myeloma
mm	millimeter
mm³	cubic millimeter
mmHg	millimeters of mercury
MMR	measles, mumps, and rubella
mod	moderate
MODM	mature-onset diabetes mellitus
mono	mononucleosis
MP	menstrual period
MR	metabolic rate
	mortality rate
MRI	magnetic resonance imaging
MS	mitral stenosis
	morphine sulfate
	multiple sclerosis
MSL	midsternal line
MSU	midstream urine specimen
MT	medical technologist
multip	multipara
MV	mitral valve
MVP	mitral valve prolapse
n	normal
NaCl	sodium chloride
NAD	no acute distress
	nothing abnormal detected
narc	narcotic
NAS	nasal
NB	newborn
NBW	normal birth weight
NC	no change
	noncontributory
N/C	no complaints
ND	natural death
	normal delivery
NED	no evidence of disease
neg	negative
NG	nasogastric
NGU	nongonococcal urethritis
NKA	no known allergies
NL	normal limits
NM	neuromuscular
NMP	normal menstrual period
noct	nocturnal
non rep	do not repeat

A

NPO	nothing by mouth
NR	nonreactive
	no refill
	normal range
NS	nonspecific
	normal saline
	not significant
	not sufficient
NSD	normal spontaneous delivery
NSR	normal sinus rhythm
NSU	nonspecific urethritis
N & T	nose and throat
N & V	nausea and vomiting
NVA	near visual acuity
NVD	nausea, vomiting, and diarrhea
NWB	non–weight-bearing
NYD	not yet diagnosed
O	oral
O₂	oxygen
OA	osteoarthritis
OB	obstetrics
OB-GYN	obstetrics-gynecology
obs	observed
OC	office call
	on call
	oral contraceptive
occ	occasionally
OD	right eye
	drug overdose
O & E	observation and examination
OGTT	oral glucose tolerance test
OH	occupational history
OHD	organic heart disease
OM	otitis media
OOB	out of bed
OP	outpatient
O & P	ova and parasites
OPV	oral poliovaccine
OR	operating room
ortho	orthopedics
OS	left eye
OT	occupational therapy
OTC	over the counter
OU	both eyes
OURQ	outer upper right quadrant
OV	office visit
P	pulse
	phosphorus
PA	posteroanterior
	physician's assistant
P & A	percussion and auscultation
PAC	premature atrial contraction
Pap	Papanicolaou (smear, test)
Para	number of pregnancies
Para I	primipara
PAT	paroxysmal atrial tachycardia
path	pathology
PBI	protein-bound iodine
PC	platelet count
pc	after meals

PCC	Poison Control Center
PCN	penicillin
PCV	packed cell volume
PD	Parkinson's disease
PDR	*Physician's Desk Reference*
PE	physical examination
peds	pediatrics
PEG	pneumoencephalography
per	by or through
peri	perineal
PERRLA	pupils equal, round, regular, react to light, and accommodation
PGH	pituitary growth hormone
PH	past history
	personal history
	public health
pH	hydrogen ion concentration
PI	present illness
	pulmonary infarction
PID	pelvic inflammatory disease
PKU	phenylketonuria
PM	after noon (post meridiem)
	post mortem (after death)
PMB	postmenopausal bleeding
PMN	polymorphonuclear neutrophils
PMP	past menstrual period
PMS	premenstrual syndrome
PMT	premenstrual tension
PNC	penicillin
PND	paroxysmal nocturnal dyspnea
PNS	parasympathetic nervous system
Pnx	pneumothorax
po	by mouth
POB	place of birth
POL	physician's office laboratory
POMR	problem-oriented medical record
pos	positive
poss	possible
postop	postoperative
PP	postprandial
PPB	positive pressure breathing
PPBS	postprandial blood sugar
PPD	purified protein derivative
PPH	postpartum hemorrhage
PPT	partial prothrombin time
PRC	packed red cells
preop	preoperative
prep	preparation
PRERLA	pupils round, equal, react to light and accommodation
primip	woman bearing first child
prn	as the occasion arises, as necessary
procto	proctoscopy
prog	prognosis
PROM	premature rupture of membranes
prox	proximal
PT	physical therapy
	prothrombin time
pt	patient
PTA	prior to admission

A

PTB	prior to birth	**SC**	subcutaneous
PTD	prior to discharge	**SCD**	sudden cardiac death
PUD	peptic ulcer disease		sudden coronary death
PVC	premature ventricular contraction	**SD**	spontaneous delivery
PVD	peripheral vascular disease		sudden death
PWB	partial weight-bearing	**S/D**	systolic to diastolic
q	each; every	**SDS**	sudden death syndrome
q AM	every morning	**sed rate**	sedimentation rate
qd	every day	**segs**	segmented neutrophils
qh	every hour	**seq**	sequela
q2(3,4)h	every 2 (3 or 4) hours	**SF**	scarlet fever
qid	four times a day		spinal fluid
qns	quantity not sufficient	**SFT**	skin-fold thickness
qod	every other day	**SG**	specific gravity
qs	of sufficient quantity	**SGA**	small for gestational age
qt	quart	**SH**	social history
R	respiration	**SIDS**	sudden infant death syndrome
r	right	**sig**	labeled
RA	right arm	**sigmoid**	sigmoidoscopy
RAF	rheumatoid arthritis factor	**sl**	slight
RAO	right anterior oblique	**SM**	simple mastectomy
RBC	red blood cell	**SOAP**	subjective data, objective data, assessment, and plan
RBC/hpf	red blood cells per high power field		
RBCM	red blood cell mass	**SOB**	shortness of breath
RBCV	red blood cell volume	**sol**	solution
RBF	renal blood flow	**solv**	solvent
RBS	random blood sugar	**SOM**	serous otitis media
RCM	right costal margin	**SOP**	standard operating procedure
RCV	red cell volume	**SOS**	if necessary
RDA	recommended daily allowance	**SP**	systolic pressure
REM	rapid eye movement	**SPA**	suprapubic aspiration
resp	respiration	**spec**	specimen
Rh	rhesus (factor)	**sp gr**	specific gravity
Rh−	rhesus negative	**spont ab**	spontaneous abortion
Rh+	rhesus positive	**SS**	signs and symptoms
RHD	rheumatic heart disease	**ss**	one-half
RHF	right heart failure	**Staph**	*Staphylococcus*
RI	respiratory illness	**stat**	immediately
RL	right leg	**STD**	sexually transmitted disease
RLE	right lower extremity	**std**	standard
RLQ	right lower quadrant	**Strep**	*Streptococcus*
RMA	Registered Medical Assistant	**subcut**	subcutaneous
RMSF	Rocky Mountain spotted fever	**sum**	to be taken
R/O	rule out	**sup**	superficial
ROM	rupture of membranes	**supp**	suppository
ROS	review of systems	**surg**	surgery
RP	radial pulse	**Sx**	signs
RQ	respiratory quotient		symptoms
rt	right	**sym**	symptoms
RUQ	right upper quadrant	**T**	temperature
RV	right ventricle	**T$_3$**	tri-iodothyronine
RVH	right ventricular hypertrophy	**T$_4$**	thyroxine
Rx	prescription	**tab**	tablet
S	subjective data (POMR)	**TB**	tuberculosis
s̄	without	**TBF**	total body fat
SA	sinoatrial	**TBLC**	term birth, living child
SBE	shortness of breath on exertion	**tbsp**	tablespoon
	subacute bacterial endocarditis	**TBW**	total body water
SBO	small bowel obstruction	**TC**	throat culture
SBP	systolic blood pressure		tissue culture

A

TC	total capacity	**URT**	upper respiratory tract
	total cholesterol	**URTI**	upper respiratory tract infection
th	thoracic	**US**	ultrasound
ther	therapy	**USP**	*United States Pharmacopoeia*
therap	therapeutic	**UT**	urinary tract
THR	total hip replacement	**UTI**	urinary tract infection
TIA	transient ischemic attack	**UV**	ultraviolet
tid	three times a day	**V**	vein
tinct	tincture	**vac**	vaccine
TLC	tender loving care	**vag**	vagina
TM	tympanic membrane		vaginal
TND	term normal delivery	**VC**	vena cava
TOP	termination of pregnancy	**VD**	venereal disease
TOPV	trivalent oral poliovirus vaccine	**VDRL**	Venereal Disease Research Laboratory
TP	total protein	**VE**	vaginal examination
TPM	temporary pacemaker	**VF**	ventricular fibrillation
TPN	total parenteral nutrition	**VH**	vaginal hysterectomy
TPR	temperature, pulse, and respiration		viral hepatitis
Tq	tourniquet	**VHD**	valvular heart disease
tr	trace	**vis**	vision
	tincture	**vit**	vitamin
Trig	triglycerides	**vit cap**	vital capacity
TSH	thyroid-stimulating hormone	**VP**	venipuncture
TSP	total serum protein		venous pressure
tsp	teaspoon	**VPC**	ventricular premature contraction
TUR	transurethral resection of the bladder	**VRI**	viral respiratory infection
tus	cough	**VS**	vital signs
TV	tidal volume	**VV**	varicose veins
	total volume	**WB**	weight bearing
	Trichomonas vaginitis		whole blood
Tx	treatment	**WBC**	white blood cell
T & X	type and crossmatch	**WC**	white cell
U	unit	**WDWN**	well developed, well nourished
UA	urinalysis	**WN**	well nourished
UC	ulcerative colitis	**WNF**	well-nourished female
U/C	urine culture	**WNL**	within normal limits
UCG	urinary chorionic gonadotropin	**WNM**	well-nourished male
UCHD	usual childhood diseases	**WO**	written order
UE	upper extremity	**w/o**	without
UGI	upper gastrointestinal	**WP**	weakly positive
ULQ	upper left quadrant	**WR**	weakly reactive
ung	ointment	**wt**	weight
UOQ	upper outer quadrant	**X**	magnification
UR	upper respiratory	**XM**	crossmatch
urg	urgent	**XR**	x-ray
URI	upper respiratory infection	**y**	years
urol	urology	**yd**	yard
URQ	upper right quadrant	**YOB**	year of birth

A

The Human Body
Highlights of Structure and Function

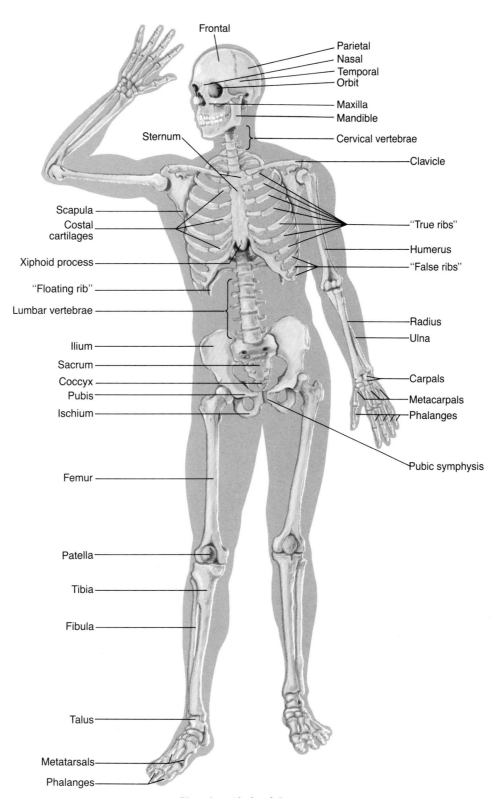

Frontal

Parietal
Nasal
Temporal
Orbit

Maxilla
Mandible

Cervical vertebrae

Sternum

Clavicle

Scapula
Costal cartilages

"True ribs"

Humerus

Xiphoid process

"False ribs"

"Floating rib"

Lumbar vertebrae

Radius
Ulna

Ilium

Sacrum

Coccyx

Carpals

Pubis

Metacarpals

Ischium

Phalanges

Pubic symphysis

Femur

Patella

Tibia

Fibula

Talus

Metatarsals

Phalanges

Plate 1 ■ **Skeletal System**

B

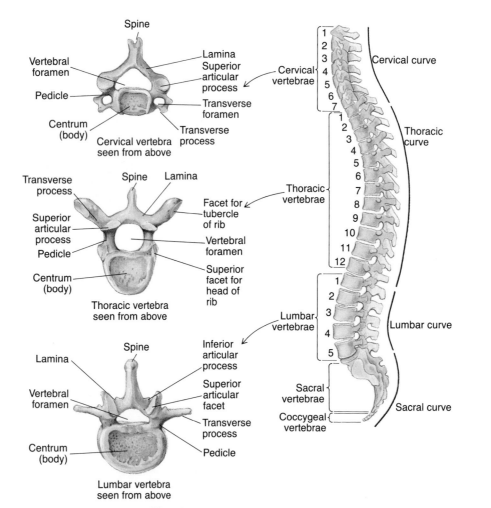

Plate 2 ■ Skeletal System *continued*

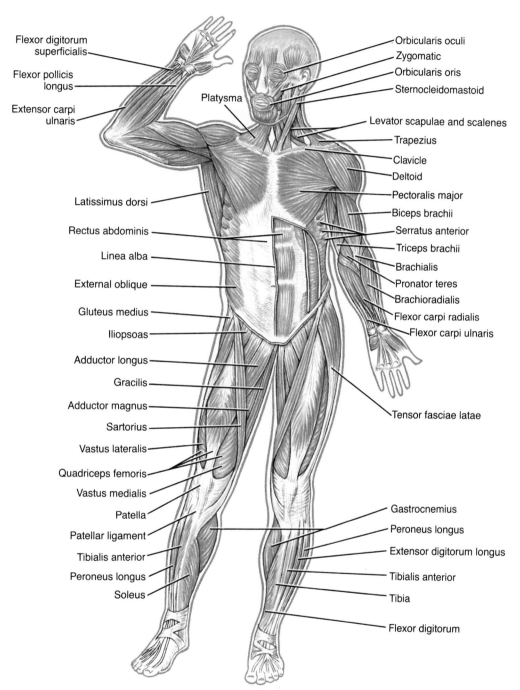

Flexor digitorum superficialis
Flexor pollicis longus
Extensor carpi ulnaris
Platysma
Latissimus dorsi
Rectus abdominis
Linea alba
External oblique
Gluteus medius
Iliopsoas
Adductor longus
Gracilis
Adductor magnus
Sartorius
Vastus lateralis
Quadriceps femoris
Vastus medialis
Patella
Patellar ligament
Tibialis anterior
Peroneus longus
Soleus

Orbicularis oculi
Zygomatic
Orbicularis oris
Sternocleidomastoid
Levator scapulae and scalenes
Trapezius
Clavicle
Deltoid
Pectoralis major
Biceps brachii
Serratus anterior
Triceps brachii
Brachialis
Pronator teres
Brachioradialis
Flexor carpi radialis
Flexor carpi ulnaris
Tensor fasciae latae
Gastrocnemius
Peroneus longus
Extensor digitorum longus
Tibialis anterior
Tibia
Flexor digitorum

Plate 3 ■ Anterior Superficial Muscles

B

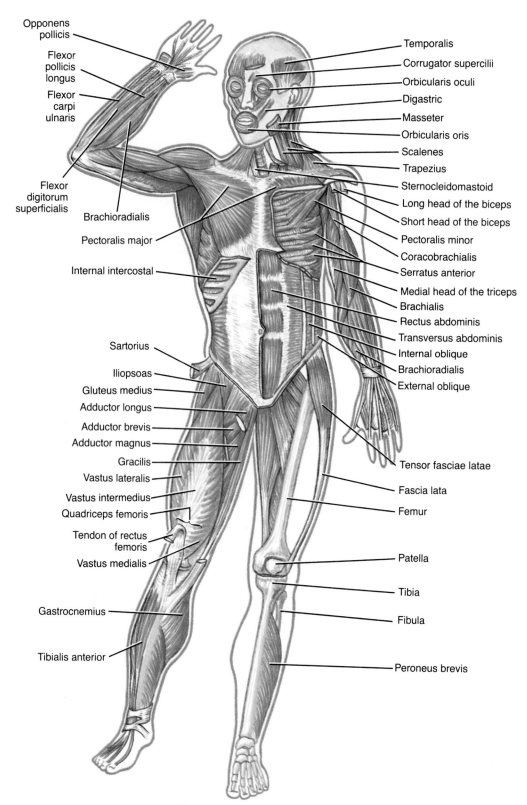

Opponens
pollicis

Flexor
pollicis
longus

Flexor
carpi
ulnaris

Flexor
digitorum
superficialis

Brachioradialis

Pectoralis major

Internal intercostal

Sartorius

Iliopsoas

Gluteus medius

Adductor longus

Adductor brevis

Adductor magnus

Gracilis

Vastus lateralis

Vastus intermedius

Quadriceps femoris

Tendon of rectus
femoris

Vastus medialis

Gastrocnemius

Tibialis anterior

B

Temporalis

Corrugator supercilii

Orbicularis oculi

Digastric

Masseter

Orbicularis oris

Scalenes

Trapezius

Sternocleidomastoid

Long head of the biceps

Short head of the biceps

Pectoralis minor

Coracobrachialis

Serratus anterior

Medial head of the triceps

Brachialis

Rectus abdominis

Transversus abdominis

Internal oblique

Brachioradialis

External oblique

Tensor fasciae latae

Fascia lata

Femur

Patella

Tibia

Fibula

Peroneus brevis

Plate 4 ■ **Anterior Deep Muscles**

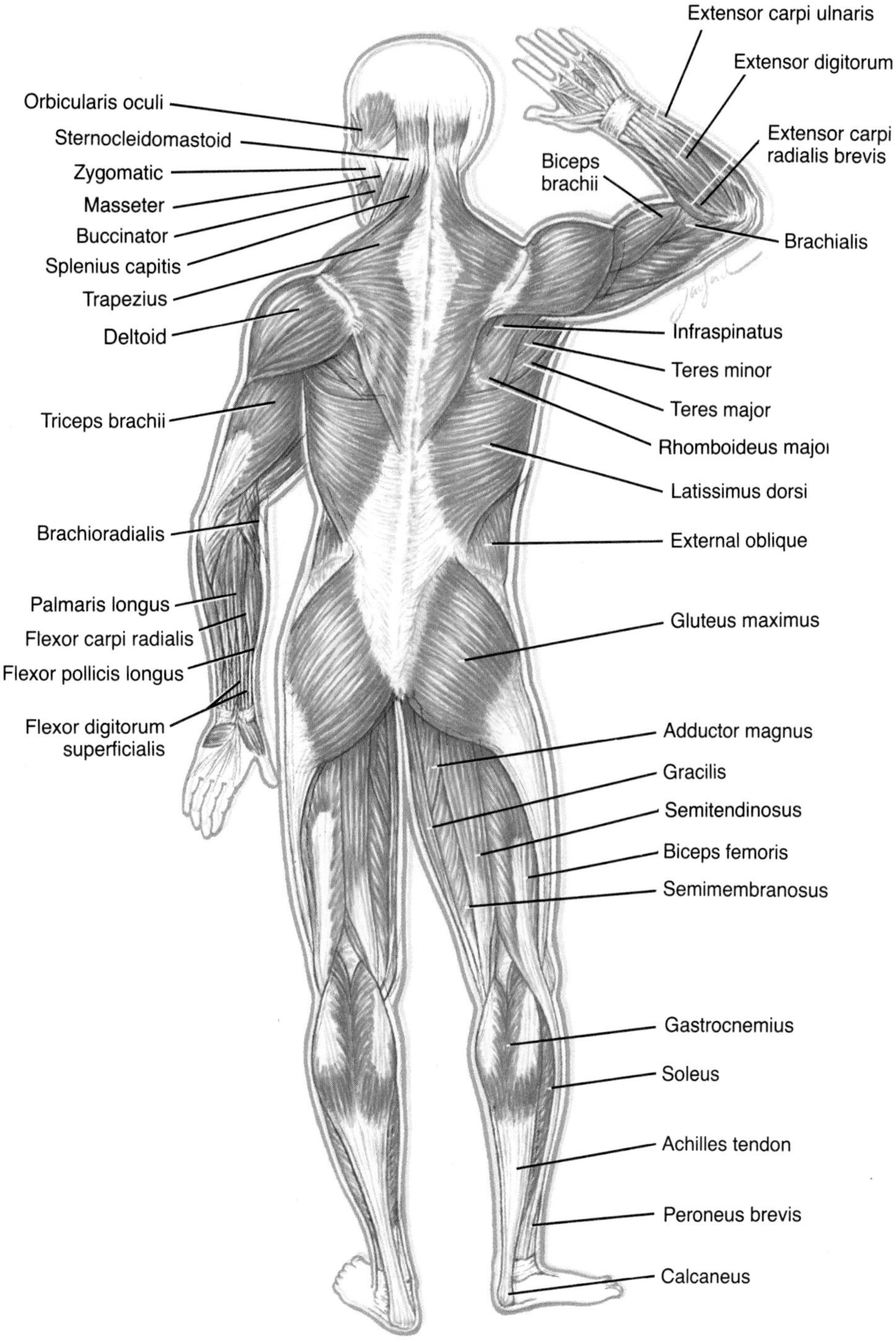

Extensor carpi ulnaris
Extensor digitorum
Extensor carpi radialis brevis
Biceps brachii
Brachialis
Orbicularis oculi
Sternocleidomastoid
Zygomatic
Masseter
Buccinator
Splenius capitis
Trapezius
Deltoid
Infraspinatus
Teres minor
Teres major
Rhomboideus major
Latissimus dorsi
Triceps brachii
External oblique
Brachioradialis
Gluteus maximus
Palmaris longus
Flexor carpi radialis
Flexor pollicis longus
Flexor digitorum superficialis
Adductor magnus
Gracilis
Semitendinosus
Biceps femoris
Semimembranosus
Gastrocnemius
Soleus
Achilles tendon
Peroneus brevis
Calcaneus

Plate 5 ■ Posterior Superficial Muscles

B

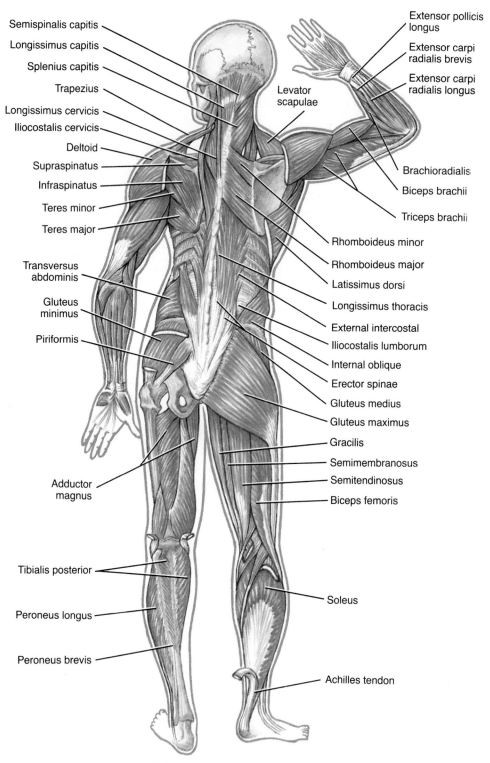

Plate 6 ■ **Posterior Deep Muscles**

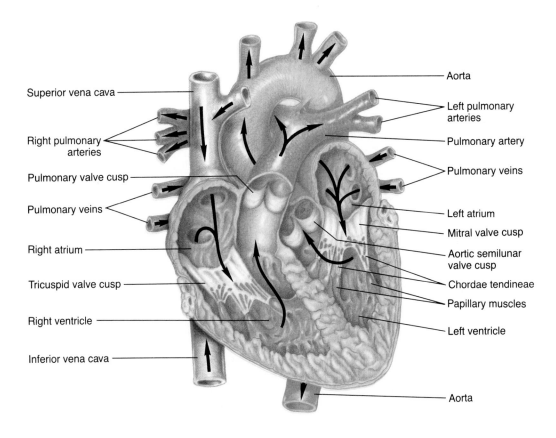

Superior vena cava

Right pulmonary arteries

Pulmonary valve cusp

Pulmonary veins

Right atrium

Tricuspid valve cusp

Right ventricle

Inferior vena cava

Aorta

Left pulmonary arteries

Pulmonary artery

Pulmonary veins

Left atrium

Mitral valve cusp

Aortic semilunar valve cusp

Chordae tendineae

Papillary muscles

Left ventricle

Aorta

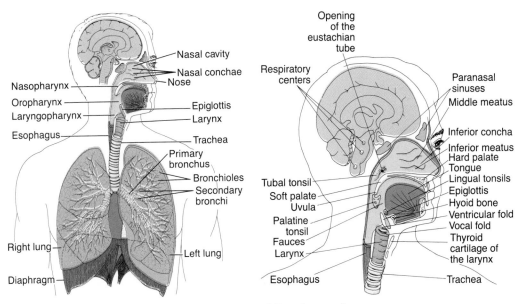

Nasal cavity

Nasal conchae

Nose

Nasopharynx

Oropharynx

Laryngopharynx

Esophagus

Epiglottis

Larynx

Trachea

Primary bronchus

Bronchioles

Secondary bronchi

Right lung

Left lung

Diaphragm

Opening of the eustachian tube

Respiratory centers

Paranasal sinuses

Middle meatus

Inferior concha

Inferior meatus

Hard palate

Tongue

Lingual tonsils

Epiglottis

Hyoid bone

Ventricular fold

Vocal fold

Thyroid cartilage of the larynx

Tubal tonsil

Soft palate

Uvula

Palatine tonsil

Fauces

Larynx

Esophagus

Trachea

Plate 7 ■ Heart and Respiratory System

B

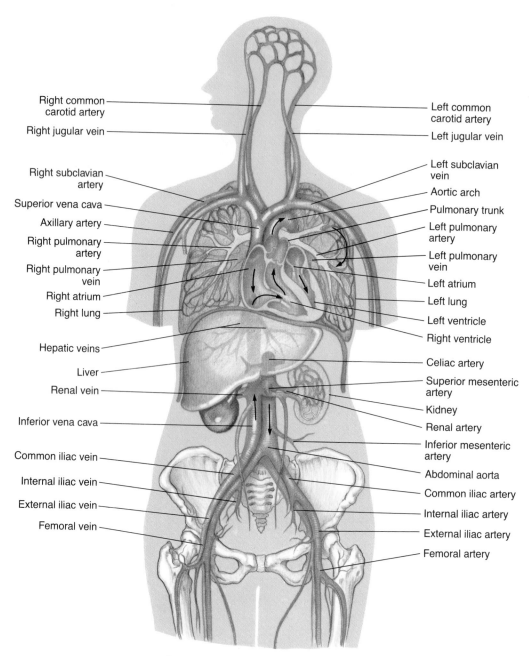

Right common carotid artery

Right jugular vein

Right subclavian artery

Superior vena cava

Axillary artery

Right pulmonary artery

Right pulmonary vein

Right atrium

Right lung

Hepatic veins

Liver

Renal vein

Inferior vena cava

Common iliac vein

Internal iliac vein

External iliac vein

Femoral vein

Left common carotid artery

Left jugular vein

Left subclavian vein

Aortic arch

Pulmonary trunk

Left pulmonary artery

Left pulmonary vein

Left atrium

Left lung

Left ventricle

Right ventricle

Celiac artery

Superior mesenteric artery

Kidney

Renal artery

Inferior mesenteric artery

Abdominal aorta

Common iliac artery

Internal iliac artery

External iliac artery

Femoral artery

Plate 8 ⬛ **Circulatory System—Blood**

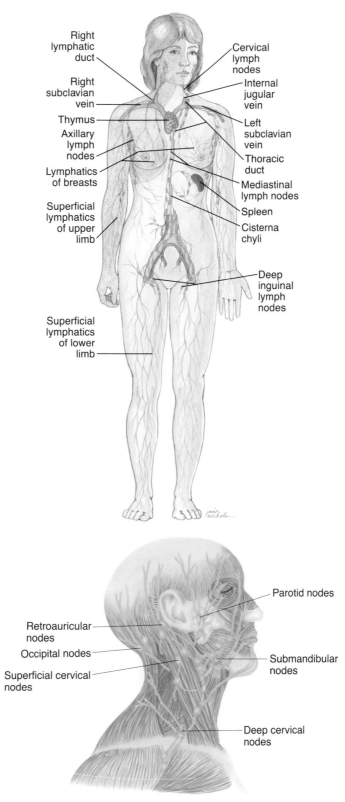

Right lymphatic duct

Right subclavian vein

Thymus

Axillary lymph nodes

Lymphatics of breasts

Superficial lymphatics of upper limb

Superficial lymphatics of lower limb

Cervical lymph nodes

Internal jugular vein

Left subclavian vein

Thoracic duct

Mediastinal lymph nodes

Spleen

Cisterna chyli

Deep inguinal lymph nodes

Parotid nodes

Retroauricular nodes

Occipital nodes

Superficial cervical nodes

Submandibular nodes

Deep cervical nodes

Plate 9 ■ Circulatory System—Lymph

B

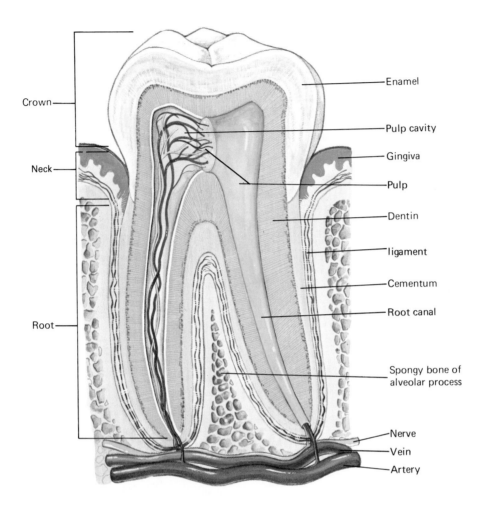

Crown

Neck

Root

Enamel

Pulp cavity

Gingiva

Pulp

Dentin

ligament

Cementum

Root canal

Spongy bone of alveolar process

Nerve

Vein

Artery

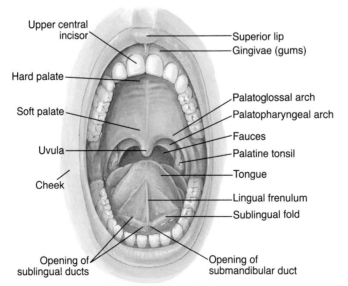

Upper central incisor

Hard palate

Soft palate

Uvula

Cheek

Opening of sublingual ducts

Superior lip

Gingivae (gums)

Palatoglossal arch

Palatopharyngeal arch

Fauces

Palatine tonsil

Tongue

Lingual frenulum

Sublingual fold

Opening of submandibular duct

Plate 10 ■ **Digestive System**

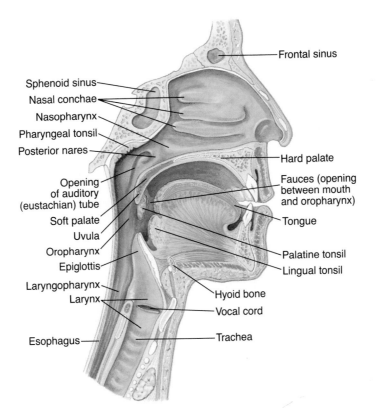

Parotid gland
Pharynx
Esophagus
Sublingual gland
Submandibular duct
Submandibular gland

Liver
Gallbladder
Ascending colon
Ileum
Cecum
Vermiform appendix
Stomach
Duodenum
Pancreas
Transverse colon
Jejunum
Descending colon
Sigmoid colon
Rectum
Anus

Frontal sinus
Sphenoid sinus
Nasal conchae
Nasopharynx
Pharyngeal tonsil
Posterior nares
Opening
of auditory
(eustachian) tube
Soft palate
Uvula
Oropharynx
Epiglottis
Laryngopharynx
Larynx
Esophagus
Hard palate
Fauces (opening
between mouth
and oropharynx)
Tongue
Palatine tonsil
Lingual tonsil
Hyoid bone
Vocal cord
Trachea

B

Plate 11 ■ **Digestive System** *continued*

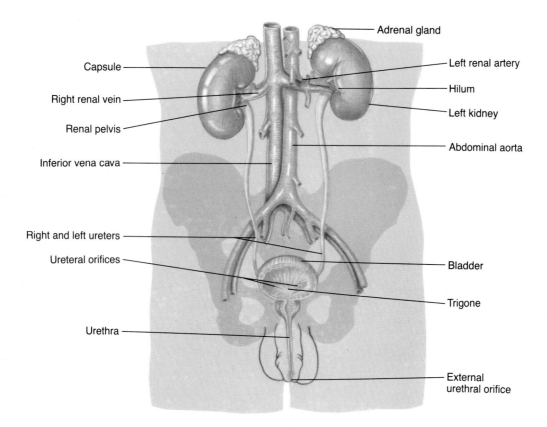

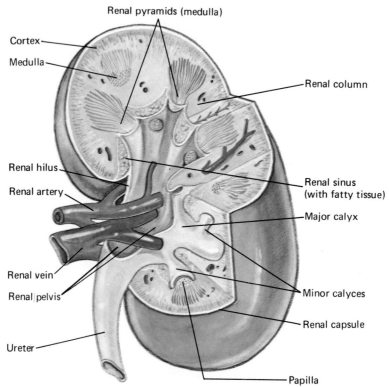

Plate 12 ▪ **Genitourinary System**

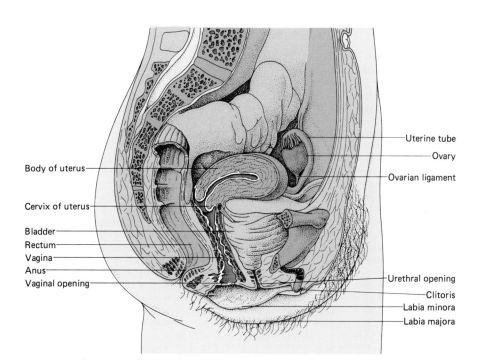

Rectum
Seminal vesicle
Urethra
Ejaculatory duct
Prostate gland

Bladder
Vas deferens
Penis
Cavernous bodies
Urethra
Testis
Prepuce
Glans penis

Anus   Bulbourethral gland   Epididymis

Pubis of pelvis   Scrotum

Body of uterus

Cervix of uterus

Bladder
Rectum
Vagina
Anus
Vaginal opening

Uterine tube
Ovary
Ovarian ligament

Urethral opening
Clitoris
Labia minora
Labia majora

Plate 13 ■ **Genitourinary System** *continued*

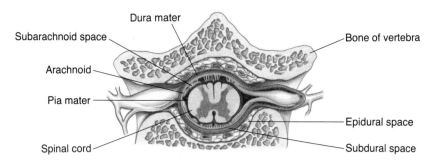

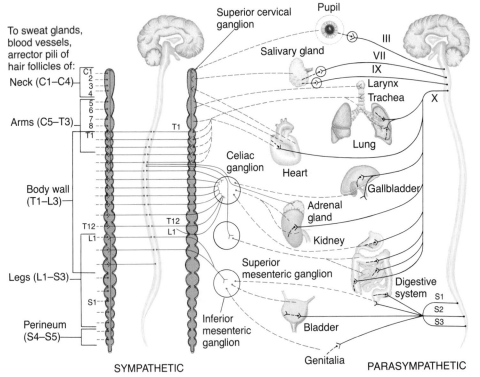

B

Plate 14 ■ **Nervous System**

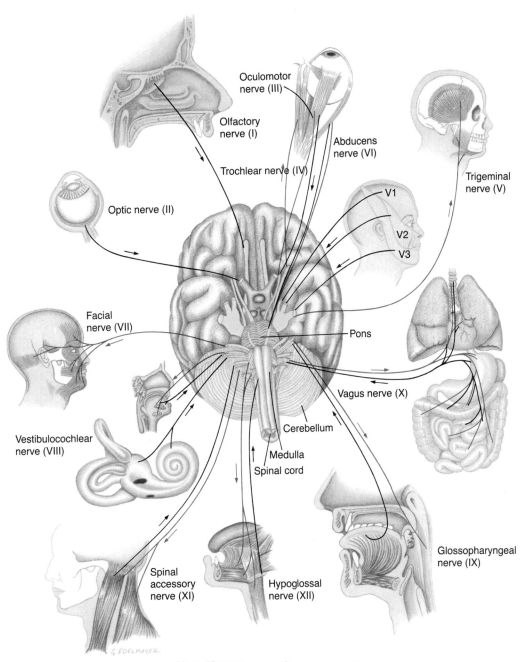

Plate 15 ■ **Nervous System** *continued*

B

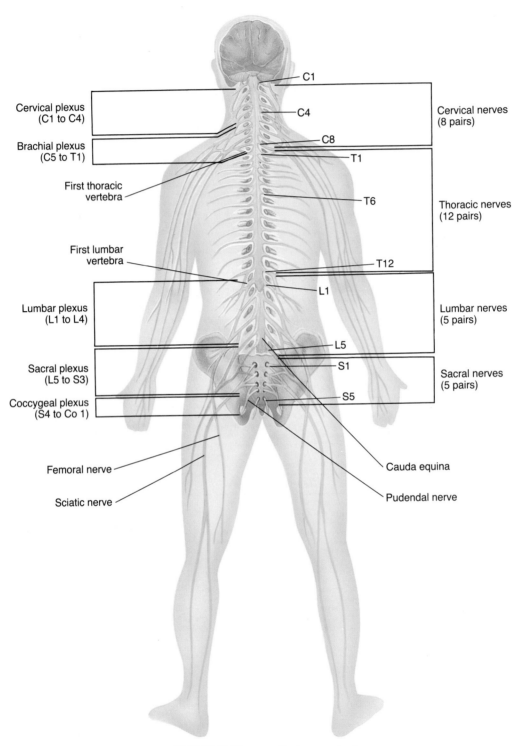

Cervical plexus (C1 to C4)

Brachial plexus (C5 to T1)

First thoracic vertebra

First lumbar vertebra

Lumbar plexus (L1 to L4)

Sacral plexus (L5 to S3)

Coccygeal plexus (S4 to Co 1)

Femoral nerve

Sciatic nerve

C1

C4

C8

T1

T6

T12

L1

L5

S1

S5

Cervical nerves (8 pairs)

Thoracic nerves (12 pairs)

Lumbar nerves (5 pairs)

Sacral nerves (5 pairs)

Cauda equina

Pudendal nerve

Plate 16 ■ **Nervous System** *continued*

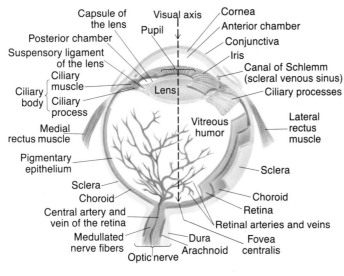

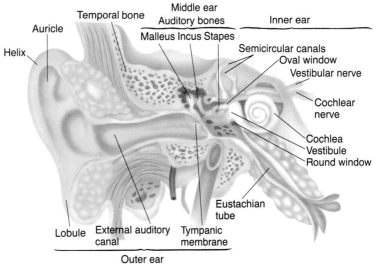

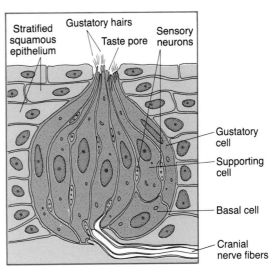

Plate 17 ■ Organs of Special Sense

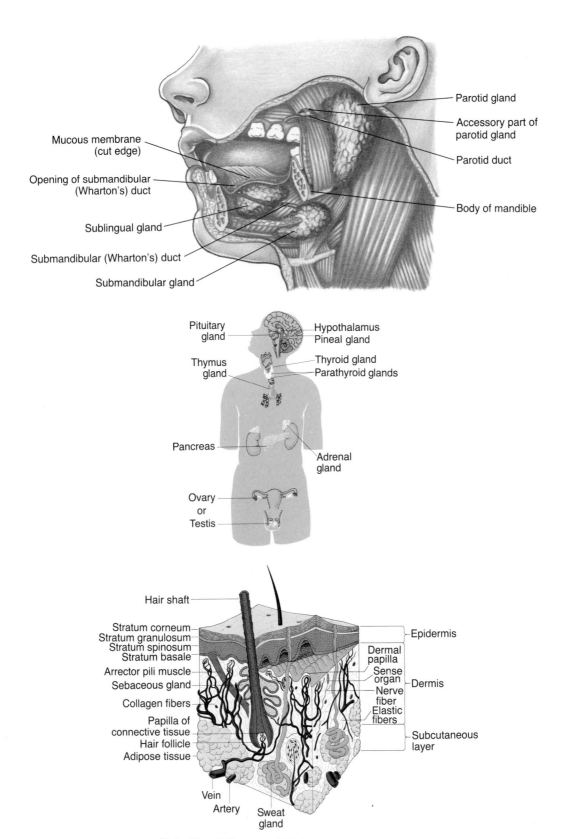

B

Plate 18 ■ **Salivary and Endocrine Glands and Skin**

Glossary

Abortion The loss of a fetus before the stage of viability.

Abrasion (Â-brâ-shun) A wound in which the outer layers of the skin are damaged; a scrape.

Abscess (AB-sess) A collection of pus in a cavity surrounded by inflamed tissue.

Absorbable suture (AB-sorb-a-bl SÛ-chur) Suture material that is gradually digested by tissue enzymes and absorbed by the body.

Adnexal (ad-NEX-al) Adjacent.

Aerobe (air-ÔB) A microorganism that needs oxygen in order to live and grow.

Afebrile (â-FÊB-ril) Without fever; the body temperature is normal.

Agglutination (a-GLÛT-in-Â-shun) The aggregation or uniting of separate particles into clumps or masses.

Allergen (AL-er-gen) A substance that is capable of causing an allergic reaction.

Allergy An abnormal hypersensitivity of the body to substances that are ordinarily harmless.

Alveolus (pl. alveoli) (al-VÊ-ô-lus) A thin-walled air sac of the lungs in which the exchange of oxygen and carbon dioxide takes place.

Ambulation (AM-bû-LÂ-shun) The ability to walk as opposed to being confined to bed.

Ameboid movement (A-mê-boyd MOVE-ment) Movement used by leukocytes that permits them to propel themselves from the capillaries out into the tissues.

Amplitude (AMP-li-TÛD) Refers to amount, extent, size, abundance, or fullness.

Ampule (AM-pûl) A small sealed glass container containing a single dose of medication.

Anaerobe (an-er-ÔB) A microorganism that grows best in the absence of oxygen.

Anemia (a-NÊ-mê-a) A condition in which there is a decrease in the number of erythrocytes or in the amount of hemoglobin in the blood.

Antecubital space (ANT-ta-CÛ-bit-al spâs) The space located at the front of the elbow.

Antibody A substance that is capable of combining with an antigen, resulting in an antigen-antibody reaction.

Anticoagulant (an-tî-KÔ-ag-û-lant) A substance that inhibits blood clotting.

Antigen A substance capable of stimulating the formation of antibodies.

Antipyretic (ANTÎ-pî-RET-ik) An agent that reduces fever.

Antiseptic (an-TÎ-sep-tik) A substance that kills disease-producing microorganisms but not their spores. An antiseptic is usually applied to living tissue.

Antiserum A serum that contains antibodies.

Aorta (â-OR-ta) The major trunk of the arterial system of the body. The aorta arises from the upper surface of the left ventricle.

Apnea (AP-nê-a) The temporary cessation of breathing.

Approximation (a-PROX-i-mâ-shun) The process of bringing two parts, such as tissue, together, through the use of sutures or other means.

Arrhythmia (â-RYTH-mê-a) An irregular rhythm. (Also termed dysrhythmia.)

Artifact Additional electrical activity, picked up by the electrocardiograph, that interferes with the normal appearance of the ECG cycles.

Asepsis Free from infection or pathogens.

Aspirate (AS-pir-âte) To remove by suction.

Atypical Deviation from the normal.

Audiometer (a-DÊ-om-it-er) An instrument used to measure hearing quantitatively for the various frequencies of sound waves.

Auscultation (AUS-kul-TÂ-shun) The process of listening to the sounds produced within the body to detect any signs of disease.

Autoclave (au-TO-klâv) An apparatus for the sterilization of materials, using steam under pressure.

Automated method (for testing laboratory specimens) A method of laboratory testing in which the series of steps in the test method is performed by an automated analyzer.

Avoirdupois (av-er-DÛ-poys) A system of weight used in English-speaking countries for weighing heavy articles. This system is not used to weigh drugs and precious stones and metals.

Axilla (AX-il-la) The armpit.

Bacilli (ba-SILL-î) (singular, bacillus) Bacteria that have a rod shape.

Bandage A strip of woven material used to wrap or cover a part of the body.

Baseline The flat horizontal line that separates the various waves of the ECG cycle.

Bilirubin (bill-ê-RÛ-bin) An orange-colored bile pigment produced by the breakdown of heme from the hemoglobin molecule.

Bilirubinuria (BILA-rû-bin-û-rê-a) The presence of bilirubin in the urine.

Biopsy (bî-OP-sê) The surgical removal and examination of tissue from the living body. Biopsies are generally performed to determine whether a tumor is benign or malignant.

Blood antibody A protein present in the blood plasma that is capable of combining with its corresponding blood antigen to produce an antigen-antibody reaction.

Blood antigen A protein present on the surface of red blood cells that determines the blood type of an individual.

Bloodborne pathogens Pathogenic microorganisms capable of causing disease that are present in human blood, such as the hepatitis B virus (HBV) and the human immunodeficiency virus (HIV), which causes AIDS.

Bounding pulse A pulse with an increased volume that feels very strong and full.

Bradycardia (BRÂ-da-car-DÊ-a) An abnormally slow heart or pulse rate (below 60 beats per minute).

755

Bradypnea (brad-IP-NÊ-a) An abnormal decrease in the respiratory rate to less than 10 respirations per minute.

Braxton Hicks contractions Intermittent and irregular painless uterine contractions that occur throughout pregnancy. They occur more frequently toward the end of the pregnancy and are sometimes mistaken for true labor pains.

Buffy coat A thin, light-colored layer of white blood cells and platelets that lies between a top layer of plasma and a bottom layer of red blood cells when an anticoagulant has been added to a blood specimen.

Burn An injury to the tissues caused by exposure to thermal, chemical, electrical, or radioactive agents.

Canthus (KAN-thus) The junction of the eyelids at either corner of the eye.

Capillary action (KAP-il-air-ê) That action which causes liquid to rise along a wick, a tube, or a gauze dressing.

Cardiac arrest A situation in which the heart has stopped beating or beats too irregularly to circulate blood effectively through the body.

Cardiac cycle One complete heart beat.

Centigrade or Celsius thermometer A thermometer on which the freezing point of water is 0 and the boiling point of water is 100 degrees.

Cerumen (se-RÛ-min) Ear wax.

Charting The process of making written entries about a patient in the medical record.

Cilia Slender hairlike projections.

Clinical diagnosis A tentative diagnosis obtained through the evaluation of the health history and the physical examination, without the benefit of laboratory or diagnostic tests.

Cocci (COCK-sî) (singular, coccus) Bacteria that have a round shape.

Colony A mass of bacteria growing on a solid culture medium that has arisen from the multiplication of a single bacterium.

Colposcope (KUL-pô-skôp) A lighted instrument with a binocular magnifying lens used for the examination of the vagina and cervix.

Colposcopy (KUL-pos-KÔ-pê) The visual examination of the vagina and cervix using a colposcope.

Compress A soft, moist, absorbent cloth that is folded in several layers and applied to a part of the body in the local application of heat or cold.

Computer-based patient record (CPR) A medical record that is stored on a computer

Conduction The transfer of energy, such as heat, from one object to another.

Conjunctiva (kun-JUNK-tiv-a) The mucous membrane that lines the eyelids and covers the eyeball, except for the cornea.

Consultation report A narrative report of an opinion about a patient's condition by a practitioner other than the attending physician.

Contagious Capable of being transmitted directly or indirectly from one person to another.

Contaminate To soil, stain, or pollute; to make impure.

Contrast medium A substance that is used to make a particular structure visible on a radiograph.

Contusion (kun-TÛ-shun) An injury to the tissues under the skin causing blood vessels to rupture, allowing blood to seep into the tissues; a bruise.

Convection The transfer of energy, such as heat, in the form of currents.

Conversion Changing from one unit of measurement to another.

Crash cart A specially equipped cart for holding and transporting medications, equipment, and supplies needed for performing life-saving procedures in an emergency.

Crepitus (KREP-it-us) A grating sensation caused by fractured bone fragments rubbing against each other.

Crisis A sudden falling of an elevated body temperature to normal.

Critical item An item that comes in contact with sterile tissue or the vascular system.

Cryosurgery (KRY-ô-SURG-er-ê) The therapeutic use of freezing temperatures to destroy abnormal tissue.

Cubic centimeter The amount of space occupied by 1 milliliter (1 ml = 1 cc).

Culture The propagation of a mass of microorganisms in a laboratory culture medium.

Culture medium A mixture of nutrients on which microorganisms are grown in the laboratory.

Cyanosis (SÎ-in-ÔS-is) A bluish discoloration of the skin and mucous membranes.

Cytology (SÎ-TOL-ô-gê) The science that deals with the study of cells, including their origin, structure, function, and pathology.

Decontamination The use of physical or chemical means to remove, inactivate, or destroy bloodborne pathogens on a surface or item to the point at which they are no longer capable of transmitting infectious particles and the surface or item is rendered safe for handling, use, or disposal.

Dermis (DUR-mis) The true skin; the main thickness of skin, with an active blood supply.

Detergent (de-TER-gent) An agent that cleanses by emulsifying dirt and oil.

Diagnosis (dî-AG-nô-sis) The scientific method of determining and identifying a patient's condition.

Diagnostic procedure A type of procedure performed to assist in the diagnosis, management, and treatment of a patient's condition.

Diapedesis (DÎ-ap-a-dis-is) The ameboid movement of blood cells (especially leukocytes) through the wall of a capillary and out into the tissues.

Diastole (DÎ-as-stol-ê) The phase in the cardiac cycle in which the heart relaxes between contractions.

Diastolic pressure (DÎ-as-STOL-ic PRESH-ur) The point of lesser pressure on the arterial walls, which is recorded during diastole.

Differential diagnosis A determination of which of two or more diseases with similar symptoms is producing the patient's symptoms.

Dilation (of the cervix) (dî-LÂ-shun) The stretching of the external os from an opening a few millimeters in size to an opening large enough to allow the passage of an infant (approximately 10 cm).

Discharge summary report A brief summary of the significant events of a patient's hospitalization.

Disinfectant (DIS-in-FEK-tant) A substance used to destroy disease-producing microorganisms but not necessarily their spores. Disinfectants are usually applied to inanimate objects.

Dislocation An injury in which one end of a bone making up a joint is separated or displaced from its normal position.

Donor One who furnishes something such as blood, tissue, or organs to be used in another person.

Dose The quantity of a drug to be administered at one time.

Dyspnea (disp-NÊ-a) Labored or difficult breathing.

ECG cycle The graphic representation of a cardiac cycle.

Echocardiogram (EK-Ô-kar-dê-ô-gram) An ultrasound examination of the heart.

EDD Expected date of delivery or due date.

Edema (a-DÊÊM-a) The retention of fluid in the tissues, resulting in swelling.

Effacement (ê-FÂS-ment) The thinning and shortening of the cervical canal from its normal length of 1 to 2 cm to a structure with paper-thin edges in which there is no canal at all. Effacement occurs late in pregnancy or during labor, or both. The purpose of effacement along with dilation is to permit the passage of the infant into the birth canal.

Electrocardiogram The graphic representation of the electrical activity of the heart.

Electrocardiograph (Ê-lek-trô-KAR-dê-ô-graf) The instrument used to record the electrical activity of the heart.

Electrode (Ê-lek-TRÔD) A conductor of electricity that is used to promote contact between the body and the electrocardiograph.

Electrolyte (Ê-lek-TRÔ-lît) A chemical substance that promotes conduction of an electrical current.

Emergency medical services (EMS) system A network of community resources, equipment, and personnel that provides care to victims of injury or sudden illness.

Endocervix (in-DÔ-serv-ix) The mucous membrane lining the cervical canal.

Endoscope (IN-dô-skôp) An instrument, consisting of a tube and an optical system, that is used for direct visual inspection of organs or cavities.

Enema An injection of fluid into the rectum to aid in the elimination of feces from the colon.

Engagement The entrance of the fetal head or the presenting part into the pelvic inlet.

Epidermis (EP-a-derm-is) The outermost, nonvascular layer of the skin.

Erythema (a-RITH-êm-a) Redness of the skin caused by congestion of capillaries in the lower layers of skin.

Erythrocyte Red blood cell.

Eupnea (ÛP-nê-a) Normal respiration.

Evacuated tube A closed glass or plastic tube containing a premeasured vacuum.

Exfoliated cells (X-FOL-ê-ât-ed SELLS) Cells that have been sloughed off from the surface of tissues into the secretions bathing those tissues.

Exhalation (X-hal-ÂSH-on) The act of breathing out.

Exposure incident A specific eye, mouth, other mucous membrane, nonintact skin, or parenteral contact with blood or other potentially infectious materials that results from an employee's duties.

External os (X-tern-al os) The opening of the cervical canal of the uterus into the vagina.

Exudate (X-û-dât) A discharge produced by the body's tissues.

Fahrenheit thermometer A thermometer on which the freezing point of water is 32 degrees and the boiling point of water is 212 degrees.

False negative A test result denoting that a condition is absent when, in actuality, it is present.

False positive A test result denoting that a condition is present when, in actuality, it is absent.

Familial (FA-mil-yel) Occurring or affecting members of a family more frequently than would be expected by chance.

Fastidious (FAS-stid-ê-us) Extremely delicate; difficult to culture, therefore involving specialized growth requirements.

Fasting Abstaining from food or fluids (except water) for a specified amount of time prior to the collection of a specimen.

Febrile (FÊ-bril) Pertaining to fever.

Fetal heart rate The number of times the fetal heart beats per minute.

Fetal heart tones The heart beat of the fetus as heard through the mother's abdominal wall.

Fetus (FÊ-tus) The child in utero, from the third month after conception to birth; during the first two months of development, it is called an embryo.

Fever A body temperature that is above normal. Synonym for pyrexia.

Fibroblast (fî-BRÔ-blast) An immature cell from which connective tissue can develop.

First aid The immediate care that is administered to an individual who is injured or suddenly becomes ill before complete medical care can be obtained.

Fluoroscope (FLOOR-ô-skôp) An instrument used to view internal organs and structures directly.

Fluoroscopy (FLOOR-os-KÔ-pê) Examination of a patient using the fluoroscope.

Forceps (FOR-seps) A two-pronged instrument for grasping and squeezing.

Fracture (FRAK-shur) Any break in a bone.

Frenulum linguae (FREN-u-lum LING-gwa) The midline fold that connects the undersurface of the tongue with the floor of the mouth.

Fundus (FUN-dus) The dome-shaped upper portion of the uterus between the fallopian tubes.

Furuncle (fur-UN-kle) A localized staphylococcal infection that originates deep within a hair follicle; also known as a boil.

Gene A unit of heredity.

Gestation (JES-tâ-shun) The period of intrauterine development from conception to birth; the period of pregnancy. The average pregnancy lasts about 280 days or 40 weeks from the date of conception to childbirth.

Glycogen (GLÎ-kô-jen) The form in which carbohydrate is stored in the body.

Glycosuria (GLÎ-ka-sur-ê-a) The presence of sugar in the urine.

Gravid (GRAV-id) Pregnant.

Gravida (GRAV-id-a) A woman who is or has been pregnant.

Gravidity (GRAV-id-i-tê) The total number of pregnancies a woman has had regardless of duration, including a current pregnancy.

Gynecology (GÎN-e-KUL-ô-jê) The branch of medicine that deals with the diseases of reproductive organs of women.

HDL cholesterol A lipoprotein consisting of protein and cholesterol, which removes excess cholesterol from the cells.

Health history report A collection of subjective data about a patient.

Hematology (HÊM-a-taul-Ô-gy) The study of blood and blood-forming tissues.

Hematoma (HÊM-a-TOME-a) A swelling or mass of coagulated blood caused by a break in a blood vessel.

Hemoconcentration (HÊM-O-kon-sen-trâ-shun) An increased nonfilterable blood components such as red blood cells, enzymes, iron, and calcium as a result of a decrease in the fluid content of the blood.

Hemoglobin (HÊM-ô-glô-bin) The iron-containing pigment of erythrocytes that transports oxygen in the body.

Hemolysis (He-maul-is-sis) The breakdown of erythrocytes with the release of hemoglobin into the plasma.

Hemostasis (HÊM-o-STÂ-sis) The arrest of bleeding by natural or artificial means.

High-risk Having an increased possibility of suffering harm, damage, or death.

Home health care The provision of medical and nonmedical care in a patient's home or place of residence.

Homeostasis (HÔM-ê-ô-STÂ-sis) The state in which the body systems are functioning normally and the internal environment of the body is in equilibrium; the body is in a healthy state.

Host An animal or plant that provides nourishment for a microorganism to grow and multiply.

Hyperglycemia (HÎ-PER-glî-sê-mê-a) An abnormal increase in the glucose level in the blood.

Hyperopia (hî-PER-op-êa) Farsightedness.

Hyperpnea (hî-PERP-nê-a) An abnormal increase in the rate and depth of respiration.

Hyperpyrexia (hî-PER-pî-REX-êa) An extremely high fever.

Hypertension (hî-PER-ten-shun) High blood pressure.

Hyperventilation (hî-PER-vent-a-LÂ-shun) An abnormally fast and deep type of breathing usually associated with acute anxiety or emotional tension.

Hypoglycemia (HÎ-PÔ-glî-sê-mê-a) An abnormally low level of glucose in the blood.

Hypopnea (hî-POP-nê-a) An abnormal decrease in the rate and depth of respiration.

Hypotension (hî-PÔ-ten-shun) Low blood pressure.

Hypothermia (hî-PÔ-THER-mê-a) A life-threatening condition in which the temperature of the entire body falls to a dangerously low level.

Hypoxia (hî-POX-ê-a) A reduction in the oxygen supply to the tissues of the body.

Immunity (IM-ûn-it-ê) The resistance of the body to the effects of a harmful agent such as a pathogenic microorganism or its toxins.

Immunization (IM-ûn-i-zâ-shun) The process of becoming immune or of rendering an individual immune through the use of a vaccine or toxoid.

Impacted Being wedged firmly together so as to be immovable.

Incision (IN-sis-shun) A clean cut caused by a cutting instrument.

Incubate (in-KÛ-bât) In microbiology, the act of placing a culture in a chamber (incubator), which provides optimal growth requirements for the multiplication of the organism, such as the proper temperature, humidity, and darkness.

Incubation period The interval of time between the invasion by a pathogenic microorganism and the appearance of first symptoms of the disease.

Induration (in-DUR-Â-shun) An area of hardened tissue.

Infant A child from birth to 1 year of age.

Infection (IN-fek-shun) The condition in which the body, or part of it, is invaded by a pathogen.

Infectious disease A disease caused by a pathogen that produces harmful effects on its host.

Infiltration (IN-fil-TRÂ-shun) The process by which a substance passes into and is deposited within the substance of a cell, tissue, or organ.

Inflammation (IN-fla-MÂ-shun) A protective response of the body to trauma and the entrance of foreign matter. The purpose of inflammation is to destroy invading microorganisms and to repair injured tissue. Local symptoms occurring at the site of inflammation include pain, swelling, redness, and warmth.

Informed consent Consent given by a patient for a medical procedure after being informed of the nature of his/her condition, the purpose of the procedure, alternative treatments or procedures available, the likely outcome of the procedure, and the risks involved with declining or delaying the procedure.

Inhalation (IN-hal-Â-shun) The act of breathing in.

Inhalation administration (in-HAL-Â-shun ad-MIN-is-trâ-shun) The administration of medication by way of air or other vapor being drawn into the lungs.

Inoculate (IN-ok-û-lâte) The introduction of microorganisms into a culture medium for growth and multiplication.

Inoculum (IN-ok-û-lum) The specimen used to inoculate a medium.

Inspection The process of observing a patient to detect any signs of disease.

Instillation The dropping of a liquid into a body cavity.

Insufflate (IN-suf-flât) To blow a powder, vapor, or gas (such as air) into a body cavity.

Intercostal (IN-ter-CAUS-tal) Between the ribs.

Internal os (in-TERN-al os) The internal opening of the cervical canal into the uterus.

Interval On an ECG, the length of a wave or the length of a wave with a segment.

Intradermal injection (in-TRA-derm-al in-JEK-shun) Introducing medication into the dermal layer of the skin.

Intramuscular injection (in-TRA-mus-kû-lar in-JEK-shun) Introducing medication into the muscular layer of the body.

Intravenous injection (in-TRA-vên-us in-JEK-shun) Introducing medication into the bloodstream directly through a vein.

In vitro (IN-VÊ-trô) Occurring in glass. Refers to tests performed under artificial conditions, as in the laboratory.

In vivo (IN-vêv-Ô) Occurring in the living body or organism.

Irrigation The washing of a body canal with a flowing solution.

Ischemia (is-KÊM-ê-a) Deficiency of blood in a part.

Ketonuria (KÊ-tô-nur-ê-a) The presence of ketone bodies in the urine.

Ketosis (KÊ-tô-sis) An accumulation of large amounts of ketone bodies in the tissues and body fluids.

Korotkoff sounds (KÔ-rot-kauf) Sounds heard during the measurement of blood pressure that are used to determine the systolic and diastolic blood pressure readings.

Laboratory test The clinical analysis and study of materials, fluids, or tissues obtained from patients to assist in diagnosing and treating disease.

Laceration (LAS-er-Â-shun) A wound in which the tissues are torn apart, leaving ragged and irregular edges.

LDL cholesterol A lipoprotein consisting of protein and cholesterol, which picks up cholesterol and delivers it to the cells.

Length A unit of linear measurement used to measure length or distance.

Leukocyte White blood cell.

Leukocytosis (lû-KÔ-sî-tô-sis) An abnormal increase in the number of white blood cells (above 11,000 per cu mm of blood).

Leukopenia (lû-KÔ-pen-ê-a) An abnormal decrease in the number of white blood cells (below 4,500 per cu mm of blood).

Ligate (LÎ-gât) To tie off and close a structure such as a severed blood vessel.

Lipoprotein (LÎ-PÔ-prô-têên) A complex molecule consisting of protein and a lipid fraction such as cholesterol. Lipoproteins function in transporting lipids in the blood.

Load The articles that are being sterilized.

Local anesthetic (LÔ-kul AN-es-THET-ik) A drug that produces a loss of feeling and an inability to perceive pain in only a specific part of the body.

Lochia (LOK-ê-a) A discharge from the uterus after delivery, consisting of blood, tissue, white blood cells, and some bacteria.

Long arm cast A cast that extends from the axilla to the fingers of the hand, usually with a bend in the elbow.

Long leg cast A cast that extends from the midthigh to the toes.

Lysis (LÎ-sis) The gradual return of the body temperature to normal.

Manometer (mun-OM-it-er) An instrument for measuring pressure.

Manual method A method of laboratory testing in which the series of steps in the test method is performed by hand.

Material safety data sheet (MSDS) A sheet that provides information regarding a chemical, its hazards, and measures to take to avoid injury and illness when handling the chemical.

Mayo tray (MÂ-ô TRÂ) A broad, flat metal tray placed on a stand and used to hold sterile instruments and supplies once it has been covered with a sterile towel.

Medical impressions Conclusions drawn by the physician from an interpretation of data. Other terms for impressions include provisional diagnosis and tentative diagnosis.

Medical record A written record of the important aspects regarding a patient, including the care of that individual and the progress of the patient's condition (also known as "the chart").

Medical record format The way a medical record is organized. The two main types of medical record formats include the source-oriented record and the problem-oriented record.

Melena (MA-lên-a) The darkening of the stool due to the presence of blood in an amount of 50 ml or greater.

Meniscus (mu-NIS-kus) The curved upper surface of a liquid in a container. The surface is convex if the liquid does not wet the container and concave if it does.

Mensuration (MEN-sa-RÂ-shun) The process of measuring the patient.

Microbiology The scientific study of microorganisms and their activities.

Microorganism A microscopic plant or animal.

Micturition (MIK-chur-ish-un) The act of voiding urine.

Mucous membrane A membrane lining body passages or cavities that open to the outside.

Multigravida (mul-TÊ-GRAV-i-da) A woman who has been pregnant more than once.

Multipara (mul-TÊ-pare-a) A woman who has completed two or more pregnancies to the age of viability regardless of whether they ended in live infants or stillbirths.

Myopia Nearsightedness.

Needle biopsy (NÊ-dle BÎ-op-sê) A type of biopsy in which tissue from deep within the body is obtained by the insertion of a biopsy needle through the skin.

Nephron (NEF-ron) The functional unit of the kidney.

Nonabsorbable suture (non-AB-sorb-a-bl SÛ-chur) Suture material that is not absorbed by the body and either remains permanently in the body tissue and becomes encapsulated by fibrous tissue or is removed.

Noncritical item An item that comes into contact with intact skin but not the mucous membranes.

Nonintact skin Skin that has a break in the surface.

Nonpathogen A microorganism that does not normally produce disease.

Normal flora Harmless, nonpathogenic microorganisms that normally reside in many parts of the body but do not cause disease.

Normal range (for laboratory tests) A certain established and acceptable parameter or reference range within which the laboratory test results of a healthy individual are expected to fall.

Normal sinus rhythm Refers to an electrocardiogram that is within normal limits.

Nullipara (nul-Ê-pare-a) A woman who has not carried a pregnancy to the point of viability (20 weeks' gestation).

Objective symptom A symptom that can be observed by an examiner.

Obstetrics (OB-stet-riks) That branch of medicine concerned with the care of the woman during pregnancy, childbirth, and the postpartal period.

Occult blood (a-KULT blud) Blood occurring in such a small amount that it is not detectable by the unaided eye.

Occupational exposure Reasonably anticipated skin, eye, mucous membrane, or parenteral contact with bloodborne pathogens or other potentially infectious materials that may result from the performance of an employee's duties.

Oliguria (au-LIG-ur-ê-a) Decreased or scanty output of urine.

Ophthalmologist (OP-tha-mall-ô-gist) A medical doctor who specializes in diagnosing and treating disorders of the eye.

Ophthalmoscope (op-THAL-ma-skôp) An instrument for examining the interior of the eye.

Opportunistic infection (OP-or-tû-nis-tik IN-fek-shun) An infection that results from a defective immune system that cannot defend the body from pathogens normally found in the environment.

Optician (OP-tish-in) A professional who interprets and fills ophthalmic prescriptions.

Optimum growth temperature The temperature at which an organism grows best.

Optometrist (OP-tom-i-trist) A licensed nonmedical practitioner who is skilled in measuring visual acuity and is qualified to prescribe corrective lenses.

Oral administration Administration of medication by mouth.

Orthopedist (orth-Ô-pêd-ist) A physician who deals with the prevention and correction of problems with the locomotor structures of the body.

Orthopnea (orth-OP-nê-a) The condition in which breathing is easier when an individual is in a standing or sitting position.

Osteochondritis (OS-tê-Ô-kun-drî-tis) Inflammation of bone and cartilage.

Osteomyelitis (OS-tê-Ô-mî-lî-tis) Inflammation of bone due to bacterial infection.

Otoscope (Ô-ta-skôp) An instrument for examining the external ear canal and tympanic membrane.

Oxyhemoglobin (ox-ê-HÊM-ô-glô-bin) Hemoglobin that has combined with oxygen.

Palpation (pal-PÂ-shun) The process of feeling with the hands to detect signs of disease.

Paper-based patient record (PPR) A medical record in paper form.

Para A term used to refer to past pregnancies that reach viability (20 weeks of gestation) regardless of whether the infant was stillborn or alive at birth.

Parenteral (pare-IN-tear-al) Taken into the body through the piercing of the skin barrier or mucous membranes, such as through needlesticks, human bites, cuts, abrasions, and so on.

Parity (PARE-it-ê) The condition of having borne offspring who had attained the age of viability (20 weeks of gestation) regardless of whether they were live infants or stillbirths.

Pathogen (PATH-ô-gen) A disease producing microorganism.

Pediatrician A medical doctor who specializes in the care and development of children and the diagnosis and treatment of diseases of children.

Pediatrics The branch of medicine dealing with the care and development of children and the diagnosis and treatment of diseases of children.

Pelvimetry (PELV-im-it-rê) Measurement of the capacity and diameter of the maternal pelvis, which helps to determine if it will be possible to deliver the infant through the vaginal route.

Percussion (per-KUSH-n) The process of tapping the body to detect signs of disease.

Percussion hammer (per-KUSH-n HAM-er) An instrument with a rubber head, used for testing reflexes.

Perinatal (PARE-ê-nâ-tul) Relating to the period shortly before and after birth.

Perineum (PER-in-ê-um) The external region between the vaginal orifice and the anus in a female and between the scrotum and the anus in a male.

Peroxidase (pur-OX-i-DÂS) (as it pertains to the guaiac slide test) A substance that is able to transfer oxygen from hydrogen peroxide to oxidize guaiac, causing the guaiac to turn blue.

pH The degree to which a solution is acidic or basic.

Phagocytosis (FÂG-ô-sî-tô-sis) The engulfing and destruction of foreign particles, such as bacteria, by special cells called phagocytes.

Phlebotomist (FLA-bot-ta-mist) A health professional trained in the collection of a blood specimen.

Phlebotomy (FLA-bot-ta-mê) Incision of a vein for the removal or withdrawal of blood; the collection of blood.

Physical examination report A report of the objective findings from the physician's assessment of each body system.

Plasma (PLAZ-ma) The liquid part of the blood consisting of a clear yellowish fluid that makes up approximately 55 percent of the total blood volume.

Poison Any substance that causes illness, injury, or death if it enters the body.

Polycythemia (paul-e-SITH-ê-mêa) A disorder in which there is an increase in the red cell mass.

Polyuria (PAUL-ê-ur-ê-a) Increased output of urine.

Position The relation of the presenting part of the fetus to the maternal pelvis.

Postoperative (post-OP-rá-tiv) After a surgical operation.

Postpartum (POST-par-tum) Occurring after childbirth.

Pre-eclampsia (PRÊ-ê-KLAMP-sê-a) A major complication of pregnancy of unknown cause characterized by increasing hypertension, albuminuria, and edema. If this condition is neglected or not treated properly, it may develop into eclampsia, which could cause maternal convulsions and coma. Pre-eclampsia generally occurs between the twentieth week of pregnancy and the end of the first week postpartum.

Prenatal (PRÊ-nâ-TUL) Before birth.

Preoperative (prê-OP-ra-tiv) Preceding a surgical operation.

Presbyopia (pres-BÊ-ôp-êa) A decrease in the elasticity of the lens due to aging, resulting in a decreased ability to focus on close objects.

Prescription (prê-SKRIP-shun) An order for a drug or other therapy written by a physician.

Presentation The part of the fetus that is closest to the cervix and will be delivered first. A cephalic presentation is a delivery in which the fetal head is presenting against the cervix. A breech presentation is a delivery in which the buttocks or feet are presented instead of the head.

Pressure point A site on the body where an artery lies close to the surface of the skin and can be compressed against an underlying bone.

Primigravida (PRÎM-i-GRAV-id-a) A woman who is pregnant for the first time (gravida I).

Primipara (PRÎM-ip-a-ra) A woman who has carried a pregnancy to viability (20 weeks of gestation) for the first time regardless of whether the infant was stillborn or alive at birth (para I).

Problem Any patient condition that requires further observation, diagnosis, management, or patient education.

Proctoscope (PROK-te-skôp) An endoscope that is specially designed for passage through the anus to permit visual inspection of the rectum.

Proctoscopy (PROK-tos-KÔ-pê) The visual examination of the rectum using a proctoscope.

Prodrome (PRÔ-drôm) A sympton indicating an approaching disease.

Profile A number of laboratory tests providing related or complementary information used to determine the health status of a patient.

Prognosis (prog-NÔ-sis) The probable course and outcome of a patient's condition and the prospects for patient recovery.

Proteinuria (PRÔ-têen-ur-ê-a) The presence of protein in the urine.

Puerperium (PURE-per-ê-um) The period of time (usually four to six weeks) in which the uterus and the body systems are returning to normal following delivery.

Pulse pressure The difference between the systolic and diastolic blood pressure.

Pulse rhythm The time interval between heart beats.

Pulse volume The strength of the heart beat.

Puncture (punk-SHUR) A wound made by a sharp pointed object piercing the skin.

Pyrexia (PÎ-rex-Ê-a) A body temperature that is above normal. Synonym for fever.

Quality control The application of methods to ensure that test results are reliable and valid and that errors are detected and eliminated.

Quickening The first movements of the fetus in utero as felt by the mother, which usually occur between the sixteenth and twentieth weeks of gestation and are felt consistently thereafter.

Radiation The transfer of energy, such as heat, in the form of waves.

Radiograph (RÂ-dê-Ô-graph) A permanent record of a picture of an internal body organ or structure produced on radiographic film.

Radiography (RÂ-dê-OG-ra-fê) The taking of permanent records (radiographs) of internal body organs and structures by passing x-rays through the body to act upon a specially sensitized film.

Radiologist (RÂ-dê-all-Ô-jist) A medical doctor who specializes in the diagnosis and treatment of disease using radiant energy such as x-rays, radium, and radioactive material.

Radiology (RÂ-dê-all-Ô-gê) The branch of medicine that deals with the use of radiant energy in the diagnosis and treatment of disease.

Radiolucent (RÂ-dê-Ô-lûs-nt) Describing a structure that permits the passage of x-rays.

Radiopaque (RÂ-dê-Ô-pâk) Describing a structure that obstructs the passage of x-rays.

Recipient One who receives something, such as a blood transfusion, from a donor.

Refraction (rê-FRAK-shun) The deflection or bending of light rays by a lens.

Refractive index The ratio of the velocity of light in air to the velocity of light in a solution.

Refractometer (rê-FRAK-tom-it-er) An instrument used to measure the refractive index of urine, which is an indirect measurement of the specific gravity of urine.

Regulated waste Any waste containing infectious materials that would pose a substantial threat to health and safety if the public were exposed to it.

Renal threshold (RÊ-nul THRESH-hold) The concentration at which a substance in the blood that is not normally excreted by the kidneys begins to appear in the urine.

Reservoir host The organism that becomes infected by a pathogen and also serves as a source of transfer of the pathogen to others.

Resident flora Harmless, nonpathogenic microorganisms that normally reside on the skin and usually do not cause disease. Also known as normal flora.

Resistance The natural ability of an organism to remain unaffected by harmful substances in its environment.

Retina (RET-in-a) The interior surface of the eye, which picks up light impulses and transmits them to the optic nerve.

Reverse chronologic order Arranging documents with the most recent document on top, which means that the oldest document is on the bottom.

Routine test Laboratory tests performed on a routine basis on apparently healthy patients to assist in the early detection of disease.

Sanitization A cleaning process to reduce the number of microorganisms to a safe level as determined by public health requirements.

Scalpel (SKAL-pul) A surgical knife used to divide tissues.

Scissors A cutting instrument.

Sebaceous cyst (sa-BÂ-shous SIST) A thin closed sac or capsule containing fatty secretions from a sebaceous gland.

Segment The portion of the ECG tracing between two waves.

Seizure (SÊ-zhur) A sudden episode of involuntary muscle contractions and relaxation, often accompanied by a change in sensation, behavior, and level of consciousness.

Semi-critical item An item that comes into contact with intact mucous membranes.

Sequela (SA-kwêl-ya) A morbid (secondary) condition occurring as a result of a less serious primary infection.

Serum (SERE-um) The clear, straw-colored part of the blood that remains after the solid elements have been separated out of it.

Shock The failure of the cardiovascular system to deliver enough blood to all the vital organs of the body.

Short arm cast A cast that extends from below the elbow to the fingers.

Short leg cast A cast that begins just below the knee and extends to the toes.

Sigmoidoscope (SIG-MÔID-ô-skôp) An endoscope that is specially designed for passage through the anus to permit visualization of the rectum and sigmoid colon.

Sigmoidoscopy (SIG-môid-OS-kô-pê) The visual examination of the rectum and sigmoid colon using a sigmoidoscope.

Smear Material spread on a slide for microscopic examination.

Soak The direct immersion of a body part in water or a medicated solution.

SOAP format A method of organization for recording progress notes. The SOAP format includes the following categories: subjective data, objective data, assessment, and plan.

Sonogram (SON-ô-gram) The record obtained by the use of ultrasonography.

Specific gravity The weight of a substance as compared with the weight of an equal volume of a substance known as the standard. In urinalysis, the specific gravity refers to the measurement of the amount of dissolved substances present in the urine, as compared with the same amount of distilled water.

Specimen (SPES-i-men) A small sample of something taken to show the nature of the whole.

Speculum (SPEK-û-lem) An instrument for opening a body orifice or cavity for viewing.

Sphygmomanometer (SFIG-mô-mun-OM-it-er) An instrument for measuring arterial blood pressure.

Spirilla (singular, spirillum) Bacteria that have a spiral shape.

Spirometer (SPÎ-rom-it-er) An instrument for measuring air taken into and expelled from the lungs.

Spirometry (SPÎ-rom-it-rê) Measurement of an individual's breathing capacity by means of a spirometer.

Splint Any item that will immobilize a body part.

Sponge A porous, absorbent pad, such as 4″ × 4″ gauze pad or cotton surrounded by gauze, used to absorb fluids, to apply medication, or to cleanse an area.

Spore A hard, thick-walled capsule formed by some bacteria that contains only the essential parts of the protoplasm of the bacterial cell.

Sprain Trauma to a joint that causes tearing of the ligaments.

Stature The height of the body in a standing position.

Sterile Free from all living microorganisms and bacterial spores.

Sterilization The process of destroying all forms of microbial life including bacterial spores.

Stethoscope (STETH-a-skôp) An instrument for amplifying and hearing sounds produced by the body.

Strain An overstretching of muscles or tendons caused by trauma.

Streaking In microbiology, the process of inoculating a culture to provide for the growth of colonies on the surface of a solid medium. Streaking is accomplished by skimming a wire inoculating loop containing the specimen across the surface of the medium, using a back-and-forth motion.

Streptolysin (STREP-tô-lî-sin) An exotoxin produced by beta-hemolytic streptococci that completely hemolyzes red blood cells.

Subcutaneous injection (sub-CÛ-tane-ê-us in-JEK-shun) Introducing medication beneath the skin, into the subcutaneous or fatty layer of the body.

Subjective symptom A symptom that is felt by the patient but is not observable by an examiner.

Sublingual administration (sub-lêng-wul ad-MIN-is-TRÂ-shun) Administration of medication by placing it under the tongue, where it dissolves and is absorbed through the mucous membrane.

Supernatant (SÛ-per-NÂ-tent) The clear liquid that remains at the top after a precipitate settles.

Suppuration (SUPP-er-Â-shun) The process of pus formation.

Surgical asepsis (SURG-i-kul Â-SEP-sis) Those practices that keep objects and areas sterile or free from microorganisms.

Susceptible Easily affected; lacking resistance.

Sutures (SÛ-churs) Material used to approximate tissues with surgical stitches.

Swaged needle (SWAGD- NÊ-dle) A needle with suturing material permanently attached to the end of the needle.

Symptom Any change in the body or its functioning that indicates that a disease is present.

Systole (SIS-tô-lê) The phase in the cardiac cycle in which the ventricles contract, sending blood out of the heart and into the aorta and pulmonary trunk.

Systolic pressure (sis-TAUL-ik PRESH-ur) The point of maximum pressure on the arterial walls, which is recorded during systole.

Tachycardia (TAK-a-CAR-dê-a) An abnormally fast heart or pulse rate (over 100 beats per minute).

Tachypnea (TAK-ip-nê-a) An abnormal increase in the respiratory rate of more than 20 respirations per minute.

Thermolabile (ther-MÔ-lâ-bill) Easily affected or changed by heat.

Thready pulse A pulse with a decreased volume that feels weak and thin.

Thrombocyte Platelet.

Topical administration Applying a drug to a particular spot, usually for a local action.

Toxemia (TOX-êm-ê-a) A pathologic condition occurring in pregnant women that includes preeclampsia and eclampsia. If preeclampsia goes undiagnosed or is not satisfactorily controlled, it can develop into eclampsia, characterized by convulsions and coma.

Toxin (TOX-in) A poisonous or noxious substance.

Toxoid (TOX-ôid) A toxin (poisonous substance produced by a bacterium) that has been treated by heat or chemicals to destroy its harmful properties. It is administered to an individual to prevent an infectious disease by stimulating the production of antibodies in that individual.

Transient flora Microorganisms that reside on the superficial skin layers and are picked up in the course of daily activities. They are often pathogenic, but can be removed easily from the skin by good handwashing techniques.

Trimester Three months, or one third, of the gestational period of pregnancy.

Tympanic membrane (tim-PAN-ik mem-BRÂN) A thin, semi-transparent membrane located between the external ear canal and middle ear that receives and transmits sound waves.

Ultrasonography (UL-TRA-sun-og-ra-fê) The use of high-frequency sound waves (ultrasound) to produce an image of an organ or tissue.

Urinalysis (YUR-in-al-is-sis) The physical, chemical, and microscopic analysis of urine.

Vaccine (VAK-sên) A suspension of attenuated (weakened) or killed microorganisms administered to an individual to prevent an infectious disease by stimulating the production of antibodies in that individual.

Venipuncture (VÊN-a-PUNK-shur) Puncturing of a vein.

Venous reflux (VÊ-nus RÊ-flux) The backflow of blood (from an evacuated tube) into the patient's vein.

Venous stasis (VÊ-nus STÂ-sis) The temporary cessation or slowing of the venous blood flow.

Vertex (VER-tex) The summit, or top, especially the top of the head.

Vesiculation (VES-ik-û-LÂ-shun) The formation of vesicles (fluid-containing lesions of the skin).

Vial A closed glass container with a rubber stopper.

Void To empty the bladder.

Volume The amount of space occupied by a substance.

Vulva (VUL-va) The region of the external genital organs in the female.

Weight The measure of heaviness of a substance.

Wheal (WHÊL) A small raised area of the skin.

Wound A break in the continuity of an external or internal surface caused by physical means.

Note: Page numbers in *italics* refer to illustrations;
page numbers followed by (t) refer to tables.

Multimedia CD-ROM
Single User License Agreement